D1195354

Critical Care
Emergency Medicine

Notice

Medicine is an ever-changing science. As new research and clinical experience broaden our knowledge, changes in treatment and drug therapy are required. The authors and the publisher of this work have checked with sources believed to be reliable in their efforts to provide information that is complete and generally in accord with the standards accepted at the time of publication. However, in view of the possibility of human error or changes in medical sciences, neither the authors nor the publisher nor any other party who has been involved in the preparation or publication of this work warrants that the information contained herein is in every respect accurate or complete, and they disclaim all responsibility for any errors or omissions or for the results obtained from use of the information contained in this work. Readers are encouraged to confirm the information contained herein with other sources. For example and in particular, readers are advised to check the product information sheet included in the package of each drug they plan to administer to be certain that the information contained in this work is accurate and that changes have not been made in the recommended dose or in the contraindications for administration. This recommendation is of particular importance in connection with new or infrequently used drugs.

DREXEL UNIVERSITY
HEALTH SCIENCES LIBRARIES
HAHNEMANN LIBRARY

Critical Care Emergency Medicine

David A. Farcy, MD, FAAEM, FACEP, FCCM
Medical Director of the Surgical Intensivist Program
Director of Emergency Department Critical Care
Mount Sinai Medical Center
Miami Beach, Florida

William C. Chiu, MD, FACS, FCCM
Associate Professor of Surgery
Director, Fellowship Programs in Surgical
Critical Care and Acute Care Surgery
R Adams Cowley Shock Trauma Center
University of Maryland School of Medicine
Baltimore, Maryland

Alex Flaxman, MD, MSE
Director, Emergency Medicine Critical Care
Emergency and Critical Care Attending
St. Joseph's Regional Medical Center
Paterson, New Jersey
Attending Intensivist
Pittsburgh Critical Care Associates, Inc
Staff Intensivist
Upper Allegheny Health System
Olean, New York

John P. Marshall, MD, FACEP
Chair
Department of Emergency Medicine
Maimonides Medical Center
Brooklyn, New York

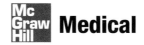

New York Chicago San Francisco Lisbon London Madrid Mexico City
Milan New Delhi San Juan Seoul Singapore Sydney Toronto

The McGraw-Hill Companies

Critical Care Emergency Medicine

WX
218
C9341
2012

Copyright © 2012 by The McGraw-Hill Companies, Inc. All rights reserved. Printed in China. Except as permitted under the United States Copyright Act of 1976, no part of this publication may be reproduced or distributed in any form or by any means, or stored in a data base or retrieval system, without the prior written permission of the publisher.

1 2 3 4 5 6 7 8 9 0   CTP/CTP   15 14 13 12 11

ISBN 978-0-07-162824-2
MHID 0-07-162824-X

This book was set in ITC Garamond by Thomson Digital.
The editors were Anne M. Sydor and Christie Naglieri.
The production supervisor was Catherine Saggese.
Project management was provided by Aakriti Kathuria, Thomson Digital.
Cover design by Pehrsson Design.
China Translation & Printing, Ltd. was the printer and binder.

Library of Congress Cataloging-in-Publication Data
Critical care emergency medicine / [edited by] David A. Farcy ... [et al.].
     p. ; cm.
  Includes bibliographical references and index.
  ISBN-13: 978-0-07-162824-2 (hardcover : alk. paper)
  ISBN-10: 0-07-162824-X (hardcover : alk. paper)
     1. Critical care medicine. 2. Emergency medical services. I. Farcy, David. A.
     [DNLM: 1. Critical Illness—therapy. 2. Critical Care—methods. 3. Emergency
Service, Hospital. 4. Emergency Treatment—methods. 5. Intensive Care Units.
WX 218]
  RC86.7.C717 2011
  616.02'8—dc23
                                                               2011017375

McGraw-Hill books are available at special quantity discounts to use as premiums and sales promotions, or for use in corporate training programs. To contact a representative please e-mail us at bulksales@mcgraw-hill.com.

To my father Dr Jean Pierre Farcy for his love and for sharing and instilling in me the passion for medicine, to Dr Thomas M. Scalea for teaching me to have compassion and to always put patients first, to Dr Amy Church and Dr John P. Marshall for believing in me. To my mother, Poe, Eve, Frederic, and Sarah for always being there for me, and all my patients and their families, who have helped me become a better doctor and believed in me during their most difficult moments.
— David A. Farcy —

To all those who have been influential to me: Terri, Anthony, Katherine, Victoria, and the extended Shock Trauma family.
— William C. Chiu —

To all those who helped, worked, and sacrificed, to get me to where I am: Mom, Dad, Sally, grandparents, great grandparents, cousins, aunts and uncles, great aunts and uncles, and great great uncle, this effort is for you.
— Alex Flaxman —

To my wife, Seriti, and my three boys, Sahm, Siahvash, and Kianoosh. Your love, patience, and support make everything possible.
—John P. Marshall —

CONTENTS

SECTION VII   HEMATOLOGIC AND ENDOCRINE DISORDERS

SECTION VIII   INFECTIOUS DISORDERS

SECTION IX   TOXICOLOGIC CONDITIONS

CONTRIBUTORS

Imoigele P. Aisiku, MD
Associate Professor
Departments of Neurosurgery and
    Emergency Medicine
University of Texas Medical School, Houston
Houston, Texas
Acute Respiratory Failure
Management of Acute Intracranial
    Hypertension

Dorothea Altschul, MD
Co-Director Department of Neuroscience
Department of Neuroscience
St. Joseph's Regional Medical Center
Paterson, New Jersey
Traumatic Brain Injury and Spinal Cord Injury

Alex M. Barrocas, MD
Director of Interventional Neuroradiology/
    Endovascular Neurosurgery
Mount Sinai Medical Center
Miami Beach, Florida
Stroke
Intracranial Hemorrhage

Selwena Brewster, MD
Attending
Internal Medicine, Emergency Medicine
St Francis Hospital
Hartford, Connecticut
Gastrointestinal Bleeding

Triminh Bui, DO
Emergency Room Resident
Miami Beach, Florida
Severe Asthma and COPD

Colleen Casey, RD, CNSC, LDN
Senior Nutrition Specialist
Department of Clinical Nutrition
R Adams Cowley Shock Trauma Center
University of Maryland Medical Center
Baltimore, Maryland
Nutritional Support in Critical Care

William C. Chiu, MD, FACS, FCCM
Associate Professor of Surgery
Director, Fellowship Programs in Surgical Critical
    Care and Acute Care Surgery
R Adams Cowley Shock Trauma Center
University of Maryland School of Medicine
Baltimore, Maryland
Vasopressors and Inotropes
Acid–Base Disorders
Electrolyte Disorders
Adrenal Insufficiency

Ari J. Ciment, MD, FCCP
Associate Professor
Mount Sinai Medical Center
Pulmonary and Critical Care
Miami Beach, Florida
Glucose Management in Critical Care

Carrie A. Cregar, MD
Clinical Instructor
Department of Emergency Medicine
University Hospitals Case Medical Center
Case Western Reserve University School of Medicine
Cleveland, Ohio
Gastrointestinal Bleeding

David W. Crippen, MD, FCCM
Professor, Department of Critical Care Medicine
University of Pittsburgh Medical Center
Co-Director, Neurovascular ICU
Presbyterian University Hospital
Pittsburgh, Pennsylvania
Alterations in Mental Status

Michael T. Dalley, DO, FAAEM
Associate Residency Director
Department of Emergency Medicine
Mount Sinai Medical Center
Miami Beach, Florida
Severe Asthma and COPD

Peter DeBlieux, MD
Professor of Clinical Medicine
Department of Medicine, Sections of Emergency
    Medicine and Pulmonary and Critical Care Medicine
LSUHSC
New Orleans, Louisiana
Mechanical Ventilation

Eitan Dickman, MD, RDMS, FACEP
Vice Chair for Academics
Director, Division of Emergency Ultrasonography
Department of Emergency Medicine
Brooklyn, New York
Ultrasound-Guided Critical Care Procedures

Therese M. Duane, MD, FACS, FCCM
Associate Professor
Department of Surgery
Division of Trauma/Critical Care
Virginia Commonwealth University
Richmond, Virginia
Transfusion in Critical Care

Marie-Carmelle Elie-Turenne, MD
Clinical Assistant Professor
Emergency Medicine
Critical Care Medicine
Hospice, Palliative Care
University of Florida
Gainesville, Florida
Gastrointestinal Bleeding

Jason A. Ellis, MD
Resident, Department of Neurological Surgery
Columbia University Medical Center
New York, New York
Traumatic Brain Injury and Spinal Cord Injury

David A. Farcy, MD, FAAEM, FACEP, FCCM
Medical Director of the Surgical Intensivist Program
Director of Emergency Department Critical Care
Mount Sinai Medical Center
Miami Beach, Florida
The Failed Airway
Mechanical Ventilation
*Extracorporeal Cardiopulmonary Membrane
    Oxygenation*
Sepsis and Septic Shock
Classification of Shock

Falk Eike Flach, MD
Clinical Assistant Professor
Department of Emergency Medicine
University of Florida
Gainesville, Florida
*Point-of-Care Echocardiography in the Emergency
    Department*

Alex Flaxman, MD, MSE
Director, Emergency Medicine Critical Care
Emergency and Critical Care Attending
St. Joseph's Regional Medical Center
Paterson, New Jersey
Attending Intensivist
Pittsburgh Critical Care Associates, Inc
Staff Intensivist
Upper Allegheny Health System
Olean, New York
Weaning and Extubation
Acute Renal Failure and Renal Replacement Therapy

Jennifer A. Frontera, MD
Assistant Professor
Neurosurgery and Neurology
Mount Sinai School of Medicine
New York, New York
*Acute Liver Failure: How to Orchestrate Emergency
    Critical Care Interventions*

David F. Gaieski, MD
Assistant Professor, University of Pennsylvania
    School of Medicine
Department of Emergency Medicine
Clinical Director, Center for Resuscitation Science
Philadelphia, Pennsylvania
*Therapeutic Hypothermia: History, Data, Translation,
    and Emergency Department Application*

Megan L. Garcia, MD
Resident Physician, Department of Surgery
University of New Mexico Health Sciences Center
Albuqueruqe, New Mexico
Acute Respiratory Distress Syndrome (ARDS)

David R. Gens, MD, FACS
Associate Professor
Department of Surgery
University of Maryland School of Medicine
Baltimore, Maryland
The Failed Airway
Deep Venous Thrombosis

Munish Goyal, MD, FACEP
Associate Professor
Department of Emergency Medicine
Georgetown University School of Medicine
Washington, District of Columbia
*Therapeutic Hypothermia: History, Data, Translation,
    and Emergency Department Application*

Lawrence E. Haines, MD, MPH, RDMS
Emergency Ultrasound Fellowship Director
Department of Emergency Medicine
Maimonides Medical Center
Brooklyn, New York
Ultrasound-Guided Critical Care Procedures

Dan Hale, RRT, RPFT
Neo Natal Pediatric Specialist
Respiratory Specialist
Department of Pulmonary Diagnostics
University of New Mexico Hospital
Albuquerque, New Mexico
Percutaneous Tracheostomy for the Intensivist

Dennis Heard, DO
Emergency Medicine Resident
Mount Sinai Medical Center
Miami, Florida
Mechanical Ventilation

Alan C. Heffner, MD
Director, Medical ICU
Director of ECMO Services
Pulmonary and Critical Care Consultants
Department of Internal Medicine
Department of Emergency Medicine
Carolinas Medical Center
Charlotte, North Carolina
Postcardiac Arrest Management
Fluid Management

Robert J. Hoffman, MD, MS
Associate Professor of Emergency Medicine
Department of Emergency Medicine
Albert Einstein College of Medicine
Bronx, New York
Approach to Poisoning
The Critically Ill Poisoned Patient

Shyoko Honiden, MD, MSc
Assistant Professor
Department of Medicine
Yale University School of Medicine
New Haven, Connecticut
Hyperglycemic Emergency

Ashika Jain, MD
Critical Care Fellow
R Adams Cowley Shock Trauma Center
University of Maryland Medical Center
Baltimore, Maryland
Ultrasound-Guided Critical Care Procedures

Timothy B. Jang, MD
Assistant Professor of Clinical Medicine
Emergency Medicine
David Geffen School of Medicine at UCLA
Harbor-UCLA Medical Center
Torrance, California
Approach to the Difficult Airway

Kevin M. Jones, MD, MPH
Department of Emergency Medicine
Department of Surgery
Albany Medical College
Albany, New York
Acid–Base Disorders
Electrolyte Disorders

Manjari Joshi, MBBS
Associate Professor of Medicine
Department of Medicine, Division of Infectious
    Diseases
University of Maryland Medical Center
R Adams Cowley Shock Trauma Center
Baltimore, Maryland
Principles of Antimicrobial Use in Critical Care

Thomas H. Kalb, MD
Associate Professor
Department of Medicine
Mount Sinai School of Medicine
New York, New York
*Acute Liver Failure: How to Orchestrate Emergency
    Critical Care Interventions*

Julio R. Lairet, DO, FACEP
Assistant Professor of Military and Emergency Medicine
Uniformed Services University of Health Sciences
Air Force Surgeon General Consultant for Critical Care
    Air Transport
San Antonio, Texas
Transportation of the Critical Care Patient

Sangeeta Lamba, MD
Assistant Professor
Department of Emergency Medicine and Surgery
UMDNJ-New Jersey Medical School
Newark, New Jersey
End-of-life Issues in Emergency Critical Care

Grace S. Lee, MD
Hospitalist Physician
Yale New Haven Hospital
New Haven, Connecticut
Hyperglycemic Emergency

Kiwon Lee, MD, FACP, FAHA
Assistant Professor of Neurology and Neurosurgery
Columbia University College of Physicians & Surgeons
Department of Neurology
New York-Presbyterian/Columbia University
    Medical Center
New York, New York
Traumatic Brain Injury and Spinal Cord Injury

Stephen J. Leech, MD
Ultrasound Director, Graduate Medical Education
Department of Emergency Medicine
Orlando Regional Medical Center
Orlando, Florida
*Point-of-Care Echocardiography in the Emergency
    Department*

Beth A. Longenecker, DO, FACOEP, FACEP
Clinical Associate Professor
Department of Family Medicine
Nova Southeastern University
College of Osteopathic Medicine
Davie, Florida
Program Director Emergency Medicine Residency
Mount Sinai Medical Center
Miami Beach, Florida
Pulmonary Embolism
Stroke
Intracranial Hemorrhage

Evie G. Marcolini, MD
Assistant Professor of Emergency Medicine
    and Critical Care
Department of Emergency Medicine
Yale University School of Medicine
New Haven, Connecticut
Adrenal Insufficiency

Jonathan L. Marinaro, MD
Assistant Professor
Department of Surgery
Department of Emergency Medicine
University of New Mexico Health Sciences Center
Albuquerque, New Mexico
Percutaneous Tracheostomy for the Intensivist

John P. Marshall, MD, FACEP
Chair
Department of Emergency Medicine
Maimonides Medical Center
Brooklyn, New York
Acute Coronary Syndrome
Vasopressors and Inotropes

Julie A. Mayglothling, MD, FACEP
Assistant Professor
Department of Emergency Medicine
Department of Surgery, Division of Trauma/Critical Care
Virginia Commonwealth University
Richmond, Virginia
Transfusion in Critical Care

Michael T. McCurdy, MD
Assistant Professor
Department of Internal Medicine, Division of
    Pulmonary & Critical Care
Department of Emergency Medicine
University of Maryland School of Medicine
Baltimore, Maryland
Nosocomial and Health Care-Associated Pneumonia

Rajeev P. Misra, DO, MS
General Surgery Resident
Department of Surgery
University of New Mexico Hospital
Albuquerque, New Mexico
Percutaneous Tracheostomy for the Intensivist

Ira Nemeth, MD, FACEP
Assistant Professor
Department of Medicine, Section of Emergency Medicine
Baylor College of Medicine
Houston, Texas
Transportation of the Critical Care Patient

H. Bryant Nguyen, MD, MS
Director, Emergency Critical Care
Associate Professor
Department of Emergency Medicine and Department
    of Medicine, Critical Care
Loma Linda University
Loma Linda, California
Hemodynamic and Perfusion Monitoring

L. Connor Nickels, MD, RDMS
Clinical Assistant Professor
Department of Emergency Medicine
University of Florida
Gainesville, Florida
*Point-of-Care Echocardiography in the Emergency
    Department*

Tiffany M. Osborn, MD, MPH, FACEP
Associate Professor
Department of Surgery
Surgical/Trauma Critical Care and Emergency Medicine
University of Washington
Barnes-Jewish Hospital
St. Louis, Mossouri
Classification of Shock

Anu Osinusi, MD, MPH
Fellow, Department of Infectious Diseases
University of Maryland
Baltimore, Maryland
Principles of Antimicrobial Use in Critical Care

Christopher M. Perry, MD
Attending Physician
Department of Emergency Medicine
North Shore University Hospital
Manhasset, New York
Hypertensive Crises

Paul L. Petersen, MD, FAAEM
Attending Physician
Department of Emergency Medicine
Mount Sinai Miami Beach
Miami, Florida
Mechanical Ventilation

Paola G. Pieri, MD, FACS
Associate Medical Director, Trauma Program
Maricopa Medical Center
Phoenix, Arizona
*Extracorporeal Cardiopulmonary Membrane
  Oxygenation*

Seth R. Podolsky, MD, MS
Attending Physician
Department of Emergency Medicine
Maimonides Medical Center
Brooklyn, New York
Acetaminophen Overdose

Mohan Punja, MD
Resident, Department of Emergency Medicine
Beth Israel Medical Center
New York, New York
Approach to Poisoning

David Rabinowitz, MS
Medical Student
Osteopathic Medical Program
Nova Southeastern University
Davie, Florida
*Extracorporeal Cardiopulmonary Membrane
  Oxygenation*

Emanuel Rivers, MD, MPH
Vice Chairman and Research Director
Department of Emergency Medicine
Attending Staff, Emergency Medicine and
  Surgical Critical Care
Henry Ford Hospital
Clinical Professor, Wayne State University
Detroit, Michigan
Sepsis and Septic Shock

Matthew T. Robinson, MD
Assistant Professor of Clinical Emergency Medicine
Department of Emergency Medicine
University of Missouri Hospitals and Clinics
Columbia, Missouri
Fluid Management

Amber Rollstin, MD
Assistant Professor of Surgery and
  Emergency Medicine
Health Sciences Center to University of
  New Mexico Health Sciences Center
Department of Surgery
University of New Mexico
Albuquerque, New Mexico
Vasopressors and Inotropes

Joseph Romero, DO
Internal Medicine Chief Resident
Osteopathic Internal Medicine
Mount Sinai Medical Center
Miami Beach, Florida
Glucose Management in Critical Care

Jonathan Rose, MD
Residency Program Director
Department of Emergency Medicine
Maimonides Medical Center
Brooklyn, New York
Acute Coronary Syndrome

Marnie E. Rosenthal, DO, MPH
Director, Infectious Disease Research
Jersey Shore University Medical Center
Department of Internal Medicine, Section
  of Infectious Diseases
Neptune City, New Jersey
Clinical Assistant Professor
University of Medicine and Dentistry New Jersey
Robert Wood Johnson Medical School
New Brunswick, New Jersey
Approach to Fever in Critical Care

Rayan A. Rouhizad, DO
Emergency Medicine Physician
Wellstar Kennestone Hospital
Marietta, Georgia
Pulmonary Embolism

Justin T. Sambol, MD
Assistant Professor of Surgery
Chief, Division of Cardiothoracic Surgery
UMDNJ-New Jersey Medical School
Newark, New Jersey
Management after Cardiac Surgery

Joseph R. Shiber, MD
Associate Professor
Departments of Emergency Medicine and Critical Care
University of Florida School of Medicine
Jacksonville, Florida
Pericardial Diseases
Infectious Endocarditis

Todd L. Slesinger, MD, FACEP, FCCM
Assistant Professor of Emergency Medicine
Hofstra North Shore-LIJ School of Medicine
Manhasset, New York
Noninvasive Ventilation
Hypertensive Crises

LaMont C. Smith, MD
Assistant Professor of Medicine
University of Pittsburgh School of Medicine
Division of Pulmonary, Allergy, and Critical
    Care Medicine
University of Pittsburgh Medical Center
Pittsburgh, Pennsylvania
Management after Cardiac Surgery

Fernando L. Soto, MD
Associate Professor
Emergency Medicine Program
University of Puerto Rico School of Medicine
San Juan, Puerto Rico
Pediatric Considerations

Deborah M. Stein, MD, MPH, FACS, FCCM
Associate Professor
Department of Surgery
University of Maryland School of Medicine
Baltimore, Maryland
Acute Renal Failure and Renal Replacement Therapy

Andrew Stolbach, MD
Assistant Professor
Department of Emergency Medicine
Baltimore, Maryland
Salicylate Overdose

Isaac Tawil, MD
Assistant Professor
Departments of Surgery and Emergency Medicine
University of New Mexico Health Sciences Center
Albuquerque, New Mexico
Acute Respiratory Distress Syndrome (ARDS)

Nestor D. Tomycz, MD
Senior Neurosurgery Resident
Department of Neurological Surgery
University of Pittsburgh Medical Center
Pittsburgh, Pennsylvania
Alterations in Mental Status

Amy Tortorich, DO
Physician, Emergency Medicine
Cheyenne Regional Medical Center
Cheyenne, Wyoming
Deep Venous Thrombosis

Claudio D. Tuda, MD, FACP
Assistant Professor
Department of Medicine, Infectious Disease Division
Program Director, Internal Medicine
Mount Sinai Medical Center
University of Miami Miller School of Medicine
Miami Beach, Florida
Clostridium difficile infection (CDI)

Jason C. Wagner, MD, FACEP
Assistant Professor of Emergency Medicine
Washington University School of Medicine
St. Louis, Missouri
Approach to the Difficult Airway

Elizabeth Lea Walters, MD
Associate Professor
Department of Emergency Medicine
Loma Linda University Medical Center
Loma Linda, California
Hemodynamic and Perfusion Monitoring

Scott D. Weingart, MD, FACEP
Director, Division of Emergency Critical Care
Mount Sinai School of Medicine
New York, New York
The Emergency Department Intensivist

Samantha L. Wood, MD
Fellow
Departments of Emergency Medicine, Internal
    Medicine, and Critical Care
University of Maryland Medical Center
Baltimore, Maryland
Electrolyte Disorders

Brian J. Wright, MD, MPH
Assistant Professor
Department of Emergency Medicine
Hofstra North Shore-LIJ School of Medicine
Manhasset, New York
Noninvasive Ventilation

John Yashou, DO
Attending Physician, Emergency Department
Memorial West Hospital
Pembroke Pines, Florida
Sepsis and Septic Shock

Dale J. Yeatts, MD
Assistant Professor
Department of Emergency Medicine
University of Maryland School of Medicine
Attending, Surgical Critical Care
R Adams Cowley Shock Trauma Center
Baltimore, Maryland
The Failed Airway

Asma Zakaria, MD
Assistant Professor
Division of Neurocritical Care
Departments of Neurology and Neurosurgery
University of Texas, Health Science Center at Houston
Houston, Texas
Management of Acute Intracranial Hypertension

(Shawn) Xun Zhong, MD
Director of ED-Critical Care
Department of Emergency Medicine
Nassau University Medical Center
East Meadow, New York
Salicylate Overdose

Qiuping Zhou, DO
Assistant Professor
Hofstra North Shore-LIJ School of Medicine
Associate Program Director
Fellowship in Critical Care Medicine
Department of Emergency Medicine
North Shore LIJ Health System
Manhasset, New York
Hypertensive Crises

FOREWORD

Critical care by its very nature is a multidisciplinary disease. Virtually every critically ill patient requires input from a multiplicity of practitioners. Physicians in the ICU provide direct care, and orchestrate and coordinate care for all other practitioners who participate. Given this complexity, it is interesting to note critical care has been a recent development. The first true multidisciplinary ICU was opened in 1958 at the Baltimore City Hospital, now named Johns Hopkins Bayview. It was also the first ICU that had 24-hour physician coverage.

Critical care was rapidly becoming its own discipline, yet lacked efficient organization. In 1970, 28 physicians met in Los Angeles and formed the Society of Critical Care Medicine. The society's leaders and first three presidents were: Peter Safar, an anesthesiologist; William Shoemaker, a surgeon; and Max Harry Weil, an internist. Throughout the 1970s, 1980s, and 1990s, these three disciplines represented the backbone of critical care in the United States.

As critical care began to develop, emergency medicine also began to develop as a real discipline. In 1961, Dr James Mills started a full-time emergency medicine practice in Alexandria, Virginia. The American College of Emergency Physicians was founded shortly after that, in 1968. Residency training began at the University of Cincinnati, followed by the Medical College of Pennsylvania, and then Los Angeles County Hospital. Finally, in 1979, the American Board of Emergency Medicine was approved. Other institutions then developed emergency medicine residencies. Today, there are over 150 accredited programs. Fellowship training followed in subspecialties such as toxicology, pediatrics, and now critical care.

The link between emergency medicine and critical care seems natural. Both require understanding of complex physiology. Practitioners in both specialties must understand a multitude of diseases, synthesize solutions for complex problems, and do this quickly. When I founded the Department of Emergency Medicine at SUNY Downstate and Kings County Hospital in 1991, we created a 4-year residency program that was heavy in critical care. However, I soon realized that emergency physicians who wanted to practice real critical care would need additional training.

Thus, when I became the Physician-in-Chief at the R Adams Cowley Shock Trauma Center, I established a critical care fellowship designed for emergency physicians. The University of Pittsburgh had been training emergency physicians for some time in its multidisciplinary critical care fellowship. There are now over 100 fellowship-trained emergency physician intensivists. Over two thirds of them are trained at either Shock Trauma or the University of Pittsburgh. Many graduates practice in major academic centers and now provide leadership roles in these institutions.

Emergency physician intensivists have become commonplace in ICUs. This will continue. Emergency physicians who wish to be leaders will need to be clinically excellent, academically productive, and superior educators. The current textbook goes a long way toward establishing emergency physicians as credible intensivists. While not every chapter is written by an emergency physician, many are. The authors are emergency physicians who most of us expect to become the leaders in critical care. The book is unique as it blends the perspective of a true intensivist with that of emergency medicine. The book is the first of its kind, and I predict it will become known as the standard reference for those emergency physicians, as well as others, who wish to understand the overlap between emergency medicine and critical care.

Despite the lack of board certification and many other local political impediments, some emergency physicians have embraced critical care clinically, academically, and now in this textbook. The role of emergency physicians in critical care remains controversial but the controversy is not as sharp as it was at the beginning. Those of us who have been there from the beginning look forward to the day that there will be no controversy left at all.

Thomas M. Scalea, MD, FACS, FCCM
Physician-in-Chief, R Adams Cowley
Shock Trauma Center
Francis X. Kelly Professor of
Trauma Surgery and Director, Program in Trauma
University of Maryland School of Medicine
Baltimore, Maryland

PREFACE

It is with great pleasure that we present the first textbook that focuses on the intersection of critical care and emergency medicine.

For the sickest patients the quality of the interface between the emergency department and the intensive care unit can literally mean the difference between life and death. As we have seen with early goal-directed therapy and postarrest hypothermia treatment, aggressive care delivered appropriately in the emergency department has been shown to decrease mortality and morbidity for critically ill patients.

Additionally, hospital overcrowding, coupled with hospital closings and an aging patient population, has resulted in a nearly 60% increase in the number of critical care patients treated in the emergency department. Increasingly, these patients are boarded for longer periods in the emergency department presenting the emergency physician with continuing care challenges that have been traditionally managed in an intensive care unit.

This book hopes to address the challenges faced by emergency medicine physicians practicing critical care on the front lines of health care on a daily basis. It is written for emergency physicians who wish to improve their knowledge base and the quality of the care they deliver. This text provides a primer on acute resuscitative care as well as continued critical care monitoring and management. Most of chapters are written by an emergency physician with critical care training or with an abiding interest in critical care. The majority of chapters are also coauthored by a fellowship-trained intensivist with a background in surgery, internal medicine, or emergency medicine. We are very thankful for the time, patience, and thoughtful work contributed generously by each of the authors.

Lastly, the editors would like to express their deep gratitude to the entire staff at McGraw-Hill and in particular to our Executive Medical Editor, Anne M. Sydor, PhD. Anne's vision, persistence, patience, and guiding hand were essential in bringing this book to reality. It literally would not have been possible without the editorial resuscitation and critical care she provided so generously. Thank you.

David A. Farcy, MD, FAAEM, FACEP, FCCM

William C. Chiu, MD, FACS, FCCM

Alex Flaxman, MD, MSE

John P. Marshall, MD, FACEP

SECTION I

Introduction

CHAPTER 1

The Emergency Department Intensivist

Scott D. Weingart

A small, but growing number of emergency physicians (EPs) have pursued fellowship training in critical care (CC).[1,2] Many of these dual-trained physicians now practice in intensive care units (ICU) or in a practice split between standard emergency department (ED) shifts and the ICU.[3] However, there is a unique role for these Emergency Medicine Critical Care (EMCC)–trained physicians: the Emergency Department Intensivist (EDI).

EPs are masters of the art of resuscitation. Resuscitation generally encompasses the diagnosis and stabilization of a critically ill patient in the first approximately 30 minutes of the ED stay. After this time period, the ED system is predicated on the patient rapidly moving upstairs to a CC unit. However, overcrowding in almost all hospitals has led to a situation in which it may be hours or, unfortunately in some cases, days before a patient may get an ICU bed. Most EDs are not designed or staffed to provide care beyond the initial resuscitation, and yet patients remain in the ED, sometimes languishing without optimal care. Even with ample staffing, the meticulous management requirements and the necessity for obsessive attention to detail in the care of the critically ill are sometimes unappealing to EPs.[4]

However, it is desirable for patients to receive the same evidence-based aggressive care regardless of their geography in the hospital. It does not make sense for there to be one standard in the ICU and a different standard for the hours spent in the ED. The EDI can bring "Upstairs Care, Downstairs©." By bringing the intensive therapies of the ICU to the bedside in the ED, the EDI can mitigate the negative effects of hospital overcrowding on the critically ill patient.

▶ TERMINOLOGY

The nascent field of EMCC has outpaced the terms needed to describe it. The following is a list of definitions:

EMCC—A subspecialty of EM dealing with the care of the critically ill both in the ED and in the rest of the hospital.

Emergency Physician Intensivist (EPI)—A physician who has completed a residency in EM and a fellowship in CC.

Emergency Department Critical Care (EDCC)—EMCC practiced specifically in the ED.

Emergency Department Intensivist (EDI)—An EPI who practices EDCC as a portion of clinical time.

Emergency Department Intensive Care Unit (ED-ICU)—A patient care unit within an ED with the same or similar staffing, monitoring, and capability for therapies as an ICU.

▶ CLINICAL SCENARIOS

Any sick patient will benefit from the presence of an EDI, but certain specific clinical scenarios are uniquely suited to their skill set.

AIRWAY MANAGEMENT

Although advanced airway techniques are the sine qua non of any EP, the EDI brings even more options to the ED. Experience with fiberoptic bronchoscope-aided intubations is possessed by only a fraction of EM programs, but most EDIs are skilled with this procedure. Many EDIs also have experience with percutaneous and open tracheostomies. In the ED, this experience allows the performance of emergent surgical airways and the management of emergencies in patients with existing tracheostomy. In some hospitals, the EDI may be an ideal practitioner to place elective bedside tracheostomies as well.

RESPIRATORY FAILURE

A large portion of CC fellowship training is spent gaining experience with the management of acute and chronic respiratory failure. This education gives the EDI knowledge of advanced modes of ventilation, salvage of acute respiratory distress syndrome (ARDS) patients, and increased exposure to noninvasive ventilation. EM offers little training in the extubation of patients, but the EDI can comfortably extubate patients who have resolved the condition that necessitated intubation.[5]

SHOCK AND SEPSIS

The early goal-directed therapy (EGDT) study by Rivers et al may have been the gateway for CC in the ED.[6] In addition to elucidating a bundle of therapies to manage the septic patient early in the hospital course, this study demonstrated that CC in the ED is possible and life-saving. EDIs possess a broader knowledge on antibiotic choices, source control, and advanced monitoring than most other EPs. An extensive knowledge of hemodynamic monitoring, vasoactive agents, and the ramifications of alterations of oxygen delivery and the microcirculation gives the EDI a unique perspective on how early actions in the ED can affect the patient's long-term outcome.

POST–CARDIAC ARREST CARE AND THERAPEUTIC HYPOTHERMIA

Aggressive treatment of the postarrest syndrome, especially with an emphasis on early and consistent maintenance of induced hypothermia, is critical for good outcome in patients after cardiac arrest.[7] This level of care is beyond the resources of many conventional EDs for longer than the first hour of care. The EDI can spearhead a hospital postarrest program or be a primary clinician in the actual clinical management of these patients.

TRAUMA

EDIs who have received their CC training in a surgical/trauma fellowship are uniquely suited to organize a trauma resuscitation program. Mastery of all aspects of the early management of the critically ill trauma patient including blood component transfusion, conservative versus operative management, timing of angiographic interventions, surgical airways, and the lethal triad of hemorrhage (acidosis, hypothermia, and coagulopathy) is in the purview of a trauma-trained EDI.

▶ PROCEDURES

The EDI is the ideal ED proceduralist, by nature of the training and experience with management of complications. While the placement of emergent central venous catheters may be routine during residency training, EDIs have a much greater appreciation for sterile technique and the value of infection control after a CC fellowship. During training in CC, EPIs learn the long-term consequences and morbidity of infectious complications.

▶ PALLIATIVE CARE

EDIs are trained to be aggressive in their care. However, this aggressive care can be directed toward a curative or a palliative path. EDIs also receive training and have experienced the intricacies of advanced directives and family discussions on palliation and withdrawal of care. All of the advanced therapies and monitoring modalities an EDI brings to the ED must be balanced with a zealous approach to palliation and end-of-life care. Training in the long-term management of the critically ill patient allows the EDI to have better insight into the outcome of resuscitating the terminally ill. Although not as glamorous as high-profile treatments, this role is another powerful reason to bring CC to the ED.

▶ PRACTICE ENVIRONMENT

ED intensive care is best performed in a dedicated area of the ED. This allows for beds with comprehensive hemodynamic monitors, a nursing staff with additional training, and the equipment necessary for advanced diagnosis and treatment. While the ideal setting may be an ED-ICU, the resuscitation area present in many EDs works well as space for EDCC.

▶ TEACHING

While some EDs can support a number of EDIs, many academic departments will benefit from a single EDI. Just as one toxicologist can elevate the toxicology-related care for an entire academic program, the addition of an EDI can allow for the development of an

EDCC program. At least at the beginning stages of bringing CC to the ED, the EDI may be the only health professional having experience with certain advanced treatment and diagnostic modalities.

In the ICU, bedside nurses may handle all of the hands-on equipment, for example, setting up pressure transduction to allow arterial line pressure monitoring. In the ED, it may be the EDI who is performing this setup in the beginnings of an EDCC program. Eventually the nursing staff may own this advanced practice, or in some EDs, CC nurses are integrated into the ED staff.

A residency program with an EDI on faculty will naturally graduate residents with a greater knowledge and appreciation of the role of CC in the ED. In my own program, both a dedicated EDCC lecture series and trauma lecture series are taught by an EDI.

▶ ADMINISTRATIVE ROLES

The EDI is well suited to provide quality improvement for ED mortalities and any discrepancies in the care of the critically ill patient. At the hospital level, he or she can act as champion for initiatives such as sepsis care, induced hypothermia, deep sedation, and advanced airway management.

▶ SUMMARY

In conclusion, the EDI is a tremendous asset to an EM program. The gratifying training path to a career as an EDI obviates any uncertainty over certification in EMCC. The EDI facilitates ED patients getting comparable care in the ED and the ICU. Through direct clinical care and program development, the EDI can bring the level of care of an entire ED up to a level beyond initial resuscitation and equivalent to an ICU.

REFERENCES

1. Osborn TM, Scalea TM. A call for critical care training of emergency physicians. *Ann Emerg Med.* 2002;39(5):562–563.
2. Huang DT, Osborn TM, Gunnerson KJ, et al. Critical care medicine training and certification for emergency physicians. *Ann Emerg Med.* 2005;46(3):217–223.
3. Mayglothling JA, Gunnerson KJ, Huang DT. Current practice, demographics, and trends of critical care trained emergency physicians in the United States. *Acad Emerg Med.* 2010;17(3):325–329.
4. Gupta R, Butler RH. Fellowship training in critical care may not be helpful for emergency physicians. *Ann Emerg Med.* 2004;43(3):420–421.
5. Weingart SD, Menaker J, Truong H, Bochicchio K, Scalea TM. Trauma patients can be safely extubated in the emergency department. *J Emerg Med.* 2011;40(2):235–239.
6. Rivers E, Nguyen B, Havstad S, et al. Early goal-directed therapy in the treatment of severe sepsis and septic shock. *N Engl J Med.* 2001;345(19):1368–1377.
7. Neumar RW, Nolan JP, Adrie C, et al. Post-cardiac arrest syndrome: epidemiology, pathophysiology, treatment, and prognostication. A consensus statement from the International Liaison Committee on Resuscitation (American Heart Association, Australian and New Zealand Council on Resuscitation, European Resuscitation Council, Heart and Stroke Foundation of Canada, InterAmerican Heart Foundation, Resuscitation Council of Asia, and the Resuscitation Council of Southern Africa); the American Heart Association Emergency Cardiovascular Care Committee; the Council on Cardiovascular Surgery and Anesthesia; the Council on Cardiopulmonary, Perioperative, and Critical Care; the Council on Clinical Cardiology; and the Stroke Council. *Circulation.* 2008;118(23):2452–2483.

SECTION II

Airway and Ventilatory Support

CHAPTER 2

Approach to the Difficult Airway

Timothy B. Jang and Jason C. Wagner

► BACKGROUND

A *difficult airway* exists in a patient when conventional face mask ventilation is problematic or tracheal intubation is difficult, requiring advanced airway skills for success. Patient factors such as micrognathia, a short neck, a large tongue, craniofacial abnormalities, pregnancy, and obesity are chronic conditions associated with a difficult airway but do not inherently define a difficult airway. Other conditions such as angioedema, epiglottitis, Ludwig's angina, retropharyngeal abscess, tracheal trauma, traumatic/expanding neck hematoma, and cervical trauma are examples of acute factors that similarly may cause a difficult airway condition to exist. When patients with any of these conditions develop dyspnea or respiratory distress, immediate action is required to avert life-threatening decompensation or permanent debility. Furthermore, these patients can present at any time: a patient with a penetrating neck injury may present to an ED without warning, or a long-term ICU patient with diffuse soft tissue edema and a beard may unexpectedly decompensate and require intubation. Therefore, in a variety of settings, clinicians must be prepared for rapid escalation of care and difficult airway management.

While either difficult bag–mask ventilation *or* difficult intubation occurs in approximately 5% of patients,[1–3] a situation in which *both* bag–mask ventilation and intubation are difficult occurs concomitantly in much fewer patients.[4] Of those, less than 1% of patients require a surgical airway for emergent management,[5] a fraction likely due to advanced airway management skills of emergency physicians and intensivists, and further aided by the development of multiple tools for managing the difficult airway.

► ANTICIPATING THE DIFFICULT AIRWAY

When new patients present in extremis, a detailed history is precluded. However, several historical factors portend a difficult airway and, if possible, should be rapidly determined:

1. History of oral, neck, or cervical spine surgery or irradiation
2. History of oral or neck tumor, cellulitis, or abscess
3. History of neck or mandibular arthritis or other joint immobility
4. Presentation as a result of oral, facial, neck, or cervical spine trauma
5. Use of anticoagulants or presence of a coagulopathy

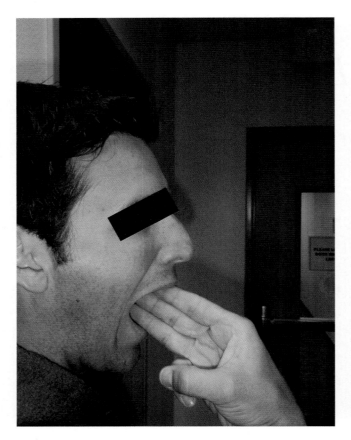

Figure 2-1. Interincisor gap or, for edentulous patients, "intergingival gap."

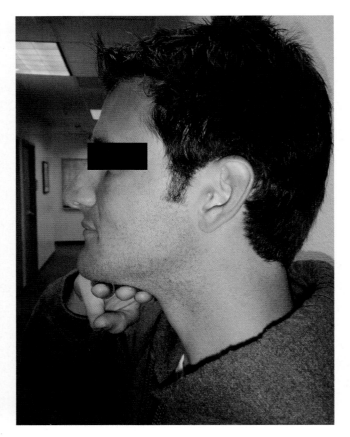

Figure 2-2. Hyomental distance.

Likewise, a focused physical exam of the head and neck should be performed. The LEMON mnemonic can help direct the physical exam to determine if the patient might have a difficult airway[6]:

1. **L**ook externally and assess factors associated with a difficult airway: obesity, micrognathia, large tongue, long upper incisors, prominent overbite with protruding maxillary incisors or underbite with large mandibular incisors, short bull neck, poor dentition that could be dislodged into the airway, or evidence of trauma.

2. **E**valuate with the 3-3-2 rule. The 3-3-2 rules states that with the mouth open the patient should be able to insert three fingers between the teeth (the interincisor gap or, for edentulous patients, the "intergingival gap"; Figure 2-1), has three finger breadths between the front of the chin and hyoid bone (the "hyomental distance"; Figure 2-2), and has two finger breadths between the hyoid bone and the thyroid cartilage (the "thyrohyoid distance"; Figure 2-3). Patients who pass the rule (i.e., meet all of the criteria) are more likely to be successfully intubated without complications, that is, are likely *not* to have a difficult airway.

3. **M**allampati score assessment: with the patient seated, mouth wide open, tongue protruding, and neck in extension, the clinician looks into the mouth to visualize the tongue, tonsils, uvula, and posterior pharynx (Figure 2-4). Class I airways allow for visualization of the entire posterior oropharynx, soft palate, uvula, fauces, and tonsils, while Class II airways allow for visualization of the soft palate, some but not all of the uvula, and fauces. Class I and II airways are associated with successful intubations. Class III airways are characterized by visualization only of the soft palate and base of the uvula, and are associated with moderate difficulty during intubation. Class IV airways do not allow for visualization of any of the posterior pharynx and are associated with severe difficulty during intubation (and may be impossible to intubate using traditional techniques).

4. **O**bstruction assessment: determine if there is an upper airway foreign body, tumor, or other obstructing factors such as epiglottitis or Ludwig's angina. Three key signs are difficulty handling secretions, stridor (which occurs when <10% of normal caliber of airway circumference is clear), and a muffled voice.

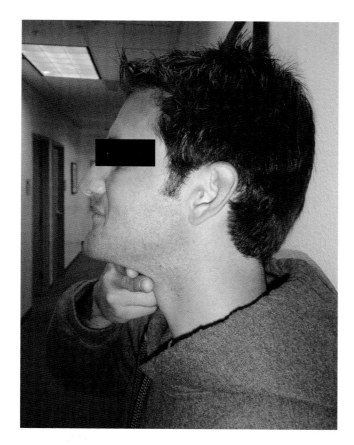

Figure 2-3. Thyrohoid distance.

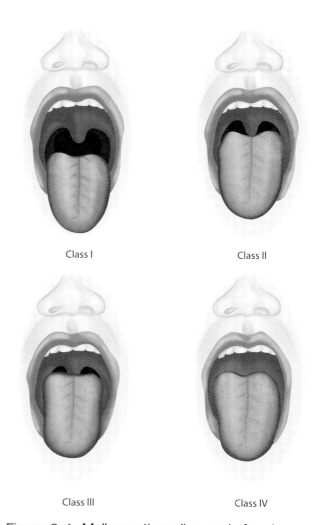

Class I

Class II

Class III

Class IV

Figure 2-4. Mallampati grading scale for airways. Class I: Faucial pillars, soft palate, and uvula can be visualized. Class II: Faucial pillars and soft palate can be visualized, but the uvula is masked by the base of the tongue. Class III: Only the base of the uvula can be visualized. Class IV: None of the three structures can be visualized. (Reproduced with permission from Tintinalli JE, Stapcyzynski JS, Cline DM, Ma OJ, Cydulka RK, Meckler GD, eds. *Emergency Medicine: A Comprehensive Study Guide*. 7th ed. McGraw-Hill Inc; 2011. Figure 30-8.)

5. **N**eck mobility assessment: neck mobility directly affects a clinician's ability to visualize the vocal cords during intubation. Normal patients should be able to touch their chin to their chest on flexion with a wide range of extension. Cervical spine trauma or immobilization can limit this mobility and subsequent visualization, as can conditions such as ankylosing spondylitis and severe rheumatoid arthritis.

The MOANS mnemonic should also be used to predict those who will be difficult to ventilate with a face mask[6]:

1. **M**ask seal should be good and not obstructed by factors such as a large beard or hindered by factors such as a large bite abnormality.
2. **O**besity with either a small jaw or mid-face can prevent a good seal.
3. **A**ge >55 years old is associated with difficult mask ventilation.
4. **N**o teeth and consequent lack of "dental tone."
5. **S**tiff necks can make it hard to position patients for proper ventilation.

For inpatients, either already in an ICU or decompensating on a regular floor, additional history may already be known. For patients who have already been intubated (such as postoperative patients, or patients who have already had an ICU stay), information may already be known about their airways. If the patient's condition allows, such information should be rapidly obtained, accepting the fact that factors since the last intubation may have negatively impacted the ability to intubate the patient (prior intubation with residual swelling, injury, or bleeding, significantly positive fluid balance leading to diffuse edema, recently reversed tracheostomy, etc.). For patients intubated in the OR, the anesthesia notes can be invaluable. Note the number of attempts, the device used, and the view

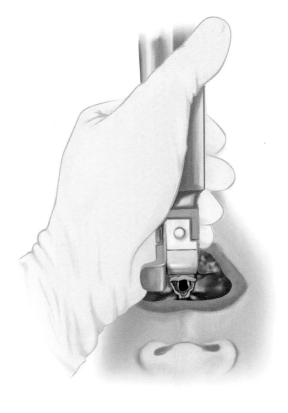

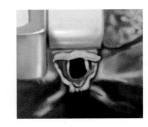

Grade I

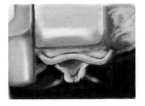

Grade II

Grade III

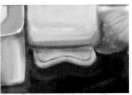

Grade IV

Figure 2-5. Cormack–Lehane grading. (Reproduced with permission from Kovacs G, Law JA, eds. *Airway Management and Emergencies.* McGraw-Hill Inc; 2007. Figure 3-11, p. 29.)

obtained (often described with the Cormack–Lehane grade) Figure 2-5.

Although predictor variables such as the Mallampati score may be highly positively correlated with descriptors such as C-L view (the Mallampati score has a positive correlation with the C-L grade of 0.8–0.9),[7] they are still only predictors. Since descriptors such as the C-L grade directly describe the laryngoscopic view, it is, perhaps, more accurate to use that information when available. Of course, C-L grades will not be available for ED patients or for many inpatients (such as nonsurgical patients). Furthermore, the C-L grade says nothing about the ease or difficulty of ventilating the patient with a bag-valve-mask.

▶ PREPARE FOR AIRWAY MANAGEMENT

Once determined that the patient needs emergent airway management, preparation should begin immediately. If possible, the ensuing events should be explained to the patient as well as reassurance provided since patient anxiety can complicate management. The patient should be positioned to align the three main axes: the laryngeal axis, the pharyngeal axis, and the oral axis

(Figure 2-6). While positioning the patient, equipment can be checked, including the following:

1. Appropriately sized face mask
2. Respiratory bag connected to oxygen
3. Suction set up and ready
4. Laryngoscope light functioning properly; backup handle available
5. Multiple types and sizes of laryngoscope blades available
6. Multiple endotracheal tubes (ETTs) available
7. ETT loaded with stylet
8. 10-cm^3 syringe
9. Confirmatory devices (end-tidal CO_2 detector, esophageal detector)

Of course, communication with staff regarding medications and other orders is imperative.

▶ OROTRACHEAL INTUBATION MANEUVERS

Even when there is concern for a difficult airway, most patients can still be orotracheally intubated with traditional direct laryngoscopy (DL). In the event that the

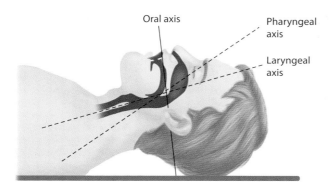

Figure 2-6. Proper patient position for endotracheal intubation showing oral, pharyngeal, and laryngeal axes. (Reproduced with permission from Tintinalli JE, Stapcyzynski JS, Cline DM, Ma OJ, Cydulka RK, Meckler GD, eds. *Emergency Medicine: A Comprehensive Study Guide.* **7th ed. McGraw-Hill Inc; 2011. Figure 30-2A.)**

initial DL attempt is unsuccessful, other maneuvers should be considered and attempted:

1. Reposition the patient to properly align the airway axes.
2. Consider the B-U-R-P maneuver, whereby the operator manipulates the thyroid cartilage with his or her right hand, providing gentle (B)ackward, (U)pward, (R)ightward (P)ressure. If this technique results in visualization of the vocal cords, an assistant can hold the thyroid cartilage in that position while the operator proceeds with intubation. The BURP maneuver is associated with improved visualization of the glottis and subsequent successful intubation.[8]
3. A different laryngoscope blade may be tried. This may involve simply changing the size of blade being used, or it may involve changing the type of blade, for instance, from a Macintosh to a Miller blade. While the Macintosh blade seems to be preferred by most clinicians, it can be difficult to use in patients with a large or "floppy" epiglottis, in which case a Miller blade may result in better visualization of the vocal cords.
4. A patient's habitus or size may preclude advancing a large-sized tube. If the vocal cords are visualized but the ETT cannot be passed, a smaller ETT may allow a successful intubation.

While these maneuvers are being attempted, preparations should simultaneously be made for one or more alternative airway control modalities. These methods can be difficult to perform under the stress of a decompensating patient. Furthermore, since the modalities often involve additional, expensive equipment, they are not part of routine practice, and skills may deteriorate. Therefore, it is important that these skills be maintained,

perhaps by semi-routine use on patients not expected to have a difficult airway, or by other means. It is reasonable that clinicians should master two or three of these "rescue" tools for use in the emergent setting.

▶ VIDEO LARYNGOSCOPE

One of the easiest difficult airway tools to use is the video laryngoscope (Figure 2-7). It has been shown to improve glottic visualization and, thus, success of intubation attempts.[9] To use a video laryngoscope, the patient is positioned, the mouth opened, and the laryngoscope placed midline into the posterior pharynx. When using the video laryngoscope, the tongue does not need to be manually displaced as with traditional laryngoscopy. Then, rather than looking into the pharynx, the clinician looks at the video monitor while advancing the laryngoscope to identify the epiglottis and then the vocal cords. On visualization of the glottis, the ETT is then placed into the pharynx under direct visualization, but then advanced into the trachea through the vocal cords under video screen visualization.

Although use of a video laryngoscope requires the clinician to go from direct visualization of the pharynx to using the video screen for visualization of the glottis to direct visualization for pharyngeal placement of the ETT and back to video screen visualization for glottic placement, this approach is easy to learn because the manual technique is similar to orotracheal intubation with traditional laryngoscopy and direct visualization. Furthermore, this technique has been associated with

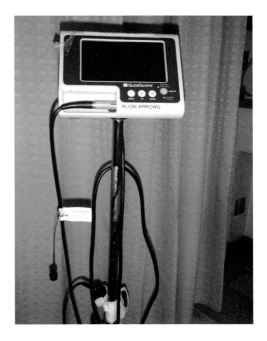

Figure 2-7. Video laryngoscope.

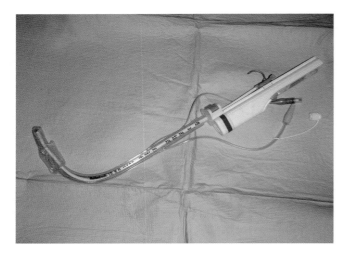

Figure 2-8. Lighted stylet (e.g., Trachlight, Surch-lite).

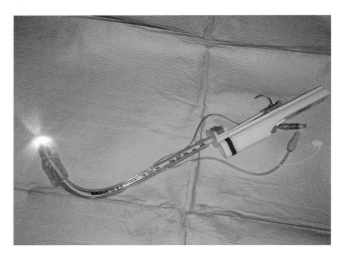

Figure 2-9. Lighted stylet, a semi-rigid stylet with a light on the end.

improved visualization of the glottis[10] and appears to be the most easy difficult airway tool to learn. This technique is also favored by many clinicians when intubating patients in cervical spine collars since the collar can be left in place, resulting in less spine movement during intubation. The biggest disadvantage, as above, is that without regular use, it remains easy to obtain good glottic visualization, but difficult to pass the ETT. These devices are also finding an increased audience in training programs, both for teaching purposes and because they allow the supervising attending to better monitor trainees.

▶ LIGHTED STYLET

The lighted stylet (e.g., Trachlight, Surch-lite; Figure 2-8) is another option for the intubation of patients with a difficult airway, especially when direct visualization is hindered due to trismus or obscuration due to copious secretions or bleeding. It involves intubation without direct visualization of the epiglottis or vocal cords, which is disconcerting to some clinicians. However, it can be more successful than traditional intubation under DL and may be used to rescue failed attempts.[11,12]

The lighted stylet is a semi-rigid stylet with a light on the end (Figure 2-9). With the patient positioned for intubation and the ETT preloaded on the stylet as with a traditional ETT, the lighted stylet is turned on and placed in the posterior pharynx, and then slowly advanced while the clinician observes the exterior, anterior neck for evidence of the light "shining" through the skin. It is important to note that the stylet is advanced without direct visualization of the pharynx or glottic structures. When the stylet is in the trachea, the light shines distinctly through the skin due to the thin tracheal membranes that allow for the transmission of light. On visualization of this light in the anterior midline of the neck, the endotracheal tube can be advanced followed by confirmation of appropriate tube placement using standard technique. If the stylet is placed in the esophagus, the light is either not seen or perceived as a diffuse "glow" rather than a distinct point of light, in which case the clinician must reposition the stylet until a distinct point of light is seen shining in the anterior midline of the neck.

Although the lighted stylet has been used as a rescue airway technique, it requires transillumination of the trachea and anterior neck that can be hindered by high levels of ambient light. Therefore, one should consider dimming the lights when performing this technique. Furthermore, clinicians must practice using the lighted stylet under controlled settings before emergent use since it is associated with an appreciable learning curve as compared with DL.[13]

▶ INTUBATING INTRODUCER

The intubating introducer (e.g., Eschmann Introducer, SunMed Flex Guide, and Frova; Figure 2-10) is a semi-rigid, long stylet (typically >60 cm) with a bent, soft tip designed for use with anterior airways or the situation when direct visualization of the glottic structures is not possible (e.g., significant bleeding from trauma). In the past, the term "bougie" was used to refer to such introducers because a bougie dilator was used as one of the first such introducers. The Frova is a particular intubating introducer that also has a fenestrated tip to allow oxygenation when used with a bag–valve–adapter.

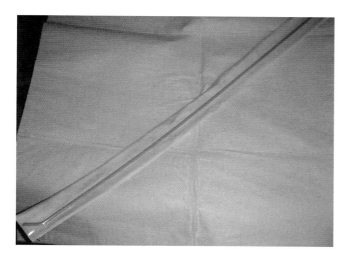

Figure 2-10. Intubating introducer (e.g., Eschmann Introducer, SunMed Flex Guide, and Frova).

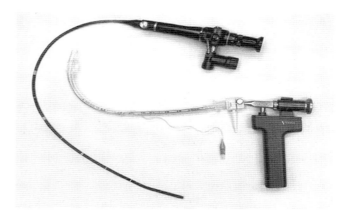

Figure 2-11. A fiberoptic laryngoscope and a Shikani endoscope (Clarus Medical LLC, Minneapolis, MN).

Once the patient is positioned for intubation, the intubating introducer is placed blindly in the posterior pharynx and slowly advanced toward the trachea, maintaining the bent tip in a midline, anterior-most position. The introducer is advanced blindly until two tactile sensations are appreciated, confirming placement in the trachea. The first is the feeling of the tracheal rings, which are appreciated as "vibrations" or "clicks" by the clinician. The second is resistance to further advancement, corresponding with arrival at the smaller airways (as opposed to the esophagus that would allow continued advancement to the stomach without resistance). Once tracheal placement is confirmed, the ETT is advanced over the bougie using the Seldinger technique, the bougie is withdrawn, and confirmation of placement can proceed using standard technique.

One technique for use as a routine rescue device is to always have an introducer immediately available, yet still in its sterile package (so if not used, there is no cost). If DL yields an airway with either visualization of only the arytenoids anteriorly or difficulty passing an ETT into an anterior airway, the operator may remain in place and simply request the bougie be opened and passed to him or her. Then under DL, the bougie can be placed, the laryngoscope removed, and the ETT passed via Seldinger technique as above.

The advantages of the intubating introducer include use for anterior airways, for those with obscured direct visualization potential for use with or without laryngoscopy, and ease of use by novice clinicians.[14] On the other hand, it may be difficult to use in cases of tracheal trauma and may be relatively contraindicated in cases of angioedema where increased edema may result from triggering of the bradykinin/complement cascade.

▶ FIBEROPTIC STYLETS

Fiberoptic stylets (FOS, e.g., Shikani Optical Stylet, Bonfils Retromolar Intubation Fiberscope, Levitan FPS scope; Figure 2-11) include a fiberoptic device at the distal end of a metal stylet, designed to move the clinician's view from the mouth and posterior pharynx to the end of the FOS near the glottis. They can be rigid or semi-rigid and may contain ancillary ports, for instance, for instillation of oxygen during intubation.

Like the lighted stylet and intubating introducers, the FOS may be placed blindly in the posterior pharynx. Then, the FOS is advanced toward the trachea while visualizing the pharyngeal anatomy through an eyepiece at the proximal end of the stylet. Once the vocal cords are visualized, the stylet is advanced into the trachea and then the ETT is advanced over the stylet with confirmation of appropriate placement using standard technique.

Alternatively, the oral, pharyngeal, and laryngeal axes may be aligned using a laryngoscope similar to traditional DL. The FOS may then be placed and advanced, using the laryngoscope to separate tissues, but with visualization via the eyepiece at the proximal end of the stylet.

One technique involves a combination of DL and fiberoptics. It may be used for routine use, or limited for use in a suspected difficult airway. The FOS is loaded with the ETT and intubation is attempted via DL. If the cords are visualized, the intubation can proceed via traditional means, utilizing the FOS like a traditional stylet to place the ETT under DL. But, if the airway turns out to be a difficult airway and the cords cannot be seen, the operator can change his or her view from one of DL to looking through the fiberoptic eyepiece of the stylet. Intubation can then proceed in a fiberoptic manner as above (advancing the FOS through the cords, and then withdrawing the FOS leaving the ETT in place). This combination of a DL approach with fiberoptic backup has several advantages: traditional DL practice is maintained (especially important in teaching programs), using a laryngoscope to separate tissue and align the axes may facilitate the fiberoptic approach, and, finally, for a difficult airway the rescue device is immediately available (in fact, already placed). The disadvantage of this technique is the cost since most patients can be intubated with routine DL, yet the FOS will still have to be sterilized.

Overall, the advantages of the FOS include use in the case of anterior airways, potential for use with or without laryngoscopy, and cost, typically thousands of dollars less than a video laryngoscope. On the other hand, it has limited use in cases where direct visualization of the glottis is hindered by secretions or hemorrhage and requires some experience before emergent use.

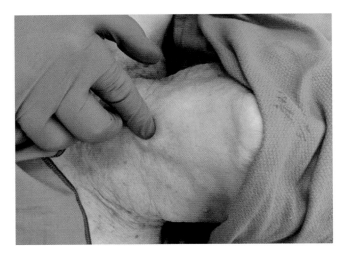

Figure 2-12. Locate the cricothyroid membrane. (Courtesy of Jennifer McBride, PhD and Michael Phelan, MD, Cleveland Clinic and Michael Smith, MD, MetroHealth.)

▶ FLEXIBLE BRONCHOSCOPE

Flexible bronchoscopes (Figure 2-11) are flexible, directable fiberoptic tools that allow for visualization of the airway anatomy with greater manual control than possible with an FOS. Unfortunately, the time required for setup and possibility of scope damage from patient biting limit the use of flexible bronchoscopes for rapid, emergent orotracheal intubation. However, when there is time to prepare for a semi-awake nasotracheal intubation, flexible bronchoscopes can be invaluable. This could be especially useful in patients with suspected epiglottitis, angioedema, or severe obstructive sleep apnea where traditional intubation would be difficult and a surgical airway challenging. It is better tolerated by patients and allows them to remain sitting up. Furthermore, for planned extubations in the ICU or OR where an emergent reintubation is possible in a suspected or known difficult airway, it is easily feasible to have all equipment set up and ready for use.

The patient can be prepared by administering intranasal, aerosolized phenylephrine and placement of a 6-0 ETT lubricated with lidocaine jelly into the nasopharynx. Then, with the patient sitting upright, the flexible bronchoscope can be advanced through the lumen of the tube into the posterior pharynx. From there, the flexible bronchoscope is advanced while visualizing the epiglottis and vocal cords with the eyepiece at the proximal end. Once the distal tip of the scope passes through the vocal cords, the ETT is then advanced, the scope removed, and placement confirmed using standard technique. If there is difficulty advancing the ETT into the trachea, it may be caught on the arytenoids, in which case rotating the flexible bronchoscope counter-

clockwise may overcome the obstruction and allow for advancement of the tube.

The main advantages of this technique are use with anterior airways, improved visualization, and ability to be performed in upright patients able to breathe on their own. Furthermore, the bronchoscope itself can be used to confirm placement, both visually and measuring amount withdrawn to determine distance from the carina, obviating the need for a postintubation chest x-ray. The main disadvantages are cost, setup time (typically 15–20 minutes), the need for greater operator/clinician skill, and need for clear visualization that can be obscured by secretions, hemorrhage, and obstructing masses.

▶ RETROGRADE WIRE INTUBATION

When other methods for tracheal intubation have failed, retrograde wire intubation can be rapidly attempted while preparing for placement of a surgical airway. The anterior neck should be quickly prepped with Betadine or ChloraPrep, followed by rapid identification of the cricothyroid membrane (Figure 2-12). Then an 18-gauge needle should be placed through the cricothyroid membrane (Figure 2-13). Placement can be confirmed by aspiration of air, and the needle repositioned aiming cephalad. A guidewire can then be advanced through the needle into the oropharynx, where Magill forceps or alligators can be used to extract the distal tip of the wire out of the mouth. Once the distal tip is obtained and firmly grasped, an ETT can be advanced over the wire into the trachea with a Seldinger-like technique and placement confirmed using standard measures.

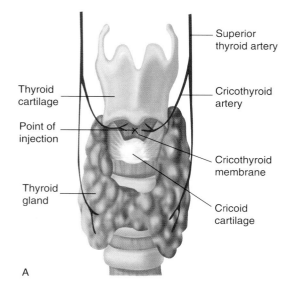

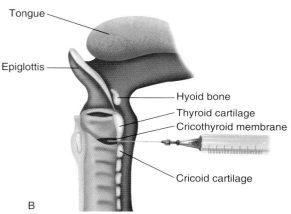

Figure 2-13. Translaryngeal anesthesia via cricothyroid puncture. Anatomy, cross-sectional view. Same landmarks as those for translaryngeal ventilation. (A) AP view and (B) lateral view. (Reproduced with permission from Tintinalli JE, Kelen GD, Stapcyzynski JS, eds. *Emergency Medicine: A Comprehensive Study Guide.* 6th ed. McGraw-Hill Inc; 2004. Figure 19-2B.)

This technique often requires two operators—one at the neck and one at the mouth—and is invasive, but has less morbidity than a surgical airway when successful. However, it can be difficult, especially in patients with upper airway obstruction or poor visualization due to blood or secretions.

► ULTRASOUND

Although never studied in the setting of the emergent, difficult airway, ultrasound can help localize the tracheal rings and cricothyroid membrane. This may

facilitate retrograde wire intubation by directing needle placement and confirming tube placement. In addition, when possible, a second operator can use ultrasound to confirm placement of the lighted stylet, intubating introducer, or FOS in the trachea prior to advancing the ETT.

► FAILED TRACHEAL INTUBATION

When the clinician is unable to perform tracheal intubation for the patient requiring emergent airway management, several tools can be used to provide oxygen while preparing to place a surgical airway (e.g., crichothyrotomy or emergent tracheostomy; see Chapter 3). However, as none of these provide definitive airway management, they should only be used to bridge patients to a definitive airway.

► LARYNGEAL MASK AIRWAY (LMA)

The LMA (Figure 2-14) is often used by anesthesiologists in the controlled setting of the operating room for elective cases, but it is not ideal for emergent settings because it does not protect the airway from secretions, aspiration, blood, or mass lesions such as expanding hematomas. Furthermore, the LMA is ineffective in situations where there is an obstruction (e.g., epiglottitis, angioedema, tracheal trauma) and should not even be attempted in such cases. The LMA works by creating a seal over the larynx with a soft mask that allows for oxygen to be blown into the lungs, in a sense moving the bag–mask apparatus from the level of the mouth to the larynx.

The LMA is inserted "backwards" into the posterior pharynx and then advanced while being rotated

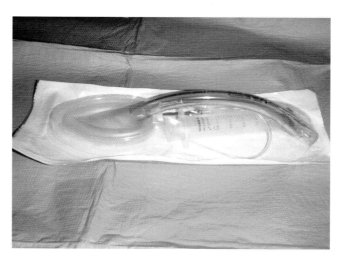

Figure 2-14. Laryngeal mask airway (LMA).

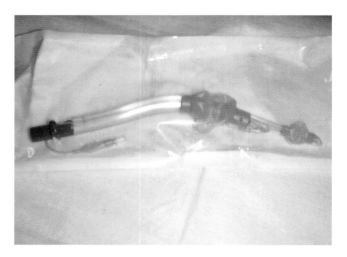

Figure 2-15. Combitube and King Airway.

forward, seating the LMA in the hypopharynx. Once this is done, the cuff is inflated and bag ventilation can be performed. Even if adequate oxygenation and ventilation can be provided with an LMA, the clinician must remember that this is not a definitive airway as the patient's airway is not protected from secretions, aspiration, blood, or mass lesions such as expanding hematomas. The LMA should only be used temporarily to provide oxygen while preparing to establish a definitive airway.

The intubating LMA (I-LMA) is a specific kind of LMA with a metal handle and an aperture in the mask that allows for passage of an ETT through the LMA into the trachea. The I-LMA is designed so that the tube aperture is above the glottis in most patients when the mask is seated in the hypopharynx. Thus, once the I-LMA is placed, a flexible ETT can be passed through the lumen into the trachea with confirmation by standard technique. However, this will not work in cases of altered anatomy or glottic obstruction.

▶ COMBITUBE OR KING AIRWAY

The Combitube and King Airway (Figure 2-15) are dual-port, double-cuffed tubes designed for use in the difficult airway. They are placed blindly into the posterior pharynx and advanced, usually resulting in an esophageal intubation. If the esophagus is intubated, the distal cuff lies in the esophagus and the proximal cuff lies in the supraglottic space. The distal cuff is inflated to prevent air from entering the stomach and help block stomach contents from aspirating into the airway. The proximal cuff is inflated to prevent air from leaking out of the mouth and help block secre-

tions from falling back into the trachea. A bag–valve setup can then be used to ventilate from the laryngeal port to laryngeal fenestrations that lie above the glottic opening between the two cuffs.

As with the LMA, even if adequate oxygenation and ventilation can be provided with a Combitube or King Airway, the clinician must remember that this is not a definitive airway because the patient's airway is not fully protected from secretions, aspiration, blood, or mass lesions. Unlike the LMA, there is no "intubating" version and, therefore, the Combitube or King Airway should only be used temporarily to provide oxygen while preparing to establish a definitive airway. The only exception is on the rare occasion when the tube is placed blindly in the trachea, in which case the pharyngeal port can be used to ventilate the trachea since it is continuous with the distal tip of the tube and essentially functioning as an ETT.

▶ NEEDLE CRICOTHYROTOMY

In the event that the clinician is unable to perform tracheal intubation and cannot provide oxygen via an LMA, Combitube, or King Airway, supplemental oxygen may be provided emergently via needle cricothyrotomy. However, by the time this is attempted, the clinician has only a few minutes in which to establish a surgical airway.

Once the anterior neck is prepped with povidone–iodine or chlorhexidine gluconate, the cricothyroid membrane is rapidly identified (Figure 2-12). An 18-gauge needle is placed through the cricothyroid membrane (Figure 2-13) into the trachea, which can be confirmed by aspiration of air using a syringe. Once this is done, the plunger is removed and a bag–valve–adapter is attached to the open end of the syringe. Then, using positive pressure, oxygen can be bagged through the needle into the lungs while preparing for a surgical airway to follow (see Chapter 3).

▶ SUMMARY

Clinicians can anticipate encountering a *difficult airway* 1–5% of the time and should be able to rapidly assess the likelihood of a patient have a difficult airway based on a directed history and physical exam. In the event that a patient has a difficult airway and requires emergent management, a number of maneuvers can be done to facilitate successful orotracheal intubation by traditional laryngoscopy. When these fail, clinicians should be familiar with available "rescue" devices and techniques to provide oxygenation and ventilation without the morbidity associated with a surgical airway.

REFERENCES

1. Langeron O, Masso E, Huraux C, et al. Prediction of difficult mask ventilation. *Anesthesiology*. 2000;92:1229–1236.

2. Kheterpal S, Han R, Tremper KK, et al. Incidence and predictors of difficult and impossible mask ventilation. *Anesthesiology*. 2006;105:885–891.

3. Burkle CM, Walsh MT, Harrison BA, Curry TB, Rose SH. Airway management after failure to intubate by direct laryngoscopy: outcomes in a large teaching hospital. *Can J Anaesth*. 2005;52:634–640.

4. Rose DK, Cohen MM. The airway: problems and predictions in 18,500 patients. *Can J Anaesth*. 1994;41:372–383.

5. Sagarin MJ, Barton ED, Chang YM, Walls RM. Airway management by US and Canadian emergency medicine residents: a multicenter analysis of more than 6,000 endotracheal intubation attempts. *Ann Emerg Med*. 2005;46:328–336.

6. Walls RM, Murphy MF. The difficult airway in adults. UpToDate.com article. Available at: http://www.uptodate.com/patients/content/topic.do?topicKey=~b3bb4xsxXjunTf. Accessed 07/06/10.

7. Cattano D, Panicucci E, Paolicchi A, et al. Risk factors of the difficult airway: an Italian survey of 1956 patients. *Anesth Analg*. 2004;99:1774–1779.

8. Lafferty KA, Kulkarni R. Tracheal intubation, rapid sequence intubation: treatment and medication. eMedicine article. Available at: http://emedicine.medscape.com/article/80222-treatment. Accessed 07/06/10.

9. Brown CA, Bair AE, Pallin DJ, Laurin EG, Walls RM. Improved glottis exposure with the video Macintosh laryngoscope in adult emergency department tracheal intubations. *Ann Emerg Med*. 2010;56:83–88.

10. Cooper RM. Cardiothoracic anesthesia, respiration, and airway: early clinical experience with a new videolaryngoscope (GlideScope) in 728 patients. *Can J Anesth*. 2005;52:191–198.

11. Hung OR, Pytka A, Morris I, et al. Clinical trial of a new lightwand device (Trachlight) to intubate the trachea. *Anesthesiology*. 1995;83:509–514.

12. Agro F, Hung OR, Cataldo R, Carassiti M, Gherardi S. Lightwand intubation using the Trachlight: a brief review of current knowledge. *Can J Anaesth*. 2001;48:592–599.

13. Soh CR, Kong CF, Kong CS, Ip-Yam PC, Chin E, Goh MH. Tracheal intubation by novice staff: the direct vision laryngoscope or the lighted stylet (Trachlight)? *Emerg Med J*. 2002;19:292–294.

14. Bair AE, Laurin EG, Schmitt BJ. An assessment of a tracheal tube introducer as an endotracheal tube placement confirmation device. *Am J Emerg Med*. 2005;23:754–758.

CHAPTER 3

The Failed Airway

David R. Gens, David A. Farcy, and Dale J. Yeatts

The airway management of unstable and critically ill patients has always been an essential skill within the emergency physician's scope of practice. The early act of inserting an artificial airway protects the lungs from aspiration in an obtunded patient, or prevents hypoxia and carbon dioxide retention in a patient who cannot spontaneously breathe. This has been shown to improve neurologic outcome when performed early during the initial phase of resuscitation, and emergency physicians are often the first clinicians to perform intubation and initiate mechanical ventilation.[1]

While direct laryngoscopy is associated with a high rate of success with few adverse events when performed by personnel skilled in its use, there are a number of clinical scenarios and presentations in which direct or indirect laryngoscopic intubation is difficult or impossible. Disruption of the normal anatomy due to body habitus, medical and surgical disease, or facial and oral trauma can result in soft tissue and bony structure distortion. Obstruction or lack of laryngeal visualization can be caused by copious amounts of blood or vomitus, facial edema, vocal cord swelling from prolonged or multiple intubation attempts, anaphylaxis, angioedema, and burns. When an emergency physician is called upon to perform urgent airway management, the approach to airway management should be standardized and similar in all contexts. Whether in the field with an emergency medical services (EMS) agency or in the hospital, a clinician should recognize when to abort further attempts at intubation through direct visualization and proceed to alternative techniques for establishing an artificial airway. As discussed in the preceding chapter, inability to identify the vocal cords should prompt the use of a "difficult airway" algorithm that includes the use of intubation adjuncts such as tracheal tube introducers, alternative intubation devices such as video laryngoscopes, flexible fiberoptic scopes, lighted stylets, retrograde approaches, or the placement of a laryngeal mask airway (LMA).

When intubation is not successful, especially after administration of neuromuscular blockade, and when adequate oxygenation or ventilation with the bag–valve–mask technique cannot be achieved, a "failed airway" has occurred. At this point, cricothyroidotomy is the emergency medicine surgical airway of choice.[2,3] It should be noted that the terms cricothyroidotomy and cricothyrotomy are synonymous and may be used interchangeably.

Fortunately, the incidence of the "failed airway" in the emergency department (ED) setting is low. Depending on the patient population and the skill level of the clinician, airway management databases report the use of a surgical airway in 0.03–1.8% of patients who require definitive airway management.[4–8] When it does occur, a "failed airway," sometimes referred to as a "cannot intubate–cannot ventilate" situation, requires a surgical airway be placed immediately. Unfortunately, when required, the establishment of an emergency surgical airway is associated with a high rate of complications, up to 14% in some reviews.[9]

Despite newer equipment and modified approaches, there remain two traditional, emergent surgical airway procedures: surgical open cricothyroidotomy and needle cricothyroidotomy. Both approaches require a firm understanding of the involved anatomy for a successful procedure, and a familiarity with the potential limitations and complications of each technique. Preparedness is the key to success.

► CONTRAINDICATIONS OF CRICOTHYROIDOTOMY

This procedure has limited contraindications. Cricothyroidotomy should not be done if oral or nasal intubation has not been attempted or if there is significant trauma to the area, such as fracture of the larynx or transection of the trachea.

The surgical approach is contraindicated in children younger than 10–14 years old due to the underdeveloped larynx; however, the exact age cutoff is not well established in the medical literature. The cricoid ring in children is the narrowest portion of the airway, much like a funnel, with the vocal cords being the widest space. This is generally the opposite in the adult. For this reason, needle cricothyroidotomy is the preferred airway in young children.

► ANATOMY

The cricothyroid membrane is located between the thyroid and cricoid cartilages (Figure 3-1A). Both structures are usually easy to palpate in a patient with normal anatomy. In the edematous intensive care unit (ICU)

patient, the anatomy can be extremely difficult to palpate. By applying pressure over the area of the larynx for several seconds, however, the edema fluid will be dispersed and the anatomic landmarks may be appreciated. Blindly, the cricothyroid membrane can be found approximately one third the distance from the manubrium to the chin, in the midline, in patients with a normal habitus (Figure 3-1B).

The thyroid cartilage is the largest cartilage on the anterior neck. Inferior to the thyroid cartilage is the beginning of the cricothyroid membrane. The superior thyroid prominence, which is often very obvious and is commonly referred to as the "Adam's apple," is the most important landmark for cricothyroidotomy. The cricothyroid artery and vein, which are branches of the superior thyroid artery and vein, run closer to the superior border of the membrane at the inferior portion of the thyroid cartilage. These vessels anastomose in the middle of the membrane (Figure 3-1C). There are usually no vessels at the lower part of the membrane near the superior aspect of the cricoid cartilage; however, a small percentage of patients may have a "thyroid ima" artery that may pass over the inferior portion of the membrane.

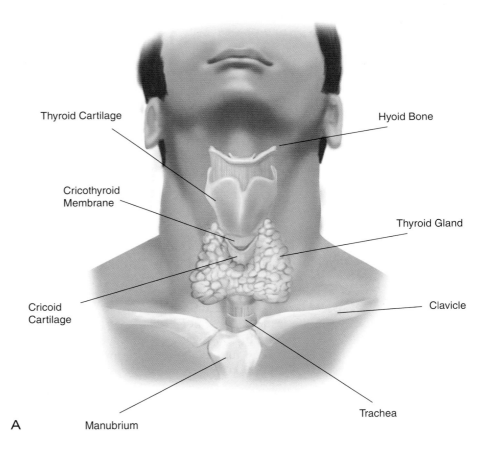

Figure 3-1. (A) Anatomy of the neck. (Reproduced with permission from Gens DR. Surgical airway management [Figure 16-2A and B]. In: Tintinalli JE, et al, eds. *Emergency Medicine: A Comprehensive Study Guide.* 5th ed. McGraw-Hill Inc; 2000:98.)

Thyroid Cartilage

Hyoid Bone

Cricothyroid Membrane

Thyroid Gland

Cricoid Cartilage

Clavicle

Trachea

Manubrium

A

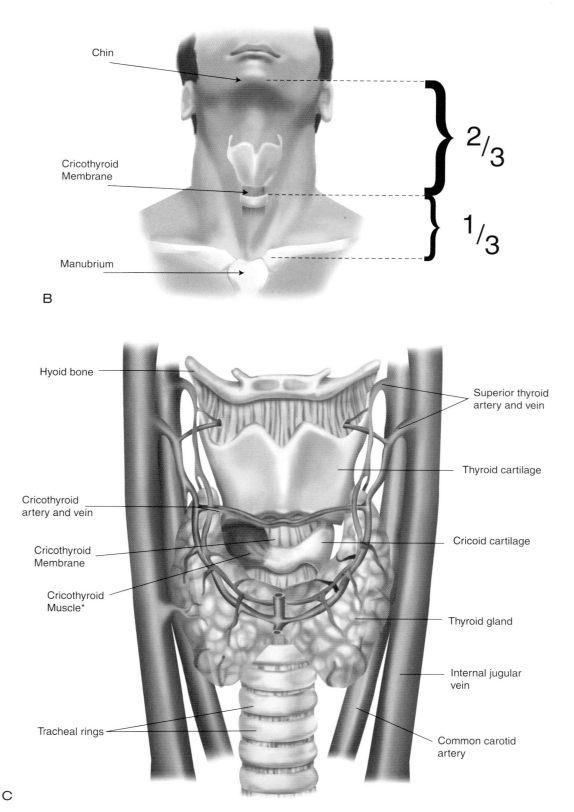

Figure 3-1. *(continued)* (B) Location of the cricothyroid membrane. (Reproduced with permission from Gens DR. Surgical airway management [Figure 16-2A and B]. In: Tintinalli JE, et al, eds. *Emergency Medicine: A Comprehensive Study Guide*. 5th ed. McGraw-Hill Inc; 2000:98.) (C) Anatomy of the cricothyroid membrane. *The cricothyroid muscle is bilateral and depicted on one side for illustrative purposes. Note the cricothyroid artery and vein. (Reproduced with permission from http://www.uptodate.com/, 2011.)

► SURGICAL CRICOTHYROIDOTOMY

In the adult size patient, a surgical cricothyroidotomy is the preferred approach. Only an open surgical crico-thyroidotomy—but *not* a needle cricothyroidotomy—establishes a definitive airway with a cuffed tube in the trachea, and provides a means for adequate artificial oxygenation and ventilation, allowing the resuscitation to continue. The needle method should only be used as a temporizing method until an open cricothyroidotomy or a tracheostomy can be performed due to the ease of catheter dislodgement and bending. The less optimal ventilation with needle cricothyroidotomy can also cause hypercapnia, which will worsen acidosis.

Cricothyroidotomy, rather than tracheostomy, is the preferred initial surgical airway of choice for the failed airway patient. Emergency tracheostomy has a more severe set of complications, such as posterior tracheal laceration, esophageal perforation, and pneumothorax. It is also technically more challenging, even in the percutaneous approach. Tracheostomy, however, is a definitive airway and should be reserved for placement under well-controlled conditions.

Although the emergent need for cricothyroidotomy usually precludes establishing optimal conditions, such as obtaining consent, everything possible should be done to use sterile technique if feasible. In every circumstance, gloves and a face shield with mask should be worn by the proceduralist. Suction should be available. Furthermore, time should be taken to position the patient in a supine position with the neck extended if no cervical injuries are suspected. The patient should remain on supplemental oxygen as long as it does not interfere with or alter the anatomic landmarks.

ICU beds are not generally suitable for any operation: the beds are wider than an operating room (OR) table or ED stretcher and the operator is further away from the patient and therefore must bend over considerably. If the procedure must be performed in an ICU bed, the patient should be moved as close to the side of the operator as possible. If time permits, prepare the neck using either povidone iodine or chlorhexidine solution. The appropriate equipment for the planned technique should be ready and available (Table 3-1).

► SURGICAL TECHNIQUE

One of the major problems with performing surgical and needle cricothyroidotomy is the lack of experience among most practitioners. Furthermore, even among those with experience, or who have practiced extensively under laboratory conditions, skills maintenance is difficult at best. There are simply too few opportunities to clinically utilize this important skill on a regular

► TABLE 3-1. EQUIPMENT FOR SURGICAL CRICOTHYROIDOTOMY

1. Povidone iodine or chlorhexidine gluconate solution
2. Personal protective equipment
3. Scalpel
4. A 6-mm ID endotracheal tube: tubes greater than 6 mm are extremely difficult to place through the cricothyroid membrane (or tracheostomy tube: size 4 or 6 cuffed)
5. Tape to secure the endotracheal tube in place (or tracheostomy tube)
6. Bag–valve–mask device or ventilator and an oxygen source

basis. A 5-year review at the Hennepin County ED found that cricothyroidotomy was performed in only 1% of intubations.[10]

Given the complexity and importance of the skill set, other techniques and equipment have been developed. The Seldinger technique for percutaneous cricothyroidotomy has many advantages over open cricothyroidotomy. First and foremost is comfort. Although open cricothyroidotomy has traditionally been taught as the airway management maneuver of last resort, the large number of other procedures done percutaneously with Seldinger technique—such as central lines and some arterial lines and chest tubes—make this approach a logical choice for many practitioners. This technique is more continuous with procedures more commonly performed. Commercial Seldinger cricothyroidotomy kits are available such as the Cook® Melker kit (Figure 3-2).

There are also good data to show that the Seldinger technique yields better outcomes when compared with open cricothyroidotomy. Schaumann et al showed that not only did the Seldinger technique result in a shorter time to successful ventilation, but it resulted in fewer

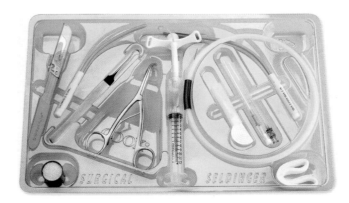

Figure 3-2. Cook® Melker Emergency Cricothyrotomy Catheter Tray. (Reproduced with permission from Cook Medical Incorporated, Bloomington, Indiana.)

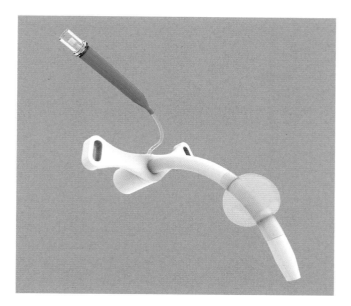

Figure 3-3. Cook® Cuffed Emergency Cricothyrotomy Catheter. (Reproduced with permission from Cook Medical Incorporated, Bloomington, Indiana.)

injuries as well.[11] It is also worth discussing the one unique piece of equipment for this procedure, a commercially available cuffed emergency cricothyroidotomy catheter (Figure 3-3) that looks similar to a tracheostomy tube but with a 5-mm diameter. Much like a tracheostomy tube, it comes with a dilator as well. One advantage of the Melker kit is that it can be used for both the Seldinger technique and the open technique, so that in the chaotic environment of the ED everything necessary is readily available. If a commercial kit is not available, it is recommended that a kit be prepared ahead of time with all the necessary equipment to prevent delay. Keep in mind that the inner diameter of the tube should not exceed 6 mm. A 6.0- or 5.0-mm ID cuffed endotracheal tube (ETT) should be used if a cuffed emergency cricothyroidotomy catheter is not available. It is important to recognize, however, that it can be difficult to secure an ETT and that there is a risk of dislodgement or right main stem bronchus intubation. Familiarity with the type of equipment available, as well as its location, is essential for the success of this procedure.

► CRICOTHYROIDOTOMY APPROACH

(A) Open technique:

1. The practitioner stands to one side of the patient at the level of the neck. A right-handed practitioner should stand on the patient's right side, a left-handed practitioner to the left.

2. The cricoid ring is located by placing the index finger at the sternal notch and palpating cephalad until the first rigid structure is felt. This is the cricoid ring. Rolling the index finger one finger breath above should locate the "hollow" between the cricoid and thyroid cartilages. This is the cricothyroid membrane. One may also choose to locate the thyroid prominence at the midline of the thyroid cartilage, holding the cartilage in place with the nondominant hand, and rolling the index finger caudally by 1 or 2 cm until a small depression or "hollow" is felt. This is the cricothyroid membrane. This may be the technique of choice in an edematous patient or a patient with a larger neck. Attention should be paid to the vessels that run at the superior border of the membrane. In severe bleeding, or whenever a landmark cannot be located, a skin incision is made and a finger should be used to locate a key landmark.

3. The thumb and middle finger of the nondominant hand are then used to stabilize the two cartilages.

4. A vertical skin incision is then made in the midline of the region between the two cartilages. A vertical skin incision is crucial because this incision can be extended if it is too high or too low, whereas a horizontal incision would require a new incision. Also, a vertical midline skin incision has less chance of cutting a vessel. The initial incision should go through the skin and subcutaneous tissues, but no deeper because of the risk of injuring the cricoid or thyroid cartilages or vascular structures.

5. With the scalpel blade now positioned horizontally, the cricothyroid membrane is perforated at the midline inferior portion of the membrane using a horizontal stabbing motion. The reason for the horizontal cut is to have a good horizontal aperture and to not cut the cricoid cartilage with the scalpel blade. The scalpel blade will slice the cricoid cartilage if inserted vertically. The blade should only enter the membrane by 1 cm in order to avoid complications.

6. Insert the back end of the scalpel handle through the cricothyroid membrane incision and rotate it 90° to widen the opening. The handle is slightly wider than the width of the blade.

7. Finally, the ETT tube can be placed in the opening and the balloon inflated as in a traditional intubation. With the practitioner holding the ETT in place, the tube can be connected to a bag–valve–mask, and tube placement should be confirmed as with a traditional intubation (auscultation, color capnometry, esophageal detector, etc.).

8. Finally, the tube is secured with a ribbon or adhesive tape.

9. As always, a portable chest x-ray should be obtained to assure proper placement of the tube relative to the carina and to check for pneumothorax.

(B) Seldinger technique: The procedure here is based on the Cook Melker kit.

1. Open the kit and insert the dilator with wire into the airway catheter (there are two dilators in the kit: one with a hole for the guidewire and one for the open technique that is blunted).

2. The cricothyroid membrane is located in same manner as with the open surgical technique.

3. Attach the needle with the sheath to the syringe and fill the syringe with a small amount of water or saline. Insert the needle into the cricothyroid membrane. With the tip of the needle pointing to the feet in a 45–50° angle, gently puncture the membrane until bubbles are apparent in the syringe. This will confirm you are in the trachea. Use slow, gentle pressure so as not to damage the posterior wall of the trachea.

4. As soon as there is a "bubble" of air in the syringe (signaling entrance into the lumen of the larynx) (Figure 3-4), the sheath is advanced over the needle and into the larynx, still at 45°. As with advancing an ETT via a surgical cricothyroidotomy, overzealous posterior advancement of the sheath may cause the sheath to get stuck on the cricoid cartilage posteriorly. In this case, the syringe with sheath should be withdrawn slightly, and readvanced taking care not to displace the sheath posteriorly.

5. Once placed, the needle can be removed leaving the sheath in place in the larynx/trachea. The wire should be advanced through the sheath (Figure 3-5). The plastic sheath is then removed leaving only the wire in place.

6. With the provided 15-blade scalpel, a 0.5-cm vertical skin incision should be made on both sides of the wire (taking care not to cut the wire). Remember that the catheter size is 0.5 cm so a slightly larger incision will be necessary.

7. Insert the external end of the wire into the dilator, which was already placed into the cricothyroidotomy catheter. Advance them as a unit, following the curvature of the dilator, through the subcutaneous tissue and into the trachea. A twisting motion may be required so as not to bend the wire. Advance until the cricothyroidotomy catheter is flush against the skin (Figure 3-6). Once in place, the dilator is removed and the cuff inflated.

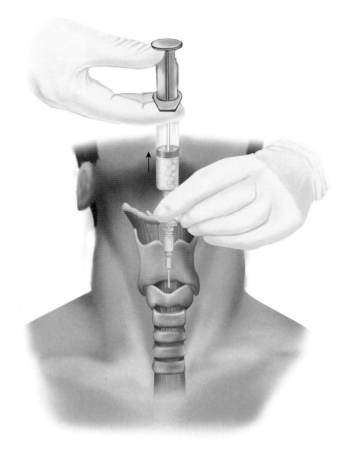

Figure 3-4. Syringe with "air bubble." (Reproduced with permission from http://www.uptodate.com/, 2011.)

8. Secure the cricothyroidotomy catheter with the provided wrap. Confirm placement as discussed in the section "Surgical Technique."

(C) Holmes et al reported a rapid four-step technique, a modified version of the open surgical technique that was found to be easier and quicker (performed in one third the time) when compared with the open technique.[12] In another variation, Hill et al found that insertion of a tracheal tube directly through the incision was challenging and modified the technique by placing a bougie through the incision. The cricothyroidotomy catheter was then advanced over the bougie. In their randomized study conducted on sheep, they found that this was easier and faster to perform.[13]

▶ NEEDLE CRICOTHYROIDOTOMY

Needle cricothyroidotomy is the preferred emergency surgical airway technique in patients under the age of 10–14 years. This is because larger endotracheal or

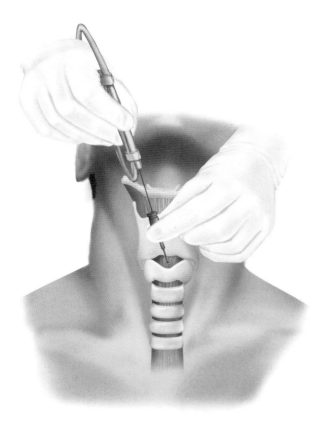

Figure 3-5. Place the guidewire through the catheter into the trachea. (Reproduced with permission from http://www.uptodate.com/, 2011.)

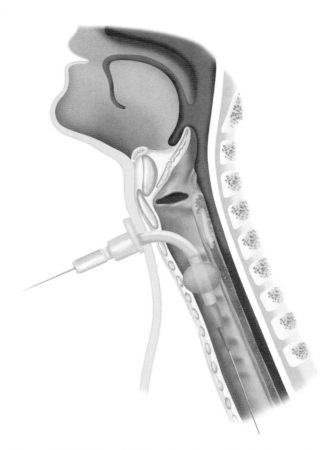

Figure 3-6. Cook® Cricothyrotomy Catheter with dilator and wire seen from a cross-sectional view. (Reproduced with permission from Cook Medical Incorporated, Bloomington, Indiana.)

tracheostomy tubes placed through the cricothyroid membrane have a high complication rate in this age group as previously discussed.[14] Ventilation may be achieved, poorly, for approximately 20–30 minutes in a patient with normal lungs, which makes this procedure an inappropriate choice in a sick ICU patient. Furthermore, the airway established by a needle cricothyroidotomy is only a temporary measure. This measure will, however, provide an additional 30 minutes or so until a more definite airway can be established. Note that even if placed correctly, there will be great resistance to ventilatory airflow because of the small lumen of the 12- or 14-gauge catheter.

See Table 3-2 for the needle cricothyroidotomy equipment.

NEEDLE CRICOTHYROIDOTOMY TECHNIQUE

1. The cricothyroid membrane is located in the same manner and, as with a surgical cricothyroidotomy, the thumb and middle finger of the nondominant hand are used to stabilize the two cartilages.

2. A sheathed 14- or 12-gauge needle with a syringe attached is placed over the location of the cricothyroid membrane at 90° to the skin. Adding water or saline will create a "bubble" once air is aspirated from the trachea. If no water is added, a "gush" of air into the syringe will confirm tracheal placement.

3. Once the needle is in the trachea, the needle should be angled 45° caudally. The sheath is then advanced and the needle is removed. As with advancing an ETT via a surgical

▶ **TABLE 3-2. EQUIPMENT FOR NEEDLE CRICOTHYROIDOTOMY**

1. Povidone iodine or chlorhexidine gluconate solution
2. Personal protective equipment
3. A 14- or 12-gauge sheathed needle catheter: 12 gauge is best
4. A 3-mL syringe
5. Adapter from the end of a 7-mm ID endotracheal tube
6. Wall oxygen source

cricothyroidotomy, overzealous posterior advancement of the sheath may cause the sheath to get stuck on the cricoid cartilage posteriorly.

4. The adapter from the end of a 3.0-mm ID ETT can be attached to the end of the catheter, and an Ambu bag or ventilator attached to the adapter. Alternately, a 3-mL syringe (without plunger) can be attached to the catheter to "step up" the size of the connection. An adaptor from the end of a 7.0-mm ID ETT can then be attached to the syringe barrel and the Ambu bag or ventilator can be attached to the adapter.

5. The catheter must be held in place manually by a provider until a proper tracheostomy is performed (which should be immediately). Because of the pressure delivered through the small lumen, the sheath cannot be secured with tape or any other device; it must be manually held in place.

6. While preparations are being made for an emergent tracheostomy, a chest x-ray should be obtained. Massive subcutaneous air could imply misplacement of the catheter into the subcutaneous tissues of the neck.

▶ CRICOTHYROIDOTOMY CONVERSION

The question frequently arises as to how long to leave a cricothyroidotomy tube in place in the larynx and at what point it should be converted to a formal tracheostomy. A tube left in place in the narrow space between the two cartilages can erode either one or both of these cartilages and bacterial chondritis may occur. This can lead to scarring and subsequent laryngeal or tracheal stenosis with loss of laryngeal function. As a rule of thumb, if the airway will be needed for more than 2 days, the cricothyroidotomy should be changed to a tracheostomy; otherwise, the cricothyroidotomy tube may be left in place. For example, in a patient who needs a surgical airway because of anaphylactic or angioedema-related airway swelling, the condition may resolve in a matter of hours, allowing for simple decannulation. If the cricothyroidotomy is to be converted to a tracheostomy, it should be done in a controlled setting with proper instruments and lighting by an appropriate practitioner, whether a surgeon in an OR or an intensivist in the ICU.

▶ COMPLICATIONS

Needle cricothyroidotomy and surgical cricothyroidotomy (whether done in an open manner or with the Seldinger technique) share some common complications.

Bleeding may occur, especially if the thyroid ima artery is injured. This artery is present in 4–10% of individuals, arises from the aorta or brachiocephalic artery, stays in the midline, and may travel cephalad as high as the thyroid cartilage.[15] Once an injury to this artery is recognized, the patient should be taken to the OR to have the artery controlled by ligation. Most bleeding, however, is from small branches of the anterior jugular veins. These veins usually have very high venous pressures due to the high airway pressure in many sick ventilated ICU patients, or in the patient trying to breathe against an obstructed airway (Valsalva). Once the airway is obtained, the intravenous pressure drops and the bleeding usually stops.

Pneumothorax from placement of a surgical airway is usually due to barotrauma from forceful ventilation and high airway pressures toward the end of the procedure. Once the airway is secure, a pneumothorax should be treated just as one that arose from any other condition, with tube thoracostomy.

In an obese or edematous neck or in one with altered anatomy from a tumor or prior surgery, it is possible to **misplace** the cricothyroidotomy catheter, ETT, or needle anterior to the larynx and trachea and into the mediastinum. Ventilation in this setting is obviously not possible. Manifestations of an incorrectly positioned tube are high airway pressures, absent breath sounds, and massive subcutaneous emphysema. When a malpositioned tube is recognized, the tube should be removed and a second attempt should be made.

Laceration or perforation of the structures of the neck, such as the trachea, esophagus, or recurrent laryngeal nerves, is extremely rare and is usually due to inadequate knowledge of the anatomy of the neck. Laceration of the thyroid ima artery, when present, may be unavoidable because it cannot be visualized through the incision.

Late airway complications may occur in up to 52% of cases. These complications include voice changes and laryngeal and/or tracheal stenosis.[16–19] They usually manifest after the course of the critical illness and are not emergent conditions, although they require evaluation and treatment as they may be debilitating for the patient.

REFERENCES

1. Chesnut RM, Marshall LF, Klauber MR, et al. The role of secondary brain injury in determining outcome from severe head injury. *J Trauma.* 1993;34:216.

2. Walls RM. The emergency airway algorithms. In: Walls RM, Murphy M, Luten RC, eds. *Manual of Emergency Airway Management.* Philadelphia: Lippincott Williams & Wilkins; 2008:14.

3. Bair AE, Filbin MR, Kulkarni RG, et al. The failed intubation attempt in the emergency department: analysis of

prevalence, rescue techniques, and personnel. *J Emerg Med.* 2002;23:131.

4. Sise MJ, Shackford SR, Sise CB, et al. Early intubation in the management of trauma patients: indications and outcomes in 1,000 consecutive patients. *J Trauma.* 2009;66:32.

5. Walls RM, Brown CA, Bair AR, et al. Emergency airway management: a multi-center report of 8937 emergency department intubations. *J Emerg Med.* 2010. Epub ahead of print.

6. Sakles JC, Laurin EG, Rantapaa AA, et al. Airway management in the emergency department: a one-year study of 610 tracheal intubations. *Ann Emerg Med.* 1998;31:325.

7. Sagarin MJ, Barton ED, Chng YM, et al. Airway management by US and Canadian emergency medicine residents: a multicenter analysis of more than 6,000 endotracheal intubation attempts. *Ann Emerg Med.* 2005;46:328.

8. Stephens CT, Kahntroff S, Dutton RP. The success of emergency endotracheal intubation in trauma patients: a 10-year experience at a major trauma referral center. *Anesth Analg.* 2009;109:866.

9. Bair AE, Panacek EA, Wisner DH, et al. Cricothyrotomy: a 5-year experience at one institution. *J Emerg Med.* 2003;24:151.

10. Erlandson MJ, Clinton JE, Ruiz E, Cohen J. Cricothyrotomy in the emergency department revisited. *J Emerg Med.* 1989;7(2):115–118.

11. Schaumann N, Lorenz V, Schellongowski P, et al. Evaluation of Seldinger technique emergency cricothyroidotomy versus standard surgical cricothyroidotomy in 200 cadavers. *Anesthesiology.* 2005;102:7.

12. Holmes JF, Panacek EA, Sakles JC, Brofeldt BT. Comparison of 2 cricothyrotomy techniques: standard method versus rapid 4-step technique. *Ann Emerg Med.* 1998;32:442–446.

13. Hill C, Reardon R, Joing S, Falvey D, Miner J. Cricothyrotomy technique using gun elastic bougie is faster than standard technique: a study of emergency medicine residents and medical students in an animal lab. *Acad Emerg Med.* 2010;17:666–669.

14. Sise MJ, Shackford SR, Cruickshank JC, et al. Cricothyroidotomy for long-term tracheal access: a prospective analysis of morbidity and mortality in 76 patients. *Ann Surg.* 1984;200:13.

15. Bergman RA, Afifi AK, Miyauchi R. *Illustrated Encyclopedia of Human Anatomic Variation: Opus II: Cardiovascular System Thyroid Ima Artery.*

16. Isaacs JH Jr, Pedersen AD. Emergency cricothyroidotomy. *Am Surg.* 1997;63:346.

17. Gleeson MJ, Pearson RC, Armistead S, et al. Voice changes following cricothyroidotomy. *J Laryngol Otol.* 1984;98:1015.

18. Kuriloff DB, Setzen M, Portnoy W, et al. Laryngotracheal injury following cricothyroidotomy. *Laryngoscope.* 1989;99:125.

19. Holst M, Hertegard S, Persson A. Vocal dysfunction following cricothyroidotomy: a prospective study. *Laryngoscope.* 1990;100:749.

CHAPTER 4

Mechanical Ventilation

David A. Farcy, Paul L. Petersen, Dennis Heard, and Peter DeBlieux

Understanding the importance of ventilator management is a crucial facet of emergency medicine. Emergency physicians are well known for their expertise in emergent airway management, but securing the airway is only a fraction of their role. Mechanical ventilation (MV) is an essential tool for critically ill patients. If not applied correctly, it can worsen the clinical course and increase morbidity and mortality.[1] In the past two decades, our understanding of ventilator-induced lung injury (VILI) has resulted in the challenging of conventional practices, such as using lower tidal volumes. With the current crisis of emergency department (ED) overcrowding, critical care patients have increased lengths of stay in the ED and, at times, are boarded for several hours or even days until a bed is available in the intensive care unit (ICU).[2,3] The emergency physician must understand critical care topics and the intricacies of MV for heterogeneous patient populations with varying pathologies—no "single setting fits all." With special consideration of each patient's needs, both patient care and outcomes will improve.

▶ INDICATIONS FOR MECHANICAL VENTILATION

Indications for intubation and institution of MV fall under three basic categories: respiratory failure, airway protection, and anticipation of the clinical course.

The most common indication for MV is respiratory failure. These patients frequently have either hypoventilation or a decreased ability to manage the work of breathing. This can lead to hypoxemia, hypercapnia, or both. Hypoxemia is often defined as a Po_2 less than 60 mm Hg. Hypercapnia is defined as an "elevated" Pco_2. In contrast to hypoxemia, hypercapnia is difficult to strictly define, as it is a component of hypoventilation directly resulting in elevation of CO_2. An exact number is less important than the clinical picture and varies in the literature. In certain populations, such as patients with COPD who chronically retain CO_2, a higher baseline Pco_2 of 45–55 mm Hg can be well tolerated. An acute rise in CO_2 from the patient's baseline will cause lethargy, sleepiness, confusion, and altered mental status. In these hypercapnic patients, the primary action of MV is the promotion of appropriate alveolar ventilation with an end goal of proper CO_2 clearance.

Another indication for the institution of MV is to protect the airway from potential aspiration of various etiologies. Common indications include acute intoxication, altered mental status from infection, or massive upper gastrointestinal hemorrhage.

Last, the predicted clinical course will often dictate securing an airway to facilitate either workup or definitive treatment. Patients in a questionable condition may need further diagnostic testing away from the critical resources of the ED, placing them at risk of sudden deterioration "in the hallway of radiology." These patients should be placed on MV prior to leaving the ED.

There are no absolute contraindications for MV. There are, however, minor adverse effects of MV. The placement of an endotracheal tube takes away the protective functions of the upper airway: gas heating, gas humidification, air filtration, and protection from

▶ TABLE 4-1. **COMMON FORMULAS FOR RESPIRATORY PHYSIOLOGY**

Minute ventilation (V_E) = tidal volume (V_T) × respiratory rate (RR)

Compliance (C) = $\Delta V/\Delta P$ or tidal volume/P_{plat} − PEEP

Predicted body weight (PBW)

Male = 50 + (2.3 × [height in inches − 60])

Female = 45.5 + (2.3 × [height in inches − 60])

aspiration. The endotracheal tube decreases effectiveness of removing secretions by expelling them through coughing. There is also loss of speech and an increase in airway resistance.

▶ BASIC PHYSIOLOGY

Appreciation of the fundamental concepts of respiration is essential for the care of a mechanically ventilated patient. The most important parameter one needs to understand and become familiar with is minute ventilation, which is the product of tidal volume and the respiratory rate (Table 4-1). Normal minute ventilation is 5–7 L/min. However, not all of the tidal volume reaches the alveoli because of dead space. Dead space can be anatomic or pathologic. Anatomic dead space exists because gas exchange does not occur in the trachea, larger airways, or ventilator tubing. It is usually estimated as 150 mL or 2.2 mL/kg lean body weight.[4] Pathologic dead space exists for reasons of ventilation/perfusion (V/Q) mismatch, shunting, and decreased diffusion across a diseased capillary–alveolar interface. The physician must be aware of the patient's approximate minute ventilation prior to instituting MV to ensure that the ordered ventilation parameters do not create a respiratory pattern that is incompatible with the patient's disease state. Lower minute ventilation will result in hypoventilation with a resulting increase in Pco_2. This will directly affect the acid–base balance resulting in an acidemia and may also lead to hypoxemia. In contrast, supranormal minute ventilation will lead to a decrease of Pco_2. This will cause an alkalemia and may cause hyperoxygenation, which has been reported to directly result in lung toxicity, although the timing of this toxicity is unclear. This underscores the importance of considering minute ventilation when ordering the initial ventilator settings. Minute ventilation should be adjusted based on the clinical picture rather than a particular number.

Compliance is a measure of the distensibility of the respiratory system. It is the inverse relationship between the change in volume (ΔV) accommodated per change in pressure (ΔP) (Table 4-1). Total compliance is a sum of the chest wall and lung compliances. Decreased compliance is seen in pulmonary/chest wall

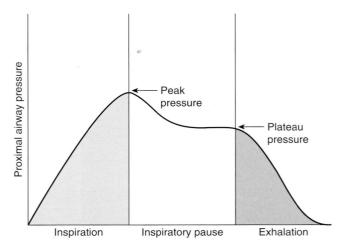

Figure 4-1. Peak inspiratory and plateau pressure.

edema, pulmonary fibrosis, pneumonia, or increased intra-abdominal pressure, whereas increased compliance is seen in emphysema and sarcoidosis. Ventilator settings should be tailored in patients with abnormal compliance to ensure adequate oxygenation and minimize the risk of VILI.

Resistance is the amount of pressure needed to achieve a given amount of airflow. It is mainly a function of the larger airways because velocity is inversely proportional to area and the smaller airways exist in parallel, rather than in series.

These concepts affect two important variables of MV: peak inspiratory pressure (PIP) and plateau pressure (P_{plat}). Both are easily measured on the ventilator (see Figure 4-1).

The PIP is a dynamic pressure measurement during maximal end inspiration. It is influenced by both airway resistance and lung compliance. This pressure only reflects upper airway pressure and not transalveolar pressure. Next, if an end-inspiratory pause is applied after maximal inflation, the airway pressure decreases and then reaches a steady state. This resulting value is the P_{plat}. Elasticity is often associated with P_{plat}, but this pressure measurement is a function of the total compliance and reflects the mean airway pressure of all of the airways. A respiratory therapist can assist the physician in obtaining these values if one does not have the expertise or time.

P_{plat} is the force the lung experiences at the alveoli, not PIP. Thus, P_{plat} has been used as marker of transalveolar pressure. This surrogate value is solely an estimation of transalveolar pressure. Elevated pressures greater than 30 cm H_2O, according to a study conducted by the Acute Respiratory Distress Syndrome (ARDS) Network, have shown a significant increase in mortality (further discussed below).[1] Consideration of the P_{plat} leads to significant changes in clinical decision making.

The PIP and P_{plat} become instrumental during ventilatory therapy. Anticipation and direct action of abnormal pressures can identify the likely cause of the problem. First, one looks at the PIP. A decrease in PIP is due to an air leak, inadvertent change of the ventilator settings, or extubation. The upper limit of normal of PIP is 35 cm H_2O. When the PIP is increased, the physician should reflexively check the P_{plat}. A normal P_{plat} indicates that there is increased airway resistance due to either bronchospasm or an obstruction reducing the endotracheal tube diameter. These obstructions can be caused by biting, kinking, or twisting of the tube. They may also be caused by blood or foreign bodies such as mucus plugs and aspiration. An elevated P_{plat} indicates decreased lung and chest wall compliance. This can be due to pneumothorax, gas trapping (also known as auto–positive end-expiratory pressure [PEEP]), atelectasis, or any of the previously mentioned medical conditions associated with decreased compliance. Careful attention and proper alarm settings for PIPs will alert the astute physician to potential problems.

▶ RISKS OF MECHANICAL VENTILATION

The primary goal of MV is oxygenation and ventilation, but of equal importance is the avoidance injury to the already compromised lung tissue. Damage caused by MV is termed VILI. VILI is a current, discrete term that encompasses and replaces older terms and misconceptions. Its mechanisms are mainly 2-fold: shear and strain stresses.

First, repetitive collapsing and inflation of alveoli produces a shear stress that can tear the thin, fragile alveolar–capillary interface (atelectrauma). It has been confirmed that high end-inspiratory pressures and volumes can lead to alveolar–capillary permeability alterations, nonhydrostatic pulmonary edema, and tissue injury similar to acute lung injury (ALI) and ARDS.[5]

Second, strain in the form of overdistension can lead to alveolar fracture and rupture (barotrauma/volutrauma). Additional effects of alveolar rupture can stem from the liberation of inspired air into the various spaces around the lung: pleural cavity (pneumothorax), mediastinum (pneumomediastinum), or simply the pulmonary parenchyma (pulmonary interstitial emphysema).

Further, the body's immune system contributes to VILI. This injury to the lung induces the production of inflammatory mediators (cytokines and products of the endothelium and arachidonic acid pathways) that infiltrate the bloodstream through the compromised alveolar–capillary interface and produce injurious effects distant to the lungs. This process of multiorgan injury is called biotrauma.[6,7]

The more severe the preventilation abnormalities are, the more severe potential VILI can be.[8] In one study, repetitive collapse and reopening of terminal units did not injure healthy lungs, although it did decrease compliance and alter gas exchange.[9] However, other studies illustrate the increased susceptibility of diseased lungs to the adverse effects of MV.

Based on animal data, P_{plat} >35 cm H_2O is concerning for VILI. This has led to the concept and strategy of "lung-protective ventilation."[10] Subsequently, the ARDS Network conducted a landmark multicenter, randomized study illustrating that a lung-protective strategy with reduced tidal volumes of 6 mL/kg predicted body weight (PBW; see Table 4-1) showed a significant decrease of days on a ventilator and decrease in mortality when P_{plat} was less than 30 cm H_2O versus traditional tidal volumes of 12–15 mL/kg PBW.[1] Tidal volumes of 12–15 mL/kg PBW are detrimental to the general population. Presently, no exact volume recommendation has been defined in the literature except in ALI/ARDS.

To ensure proper minute ventilation with lower tidal volumes, higher respiratory rates should be used and then adjusted. Clear benefit to the patient was demonstrated in spite of hypoventilation, introducing the concept of permissive hypercapnia. Permissive hypercapnia is the acceptance of hypoventilation and resultant CO_2 retention caused by reduced tidal volumes selected to prevent VILI. The retention and breakdown of CO_2 then leads to acidemia. A pH greater than 7.2 has been shown to be well tolerated.[11] Although hypercapnia as a beneficial lung-protective strategy is clear in animal studies, the precise contribution of hypercapnia in human populations remains heavily debated.

▶ MODES OF MECHANICAL VENTILATION

After the airway has been secured, physicians must decide on the mode, target, and variable settings in their orders. This discussion will begin with the four common basic modes of ventilation that most ventilators can deliver: assist/control (A/C), intermittent mandatory ventilation (IMV), pressure support ventilation (PSV), and continuous positive airway pressure (CPAP), all of which can be volume or pressure targeted. Figure 4-2 provides a graphic representation of how the patient and ventilator interact with the different modes of ventilation.

A/C is a combination of two types of MV. Assist mode allows the patient to spontaneously initiate a fully assisted, machine-delivered tidal volume, whereas control mode (or control mechanical ventilation [CMV]) provides ventilation without regard to patient effort. CMV alone has an application solely in deeply sedated or paralyzed patients.

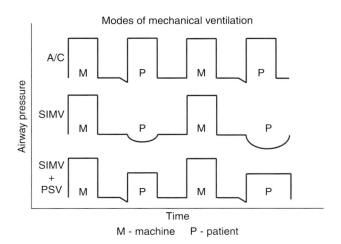

Figure 4-2. Modes of ventilation.

In A/C mode, the ventilator monitors the circuit for the patient to trigger a ventilator-assisted spontaneous breath. In the absence of that trigger, the ventilator automatically cycles, delivering set tidal volume machine breaths at a predetermined rate (Figure 4-3). All breaths in A/C mode receive the set tidal volume; the patient can have a varying rate but the tidal volume is always the set TV. A/C mode is appropriate for apneic, pharmacologically paralyzed and deeply sedated patients, as well as patients with hypoventilation, respiratory muscle fatigue, and those requiring therapeutic hyperventilation.

Settings: For A/C mode, the primary settings are respiratory rate, tidal volume, and fraction of inspired oxygen (FiO$_2$), with or without PEEP.

IMV combines periods of control ventilation with spontaneous breathing. Spontaneous breaths generate a tidal volume proportional to the patient's efforts, that is, no ventilator assistance. The intermittent mandatory breaths are the set amount (rate) of fully assisted breaths delivered by the machine. Currently, IMV has been replaced by synchronized IMV (SIMV). In SIMV, intermittent mandatory breaths are synchronized with spontaneous breaths to preclude breath stacking (Figure 4-4). In patients who are not spontaneously breathing, SIMV is identical to A/C ventilation (Figure 4-5). For each of the nonmandatory, spontaneous breaths, the patient is forced to generate the entire work of breathing. For this reason, it is the authors' opinion that SIMV should always be paired with PSV (discussed next) to decrease the work of breathing.

Settings: Similar to A/C mode, the physician sets an IMV rate, tidal volume, and FiO$_{2s}$ to determine a minimum minute ventilation as well as the optional PEEP and PSV.

PSV augments spontaneous breathing with a set inspiratory pressure while the patient determines the tidal volume and respiratory rate; thus, PSV is a mode of partial ventilator support. The negative pressure generated by the patient opens a valve that delivers a preset pressure. To keep the pressure constant, the ventilator adjusts the flow rate. When the machine detects the end of inspiration, the pressure support terminates and the

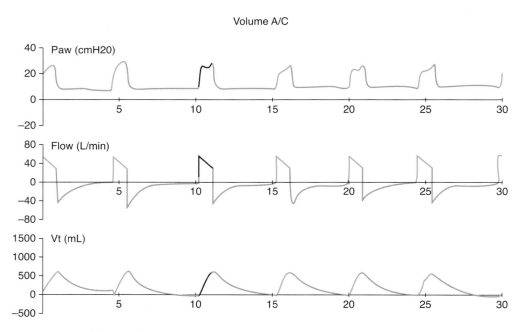

Figure 4-3. A/C mode.

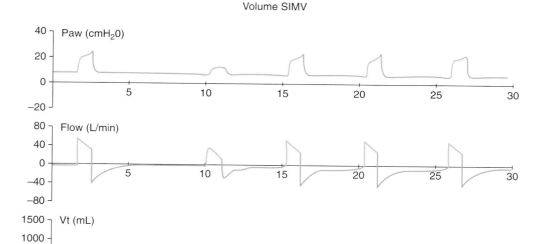

Figure 4-4. SIMV mode.

patient is allowed to exhale spontaneously. As well as augmenting spontaneous breathing, PSV provides assistance to overcome the resistance of the tubing of the ventilator circuit. It is the authors' recommendation that PSV always be added to SIMV.

Settings: The physician sets the PSV generally between a range of 0 and 35 cm H_2O with an average starting value of 5–10 cm H_2O and FiO_2, with or without PEEP. It is essential to set a rate alarm in those patients who are ventilated by PSV alone because there is no guaranteed minute ventilation.

CPAP is another mode for spontaneous breathing patients. Patients who are able to generate an acceptable minute ventilation can undergo a trial of CPAP. It

is frequently used as a weaning mode. CPAP should equal the amount of PEEP, between 2 and 5 cm H_2O, to prevent loss of alveolar recruitment, atelectasis, and hypoxia. CPAP is also added to decrease the work of breathing (Figure 4-6). The recommended CPAP is 5–10 cm H_2O.

▶ TARGET OF VENTILATION

After a mode has been selected, the mechanism of breath delivery must be determined: inflating the lungs to a predetermined either volume or pressure. Over the years, various terms have been used for the type of

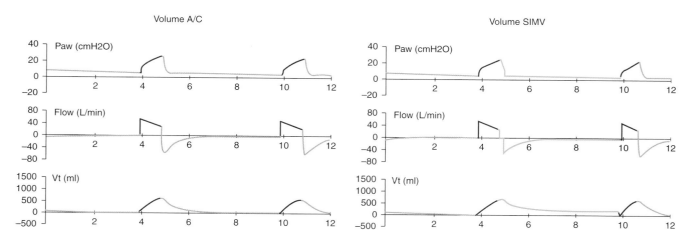

Figure 4-5. Comparison of A/C and SIMV in nonspontaneously breathing patients.

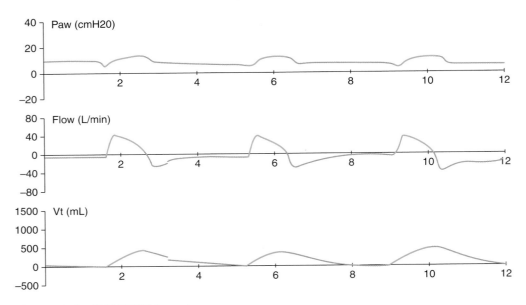

Figure 4-6. CPAP/PSV mode.

mechanically delivered breath: targeted, controlled, and cycled. These terms are all interchangeable. For ease of discussion, the term "target" will be used hereafter.

Volume-targeted MV delivers a set tidal volume regardless of the pressures needed to do so. Throughout lung inflation, the gas in a volume-assisted breath exerts different pressures in the proximal airways than in the alveoli. The pressure in the proximal airways is a function of resistance; the higher the resistance, the more the pressure needed to deliver the set volume to the lungs. In disease states where compliance is decreased, increased pressures are required to achieve the desired tidal volume.

The other option is pressure-targeted ventilation. The ventilator will deliver variable or intermittent flow to maintain a predetermined inspiratory pressure that is generally equivalent to or lower than P_{plat} to achieve gas delivery. This setting aims to distribute adequate pressures and reduce alveolar overdistension. This can be achieved through precise tailoring.[12] Given that the pressure is constant resulting in variable tidal volumes, the patient may experience hypoventilation due to variations in minute ventilation. Hence, any alteration in the respiratory circuit such as endotracheal tube/airway resistance or lung compliance can lead to hypoventilation. This variability requires more monitoring such as tidal volume and minute ventilation alarms, evaluation of respiratory circuit, and decision making by the physician.

Pressure-targeted ventilation is mainly reserved for patients with increased P_{plat} and is recommended to limit VILI or allow healing in ALI/ARDS. All things considered, pressure-targeted ventilation is an option worth considering for specific scenarios. Currently, no study exists stating that one mode is superior to another; however, physician familiarity with a specific mode is more important than modality.

► OXYGENATION VERSUS VENTILATION

Oxygenation is mainly a function of FiO_2 and PEEP. Increasing the PEEP decreases intrapulmonary shunting and increases alveolar recruitment. An increase in FiO_2 supplies the substrate for those two advantages. One approach is to set the FiO_2 at 1.0 and increase the PEEP in increments of 2–3 cm H_2O every 10–15 minutes until oxygenation goals are met.

The role of ventilation is to maintain adequate Pco_2 and, therefore, pH. This is manipulated primarily by controlling respiratory rate and tidal volume. The goal is to keep the pH between 7.3 and 7.4. Rate has a greater influence on Pco_2 than tidal volume; however, an increase in either will cause a decrease in the pH.

► INITIAL SETTINGS

Finally, the physician must determine the remaining variables. These variable settings most commonly found on a ventilator are PEEP, FiO_2, respiratory rate, tidal volume, and inspiration flow rate and time. Although recommendations will be made regarding *initial* settings, there are numerous scenarios in which variations should be considered (discussed later in this chapter). As the patient's condition changes, the settings may need to be adapted as well.

Positive pressure applied at the end of expiration is PEEP. Its main function is to overcome the tendency of alveolar collapse, especially in states of decreased compliance. It is usually set between 3 and 8 cm H_2O, which has become a standard setting for some. However, PEEP can have adverse consequences as well, since it increases the intrathoracic pressure. Increased intrathoracic pressure impedes venous return and decreases preload, leading to systemic hypotension. Thus, caution should be exercised with PEEP values greater than 8 cm H_2O. At times, however, greater values are needed for adequate oxygenation.

FiO_2 is usually set at 1.0 (100% oxygen) initially, but the general recommendation is to titrate it down shortly thereafter to maintain a Pao_2 greater than 60 mm Hg or SpO_2 greater than 92% to prevent the theoretical risk of oxygen toxicity.

Normal respiratory rate is 8–12 breaths/min but ventilators are usually set at 10–14 breaths/min. This may need to be increased when utilizing reduced tidal volumes. Normal tidal volume in a healthy adult without respiratory distress is 5–8 mL/kg PBW (Table 4-1). Tidal volumes have historically been set at 10–15 mL/kg PBW. In a 70-kg patient, this is 700–1,050 mL. Assuming a 1 L tidal volume, the first 150 mL goes to the dead space and 850 mL to the patient's alveoli. If the respiratory rate is 10, this produces a minute ventilation of 8.5 L/min. In the ARDS Network trial, it was learned that lower tidal volumes decreased the incidence of VILI and barotrauma. In that study, the tidal volume goal for lung-protective ventilation was 4–6 mL/kg PBW. In another study, it was shown that tidal volumes greater than 9 mL/kg PBW are a risk factor for development of VILI.[13] The ideal tidal volume should lie somewhere in between the old logic and the ARDS Network trial. Thus, the authors recommend an initial value of 8–10 mL/kg PBW as needed.

Normal physiologic inspiratory to expiratory (I:E) ratio is approximately 1:3, whereas patients on MV typically are set to 1:2. This can be manipulated by changing the respiratory rate, tidal volume, and the inspiration time or flow rate. This becomes important in reactive airway diseases.

An assisted breath can be triggered by a timer on the ventilator or by patient effort. One of the two factors can be used to sense patient effort. A decrease in airway pressure can be the trigger detected by the ventilator that causes a breath to be given. This threshold pressure is usually set at a level of −1 to −2 cm H_2O and is commonly used in MV today. It is worth noting that most patients on MV have PEEP. This adds to the total amount of force needed to trigger a breath. For example, if the trigger pressure is −2 cm H_2O and the

PEEP is 5 cm H_2O, the patient must generate a pressure of −7 cm H_2O, a considerable amount of force from a patient in respiratory failure. Ventilators can also deliver a breath based on the amount of inspiratory flow. Generally a setting of 2 L/min is used because this amount does not generate significant airway pressures and should require less effort by the patient.[14]

▶ SPECIFIC SCENARIOS

Although respiratory failure is the most common indication for MV, its causes are numerous, and thus it is optimally treated in various ways based on the specific etiology.

Obstructive lung diseases such as asthma and COPD are commonly encountered in the ED. When medical therapy fails or the clinical condition deteriorates (severe hypoxia, hypercapnia, or acidosis), intubation and MV may be the only life-saving options. The specifics of MV in these patients primarily revolve around the prevention of a gas trapping phenomenon called intrinsic PEEP (also termed auto-PEEP or dynamic hyperinflation). By definition, obstructive lung disease involves problems that result in prolonged exhalation exhibited by their decreased FEV_1. If the ventilator delivers a breath before the patient is able to exhale back down to baseline, breath stacking occurs. This breath stacking phenomenon increases lung volumes, placing the patient at risk of pneumothorax. The gas trapping of intrinsic PEEP results in a higher alveolar pressure. In a patient not on MV, this increases the work required by the respiratory muscles to generate the negative intrathoracic pressure for inhalation that leads to worsening respiratory failure. Regardless of MV, intrinsic PEEP also causes decreased venous return that leads to hypotension, thereby increasing morbidity and mortality.

To begin, outcomes can be improved by optimizing preintubation volume status. Induction agents as well as auto-PEEP from bag–mask ventilation for preoxygenation can lead to hypotension. A 500-mL to 1-L crystalloid bolus can abate these adverse issues.[15] Also, ventilator settings can be adjusted to prevent auto-PEEP. To prevent breath stacking, a lower respiratory rate (6–10 breaths/min), an increased flow rate (around 80–100 L/min initially), and lower tidal volumes (5–7 mL/kg PBW) should be employed to increase the I:E ratio. However, these changes are not without consequences. The reduction in minute ventilation with a decreased respiratory rate and tidal volume does lead to hypercapnia, which in turn leads to a respiratory acidosis. The consequences of hypercapnia can be increased cerebral blood flow (and subsequent increase in intracranial pressure [ICP]), myocardial depression, arrhythmias, and abnormal cellular metabolism. Overall, these decreases in arterial pH are generally well tolerated and much less harmful than the complications of auto-PEEP. The pH may require intervention when it is less than 7.15–7.20 with sodium bicarbonate or tromethamine (an alternative alkalinizing agent known as THAM), but some physicians tolerate these values and continue to monitor for adverse consequences of the acidosis. Hypercapnia can be a powerful central stimulus to increase respiratory rate. This response is usually blunted with medications such as opiates or other sedatives. The response may be so strong as to require chemical paralysis. However, paralytics should be used with caution in conjunction with steroids because of the relation of the steroid-induced neuropathies.[16]

Another cause of shortness of breath that usually requires MV in the ED is ARDS and the similar ALI. The American–European Consensus Conference, in the absence of a biopsy, defines these diseases with four criteria: (1) acute onset, (2) bilateral patchy airspace disease on chest x-ray, (3) without evidence of increased left atrial pressures (pulmonary capillary wedge pressure <18 mm Hg), and (4) $Pao_2/FIO_2 \leq 200$ for ARDS or $Pao_2/FIO_2 \leq 300$ for ALI. As previously discussed, the ARDS Network trial utilized "lung-protective ventilation" with a lower TV of 6 mL/kg PBW; respiratory rates of 18–22 breaths/min and oxygenation goals were met by initially setting the FiO_2 and PEEP high (1.0 and 24, respectively) and decreasing them incrementally. If oxygenation suffers at any point, there is a mortality benefit to increase PEEP before the FiO_2 is augmented.

MV has hemodynamic consequences, as well as apparent pulmonary effects. The following properties are important in patients with cardiogenic shock and severe pulmonary edema, when PEEP should be used judiciously to titrate oxygen concentrations. The positive pressure generated by MV increases intrathoracic pressure. This increased intrathoracic pressure decreases preload by decreasing venous return to the heart and compressing the right atrium. This decreases cardiac distensibility, inhibiting ventricular filling and compressing the pulmonary artery. The resulting increased pulmonary artery resistance dilates the right ventricle and inhibits the filling of the left ventricle as well. Inversely, the extrinsic pressures decrease afterload, improving cardiac output by assisting ventricular emptying. The exact mechanisms of these effects remain controversial.[17] The variable that determines which effect predominates is the intravascular volume. If a patient has a decreased intravascular volume, the preload effects dominate, decreasing cardiac output. If the volume is within normal limits, the afterload effects dominate, increasing cardiac output.[4] These properties are important in MV of patients with cardiogenic shock and severe pulmonary edema, when PEEP should be used judiciously to titrate oxygen concentrations.

Patents with brain injury, encephalopathy, and increased ICP commonly need MV due to respiratory failure and for airway protection. The goal with these patients is to maintain adequate cerebral perfusion pressure. Although hypercapnia and acidosis can compromise cerebral blood flow, prophylactic hyperventilation has been shown to be deleterious in patients with head injuries and is no longer recommended.[18] Settings should focus on adequate oxygenation, normalizing pH, and hemodynamic stability. If a patient deteriorates secondary to worsening neurologic pathology, hyperventilation can be instituted briefly to allow time for other therapies to take effect. This application of hyperventilation should not extend past 1–2 hours.

▶ TROUBLESHOOTING MECHANICAL VENTILATION

It is essential to establish a quick and logical approach to the unstable patient on MV when the ventilator alarms are sounding and the patient is hemodynamically compromised. VILI, MV-induced cardiovascular collapse, and patient-ventilator dyssynchrony are the primary concerns.

The first critical action is to disconnect the ventilator tubing from any patient in the presence of ventilator alarms and cardiovascular collapse. Removing the ventilator from the equation limits the number of variables in solving this life-threatening challenge and immediately eliminates it as a primary culprit. Ventilations with a bag–valve system can confirm endotracheal tube placement with an end-tidal CO_2 device, estimate the degree of airway resistance, and observe the chest or abdomen rise with each ventilation. These steps eliminate immediate threats of extubation, endotracheal tube obstruction, and increased airway resistance. If an end-tidal CO_2 device and auscultation are not sufficient in detecting appropriate tube placement, direct visualization is the gold standard. If evidence of extubation is discovered, the tube should be removed and the patient must be ventilated with bag–valve mask applying high-flow oxygen to achieve appropriate oxygenation prior to reintubation.

Endotracheal tube obstructions due to mucus plug, blood clot, or aspirate are quickly deduced utilizing airway intubating stylets (gum elastic bougie) and require prompt extubation and reintubation. Increased airway resistance and difficulty during bag–valve ventilations are linked to increased airway resistance and reduced compliance. The differential in these cases includes elevation in intrinsic PEEP, pneumothorax, main stem intubation, and worsening reactive airway disease. Utilization of bedside ultrasound or portable chest x-ray can quickly identify the etiology of the reduced compliance in most of these cases. Emergent diagnosis of tension pneumothorax and immediate intervention with needle thoracostomy can be life saving.

Caution should be maintained for patients with reactive airway disease and dynamic hyperinflation or intrinsic PEEP. Rescue ventilations can further exacerbate this condition if ventilations are too fast (greater than 10 breaths/min), or too large (more than 500 mL tidal volume). Limiting the rate and size of the tidal volume breaths increases the expiratory time and permits enhanced lung emptying of trapped volume present in intrinsic PEEP. As previously stated, a crystalloid bolus of 500 mL to 1 L should be administered over 5–15 minutes with consideration for appropriate sedation.

It is critical for providers to understand that the diagnosis of patient agitation causing patient-ventilator dyssynchrony should be one of the exclusions. Treating the unstable, agitated patient on MV with paralysis or heavy sedation without applying a quick and logical approach to exclude other life-threatening causes can be a preterminal event. When the respiratory demands of the patient are not met by MV, patient-ventilator dyssynchrony occurs, and it is one of the more common problems of MV.[19] Physiologic issues, such as neurologic derangements, hypoxia, and hypercapnia, need to be investigated primarily. Lastly, dyssynchrony can also be an issue of inadequate sedation—again a diagnosis of exclusion. One study has shown that adequate postintubation anxiolysis and analgesia is commonly overlooked by emergency physicians.[20]

REFERENCES

1. The Acute Respiratory Distress Syndrome Network. Ventilation with lower tidal volumes as compared with traditional tidal volumes for acute lung injury and the acute respiratory distress syndrome. *N Engl J Med.* 2000;342:1301–1308.

2. Lambe S, Washington DL, Fink A, et al. Trends in the use and capacity of California's emergency departments, 1990–1999. *Ann Emerg Med.* 2002;39(4):389–396.

3. McCaig LF, Burt CW. National Hospital Ambulatory Medical Care Survey: 2002 emergency department summary. *Adv Data.* 2004;(340):1–34.

4. Roberts J, Hedges J. *Clinical Procedures in Emergency Medicine.* Philadelphia: Elsevier; 2010.

5. Ricard JD, Dreyfuss D, Saumon G. Ventilation-induced lung injury. *Eur Respir J.* 2003;22(suppl 42):2s–9s.

6. Dos Santos CC, Slutsky AS. Mechanotransduction, ventilator-induced lung injury and multiple organ dysfunction syndrome. *Intensive Care Med.* 2000;26:638–642.

7. Held HD, Boettcher S, Hamann L, Uhlig S. Ventilation-induced chemokine and cytokine release is associated with activation of nuclear factor-kappaB and is blocked by steroids. *Am J Respir Crit Care Med.* 2001;163 (3 pt 1):711–716.

8. Dreyfuss D, Soler P, Saumon G. Mechanical ventilation-induced pulmonary edema. Interaction with previous lung alterations. *Am J Respir Crit Care Med.* 1995;151: 1568–1575.

9. Taskar V, John J, Evander E, Robertson B, Johnson B. Healthy lungs tolerate repetitive collapse and reopening during short periods of mechanical ventilation. *Acta Anaethesiol Scand.* 1995;39:370–376.

10. Slutsky AS. Mechanical ventilation. American College of Chest Physicians' Consensus Conference. *Chest.* 1993;104:1833–1859.

11. Peltekova V, Engelberts D, Otulakowski G, Uematsu S, Post M, Kavanagh BP. Hypercapnic acidosis in ventilator-induced lung injury. *Intensive Care Med.* 2010;36(5): 869–878. Epub March 6, 2010.

12. Rappaport SH, Shpiner R, Yoshihara G, Wright J, Chang P, Abraham E. Randomized, prospective trial of pressure-limited versus volume-controlled ventilation in severe respiratory failure. *Crit Care Med.* 1994;22(1):22–32.

13. Gajic O, Dara SI, Mendez JL, et al. Ventilator-associated lung injury in patients without acute lung injury at the onset of mechanical ventilation. *Crit Care Med.* 2004;32:1817.

14. Leung P, Jurban A, Tobin MJ. Comparison of assisted ventilator modes on triggering, patient's efforts, and dyspnea. *Am J Respir Crit Care Med.* 1997;155:1940–1948.

15. Santanilla J, Daniel B, Yeow M. Mechanical ventilation. *Emerg Med Clin North Am.* 2008;26:849–862.

16. Behbehani NA, Al-Mane F, D'yachkova Y, Paré P, FitzGerald JM. Myopathy following mechanical ventilation for acute severe asthma: the role of muscle relaxants and corticosteroids. *Chest.* 1999;115(6):1627–1631.

17. Pinsky MR. The hemodynamic consequences of mechanical ventilation: an evolving story. *Intensive Care Med.* 1997;23(5):493–503.

18. Muizelaar JP, Marmarou A, Ward JD, et al. Adverse effects of prolonged hyperventilation in patients with severe head injury: a randomized clinical trial. *J Neurosurg.* 1991;75(5):731–739.

19. Thille AW, Rodriguez P, Cabello B, et al. Patient-ventilator asynchrony during assisted mechanical ventilation. *Intensive Care Med.* 2006;32:1515.

20. Bonomo JB, Butler AS, Lindsell CJ, Venkat A. Inadequate provision of postintubation anxiolysis and analgesia in the ED. *Am J Emerg Med.* 2008;26:469–472.

CHAPTER 5

Weaning and Extubation

Alex Flaxman

▶ INTRODUCTION

Mechanical ventilation consists of two parts: the ventilator and the delivery device, most commonly an endotracheal tube (ETT). Similarly, there are two parts to liberation from mechanical ventilation: reducing and then eliminating the assistance provided by the ventilator and removing the ETT.

Although much attention is paid to when to intubate patients, significantly less attention is paid to when and how to extubate them. For those accustomed to literature searches using databases such as Ovid, there is not even a MeSH heading for "extubate" or "extubation." There is similarly less guidance on how to reduce the patient's reliance on the ventilator, that is, weaning. While weaning is—or should be—a precursor to extubation, the reverse is not always true, that is, a patient not ready for extubation still may be weaned. For example, a patient with a penetrating neck injury with a rapidly expanding hematoma requires an ETT for airway protection, but may only require minimal, if any, support from the ventilator. Either way, given the risk and expense of intubation and mechanical ventilation,[1,2] there should be no delay in ventilator weaning and patients should be extubated as soon as possible.

Before deciding on whether to wean or extubate a particular patient, one must recall why the patient was intubated in the first place. Many patients are intubated for respiratory failure, either for a primary pulmonary problem (e.g., pneumonia), a problem with another organ system (e.g., myocardial infarction, fluid overload from renal failure), or a systemic problem (e.g., sepsis). Other patients are intubated for airway protection, either from altered mental status (e.g., drug overdose) or because of impending airway collapse (e.g., anaphylaxis, smoke inhalation, trauma). The reason for intubation will have a direct bearing on when, and if, a patient may be weaned or extubated.

▶ CURRENT PRACTICE— EXTUBATION IN THE EMERGENCY DEPARTMENT

The majority of patients extubated in the ED are those who either self-extubate or were intubated for a state reversed with time in the ED, for example, drug overdose. A recent study showed that ED extubation in such conditions can be safe and can successfully reduce the need for additional resources such as an ICU bed, or even admission altogether.[3] Otherwise, it falls to the intensivist to wean and extubate the patient.

▶ THE GOAL

Clinical progress and, in fact, early research in the area support the progression from weaning to extubation. Although recent efforts have questioned the approach albeit with equivocal results,[4–6] traditionally extubation is the last step in liberating a patient from mechanical ventilation.

Since a failed extubation (defined as an extubation followed by an unplanned reintubation) carries significant mortality and morbidity,[7,8] an assessment should be taken to determine which patients will remain extubated and which will fail and require emergent reintubation. For the latter, instead of extubation, further treatment of the patient's underlying condition(s) or additional weaning steps should be undertaken, with continual reassessment for readiness to extubate. The former group should be extubated as soon as possible. So how, then, can a patient's readiness for extubation be ascertained?

The first step is to recall why the patient was intubated. For patients intubated to protect their airway or facilitate evaluation such as physical exam and imaging studies during an altered mental state, it seems reasonable to wait until the patients have had return of their baseline mental status. These patients, generally intubated for only short periods of time, may not need any assessment of their readiness to extubate other than an assessment to ensure return of their baseline mental status. These are the patients most commonly electively extubated in the ED.[3]

Except for those few patients extubated in the ED, a significant amount of time may elapse before a patient's clinical condition improves to the point where he or she may tolerate weaning and extubation. A variety of different parameters have been studied to determine which, if any, predicted a successful extubation.[9] Depending on the reason for intubation, one test with one parameter has generally been shown superior to other tests. For those patients intubated for respiratory failure, the spontaneous breathing trial (SBT) with calculation of the rapid spontaneous breathing index (RSBI) has been shown to most closely correlate with successful liberation from mechanical ventilation. For those patients intubated for airway protection, the cuff-leak test has similarly been shown to be predictive. Furthermore, many practitioners routinely perform both tests: an SBT to assess the patient's ability to breathe without artificial support and then a cuff-leak test to assess the patient's natural airway.

▶ SPONTANEOUS BREATHING TRIAL AND THE RAPID SHALLOW BREATHING INDEX

An SBT is, just as its name implies, a clinically applied test to see if and how a patient will breathe on his or her own. Artificial ventilatory support (but *not* the ETT) is removed, and the pattern of the patient's ventilation is observed. A "successful" test is one that predicts successful extubation, where "successful extubation" means a patient does not require reintubation for the same condition within 24 hours.

Over time, many parameters have been investigated to see which best defines a successful SBT. In other words, which parameter during an SBT best

predicts successful extubation. The RSBI (often pronounced "risby"), also referred to as the Yang–Tobin Index or, simply, the Tobin Index, has been consistently proven to be the best predictor of which patients may be successfully extubated. The RSBI is the respiratory frequency divided by the tidal volume (TV) while a patient is breathing spontaneously, as follows:

$$\text{RSBI} = \frac{f}{V_T}$$

where f is the number of breaths per minute, V_T the average TV per breath in liters, and the RSBI expressed in breaths per minute per liter. It can be seen from the equation that rapid, shallow breaths ("panting") such as occur with respiratory distress would result in a very high RSBI. Conversely, fewer, deeper breaths result in a lower RSBI. In a neurologically intact patient, therefore, lower scores are better.

A RSBI of ≤105 predicts successful extubation with a sensitivity of 97%, specificity of 65%, positive predictive value of 78%, and a negative predictive value of 95%. That means patients ready for extubation have a 97% chance of having a RSBI ≤105 (in other words, almost every patient ready to be extubated will have a RSBI ≤105). Unfortunately, the specificity of 65% means that 35% of patients who have RSBI <105 will still fail extubation. And therein lies the rub. Even the RSBI—the best proven predictor to date—will lead clinicians to extubate many patients who will fail, and to leave intubated a few patients who could otherwise be liberated from mechanical intubation.

Subsequent investigations into the RSBI have yielded varying thresholds, but in general a value ≤105 correlates with an 80% chance of successful extubation (extubation not requiring reintubation for the same cause within 24 hours) and a value >105 correlates with a 95% chance of the patient failing extubation.[10] Some practitioners prefer to use a RSBI value of 100 considering it an easier number to remember.

It is important to keep in mind a RSBI is only valid during an SBT. Historically, SBTs were performed by disconnecting the patient from the ventilator and placing them on a respiratory circuit, often referred to as a T-piece due to the circuit's shape (see Figures 5-1 and 5-2). This setup, however, is rarely, if ever, still encountered in clinical practice. There are two reasons for this, one physiologic and one practical.

Physiologically, the T-piece circuit increases the amount of dead-space ventilation (see Figure 5-1). Unlike in vivo dead space, the "bleeding" of oxygen into the T-piece circuit ensures that the circuit's dead space does not adversely affect fraction of inspired oxygen (FiO_2) actually reaching the alveoli. That is to say, the oxygen bled into the T-piece circuit clears out expired gases and provides a reservoir for inhalations faster than oxygen can be delivered. However, exactly

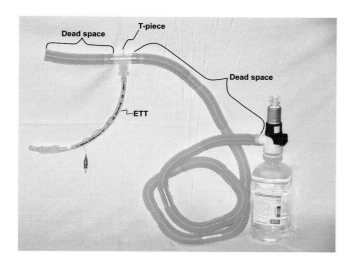

Figure 5-1. T-piece setup, historically used for weaning and readiness-to-extubate trials, is still in use in some facilities today. The blue tubing from the right supplies humidified oxygen. The long tube is necessary to reach the patient from the wall oxygen adaptor. The great length also provides a large oxygen reservoir to ensure adequate humidified oxygen in the circuit for when the patient inhales. However, the greater length increases resistance and therefore work of breathing. Since this length of the respiratory circuit does not participate in gas exchange, this is analogous to in vivo dead space. The blue tubing on the left also has two purposes. It, too, functions as a small oxygen reservoir for when the patient inhales and contributes a small amount of dead space. However, the practitioner can also visually inspect the end to make sure mist emerges. There should be a small, steady amount of mist when the patient is between respiratory cycles, no mist when the patient inhales, and a brief, rapid, efflux of mist when the patient exhales.

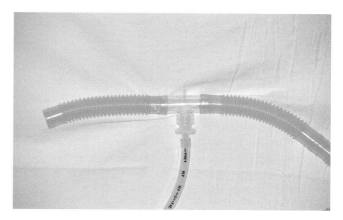

Figure 5-2. Close-up of the T-piece itself. Oxygen is fed into the circuit from the blue tubing on the right. Exhaled gases leave the circuit to the left. And the bottom of the T-piece affixes to an ETT.

like in vivo dead space, the T-piece circuit adds resistance to gas flow that increases the work of breathing.

In one respect, this can be seen as an advantage. A patient capable of breathing through a T-piece circuit—which requires more effort than if not intubated at all—should successfully tolerate extubation. Conversely, this means there are patients who cannot tolerate breathing through a T-piece but who would tolerate extubation. Further proving this point, during investigation into shorter-duration SBTs, Esteban et al showed that patients subjected to longer durations breathing through a T-piece circuit actually had longer ICU and hospital LOS.[11] In other words, the "bar" of this test is set too high, so high, in fact, that the test itself is harmful.

The practical disadvantage of T-piece trials involves the T-piece circuit itself. First, it requires extra equipment. Second, it requires disconnection from the ventilator. Given the built-in monitoring and safety features of modern ventilators (e.g., apnea monitoring), discon-

nection from the ventilator in favor of a circuit with no intrinsic monitoring introduces risk and a chance for medical error.

Therefore, in clinical practice, T-piece breathing trials have been eliminated in favor of SBTs with the patient still connected to the ventilator. This allows the same RSBI to be calculated while maintaining the monitoring and safety features of the modern-day ventilator. Moreover, most modern ventilators will automatically calculate the patient's RSBI, although care must be taken to ensure the RSBI is calculated over the desired time period, and is not "just a number" that the ventilator calculates for some preceding, random time period (such as over only the preceding minute).

Note that a RSBI is only valid if the patient is breathing completely spontaneously. If the patient is still receiving machine-delivered breaths, the RSBI is not valid, even if the ventilator reports a score.

▶ MODERN ADVANCES

Given that SBTs are better conducted with the patient remaining connected to the ventilator, an improvement would be if the ventilator could also be used to overcome the physiologic disadvantage of increased dead space causing increased resistance and therefore work of breathing. By setting a low level of pressure support (PS), the ventilator can, indeed, assist in making the test better by helping to overcome the extra work of breathing imposed by the ventilator circuit.[12,13]

Some ventilators, in fact, have a feature to do this automatically. For ventilators so equipped, "automatic tube compensation" (ATC) allows the ventilator to automatically and dynamically adjust its own support of a patient's breathing to provide the exact amount of support necessary to overcome the circuit. This may, in fact, be more accurate than simply setting a static level of support since resistance of the ventilator circuit is a function not only of length and cross-section (which are relatively constant) but also of velocity (flow) and acceleration (change in flow), both of which vary across the respiratory cycle itself, from breath to breath, and as the patient's clinical condition improves.

The remaining question is for how long to perform an SBT. Traditionally SBTs were performed for 120 minutes.[2,14,15] Subsequent investigation showed that for patients who have not yet been given a weaning or extubation trial, if a patient was to fail a 120-minute SBT, the failure was going to occur within 30 minutes; contrapositively, successful completion of a 30-minute SBT predicted successful completion of a 120-minute SBT and therefore successful extubation.[11]

Furthermore, 15% of patients of Esteban et al who required reintubation did so because of upper airway obstruction, for which there is now a good test, the cuff-leak test, which is detailed later in this chapter. Had patients of Esteban et al with upper airway obstruction been identified and not extubated, SBTs would have been shown to be even more successful.[11]

► WEANING

Weaning is the act of reducing ventilatory support in preparation for liberation from mechanical ventilation. Now that specific, objective criteria (RSBI ≤105) have been described, attention must be given to the methods to bring the patient to that state, specifically, to the ventilatory and adjunct strategies that can be employed to improve a patient's respiratory status to one with a RSBI ≤105, when the patient does not require any additional ventilatory assistance.

First consider, independently, the FiO_2, and when, after intubation, it may be reduced. Until the mid-1990s, the variables commonly available to evaluate artificial ventilation were those obtained by an arterial blood gas (ABG): pH, PaO_2, and $PaCO_2$. When considering how much oxygen was being delivered to the systemic arteries and whether or not FiO_2 can be reduced, the salient value was the PaO_2. But with the widespread use of pulse oximetry, it is now possible to know how much oxygen is being delivered to the systemic arteries by the continuous, noninvasive, bedside measurement of the oxygen saturation of arterial hemoglobin (SaO_2). Recall the equation of oxygen content of arterial blood[16]:

$$CaO_2 = [1.34 \times Hgb \times SaO_2] + [0.003 \times PaO_2]$$

where 1.34 is the oxygen binding capacity of hemoglobin (mL O_2/g Hgb), hgb the concentration of hemoglobin in blood (g/dL), SaO_2 the percent hemoglobin saturated with oxygen, 0.003 the solubility coefficient of oxygen in water at PO_2 of 1 mm Hg (mL O_2/100 mL

water/mm Hg), PaO_2 the partial pressure of oxygen (mm Hg), and CaO_2 the oxygen content of arterial blood (g O_2/dL plasma).

From the above equation, it can be seen that, except in cases of hyperbaric oxygen therapy, the partial pressure of oxygen is only a minimal contributor to the oxygen content of arterial blood and the term, therefore, may be removed from the equation. The equation then simplifies to:

$$CaO_2 = 1.34 \times hemoglobin \times SaO_2$$

From the above equation, it can be seen that for a given hemoglobin concentration, the amount of oxygen in arterial blood is directly and completely measured by pulse oximetry. It also shows that SaO_2 (as determined by a pulse oximeter) is, in fact, a better measure of oxygen content than PaO_2 (as reported on a blood gas result). For blood gas instrumentation that reports oxygen saturation results, it must be kept in mind that frequently the saturation number is calculated from the PaO_2, and not measured directly as is done by a pulse oximeter.

Since SaO_2 is a dynamic measure of the oxygen content of arterial blood, the ventilator's FiO_2 can be titrated by monitoring pulse oximetry. In fact, given the dangers of hyperoxia[17,18] and the ease, safety, and rapidity with which SaO_2 is measured, FiO_2 should be reduced as soon as possible after intubation, as tolerated, by monitoring the pulse oximeter.

The remaining parameters to wean will be the amount and frequency of ventilator support as well as how the ventilator delivers that support (i.e., the mode). The first two parameters determine minute ventilation, the adequacy of which can only be objectively ascertained by the ABG: specifically, the pH and $PaCO_2$. Still, unlike a continuous bedside pulse oximeter, ABGs are only snapshots in time. Fortunately, there is a monitor capable of continually measuring the patient's pH and, thereby, $PaCO_2$: the patient's own respiratory center.

It follows, then, as soon as a patient's condition sufficiently improves, sedation should be lightened enough to ensure comfort and cooperation with the ventilator (ventilatory synchrony) yet allow normal ventilatory drive. All that remains is to use a ventilatory mode that allows the patient to regulate his or her minute volume. This suggests that modes that allow the patient to both breathe spontaneously and regulate the volume of his or her spontaneous breaths will facilitate weaning.

Once a patient has achieved an adequate and comfortable respiratory status on the ventilator, parameters can then be reduced (e.g., fewer mandatory breaths per minute), to allow the patient to take over more and more of his or her own breathing. Finally, the patient can be moved to an entirely patient-controlled ventilatory mode, providing just enough support to overcome the resistance of the ETT and ventilator support.[12,13]

To achieve this goal is to achieve the maximal level of ventilatory weaning, proving the patient's pulmonary, cardiovascular, and other organ systems can tolerate extubation. Of course, this goal says nothing about extubation as a function of the patient's airway—itself reliant on airway anatomy and physiology (e.g., no swelling)—or the patient's ability to protect the airway, but it is the end point of weaning after which no further decrease in ventilatory support is either meaningful or appropriate.

Finding the optimal way to move a patient from initial ventilator settings to a state where the patient is ready for extubation is not trivial. Indeed, much work has been done on the topic.[15]

WEANING METHODS

It would seem that the logical way to eventually remove support of any kind would be to decrease the amount of support and evaluate whether the subject tolerates the loss. With regards to ventilatory support, it is possible to decrease either, or both, the amount or frequency, of support, as well as additional parameters. Some approaches to weaning have involved simply removing the patient from the ventilator for a short period of time and, if tolerated, gradually increasing the length of time. One then establishes some value for time off the ventilator that, once reached, is assumed to indicate that the patient can function off the ventilator permanently. Often a cutoff of 2 hours has been used, but periods as long as 24 hours have been reported. This process, however, involves removing the patient from the ventilator, which, as discussed above, is not desirable. By using the ventilator for assistance, support can be gradually reduced or removed to facilitate a faster weaning.

The first consideration when using the ventilator to assist in weaning is the mode of ventilation. In 1994, Brochard et al were the first to examine the question of the optimal mode for weaning in a prospective randomized controlled trial (RCT).[14] After excluding all patients who passed a single 2-hour T-piece SBT and were successfully extubated, they randomized patients to be weaned via gradually increasing SBTs on T-piece, synchronized intermittent mandatory ventilation (SIMV), or pressure support ventilation (PSV). They found that patients weaned fastest and most successfully using PSV. Furthermore, PSV yielded a shorter length of stay in the ICU and a trend toward lower all-cause mortality.

Conversely, in 1995, Esteban et al found that PSV actually increased weaning time,[15] with SIMV being better, and once-daily SBTs on T-piece the best. However, unlike Brochard who only studied patient's who failed their first SBT or extubation attempt, Esteban studied all comers. This means Esteban's results are colored by the fact that 76% of his patient population was successfully extubated on the first attempt, suggesting a majority of his patients did not require weaning, per se, merely identification of those patients ready to be extubated on their first attempt. This crucial point was proven in a 1996 study by Ely et al that demonstrated that many patients who can be successfully extubated are not identified by the intensivist as such,[2] and thus require objective evaluation and action based on positive performance on the evaluative measures. The only firm conclusion that can be drawn is that SBT is not the best weaning method, but rather is an indispensable test to identify patients as soon as they are ready for extubation.

Although denied in the discussion, Brochard's approach to SIMV potentially blunted the performance of SIMV or T-piece by using a protocol that limited how fast patients could be weaned on various modes. In other words, if SIMV did, in fact, lead to faster weaning in this study, it would not be apparent since the speed with which a patient could be weaned was limited by the study's protocol.

Finally, in both studies continuous positive airway pressure (CPAP) was allowed, but not required, which may confound the results of both studies. Since positive end-expiratory pressure (PEEP) of 5 cm H_2O is generally considered physiologic, it would seem a possible methodological bias to have not included PEEP on all patients, or at least have it set and titrated based on protocol. Brochard does note that CPAP was set in most patients with chronic obstructive pulmonary disease (COPD) to facilitate patient triggering of the ventilator by ensuring pressure in the circuit equaled the patient's intrinsic PEEP, which decreases the inspiratory effort needed to drop the pressure sufficiently to trigger the ventilator.

For other less traditional modes, the mode itself may either not lend itself to weaning via eventual conversion to CPAP and PS or lend itself to a distinctive weaning methodology. As opposed to SIMV, which is usually programmed with volumes (e.g., volumes of 6–8 mL/kg), pressure-regulated modes function by lessening the pressures applied before lowering the mandatory rate. This can be done by lowering the mandatory-breath pressure and monitoring to ensure that adequate volumes are maintained. As pulmonary compliance, and therefore resultant volumes, increases, the pressure may be again reduced. At lower pressures, the mandatory rate can eventually be lowered.

In airway pressure release ventilation (APRV), it seems prudent to first lower P_{high} until it is in a safe range below 20 mm Hg. At that point, T_{high} may be increased, therefore increasing the time the patient remains at P_{high}, which also decreases the number of releases, or mandatory breaths, per minute.[19] This method is commonly known as the "drop and stretch" method, referring to dropping, or lowering, P_{high} and stretching, or increasing, T_{high}. In general, P_{high} can be dropped in increments of 2 mm Hg, while T_{high} can be increased in 0.5- to 2-second increments. Eventually P_{high} will end up at levels of 5–12 mm Hg and, as T_{high} is increased, CPAP is approximated. Of course, PS or ATC should also be applied, assisting the patient's spontaneous breaths in overcoming the resistance of the circuit, as in more traditional modes. Once these settings are achieved, the patient may be extubated directly from APRV or may be converted to CPAP/PS to calculate a RSBI.

▶ EXTUBATION

Extubation is the act of removing the artificial ventilatory delivery device, which usually means removing the ETT. Traditionally ETTs are removed and the patients are left on room air, oxygen via nasal cannula or mask, or, more commonly, humidified oxygen via a simple mask. Recently, consideration has been given to extubating patients—earlier than once thought—and immediately applying noninvasive ventilation (NIV).

EXTUBATION TO NONINVASIVE VENTILATION

When considering application of NIV, a distinction must be made between applying NIV after extubation immediately and applying NIV to a patient recently extubated but who is now having respiratory distress.

PLANNED EXTUBATION TO NIV

The mechanisms and advantages of NIV are discussed elsewhere in this text, and will not be repeated here. It should be noted that in most cases of home, ED, or other uses of NIV, the predominant modes do not include a mandatory rate. In other words, CPAP or CPAP/PS (which is also known as bilevel positive airway pressure [BiPAP]) is usually applied via face or nasal-only mask, but relies on a patient's own respiratory effort to determine the respiratory rate. Despite the fact that almost any mode applied via an ETT may be applied via NIV—including SIMV, SIMV/PS, PRVC, APRV, and others—current research into, and experience with, extubation and immediate application of NIV tends to utilize CPAP or CPAP/PS via face mask. The future may very well show that NIV via a nasal-only mask may be sufficient, facilitating feeding and oral care. Or perhaps NIV with the application of a mandatory rate may help achieve earlier extubation in all or a subset of patients. Furthermore, all of these modalities can also be applied to patients with a tracheostomy, allowing the patients to entirely determine their own TV and respiratory rate,

but the concern is less for these patients who maintain a secured airway of a cuffed tube in the trachea.

In a review article, Epstein[4] cites several uncontrolled studies of extubation directly to NIV. Many seem to show benefit but the studies suffer from several problems. First, none were RCTs. Second, many trials dealt with only a subset of patient pathology.[5] While that is not an inherent problem, caution must be used when trying to generalize the results to all patients, or other subsets of patients. Of course, such results unmask benefits in certain subgroups—such as patients with COPD where there appears to be an exponential benefit—that might not be uncovered in larger studies with heterogeneous populations. Third, the specific NIV technique, as well as modality (face vs. nasal mask), was not standardized. Finally, each of the centers had experience in use of, and monitoring of patients on, NIV. These factors should be considered when applying the results of these studies to the extubation of a patient directly to NIV. Consider also that, while NIV has been growing in popularity in the ED, few emergency physicians apply NIV to the recently extubated patient. The initial settings and titrating of NIV as part of weaning program are not necessarily the same as those ordinarily used for the ED management of patients who receive NIV as part of their acute treatment for acute pulmonary edema or COPD.

Perhaps one of the most intriguing observations involves a rediscovery of conclusions drawn by Ely et al[2] that part of the benefit of extubating patients and applying NIV may be artificially elevated by applying NIV to patients who might otherwise have been ready for extubation even without NIV.[4,20] This correlates with several of Tobin's observations of the heuristics of extubation science.[9] That effect, however, cannot account for all of the benefit. Additional benefit is also realized via the reduction of the risks of receiving mechanical ventilation: most notably ventilator-associated pneumonia. Furthermore, once an ETT is removed, there is no further indication for even mild amounts of sedation. Epstein concludes with an opinion of the criteria necessary to consider extubating a patient, earlier than might otherwise be considered, for immediate application of NIV[4] (see Table 5-1).

Further recommendations for planned extubation to NIV are as follows:

1. The underlying condition necessitating the initial intubation should be resolved or, at least, resolving, with minimal remaining effect on respiratory status.
2. A large cuff leak with the balloon deflated, which is further described below.
3. Until further studied, a patient who has been extubated to NIV should remain in the ICU until no further assisted ventilation is required. In terms of acuity, monitoring, and management, a patient extubated to NIV still requires critical care.

▶ **TABLE 5-1. CRITERIA FOR EXTUBATING A PATIENT DIRECTLY TO NIV**

Parameter	Recommendation
Spontaneous respiration	The patient must be able to breathe unassisted for 5–10 min since the application of NIV may require 10 min to allow for the adjustment of settings and the delivery device (face or nasal mask)
Secretions	The patient should require suctioning less frequently than every 2 h
Cough	The patient's cough should be strong in order to protect the airway
Mental status	The patient must be alert enough to cooperate with NIV
Interface	The patient must be able to tolerate the interface. This may preclude certain facial anatomy or facial injuries

Data adapted from Epstein SK. Noninvasive ventilation to shorten the duration of mechanical ventilation. *Respir Care.* 2009;52(2):203.

In conclusion, the data do not, as of yet, support planning to extubate a patient and immediately placing him or her on NIV. There is, however, cause for optimism that this therapy may shorten the time patients spend sedated on a ventilator with an ETT and, perhaps, in the ICU overall. For now, though, this therapy should not be thought of as assisting an otherwise weaned patient, but rather as part of weaning. Patients receiving NIV after extubation should be monitored and receive critical care until they are fully weaned from the NIV. In fact, such patients may be even more tenuous than an otherwise similar patient who still has a cuffed tube in the trachea.

NIV AS TREATMENT FOR RESPIRATORY INSUFFICIENCY FOLLOWING EXTUBATION

As opposed to planning on applying NIV to patients immediately after extubation, consideration has been given to only applying NIV to patients who develop respiratory distress after extubation in an attempt to avoid reintubation. Unfortunately, there is significantly less investigation into this approach and the data have yielded conflicting results. In one of the earlier works, Keenan et al[21] noted no benefit in the application of NIV when applied to patients only *after* they develop respiratory distress. One notable caveat is that after the first of their 3-year enrollment period, they stopped randomizing COPD patients since they believed, at that time, that the literature strongly favored extubating those patients to NIV.

Further confusing the data are findings perhaps best seen in the study by Nava et al: although NIV was associated in a 16% decreased risk for reintubation, those patients requiring reintubation had a 60% higher mortality risk.[5] However, it is possible that confounding factors have obscured the benefits of extubation to NIV. First, subgroup analyses suggest the modality *is* beneficial to certain subgroups, such as those with CHF

or COPD. Second, it may be that once patients are extubated to NIV, they may be thought to be more stable than they actually are, and may receive less therapy and monitoring than if they were intubated.

Therefore, as of now, the data do *not* support utilizing NIV for patients who develop respiratory distress after intubation. However, for the subset of patients with COPD, the data are not clear. The reasons for this are probably 2-fold. First, although not yet proven, patients with COPD benefit from NIV more so than other patients, so it is likely that some of these patients with postextubation respiratory distress will respond in the same manner as the *tendencies* shown thus far in COPD patients extubated directly to NIV. Second, because patients with COPD have shown a *trend* to decreased mortality and morbidity when extubated directly to NIV, many studies have either excluded COPD patients or been hesitant to randomize them due to ethical considerations. This means that current study results may not be necessarily applicable to COPD patients. Therefore, a large, prospective randomized controlled study is required to study the outcome of application of NIV to COPD patients who develop respiratory distress after extubation. For all other patients, however, the data support early reintubation of patients who develop respiratory distress after extubation.

POSTEXTUBATION STRIDOR

A major cause of postextubation respiratory failure is upper airway pathology. Various studies have reported the frequency between 2% and 16%.[22] Usually resulting from laryngeal edema, physiologic causes include local damage, release of inflammatory mediators, and systemic third spacing. This is demonstrated by studies showing that risk factors for postextubation stridor include severity of illness (as indicated by the Simplified Acute Physiology Score), medical admission, traumatic intubation, self-extubation, duration of intubation, balloon pressure of the ETT balloon,[22] intubation without sedation or paralysis, neurologic deficit as determined by a decreased GCS, and female gender.[23] Interestingly enough, with respect to "traumatic intubation," no association has been found between the primary training or experience of the intubator (prehospital, resident, nurse anesthetist, nonanesthesia attending, or anesthesia attending) and the incidence of postextubation airway obstruction,[23] further confirming that postextubation respiratory distress is a result of the chronic course and treatment of a patient's disease, rather than of any single, acute event.

Attention must then be turned to ways of predicting and treating postextubation airway obstruction. As discussed above, NIV has been shown to be an ineffective treatment. Although depending on how the data are examined, it is theoretically possible that an attempt does not confer additional harm. Overall, reintubation carries such high mortality and morbidity that it is better to not extubate these patients until postextubation airway problems will not occur.

A test, called cuff-leak test, has been postulated to accurately detect the incidence of postextubation respiratory distress. The concept of the test is straightforward: measure the TV with the ETT balloon inflated and deflated. The difference is the "cuff leak." With the ETT balloon inflated, all air should exhale through the ETT, allowing measurement by the ventilator. With the ETT deflated, some air will go through the ETT and be measured by the ventilator. The rest will go around the ETT, or "leak" out, and this quantity will not be measured by the ventilator. A larger leak volume is good and indicates a less occluded or swollen airway.

Several methods for performing the cuff-leak test have emerged, but none have become standard in the literature. Measuring the nonleak volume is trivial; simply note the TV before deflating the ETT balloon. Many studies use the average over four to six breaths. Prior to measurement of the leak volume, it is prudent to suction the ETT as well as the pharynx and upper larynx. The balloon is then deflated, whereupon the patient will generally cough. After the patient ceases coughing, the measured TV can be recorded or, as above, the mean over four to six breaths can be calculated. At that point, the balloon is reinflated.

Originally the cuff leak was expressed as an absolute number of milliliters of air. However, in attempts to standardize reporting, and to make results generalizable to patients and ETTs of all sizes, Sandhu et al assert that cuff leak should always be expressed as a percentage of TV.[24] To accomplish this, one simply divides the absolute cuff-leak volume by the TV obtained with the cuff inflated.

Sandhu does not consider cases where the cuff-leak value may be misleading. For patients with large TVs and large ETTs, a cuff leak might be small because the ETT takes up most of the airway, forcing all air through the ETT whether the cuff is inflated or not. This would result in a small leak in a patient whose airway is fine. Conversely, with an ETT smaller than that usually used for patients taking a given TV, there are lower limits below which even a large relative leak (i.e., a large percentage leak) would not negate the possibility of severe, immediate respiratory distress. This is because, in this case, the maximal cross-sectional area of a partially occluded trachea may still be larger than that of a small ETT and yet could still be too small for sufficient flow without the ETT. To date, there are no studies suggesting values for concern, so it falls to the provider to exercise due diligence without guidance from the literature. Furthermore, for naturally small airways (tracheal malacia, airway trauma or growths, prolonged or multiple prior intubations with possible scar tissue formation), it seems prudent to take additional precautions in the periextubation period with a low threshold for reintubation if the patient exhibits any signs of respiratory distress.

Given the various works in the area, and barring extremes of patient size compared with ETT size, it seems that a cuff leak of 10–12% is a reasonable cutoff for extubation. Patients with cuff leaks below 10–12% are at high risk for postextubation respiratory distress requiring reintubation.[22–24]

A FINAL WORD ABOUT CUFF LEAK

Prinianakis et al did an extensive and elegant study to further delineate the etiology of cuff leaks.[25] They noted that when the TV for a cuff leak is measured, the ETT balloon is deflated and left deflated throughout the entire respiratory cycle, allowing air to "leak" during both the inspiratory and expiratory phases. Although leak during the expiratory phase is the desired quantity, what actually may be measured by this test is leak during both phases. This is because when the ventilator applies a breath with the ETT balloon deflated, some air will exit the ETT tube into the trachea and immediately go up, around the ETT, into the mouth, and out of the body. Yet the ventilator measurement will assume that the entire volume has been delivered to lungs. Prinianakis therefore asserts that the traditional approach overestimates the expiratory leak by a factor of two or more.

In order to isolate the inspiratory and expiratory components, during the "leak assessment" ventilations, Prinianakis et al deflated the ETT balloon only during the expiratory phase. However, to ensure isolation of the expiratory from inspiratory phase, patients were heavily sedated with propofol and fentanyl and then paralyzed with cis-atracurium. Furthermore, the TV was set at 10 mL/kg, which is much higher than the generally recommended 6–8 mL/kg. Finally, no PEEP was applied, again different from most patient treatment regimens. Under these parameters, patients were found to have a significantly higher cuff leak when the ETT balloon was deflated for the entire respiratory cycle when compared with deflation only during the expiratory cycle, suggesting a significant component of inspiratory phase leak, possibly obscuring the "true" expiratory cuff leak. Although the protocol used by Prinianakis should not be routinely performed in all patients, especially those in whom extubation is being planned, the study does suggest that the cuff-leak test as is usually performed is insufficient, and further study may yield a more accurate test providing different values.

TREATMENT PRE-EXTUBATION AND POSTEXTUBATION

Whether a patient is suspected to have postexpiratory airway occlusion, or a cuff-leak test has demonstrated the possibility, attention must be given to treatments to prevent postextubation stridor. These treatments fall into two categories: *pretreatment* given pre-extubation to decrease the possibility of postextubation stridor and *post-treatment* given after extubation as prophylaxis or if stridor develops.

Pre-extubation treatment has generally focused on steroids. While studies have considered different steroids, most work has been done with either hydrocortisone or dexamethasone. However, as with other investigations into periextubation treatment, the regimens have not been standardized. One of the most successful studies by Cheng et al not only delineated cuff-leak thresholds predictive of postextubation stridor, but also established that the timing of IV steroids (>6 hours before extubation) is probably more important than the specific medication used or the number of doses given.

Other treatment modalities such as diuretic therapy for 24 hours before extubation, inhaled racemic epinephrine, heliox, and anesthetic gases have all been shown to contribute to the reduction of postextubation stridor. The literature has yet to delineate which treatments are the most beneficial and in exactly which patient populations but it is important for the practitioner to keep these modalities in mind when considering extubating a patient with a concerning cuff-leak test. Currently the data show a single dose of 40 mg of methylprednisolone IV 24 hours prior to extubation reduces the incidence of postextubation stridor.

THE PHYSICAL ACT OF EXTUBATION

Once the patient has been weaned, consideration may be turned to removing the artificial airway. Unfortu-

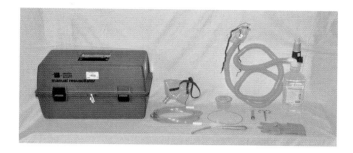

Figure 5-3. Equipment needed for extubation.

nately, the act itself is an unpleasant one for the patient. Care must be taken in the process, not only to reduce patient discomfort but also because the procedure itself as well as the patient's involuntary reactions, such as gagging, may be harmful.

Before beginning, all necessary equipment should be assembled (see Figures 5-3 and 5-4), including postextubation treatment modalities such as humidified oxygen. Note that the equipment list includes reintubation equipment and, depending on the patient, may also include difficult airway devices as well. Although not pictured, some practitioners like to place a folded-up sheet, absorbent pad, or water-impermeable barrier (such as a blue underpad or "Chux") on the patient's chest to catch any secretions. This also provides a convenient location to quickly place the ETT once removed (while keeping the patient clean) so attention can be immediately turned to the rest of the procedure.

Since secretions pool in the posterior oropharynx, the oral cavity should be suctioned down to the posterior oropharynx using a soft suction device prior to extubation. Furthermore, secretions also pool in the ETT so that, too, should be suctioned. While preoxygenating a patient prior to suctioning is widely practiced, some authorities also advocate preoxygenating with 100% oxygen for 1–2 minutes prior to extubation.

When ready to extubate, the procedure involves deflating the ETT balloon and removing the ETT. Some advocate actually cutting the pitot tube so the balloon will deflate on its own. However, the balloon may not empty entirely, and withdrawing it through the vocal cords may damage or inflame the cords, causing damage or swelling. If the pitot tube is to be cut, it is reasonable to first use a syringe to deflate the balloon as much as possible.

Once the balloon is deflated, patients will usually start coughing for a variety of reasons. First, the pressure sensation in the trachea changes, which can stimulate coughing. Second, airflow changes when the balloon is deflated that may make it harder for patients to move air. Third, secretions in the trachea from above

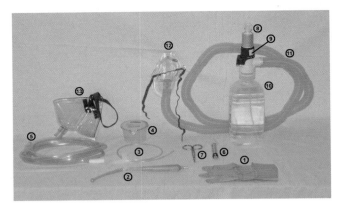

1. Gloves. Some practitioners also choose to wear a mask (not pictured) for face and eye protection from respiratory secretions.
2. Rigid (Yankauer) suction catheter for suctioning the oropharynx before and after extubation.
3. Soft suction catheter for suctioning the ETT before extubation. Some also use this catheter to suction the oropharynx after extubation in addition to, or in place of, a rigid suction device.
4. Water for use with the soft suction catheter.
5. Suction tubing.
6. Syringe 10 ml for deflating ETT balloon.
7. Scissors for cutting ETT balloon (if desired).
8. Adapter for humidification system to plug into oxygen wall adapter.
9. FiO_2 selector knob (see Figure 5-6 for magnified view).
10. Sterile water for humidification.
11. Corrugated oxygen tubing.
12. Aerosol mask.
13. Face tent.

Not pictured:

1. Rolled-up sheet or pad of absorbent material with impermeable barrier ("Chux") to place on patient's chest and abdomen for placement of the ETT and suctioning apparatuses
2. Oxygen wall adaptor
3. Other aerosol therapy such as racemic epinephrine and delivery device
4. Intubation kit (shown in Figure 5-3)
5. Difficult airway equipment (if indicated)

Figure 5-4. Close-up of equipment needed for extubation.

the balloon or in the posterior oropharynx may drip down into the patient's airway, causing a cough. Finally, movement of the ETT as it is extracted presses on the throat and can, itself, directly cause a cough.

To actually remove the tube, have the patient take a deep breath, deflate the ETT balloon, and have the patient forcefully exhale, removing the ETT as the patient exhales. Having the patient exhale prevents aspiration and reduces the likelihood of causing vocal cord damage by removing the tube during maximal vocal cord abduction.

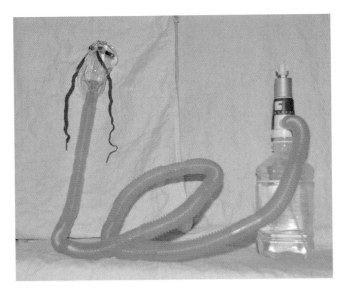

Figure 5-5. Humidified oxygen setup (attachment to oxygen not shown).

For patients who have concomitant orogastric, nasogastric, or jejunal tubes, those tubes may be removed simultaneously with the ETT. For gastric tubes, many practitioners place them on suction for some time before extubation to prevent aspiration. Regardless, make sure the tube is not to suction during the removal or extubation.

Once the ETT has been removed, suction the oropharynx for any secretions dislodged by removal of the ETT and apply humidified oxygen (Figure 5-5). Use cool mist since heated mist may increase swelling. Note that the patient may require a higher FiO_2 than just before extubation. Humidified systems allow almost any FiO_2 to be set but 40% is a typical value used (Figure 5-6). If indicated, consider nebulized racemic epinephrine to combat postextubation edema.

Although humidified oxygen is most commonly applied using an aerosol mask, some practitioners prefer to place a face tent (Figure 5-4, item #13). Furthermore, some patients find the aerosol mask uncomfortable but tolerate a face tent better. Finally, for patients with a history of facial trauma, an aerosol mask may be contraindicated in which case a face tent should be used.

It is important to reassess the patient after extubation. In particular, check for stridor, bilateral and equal breath sounds, and significant changes in vital signs. Note that because of the noxious nature of the procedure, a slight elevation in pulse and blood pressure is common and usually will resolve without treatment. Extreme changes in vital signs should prompt a full reassessment of the patient.

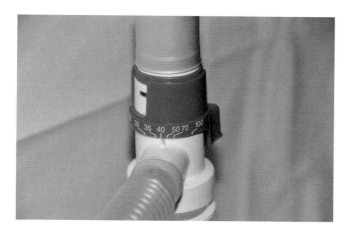

Figure 5-6. Close-up of humidified oxygen valve that allows selection of FiO$_2$.

COMPLICATIONS OF EXTUBATION

There are very few immediate complications of extubation. When present, however, they can be devastating.

Laryngeal spasm, though rare, can be an immediately life-threatening complication of extubation. While most laryngospasms spontaneously subside within seconds, any laryngospasm lasting longer than a few seconds demands immediate action. Reintubation using neuromuscular blockade will almost certainly be required, with simultaneous preparations for an emergency cricothyrotomy if the spasm prevents intubation through the vocal cords.

Vocal cord edema from irritation by ETT removal may be immediate or delayed. Ensuring that the ETT balloon is fully deflated should make this an infrequent occurrence. If it does occur, adjunct modalities such as humidified oxygen, racemic epinephrine, or even NIV may help. If not, the airway is in danger and reintubation or even cricothyrotomy might be required.

The most common complication is respiratory distress. This may resolve or may necessitate reintubation. Postextubation respiratory distress may be treated with racemic epinephrine and/or NIV as discussed earlier. Unfortunately, most patients requiring reintubation are fine in the periextubation period, but fail minutes to hours later. This indicates that recently extubated patients must continue to be monitored in an appropriate setting.

A FINAL WORD ON PREDICTING SUCCESSFUL EXTUBATION

The best parameter currently known to predict successful extubation is the RSBI. But given its imperfect specificity, and the desire to, as soon as possible, extubate patients that will or even *may* tolerate extubation, the most important safety parameter may be the intensivist's comfort with dealing with the complications of failure: specifically, the need for reintubation.

This places the emergency physician in the position of being among the best specialties to practice as intensivists. Although practitioners of other specialties can pursue and master the art of intubation, except for anesthesiology, no other specialty encompasses—and trains for—the need for emergent intubation like emergency medicine. In the emergency department, patients who require airway management require intubation regardless of airway anatomy, last meal eaten, or any of the other factors controlled for with elective procedures. It is perhaps this mindset that stands practitioners of emergency medicine in good stead.

Since extubating a patient carries a risk of reintubation, the best plan is to perform a 30-minute SBT and a cuff-leak test. If the patient passes both, extubation may proceed. Obviously, the practitioner must always be ready to reintubate should the patient decompensate clinically.

Other considerations involve the resources necessary to reintubate a patient. Since staffing levels vary with time of day, it seems reasonable to limit elective extubations to those times when maximal resources are available. For instance, one should consider not extubating patients at night.

Furthermore, for patients known or suspected to be a difficult intubation, it would seem prudent to make sure maximal resources are immediately available prior to extubating the patient. This may mean having fiberoptic or other rescue equipment at the bedside or perhaps planning for extubation in the OR with a double setup for cricothyroidotomy. Some patients for whom this may be required include known difficulty when originally intubated, history of airway trauma, airway masses, prior tracheostomy, or other airway surgical procedures.

▶ SUMMARY

To wean patients on mechanical ventilation, the following points would seem to be supported:

- Weaning should take place as soon as possible; in many cases, weaning can and should be started immediately on initiation of mechanical ventilation.
- FiO$_2$ may be titrated independently of ventilation, using pulse oximetry.
- Protocols should be instituted so that once- or twice-daily SBTs are performed automatically by the respiratory therapist or critical care nurse with calculation of the RSBI.
- Modes that allow patient to control minute ventilation are superior. SIMV is preferable to CMV

since CMV requires the patient who initiates an extra breath to take the full programmed TV.

- Modes should always be applied with PS or ATC so that additional, patient-initiated breaths are provided at a level comparable to what a patient would experience if not intubated.
- Modes, including TV and rate, should be titrated down based on patient comfort, allowing the patient to "take over" more and more of his or her own respiratory effort.
- For alternate ventilatory modes, weaning should proceed in a manner best suited to that mode, with extubation directly from that mode or conversion to CPAP/PS and progressed as above. For specific weaning parameters for each mode (SIMV/PS, APRV), see above.
- When at a minimum level of support, the ventilatory mode should be changed to CPAP/PS with levels similar to those provided to the patient while on SIMV/PS.
- When the patient is at CPAP level of 5, or a CPAP/PS level of 5/10, a RSBI should be calculated for 30 minutes.
- If the RSBI is ≤105, the patient should be considered for extubation and cuff-leak test performed. If the patient has a tracheostomy and has a RSBI ≤105, the patient should be considered for removal from the ventilator to be placed on a tracheostomy collar.
- For those with laryngeal swelling as evidenced by a concerning cuff-leak test, consider pre-extubation steroids, diuretic therapy, and/or NIV.
- For those with RSBI ≤105 and a cuff leak >10–12%, consider extubation as soon as is practical and safe.

► ACKNOWLEDGMENTS

The author would like to extend his gratitude to Reneé Rainey, RRT, RN, for assistance with the equipment pictured in Figures 5-1 to 5-6 and to Zev Perlmutter for technical assistance and postprocessing of Figures 5-1 and 5-4.

REFERENCES

1. Coplin WM, Pierson DJ, Cooley KD. Implications of extubation delay in brain-injured patients meeting standard weaning criteria. *Am J Respir Crit Care Med.* 2000;161:1520.
2. Ely EW, Baker AM, Dunagan DP, et al. Effect on the duration of mechanical ventilation of identifying patients capable of breathing spontaneously. *N Engl J Med.* 1996;335(25):1864.
3. Weingart SD, Menaker J, Truong H, et al: Trauma patients can be safely extubated in the emergency department. *J Emerg Med.* 2011 Feb;40(2):235–239.
4. Epstein SK. Noninvasive ventilation to shorten the duration of mechanical ventilation. *Respir Care.* 2009;52(2):198.
5. Nava S, Gregoretti C, Fanfulla F, et al. Noninvasive ventilation to prevent respiratory failure after extubation in high-risk patients. *Crit Care Med.* 2005;33(11):2465.
6. Girault C, Daudenthun I, Chevron V, et al. Noninvasive ventilation as a systematic extubation and weaning technique in acute-on-chronic respiratory failure. *Am J Respir Crit Care Med.* 1999;160:86.
7. Epstein SK, Ciubotaru RL. Independent effects of etiology of failure and time to reintubation on outcome for patients failing extubation. *Am J Respir Crit Care Med.* 1998;158:489.
8. Mort TC. Unplanned tracheal extubation outside the operating room: a quality improvement audit of hemodynamic and tracheal airway complications associated with emergency tracheal reintubation. *Anesth Analg.* 1998;86:1171.
9. Tobin MJ. Remembrance of weaning past: the seminal papers. *Intensive Care Med.* 2006;32:1485.
10. Yang KL, Tobin MJ. A prospective study of indexes predicting the outcome of trials of weaning from mechanical ventilation. *N Engl J Med.* 1991;324(21):1445.
11. Esteban A, Alía I, Tobin MJ, et al. Effect of spontaneous breathing trial duration on outcome of attempts to discontinue mechanical ventilation. *Am J Respir Crit Care Med.* 1999;159:512.
12. Fiastro JF, Habib MP, Quan SF. Pressure support compensation for inspiratory work due to endotracheal tubes and demand continuous positive airway pressure. *Chest.* 1998;93;499–505.
13. Brochard L, Rua F, Lorino H, et al. Inspiratory pressure support compensates for the additional work of breathing caused by the endotracheal tube. *Anesthesiology.* 1991;75:739–745.
14. Brochard L, Rauss A, Benito S, et al. Comparison of three methods of gradual withdrawal from ventilatory support during weaning from mechanical ventilation. *Am J Respir Crit Care Med.* 1994;150:896.
15. Esteban A, Frutos F, Tobin MJ, et al. A comparison of four methods of weaning patients from mechanical ventilation. *N Engl J Med.* 1995;332(6):345.
16. Oxygen and Carbon Dioxide Transport in The ICU Book. 3rd ed. In: Marino PL, ed. Philadelphia: Lippincott Williams & Williams:23.
17. Devaskar SU. The role of oxygen in health and disease—a series of reviews. *Pediatr Res.* 2009;66(2):121.
18. Altemeiera WA, Sinclair SE. Hyperoxia in the intensive care unit: why more is not always better. *Curr Opin Crit Care.* 2007;13:73.
19. Frawley PM, Habashi NM. Airway pressure release ventilation: theory and practice. *AACN Clin Issues.* 2001;12(2):234.
20. Calfee CS, Matthay MA. Recent advances in mechanical ventilation. *The American Journal of Medicine.* 118:584, 2005.

21. Keenan SP, Powers C, McCormack DG. Noninvasive positive-pressure ventilation for postextubation respiratory distress: a randomized controlled trial. *JAMA.* 2002;287(24):3238.

22. Jaber S, Chanques G, Matecki S, et al. Post-extubation stridor in intensive care unit patients: risk factors evaluation and importance of the cuff-leak test. *Intensive Care Med.* 2003;29:69.

23. Cheng KC, Hou CC, Huang CC, et al. Intravenous injection of methylprednisolone reduces the incidence of postextubation stridor in intensive care unit patients. *Crit Care Med.* 2006;34(5):1345.

24. Sandhu R, Pasquale M, Miller K, et al. Measurement of endotracheal tube cuff leak to predict postextubation stridor and need for reintubation. *J Am Coll Surg.* 2000;190(6):682.

25. Prinianakis G, Alexopoulou C, Mamidakis E, et al. Determinants of the cuff-leak test: a physiologic study. *Crit Care.* 2005;9(1):R24.

CHAPTER 6

Noninvasive Ventilation

Brian J. Wright and Todd L. Slesinger

▶ INTRODUCTION

Acute respiratory distress is a frequent problem encountered by emergency physicians and intensivists. Often the clinician must act to ensure adequate oxygenation and ventilation before a definitive diagnosis is achieved. The treatment of acute respiratory distress requires an aggressive approach that entails use of medications, oxygen, and often positive pressure ventilation. Historically, patients who required positive pressure ventilation underwent endotracheal intubation (ETI) and were placed on a mechanical ventilator. However, over the past decade there has been an increased use of noninvasive positive pressure ventilation (NIV).[1,2] As opposed to ETI, NIV uses an external mask interface to deliver positive pressure to the patient.

NIV and ETI with conventional ventilation are not synonymous alternatives; NIV is not warranted when the airway needs to be secured. Rather, NIV should be considered an additional tool that can augment medical care to possibly prevent ETI. This chapter will discuss the use of NIV in the emergency medicine patient with acute respiratory distress.

▶ PHYSIOLOGY OF NIV

NOMENCLATURE

There are two major types of NIV (or noninvasive positive pressure ventilation) that are used in the pre-hospital and emergency medicine setting: continuous positive airway pressure (CPAP) and bilevel positive airway pressure (BiPAP).

CPAP provides continuous positive airway pressure throughout the entire respiratory cycle (see Figure 6-1).

There are small variations in pressure that are dependent on patient respiratory effort: a drop in pressure that occurs with each spontaneous inspiration and a rise in pressure that occurs with each exhalation. The set pressure will very closely approximate mean airway pressure (Pma). The amount of flow or tidal volume (Tv) will depend on patient effort, lung compliance, and the fit of the mask.

BiPAP consists of two applied pressures: inspiratory positive airway pressure (IPAP) and expiratory positive airway pressure (EPAP) (see Figure 6-2). EPAP is similar to applied positive end-expiratory pressure (PEEP) on the mechanical ventilator, maintaining positive pressure throughout the expiratory cycle. IPAP provides a higher positive pressure during inspiration to support the work of breathing and augment ventilation.

CPAP AND EPAP: OPENING THE LUNG AND KEEPING IT OPEN

CPAP and EPAP (in BiPAP) are analogous to applied PEEP in the mechanically ventilated patient, applying pressure above that of atmospheric pressure during the expiratory cycle. The addition of positive pressure during the expiratory cycle can have multiple physiologic effects, and depending on particular patient pathophysiology, these effects can be beneficial or harmful.

The addition of CPAP and EPAP (applied PEEP) is helpful in the treatment of hypoxic respiratory failure that is refractory to supplemental oxygen. The beneficial effects of applied PEEP in hypoxic respiratory failure occur primarily through the opening of collapsed, atelectatic, or fluid-filled alveoli that have a low ventilation to perfusion (V/Q) ratio. In these alveoli, there is absent or inadequate ventilation and blood shunts

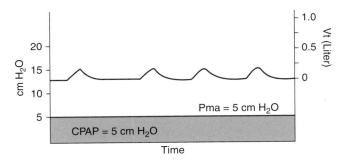

Figure 6-1. Continuous positive airway pressure (CPAP). CPAP set at 5. Patient breathing spontaneously, with approximately 200 cm³ tidal volume (Vt). Mean airway pressure (Pma) is approximately 5 cm H_2O. Pressure and Vt tracings are ideal.

from the right side of the circulation to left side without unloading carbon dioxide or oxygenating hemoglobin. Some of these fluid-filled or collapsed alveoli are "recruitable" and have the potential to be "opened" and take part in gas exchange, depending on the underlying disease process and severity of illness. "Recruitable" alveoli can open and close during the respiratory cycle or remain closed throughout the entire cycle. Applied PEEP can help limit expiratory collapse by providing positive pressure during exhalation that splints the alveoli open, or it can serve as a pressure head that opens collapsed alveoli. Opening collapsed alveoli decreases the shunting of venous blood and leads to an improvement of hypoxemia.[3-5]

At higher pressures, applied PEEP has negative effects that may outweigh the benefits of recruitment. First, some diseased alveoli are not "recruitable" and increasing levels of applied PEEP will not improve shunt effect.[4] Second, high alveolar pressures can cause overdistention of healthy alveoli leading to barotrauma and the release of inflammatory cytokines, propagating pulmonary and nonpulmonary organ injury.[4] Third, high PEEP can have negative effects on venous return and cardiac output in preload-dependent states (e.g., sepsis,

hypovolemic shock), leading to decreased oxygen delivery and tissue perfusion.[4] Finally, high PEEP can paradoxically worsen V/Q mismatch by overdistending alveoli and decreasing blood flow to previously perfused healthy lung segments.[3-5]

The level of applied PEEP provided in NIV is usually beneficial to patient oxygenation. Provided that the patient is not in a preload-dependent state, the negative effects of applied PEEP usually occur at higher pressures that are not well tolerated by patients because of discomfort and air leaks from the mask interface.

If a patient requires higher levels of CPAP or EPAP (greater than 12 or 15 cm H_2O) to maintain oxygenation, this should signal that the clinical status is worsening and that the disease state is not amenable to NIV. Conventional ETI with mechanical ventilation should be strongly considered in these situations.

FLOW AND TIDAL VOLUME: GETTING AIR IN AND OUT OF THE LUNGS

Airflow and ventilation are directly dependent on the pressure gradient and inversely related to airway resistance from the atmosphere to the alveolus. This can be conceptually explained as Ohm's law:

(1) $V = IR$

Rearranging Ohm's law for flow gives you the following:

(2) $\text{Flow} = \dfrac{\Delta\text{Pressure}}{\text{Resistance}}$ or $\text{Flow} = \dfrac{\text{Patm} - \text{Palv}}{R}$

Airway resistance is important in many different disease states (e.g., chronic obstructive pulmonary disease [COPD] and asthma), and it is essential that the clinician optimize treatment (i.e., steroids and β-agonists) to decrease resistance and maximize potential flow when indicated. From a schematic standpoint, we will assume airway resistance remains relatively constant from one breath to another, and that the pressure gradient between the atmosphere and the alveolus becomes the major determinant of air flow.

Figure 6-2. Bilevel positive airway pressure (BiPAP). Inspiratory positive airway pressure (IPAP) set at 10 cm H_2O. Expiratory positive airway ressure (EPAP) set at 5 cm H_2O. Pressure support (PS), IPAP – EPAP is 5 cm H_2O. Mean airway pressure (Pma) is approximately 7 cm H_2O. Patient breathing spontaneously; Vt is approximately 300 cm³. Pressure and Vt tracings are ideal.

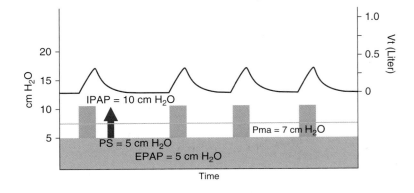

In the spontaneously breathing individual, the pressure gradient between the alveolus and the atmosphere is accomplished by creating negative pressure in the thorax. At the onset of inspiration, the diaphragm and intercostal muscles contract, increasing intrathoracic volume and decreasing intrathoracic pressure. Relative to the atmosphere, the alveolus is at a negative or lower pressure and air flows through the airways down a pressure gradient into the alveolus. At the end of inspiration, the elastic recoil of the chest wall increases alveolar pressure, creating a positive pressure relative to the atmosphere; air flows out of the lungs down a pressure gradient.[3,5]

The same principle of air flowing down a pressure gradient applies to NIV and other forms of positive pressure ventilation. In both cases, during inspiration the ventilator provides support in the form of positive pressure at the airway to create a pressure gradient for air to flow from the atmosphere (or ventilator) into the alveolus. Atmospheric pressure is made more positive (as opposed to alveolar pressure becoming more negative) to create the pressure gradient necessary for inspiratory flow to occur. Exhalation is similar to the nonventilated patient in that it is a passive phenomenon where the elastic recoil of the chest wall is used to exhale air down a pressure gradient.

Ensuring adequate tidal volume and minute ventilation is necessary for carbon dioxide elimination. Assuming a constant airway resistance, tidal volume is dependent on the pressure gradient between the alveolus and the atmosphere. Understanding this concept is helpful when manipulating the noninvasive ventilator. Rearranging Eq. (2) to noninvasive parameters yields the following:

$$(3) \text{ Tidal volume (Tv)} \approx \frac{\text{IPAP} - \text{EPAP}}{R}$$

Tv and flow are dependent on the level of pressure support provided by the BiPAP. Pressure support equals the difference between IPAP and EPAP. Increasing pressure support, provided that the patient has an adequate respiratory rate (RR), will increase Tv and minute ventilation.

▶ SETUP AND PRACTICAL APPLICATIONS

PATIENT SELECTION

The appropriate selection of patients with respiratory distress for application of either NIV versus ETI and conventional ventilation is critical to minimize additional morbidity and mortality.[6] First, the patient should have a derangement in pulmonary physiology that requires positive pressure respiratory support. Clinically, the patient should have moderate to severe respiratory distress with evidence of tachypnea, accessory muscle use, or paradoxical abdominal muscle use. Supplemental or laboratory evidence of moderate to severe respiratory distress includes a respiratory acidosis (pH <7.35 with a $Paco_2$ >45 mm Hg) or severe hypoxemia (oxygen saturation <92% despite supplemental oxygen or a Pao_2/FiO_2 ratio [P/F] <300), and can also be used to guide the physician in selecting patients for NIV. However, the physician should interpret laboratory data appropriately given the clinical scenario: a $Paco_2$ of 40 mm Hg and oxygen saturation of 92% in an asthmatic can have a significantly different meaning than the same blood gas value in a patient with a COPD or CHF exacerbation. Second, the patient should have a disease process that is amenable to treatment with NIV and has a high likelihood of reversibility, for example, exacerbations of COPD or CHF. In these patients, NIV should be started as soon as possible to prevent fatigue, further organ dysfunction, and worsening respiratory distress. Finally, contraindications and predictors of failure to NIV, such as apnea or respiratory arrest, medical instability, inability to protect airway or manage secretions, excessive agitation, poor mask fit, or recent upper airway or gastrointestinal surgery, should be absent.[7] An exception to this rule is patients that have a Do-Not-Intubate (DNI) order. Acute respiratory distress and failure are often multifactorial, and the emergency medicine clinician is frequently required to treat and stabilize with incomplete patient data. Provided that contraindications are not present, a 1- to 2-hour trial of NIV may be warranted if the clinician deems NIV appropriate.[6,7] If there is improvement in the patient's clinical status and blood gas parameters, NIV should be continued or weaned if applicable. However, if the patient's status does not improve, deteriorates, or it is determined that the patient has a disease process that is not amenable to NIV, the plan of action should be reassessed and therapy should be adjusted. In select patients who are DNI or DNR, palliative care measures should be initiated. A major risk of NIV is delaying ETI in patients who require mechanical ventilation, and there is a potential for an increased morbidity and mortality in those patients who "linger" on NIV.[8] If there is no improvement after a trial period, or any deterioration, ETI should be conducted to prevent intubation under "crash" conditions.

PATIENT AND NONINVASIVE VENTILATION INTERFACE

There are three basic interfaces or masks that the clinician can use to provide NIV: helmet, nasal mask, and full face mask. Each has its own strengths and weaknesses.

The helmet interface encases the patient's entire head. There is some concern that with the helmet interface patients can rebreathe carbon dioxide, particularly if the ventilator becomes disconnected from the patient.[6,9] The helmet interface can also be louder than the oral or nasal interface.[6,9] However, there is less risk of skin breakdown and this interface may be more comfortable for prolonged NIV use.[6,9] The majority of clinical studies did not use a helmet interface, and the experience with this type of interface in US centers is limited.[6]

The nasal mask is a partial mask that goes around the nose of the patient. The patient's mouth is not covered. This type of interface is commonly used in chronic conditions such as obstructive sleep apnea. The nasal mask may be more comfortable than the standard full face mask and provokes less claustrophobia. However, it is not particularly suited for the acute setting because of the potential for large air leaks and loss of pressure when the patient opens or breaths through his or her mouth.[6,7,9]

The most commonly used interface in the emergency department (ED) and critical care setting is the full face mask.[6,7,9] The full face mask covers the nasal bridge, goes around the nose, and then forms a seal around the chin and mouth. When using the full face mask, it is important that there is no leak of air around the face mask. An air leak will limit the amount of pressure and volume provided to the patient. Extended use or an overly tight fit can lead to pressure sores on the face. Some patients experience discomfort and a sensation of claustrophobia with the full face mask and positive pressure ventilation.[6,7,9] It is often necessary for the clinician to be at the bedside to provide reassurance and make adjustments to the ventilator and face mask. The clinician may decide to provide the patient with analgesia or anxiolysis; however, the negative effects and risks of respiratory and mental status depression must be taken into consideration.

INITIAL SETTINGS AND PATIENT MONITORING

When choosing initial NIV settings, it is important to consider the patient's underlying disease process, the need for positive pressure support, and patient comfort and compliance. Increased patient compliance at lower pressures must be weighed against improved respiratory mechanics, ventilation, and oxygenation at higher pressures. A common BiPAP starting point for many emergency medicine physicians is to begin with an IPAP of 10 cm H_2O and an EPAP of 5 cm H_2O—"10 and 5." This is an acceptable starting point, and lower initial pressures may help facilitate patient compliance. However, "10 and 5" provides a pressure support of about 5 cm H_2O, slightly less than or equal to the amount of pressure

▶ **TABLE 6-1. NIV MONITORING**

Subjective
- Dyspnea
- Mental status
- Airway maintenance
- Patient comfort
- Patient-ventilator synchrony
- Accessory muscle use
- Air leak

Objective
- Heart rate
- Oxygen saturation
- Blood pressure
- Respiratory rate
- Tidal volume (6–8 cm³/kg)
- ABG: pH, $Paco_2$, Pao_2 (baseline and at 1–2 hours)

support utilized in weaning trials. There is a subtle yet important difference in nomenclature when describing pressure support in BiPAP and conventional mechanical ventilators. "10 and 5" on the BiPAP translates to an IPAP of 10 cm H_2O and an EPAP of 5 cm H_2O. The "10 and 5" on the conventional mechanical ventilator utilized during a pressure support wean is actually "10 over 5"—an inspiratory pressure of 15 cm H_2O and expiratory pressure of 5 cm H_2O. It is therefore critical that the clinician monitors response and titrates pressures appropriately to ensure adequate gas exchange and decrease work of breathing. Inadequate pressure support or PEEP (EPAP) may increase work of breathing.[6,7]

When monitoring patients on NIV, it is important to look for certain subjective and objective criteria (see Table 6-1). First, examine the patient–ventilator interface for air leaks. Air leaks may be audible. You can also place your hands around the mask to feel for air leaking. Air leaks decrease the amount of support provided to the patient and can lead to NIV failure. One method to compensate for air leaks is to increase the applied pressures to increase the actual support that the patient receives. However, increasing the applied pressures can lead to increased air leak. The best way to overcome air leaks is to readjust the mask or change to a different interface. Second, the clinician should look at clinical parameters, such as the patient's mental status, use of accessory muscles, comfort level, and presence of subjective dyspnea or chest pain. Worsening mental status can imply a worsening respiratory status, worsening $Paco_2$, and an increased risk of aspiration, and should signal the end of the NIV trial. The patient should report an improvement in dyspnea, and the clinician should look for decreased accessory muscle use and good patient and NIV synchrony. Third, objective clinical data such as Tv on the NIV, RR, heart rate (HR), oxygen saturation (SaO_2), and blood pressure (BP) should be monitored continuously, and a baseline arterial blood gas (ABG) and 1- to 2-hour ABG should be obtained to measure pH, $Paco_2$, and Pao_2.

CLINICAL EXAMPLE: VENTILATION AND WORK OF BREATHING

To give a clinical example, a patient is placed on BiPAP for hypercarbic respiratory failure secondary to a COPD exacerbation. This particular patient has inadequate ventilation, respiratory acidosis, and elevated work of breathing. The clinician selects a "standard" setting of IPAP 10 cm H_2O and EPAP 5 cm H_2O, adjusting the FiO_2 to maintain SaO_2 between 88% and 92%. Additional SaO_2 is not required, and can run the risk of inhibiting respiratory drive. An EPAP of 5 cm H_2O is a good starting point to decrease the work of breathing needed to overcome the inspiratory threshold created by intrinsic PEEP. An IPAP of 10 cm H_2O provides a pressure support of 5 cm H_2O. This is minimal, but patient compliance is a concern so the clinician begins with lower pressures. After a trial period, the clinician finds that the patient is not pulling enough Tv on the BiPAP and the $Paco_2$ level is not dropping appropriately. A decision is made to continue the BiPAP and increase pressure support. Rather than increase both the IPAP and EPAP together, the clinician should only increase the IPAP (see Figure 6-3). Increasing the IPAP and EPAP equally together will maintain the same pressure gradient between the alveolus and the ventilator and the same tidal volume and ventilation. By selectively increasing the IPAP, the clinician increases the pressure gradient between the atmosphere and ventilator and therefore will increase the flow of air and tidal volume.

CLINICAL EXAMPLE: HYPOXIA

In the second clinical example, a patient with a CHF exacerbation and hypoxic respiratory failure is placed on BiPAP. Again the clinician selects a "standard" setting of IPAP 10 cm H_2O over EPAP of 5 cm H_2O, and applies supplemental FiO_2. Initially the clinician will increase the level of FiO_2. Often, 100% FiO_2 will not completely correct hypoxia. If the patient does not adequately improve, the clinician must improve Pma (see the following equation) and alveolar recruitment to improve V/Q mismatch, reduce shunt, and effectively treat hypoxia.[10]

(4) Mean airway pressure (Pma) $\approx \dfrac{p_1 t_1 + p_2 t_2 + \cdots + p_\infty t_\infty}{time}$

This is best accomplished by increasing the EPAP (or PEEP) level of support as this will have a greater impact on the mean airway pressure than increasing pressure support. Both IPAP and EPAP are increased equally

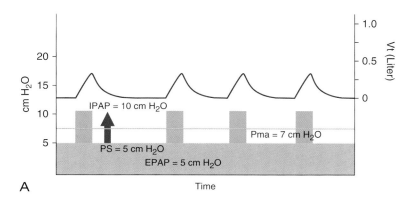

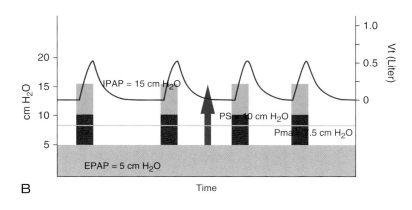

Figure 6-3. Ventilation and pressure support (PS). (A) Patient placed on BiPAP of 10 and 5, corresponding to IPAP of 10 cm H_2O and EPAP of 5 cm H_2O. Patient pulling minimal Tv because PS is only 5 cm H_2O. (B) To increase PS, IPAP is increased to 15 cm H_2O and EPAP is kept same. PS is now 10 cm H_2O and patient's Tv has improved. Mean airway pressure (Pma) has increased minimally. Pressure and Vt tracings are ideal.

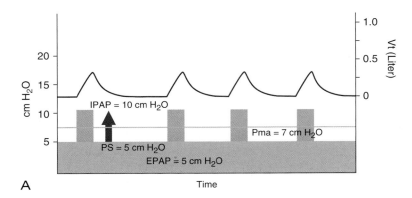

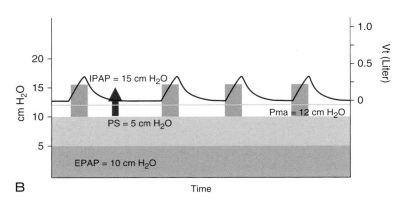

Figure 6-4. Oxygenation and mean airway pressure. (A) Patient placed on BiPAP of 10 and 5, corresponding to IPAP of 10 cm H_2O and EPAP of 5 cm H_2O. However, patient is still hypoxic on 100% FiO_2. (B) To increase mean airway pressure (Pma), IPAP and EPAP are increased together to IPAP of 15 cm H_2O and EPAP of 10 cm H_2O. Pma increases from 7 to 12 cm H_2O. PS remains at 5 cm H_2O and Tv stays the same. Pressure and Vt tracings are ideal.

together (see Figure 6-4). This will provide the same level of inspiratory support while increasing Pma and oxygenation.

► CLINICAL SCENARIOS AND EVIDENCE BEHIND USE

Before examining the different articles studying NIV use, it is important to discuss their validity and application to bedside care. The respective studies, in addition to being conducted in centers with extensive experience with NIV, had strict inclusion and exclusion criteria. The majority of studies excluded patients with hemodynamic instability, multiorgan dysfunction, altered mental status, difficulty in maintaining their airway, or excessive secretions. In addition, the sickest patients were intubated before randomization, and were not included. NIV is appropriate for only a select subgroup of patients with acute respiratory distress.

COPD AND HYPERCARBIC RESPIRATORY FAILURE

The use of NIV in acute COPD exacerbations and hypercarbic respiratory failure is well supported by multiple clinical trials.[11–14] NIV is believed to help improve respiratory mechanics and symptoms in patients with COPD

exacerbations through a number of mechanisms. First by providing pressure support, BiPAP can partially offload the work of breathing of the diaphragm and other respiratory muscles. Second, providing extrinsic PEEP in certain scenarios may reduce air trapping and dynamic hyperinflation and overcome intrinsic PEEP, leading to improved pulmonary function. Finally, NIV can decrease the cost of breathing. Normal breathing utilizes approximately 2% of cardiac output; this can increase to 20% in patients with acute respiratory distress. By improving $Paco_2$ and pH, NIV can improve mental status and respiratory muscle function, improving the efficiency of breathing.[4]

The use of NIV in COPD, as in other disease states, is intended to bridge the patient through the exacerbation until medical therapy can ameliorate and reverse the disease process. For the appropriately selected patient without exclusion criteria, NIV should be considered first-line therapy for the patient with respiratory distress from COPD exacerbations. NIV success rates have been cited near 80–85%.[11,12] The beneficial effects of NIV can be attributed to decreasing the complications associated with ETI and conventional mechanical ventilation—for example, oversedation, ICU-associated weakness, ventilator-associated pneumonia (VAP), and pneumothorax.[6,7,11–14] In addition, patients on NIV "wean" faster than patients on standard mechanical ventilation.[6,7,11–14]

In 1995, Brochard et al[12] published the results of a randomized multicenter trial on the use of NIV in patients with acute exacerbations of COPD. In this study, the authors compared standard medical therapy alone with a combination of standard medical therapy and NIV in 85 patients with an acute exacerbation of COPD. The NIV group had a lower rate of ETI (26% vs. 74%, $P < .001$), frequency of complications (16% vs. 48%, $P < .001$), hospital length of stay (LOS) (23 ± 17 days vs. 35 ± 33 days, $P = .005$), and in-hospital mortality (9% vs. 29%, $P = .02$). Importantly, the sickest patients (approximately 30%), who required emergent intubation or were hemodynamically unstable, were *excluded* from the trial. This study was conducted in an ICU setting.

In 2000, Plant et al[13] conducted a similar but larger multicenter trial on the use of NIV in acute exacerbations of COPD. The authors included patients with COPD exacerbations that had tachypnea, hypercarbia, and mild to moderate acidosis (defined as pH 7.25–7.35). This study differed from the earlier study by Brochard in that it was conducted in a general respiratory ward and not in an ICU—still not a busy ED but in theory closer to the functioning and staffing of the ED than an ICU. Plant found similar results to the prior work of Brochard. In 236 randomized patients, NIV was associated with a reduced need for intubation (15% vs. 27%, $P = .02$), lower in-hospital mortality (10% vs. 20%, $P = .05$), and a more rapid improvement in breathlessness and RR.[13]

In general, the beneficial results demonstrated by Brochard and Plant have been reproduced in multiple studies examining the use of NIV in acute COPD exacerbations. Ram et al,[14] in 2001 and then again in 2004, conducted a systematic review of the literature for the *Cochrane Database* on the use of NIV in acute COPD exacerbations. In a pooled analysis, the use of NIV was associated with decreased mortality (RR 0.52; 95% CI 0.35–0.76), decreased need for intubation (RR 0.41; 95% CI 0.33–0.53), reduction in treatment failure (RR 0.48; 95% CI 0.37–0.63), less complications with associated treatment (RR 0.38; 95% CI 0.24–0.60), and shorter LOS (weighted mean difference [WMD] −3.24 days; 95% CI −4.42 to −2.06). In addition, NIV showed beneficial effects on physiologic respiratory parameters such as pH, $Paco_2$, and RR. The authors concluded that data from good-quality randomized controlled trials (RCT) support the benefit of NIV as first-line therapy in conjunction with medical care in suitable patients with respiratory failure secondary to an acute exacerbation of COPD. In addition, they further recommend that NIV should be considered early in the course of respiratory failure, before severe acidosis ensues, as a means of reducing the likelihood of ETI, treatment failure, and mortality.[14]

The use of NIV in hypercarbic narcosis is controversial. Altered mental status has classically been an exclusion criteria or contraindication to the use of NIV. However, two studies suggest that NIV may be effective in patients with encephalopathy secondary to hypercarbic respiratory failure. Díaz et al[15] conducted a prospective observational study comparing the use of NIV in patients with acute hypercapnic respiratory failure and a Glasgow Coma Scale (GCS) ≤8 ($n = 76$) versus those with a GCS >8 ($n = 605$). Their group found similar results between the two groups with regards to in-hospital mortality (33.2% in "No Coma" group vs. 26.3% in "Coma" group, $P = .17$) and success with avoidance of ETI (70.1% in "No Coma" group vs. 80% in "Coma" group, $P = .04$). In the subgroup with COPD, the results were even more encouraging with 89% of patients without coma avoiding intubation and 86.3% of patients with coma avoiding intubation. Improvement of GCS within 1 hour of therapy predicted NIV success (OR 2.32, 95% CI 1.53–3.53), again highlighting the need for the clinician to *reassess* the patient's response to NIV, search for objective criteria of success or failure, and appropriately escalate therapy if necessary. The major weakness of the Díaz study is the lack of a control group, but the results suggest that a trial of NIV may be warranted in patients with hypercarbic narcosis and especially in COPD patients with hypercarbic narcosis. There was only one episode of aspiration pneumonia in 76 patients. Scala et al[16] conducted a case-controlled study of 80 individuals, matching comatose and noncomatose COPD patients. They found similar results to Díaz's group. However, patients with worsening mental status depression had higher failure rates and higher mortality than matched controls with normal mental status. There were no cases of aspiration in the selected patients. Patients who improved usually did so within the first hour, and the majority of cases of NIV failure were secondary to hemodynamic instability and need for vasopressors. Again the authors suggest that a trial of NIV may be warranted in patients with hypercarbic narcosis.

In 2009, the Global Initiative for Chronic Obstructive Lung Disease (GOLD) recommended NIV for use in COPD exacerbations in patients with moderate to severe disease, defined by dyspnea with use of accessory muscles, tachypnea (RR >25 breaths/min), acidosis (pH ≤7.3), or hypercapnia ($Paco_2$ >45).[11] NIV in multiple clinical trials has consistently improved respiratory acidosis and decreased RR, sensation of breathlessness, hospital LOS, complication rate, need for intubation, and mortality. It should be considered in all patients with moderate to severe dyspnea from a COPD exacerbation who do not require immediate intubation. It is probably prudent to institute NIV as early as possible in the disease course. An altered level of consciousness is usually a contraindication to NIV; however, if the depressed mental status is secondary to CO_2 retention, the clinician can consider a trial of NIV. The patient should be closely monitored for evidence of hemodynamic instability, worsening mental status, respiratory failure, apnea, and aspiration. If the patient does not improve clinically within 1–2 hours, therapy should be escalated. It is probably prudent to place a nasogastric tube in patients with depressed level of consciousness to decrease gastric distention and the incidence of aspiration, although this statement has been both supported[15] and disavowed[16] by different authors. Furthermore, a nasogastric tube can worsen an air leak.

ACUTE CARDIOGENIC PULMONARY EDEMA

The use of NIV and CPAP in patients with respiratory distress secondary to acute cardiogenic pulmonary edema (ACPE) is generally well supported in the literature. BiPAP and CPAP are thought to benefit in ACPE by decreasing both preload and afterload, reducing the sensation of breathlessness, decreasing CO_2 retention when present, and, when BiPAP is used, decreasing the work of breathing.[4] The application of external PEEP increases intrathoracic pressure. This increase in intrathoracic pressure is believed to decrease venous return to right side of the heart, dropping preload and placing the heart on a more favorable part of the Starling curve. Some studies have called this theory into question however. Venous return is based largely on the gradient between right atrial pressure (RAP) and the mean systemic pressure (MSP) of the peripheral circulation. Jellinek et al[17] showed that RAP and MSP increased equally with the application of PEEP. The gradient for venous return stayed the same while venous return decreased. Therefore, the drop in venous return that accompanies the application of PEEP is likely related to both an increase in intrathoracic pressure and more complicated interactions between the right side of the heart and the peripheral circulation.[4,17]

Venous return and cardiac output over any given time period are equivalent. In preload-responsive states, this drop in venous return is more pronounced, leading to a potentially dangerous drop in cardiac output, BP, and tissue perfusion. In conditions where the heart is adequately fluid resuscitated or volume overloaded (e.g., ACPE), this drop in cardiac output is negligible.[4]

The application of PEEP, via BiPAP or CPAP, is also believed to be beneficial in patients with ACPE through a reduction in afterload. Afterload is the force opposing ventricular contraction. This force is determined by two major variables: systemic arterial resistance and the left ventricular transmural pressure. The left ventricular transmural pressure is equal to the difference between the systolic BP and the intrathoracic pressure.[4] In patients with ACPE, the clinician administers nitrates and vasodilators, decreasing afterload by reducing systemic arterial resistance and also reducing transmural pressure by reducing systolic BP. The application of PEEP through BiPAP or CPAP raises intrathoracic pressure that leads to a decrease in left ventricular transmural pressure and left ventricular afterload, leading to a decrease in edema formation in the lungs.[4]

Numerous studies have compared the use of BiPAP and CPAP in ACPE, with mixed results.

In 2008, Vital et al[18] published a systematic review in the *Cochrane Database* examining the use of BiPAP or CPAP in ACPE. They included a total of 21 trials with 1,071 patients. Their results suggest that BiPAP or CPAP significantly reduced hospital mortality (RR 0.6, 95% CI 0.45–0.84) and ETI (RR 0.53, 95% CI 0.34–0.83). The number needed to treat (NNT) to prevent one death was 13 and to prevent one intubation was 8. ICU LOS was reduced by 1 day (WMD −1.07 days, 95% CI −1.60 to −0.53). No significant increases in acute myocardial infarction with BiPAP during (RR 1.24, 95% CI 0.79–1.95) or after (RR 0.82, 95% CI 0.09–7.54) its application were observed.

The validity of the systematic review in critical care medicine has recently been called into question.[19] Lumping together populations from multiple studies will increase the sample size, tighten the confidence interval, and decrease the chance of random error, but unfortunately these populations are often heterogeneous. Analyzing heterogeneous study populations together can serve to amplify systematic errors, threatening accuracy or usefulness of the evidence for the clinician at the patient's bedside.[19] Furthermore, meta-analyses fail to predict the outcomes of future large multicenter randomized trials 35% of the time.[20]

In 2008, Gray et al[21] published the Three Interventions in Cardiogenic Pulmonary Oedema (3CPO) trial, examining NIV in cardiogenic pulmonary edema. This trial was a large, randomized multicenter trial involving 1,069 ED patients with ACPE. Patients were randomized to standard care (supplemental oxygen) versus CPAP or BiPAP. The 3CPO trial found that CPAP and BiPAP were better than standard care in relieving dyspnea, improving HR, RR, hypercapnia, and acidosis at 1 hour. Unfortunately, these benefits did not translate into a lower hospital mortality rate (9.8% vs. 9.5%, $P = .87$) or intubation rate (2.8% vs. 2.9%, $P = .90$). CPAP and BiPAP were equally effective, and there was no associated increase in the incidence of acute myocardial infarction with BiPAP (27.2% vs. 26.8%, $P = .90$). The authors recommend that NIV be used as an adjunctive therapy in patients with ACPE with severe respiratory distress or in patients who do not improve with standard pharmacologic therapy (nitrates, diuretics, and possibly afterload-reducing agents).

There are some important critical elements and controversies to point out about the 3CPO trial. First, the sickest patients, those who required immediate life-saving interventions (i.e., intubation), were excluded. This exclusion possibly selected a "healthier" group of patients. The intubation rate in the 3CPO trial was approximately 3%.[21] In all other trials besides 3CPO, the intubation rate was around 27% in the control groups.[17,22] It is harder to find a difference in outcomes (i.e., intubation and mortality) when these outcomes are rare to begin with.

Second, this trial was conducted as an open trial with an "intention-to-treat" analysis. Briefly, intention to treat means that regardless of the actual treatment given, a particular patient is analyzed in the group to which he or she is randomized. With regards to this trial, if a patient was randomized to receive standard care, but shortly after randomization was deemed to need additional support and crossed over to an NIV arm, he or she was still analyzed in the standard care arm (and vice versa). From a research standpoint, the intention-to-treat study design is critical to protect the randomization process but from a practical standpoint it can make the results difficult to interpret and apply at the patient's bedside. Researchers attempt to minimize confounding results from crossover among treatment groups. This is not always practically or ethically possible. In the 3CPO trial, between 15% and 24% of patients did not complete the trial in the group they were randomly assigned.[21] This high rate of crossover serves as a confounding variable because some patients treated with standard medical treatment likely benefited from NIV application, yet were analyzed as successes in the standard treatment group. Approximately 15.5% of the patients treated with standard therapy were put on NIV because of worsening respiratory distress or deterioration in blood gas values.[21] Similarly, 5.2–8.4% of patients treated with NIV did not complete the trial because of discomfort with the mask and ventilator.[21] A major determinant of NIV success or failure is patient compliance and tolerance of treatment.

The aggregated data on the use of NIV in ACPE suggest that there is a definite benefit in terms of physiologic and clinical parameters. This seems to support its use in the care of patients with ACPE. However, this does not necessarily translate statistically into a reduction in mortality and the reduced need for intubation. Weng et al[22] conducted another systematic review and included the data of the 3CPO trial investigators. They concluded that even with the equivocal results of the 3CPO trial, the previous assessments that the use of CPAP reduces mortality and intubation rates in patients with ACPE and that BiPAP reduces the need for intubation compared with standard therapy still appear to be true.

Perhaps the most useful information from these, at times, conflicting data is that the use of NIV in ACPE does not cause harm. One of the first studies published by Mehta et al[23] in 1997 found an increased rate of myocardial infarction in the BiPAP group (71%) when compared with the CPAP group (31%), leading to an early termination of their study. However, the patients in the BiPAP group had a higher percentage of chest and jaw pain, and likely presented with myocardial infarction rather than developing one on BiPAP. In addition, this study had a small sample size. The 3CPO trial[21] and multiple systematic reviews[18,22] did not find an increased incidence of myocardial infarction with the use of NIV, particularly BiPAP.

The question of whether to use CPAP or BiPAP in ACPE is controversial. From a purely statistical standpoint, it would appear that CPAP has a slight advantage. From the studies of Vital et al[18] and Weng et al,[22] CPAP was associated with a statistically significant decrease in hospital mortality and reduced need for intubation. BiPAP was associated with a less robust decrease in mortality and intubation.[18,22] From a physiologic standpoint, BiPAP would seem to be more logical. BiPAP provides all the benefits of CPAP as the EPAP is essentially the same as CPAP. Plus BiPAP better offloads the respiratory muscles and work of breathing, better augments ventilation and improves hypercarbia and respiratory acidosis when present, and better improves dyspnea, HR, hypoxemia, and RR.[18,21] When compared directly with one another, CPAP and BiPAP perform identically in terms of mortality and need for intubation.[21,24] The difference appears to be statistical rather than actual. For ACPE, the use of CPAP and BiPAP appears to be equally effective. However, patients with coexisting COPD or any degree of hypercapnia or respiratory acidosis may benefit more from BiPAP over CPAP.

NIV, in addition to aggressive medical management, should be considered *first-line* therapy for the appropriately selected patient with ACPE. The patient should not be hypotensive, in shock, or otherwise hemodynamically unstable. In addition, active ischemia, STEMI requiring emergent intervention, or an unstable arrhythmia should not be present. These patients are better managed by ETI and mechanical ventilation. The BiPAP should be set with an emphasis on a higher EPAP to increase mean airway pressure and lung recruitment that can be used to improve oxygenation, along with supplemental oxygen. Alternatively, CPAP can be used alone. Pressure support, if used, should be adjusted by raising the IPAP to decrease the work of breathing and improve ventilation, hypercapnia, and respiratory acidosis as needed. As with all patients on NIV, they should be monitored closely for signs of NIV failure, and the clinician should be prepared to escalate care and perform ETI if necessary. Objective data from ABGs, and other clinical parameters such as HR, RR, SaO$_2$, and dyspnea, should be frequently reassessed. After 1–2 hours of NIV, clinical improvement should be evident. If there is no improvement, or deterioration occurs at any time, intubation should strongly be considered.

THE IMMUNOCOMPROMISED PATIENT

ETI and conventional mechanical ventilation are associated with a risk of VAP and other nosocomial infections. VAP can have a 20–50% mortality rate.[25] NIV has been shown to benefit immunocompromised patients by reducing mortality, mainly secondary to prevention of VAP and other nosocomial infections and complications such as pneumothorax.

In a case-controlled study looking at NIV in 48 acquired immunodeficiency syndrome (AIDS) patients admitted to the ICU with acute respiratory failure secondary to *pneumocystis carinii pneumonia* (PCP), Confalonieri et al[26] showed a decrease in ICU mortality in patients treated with NIV (75% vs. 38%), a reduction in the need for intubation in the NIV group (67% avoided intubation), and a decreased ICU LOS (7 ± 4 days vs. 10 ± 4 days) as compared with controls who were intubated on presentation of acute respiratory failure. The retrospective nature of the study makes it difficult to draw complete conclusions. It is very possible that those initially intubated were sicker and destined to do worse, but the fact that intubation was prevented in approximately two thirds of the patients treated with NIV suggests that a trial of NIV *is warranted* in AIDS patients with acute respiratory failure secondary to PCP pneumonia. Hilbert et al[27] compared NIV with standard treatment (supplemental oxygen) in 52 patients with evidence of immunocompromise, acute hypoxic respiratory failure, pulmonary infiltrates, and fever. They found a decrease in the need for intubation (12 vs. 20, P = .03), fewer serious complications (13 vs. 21, P = .02), fewer ICU deaths (10 vs. 18, P =0.03), and fewer hospital deaths (13 vs. 21, P = .02). Again, it is important to emphasize that this study did not compare NIV with intubation, but rather NIV with standard oxygen therapy. The benefits of NIV may be most pronounced when used early in the disease process. All of the patients who were intubated died, regardless of initial treatment, highlighting the severity of underlying illness and poor prognosis associated with respiratory failure in the immunocompromised population. Similar results were found by Antonelli et al[28] in immunocompromised patients with acute respiratory failure after solid organ transplantation. In 51 patients with acute respiratory failure after solid organ transplantation, the use of NIV was associated with a significant reduction in the rate of ETI (20% vs. 70%, P = .002), a lower rate of fatal complications (20% vs. 50%, P = .05), decreased LOS in the intensive care unit by survivors (mean [SD] days, 5.5 [3] vs. 9 [4], P = .03), and lower intensive care unit mortality (20% vs. 50%, P = .05). An initial trial of NIV *is warranted* in immunocompromised patients with acute respiratory failure as it may prevent ETI and the complications associated with standard mechanical ventilation.

ASTHMA

Clinicians can consider the use of NIV for the treatment of acute asthma exacerbations. However, the evidence behind the use of NIV for acute asthma exacerbations is not as strong as other disease states such as COPD or ACPE. Asthma-induced acute respiratory failure is secondary to airflow obstruction and dynamic hyperinflation, leading to increased intrinsic PEEP and an increased work of breathing. An early study by Meduri et al[29] studied the use of NIV in 17 patients with status asthmaticus admitted to the intensive care unit, and showed that NIV improved clinical and physiologic parameters (pH, Paco$_2$, RR). Only two of the patients required intubation. This was a case series and was therefore unable to show if NIV can prevent intubation. However, it did demonstrate that a trial of NIV may be safe in status asthmaticus. In a study conducted in an ED, Soroksky et al[30] compared BiPAP with medical therapy alone in 30 patients with severe asthma exacerbations. They found a reduction in the need for hospital admission, more rapid improvement in FEV$_1$, and a greater percentage of patients who improved their FEV$_1$ to greater than 50%. This study was mainly limited by size, and only patients with moderate to severe disease were included. It is difficult to apply these data to status asthmaticus patients with acute respiratory failure because there were no intubations or morbidity in either group. Except for FEV$_1$ and PEFR, other clinically important variables such as ICU admission and ICU LOS were not commented on. However, applying NIV *early* as opposed to waiting for ICU admission in status asthmaticus patients may explain the very positive results of this trial. A *Cochrane* meta-analysis by Ram et al[31] found the use of NIV in asthma exacerbations to be "promising" but also still "controversial" because of lack of evidence. The meta-analysis included only the aforementioned Soroksky study, as no other trials were adequately designed for inclusion in this analysis. More evidence is needed to develop evidenced-based recommendations, but it is generally agreed that a trial of NIV is warranted in select patients with severe asthma exacerbation provided that there are no contraindications present.[32] Again it must be emphasized that NIV is not a treatment for status asthmaticus, but rather a means of respiratory support. The clinician should optimize medical treatment and aggressively treat the patient with β-agonists, corticosteroids, and magnesium sulfate. Intubation and conventional mechanical ventilation in the status asthmaticus patient are sometimes necessary. If a trial of NIV is to be attempted, it should be done early and the patient should be monitored closely. If there are signs of worsening fatigue or respiratory failure, support should be escalated. Intubation should strongly be considered if the patient fails the NIV trial.[32]

PNEUMONIA

The use of NIV in pneumonia is controversial, but in a carefully selected patient, a trial of NIV may be attempted. Even with optimal antibiotic therapy and aggressive medical management, the course of pneumonia is usually not rapidly correctable. Therefore, standard mechanical ventilation may be a better option than NIV. Multiple studies have looked at acute respiratory failure and pneumonia either directly or via subgroup analysis, often with differing results.

One of the larger studies looking specifically at pneumonia patients, conducted by Confalonieri et al,[33] compared 56 patients with acute respiratory failure secondary to severe community-acquired pneumonia (CAP) with NIV versus conventional therapy. They found a decreased need for ETI (21% vs. 50%, $P = .03$) and duration of ICU stay (1.8 ± 0.7 days vs. 6 ± 1.8 days, $P = .04$). However, there was no decrease in ICU mortality or 60-day mortality. Furthermore, the applicability of this benefit may be limited to patients with COPD. A post hoc analysis suggested that the subset of CAP patients with underlying COPD benefited the most from a trial of NIV. In this study, patients with COPD treated with NIV versus conventional therapy had a decreased need for intubation (0% vs. 55.5%), duration of ICU LOS (0.25 ± 2.1 days vs. 7.6 ± 2.2 days, $P = .02$), and 60-day mortality (11.1% vs. 62.5%, $P = .05$). A reduction in intubation, duration of ICU stay, and mortality was *not* seen in patients without COPD.

In an observational study looking at NIV in 24 patients with severe CAP, Jolliet et al[34] found that NIV was associated with a moderate improvement of P/F and a decrease in RR. A large proportion (66%) of patients eventually required intubation and eight of those patients expired. Likewise, those patients who did not require intubation had a shorter ICU stay (6 days vs. 16 days) and hospital stay (9.5 days vs. 23 days).

Studies looking at all-comers with hypoxic respiratory failure have found conflicting results with regards to the use of NIV in patients with pneumonia. In a study of 64 patients with acute respiratory failure from multiple different causes by Honrubia et al,[35] a small subset of 8 patients with pneumonia all failed an NIV trial and required mechanical ventilation. In the Antonelli et al[36]

study of 354 patients with acute hypoxemic respiratory failure, the presence of CAP was an independent predictor of NIV failure, with 50% requiring intubation. Ferrer et al,[37] looking at the use of NIV versus conventional therapy in 105 patients with acute hypoxemic respiratory failure, showed a decreased need for intubation (26% vs. 73%, $P = .017$) and ICU mortality (15.7% vs. 53%, $P = .030$) in a subset of 34 patients with acute hypoxemic respiratory failure from pneumonia.

The evidence surrounding the use of NIV in acute hypoxemic respiratory failure secondary to pneumonia does not provide a clear signal to the clinician. Although patients who avoid intubation do better, this effect may not be related to the efficacy of NIV but may rather suggest the obvious—sicker patients do worse. To complicate matters, with the exception of the sickest pneumonia patients, it may be difficult to initially differentiate the subset of pneumonia patients who may benefit from a trial of NIV from those who should be immediately intubated. The American Thoracic Society (ATS) and Infectious Disease Society of America (IDSA) in their 2007 guidelines for the management of CAP recommend a "cautious trial" of NIV in patients with CAP who have signs of respiratory distress and/or hypoxemia unless they are candidates for immediate intubation as evidenced by severe disease, bilateral infiltrates, or a P/F ≤150.[38] The ATS/IDSA guidelines note that severe CAP and acute respiratory distress syndrome (ARDS) may be hard to distinguish clinically early in the disease process, and NIV has poor efficacy in ARDS (see below), further decreasing the benefit of NIV in these patients.[38]

A short trial (1 or 2 hours) looking objectively for signs of improvement or failure of NIV (fatigue, accessory muscle use, change in Pao_2, and $Paco_2$) may be warranted in the appropriately selected patient with pneumonia. Similar to COPD and CHF, NIV may be most useful in pneumonia patients *earlier* in the disease course. The clinician should anticipate that there is a possibility that the patient with CAP will fail his or her NIV trail and should take the appropriate steps to be prepared to endotracheally intubate the patient in the event of decompensation or failure to improve. However, if intubation can be avoided, there is a higher likelihood of favorable outcomes and decreased associated morbidity and health care costs. Again, patients with evidence of severe disease or any evidence of hemodynamic instability, septic shock, or additional nonpulmonary organ failure should *not* be considered for NIV.

ARDS/ALI

The use of NIV in ARDS and acute lung injury (ALI) draws many parallels to the previously discussed use of NIV in pneumonia. Similar to pneumonia, the evidence for the benefit of NIV in ARDS and ALI is not straightforward. Studies looking at the use of NIV in ARDS and ALI have shown rates of intubation or failure of NIV ranging from 46% to 85%.[36,37,39,40] NIV may not be as efficacious at preventing intubation in ARDS/ALI when compared with COPD, CHF, and other disease processes. With regards to the following research studies, all included patients were relatively stable and not in shock. In addition, the sickest patients were endotracheally intubated immediately, before they had a chance of enrolling in the respective studies. Looking at patients with ARDS in multiple studies, NIV could be applied to only about 30% of patients with ARDS, and only succeeded in half, or about 16%, of total ARDS patients. Therefore, it should be clear that the use of NIV in ARDS applies to only a very specific, and small, subset of the ARDS population.

Looking at 354 patients with acute hypoxemic respiratory failure, and in particular 86 patients with ARDS, Antonelli et al[36] found the presence of ARDS and P/F ≤146 to be predictors of NIV failure. Patients with pulmonary and nonpulmonary causes of ARDS required intubation about 46% and 54% of the time, respectively. Stated differently, NIV was successful in preventing intubation in ARDS patients approximately half of the time. Half of the ARDS patients who avoided intubation survived versus 9.5% of ARDS patients who were intubated. It is difficult to make conclusions about mortality benefit from this study because of its uncontrolled nature; rather the mortality difference may simply prove that sicker patients do worse.

In the study of Ferrer et al[37] of 105 patients with acute hypoxemic respiratory failure, 15 patients met the criteria for ARDS. Nearly all of the patients who required intubation, in both the NIV and supplemental oxygen groups, expired. The results from both groups were equally dismal from a clinical standpoint and not statistically different. It is difficult to draw useful conclusions from such a small group of patients; however, these results suggest that NIV is less helpful in the treatment of ARDS than other disease states.

Rana et al in 2006[39] conducted an observational cohort study examining the use of NIV in patients with ALI. In analysis of 54 patients, 70.3% failed therapy with NIV and required intubation and standard mechanical ventilation. All 19 patients in shock failed the NIV trial. Additionally, patients with severe hypoxemia as evidenced by a median P/F <112 (70–157) and metabolic acidosis (base excess −4.0, range −7 to 0.2) had a higher incidence of NIV failure. While there was no control group in this study, it seems prudent to bypass an NIV trial and proceed directly to ETI and standard mechanical ventilation in patients with evidence of shock and metabolic acidosis.[40]

Antonelli et al[41] in 2007 looked at the use of NIV as first-line therapy in 147 patients with ARDS who were not intubated. NIV was successful in avoiding intubation in 79 patients (54%). Multivariate analysis showed that a Simplified Acute Physiology Score (SAPS II) >34 (OR 3.6, 95% CI 1.66–7.7) and a P/F ≤175 (OR 2.34, 95% CI 1.1–5.15) after 1 hour of NIV were independently associated with NIV failure and the need for ETI. The ICU mortality rate was 28%, but ICU mortality was significantly higher in those who required ETI, 5% versus 36% (OR 21, 95% CI 6.4–76.5, P < .001). Patients requiring intubation developed severe sepsis or septic shock and VAP more often. Mortality was higher in those who failed the trial of NIV and required intubation (54% vs. 19%, P < .01). The authors recommend that patients with less severe disease (SAPS II <34) and with a P/F >175 after 1 hour of NIV will likely benefit from continuation of NIV, but those who fail to show substantial improvement in oxygenation after a 1-hour trial of NIV should be closely monitored with a *low* threshold for ETI.

In conclusion, there are two important factors that the clinician must consider before placing a patient with ARDS/ALI on NIV. First, patients with severe disease as evidenced by a severe hypoxemia (P/F ≤ 150), additional nonpulmonary organ failure, or hemodynamic instability with the need for vasopressors or significant fluid resuscitation should *not* be considered candidates for NIV as they have a very high likelihood of failure and may do worse with a trial of NIV.[40] Second, if the patient does not show improvement within 1–2 hours of NIV, it is important that the clinician not permit the patient to linger on NIV, but rather escalate therapy.[40] A cautious trial of NIV can be attempted in a certain subset of ARDS/ALI with less severe disease that does not have any of the aforementioned high-risk factors for failure.

DO-NOT-INTUBATE

When considering the use of NIV in patients with a DNI, it is important for the clinician to have an understanding of the patient's goals of care as well as the underlying disease process responsible for respiratory distress. Some patients and their families may be amenable to an attempt of NIV; however, some may consider NIV to be unnecessary "life support" that merely prolongs suffering. The treating physician should explain the risks and benefits of NIV and determine the patient's and family members' wishes. NIV may alleviate dyspnea and air hunger *or* may worsen discomfort. As with any other patient placed on a trial of NIV, the clinician should frequently reassess the patient for evidence of NIV failure or success. In DNI patients, failure of NIV trial warrants escalation of opiate and other palliative measures in conjunction with the patient's and family members' wishes.

Similar to other patients placed on NIV, DNI patients with more reversible disease processes causing respiratory distress (i.e., COPD and CHF exacerbations) have more success with NIV than disease states such as pneumonia or ARDS.

Levy et al[42] in 2004 looked at the use of NIV in 114 patients with DNI status. Forty-three percent of these patients survived to hospital discharge. The presence of a strong cough (OR 0.16, 95% CI 0.05–0.51), being awake (OR 0.18, 95% CI 0.05–0.62), having a high baseline Paco$_2$ (OR 0.01, 95% CI 0.01–0.93), having COPD (OR 0.31, 95% CI 0.10–0.90), or having CHF (OR 0.14, 95% CI 0.02–0.75) as the underlying cause of respiratory failure had better outcomes in terms of hospital mortality. Patients with CHF and COPD survived to hospital discharge approximately 75% and 50% of the time, respectively. Patients with pneumonia, cancer, and other diagnosis did poorly, with less than 30% surviving to hospital discharge.

Schettino et al[43] in 2005 found similar results in their observational trial of NIV in 131 patients with DNI status. Patients treated with NIV for COPD exacerbations had a hospital mortality rate of 37.5%, and those treated for an exacerbation of ACPE had a hospital mortality rate of 39%. However, patients had significantly higher mortality rates when treated with NIV for other conditions such as non-COPD hypercapnic respiratory failure (68%), postextubation respiratory failure (77%), advanced cancer (85%), and hypoxemic respiratory failure (86%). In addition, Schettino et al[43] found that a baseline albumin ≤2.5 g/dL or a SAPS II score >35 also predicted mortality.

In 2007, the Society of Critical Care Medicine Palliative Noninvasive Positive Pressure Ventilation Task Force[44] put forth a stratification system for the use of NIV in DNI and palliative care patients. They proposed three broad classifications of patients with acute or chronic respiratory failure that NIV can be used in: (1) patients without preset limits for life support, (2) patients with a preset limit for life support (i.e., a DNI order), or (3) patients who desire comfort care only. Each separate category should have different goals of care, definitions of success, type of escalation in case of failure, and the appropriate clinical setting where NIV may be used.

The first category, patients without preset limits for life support, is the standard group of critical care patients with respiratory failure who have no restrictions on care and therefore require all appropriate life-sustaining measures. In this group, the goal of care is to restore health. NIV can be used for these patients as a means to assist with ventilation and oxygenation as well as to prevent intubation. If NIV fails, patients in this category should be endotracheally intubated. According to

the task force, these patients should be cared for in an ICU or step-down unit setting.[44]

The second category, patients who request life support but place a limit on care (in this particular situation ETI), comprises patients with respiratory failure where the use of NIV may prove to be beneficial. The goal in this group of patients is also to restore health if possible, with a secondary goal of minimizing discomfort. If NIV fails in this category of patients, palliative measures should be initiated, and NIV should be discontinued. These patients should also be cared for in an ICU or step-down unit setting; however, local institutional practice and resource availability should be taken into consideration.[44]

The final category involves patients who desire comfort care and palliation of symptoms. The use of NIV in this group is controversial, and there are little data to support the use of NIV in this situation.[44] However, NIV may be helpful in improving dyspnea and cognition. In these situations, the use of NIV can be discussed with the patient and family members. If NIV fails to improve dyspnea, or the patient loses consciousness, NIV should be discontinued as other palliative measures are pursued. These patients can be cared for in an ICU or step-down setting, but a more appropriate locale is probably a hospice or palliative care unit with properly trained personnel.

The delineation of these categories is helpful when discussing treatment options and goals of care with patients and family members in order to ensure that the proposed treatment is congruent with their wishes.

In conclusion, the use of NIV can be considered in select patients who have a DNI status. An honest discussion should take place between the clinician and patient or family members to ensure that this level of treatment is acceptable. Patients who have respiratory failure secondary to a COPD or CHF exacerbation are most likely to benefit from NIV. As with all patients on NIV, they should be closely monitored for signs of NIV failure. If NIV failure occurs, care should focus on comfort and NIV should be discontinued.

► CONCLUSION

The use of NIV to assist in the treatment of ED patients with acute respiratory failure has increased in the past decade. Patients should be appropriately selected for NIV—individuals who are hemodynamically unstable or are unable to protect their airway are *not* candidates for NIV. NIV works best in disease processes that are easily reversible. Good clinical evidence supports the use of NIV in exacerbations of COPD, ACPE, and acute respiratory failure in the immunocompromised, with weaker evidence for its use in asthma patients. A trial of NIV may be attempted in a very select subgroup of patients with hypoxemic respiratory failure secondary to pneumonia or ARDS, but there is a higher rate of failure. Regardless of the etiology of respiratory distress, aggressive medical management should be used in tandem with NIV. Patients on NIV should be monitored closely for signs of improvement or failure, and NIV therapy should be titrated appropriately to assist the patient with work of breathing, oxygenation, and ventilation. If improvement is not apparent within 1–2 hours, or any deterioration occurs, the patient should be endotracheally intubated, placed on conventional mechanical ventilation, and not allowed to *linger* on NIV. Patients placed on NIV should be admitted to an ICU or a respiratory care unit depending on disease etiology and severity, as well as local hospital resources and experience.

▶ ACKNOWLEDGMENTS

The authors would like to thank Lauren Houdek, B.S., David Ozimek, B.A., Elizabeth Barton, B.A., Richard Tan, B.A., and Sue Hahn, B.S., for their help with the creation of the manuscript.

REFERENCES

1. Mehta S, Hill NS. Noninvasive ventilation: state of the art. *Am J Respir Crit Care Med*. 2001;163:540–577.
2. Liesching T, Kwok H, Hill NS. Acute applications of noninvasive positive pressure ventilation. *Chest*. 2003;124:699–713.
3. West JB. *Pulmonary Pathophysiology: The Essentials*. 8th ed. New York: Wolters Kluwer Lippincott Williams & Wilkins; 2008:19.
4. Navalesi, P, Maggiore, SM. Positive end-expiratory pressure. In: Tobin M, ed. *Principles and Practices of Mechanical Ventilation*. New York: McGraw-Hill; 2006.
5. West JB. *Respiratory Physiology: The Essentials*. 8th ed. New York: Wolters Kluwer Lippincott Williams & Wilkins; 2008:176–177.
6. Garpestad E, Brennan J, Hill NS. Noninvasive ventilation for critical care. *Chest*. 2007;132;711–720.
7. Hill NS, Brennan J, Garpestad E, Nava S. Noninvasive ventilation in acute respiratory failure. *Crit Care Med*. 2007;35:2402–2407.
8. Esteban A, Frutos-Vivar F, Ferguson ND, et al. Noninvasive positive-pressure ventilation for respiratory failure after extubation. *N Engl J Med*. 2004;350:2452–2460.
9. Hill NS. Noninvasive positive pressure ventilation. In: Tobin M, ed. *Principles and Practices of Mechanical Ventilation*. New York: McGraw-Hill; 2006.
10. Marini JJ, Ravenscraft SA. Mean airway pressure: physiologic determinants and clinical importance—part 1: physiologic determinants and measurements. *Crit Care Med*. 1992;20:1461–1472.
11. Global Initiative for Chronic Obstructive Lung Disease: GOLD Report, Global Strategy for Diagnosis, Management, and Prevention of COPD. May 15, 2011. Available at: http://www.goldcopd.com/Guidelineitem.asp?l152&l251&intId52003. 2009.
12. Brochard L, Mancebo J, Wysocki M, et al. Noninvasive ventilation for acute exacerbations of chronic obstructive pulmonary disease. *N Engl J Med*. 1995;333:817.
13. Plant PK, Owen JL, Elliott MW. Early use of non-invasive ventilation for acute exacerbations of chronic obstructive pulmonary disease on general respiratory wards: a multicentre randomised controlled trial. *Lancet*. 2000;355:1931.
14. Ram F, Picot J, Lightowler J, Wedzicha JA. Non-invasive positive pressure ventilation for treatment of respiratory failure due to exacerbations of chronic obstructive pulmonary disease [review]. *Cochrane Database Syst Rev*. 2009:CD004104.
15. Díaz GG, Alcaraz AC, Talavera JCP, et al. Noninvasive positive-pressure ventilation to treat hypercapnic coma secondary to respiratory failure. *Chest*. 2005;127:952.
16. Scala R, Naldi M, Archinucci I, et al. Noninvasive positive pressure ventilation in patients with acute exacerbations of COPD and varying levels of consciousness. *Chest*. 2005;128:1657.
17. Jellinek H, Krenn H, Oczenski W, et al. Influence of positive airway pressure on the pressure gradient for venous return in humans. *J Appl Physiol*. 2000;88:926–932.
18. Vital FMR, Saconato H, Ladeira MT, et al. Non-invasive positive pressure ventilation (CPAP or bilevel NPPV) for cardiogenic pulmonary edema [review]. *Cochrane Database Syst Rev*. 2008;(3):CD005351.
19. Tobin MJ, Jubran A. Meta-analysis under the spotlight: focused on a meta-analysis of ventilator weaning. *Crit Care Med*. 2008;36:1–7.
20. LeLorier J, Gregoire G, Benhaddad A, et al. Discrepancies between meta-analyses and subsequent large randomized, controlled trials. *N Engl J Med*. 1997;337:536.
21. Gray A, Goodacre S, Newby DE, et al. Noninvasive ventilation in acute cardiogenic pulmonary edema. *N Engl J Med*. 2008;359:142.
22. Weng CL, Zhao YT, Liu QH, et al. Meta-analysis: noninvasive ventilation in acute cardiogenic pulmonary edema. *Ann Intern Med*. 2010;152:590.
23. Mehta S, Jay GD, Woolard RH, et al. Randomized, prospective trial of bilevel versus continuous positive airway pressure in acute pulmonary edema. *Crit Care Med*. 1997;25:620–628.
24. Mortiz F, Brousse B, Gellée B, et al. Continuous positive airway pressure versus bilevel noninvasive ventilation in acute cardiogenic pulmonary edema: a randomized multicenter trial. *Ann Emerg Med*. 2007;50:666.
25. Davis KA. Ventilator-associated pneumonia: a review. *J Intensive Care Med*. 2006;21;211.
26. Confalonieri M, Calderini E, Terraciano S, et al. Noninvasive ventilation for treating acute respiratory failure in AIDS patients with pneumocystis carinii pneumonia. *Intensive Care Med*. 2002;28:1233.
27. Hilbert G, Gruson D, Vargas F, et al. Noninvasive ventilation in immunosuppressed patients with pulmonary

infiltrates, fever, and acute respiratory failure. *N Engl J Med.* 2001;344:481.

28. Antonelli M, Conti G, Bufi M, et al. Noninvasive ventilation for treatment of acute respiratory failure in patients undergoing solid organ transplantation: a randomized trial. *JAMA.* 2000;283:235.

29. Meduri GU, Cook TR, Turner RE, et al. Noninvasive positive pressure ventilation in status asthmaticus. *Chest.* 1996;110:767.

30. Soroksky A, Stav D, Shpirer I. A pilot prospective, randomized, placebo-controlled trial of bilevel positive airway pressure in acute asthmatic attack. *Chest.* 2003;123:1018.

31. Ram FSF, Wellington SR, Rowe BH, et al. Non-invasive positive pressure ventilation for treatment of respiratory failure due to severe acute exacerbations of asthma. *Cochrane Database Syst Rev.* 2005;(3):CD004360.

32. Nowak R, Corbridge T, Brenner B. "Noninvasive ventilation." Joint Task Force Report: Supplemental Recommendations for the Management and Follow-up of Asthma Exacerbations. *J Emerg Med.* 2009;37(2, suppl 1):S18–S22.

33. Confalonieri M, Potena A, Carbone G, et al. Acute respiratory failure in patients with severe community-acquired pneumonia. *Am J Respir Crit Care Med.* 1999;160:1585.

34. Jolliet P, Abajo B, Pasquina P, Chevrolet JC. Non-invasive pressure support ventilation in severe community-acquired pneumonia. *Intensive Care Med.* 2001;27:812–821.

35. Honrubia T, López FJG, Franco N, et al. Noninvasive vs conventional mechanical ventilation in acute respiratory failure. *Chest.* 2005;128:3916.

36. Antonelli M, Conti G, Moro ML, et al. Predictors of failure of noninvasive positive pressure ventilation in patients with acute hypoxemic respiratory failure: a multi-center study. *Intensive Care Med.* 2001;27:1718.

37. Ferrer M, Esquinas A, Leon M, et al. Noninvasive ventilation in severe hypoxemic respiratory failure: a randomized clinical trial. *Am J Respir Crit Care Med.* 2003;168:1438.

38. Mandell LA, Wunderink RG, Anzueto AA, et al. Infectious Diseases Society of America/American Thoracic Society consensus guidelines on the management of community-acquired pneumonia in adults. *Clin Infect Dis.* 2007;44:S27–S72.

39. Rana S, Jenad H, Gay PC, et al. Failure of non-invasive ventilation in patients with acute lung injury: observational cohort study. *Crit Care.* 2006;10:R79.

40. Garpestad E, Hill N. Noninvasive ventilation for acute lung injury: how often should we try, how often should we fail? *Crit Care.* 2006;10:147.

41. Antonelli M, Conti G, Esquinas A, et al. A multiple-center survey on the use in clinical practice of noninvasive ventilation as a first-line intervention for acute respiratory distress syndrome. *Crit Care Med.* 2007;35(1):18–25.

42. Levy M, Tanios MA, Nelson D. Outcomes of patients with do-not-intubate orders treated with noninvasive ventilation. *Crit Care Med.* 2004;32(10):2002–2007.

43. Schettino G, Altobelli N, Kacmarek RM. Noninvasive positive pressure ventilation reverses acute respiratory failure in select "do-not-intubate" patients. *Crit Care Med.* 2005;33(9):1976–1982.

44. Curtis JR, Cook DJ, Sinuff T, et al. Noninvasive positive pressure ventilation in critical and palliative care settings: understanding the goals of therapy. *Crit Care Med.* 2007;35(3):932–939.

CHAPTER 7

Extracorporeal Cardiopulmonary Membrane Oxygenation

David A. Farcy, David Rabinowitz, and Paola G. Pieri

▶ INTRODUCTION

Despite the advances in lung-protective strategies and cardiac assist devices, severe pulmonary and cardiac failure continue to be associated with high mortality. Acute respiratory distress syndrome (ARDS) still maintains a mortality rate as high as 30–40%, 50% for patients with cardiogenic shock.[1] Patients with failing conventional or advanced methods of therapy or patients who are worsening clinically have few rescue therapy options. Early referral to an extracorporeal membrane oxygenation (ECMO) center might be the only option. This chapter will review the clinical indications, contraindications, types of ECMO, and the complications of ECMO use.

▶ HISTORY OF ECMO

ECMO is a term used to describe a form of partial cardiopulmonary bypass used for temporary, albeit prolonged, support of respiratory and/or cardiac function. Cardiopulmonary bypass was initially developed for use in the operating room to provide short-term cardiopulmonary support (CPS) during cardiac surgery procedures. Extracorporeal membrane oxygenation is more commonly known as and referred to by the acronym ECMO. Other names synonymous with ECMO include extracorporeal lung assist (ECLA), extracorporeal CO_2 removal (ECCOR), CPS, and extracorporeal cardiopulmonary resuscitation (ECPR).

Currently ECMO is utilized in the critical care setting for patients with acute, severe, potentially lethal *but reversible* respiratory or cardiac failure unresponsive to conventional medical management. It is occasionally used in patients with irreversible cardiac or respiratory disease under the circumstances that the patient is a candidate for a heart or lung transplant. In these cases, ECMO may be used as a "bridge" before or after transplantation. ECMO is reserved for patients with potentially reversible disease who are unlikely to survive with conventional medical management. It is important to remember that the primary medical indication for ECMO therapy must be a potentially reversible condition, with possibility for other treatments such as revascularization or transplant.

ECMO was developed in the 1970s from a modification of cardiopulmonary bypass. It uses a modified heart–lung bypass machine to provide gas exchange, and systemic perfusion if necessary, which can provide pulmonary and cardiac support. Unlike standard cardiopulmonary bypass, which is used for short-term support measured in hours, ECMO can provide longer support ranging from days to weeks in the intensive care unit (ICU). Additionally, the purpose of ECMO is to compensate for further harm or allow for intrinsic recovery of the heart and lungs, unlike standard cardiopulmonary bypass, which provides support during various cardiac surgical procedures.

ECMO functions by providing membrane oxygenation to temporarily take over the role of the lung or the heart. It provides for gas exchange while mechanical ventilation settings are adjusted to prevent a high-pressure environment. This minimizes ventilator-induced lung injury (VILI) and maximizes lung recruitment of the functional residual capacity. By providing support without reliance on mechanical ventilation for gas exchange, the native lung has time to heal and potentially recover. Additionally, some believe that the injured lung activates the release of inflammatory mediators, which may precipitate renal failure, liver failure, cardiac failure, and other systemic consequences. Release of these inflammatory mediators may be significantly decreased with ECMO support compared with high-pressure mechanical ventilation.[2]

There is clear evidence of the efficacy of respiratory ECMO for neonates. In 1996, a randomized controlled trial involving 185 neonates with respiratory failure showed a mortality reduction from 59% to 32%.[3] Subsequently, ECMO has been a common medical therapy in neonatal ICUs around the globe for specific conditions including meconium aspiration syndrome, primary pulmonary hypertension of the newborn, myocarditis, congenital diaphragmatic hernias, and other reversible lung injuries. The use of ECMO in the aforementioned pathologies has yielded survival rates as high as 80%.[4,5] Similar data have supported the use of ECMO in the pediatric population, with survival rates as high as 73% in pediatric patients suffering from respiratory failure.[6] The data for cardiac failure in both the neonate and pediatric populations result in a much lower rate of survival than for lung disease with a quoted rate ranging from 38% to 43%. However, recently a very large retrospective review of ECMO for myocarditis in infants, children, and young adults with 255 patients found a 61% survival at discharge.[7]

Unfortunately, the efficacy and safety of ECMO for adults has been less clear and has been debated in the literature. ECMO has been subject to a wide range of opinions in the medical literature since the 1970s and has shown that use in adults with ARDS is invasive, expensive, and without any morbidity improvement as compared with mechanical ventilation.[8] In 2004, one large study of 255 adults with severe ARDS who received ECMO revealed a 52% survival rate.[9] The first multicenter randomized controlled trial in ARDS looking at ECMO versus conventional mechanical ventilation was evaluated in a recently published trial. Efficacy and economic assessment of conventional ventilatory support versus extracorporeal membrane oxygenation for severe adult respiratory failure (CESAR) trial.[10] A total of 180 patients with ARDS were enrolled; they were either randomized to a tertiary care center or transferred and managed at a single ECMO center. Of the 90 patients who were due to transfer to the ECMO center, only 68 patients actually received ECMO therapy; there was an overall survival at 6 months of 63% for the ECMO group and 47% for the conventional group. This trial has, appropriately, come under scrutiny due to the lack of standardized treatment management in the control group and because the only ECMO center observed happened to be one of the most experienced in the world. One can conclude that early transfer to a specialized ECMO center might increase survivability but well-randomized controlled trials still need to be conducted.

Interestingly, due to the arrival of the H1N1 influenza epidemic, there has been a resurgence of small trials and case reports favoring the use of ECMO in adults[11] (a large observational study of 68 patients suffering with the 2009 influenza [H1N1]–associated ARDS, who received ECMO therapy in Australia and New Zealand). The ECMO group had severe hypoxemia that was defined by a mean $Pao_2/FiO2$ ratio of less than 60. The ECMO group had originally posted a survival rate of 79% but, in an update of their data, the authors quoted a survival rate of 75% at time of discharge.[12]

ECMO may have a role in certain disease processes, but it is not considered the standard of care. Recent studies suggest a mortality benefit when used early if proven ventilation techniques have failed. ECMO is best left to centers that are specialized with ideal resources.[13]

▶ INDICATIONS

ECMO can be utilized for mechanical assistance during pulmonary or cardiac failure in newborn infants, children, or adults.

NEONATAL

ECMO, as described above, is a routine part of neonatal care used in newborn infants for severe respiratory failure commonly associated with primary pulmonary hypertension, meconium aspiration syndrome, congenital diaphragmatic hernia, respiratory distress syndrome, group B streptococcal sepsis, and asphyxia.

PEDIATRIC

Pediatric ECMO is used for respiratory distress syndrome and in low cardiac output situations such as right, left, or biventricular failure following repair of congenital heart defects and with pulmonary vasoreactive crises that can occur following these surgeries. Sometimes ECMO is used as a bridge to cardiac transplant or as a bridge to recovery in temporary cardiomyopathy secondary to renal failure, myocarditis, and burns.

ADULT

Common etiologies of adult pulmonary and cardiac failure requiring ECMO support include:

1. Respiratory failure, characterized by the severity of hypoxemia or impaired ventilation:
   a. Adult respiratory distress syndrome due to:
      - Pneumonia—viral, bacterial, and aspiration
      - Sepsis
      - Multisystem trauma
      - Pulmonary contusion
      - Pancreatitis
      - Disseminated intravascular coagulation (DIC)
      - Intestinal infarction
      - Vasculitis
2. Cardiac failure:
   a. Acute cardiomyopathy
   b. Massive pulmonary embolus
   c. Congenital heart disease
   d. Right ventricular failure
   e. Biventricular failure
   f. "Bridge" to transplant

Unfortunately, patients who are sick enough to require ECMO but do not have access to this therapy often have a mortality rate approaching near 100% despite maximizing all other forms of available medical treatment. Early referral to a specialized ECMO center may provide a survival advantage in the adult.

▶ PATIENT SELECTION

Patient selection criteria for ECMO vary from center to center. The usual criteria include patients with a severe reversible process that would otherwise result in a very high predicted mortality with conventional medical support. See Table 7-1 for indications and Table 7-2 for contraindications.

▶ TECHNIQUE & METHODS

ECMO is simply the use of a modified heart–lung bypass machine to provide gas exchange and systemic perfusion. The technique can be performed one of the following two ways: by venovenous (V-V) (Figure 7-1) or venoarterial (V-A) (Figure 7-2) bypass. V-A ECMO can support respiratory and cardiac function. A large (23–30 French) catheter is inserted into the inferior vena cava via the femoral vein or the right atrium via the right internal jugular vein. This is the drainage catheter. The ECMO circuit requires high flow, typically 100 mL/kg/min requiring placement of such large-diameter catheters.

▶ **TABLE 7-1. INDICATIONS FOR ECMO**

- Refractory cardiogenic shock
- Pao_2/FIO_2 ratio less than 100 on FIO_2 of 1.0
- Cardiac arrest
- Hypercapnic respiratory failure w/ arterial pH of less than 7.2
- Unable to come off cardiopulmonary bypass from operating room
- Bridge to cardiac transplant or ventricular assist device

Data adapted from *ECMO: Extracorporeal Cardiopulmonary Support in Critical Care.*[2]

The ECMO catheters, or cannulas as they are also called, are typically placed by direct cutdown on vessels or by percutaneous introduction of the cannula using sequential dilators and a guidewire similar to the technique used in standard central line placement.

A second catheter, from which blood is returned to the patient's arterial circulation, returns blood to the descending aorta via a cannula placed in the femoral artery or the aortic arch via a cannula placed in the right carotid artery. Since blood flow through the patient's native heart and lungs is diverted to the ECMO circuit, the patient's cardiac output is controlled by the amount of blood that travels through the circuit. In V-A ECMO, the ECMO flow determines the cardiac output and oxygen delivery. Thus, V-A ECMO can provide pulmonary and cardiac support.

V-V bypass is physiologically different from V-A ECMO. Whereas V-A ECMO supports both respiratory and cardiac function, V-V ECMO supports only respiratory function. V-V ECMO diverts the patient's blood from the venous circulation and returns it to the venous circulation. It utilizes two venous catheters: A drainage catheter is placed in the right atrium via the right internal jugular vein in the same manner as performed for

▶ **TABLE 7-2. CONTRAINDICATIONS TO ECMO**

The following parameters describe a patient population with a greater than 80% predicted mortality risk from ARDS

- Mechanical ventilation for more than 7 days
- Irreversible cardiac or respiratory failure
- Morbid obesity
- Active bleeding, recent surgery, or any other situation in which anticoagulation is contraindicated
- Neurologic dysfunction
- Poor preexisting functional status
- Patients where ventricular assist device is contraindicated (cardiac patients)
- Age >60 years (relative contraindication)

Data adapted from *ECMO: Extracorporeal Cardiopulmonary Support in Critical Care.*[2]

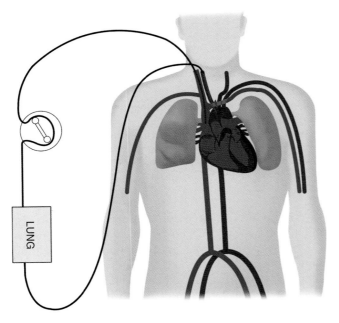

Figure 7–1. V-V ECMO. Venous drainage occurs through right internal jugular vein. Venous return occurs via the R femoral vein to the right atrium. (Data adapted from *ECMO: Extracorporeal Cardiopulmonary Support in Critical Care.*[2])

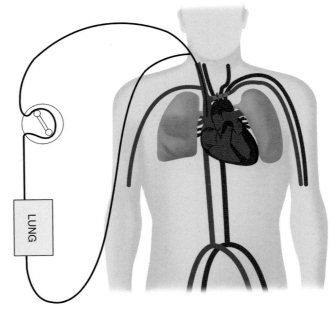

Figure 7–3. V-V double-lumen ECMO. Drainage and return occur via the IJ into the SVC. (Data adapted from *ECMO: Extracorporeal Cardiopulmonary Support in Critical Care.*[2])

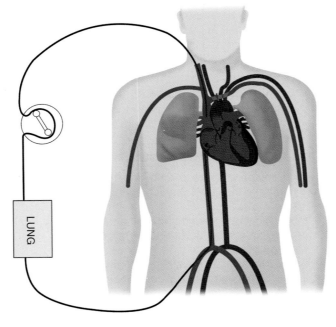

Figure 7–2. V-A ECMO. Venous drainage occurs through right internal jugular vein. Arterial return occurs through the common carotid artery into the aortic arch. (Data adapted from *ECMO: Extracorporeal Cardiopulmonary Support in Critical Care.*[2])

V-A ECMO and a second cannula, the return venous catheter, is placed in the femoral vein. Additionally, a double-lumen cannula inserted into the right internal jugular vein and guided to the right atrium may be utilized; however, these catheters are smaller in size and may not be adequate for adult patients (Figure 7-3).

When catheter access has been obtained, the patient is connected to the ECMO circuit. Often, the circuit may be primed with blood to avoid hypotension from acute changes in hemoglobin that can occur with crystalloid primed circuits. Venous blood is removed from the patient via the drainage catheter and pumped through an artificial lung called a membrane oxygenator. It is in the oxygenator that oxygen diffusion occurs because of a pressure gradient between the partial pressure of oxygen in the patient's venous blood being pumped through the circuit and the partial pressure of oxygen perfusing the membrane oxygenator.

Venous saturation is the monitor used to assess the adequacy of oxygen delivery from the ECMO circuit. It is usually kept between 70% and 75%. This is accomplished by titrating the ECMO circuit's pump flow rate. Increasing the flow increases the oxygen delivery and directly affects the venous saturation.

Carbon dioxide diffusion across the membrane is a function of the gradient from the patient's blood to the ECMO circuit's gas, that is, the gas ventilating the membrane oxygenator. The $PaCO_2$ is isolated by titrating the amount of gas used to ventilate the oxygenator (sweep

▶ TABLE 7–3. **SUMMARY OF DIFFERENCES BETWEEN V-A AND V-V ECMO**

Parameter	Venoarterial ECMO	Venovenous ECMO
PaO_2	Higher PaO_2 is achieved	Lower PaO_2 is achieved
Perfusion rate	Lower perfusion rates are needed	Higher perfusion rates are needed
Pulmonary circulation	Bypasses pulmonary circulation	Maintains pulmonary blood flow
	Decreases pulmonary artery pressures	Elevates mixed venous PO_2
Affect on cardiac support	Provides cardiac support to assist systemic circulation	Does not provide cardiac support to assist systemic circulation
Cannulation system	Requires arterial cannulation	Requires only venous cannulation

Data from http://surgery.med.umich.edu/pediatric/research/section/ecmo.shtml.

gas). Increasing the sweep will decrease CO_2 removal, while decreasing the sweep will increase the CO_2.

After having been pumped through the oxygenator, the oxygenated blood, under pressure, is pumped through a heat exchanger that maintains the patient's body temperature at a set desired temperature, usually 37.0°C. The blood is pumped either to the arterial circulation via the aorta in V-A ECMO or back into the venous circulation via the right atrium in V-V ECMO.

Currently ECMO circuits require the use of systemic anticoagulation with heparin to keep the system patent. The surfaces of the ECMO circuit and devices are plastic and therefore thrombogenic. It is necessary to provide anticoagulant prophylaxis to the patient's blood with a continuous infusion of heparin. The level of anticoagulation is measured by whole-blood activated clotting times (ACT) performed at the patient's bedside by the ECMO specialist. The ACT is usually maintained at approximately 180–240 seconds.

During ECMO therapy, the patient's ventilator settings are gradually weaned to allow lung "rest," keeping peak inspiratory pressures around 20 mm Hg. Patients are diuresed to dry weight. Hemoglobin levels are kept above 10 g/dL and platelet counts above 100,000/mL.

For summary of differences between V-A and V-V ECMO, see Table 7-3.

▶ ECMO COURSE AND WEANING

The average adult ECMO course can vary from days to weeks. During the first 24–48 hours, the condition of a patient's lungs will likely worsen as evidenced by increased radiographic opacification, which is thought to be due to the sudden decreasing airway pressure in response to diversion of pulmonary flow by ECMO. Additionally, it is thought that various vasoreactive substances are released and activated from the patient's blood reacting to the ECMO circuit surface. Improvement of lung function and compliance usually begin to occur within 1–3 days.

As lung function improves, the patients are weaned from ECMO by decreasing the circuit flow. When evidence of improved lung compliance and adequate gas exchange without excessive ventilatory support has been demonstrated, a "trial of" ECMO is performed. Good indicators of lung recovery include improving chest radiographs, increasing lung compliance, increasing PaO_2, or decreasing $PacO_2$ on resting ventilator settings. Eventually the patient is removed from ECMO support and the catheters are removed.

▶ COMPLICATIONS

As with any invasive procedure, ECMO has many potential life-threatening complications that can occur. These can be categorized into mechanical complications and patient complications (Tables 7-4 and 7-5). Mechanical complications are related to cannula placement and the ECMO circuit itself. Patient complications may be attributed to physiologic complications that occur due to ECMO therapy.

MECHANICAL COMPLICATIONS

The required placement of large-bore ECMO cannulas can cause several complications. As with placement of any type of central line, pneumothorax, line infection, and bleeding may occur. In addition, due to the larger

▶ TABLE 7–4. **MECHANICAL COMPLICATIONS OF ECMO**

Source of Complication	Nature of Complication
Cannula	Vascular injuries, bleeding, pneumothorax, infection, emboli
ECMO circuit	Air emboli, thrombocytopenia, hypothermia, clot development (oxygenator failure, consumptive coagulopathy, pulmonary or systemic emboli)

Data adapted from *ECMO: Extracorporeal Cardiopulmonary Support in Critical Care*.[2]

▶ TABLE 7-5. **PATIENT COMPLICATIONS OF ECMO**

Systemic Source of Complication	Nature of Complication
Neurologic	Seizures, intracranial bleed, infarction, paralysis
Hemotologic	Hemolysis, hemorrhage, coagulopathy, thrombocytopenia
Pulmonary	Pneumothorax, pulmonary hemorrhage
Metabolic	Acidosis/alkalosis, hyponatremia/hypernatremia, hypokalemia/hyperkalemia, hypoglycemia/hyperglycemia, hypocalcemia/hypercalcemia
Renal	Acute tubular necrosis, oliguria
Cardiac	Myocardial stunning, pericardial tamponade
Gastrointestinal	Hemorrhage, biliary calculi, elevated direct hyperbilirubinemia

Data adapted from *ECMO: Extracorporeal Cardiopulmonary Support in Critical Care.*[2]

size of the cannula required with ECMO, direct damage to the internal jugular vein can cause massive mediastinal bleeding. Cannulation of the carotid artery can cause dissection of the carotid arterial intima, leading to aortic dissection. In addition, any potential for bleeding from the placement of the cannulas is increased due to the requirement of systemic heparinization to maintain the ECMO circuit. The cannulas may also serve as a nidus for thrombus formation and emboli.

The ECMO circuit has potential to cause numerous complications. Because the surfaces of the ECMO circuit and devices are plastic, it is necessary to provide anticoagulant prophylaxis to the patient's blood with a continuous infusion of heparin. The most common mechanical complication is the development of clots within the circuit. These develop due to the platelets adhering to the plastic surface of the circuit, becoming activated, recruiting more platelets, and growing into platelet aggregates. Eventually these platelet aggregates break off. These clots can cause failure of the ECMO circuit's oxygenator. Larger clots can cause pulmonary or systemic emboli. Thrombocytopenia and a consumptive coagulopathy may also occur due to a large clot burden in the circuit.

Air can enter the ECMO circuit from dislodgement of a cannula, which then sucks in air, a small tear in the membrane oxygenator, compromised integrity in any of the connections in the circuit tubing, or high partial pressure of oxygen in the blood. Small bubbles in the circuit can be easily removed and have low potential for harm. A large bolus of air can be fatal.

Malfunction of the circuit heat exchanger can lead to significant patient hypothermia that may cause or exacerbate any coagulopathy that already exists.

PATIENT COMPLICATIONS

Patients undergoing ECMO therapy can suffer complications in any organ system. Many of these complications are due to the need for systemic anticoagulation.

Neurologically, patients may have spontaneous intracranial bleeding due to anticoagulation. This is more commonly seen in the neonatal ECMO population. Infarction from emboli may occur, and seizures induced by bleeding, infarction, or hypoxemia are also a threat.

Hemolysis from clot development typically manifests itself as renal dysfunction and rising serum haptoglobin levels. Coagulopathy and thrombocytopenia occur due to platelet consumption from activation by the circuit's plastic surface. Moreover, a dilutional coagulopathy can occur. Hemorrhage at any surgical site or cannula site, or into the site of previous invasive procedures is a frequent complication because of the required systemic heparinization. Intrathoracic, abdominal, or retroperitoneal hemorrhage may also occur. Exsanguination from circuit disruption, while uncommon, can be fatal.

Pericardial tamponade can occur due to cannula placement in the face of systemic anticoagulation. Myocardial stunning, which is defined as a decrease of left ventricular ejection fraction by more than 25% with the initiation of ECMO, may occur, requiring further V-A-ECMO support or vasopressor and inotropic support. Fortunately, stunning is a temporary effect and cardiac ejection function returns to normal within 48 hours of ECMO initiation.

Pulmonary hemorrhage, and spontaneous and iatrogenic pneumothorax may occur, as well. Oliguria is common during early ECMO therapy, and acute tubular necrosis and renal failure may occur from hemolysis, hypovolemia, or decreased perfusion.

Gastrointestinal hemorrhage may occur due to physiologic stress response, ischemia, embolic, or systemic anticoagulation. Elevated direct bilirubin and the development of biliary calculi occur secondary to prolonged fasting, use of parenteral nutrition, hemolysis, and diuretics.

Last, due to the ECMO circuit functioning as a large intravascular foreign body, numerous metabolic complications of either acidosis or alkalosis in response to any electrolyte disturbances may develop.

Due to the highly invasive nature of ECMO and the potential for numerous complications, a trained ECMO technician is usually present at all times, 24 hours per day, at the patient's bedside to monitor the circuit and the patient for potential complications. This is in addition to the patient's usual nursing personnel.

► CONCLUSION

ECMO is an effective, cutting-edge technology capable of providing pulmonary and cardiac life support in patients with severe respiratory failure. Often these patients have a high mortality risk despite optimal conventional medical care. While ECMO treatment is not without its risks and complications, it is a reasonable treatment modality that will allow for the recovery of injured native lung and improved survival in a patient population with a previously poor predicted outcome.

REFERENCES

1. Schuerer DJE, Kolvos NS, Boyd KV, Coopersmith CM. Extracorporeal membrane oxygenation, current clinical practice, coding, and reimbursement. *Chest.* 2008;134:179–184.
2. Van Meurs K, Lally KP, Peek G, Zwischenberger JB. *ECMO: Extracorporeal Cardiopulmonary Support in Critical Care (The "Red Book").* 3rd ed. Michigan: Extracorporeal Life Support Organization; 2005.
3. UK Collaborative ECMO Trial Group. UK collaborative randomized trial of neonate extracorporeal membrane oxygenation. *Lancet.* 1996;348:75–82.
4. Bartlett RH, Gazzaniga AB, Toomasian J, et al. Extracorporeal membrane oxygenation (ECMO) in neonatal respiratory failure. 100 cases. *Ann Surg.* 1986;204(3):236–245.
5. Shanley CJ, Hirschl RB, Schumacher RE, et al. Extracorporeal life support for neonates respiratory failures: a 20 years experience. *Ann Surg.* 1994;220:269–280.
6. Swaniker F, Kolla S, Moler F, et al. Extracorporeal life support outcome for 128 pediatric patients with respiratory failure. *J Pediatric Surg.* 2000;35:197–202.
7. Rajagopal S, Almond C, Laussemn P, et al. Extracorporeal membrane oxygenation for the support of infants, children and young adults with acute myocarditis: a review of the Extracorporeal Life Support Organization registry. *Crit Care Med.* 2010;38:382–387.
8. Morris AH, Wallace CJ, Menlove RL, et al. Randomized clinical trial of pressure controlled inversed ratio ventilation and extracorporeal CO_2 removal for adult respiratory distress. *Am J Respir Crit Care Med.* 1994;149(2 pt 1):295–305.
9. Hemmila M, Rowe S, Boules T, et al. Extracorporeal life support for severe acute respiratory distress syndrome in the adults. *Ann Surg.* 2004;240:595–607.
10. Peek GJ, Mugford M, Tiruvoipati R, et al. Efficacy and economic assessment of conventional ventilatory support versus extracorporeal membrane oxygenation for severe adult respiratory failure (CESAR): a multicentre randomised controlled trial. *Lancet.* 2009;374:1351–1363.
11. The Australia and New Zealand Extracorporeal Membrane Oxygenation (ANZ ECMO) Influenza Investigators. Extracorporeal membrane oxygenation for 2009 influenza A (H1N1) acute respiratory distress syndrome. *JAMA.* 2009;302(17):1888–1895.
12. Davies D, Jones J, Gattas D. Extracorporeal membrane oxygenation for ARDS due to 2009 influenza A (H1N1)—author reply. *JAMA.* 2010;303:942.
13. Bartlett RH. Extracorporeal life support in the management of severe respiratory failure. *Clin Chest Med.* 2000:21(3):555–561.

SECTION III

Pulmonary Disorders

CHAPTER 8

Acute Respiratory Failure

Imoigele P. Aisiku

► INTRODUCTION

Acute respiratory failure (ARF) is one of the leading causes of admission to the intensive care unit (ICU). Recently, incidence ranges for ARF, acute lung injury (ALI), and acute respiratory distress syndrome (ARDS) in adults were found to be 77.6–88.6, 17.9–34.0, and 12.6–28.0 cases/100,000 population per year, respectively.[1,2] Mortality rates of approximately 40% were reported for patients with ARF, and similar or slightly lower rates for those with ALI and ARDS.[3,4]

The respiratory system primarily functions to provide adequate blood oxygenation and carbon dioxide elimination for the purposes of sustaining aerobic metabolism and pH homeostasis, respectively. Although the etiologies of respiratory failure are far too numerous to list, the underlying pathophysiologic mechanisms are similar and usually lead to a final common pathway. A consensus definition has not been established for ARF; however, several large studies have defined ARF as a Pao_2/FiO_2 ratio <200, or Pao_2 <60 with either an FiO_2 of >0.6 (hypoxemic) or a $Paco_2$ >50 (hypercapnic). Irrespective of the criterion used to establish ARF, it can generally be stated that all patients with respiratory impairment will have either primary ventilatory or primary oxygenation impairment (Figure 8-1).

This chapter will discuss the basic pathophysiologic mechanisms of respiratory failure and the approach to the management of these patients. The most common diseases for respiratory failure are discussed in other chapters and will not be discussed in great detail here. However, two disease processes not discussed elsewhere will be covered in greater detail here as they present their own unique challenges that is, cervical spinal cord injury (SCI) and neuromuscular diseases.

► HYPOXEMIC RESPIRATORY FAILURE

Hypoxemic respiratory failure is usually the result of hypoventilation, a disorder of alveolar oxygen diffusion, shunting of systemic venous blood to the arterial circuit, or a ventilation–perfusion (V/Q) mismatch. These descriptions provide an accurate depiction of the physiologic mechanisms for hypoxemic respiratory failure and are most useful for understanding how a particular disease causes hypoxemia.[5] In a large multicenter international prospective cohort study of patients requiring mechanical ventilation (MV), the most common reported causes of ARF were postoperative respiratory failure, pneumonia, congestive heart failure, sepsis, and trauma.[6] In a small prospective cohort study that included 41 patients with hypoxemic respiratory failure, chronic obstructive pulmonary disease and pneumonia were the most common causes.[7] Other data from small, randomized controlled trials of noninvasive ventilation identified congestive heart failure, pneumonia, trauma, ARDS, and mucous plugging as the most common causes of respiratory failure.[8,9]

HYPOVENTILATION

Hypoventilation is a reduction in the volume of gas delivered to the alveoli per unit time (alveolar ventilation). Assuming oxygen consumption remains unchanged, hypoxia then results. Hypoventilation always causes a rise in $Paco_2$. Alveolar hypoventilation of a nonpulmonary etiology is typically characterized by hypercapnia with a normal alveolar–arterial oxygen gradient (A–a gradient) and therefore differs from the other three mechanisms of hypoxemia.[10] Hypoventilation or apnea causes the partial pressure of alveolar

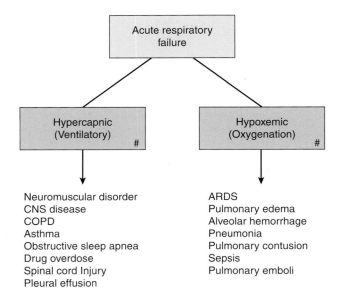

Figure 8-1. Common causes of acute respiratory failure in the ICU.

oxygen to fall faster than the rise of the partial pressure of carbon dioxide. The other three mechanisms are typically characterized by a widening A–a gradient, which is normally less than 20 mm Hg.[10]

DIFFUSION

Diffusion typically refers to oxygen transport across the alveolar capillary membrane. In nondiseased states, oxygen transport is diffusion and perfusion limited. The diffusion properties of the alveolar membrane depend on its thickness and area. Thus, the diffusing capacity is reduced by diseases in which the thickness is increased, including acute conditions such as pulmonary edema, or chronic conditions such as diffuse interstitial pulmonary fibrosis, asbestosis, and sarcoidosis (Figure 8-2A). It is also reduced when the area is decreased, for example, by emphysema or pneumonectomy. Theoretically impaired diffusion prevents complete equilibration of alveolar gas with pulmonary capillary blood. The clinical relevance of this, however, is often questioned since most transport is more perfusion limited than diffusion limited. Therefore, in the ICU setting, this mechanism is rarely specifically addressed.

SHUNT

The term shunt refers to the percentage of the total systemic venous blood flow that bypasses the gas-exchanging membrane or the lung and transfers venous blood unaltered to the systemic arterial system (Figure 8-2B). Shunting can be intracardiac, as in cyanotic right to left congenital heart disease, opening of a patent foramen ovale due to right ventricular overload, or result from passage of blood through pulmonary arteriovenous malformations. But the most common cause of shunting is pulmonary disease. In lung disease, there may be gas-exchanging units that are completely unventilated because of airway obstruction, atelectasis, or alveolar filling with fluid or cells.

VENTILATION–PERFUSION

Even in normal subjects, relative ventilation and perfusion in different areas of the lung are unequal, resulting in inefficient gas exchange (Figure 8-2B). This leads to V/Q mismatch. Areas of low ventilation relative to perfusion contribute to hypoxemia and are the most

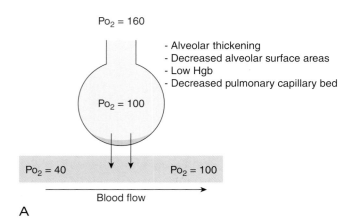

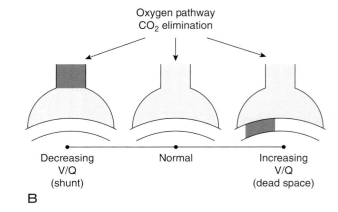

Figure 8-2. (A) Oxygen diffusion; (B) ventilation/perfusion mismatching.

common cause of hypoxemia in lung disease. Furthermore, this is an important cause of hypoxemia affecting patients in the ICU.

The distribution of ventilation even in normal subjects varies depending on the mode of ventilation and position, but even in nonpathologic disease states ventilation is not uniform. The right lung developmentally is larger and therefore receives greater ventilation. The position of the subject also influences ventilation, with the apices of both lungs receiving a greater percentage of ventilation than the bases in the upright position while the lower lung is preferentially ventilated when laying in any horizontal position, irrespective of which side is lain upon (supine, prone, or on a side). This is due to the dependent diaphragm lying higher in the thorax, with increased length of muscle fibers providing more efficient contraction during inspiration. In the sedated and paralyzed patient, however, irrespective of the mode of ventilation, the upper lung receives more gas flow.

Conversely, the bases of both lungs receive more pulmonary blood flow than the apices in the erect subject. Furthermore, the distribution of flow through the lung is uneven due to the relatively low pressures in the pulmonary circulation, so gravity assumes a greater role than in the systemic circulation. While supine or prone gravity assumes a more constant role throughout the lungs, though in a lateral position, the dependent lung is perfused more than the upper lung.

Although both perfusion and ventilation increase from the apices to the bases in a subject lying horizontally, the increase in ventilation is less than that of perfusion. The relationship between the two is described as the V/Q ratio. Resting values are approximately 4 L/min for ventilation and 5 L/min for pulmonary blood flow, giving an overall ratio of 0.8 throughout the whole lung (assuming ventilation and perfusion of all alveoli are equal).

V/Q mismatch is responsible for the hypoxemia seen in pulmonary edema, chronic obstructive airways disease, pulmonary embolism, and interstitial lung disease. The hypoxemia worsens with increasing V/Q mismatch for two reasons. First, with V/Q mismatch, a greater percentage of the cardiac output passes through lung units with lower V/Q ratios (perfusion > ventilation) so that less well-saturated blood makes a greater contribution to total pulmonary blood flow.[11] Second, as mentioned above in relation to shunts, the oxygen content of blood from lung units with low V/Q ratios exerts a greater effect on the saturation of blood flowing to the left side of the circulation because of the shape of the oxygen dissociation curve.[11] Hypoxic pulmonary vasoconstriction (HPV) is a potent regulator of the distribution of blood flow to match areas of ventilation. It normally acts to improve gas exchange by reducing the blood flow to lung regions with low V/Q ratios.

In conditions producing inflammatory mediators—such as sepsis and trauma—HPV is impaired, resulting in blood flowing to poorly ventilated lung, thus causing hypoxia.[11] Drugs such as sodium nitroprusside and nitroglycerine can also impair HPV by indiscriminately causing vasodilation. HPV can also be abolished in the presence of raised pulmonary artery pressures leading to V/Q mismatch and hypoxia.

▶ HYPERCAPNIC RESPIRATORY FAILURE

Alveolar ventilation becomes inadequate in relation to carbon dioxide production when either ventilatory demand exceeds the patient's capability (pump failure) or the patient's ventilatory effort is insufficient (drive failure).[12-14] These two mechanisms are distinct in their clinical presentation: patients with acute failure of the ventilatory pump are dyspneic and tachypneic with other signs of distress and sympathetic nervous system activation, whereas patients with failure of ventilatory drive are not short of breath and typically demonstrate bradypnea or apnea.

Although acute ventilatory failure is primarily a disorder of alveolar ventilation—as demonstrated by increasing P_{CO_2} and decreasing pH—hypoxemia is also usually present. More than one mechanism may coexist in a given patient at a given time, producing a life-threatening condition even when the individual processes are only moderate in severity.[15] For example, in decompensated obesity hypoventilation syndrome, a patient whose underlying respiratory drive is reduced and whose obesity poses an increased elastic load on the ventilatory pump may develop acute-on-chronic ventilatory failure in the presence of a relatively modest increase in the work of breathing (WOB) from the additional restrictive effects of cardiomegaly and pleural effusions.[16]

In the ICU setting, the most common disorders encountered are:

1. Impairment of ventilatory drive due to sedative drugs
2. Acquired neuromuscular disorders such as cervical SCI, Guillain–Barré syndrome (GBS), acute stroke, or amyotrophic lateral sclerosis (ALS)
3. Restrictive and obstructive diseases such as pulmonary fibrosis, chest wall burns, COPD, and asthma

CERVICAL SPINAL CORD INJURY

Cervical SCI effectively disrupts the transmission of neurologic input from the respiratory centers to the ventilatory muscles needed for respiration. The diaphragm is innervated by the phrenic nerve whose root segments originate from C3–C5; therefore, high cervical SCI may result in a permanent need for MV. Although patients with lower cervical SCI may initially require MV, with rehabilitation they may progress to a ventilator-independent lifestyle.

The subacute management phase of cervical SCI may resemble that of most neuromuscular disease patients. The unique aspects are related to the acute management and the impact on the rehabilitation potential. Adverse physiologic effects of cervical SCI in the initial days or weeks after the injury include loss of lung volumes and inability to take deep breaths (which predisposes to atelectasis), inability to cough normally (which predisposes to the development of pneumonia and complicates its management), and impaired HPV (which predisposes to severe and often refractory hypoxemia when atelectasis or pneumonia occurs). Retrospective studies have shown that both mortality[17] and ICU length of stay[18] for patients with cervical SCI are more strongly influenced by the development of pneumonia and other respiratory complications than by the specific cord injury level.[19]

In the unintubated patient, initial management should include frequent assessment of forced vital capacity (FVC) and negative inspiratory forces (NIF). A vital capacity (VC) less than 1 L or an NIF >−20 (e.g., −10) despite normal blood gases and oxygenation should warrant early intubation.

Ventilator management principles are also different in these patients. Retrospective studies have demonstrated that high tidal volume ventilation or lung expansion ventilation may impact the duration for which MV is required and decrease the incidence of atelectasis and pneumonia.[20] Contradictory to the lung-protective strategies of ARDS/ALI, patients are managed with tidal volumes of 15–20 cm^3/kg while maintaining peak inspiratory pressures less than 40 cm H_2O. Exceptions to this mode of ventilation include severe traumatic brain injury, chest trauma, bilateral pulmonary contusions, flail chest, pneumothorax/hemothorax, or bullous emphysema. In a recent retrospective study, NIF and FVC were shown to be the best predictors of ventilator weaning in this patient population.[21]

NEUROMUSCULAR DISORDERS

Neurologic patients can develop respiratory failure from neuromuscular weakness, decreased central respiratory drive, or associated pulmonary complications. In patients with neuromuscular disease, respiratory failure can present as a consequence of progression of a chronic condition such as ALS, exacerbation of a fluctuating disorder such as myasthenia gravis (MG), or sudden onset and fulminant course of an acute illness such as GBS.[22] In all these cases, respiratory failure can result

from worsening weakness affecting respiratory muscles or from an intercurrent pulmonary complication, typically aspiration, facilitated by concomitant weakness of oropharyngeal musculature or inability to cough up large regurgitated gastric contents.

GBS is the leading cause of nontraumatic acute paralysis in industrialized countries.[23] About 30% of the patients have respiratory failure requiring ICU admission and invasive MV.[24] The underlying mechanism is progressive weakness of both the inspiratory and expiratory command systems. Several factors that, if present either at admission or during the patient's hospital stay, predict a need for invasive MV; they include rapidly progressive motor weakness, involvement of both the peripheral limb and the axial muscles, ineffective cough, bulbar muscle weakness (dysarthria, dysphagia, impaired gag reflex), or a rapid drop in VC or respiratory pressures.[25]

Upper airway muscle dysfunction is related to cranial nerve involvement and deserves special attention because impaired coughing is common and increases the risk of aspiration and therefore of aspiration-related complications such as atelectasis and pneumonia. Most commonly, the seventh cranial nerve and the ninth and tenth cranial nerves are involved, manifesting as facial paralysis and swallowing impairment, respectively.[26,27] If present, tongue weakness may contribute to the development of respiratory failure by causing upper airway obstruction during sleep, and aspiration during the initial phase of swallowing.[28] The result is a combination of inadequate neuromuscular strength leading to alveolar hypoventilation, low tidal volume breathing, and diffuse atelectasis.

MV is frequently required when VC falls below 4–5 mL/kg body weight and there is progressive worsening of bulbar functions.[29,30] Therefore, patients with neuromuscular respiratory failure should be closely monitored with frequent measurements of VC, NIF, arterial blood gases, clinical evaluation of their swallowing mechanisms, ability to handle secretions, and presence and strength of cough mechanism.

▶ APPROACH TO THE PATIENT WITH ARF

As with all aspects of acute management of patients, airway, breathing, and circulation should be addressed. After assessing and securing, if necessary, the airway, the next step is to manage and diagnose the etiology of the respiratory failure.

If intubating is not emergently required, evaluation continues with a high clinical suspicion for impending respiratory failure. Early recognition allows for greater therapeutic options. An often underappreciated concept in respiratory system mechanics relates to WOB.

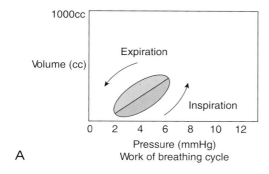

A

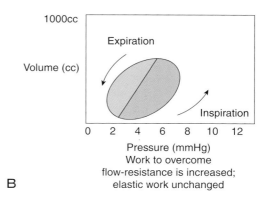

B

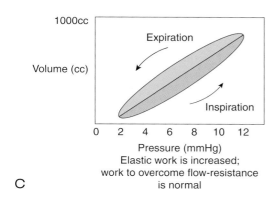

C

Figure 8-3. Work of breathing (pressure–volume diagram during one respiratory cycle). (A) Normal; (B) obstructive lung disease; (C) restrictive lung disease.

The WOB in normal resting state accounts for approximately 5% of oxygen consumption but dramatically increases in diseased states. Although an oversimplification, WOB typically constitutes airway resistance and chest wall and lung compliance. Airway resistance is a function of airway caliber and flow. Compliance is the change in pressure over volume and encompasses the compliance of both the lungs and chest wall. Therefore, WOB is comprised of the amount of work necessary to overcome resistance of the airways to flow (Figure 8-3) and the elastic recoil of the lungs and chest wall.

Signs of increased WOB include dysconjugate breathing, accessory muscle use, and tachypnea. These signs are compensatory mechanisms and, as such, often exist prior to oxygen desaturation. Systemic signs and symptoms that accompany an increased WOB include restlessness, anxiety, diaphoresis, confusion, seizures, somnolence, tachycardia, bradycardia, and arrhythmias. The key is to suspect and treat the increased WOB prior to the appearance of systemic signs and symptoms.

The goal of managing respiratory failure is to reduce the workload on the pulmonary system while the underlying etiology is resolved. The practitioner must consider early the possibility of respiratory failure. Otherwise a common pitfall is to treat the signs and symptoms and miss the underlying etiology until full respiratory failure has ensued and MV becomes the only treatment option.

Once the respiratory distress/failure has been addressed, the next step is to evaluate the underlying etiology of the respiratory failure through the use of diagnostic aids. An arterial blood gas and a chest x-ray should be the first diagnostic step in addressing a patient in respiratory distress. The ABG (Figure 8-4) and chest x-ray will provide important data as to the potential mechanism for respiratory failure, that is, a primary oxygenation problem (widened A–a gradient), a primary ventilator problem (elevated Pco_2 and acidemia), or a combination of both. As respiratory failure ensues and progresses inevitably, the picture is a mixed picture, particularly in the critically ill patient.

Etiology	pH	PaCO$_2$	PaO$_2$	PAO$_2$ - PaO$_2$
Central nervous system	↓	↑	nl or ↓	nl or ↑
Peripheral nervous system	↓	↑	nl or ↓	nl or ↑
Asthma*	↑	↓	nl	↑
COPD#	↓	⇑	⇓	↑
Pneumonia*#	↑	↓	⇓	⇑

*Early phase, pH & PaCO$_2$ may normalize as severity increases which is ominous
Acute on chronic exacerbation
*# Early in course before ventilatory failure

Figure 8-4. Arterial blood gas analysis in acute respiratory failure.

TREATMENT OPTIONS

ARF of hypoxemic nature can be addressed with MV but may not be necessary. It is common for practitioners to resolve ARF with noninvasive positive pressure ventilation (NPPV) or conventional MV, but securing the airway and initiating MV has significant complications. Furthermore, prolonged MV increases the incidence of ventilator-associated pneumonia, critical illness polyneuropathy, and ICU morbidity and mortality.

Instead, if the patient's condition allows sufficient time, attempts may be made to maximize all medical options before considering intubation. For instance, supplemental oxygen therapy should be maximized. Supplemental oxygen in excess of 70% oxygen can be provided without the use of a ventilator. Nasal cannula, venturi mask, partial non-rebreather, non-rebreather, and complex air entrapment high-flow systems can be set up to deliver high FiO_2. In instances where airway resistance is increased such as COPD or asthma or in upper airway obstructive scenarios such as postextubation stridor, heliox (70:30 or 80:20 mixtures) may facilitate delivery of supplemental oxygen.[31]

Of course, progressive hypoxic failure will lead to ventilatory failure secondary to fatigue. ARF of a primary ventilator disorder may be managed with close observation in the ICU and NPPV. NPPV has the advantage of improving tidal volume and minute ventilation while delivering high FiO_2 without the ventilator circuitry but may be of limited use in some neuromuscular disorders. Relative contraindications to NPPV include decreased mental status and ability to clear secretions since NIV still requires that a patient maintain his or her own airway.

Still, when there is concern for the patient's ability to maintain his or her airway, the primary objective is to protect and maintain the airway and traditional endotracheal intubation and conventional MV should be employed. The decision to intubate and provide MV should not be the first treatment option but should never be delayed and allow for an uncontrolled clinical scenario if avoidable. MV should always be regarded as a temporizing measure while the underlying cause of respiratory failure is addressed.

REFERENCES

1. Lewandowski K. Contributions to the epidemiology of acute respiratory failure. *Crit Care*. 2003;7:288–290.
2. Luhr OR, Antonsen K, Karlsson M, et al. Incidence and mortality after acute respiratory failure and acute respiratory distress syndrome in Sweden, Denmark, and Iceland. *Am J Respir Crit Care Med*. 1999;159:1849–1861.
3. Flaatten H, Gjerde S, Guttormsen AB, et al. Outcome after acute respiratory failure is more dependent on dysfunction in other vital organs than on the severity of the respiratory failure. *Crit Care*. 2003;7:R72–R77.
4. Bersten AD, Edibam C, Hunt T, et al. Incidence and mortality of acute lung injury and the acute respiratory distress syndrome in three Australian states. *Am J Respir Crit Care Med*. 2002;165:443–448.
5. Mathay M. *Acute Hypercapnic Respiratory Failure: Neuromuscular and Obstructive diseases. Chest Medicine: Essentials of Pulmonary and Critical Care Medicine*. 3rd ed. Williams and Wilkins, Baltimore, Maryland; 1995:578–608.
6. Esteban A, Anzueto A, Frutos F, et al. Characteristics and outcomes in adult patients receiving mechanical ventilation: a 28-day international study. *JAMA*. 2002;287:345–355.
7. Meduri GU, Turner RE, Abou-Shala N, et al. Noninvasive positive pressure ventilation via face mask: first-line intervention in patients with acute hypercapnic and hypoxemic respiratory failure. *Chest*. 1996;109:179–193.
8. Antonelli M, Conti G, Rocco M, et al. A comparison of noninvasive positive-pressure ventilation and conventional mechanical ventilation in patients with acute respiratory failure. *N Engl J Med*. 1998;339:429–435.
9. Delclaux C, L'Her E, Alberti C, et al. Treatment of acute hypoxemic nonhypercapnic respiratory insufficiency with continuous positive airway pressure delivered by a face mask: a randomized controlled trial. *JAMA*. 2000;284:2352–2360.
10. West J, Wagner PD. *Ventilation, Blood Flow, and Gas Exchange. Textbook of Respiratory Medicine*. 3rd ed. Philadelphia: WB Saunders; 2000:55–90.
11. Hall JB, Schmidt GA, Wood LDH. *Acute Hypoxemic Respiratory Failure. Textbook of Respiratory Medicine*. 3rd ed. Philadelphia: WB Saunders; 2000:2413–2442.
12. Pierson DJ, Kacmarek RM. Respiratory failure: introduction and overview. In: Pierson DJ, ed. *Foundations of Respiratory Care*. New York: Churchill Livingstone; 1992:295–302.
13. Roussos C, Macklem PT. The respiratory muscles. *N Engl J Med*. 1982;307:786–797.
14. Roussos C, Koutsoukou A. Respiratory failure. *Eur Respir J*. 2003;47:3s–14s.
15. Grippi M. *Respiratory Failure: An Overview. Fishman's Pulmonary diseases and Disorders*. 4th ed. McGraw-Hill; New York, NY; 2008:2509–2521.
16. Schmidt GA, Hall JB, Wood LDH. *Ventilatory Failure. Textbook of Respiratory Medicine*. 3rd ed. Philadelphia: WB Saunders; 2000:2443–2470.
17. Claxton AR, Wong DT, Chung F, et al. Predictors of hospital mortality and mechanical ventilation in patients with cervical spinal cord injury. *Can J Anaesth*. 1998;45:144–149.
18. Winslow C, Bode RK, Felton D, et al. Impact of respiratory complications on length of stay and hospital costs in acute cervical spine injury. *Chest*. 2002;121:1548–1554.
19. Berlly M, Shem K. Respiratory management during the first five days after spinal cord injury. *J Spinal Cord Med*. 2007;30:309–318.
20. Peterson WP, Barbalata L, Brooks CA, et al. The effect of tidal volumes on the time to wean persons with high tetraplegia from ventilators. *Spinal Cord*. 1999;37(4):284–288.

21. Chiodo AE, Scetza W, Forchheimer M. Predictors of ventilator weaning in individuals with high cervical spinal cord injury. *J Spinal Cord Med.* 2008;31:72–77.

22. Rabinstein AA, Wijdicks EF. Warning signs of imminent respiratory failure in neurological patients. *Semin Neurol.* 2003;23:97–103.

23. Hughes RA, Cornblath DR. Guillain–Barré syndrome. *Lancet.* 2005;366:1653–1666.

24. Ropper AH, Kehne SM. Guillain–Barré syndrome: management of respiratory failure. *Neurology.* 1985;35:1662–1665.

25. Chevrolet JC, Deléamont P. Repeated vital capacity measurements as predictive parameters for mechanical ventilation need and weaning success in the Guillain–Barré syndrome. *Am Rev Respir Dis.* 1991;144:814–818.

26. Raphael JC, Masson C, Morice V, et al. The Landry–Guillain–Barré syndrome. Study of prognostic factors in 223 cases. *Rev Neurol (Paris).* 1986;142:613–624.

27. Ropper AH, Wijdicks EFM, Truax BT. *Clinical Features of the Typical Syndrome, Guillain–Barré Syndrome.* Philadelphia: FA Davis; 1991:73–105.

28. Orlikowski D, Terzi N, Blumen M, et al. Tongue weakness is associated with respiratory failure in patients with severe Guillain–Barré syndrome. *Acta Neurol Scand.* 2009;119:364–370.

29. Moore P, James O. Guillain–Barré syndrome: incidence, management and outcome of major complications. *Crit Care Med.* 1981;9:549–555.

30. Eisendrath SJ, Matthay MA, Dunkel J, et al. Guillain–Barré syndrome: psychosocial aspects of management. *Psychosomatics.* 1983;24:465–475.

31. JW Berkenbosch, RE Grueber, GR Graff, et al. Patterns of helium–oxygen (heliox) usage in the critical care environment. *J Intensive Care Med.* 2004;19(6):335–344.

CHAPTER 9

Acute Respiratory Distress Syndrome (ARDS)

Isaac Tawil and Megan L. Garcia

► DIAGNOSIS

The acute respiratory distress syndrome (ARDS), first identified by Ashbaugh et al in 1967, described a constellation of findings in 12 patients who had experienced acute onset of tachypnea, hypoxemia, loss of lung compliance, cyanosis refractory to oxygen therapy, and diffuse alveolar infiltration on chest x-ray. Pathologic examination from seven of these patients found atelectasis, vascular congestion with hemorrhage, hyaline membranes, and pulmonary edema.[1]

Decades later, in an effort to better define the syndrome using specific and measurable criteria, Murray et al developed a lung injury scoring system. The components of the score quantified alveolar consolidation measured by chest x-ray, hypoxemia measured by Pao_2/FiO_2 ratios, levels of required positive end-expiratory pressure (PEEP), and pulmonary compliance.[2]

In 1994 the American–European Consensus Committee (AECC) on ARDS implemented new criteria, identifying two different levels of severity of lung injury. It allowed for those with less severe hypoxemia to be classified as having acute lung injury (ALI) and those with more severe hypoxemia to be defined as having ARDS.[3]

The AECC defined ALI as the acute onset of respiratory distress with Pao_2/FiO_2 <300 mm Hg, bilateral, patchy infiltrates on chest radiograph, and a pulmonary artery occlusion pressure (PAOP) <18 mm or absent clinical evidence of left atrial hypertension (indicating presumptive noncardiac etiology of pulmonary edema). ARDS was given similar diagnostic criteria, but with Pao_2/FiO_2 <200 mm Hg.

Achieving diagnostic accuracy using clinical definitions is imperative so as not to underdiagnose or overdiagnose the pathology and to assure that clinical trials are in fact targeting the correct disease process. However, the subjective nature of describing chest x-ray morphology, the limitations of PAOP to evaluate cardiac dysfunction, and the impact of mechanically delivered airway pressures on oxygenation are just a few of the limitations of the standard ARDS definitions.[4]

Pathologic examination is perhaps the gold standard for ALI/ARDS diagnosis with the key lesion identified being diffuse alveolar damage (DAD).[5] While not typically performed to diagnose ARDS, one retrospective study concluded that open lung biopsy may be safely done for the diagnosis of ALI/ARDS and that in many cases (60% in their series) it produced alternative diagnoses such as pneumonia, pulmonary hemorrhage, and interstitial fibrosis, among others.[6]

Several studies have attempted to clarify the diagnostic accuracy of the arguably subjective clinical definitions. One such study by Ferguson et al compared the accuracy of the three different commonly used clinical definitions (Table 9-1) with autopsy results and with

▶ **TABLE 9-1. LUNG INJURY SCORING, AECC CRITERIA, AND THE DELPHI DEFINITION**

Score	Hypoxemia, Pao_2/FiO_2	Consolidation on Chest Radiograph	PEEP (When Ventilated)	Compliance (When Available) (mL/[cm H_2O])
Lung injury score[a]				
0	≥300	No alveolar	≤5 cm H_2O	≥80
1	225–299	1 quadrant	6–8 cm H_2O	60–79
2	175–224	2 quadrants	9–11 cm H_2O	40–59
3	100–174	3 quadrants	12–14 cm H_2O	20–39
4	<100	4 quadrants	≥15 cm H_2O	<20
	Hypoxemia	**Chest Radiograph**	**Onset**	**Pulmonary Artery Occlusion Pressure**
American–European Consensus Conference Definition[b]	Pao_2/FiO_2 ≤300 (ALI)	Bilateral infiltrates	Acute onset	≤18 mm Hg or no clinical suspicion of left atrial hypertension
	1. Hypoxemia	**2. Chest Radiograph**	**3. Onset**	**4. Noncardiogenic—Subjective**
Delphi definition[c]	Pao_2/FiO_2 ≤200 with PEEP ≥10	Bilateral airspace disease	Within 72 h	No clinical evidence of congestive heart failure
	5a. Noncardiogenic—Objective			**5b. Predisposition**
	PAWP ≤18 mm Hg or LV ejection fraction ≥40%			Presence of a recognized risk factor for ARDS

PEEP, positive end-expiratory pressure; ARDS, acute respiratory distress syndrome; LIS, lung injury score; ALI, acute lung injury; PAOP, pulmonary artery occlusion pressure; LV, left ventricle. (Reproduced with permission from Ferguson ND, et al. Acute respiratory distress syndrome: underrecognition by clinicians and diagnostic accuracy of three clinical definitions. *Crit Care Med.* 2005;33(10):2228–2234. Table 1. Copyright © Lippincott Williams & Wilkins.)
[a]Sum scores from each domain and divide by number used (ARDS = LIS >2.5).
[b]Diagnose ARDS when all four criteria are present.
[c]Diagnose ARDS when criteria 1–4 and 5a and/or 5b are present.

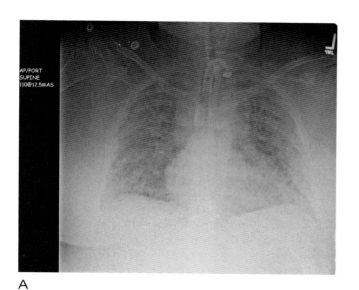

A

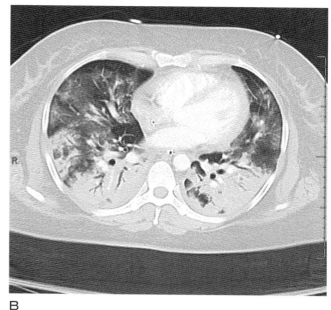

B

Figure 9-1. (A) Chest x-ray demonstrates diffuse alveolar infiltrates of ARDS. (B) On CT, diffuse alveolar infiltrates with predominance in the dependent lung zones can be seen.

each other, in 138 subjects.[7] They found that clinicians diagnosed ARDS in only 48% of autopsy-confirmed disease and their clinical diagnoses were 91% specific. Agreement between the Delphi and lung injury score definitions was good. Both showed significant disagreement with the AECC definition. The AECC definitions had the highest sensitivity (83%) and lowest specificity (51%), while the Delphi definition had the lowest sensitivity (69%) and highest specificity (82%). Lung injury scores had a 74% sensitivity and 77% specificity. These limited diagnostic accuracies which have been corroborated in several studies, have important implications for clinical practice, and may be problematic for subject recruitment into clinical trials.

▶ PATHOPHYSIOLOGY

ALI and ARDS describe a hypoxemic state caused by noncardiogenic pulmonary edema. The pathophysiology is complex, mediated by many cell types and cytokines, but ultimately culminates in diffuse damage to the alveolar capillary membrane (ACM). The ACM consists of the capillary endothelium and alveolar epithelium. The alveolar epithelium is made up of type 1 and type 2 alveolar epithelial cells. Type 1 epithelial cells are the most common and allow for gas exchange from the vascular endothelium. Type 2 cells play a role in the resorption of airspace fluid and surfactant production.[8]

In ALI/ARDS, the capillary endothelium is activated by cytokines. The cells swell and intercellular junctions widen that beget capillary leakage. Damaged type 1 cells impair gas exchange, and damaged type 2 alveolar epithelial cells impair fluid resorption and surfactant production. The resultant endothelial-capillary permeability leads to alveolar flooding with proteinaceous material.

Two phases are regularly described in ARDS. The acute or exudative phase is clinically characterized by rapid-onset respiratory failure and hypoxemia often refractory to supplemental oxygen. The chest x-ray during this phase typically reveals bilateral patchy infiltrates (Figure 9-1a) and computed tomography (CT) further elucidates increased density within the dependent lung zones (Figure 9-1b).[9] Pathologic examination during this stage reveals DAD characterized by a disruption of the alveolar epithelium, capillary injury, microvascular thrombi, and the presence of inflammatory cells within the alveoli. The DAD results in replacement of pneumocytes with hyaline membranes and decreased surfactant production.[10] These pathologic changes result in alveolar collapse and decreased lung compliance.

ALI and ARDS may completely resolve after this acute exudative phase. A subset of patients, however, progresses with persistent hypoxemia, increased alveolar dead space with continued ventilation/perfusion mismatch, and, ultimately, fibrosing alveolitis. This fibroproliferative phase occurs 5–7 days after the onset of ARDS and begins after resolution of the acute exudative phase.[8] Progression to fibrosing alveolitis is also associated with a higher mortality rate.[6] CT findings during this phase reveal reticular opacities, diffuse ground glass opacities, and bullae.[9] Eventually, type 2 pneumocytes begin resorption of pulmonary edema and organize the hyaline membranes. They also repair the alveolar epithelium and differentiate into type 1 pneumocytes. With this repair comes interstitial pulmonary fibrosis with permanent disruption of the normal alveolar architecture.

A critical component contributing to increased pulmonary inflammation in ALI/ARDS is often iatrogenic. Ventilator-induced lung injury (VILI) is the term used to describe the microscopic and macroscopic pulmonary sequela of mechanical ventilation (MV).[11] It has been long accepted that high fractions of inspired oxygen exacerbate lung injury. Additionally, it is now known that high tidal volumes (volutrauma) and pressures (barotrauma) significantly contribute to lung injury. Furthermore, the cyclic opening and closing of alveoli during tidal ventilation often translates to alveolar overdistension and complete collapse throughout the respiratory cycle. This creates shear forces on the alveoli that increase pro-inflammatory cytokines that worsens the capillary leak and alveolar edema described above. Research in this area has lead to lung-protective ventilatory strategies that seek to limit the injurious repetitive alveolar overdistension and collapse.

► INCIDENCE/RISK FACTORS

The incidence of ARDS was initially found to be approximately 150,000 cases per year in the United States.[3] Studies now estimate the incidence at 13.5–58.7 per 10^5 person-years.[5] ALI affects approximately 200,000 people in the United States and accounts for 10–15% of all ICU admissions.[12]

Risk factors for ALI and ARDS are numerous and are divided into two groups, direct (pulmonary) and indirect (extra-pulmonary), depending on their mode of injury to the lung. Examples of direct causes include aspiration, pneumonia, near drowning, toxic inhalation, lung contusion, and fat or amniotic emboli. Indirect causes or ARDS include sepsis, severe trauma, blood product transfusion, drug overdose, acute pancreatitis, cardiopulmonary bypass, and disseminated intravascular coagulation. The most common causes of ARDS include direct lung injury, sepsis, and multiple transfusions.[13] Other potential predisposing conditions include renal transplant and alcoholism. One theory asserts that renal transplantation increases the risk for ARDS because immunosuppression increases the risk for pneumonia and sepsis; however, similar associations were not found for liver or pancreas transplant recipients.[14] Similarly, alcoholism has been linked to increased ARDS susceptibility; however, this may be due to the fact that these patients are increasingly predisposed to trauma, sepsis, aspiration pneumonia, and transfusion from gastrointestinal bleeding. Lastly, studies suggest a possible genetic susceptibility to ARDS along with other demographic factors (age, sex, and race) further influencing the risk of developing the disease and the resultant mortality.[9]

► MORTALITY/PROGNOSIS

Initially the mortality from ARDS was thought to be from respiratory failure. More recent studies report that respiratory failure is the cause in only 9–16% of ARDS deaths. The most common cause of death is multiple organ failure and sepsis.[14] ARDS mortality was initially reported to be as high as 70% but has steadily decreased over time. Recent reports suggest that mortality has leveled off between 36% and 44% since 1994.[15] Many factors are thought to increase mortality in patients with ARDS. These include old age, presence of nonpulmonary organ dysfunction, shock, hepatic failure, and blood transfusion. There does not appear to be a mortality difference between pulmonary and extrapulmonary causes of ARDS.[8]

Patients who survive ARDS do appear to regain pulmonary function within 12 months from ICU discharge, but with measurable functional disability. An evaluation of 109 ARDS survivors at 1 year found them to have mild restrictive lung disease on pulmonary function testing. None of these patients required the use of supplemental oxygen at 12 months and only 6% of patients had arterial oxygen saturations below 88% with exercise.[16] Yet, at 1 year from ICU discharge, only 49% of patients had returned to work, and quality of life assessments were below average. Interestingly, the functional limitations experienced were largely a consequence of persistent neuromuscular weakness and muscle wasting and to a lesser extent their persistent pulmonary dysfunction.

► ARDS TREATMENT

As the etiologies and contributing factors to the development of ARDS are diverse, so too are the approaches to both the supportive care and directed treatment of the lung-injured patient. The following section reviews treatment strategies supported by varying levels of evidence. Some strategies such as protective ventilatory strategies are supported by class 1 evidence, while others such as prone position ventilation or steroid therapy are still hotly debated. Because of the heterogeneous nature of critically ill patients as well as the heterogeneity of lung injury itself, the limitations of outcome studies using mortality endpoints must be recognized. Even the most well-done studies of ventilatory and pharmacologic strategies are impacted by many variables including patient selection, etiology of lung injury, timing of therapy, and concomitant treatments, to name a few. Thus, it is important to recognize strategies that are not supported by class 1 evidence, but may play a key role in ARDS treatment if considered within the context of the individualized care of the lung-injured patient.

▶ SUPPORTIVE SYSTEMIC CARE

The importance of the many aspects of general supportive critical care in the treatment of the ARDS patient cannot be overstated. For example, a fluid-restrictive strategy (discussed later) that has been shown to improve ARDS outcome would be futile and likely harmful if this diverted attention from a targeted resuscitation to minimize the patient's degree of shock. The benefits of proven ventilatory strategies will be unrealized if appropriate treatment of infections are not delivered, and even best practices regarding MV will not limit ventilator days without judicious use of sedatives, blood product transfusions, and nutritional supplementation.

Supportive care starts with treatment of the predisposing disease process. Advances in the care of these pulmonary and extrapulmonary conditions are responsible for the decreasing ARDS mortality over the years.[17] Best care practices for sepsis, trauma, and other predisposing conditions must be followed if ARDS outcomes are to be optimized. ALI/ARDS is rarely an isolated organ system failure in ICU patients and mortality is more often associated with the accompanying multiorgan dysfunction syndrome.[18] Thus, it is unlikely that any lung-directed treatment on its own will impact outcome without care directed to the cardiovascular, renal, and central nervous systems, as well.

▶ FLUID & HEMODYNAMIC MANAGEMENT

The optimization of hemodynamics and intravascular volume in the setting of ALI/ARDS is a most challenging task. Since patient survival is tied to extrapulmonary organ function, the overriding goal is to reverse any shock state and optimize organ perfusion while minimizing volume overload. Underresuscitation potentiates ongoing hypoperfusion that contributes to the inflammatory cascade and worsening lung injury. Conversely, once resuscitated, a fluid-restrictive strategy has been shown to improve pulmonary function in patients with ALI/ARDS.[19,20] The ARDS Clinical Trials Network performed a prospective randomized trial of a fluid-restrictive strategy versus a liberal fluid strategy in ventilated patients with ALI. They found that targeting lower filling pressures (central venous pressure [CVP] and PAOP) and tolerating lower urine outputs in the

study group significantly lowered the amount of fluids administered and in turn improved oxygenation indices and lung injury scores and minimized ventilator and ICU days as compared with control subjects.[19] In this study, the fluid-restricted patients did not suffer any increased incidence of cardiovascular or renal dysfunction, although they did not realize any mortality benefit either. Similar conclusions were reached in a separate post hoc analysis of the surgical patient cohort from the larger trial.[20] Hence, the paradigm of care is to first assure that patients are resuscitated to the point of optimal organ perfusion and reversal of any shock state, but to not overresuscitate them, as restricting further fluids and decreasing the overall hydrostatic pressure will lead to net negative fluid balances and improved pulmonary outcomes.

Another ALI treatment strategy with similar goals—using albumin repletion to increase colloid osmotic pressure in hypoproteinemic patients combined with furosemide diuresis to decrease hydrostatic pressure—has shown promise.[21,22] Martin et al evaluated this furosemide plus albumin regimen in a randomized, placebo-controlled trial and found improved oxygenation while reducing hypotension and shock, as compared with furosemide monotherapy.[22] While the exact mechanisms require further elucidation, the authors contend that the addition of albumin to a diuretic strategy stabilizes hemodynamics—presumably through the maintenance of effective circulating blood volume—while promoting egress of pulmonary edema fluid from the alveolar space.

Of course, even if one subscribes to a particular endpoint of fluid therapy (dryer vs. wetter), targeting that endpoint of intravascular fluid repletion is no easy task. Since the general parameters of intravascular volume status such as urine output, heart rate, and blood pressure do not accurately predict volume responsiveness, clinicians have advocated for other hemodynamic monitoring tools to better titrate fluid therapy. The use of pulmonary artery catheters (PAC), for example, is the source of continuous debate, and their efficacy in guiding treatment in the ALI patient has recently been evaluated. The recent ARDS network trial of 1,000 ALI patients concluded that PAC-guided therapy did not improve survival or organ function, but was associated with more complications than central venous catheter (CVC)–guided therapy.[19] Others further argue that both the PAOP and the CVP are confounded by too many variables for these static filling pressures to be useful guides of volume therapy and that functional hemodynamic parameters are more accurate and preferable. A growing body of literature supports the use, during MV, of dynamic arterial waveform-derived parameters—such as stroke volume variation (SVV) or pulse pressure variation (PPV)—to more accurately predict volume responsiveness in the critically ill.[23] These techniques, however, are limited to patients receiving controlled ventilation and not breathing spontaneously. Another limitation may be that tidal volumes (Vt) of 8–10 cm³/kg are required to identify the cyclic variations in stroke volume indicative of fluid responsiveness. This would be problematic in ARDS patients who benefit from low Vt ventilation. Recently, however, PPV was found to accurately predict fluid responsiveness in ARDS patients ventilated with low Vt and high PEEP, albeit in a small study.[24] Further evaluation of these functional hemodynamic parameters in ALI/ARDS patients is needed. These tools may help the clinician judiciously provide volume expansion to only those who stand to increase their cardiac output without worsening pulmonary function.

► NUTRITION

The goals of nutritional support for the lung-injured patient are to meet the patient's caloric requirements and resting energy expenditure and replete deficiencies of various nutrients, while minimizing overfeeding and other complications associated with the way nutrition is delivered. Enteral feeding is preferable to parenteral nutrition as it has a beneficial impact on gastrointestinal immune function and reducing infectious complications.[25] In addition to meeting the patient's metabolic needs, certain nutrients may actually modulate the inflammatory response in lung-injured patients that may have beneficial effects on pulmonary alveolar–capillary permeability, and hence lung and other organ function. The most promising dietary additives studied include fish oils rich in omega-3 polyunsaturated fatty acids (PUFA). The anti-inflammatory properties of such supplements are well studied in in-vitro and animal models. Several prospective, randomized controlled trials reported that patients receiving nutritional formulas rich in fish oil PUFAs had improved oxygenation, fewer ventilator and ICU days, and fewer nonpulmonary organ failures.[26–28] A meta-analysis of the pooled data from these trials confirmed the positive outcomes correlation with use of fish oil–based formulas.[29] Lastly, another meta-analysis evaluating immune-modulating diets in more heterogeneous ICU patients supported the beneficial effects of fish oil–derived omega-3 PUFAs, but only in patients with septic shock and ARDS.[30] This analysis found these formulas to be of no clinical benefit to general ICU, burn, or trauma patients and further suggested that the failure of some previous studies to show a benefit from fish oil derivatives is likely due to excessive arginine supplementation. These omega-3 PUFA-enriched formulas are currently recommended for ARDS patients by the American Society of Parenteral and Enteral Nutrition (ASPEN) as well as the Society for Critical Care Medicine (SCCM).

► PHARMACOTHERAPY

A variety of pharmacologic agents have been investigated in ARDS including surfactant replacement, ketoconazole, nitric oxide, lisofylline, N-acetylcysteine, glucocorticoids, and β-agonist therapy. None of these therapies have emerged as accepted treatments for lung injury, but some show more promise than others. Much controversy surrounds the most studied drugs in ARDS: glucocorticoids.

Proponents assert that steroids hasten the resolution of the fibroproliferative stage of ARDS. There are many small studies using variable steroid regimens differing in therapy timing, dosage, formulation, treatment duration, and tapering regimens. A recent ARDSNet study did not support the use of methylprednisolone therapy in ARDS and cautions that steroid therapy started more than 2 weeks after ARDS onset may increase mortality.[31] Conversely, the most recent meta-analysis concluded that low-dose corticosteroids were associated with improved mortality and morbidity outcomes and are an effective treatment for ARDS.[32] However, they note that a well-powered randomized trial is still needed to clarify the aforementioned variables in steroid protocols.

β-Agonists in ARDS are an intriguing potential therapy that target the alveolar–capillary barrier. In vitro and animal data identified that catecholamines upregulate aquaporin channels on alveolar cells and increase alveolar water clearance. A randomized clinical trial of intravenous salbutamol for ARDS concluded that β-agonist therapy decreased extravascular lung water and improved plateau pressures.[33] Further research may clarify the efficacy of β-agonist treatment in lung injury.

► MECHANICAL VENTILATION

Strategies of mechanical ventilatory support are central to the care of the ALI/ARDS patient. The overriding goals of MV are to maintain sufficient oxygenation and ventilation and decrease the patient's work of breathing while mitigating further VILI. This last goal is paramount to understanding why the strategy of lung-protective/low Vt ventilation improved mortality in the landmark ARDSNet study known as the Respiratory Management in ALI/ARDS trial (ARMA).[19] It is equally important to understand that there are many other ways to provide lung protection. While not yet supported by large randomized controlled trials like those performed by the ARDSNet investigators, some alternative strategies that will be discussed have face validity when considering the underlying pathophysiology of the disease, as well as support from prospective evaluation. In addition to the strategy touted by the ARDS Network, there are also merits of prone position ventilation and "open lung" strategies using airway pressure release ventilation (APRV) or high-frequency oscillatory ventilation (HFOV). Additionally, independent of the mode of delivering ventilatory support are the challenges of how to best target the optimal distending airway pressure as well as how to address the permissive hypercapnia that accompanies strategies of lung protection.

Understanding the importance of limiting alveolar stretch and barotrauma, the ARMA trial randomized 861 patients to either conventional Vt of 12 mL/kg or low Vt of 4–6 mL/kg of predicted ideal body weight. The low Vt group had their tidal volumes adjusted (between 4 and 6 mL/kg) to maintain plateau pressures ≤30 cm H_2O. The lower Vt strategy resulted in a 9% absolute mortality reduction (from 39.8% to 31.0%) and reduced ventilator-dependent days.[19] The low Vt group also had lower plasma IL-6 levels, suggesting less lung inflammation that may have contributed to the lower rate of nonpulmonary organ dysfunction. Both arms of this trial used the assist control (AC) mode of ventilation and a predetermined PEEP strategy based on the patient's required FiO_2. The low Vt group required higher PEEP levels to maintain oxygenation, and some argue this contributed to the protection against cyclic alveolar opening and closing, a key component of VILI. The PEEP and FiO_2 strategy used by the ARDSNet investigators in ARMA remains unvalidated and is the source of continued controversy and investigation in lung injury. Studies supporting higher versus lower PEEP strategies are conflicting.[34,35] Likewise, while many clinicians have adopted the entire ARDSNet strategy from this landmark study, the AC mode of delivery has also not been proven to be the optimal ventilator mode.

Some level of PEEP is required to prevent low-volume lung injury and alveolar collapse during exhalation. Too much may lead to lung overinflation, barotrauma, and hemodynamic compromise. The challenge is to target the level of PEEP that keeps the patient breathing between the lower and upper inflection points of the pressure volume (P–V) curve (Figure 9-2). This is particularly difficult given the heterogeneous pattern of aeration and alveolar collapse in the ARDS patient so that different lung units have different P–V curves. Several techniques or guides to find the "best PEEP" exist including trending measures of pulmonary compliance along with oxygen delivery indices as one manipulates the PEEP,[36] using esophageal pressure measurements to estimate transpulmonary pressures to optimize PEEP,[37] CT lung morphology assessment to guide PEEP levels,[38] or using the continuous flow method to measure bedside P–V relationships.[39]

Optimizing the PEEP during lung-protective ventilation is one challenge. Another important element is

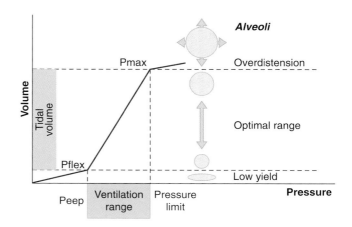

Figure 9-2. The lower and upper inflection points indicate the pressures at which lung recruitment begins and ends. The optimal pressure–volume relationship is between Pflex and Pmax. The slope of the curve represents the potential for alveolar recruitment. (Used with permission from Patrick Neligan, MD.)

the hypercapnia resulting from a low Vt strategy. The discussed ARMA trial used increased respiratory rates and bicarbonate infusions to limit the hypercarbia and resultant acidosis. Both of these strategies are potentially problematic as high ventilatory rates may exacerbate auto-PEEP and overdistension, while bicarbonate infusions arguably increase the resultant CO_2 load and may worsen intracellular acidosis. Interestingly, a growing body of literature supports that hypercapnia and moderate acidosis are not only well tolerated but may also be protective against lung and extrapulmonary organ dysfunction independent of the particular ventilator strategy. However, at this time, there are insufficient data to suggest that hypercapnia should be independently induced outside of the context of a protective ventilatory strategy.[40]

▶ ALTERNATIVE VENTILATORY STRATEGIES

In ARDS patients in the supine position, alveolar aeration is greater in the anterior/nondependent lung regions. Without PEEP, the ratio of ventilated nondependent to dependent lung zones approximates 2.5:1. At higher levels of PEEP, the distribution of ventilation becomes more homogenous but at the expense of overdistending and reducing the compliance of the nondependent (anterior) lung zones.[41] Ventilating a patient in the prone position may homogenize alveolar inflation and the distribution of ventilation. This is just one mechanism responsible for the favorable effects of prone position ventilation. In addition to reducing the physiologic dead space and the resulting ventilation–

perfusion mismatch, the prone position has been shown to consistently improve oxygenation in many retrospective and prospective studies.[42–45] Other benefits include reducing right ventricular pressures in ARDS patients with cor pulmonale,[46] facilitating drainage of secretions, and improving respiratory mechanics. Yet despite significant improvements in gas exchange shown across most studies, mortality benefits have not been seen in larger evaluations.[47]

Various subgroup analyses, however, have revealed mortality benefits in specific patient subgroups that depend on intervention timing, the particular CT lung morphology, and/or the etiology of the lung injury. Still other trials have reported the prone position to be synergistic with other ventilatory strategies (APRV or HFOV). Many experts have accordingly called for future prospective evaluation to clarify which patients may benefit from prone positioning as well as the optimal timing, frequency, duration of the intervention, and concomitant ventilator management.

Since ongoing VILI or atelectrauma results from cyclic opening and closing of lung units, ventilatory modes designed to keep the lung opened more continuously have received considerable attention. Ventilator modes such as HFOV and APRV are two modalities that achieve "open lung ventilation" via different mechanisms.

HFOV delivers very small tidal volumes at frequencies ranging from 3 to 15 Hz that limits alveolar distension, while maintaining a continuous distending pressure throughout inspiration and expiration, preventing alveolar collapse. Thus, HFOV proponents assert that this modality achieves the goals of a lung-protective strategy while improving continuous alveolar recruitment.[48] One shortcoming is that patients generally require deep sedation and neuromuscular blockade to tolerate HFOV. There are many studies evaluating HFOV in adults with ARDS, none of which reported mortality benefits. However, many of them have shown improved physiologic endpoints such as oxygenation indices and decreased ventilator days. Similar to limitations in the trials of prone position ventilation, many of the HFOV trials used this modality as a rescue therapy once conventional ventilation had failed. Proponents argue that such delays limit the efficacy of the therapy.

Another modality that can be tailored to accomplish the goals of lung protection along with the benefit of continuous alveolar recruitment is APRV. APRV essentially provides continuous positive airway pressure (CPAP) with very brief (typically <1 second) releases of this pressure to augment CO_2 clearance. Maintaining CPAP above the alveolar closing pressure provides near-continuous alveolar recruitment. This improves oxygenation as well as ventilation via improved alveolar ventilation/passive gas exchange versus depending on tidal ventilation using conventional modes. Another advantage unique to APRV is maintenance of patients' spontaneous breathing. Allowing for spontaneous respiration improves the ventilation and perfusion distributions to a more physiologic pattern.[49] Maintenance of spontaneous breathing also improves the overall hemodynamic profile, cardiac performance, and blood flow to end organs. Lastly, patients spontaneously breathing on APRV have been consistently shown to have lower sedative and paralytic requirements.[50] But here again, the existing clinical trials have not demonstrated mortality reduction and the current successes are limited to physiologic endpoints.

In summary, the relative success of any new ventilatory strategy depends on the control ventilatory strategy with which it is compared. Larger trials in the future should test these alternatives to the well-accepted ARDSNet protocol. Nevertheless, the improved physiologic endpoints seen with these modalities, combined with sound understanding of physiology, make these alternatives viable and perhaps preferable to the conventional dogma of controlled ventilation in the supine position.

REFERENCES

1. Ashbaugh DG, Bigelow DB, Petty TL, et al. Acute respiratory distress in adults. *Lancet*. Aug 12 1967;2(7511): 319–323.
2. Murray JF, Matthay MA, Luce JM, et al. An expanded definition of the adult respiratory distress syndrome. *Am Rev Respir Dis*. Sep 1988;138(3):720–723.
3. Bernard GR, Artigas A, Brigham KL, et al. The American–European Consensus Conference on ARDS. Definitions, mechanisms, relevant outcomes, and clinical trial coordination. *Am J Respir Crit Care Med*. Mar 1994;149(3 pt 1): 818–824.
4. Meade MO, Cook RJ, Guyatt GH, et al. Interobserver variation in interpreting chest radiographs for the diagnosis of acute respiratory distress syndrome. *Am J Respir Crit Care Med*. Jan 2000;161(1):85–90.
5. Avecillas JF, Freire AX, Arroliga AC. Clinical epidemiology of acute lung injury and acute respiratory distress syndrome: incidence, diagnosis, and outcomes. *Clin Chest Med*. Dec 2006;27(4):549–557; abstract vii.
6. Patel SR, Karmpaliotis D, Ayas NT, et al. The role of open-lung biopsy in ARDS. *Chest*. Jan 2004;125(1): 197–202.
7. Ferguson ND, Davis AM, Slutsky AS, et al. Development of a clinical definition for acute respiratory distress syndrome using the Delphi technique. *J Crit Care*. Jun 2005;20(2):147–154.
8. Suratt BT, Parsons PE. Mechanisms of acute lung injury/ acute respiratory distress syndrome. *Clin Chest Med*. Dec 2006;27(4):579–589; abstract viii.
9. Ware LB, Matthay MA. The acute respiratory distress syndrome. *N Engl J Med*. May 4 2000;342(18): 1334–1349.

10. Penuelas O, Aramburu JA, Frutos-Vivar F, et al. Pathology of acute lung injury and acute respiratory distress syndrome: a clinical–pathological correlation. *Clin Chest Med*. Dec 2006;27(4):571–578; abstract vii–viii.

11. Ricard JD, Dreyfuss D, Saumon G. Ventilator-induced lung injury. *Curr Opin Crit Care*. Feb 2002;8(1):12–20.

12. Erickson SE, Martin GS, Davis JL, et al. Recent trends in acute lung injury mortality: 1996–2005. *Crit Care Med*. May 2009;37(5):1574–1579.

13. Hudson LD, Milberg JA, Anardi D, et al. Clinical risks for development of the acute respiratory distress syndrome. *Am J Respir Crit Care Med*. Feb 1995;151(2 pt 1):293–301.

14. Frutos-Vivar F, Nin N, Esteban A. Epidemiology of acute lung injury and acute respiratory distress syndrome. *Curr Opin Crit Care*. Feb 2004;10(1):1–6.

15. Phua J, Badia JR, Adhikari NK, et al. Has mortality from acute respiratory distress syndrome decreased over time? A systematic review. *Am J Respir Crit Care Med*. Feb 1 2009;179(3):220–227.

16. Herridge MS, Cheung AM, Tansey CM, et al. One-year outcomes in survivors of the acute respiratory distress syndrome. *N Engl J Med*. Feb 20 2003;348(8):683–693.

17. Milberg JA, Davis DR, Steinberg KP, et al. Improved survival of patients with acute respiratory distress syndrome (ARDS): 1983–1993. *JAMA*. Jan 25 1995;273(4):306–309.

18. Vincent JL, Zambon M. Why do patients who have acute lung injury/acute respiratory distress syndrome die from multiple organ dysfunction syndrome? Implications for management. *Clin Chest Med*. Dec 2006;27(4):725–731; abstract x–xi.

19. Ventilation with lower tidal volumes as compared with traditional tidal volumes for acute lung injury and the acute respiratory distress syndrome. The Acute Respiratory Distress Syndrome Network. *N Engl J Med*. 2000;342(18):1301–1308.

20. Stewart RM, Park PK, Hunt JP, et al. Less is more: improved outcomes in surgical patients with conservative fluid administration and central venous catheter monitoring. *J Am Coll Surg*. May 2009;208(5):725–735; discussion 735–737.

21. Martin GS, Mangialardi RJ, Wheeler AP, et al. Albumin and furosemide therapy in hypoproteinemic patients with acute lung injury. *Crit Care Med*. Oct 2002;30(10):2175–2182.

22. Martin GS, Moss M, Wheeler AP, et al. A randomized, controlled trial of furosemide with or without albumin in hypoproteinemic patients with acute lung injury. *Crit Care Med*. Aug 2005;33(8):1681–1687.

23. Marik PE, Cavallazzi R, Vasu T, et al. Dynamic changes in arterial waveform derived variables and fluid responsiveness in mechanically ventilated patients: a systematic review of the literature. *Crit Care Med*. Sep 2009;37(9):2642–2647.

24. Huang CC, Fu JY, Hu HC, et al. Prediction of fluid responsiveness in acute respiratory distress syndrome patients ventilated with low tidal volume and high positive end-expiratory pressure. *Crit Care Med*. Oct 2008;36(10):2810–2816.

25. Heyland DK, Cook DJ, Guyatt GH. Enteral nutrition in the critically ill patient: a critical review of the evidence. *Intensive Care Med*. 1993;19(8):435–442.

26. Gadek JE, DeMichele SJ, Karlstad MD, et al. Effect of enteral feeding with eicosapentaenoic acid, gamma-linolenic acid, and antioxidants in patients with acute respiratory distress syndrome. Enteral Nutrition in ARDS Study Group. *Crit Care Med*. Aug 1999;27(8):1409–1420.

27. Pontes-Arruda A, Aragao AM, Albuquerque JD. Effects of enteral feeding with eicosapentaenoic acid, gamma-linolenic acid, and antioxidants in mechanically ventilated patients with severe sepsis and septic shock. *Crit Care Med*. Sep 2006;34(9):2325–2333.

28. Singer P, Theilla M, Fisher H, et al., Benefit of an enteral diet enriched with eicosapentaenoic acid and gamma-linolenic acid in ventilated patients with acute lung injury. *Crit Care Med*. Apr 2006;34(4):1033–1038.

29. Pontes-Arruda A, Demichele S, Seth A, et al. The use of an inflammation-modulating diet in patients with acute lung injury or acute respiratory distress syndrome: a meta-analysis of outcome data. *JPEN J Parenter Enteral Nutr*. Nov–Dec 2008;32(6):596–605.

30. Marik PE, Zaloga GP. Immunonutrition in critically ill patients: a systematic review and analysis of the literature. *Intensive Care Med*. Nov 2008;34(11):1980–1990.

31. Steinberg KP, Hudson LD, Goodman RB, et al. Efficacy and safety of corticosteroids for persistent acute respiratory distress syndrome. *N Engl J Med*. Apr 20 2006;354(16):1671–1684.

32. Tang BM, Craig JC, Eslick GD, et al. Use of corticosteroids in acute lung injury and acute respiratory distress syndrome: a systematic review and meta-analysis. *Crit Care Med*. May 2009;37(5):1594–1603.

33. Perkins GD, McAuley DF, Thickett DR, et al. The beta-agonist lung injury trial (BALTI): a randomized placebo-controlled clinical trial. *Am J Respir Crit Care Med*. Feb 1 2006;173(3):281–287.

34. Amato MB, Barbas CS, Medeiros DM, et al. Effect of a protective-ventilation strategy on mortality in the acute respiratory distress syndrome. *N Engl J Med*. Feb 5 1998;338(6):347–354.

35. Meade MO, Cook DJ, Guyatt GH, et al. Ventilation strategy using low tidal volumes, recruitment maneuvers, and high positive end-expiratory pressure for acute lung injury and acute respiratory distress syndrome: a randomized controlled trial. *JAMA*. Feb 13 2008;299(6):637–645.

36. Suter PM, Fairley B, Isenberg MD. Optimum end-expiratory airway pressure in patients with acute pulmonary failure. *N Engl J Med*. Feb 6 1975;292(6):284–289.

37. Talmor D, Sarge T, Malhotra A, et al. Mechanical ventilation guided by esophageal pressure in acute lung injury. *N Engl J Med*. Nov 13 2008;359(20):2095–2104.

38. Rouby JJ, Puybasset L, Nieszkowska A, et al. Acute respiratory distress syndrome: lessons from computed tomography of the whole lung. *Crit Care Med*. Apr 2003;31(4 suppl):S285–S295.

39. Lu Q, Rouby JJ. Measurement of pressure–volume curves in patients on mechanical ventilation: methods and significance. *Crit Care*. 2000;4(2):91–100.

40. O'Croinin D, Ni Chonghaile M, Higgins B, et al. Bench-to-bedside review: permissive hypercapnia. *Crit Care.* Feb 2005;9(1):51–59.

41. Pelosi P, Brazzi L, Gattinoni L. Prone position in acute respiratory distress syndrome. *Eur Respir J.* Oct 2002; 20(4):1017–1028.

42. Davis JW, Lemaster DM, Moore EC, et al. Prone ventilation in trauma or surgical patients with acute lung injury and adult respiratory distress syndrome: is it beneficial? *J Trauma.* May 2007;62(5):1201–1206.

43. Gattinoni L, Tognoni G, Pesenti A, et al. Effect of prone positioning on the survival of patients with acute respiratory failure. *N Engl J Med.* Aug 23 2001;345(8):568–573.

44. Fernandez R, Trenchs X, Klamburg J, et al. Prone positioning in acute respiratory distress syndrome: a multicenter randomized clinical trial. *Intensive Care Med.* Aug 2008;34(8):1487–1491.

45. Mancebo J, Fernandez R, Blanch L, et al. A multicenter trial of prolonged prone ventilation in severe acute respiratory distress syndrome. *Am J Respir Crit Care Med.* Jun 1 2006;173(11):1233–1239.

46. Vieillard-Baron A, Charron C, Caille V, et al. Prone positioning unloads the right ventricle in severe ARDS. *Chest.* Nov 2007;132(5):1440–1446.

47. Abroug F, Ouanes-Besbes L, Elatrous S, et al. The effect of prone positioning in acute respiratory distress syndrome or acute lung injury: a meta-analysis. Areas of uncertainty and recommendations for research. *Intensive Care Med.* jun 2008;34(6):1002–1011.

48. Downar J, Mehta S. Bench-to-bedside review: high-frequency oscillatory ventilation in adults with acute respiratory distress syndrome. *Crit Care.* 2006; 10(6):240.

49. Putensen C, Mutz NJ, Putensen-Himmer G, et al. Spontaneous breathing during ventilatory support improves ventilation–perfusion distributions in patients with acute respiratory distress syndrome. *Am J Respir Crit Care Med.* Apr 1999;159(4 pt 1):1241–1248.

50. Habashi NM. Other approaches to open-lung ventilation: airway pressure release ventilation. *Crit Care Med.* Mar 2005;33(3 suppl):S228–S240.

CHAPTER 10

Severe Asthma and COPD

Michael T. Dalley and Triminh Bui

► INTRODUCTION

Obstructive airway disease is the most common chronic pulmonary pathology encountered in emergency medicine. Its most common etiology, asthma, is characterized by bronchoconstriction and airway hyperresponsiveness to certain stimuli. These stimuli trigger inflammatory mediators that lead to airway inflammation, mucosal edema, and, ultimately, reversible bronchospasm.[1]

Conversely, chronic obstructive pulmonary disease (COPD) is a disorder characterized by abnormal tests of expiratory flow demonstrating air flow obstruction that becomes fixed and does not change markedly over a period of months. It is a multifocal pathology encompassing the triad of emphysema, chronic bronchitis, and asthma.[2] The increasing prevalence and the large burden these disease entities impose on emergency medical care make the diagnosis and management of acute exacerbations vital to any health care provider.

► EPIDEMIOLOGY

Approximately 22.5 million Americans had asthma in 2005, conferring an estimated financial burden of $19.7 billion in annual health care costs.[3] In the United States, there are approximately 2 million emergency department visits per year for acute asthma, with 12 million people reporting having had asthma "attacks" in the past year.[4] Approximately 2–20% of all ICU admissions are attributed to severe asthma, with intubation and mechanical ventilation necessary in up to one third of

ICU admissions[5] and mortality rates in patients receiving intubation ranging from 10% to 20%.[6]

COPD is the fourth most common cause of death in the United States, the third most common cause of hospitalization, and the only cause of death that is increasing in prevalence. The mortality of all patients while hospitalized for a COPD exacerbation is approximately 5–14%,[7] while mortality of COPD patients admitted to an ICU for an exacerbation is 24%. For patients 65 years or older and discharged from the ICU after treatment of a COPD exacerbation, the 1-year mortality is 59%.[7]

► PATHOPHYSIOLOGY

Asthma is characterized by airway inflammation with an abnormal accumulation of inflammatory mediators in response to various stimuli. Acutely this accumulation leads to a reversible reduction of airway diameter caused by smooth muscle contraction, vascular congestion, bronchial wall edema, and thickened secretions.

Chronic asthma can lead to airway remodeling, with subepithelial collagen deposition and increased airway resistance that manifests as a progressive decline in forced expiratory volume in 1 second (FEV1) measurements. Once airway remodeling has occurred, the pathologic changes may become irreversible.

Pathologic findings in patients with chronic asthma include bronchial wall thickening due to inflammation and edema, bronchial narrowing or obstruction, and the presence of mucus plugs that at times may be large and thick. This airway narrowing leads to alveolar

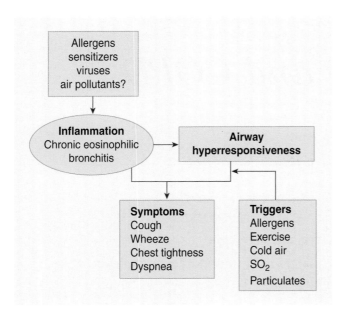

Figure 10-1. Inflammation in the airways of asthmatic patients leading to airway hyperresponsiveness and symptoms. (Reproduced with permission from Fauci AS, Kasper DL, Braunwald E, et al. *Harrison's Principles of Internal Medicine*. 17th ed. New York, NY: McGraw-Hill Inc; 2008. Figure 248-2.)

hyperinflation and, in a subset of patients, may lead to the formation of bullae, the potential for bullae rupture, and the development of pneumothoraces (Figures 10-1 and 10-2).

COPD is a triad of disease entities that includes the pathophysiology of asthma as well as incorporates the irreversible changes associated with both chronic bronchitis and emphysema. Chronic bronchitis is defined by excessive mucus production resulting in airway obstruction and hyperplasia of mucus-producing glands. Damage to the endothelium impairs mucociliary function that inhibits the clearance of bacteria and mucous. Inflammation and secretions, worse because of the decreased mucus clearance, provide the obstructive component of this disease. Emphysematous changes (described below) may be present to a variable degree and are usually centrilobar rather than pan lobar. This leads to increased cardiac output in an attempt to compensate for decreased ventilation. The resulting rapid circulation through a poorly ventilated lung represents a V/Q mismatch with hypoxemia and polycythemia. Eventually, hypercapnia and respiratory acidosis develop that lead to cor pulmonale. The development of cor pulmonale ultimately produces clinical evidence of right heart failure and produces the classic "Blue Bloater" appearance.

Emphysema is defined by destruction of airways distal to the terminal bronchiole. Pathologically, this disease involves the gradual destruction of alveolar septae and of the pulmonary capillary bed, leading to decreased ability to oxygenate blood. The body compensates with hyperventilation and the lowering of cardiac output. This V/Q mismatch results in relatively limited blood flow through a fairly well-oxygenated lung (as opposed to chronic bronchitis where there is rapid circulation through a poorly ventilated lung). The low cardiac output ultimately leads to systemic tissue hypoxia and pulmonary cachexia. Eventually these patients develop muscle wasting and weight loss and are identified as "pink puffers."

The diagnosis, severity, clinical course, and response to treatment of all obstructive lung diseases (OLDs) can best be evaluated objectively by testing pulmonary function. OLD causes a delay in emptying lung volume. Normally, an individual can forcefully expel all of the air in the lungs (the vital capacity) within 4–6 seconds. In established OLD, patients may continue to expire during a forced expiratory maneuver for 10–20 seconds or more.

While all individuals have flow limitation during a forced expiration, those with obstructive airway disease demonstrate flow limitation with less effort and at lower airflow. The three lung abnormalities that reduce flow during forced expiration are decreased lung recoil pressure, increased resistance of the airways, and increased tendency of airways to collapse. Decreased lung recoil pressure causes a lower distending pressure between the airway and the surrounding pleural pressure, promoting a tendency for the airways to narrow. Increased resistance of the airways, especially in the periphery of the lung, creates increased pressure drops along the airways during expiration, thus promoting the tendency of the airways to constrict before the entire tidal volume is expelled. Bronchial smooth muscle constriction, inflammatory products encroaching upon the airway lumen, and decreased tethering of the airway by the alveolar septa also cause airways to collapse more easily.[8]

The airflow limitation in emphysema can be attributed to the decreased elastic recoil of the lung, in chronic bronchitis to the increased peripheral airway resistance, and in asthma to the increased tendency of airways to collapse.[8]

► CLINICAL PRESENTATION

Asthma classically presents with a triad of symptoms that include cough, wheeze, and shortness of breath. However, certain patients may present with only one or two of these symptoms. Patients may complain of chest tightness or bandlike constriction across their chest. The cough may be dry or productive with pale yellow sputum. Wheezing may be subjective in

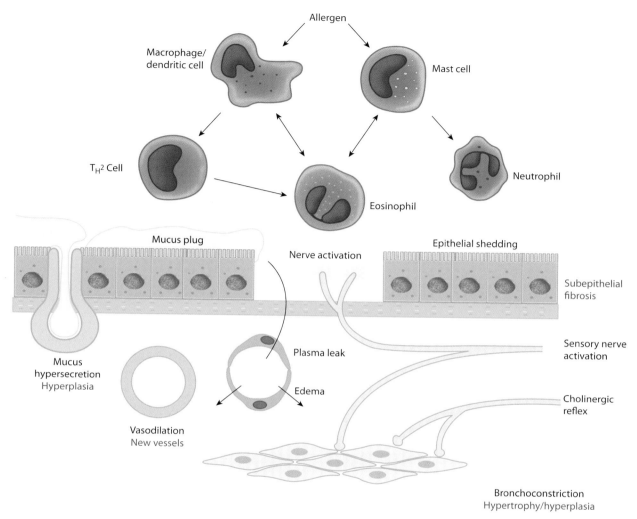

Figure 10-2. Pathophysiology of asthma showing participation of several interacting inflammatory cells and resulting in acute and chronic inflammatory effects on the airway. (Reproduced with permission from Fauci AS, Kasper DL, Braunwald E, et al. *Harrison's Principles of Internal Medicine*. 17th ed. New York, NY: McGraw-Hill Inc; 2008. Figure 248-3.)

patients familiar with the term and used to describe a variety of sounds including upper airway noises from the throat or nares. Since many of these complaints are consistent with many pulmonary pathologies, it can be hard to diagnose asthma based on chief complaint alone. However, certain historical clues such as episodic symptoms, characteristic triggers, and personal or family history of atopy or asthma as a child raise the likelihood.

In terms of how and why COPD patients present, there are four major causes of acute decompensation in COPD patients: (1) superimposed respiratory illness, (2) noxious environmental exposure, (3) noncompliance with medications, and (4) continued cigarette smoking. Patients complain of dyspnea, cough, and increased sputum production. During acute exacerbations, patients may also present with wheezing, particularly with exertion. As the disease becomes more chronic, intervals between acute exacerbations lessen. Patients may also complain of morning headaches, which are attributed to increased hypercapnia while asleep leading to worsening respiratory acidosis.

► HISTORY AND PHYSICAL EXAMINATION

The spectrum of disease that presents to the emergency department is vast and the severity of exacerbation can progress in minutes. Caregivers should be familiar with

Asthma history

Previous severe exacerbation (e.g., intubation or ICU admission for asthma)
Two or more hospitalizations for asthma in the past year
Three or more ED visits for asthma in the past year
Hospitalization or ED visit for asthma in the past month
Using >2 canisters of SABA per month
Difficulty perceiving asthma symptoms or severity of exacerbations
Other risk factors: lack of a written asthma action plan, sensitivity to *Alternaria*

Social history

Low socioeconomic status or inner-city residence
Illicit drug use
Major psychosocial problems

Comorbidities

Cardiovascular disease
Other chronic lung disease
Chronic psychiatric disease

Key: ED, emergency department; ICU, intensive care unit; SABA, short-acting beta$_2$-agonist

Sources: Abramson et al. 2001; Greenberger et al. 1993; Hardie et al. 2002; Kallenbach et al. 1993; Kikuchi et al. 1994; O'Hollaren et al. 1991; Rodrigo and Rodrigo 1993; Strunk and Mrazek 1986; Suissa et al. 1994

Figure 10-3. Risk factors for death from asthma. (US Department of Health and Human Services, National Institute of Health, National Heart, Lung, and Blood Institute. *Expert Panel Report 3: Guidelines for the Diagnosis and Management of Asthma.* Figure 5-2a, p. 377.)

the risk factors for death from asthma (Figure 10-3),[9] and if there is only time for an abbreviated history, it should be focused on the predictors of fatal outcomes: a prior asthma attack severe enough to require intubation and mechanical ventilation, prior ICU admissions/hospitalizations, and an increased frequency and use of rescue inhalers.

On physical examination, widespread, high-pitched, musical wheezes are characteristic of asthma; however, these findings are nonspecific and may be absent in severe obstruction. The most concerning physical findings suggestive of air flow obstruction include conversational dyspnea or inability to speak at all, tachypnea (RR >30), tachycardia (HR >130), and a prolonged expiratory phase of respiration (decreased I:E ratio). More ominous signs include tripod positioning, retractions, and pulsus paradoxus (a fall in systolic blood pressure greater than 12 mm Hg during inspiration).

Signs indicating impending respiratory failure include a silent chest (no wheezing is worse than wheezing), inability to recline or lay supine in the stretcher, altered mental status, and paradoxical respirations (Figure 10-4).[1]

► ASSESSMENT OF LUNG FUNCTION

Pulmonary function tests are critical tools in the diagnosis and management of OLD exacerbations. Measurement of peak expiratory flow rate (PEFR) and spirometry are the tests most often used in the diagnosis of asthma or an exacerbation and the best objective evaluation for risk stratifying patients, monitoring response to therapy, and determining final disposition in exacerbations of OLD.

The PEFR, or "peak flow," is measured during a brief, forceful exhalation. The resulting measurements are highly dependent on the patient's expiratory effort and technique. Serial measurements performed at presentation and 30–60 minutes after initial treatment are recommended.[10] However, in patients experiencing a severe or life-threatening exacerbation with impending respiratory failure, PEFR testing is not warranted and should not preclude immediate therapy.

Spirometry, which includes measurement of FEV1 and forced vital capacity (FVC), provides additional objective information in the diagnosis and management of OLD. Variable/reversible airflow obstruction is the hallmark of asthma. Progressively worsening fixed airflow obstruction is the hallmark of COPD. Since bronchospasm is not the major pathologic mechanism behind COPD, the improvement in pulmonary function measurement during therapy is less than that of asthmatics.

Indicators for admission to the hospital include PEFR less than 100 mL/min or FEV1 less than 1 L prior to treatment, PEFR or FEV1 less than 40% baseline/predicted, failure of PEFR to increase greater than 10% following initial treatment, and PEFR that does not reach 80% of predicted following aggressive therapy.[9]

	Mild	Moderate	Severe	Subset: Respiratory arrest Imminent
Symptoms				
Breathlessness	While walking	While at rest (infant—softer, shorter cry, difficulty feeding)	While at rest (infant—stops feeding)	
	Can lie down	Prefers sitting	Sits upright	
Talks in	Sentences	Phrases	Words	
Alertness	May be agitated	Usually agitated	Usually agitated	Drowsy or confused
Signs				
Respiratory rate	Increased	Increased Guide to rates of breathing in awake children: Age <2 months 2–12 months 1–5 years 6–8 years	Often >30/minute Normal rate <60/minute <50/minute <40/minute <30/minute	
Use of accessory muscles; suprasternal retractions	Usually not	Commonly	Usually	Paradoxical thoracoabdominal movement
Wheeze	Moderate, often only end expiratory	Loud; throughout exhalation	Usually loud; throughout inhalation and exhalation	Absence of wheeze
Pulse/minute	<100	100–120 Guide to normal pulse rates in children:: Age 2–12 months 1–2 years 2–8 years	>120 Normal rate <160/minute <120/minute <110/minute	Bradycardia
Pulsus paradoxus	Absent <10 mmHg	May be present 10–25 mmHg	Often present >25 mmHg (adult) 20–40 mmHg (child)	Absence suggests respiratory muscle fatigue
Functional Assessment				
PEF percent predicted or percent personal best	≥70 percent	Approx. 40–69 percent or response lasts <2 hours	<40 percent	<25 percent Note: PEF testing may not be needed in very severe attacks
PaO_2 (on air)	Normal (test not usually necessary)	≥60 mmHg (test not usually necessary)	<60 mmHg: possible cyanosis	
and/or PCO_2	<42 mmHg (test not usually necessary)	<42 mmHg (test not usually necessary)	<42 mmHg: possible respiratory failure (See pages 393–394, 399.)	
SaO_2 percent (on air) at sea level	>95 percent (test not usually necessary)	90–95 percent (test not usually necessary)	<90 percent	
	Hypercapnia (hypoventilation) develops more readily in young children than in adults and adolescents.			

Key: PaO_2, arterial oxygen pressure; PCO_2, partial pressure of carbon dioxide; PEF, peak expiratory flow; SaO_2, oxygen saturation

Notes:

■ The presence of several parameters, but not necessarily all, indicates the general classification of the exacerbation.

■ Many of these parameters have not been systematically studied, especially as they correlate with each other. Thus, they serve only as general guides (Cham et al. 2002; Chey et al. 1999; Gore lick et al. 2004b; Karras et al. 2000; Kelly et al. 2002b and 2004; Keogh et al. 2001; McCarren et al. 2000; Rodrigo and Rodrigo 1998b; Rodrigo et al. 2004; Smith et al. 2002).

■ The emotional impact of asthma symptoms on the patient and family is variable but must be recognized and addressed and can affect approaches to treatment and followup (Ritz et al. 2000; Strunk and Mrazek 1986; von Leupoldt and Dahme 2005).

Figure 10-4. Formal evaluation of asthma exacerbation severity in the urgent or emergency care setting. (US Department of Health and Human Services, National Institute of Health, National Heart, Lung, and Blood Institute. *Expert Panel Report 3: Guidelines for the Diagnosis and Management of Asthma.* Figure 5-3, p. 380.)

Pulse oximetry measurement is desirable in all patients with acute exacerbations of OLD to exclude hypoxemia. However, an isolated pulse oximetry reading at triage is not predictive in most cases, and serial monitoring can provide more subtle evidence for or against the need for hospital admission.

▶ LABORATORY STUDIES

Routine laboratory studies are not contributory in the evaluation of exacerbations of OLD, but are used to diagnose or exclude other conditions, detect or confirm impending respiratory failure and theophylline toxicity, and diagnose comorbid conditions that might compromise therapy.

Arterial blood gas (ABG) measurement provides important information in severe asthma exacerbations. The test may reveal dangerous levels of hypercapnia secondary to poor ventilation due to exhaustion. ABGs are indicated in patients with fatigue or exhaustion, suspected hypoventilation, SaO_2 <90%, or PEFR <25% predicted after aggressive therapy. In COPD patients, ABG values are helpful in determining whether inadequacy of ventilation (hypercapnia) is an acute decompensation or a chronic compensation.

Chest radiographs in exacerbations of obstructive disease are usually nondiagnostic, but are indicated to rule out secondary causes of wheezing (i.e., congestive heart failure, pneumothorax, pneumomediastinum, pneumonia, etc.).

▶ TREATMENT

The goals of therapy for acute exacerbations of OLD remain constant throughout the spectrum of the disease process: improving hypoxemia, reversal of acute bronchospasm, and prevention of post-therapy relapse. The primary treatment consists of the administration of oxygen, inhaled β_2-agonists, and systemic corticosteroids; these should be given to all patients with acute exacerbations requiring medical evaluation. The severity of the asthma exacerbation determines the intensity of treatment and the frequency of patient monitoring (Figure 10-5).[9]

In addition to the primary treatments, therapy with inhaled ipratropium bromide is typically added to the other agents. Ipratropium bromide competitively inhibits muscarinic cholinergic receptors to produce bronchodilation. It works synergistically with β_2-agonists and has been shown to reduce hospitalizations in patients with severe airflow obstruction.[10] It reduces bronchoconstriction in the central airways that may explain the better therapeutic outcomes when treating COPD—as opposed to asthma—exacerbations.

▶ IMPENDING RESPIRATORY FAILURE

Intensive therapy with inhaled bronchodilators and systemic corticosteroids is usually sufficient to reduce airflow obstruction and alleviate symptoms in patients with exacerbations of OLD. A small percentage of patients, however, will show signs of worsening ventilation. It is recommended that intubation not be delayed once it is deemed necessary,[10] and it is this subset of patients that the rest of the chapter will focus on.

Intubation and mechanical ventilation in OLD is complex and fraught with potential complications. Therefore, prevention of intubation is an important goal in the treatment of severe, acute OLD. Various second-line therapies have been suggested and bear consideration for critically patients who would otherwise require intubation.

Intravenous magnesium sulfate can be considered in patients with life-threatening exacerbations and those whose exacerbations remain severe after 1 hour of intensive conventional treatment.[11,12] Magnesium sulfate is thought to inhibit bronchial smooth muscle contraction by inhibiting intracellular influx of calcium. The dose is usually 2 g over 20 minutes in adults and 25–75 mg/kg in children (up to a maximum of 2 g), and its selective use is common.[13]

Heliox is a mixture of oxygen and helium that decreases airway resistance by reducing airflow turbulence in the lungs, thus reducing the work of breathing. It is available in a variety of percentages. An 80:20 mix (80% helium, 20% oxygen) contains about the same amount of oxygen as room air, but mixes with higher percentages of oxygen are available. The higher the helium content, the less viscous the mixture, so the greater the tendency toward laminar flow and a lower work of breathing. However, the higher the helium content, the lower the oxygen content, and the greater the tendency toward hypoxia. For patients with severe exacerbations of their disease, the National Asthma Education and Prevention Program Expert Panel Report 3 calls this form of therapy promising but gives it a conditional recommendation citing the need for a large multicenter study.[10]

▶ NONINVASIVE VENTILATION

Noninvasive positive pressure ventilation (NPPV) is a respiratory assist therapy in which positive airway pressure is delivered throughout the entire respiratory cycle. There are two principal forms used: continuous positive airway pressure (CPAP) and bilevel positive airway pressure (BiPAP). BiPAP differs from CPAP in that the pressure support is "bilevel," or biphasic, with a higher pressure offered during inhalation than during exhalation or between cycles.

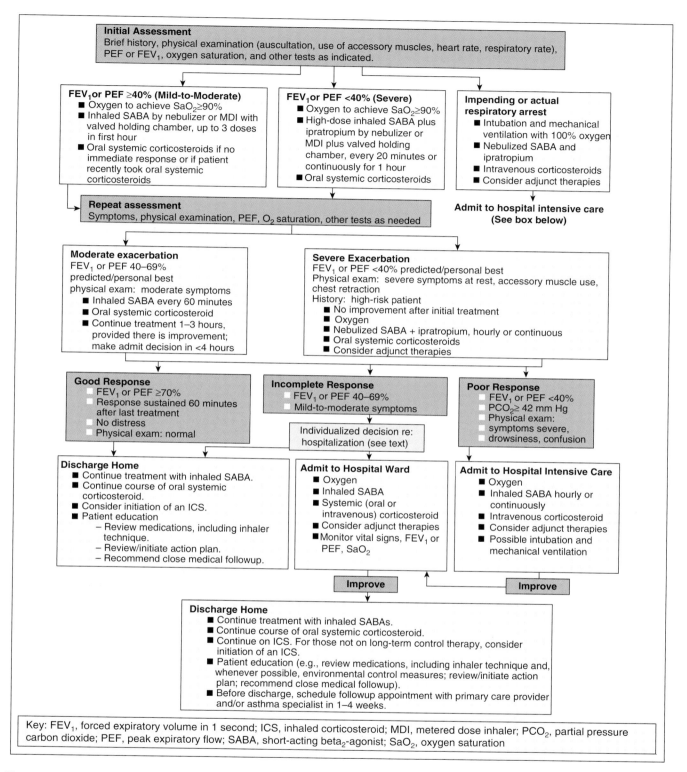

Figure 10-5. Management of asthma exacerbations: emergency department and hospital-based care. (US Department of Health and Human Services, National Institute of Health, National Heart, Lung, and Blood Institute. *Expert Panel Report 3: Guidelines for the Diagnosis and Management of Asthma.* Figure 5-6, p. 388.)

In OLD, some gas remains trapped in alveoli at end expiration causing levels of positive end-expiratory pressure (PEEP) above those seen in normal physiology. Since this PEEP comes from within the lung itself, it is termed "auto-PEEP." It may seem counterintuitive to then apply additional external PEEP, but studies have shown that a low level of applied CPAP may offset the deleterious effects of auto-PEEP.[14] The proposed mechanism is externally applied PEEP both delays or prevents airway collapse (reducing or relieving airway obstruction) and lessens the work of breathing (allowing extra time for other modalities to exert their effect). The addition of inspiratory pressure support to CPAP (aka BiPAP) improves tidal volume in proportion to the amount of pressure applied.

NPPV has prevented intubations in a variety of respiratory conditions in addition to OLD exacerbations. Randomized control trials have demonstrated that NPPV decreases respiratory rate, dyspnea, $Paco_2$, length of stay, and rates of intubation as well as improves mortality in COPD exacerbations.[15] Pathophysiologically, acute asthma exacerbations are similar in mechanism but there is less literature supporting NPPV in the treatment of asthma exacerbations.[16]

According to the National Asthma Education and Prevention Program Expert Panel Report 3, a trial of NPPV before intubation and mechanical ventilation should be considered in select patients with acute asthma exacerbation and respiratory failure, provided they are alert and can tolerate and cooperate with the therapy.[16] Initial settings call for an initial expiratory pressure of 3 cm H_2O increased every 15 minutes to a maximum of 5 and an initial inspiratory pressure of 8 cm H_2O increased every 15 minutes to a maximum pressure of 15 or until the respiratory rate is less than 25 breaths/min.[17] Nebulizer therapy should be continued throughout the administration of NPPV. Many facilities use a dedicated NPPV machine, although some practitioners prefer to administer NPPV using a traditional ventilator; this way, if the patient fails NPPV therapy and requires intubation, the ventilator is already in place.

► INTUBATION AND MECHANICAL VENTILATION IN RESPIRATORY FAILURE

CRITERIA FOR INTUBATION

In spite of all efforts for prevention of intubation, patients may still decompensate and require intubation and mechanical ventilation. Clinically, there are four major indications for intubation: (1) cardiac arrest, (2) respiratory arrest or profound bradypnea, (3) physical exhaustion, and (4) altered mental status such as lethargy or agitation. Patients may tell you, "I am too tired

to breathe," or "I can't go on any more"; these statements alone are ominous and should trigger a consideration for intubation.

Objectively, an ABG may be helpful and indicate failed noninvasive therapy and the need for intubation. An ABG showing progressive hypoxemia, hypercapnia, and respiratory acidosis in a patient who has changes in mental status should immediately trigger airway intervention.[18] Even a normal pH or Pco_2 should prompt consideration of intubation since normalization of these values may indicate tiring of the respiratory muscles.

INTUBATION TECHNIQUE

Intubation with a rapid sequence of sedation followed by muscle paralysis is the preferred method for airway control in the emergency department setting.[19] Airway control should be obtained by an experienced care provider because even minor manipulation of the airway during an acute OLD exacerbation can lead to laryngospasm and worsen bronchospasm.

Of the available sedatives used during RSI, ketamine and propofol offer the best therapeutic advantages during an OLD exacerbation. Ketamine stimulates the release of catecholamines and may have a direct relaxation effect on bronchial smooth muscle, leading to bronchodilation.[20] Side effects include hypersecretion, hypertension, arrhythmias, and hallucinations, although pretreatment with atropine may reduce or eliminate some of these. It is contraindicated in patients with ischemic heart disease, hypertension, preeclampsia, and increased intracranial pressure.

Propofol is a short-acting sedative with bronchodilatory effects. It has a rapid onset of action and is very short acting which allows for rapid awakening. It is an excellent alternative for patients with elevated blood pressure during the peri-intubation period. Some practitioners also prefer propofol because it can be easily used for ongoing sedation.

SETTING THE VENTILATOR

The physiology of patients with OLD exacerbations presents a unique and complex challenge when these patients are placed on mechanical ventilation. Inhalation, controlled by the ventilator, is unchanged or even improved. But exhalation becomes an entirely passive process dependent only on patient variables. Since the patient's condition is one of airway obstruction, air can easily get into the patient, but may not be able to get out. This can lead to severe lung hyperinflation (auto-PEEP), which can ultimately lead to hypotension and barotrauma.[21] Therefore, ventilatory strategies that reduce hyperinflation are crucial.

► **TABLE 10-1. INITIAL VENTILATOR SETTINGS FOR THE INTUBATED ASTHMATIC PATIENT**

Controlled mechanical ventilation at 10 breaths/min
Tidal volume at 7–8 mL/kg (ideal body weight)
Peek inspiratory flow at 60 L/min (constant flow) or
    80–90 L/min (decelerating flow)
Fraction of inspired oxygen at 1.0

Reproduced with permission from Brenner B, Corbridge T, Kazzi A. Intubation and mechanical ventilation of the asthmatic patient in respiratory failure. *J Emerg Med.* 2009;37(2 suppl):S29.

There are three ventilator strategies used to reduce hyperinflation and auto-PEEP in the intubated asthmatic patient (Table 10-1): (1) reduction of the respiratory rate, (2) reduction of tidal volume, and (3) shortening of inspiration by increasing the inspiratory flow rate to allow more time for exhalation during each respiratory cycle.

Reduction of tidal volume is limited by the progressive effect on the amount of dead space in the lung, so increasing the pressure limitation (up to 100 cm H_2O) may be necessary to ensure delivery of a full tidal volume.[22] Typically a reduction to an acceptable level of auto-PEEP (10–15 cm H_2O) can be obtained by tweaking the first two strategies. But if the respiratory rate cannot be sufficiently lowered to reduce hyperinflation, inspiratory time can be shortened to allow for more time in the exhalation phase. Furthermore, increasing the flow rate and using a square wave flow pattern shorten inspiratory time, do not represent a significant danger for barotrauma, and reduce the possibility of auto-PEEP.[22]

Of course, decreasing the respiratory rate can cause hypercapnia. In this subset of patients, hypercapnia is usually well tolerated and safer than (over)ventilating to a normal $Paco_2$ and causing harmful hyperinflation. This strategy is termed "permissive hypercapnia." Anoxic brain injury and severe myocardial dysfunction are contraindications to permissive hypercapnia because of the potential for hypercapnia to dilate cerebral vessels, constrict pulmonary vessels, and decrease myocardial contractility.[22]

Having objective data to help determine the severity of lung hyperinflation is central to assessing patients and adjusting ventilator settings. In practice, two relatively easy to measure pressures are used as surrogate markers of lung inflation: auto-PEEP and plateau pressure (Pplat). Accurate measurements of Pplat and auto-PEEP require patient–ventilator synchrony and absence of patient effort, although paralysis is generally not required. Neither parameter has been validated as a predictor of complications of mechanical ventilation, but experts agree that complications are rare when Pplat is less than 30 cm H_2O and auto-PEEP is less than 15 cm H_2O.[23]

MEDICAL MANAGEMENT

As with all intubated patients, effective sedation is paramount. Sedation allows for synchrony between the patient and the ventilator and prevents self-extubation and auto-PEEP from a rapid spontaneous respiratory rate. Propofol is a good sedative because not only can it be easily titrated, but it possesses bronchodilatory properties as well.[22]

Neuromuscular blockade during mechanical ventilation might reduce the risk of barotrauma, avoid coughing and dyssynchronous breathing, and allow the respiratory muscles to rest. However, prolonged use can cause myopathy, particularly when used in conjunction with corticosteroids, and so is only recommended in patients in whom deep sedation alone does not allow synchrony with the ventilator.

Systemic corticosteroids and inhaled β-agonists are the mainstay of asthma therapy prior to intubation, and should be continued while on mechanical ventilation, as well. High flow aerosolized (HFA, aka multidose inhaler [MDI]) or nebulizer treatments should be added to the ventilator circuit.[23]

TREATMENT COMPLICATIONS

Persistent or worsening hypoxemia suggests the development of a complication from mechanical ventilation. Complications that must be considered include right mainstem intubation, pneumothorax, gastric distention, endotracheal tube dislodgement, tube blockage, aspiration, bronchospasm, and ventilatory malfunction. Each of these must be considered and the patient reassessed after any intervention.

Hypotension can be caused directly by the physiology of mechanical ventilation. The increase in intrathoracic pressure caused by mechanical ventilation leads to a reduction in preload and a decrease in cardiac output. These effects can be avoided by preventing complications caused by elevated intrathoracic pressure such as hyperinflation, gastric distention, and pneumothoraces. Medications used for sedation and neuromuscular blockade can also be a culprit. A fluid bolus is useful if not contraindicated. Adjusting the ventilator to prevent ventilator causes of hypotension as well as an apnea trial for 30–60 seconds in a preoxygenated patient may be prudent in helping differentiate the cause of hypotension. If no reversible cause is found and hypotension remains critical, then inotropic support is indicated.

Critical lung hyperinflation can produce deleterious effects such as decreasing preload to the right ventricle, increasing pericardial pressure causing tamponade physiology, and predisposing to a tension pneumothorax. If cardiac arrest presents with pulseless electrical activity

(PEA), all potential causes of PEA should be considered, recognizing the increased risk of pneumothorax and tamponade physiology. If clinical signs of tension pneumothorax are present (unequal breath sounds, tracheal deviation, subcutaneous emphysema), needle decompression should be performed followed by tube thoracostomy. Note that puncturing a hyperinflated lung during chest tube insertion can produce a rush of air similar to releasing a tension pneumothorax but will not improve ventilation.[22] In this case, the tube should be repositioned or another tube inserted.

Barotrauma is a well-known complication of mechanical ventilation, but the issue of development of barotrauma in relation to airway pressure, PEEP, and tidal volume is controversial. In asthmatic patients, a VEI (total exhaled volume over 20–60 seconds, after a machine-delivered breath) of greater than 20 mL/kg correlates with barotrauma[24]; however, this measurement is not routinely obtained in most ICU settings.

Weaning and extubation criteria have not been validated for patients with acute exacerbations of OLD. A recommended approach is to perform a spontaneous breathing trial in an awake patient once $Paco_2$ normalizes, airway resistance is less than 20 cm H_2O, and neuromuscular weakness has not been identified.[22] After extubation, observation in an ICU setting is recommended for an additional 12–24 hours. Once the patient is stable enough for discharge, patient education, systemic corticosteroids, and proper use of β-agonist therapy must be reinforced along with timely follow-up with a pulmonologist or his or her primary care provider to help prevent further exacerbations.

REFERENCES

1. Barnes Peter J. Asthma. Kasper DL, Braunwald E, Fauci AS, Hauser SL, Longo DL, Jameson JL, Loscalzo J. eds. Harrison's. *Principals of Internal Medicine*. 17th ed., New York, NY: McGraw-Hill; 2008:1596–1607.

2. American Thoracic Society. Standards for the diagnosis and care of patients with chronic obstructive pulmonary disease. *Am J Respir Crit Care Med*. 1995;152:s77.

3. American Lung Association Asthma in Adults fact sheet. Available at: http://www.lungusa.org.

4. Environmental Protection Agency. Asthma facts. Available at: http://www.epa.gov/asthma/pdfs/asthma_fact_sheet_en.pdf.

5. McFadden ER Jr. Acute severe asthma. *Am J Respir Crit Care Med*. 2003;168:740–759.

6. Shapiro JM. Intensive care management of status asthmaticus. *Chest*. 2001;120:1439–1441.

7. Connors AF Jr, Dawson NV, Thomas C, et al. Outcomes following acute exacerbation of severe chronic obstructive lung disease. The SUPPORT investigators. *Am J Respir Crit Care Med*. 1997;155:386.

8. Wise RA, Liu MC. Obstructive airway diseases: Asthma and COPD. In: Barker R. *Principles of Ambulatory Medicine*. 6th ed. Philadelphia: Lippincott Williams & Wilkins; 2003:808–841.

9. US Department of Health and Human Services, National Institute of Health. *Expert Panel Report 3: Guidelines for the Diagnosis and Management of Asthma*. Bathesda, MD: National Heart, Lung, and Blood Institute, 2007. NIH publication no. 4008-4051.

10. Camargo CA Jr, Rachelefsky, G, Shatz M. et al. Managing asthma exacerbations in the emergency department: summary of the National Asthma Education and Prevention Program Expert Panel report 3 guidelines for the management of asthma exacerbations. *J Emerg Med*. 2009;37(2 suppl 1):S6–S17.

11. Cheuk DK, Chau TC, Lee SL. A meta-analysis on intravenous magnesium sulphate for treating acute asthma. *Arch Dis Child*. 2005;90:74–77.

12. Rowe BH, Bretzlaff JA, Bourdon C, et al. Intravenous magnesium sulfate treatment for acute asthma in the emergency department: a systematic review of the literature. *Ann Emerg Med*. 2000;36:181–190.

13. Rowe BH, Carmargo CA Jr. The use of magnesium sulfate in acute asthma: rapid uptake of evidence in North American emergency departments. *J Allergy Clin Immunol*. 2006;117:53–58.

14. Appendini L, Patessio A, Zanaboni S, et al. Physiologic effects of positive end-expiratory pressure and mask support during exacerbations of COPD. *Am J Respir Crit Care Med*. 1994;149:1069–1076.

15. Mehta S, Hill NS. State of the art. *Am J Respir Crit Care Med*. 2001;163:540–577.

16. Nowak R, Corbridge T, Brenner B. Non-invasive ventilation. *J Emerg Med*. 2009;37(2s):S18–S22.

17. Sorosky A, Stav D, Shpirer I. A pilot prospective, randomized placebo-controlled trial of bilevel positive airway pressure in acute asthma attack. *Chest*. 2003;123:1018–1025.

18. Kohn MS. Intubation of the asthma patient. *Clin Allergy Immunol*. 1999;13:419–428.

19. Nee Pa, Benger J, Walls RM. Airway management. *Emerg Med J*. 2008;25:98–102.

20. L'Hommediu CS, Arens JJ. The use of ketamine for the emergency intubation of patients with status asthmaticus. *Ann Emerg Med*. 1987;16:568–571.

21. Lougheed MD, Fisher T, O'Donnell DE. Dynamic hyperinflation during bronchoconstriction in asthma: implications for symptom perception. *Chest*. 2006;130:1072–1081.

22. Brenner B, Corbridge T, Kazzi A. Intubation and mechanical ventilation of the asthmatic patient in respiratory failure. *J Emerg Med*. 2009;37(2 suppl):S23–S33.

23. Corbridge T, Corbridge S. Severe asthma exacerbation. In: Fink M, Abraham E, Vicent JL, Kochanek PM, eds. *Textbook of Critical Care*. 5th ed. Philadelphia: Elsevier Saunders; 2005:587–597.

24. Tuxen DV, Lane S. The effects of ventilator pattern on hyperinflation, airway pressures, and circulation in mechanical ventilation of patients with severe air-flow obstruction. *Am Rev Respir Dis*. 1987:136:872–879.

CHAPTER 11

Pulmonary Embolism

Rayan A. Rouhizad and Beth A. Longenecker

▶ PULMONARY EMBOLISM

Approximately 600,000 patients per year are diagnosed with pulmonary embolism (PE).[1] By far, most pulmonary emboli are thromboembolic in nature, although other causes, such as air, fat, amniotic fluid, tumor, and septic emboli, do occur.

▶ THROMBOEMBOLIC PULMONARY EMBOLISM

The risk factors for thromboembolic PE mirror those for deep venous thrombosis (DVT) and include recent surgery, malignancy, confinement to a hospital or nursing home, confinement to a bed ("bed rest"), immobility, oral contraceptives or hormone replacement therapy, and paresis of an extremity.[2] The mortality rate is high. In a large observational study of 2,388 hospitalized patients that evaluated cause of death, it was found that approximately 10% of all deaths were due to PE.[3] With prompt diagnosis and treatment, mortality can be significantly impacted and the incidence of long-term complications such as chronic thromboembolic pulmonary hypertension and cor pulmonale can be reduced.

▶ CLINICAL FEATURES

The clinical diagnosis of PE can be very challenging. The classic findings—or triad—of dyspnea, pleuritic chest pain, and tachycardia can be found in up to 95% of patients with confirmed PE. However, they are very nonspecific and could be indicative of any number of disorders. Furthermore, the first two, being symptoms, are difficult or impossible to evaluate in patients who are intubated and/or sedated, such as many ICU patients. Still, PE should be considered in any patient with any of these signs or symptoms.

Dyspnea is the most common symptom related to PE and is caused by a ventilation–perfusion (V/Q) mismatch. Chest pain is the second most common symptom, although up to one third of patients with PE deny chest pain or complain only of a vague chest discomfort. Hemoptysis secondary to PE is due to pulmonary infarction and is an uncommon and late finding. When present, it should significantly raise clinical suspicion. Fever is also rare but, if present, is usually "low grade" (<102°F), and appears more commonly when hemoptysis is present. Tachycardia is due to the cardiopulmonary stress created by the PE, but lacks sensitivity. Approximately 50% of all patients ultimately diagnosed with PE never demonstrated a persistent heart rate above 100 beats/min.[3] Furthermore, patients on chronic β-blocker therapy will likely not develop a tachycardic response. Other clinical findings include diaphoresis, anxiety, cough, rales, murmur, syncope, cyanosis, and altered mental status. Cardiac arrest occurs in approximately 2% of patients suffering an acute PE, with pulseless electrical activity the initial rhythm in 60% of patients and asystole in 33%.[4]

Patients presenting with any of the above clinical findings along with unilateral arm or leg swelling have a significant risk for both DVT and PE; yet the finding of a single swollen limb is often overlooked. In the previously mentioned study, of the 2,388 autopsies performed, 83% of the patients with confirmed PE had evidence of DVT in their lower extremities but only 19% of them had reported symptoms of DVT prior to death.[2]

▶ DIAGNOSTIC TESTING

The clinical presentation of PE can be very nonspecific and the consequences of misdiagnosis can be dire. Therefore, clinicians should have a low threshold for ordering diagnostic testing. Because the diagnosis of PE is often elusive, a large body of current research focuses on diagnostic strategies to assist in accurately identifying patients with an embolism.

Any patient complaining of chest pain should have an electrocardiogram (EKG) and chest x-ray (CXR). These tests are nonspecific, however, and are more useful for ruling out other diagnoses than for diagnosing PE, per se.

The most commonly seen EKG abnormalities are sinus tachycardia and nonspecific ST-segment and T-wave changes.[4] The classic EKG pattern of S1Q3T3, often quoted as "pathognomonic" for PE, is infrequently found. Furthermore, S1Q3T3 is not a specific finding for PE, so even when the pattern does appear, the diagnosis may still be other than PE. When it is found in the setting of PE, it is most commonly seen with massive acute PE and cor pulmonale. Overall, the EKG is best used to rule out other pathology, such as myocardial infarction and pericarditis.

Similarly, CXR is not sensitive for PE. Up to 25% of CXRs in patients with confirmed PE are normal. Nonspecific findings seen in patients with PE include atelectasis and pleural effusion, but these findings are equally common in patients without embolism.[5] The classic CXR findings of Hampton's Hump (a wedge-shaped consolidation in a peripheral lung field) and Westermark's sign (dilation of proximal pulmonary veins with decreased vascular markings in the periphery) are also very uncommon; however, when present, they should raise clinical suspicion significantly. Like the EKG, the CXR is best done to rule out other pathology such as pneumonia or pneumothorax, or to diagnose or lend weight to an alternate diagnosis such as aortic dissection or esophageal rupture that would alter the diagnostic workup.

Oxygen saturation (SaO_2) is an important tool when assessing for the possibility of a PE, and any degree of hypoxemia must be investigated. Conversely, an SaO_2 of 100% while breathing room air tends to favor the absence of a PE. It may also be useful to obtain an ABG to further assess the Pao_2 and $Paco_2$, and calculate the alveolar–arterial (A–a) gradient, as the sensitivity of an abnormal Pao_2 and/or A–a gradient is 90%.[7] Furthermore, for those patients with PE, an ABG may help risk stratify and guide treatment as the Pao_2 appears to correlate well with the extent of pulmonary vascular occlusion. However, a normal SaO_2 and/or ABG alone cannot exclude PE, as up to 18% of patients with this diagnosis will still have an SaO_2 of 100% and a Pao_2 between 85 and 105 mm Hg.[6]

Compared with the above testing modalities, the concept of testing for D-dimers is relatively new. As a thrombus is forming, natural anticoagulation systems within the body begin to break it down. A degradation product of cross-linked fibrin, D-dimers are released as a thrombus is broken down. Many studies have evaluated the utility of D-dimer levels for predicting the likelihood of PE. It was found that among patients with a low pretest probability, a normal D-dimer was associated with at least a 99% likelihood of not having a PE. Conversely, approximately 95% of patients with confirmed PE had an abnormal D-dimer. Current evidence indicates that D-dimer analysis using enzyme-linked immunosorbent assays (ELISA) yields the best results with >95% sensitivity. A negative quantitative ELISA result (<500 ng/mL) is generally felt to have a sufficient negative predictive value for PE when the pretest probability of a patient is low. Further complicating the assessment, however, is the multitude of D-dimer assays available, each with its own sensitivity and specificity. It is therefore important to be aware of the parameters of the assay available at a particular institution, as well as the threshold used for diagnosing a positive result. In general, however, D-dimer assays are only useful when negative and then only in the setting of a low-risk patient.[7–10]

The traditional test for evaluating for PE was a V/Q scan. A V/Q scan can be useful for the evaluation of a PE, and the PIOPED study published in 1990 had much to do with its widespread use. The study, which enrolled almost 1,000 patients across six centers, included inpatients and outpatients, although neither the number of each nor, for inpatients, floor versus ICU status was reported.

In the study, clinicians determined the probability of PE prior to a V/Q scan being performed. It was found that patients with a high clinical probability and high-probability V/Q scan had a 95% likelihood of having a PE. Patients with a low clinical probability and low-probability V/Q scan had only a 4% likelihood of having a PE. Perhaps most useful, a V/Q scan read as "normal" virtually excluded PE[11] (Note: "normal," *not* "low probability"). Unfortunately, in the ED, only approximately 33% of patients will have a normal V/Q scan and only another 10% will have a high-probability V/Q scan, leaving a large percentage of patients for whom this test cannot be considered diagnostic. These patients require further diagnostic studies to rule out PE. Therefore, many institutions have not made this their initial study of choice.

Pulmonary angiography has long been considered the "gold standard," and in some institutions it is the next study of choice in patients with nondiagnostic V/Q scans. However, due to the invasiveness of this procedure and the exposure to a significant contrast load, as well as the need for interventionalists to perform this study, it is reserved for patients in whom noninvasive

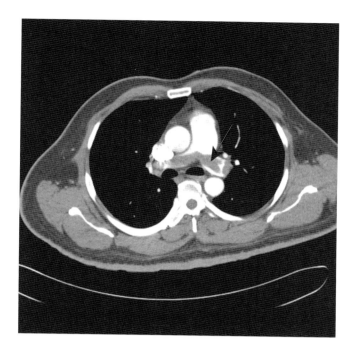

Figure 11-1. CT angiography with large bilateral central filling defects (arrow shows left pulmonary artery filling defect).

studies are either equivocal or discordant with strong clinical suspicion. It may also be considered in patients for whom treatment of a PE is highly risky (e.g., metastatic disease of the brain and CNS) and the practitioner desires to be "as sure as possible" in weighing the risks and benefits of treatment.

CT pulmonary angiography has become the diagnostic modality of choice in most institutions across the United States. It is easily available and it has the benefit of detecting alternative pulmonary abnormalities.[2-14] In one study, approximately 7% of CTs negative for PE found other abnormalities that required immediate attention, and another 10% required follow-up attention. In a large study of 824 patients, 83% of patients with a PE had a positive study (Figure 11-1), and 96% of patients without a PE had a negative study. CT angiography is also the study of choice in patients with an infiltrate on CXR or a history of emphysema, situations in which a V/Q scan is unlikely to be normal. There is great variation in sensitivity from institution to institution; this variability is dependent on the experience of the person reading the study, study quality, and resolution of the CT scanner. Furthermore, a pulmonary CT angiogram subjects the patient to radiation, high-pressure injection of nephrotoxic contrast medium, and transport out of the controlled environment of the ED or ICU. The clinician should take these concerns into consideration when ruling out PE as a diagnosis.

Echocardiography may be useful in unstable patients who cannot be transported, or for further

confirmatory data in patients with suspected PE and equivocal results. It may reveal abnormalities such as increased right ventricular size, decreased right ventricular function, or tricuspid regurgitation.

PREGNANCY AND PE

It has long been acknowledged that pregnancy increases the risk of venous thrombosis and thromboembolism, and that PE is a leading cause of maternal death.[15] This population presents a unique set of diagnostic challenges. D-dimer levels naturally increase during normal pregnancy, rendering the test relatively useless in ruling out thromboembolism if routine thresholds of 0.4–0.5 mg/L are used as a screening tool.[16]

Controversy still exists as to imaging modalities to utilize in pregnant patients with suspected PE. While lower extremity US may be useful if positive, there are many issues that may negatively impact sensitivity in pregnant females (increased diameter of lower extremity veins, decreased lower extremity venous flow velocity, nonpathologic leg swelling common in pregnancy).[17] Therefore, this test is helpful only if positive. Ultrasound, however, does not expose the fetus to ionizing radiation and therefore is often recommended for initial screening in this population.

V/Q scan is less likely to be equivocal among pregnant patients than in the general populace, but the negative predictive value of CT angiography remains higher than that of the V/Q scan.[18] Also, radiation dosages to the fetus are actually lower with CT angiography.[19] In spite of this, many physicians still prefer to order V/Q scans in their pregnant patients due to a misconception that this test exposes the fetus to less radiation.[20]

RISK STRATIFICATION AND PRETEST PROBABILITY

As noted above, the majority of diagnostic testing available for the diagnosis of PE has significant limitations or risks. Therefore, it has been suggested that decision making and diagnostic testing should also incorporate a pretest clinical probability score. In 2004, the PIOPED II study was published evaluating the utility of CT for a suspected PE. Patients were classified as low, moderate, or high probability using the Well's criteria for PE (Table 11-1). In patient groups with an intermediate or high pretest probability, a CT positive for PE was found in 89% and 99% of patients, respectively. In patient groups with a low or intermediate pretest probability, a CT positive for PE was found in 0.5% and 7% of patients, respectively.[21] One cost-effective approach in institutions where an ELISA D-dimer is rapidly available is to initially obtain a D-dimer on all patients deemed

▶ **TABLE 11-1. WELL'S CRITERIA FOR PULMONARY EMBOLUS**

Clinical Feature	Score
Clinical suspicion for DVT	3.0
Other diagnosis less likely than PE	3.0
Heart >100	1.5
Immobilization (3 or more days) or surgery in the previous 4 weeks	1.5
Previous DVT or PE	1.5
Hemoptysis	1.0
Malignancy (within 6 months or palliative treatment)	1.0
High probability	>6.0
Moderate probability	2.0–6.0
Low probability	<2.0

low risk based on their pretest probability. If negative, a CT does not need to be performed. If the patient has a moderate or high pretest probability for PE, D-dimer testing is not rapidly available, or clinical suspicion remains high despite low pretest probability, a CT pulmonary angiogram is recommended as the initial diagnostic modality. Patients with a CT negative for PE with a high clinical suspicion should undergo further diagnostic testing, likely with pulmonary angiography.

The above approach still yields a significant population that has a low score on the Well's criteria, a positive D-dimer, and, ultimately, a CT angiogram negative for PE. This has prompted further research in an attempt to determine if it is possible to establish criteria that place a patient at such low risk that even laboratory evaluation is not necessary. The pulmonary embolism rule-out criteria ("PERC criteria"), first published in 2004, is such an attempt (Table 11-2). In this study, patients felt to be at risk for PE who met none of the PERC criteria had a 1.6% chance of having an embolism. None of the patients clinically considered unlikely to have PE and who "ruled out" per PERC actually had a PE.[22] This study has been prospectively

▶ **TABLE 11-2. PULMONARY EMBOLISM RULE-OUT CRITERIA**

Age >50 years
Tachycardia (HR <100)
Pulse oximetry <95% on room air
Presence of hemoptysis
Patient taking exogenous estrogen
Patient has prior history of DVT or PE
History of recent surgery or trauma (in the preceding weeks)
Unilateral leg swelling
If any of the above applies, the patient is no longer at low risk for PE and requires further evaluation

validated with similar results.[23] Many clinicians now utilize a combination of "gestalt" and the PERC to determine a threshold for diagnostic testing; if the PERC is negative and the clinician has a low index of suspicion of PE in a particular patient, the risk of further testing outweighs benefit to the patient and no further testing is required to eliminate the diagnosis of PE.[24] It is important to remember that the PERC rule was not studied or validated for inpatients either on the floor or in the ICU.

TREATMENT

The main goal of treatment of PE is to maintain hemodynamic stability, reduce clot burden, and prevent extending or recurrent thrombosis. Initiating treatment early also helps decrease the incidence of the delayed complications of PE, such as chronic thromboembolic pulmonary hypertension and cor pulmonale. If treatment is not initiated early, the mortality rate reaches 30%, with the majority of these patients dying within the first few hours due to continued or recurrent thrombosis.[25]

As with all conditions, initial care of any patient presenting with suspected or diagnosed PE should focus on the status of the airway, breathing, and circulation. Hypoxic patients not needing ventilatory support should be placed on supplemental oxygen, but patients unable to maintain their airway, or who are in respiratory distress, should be intubated. Intravenous fluid (IVF) may be beneficial, but should be administered cautiously because large volumes may precipitate right ventricular failure. If a patient with hypotension does not respond to 500–1,000 cm³ of IVF, consider initiating vasopressor therapy.

The classic approach to treatment has been with unfractionated heparin (UFH) and should mirror dosages seen in the treatment of DVT. It may be prudent to initiate anticoagulation therapy prior to the diagnosis of PE in any patient with a high pretest probability, clinically high suspicion for massive PE, or unstable vital signs, especially if imaging is expected to be delayed.

LMWH has been shown to have similar efficacy and safety profiles as UFH in patients with PE and may be used in the treatment of acute PE. Some studies suggest it may also have a greater inhibition of in vivo thrombin generation.[26] Since all LMWHs are cleared by the kidneys, care must be taken when administering the drug to patients with renal insufficiency; do not use LMWH in patients with a creatinine greater than 2.0 mg/dL. The recommended dosing is 1 mg/kg subcutaneously every 12 hours or 1.5 mg/kg subcutaneously once per day. Although no large studies have shown any mortality benefit, thrombolytic therapy does improve other important parameters such as right ventricular function and pulmonary perfusion. Most studies advocate the use of thrombolytic therapy in any patient with persistent hypotension or hemodynamic instability and proven or clinical suspicion of a massive PE. Other clinical circumstances that may also benefit include severe hypoxemia, large perfusion defects, severe right ventricular dysfunction, free-floating right ventricular thrombus, and a patent foramen ovale.[27] The contraindications for thrombolysis for PE are the same as those when used for acute myocardial infarction or stroke. The most commonly used agents are alteplase (tPA) and urokinase.

Patients with contraindications for thrombolytics or who fail thrombolytic therapy may benefit from embolectomy. The procedure can be performed surgically or under fluoroscopic guidance with catheter fragmentation. These modalities of treatment are obviously very invasive and are limited only to institutions that have specialists experienced in these treatment modalities. Intraoperative mortality remains high, and there are no large studies available to guide decision making for transfer to tertiary care centers. It is likely that the high mortality is due to the extensive clot burden and hemodynamic compromise in patients considered for such interventions, rather than the actual procedure.[28]

Although not crucial in the acute setting (ED or ICU), at some point a decision must be made as to the optimal outpatient therapy. For cost considerations or because of patient ability, compliance, or preference, few patients maintain their therapy with outpatient injections of LMWH. For those patients who will not continue LMWH outside of the hospital, warfarin therapy should begin soon after the initiation of either UFH or LMWH. Once the INR is within 2.0–3.0 for 2 consecutive days, UFH or LMWH is discontinued. The patient should remain on warfarin for 3–6 months or indefinitely depending on his or her risk factors. Pregnant patients must be maintained on LMWH since warfarin is contraindicated as teratogenic and potentially lethal to the fetus, having been implicated in fatal fetal hemorrhage.

▶ VENOUS AIR EMBOLISM

Venous air emboli are usually iatrogenic in nature, usually occurring during central line insertion (although they have been reported after peripheral IV insertion). For patients who decompensate during or immediately after central line placement or manipulation, a venous air embolus should be strongly considered. For subclavian and internal carotid lines, immediate aspiration from the central line is warranted since, if the catheter is in the right atrium, remaining air may be aspirated. If the procedure was a femoral central line or peripheral

IV where the catheter does not extend to the heart, or if the procedure was a subclavian or internal carotid central line but aspirating does not help, a pulmonary artery catheter (PAC) may be placed and an attempt made to aspirate once the PAC is known to be in the right atrium. The patient should also be placed in the left lateral decubitus position as this position may "trap" the air in the right atrium, preventing further embolization to the lungs or beyond.

For patients who present after hyperbaric oxygen exposure (underwater divers, patients receiving hyperbaric oxygen therapy), the patient should be placed in the left lateral decubitus position. A PAC may similarly be placed and an attempt made at aspiration.

For female patients, especially if pregnant, who present to an emergency department with a history, symptoms, and signs consistent with PE along with a recent history of recipient orogenital intercourse, vaginal insufflation resulting in air emboli should be strongly considered. Therapy is the same as above.

For all patients with suspicion of air emboli, along with the above maneuvers, hyperbaric oxygen therapy may be considered if available and the patient may be safely moved to a chamber. For all patients in cardiac arrest unresponsive to CPR and ACLS, thoracotomy and needle aspiration of intracardiac air are appropriate.

▶ FAT OR BONE MARROW EMBOLISM

Fat, or bone marrow, PE is a risk after any bone fracture or surgery, but most often occurs following long bone fracture or surgery. Unfortunately, while corticosteroids before surgeries such as intramedullary nailing have been shown to decrease the incidence, no therapy has been shown to adequately treat fat emboli once they occur. Since it can be difficult to differentiate a thromboembolic from fat PE, and since thromboembolic PE is more common, it is reasonable to treat for thromboembolic PE as above, and provide other supportive therapy as necessary. For severe hemodynamic collapse, consideration may be given to placing the patient on cardiopulmonary bypass.

▶ AMNIOTIC FLUID EMBOLISM

Although amniotic fluid embolism is a consideration in the peripuerperal period, given the hypercoagulable state of pregnancy and increased risk of being bed bound before, during, and after vaginal delivery or C-section, thromboembolic PE is still more common. Therefore, since there has been no proven therapy for amniotic fluid embolism, and since thromboembolic PE is more common, as with fat embolism a reasonable approach is to treat for thromboembolic PE and provide other supportive therapy as indicated. As with antepartum patients discussed above, warfarin is teratogenic and should not be started until after delivery.

For septic emboli, the reader is referred to Chapter 38.

REFERENCES

1. Hirsh J, Hoak J. Management of deep vein thrombosis and pulmonary embolism. A statement for healthcare professionals. Council on Thrombosis (in consultation with the Council on Cardiovascular Radiology), American Heart Association. *Circulation*. 1996;93:2212.

2. Heit JA, Silverstien MD, Mohr DN, et al. Risk factors for deep venous thrombosis and pulmonary embolism: a population-based, case-controlled study. *Arch Int Med*. 2000;160:810–815.

3. Sandler DA, Martin JF. Autopsy proven pulmonary embolism in hospital patients: are we detecting enough deep vein thrombosis? *J R Soc Med*. 1989;82:203.

4. Courtney DM, Sasser H, Pincus B, et al. Pulseless electrical activity with witnesses arrest as a predictor of sudden death from massive pulmonary embolism in outpatients. *Resuscitation*. 2001;49:265.

5. Stein PD, Saltzman HA, Weg JG. Clinical characteristics of patients with acute pulmonary embolism. *Am J Cardiol*. 1991;68:1723.

6. Stein PD, Terrin ML, Hales CA, et al. Clinical, laboratory, roentgenographic and electrocardiographic findings in patients with acute pulmonary embolism and no pre-existing cardiac or pulmonary disease. *Chest*. 1991;100:598.

7. Kline JA, Nelson RD, Jackson RE, et al. Criteria for the safe use of d-dimer testing in emergency department patients with suspected pulmonary embolism: a multicenter Untied States study. *Ann Emerg Med*. 2002;39:144.

8. Kline JA, Johns KL, Coluciello SA, et al. New diagnostic tests for pulmonary embolism. *Ann Emerg Med*. 2000;35:168.

9. Kearon C, Ginsberg JS, Douketis J, et al. An evaluation of D-dimer in the diagnosis of pulmonary embolism: a randomized trial. *Ann Intern Med*. 2006;144:812.

10. Stein PD, Hull RD, Patel KC, et al. D-dimer for the exclusion of acute venous thrombosis and pulmonary embolism: a systematic review. *Ann Intern Med*. 2004;140:589.

11. Value of the ventilation/perfusion scan in acute pulmonary embolism. Results of the prospective investigation of pulmonary embolism diagnosis (PIOPED). The PIOPED Investigators. *JAMA*. 1990;263:2753.

12. Kim KI, Muller NL, Mayo JR. Clinically suspected pulmonary embolism: utility of spiral CT. *Radiology*. 1999;210:693.

13. Stein PD, Fowler SE, Goodman LR, et al. Multidetector computed tomography for acute pulmonary embolism. *N Engl J Med*. 2006;354:2317.

14. Richman PB, Courtney DM, Wood J, et al. Chest CT angiography (CTA) to rule out pulmonary embolism (PE) frequently reveals clinically significant ancillary findings—a multi-center study of 1025 emergency department patients. *Acad Emerg Med*. 2003;10:564.

15. Pabinger A, Grafenhofer H. Thrombosis during pregnancy: risk factors, diagnosis and treatment. *Pathophysiol Haemost Thromb*. 2002;32:322–323.

16. Kline JA, Williams GW, Hernandez-Nino J. D-dimer concentrations in normal pregnancy: new diagnostic thresholds are needed. *Clin Chem*. 2005;51:825–829.

17. Chan W-S, Ginsberg JS. Diagnosis of deep vein thrombosis and pulmonary embolism in pregnancy. *Thromb Res*. 2002;107:85–91.

18. Mathews S. Imaging pulmonary embolism in pregnancy: what is the most appropriate imaging protocol? *Br J Radiol*. 2006;79:441–444.

19. Winer-Muram HT, Boone JM, Brown HL, et al. Pulmonary embolism in pregnant patients: fetal radiation dose with helical CT. *Radiology*. 2002;224:487–490.

20. Groves AM, Yates SJ, Win T, et al. CT pulmonary angiography versus ventilation–perfusion scintigraphy in pregnancy: implications from a UK survey of doctors' knowledge of radiation exposure. *Radiology*. 2006;240:765–770.

21. Horlander KT, Mannino DM, Leeper KV. Pulmonary embolism mortality in the United States, 1979–1998: an analysis using multiple-cause mortality data. *Arch Intern Med*. 2003;163:1711.

22. Kline JA, Mitchell AM, Kabrhel C, et al. Clinical criteria to prevent unnecessary diagnostic testing in emergency department patients with suspected pulmonary embolism. *J Thromb Haemost*. 2004;2:1247–1255.

23. Kline JA, Courtney DM, Kabrhel CL, et al. Prospective multicenter evaluation of the pulmonary embolism rule-out criteria. *J Thromb Haemost*. 2006;6:772–780.

24. Lessler AL, Isserman JA, Agarwal R, et al. Testing low-risk patients for suspected pulmonary embolism: a decision analysis. *Ann Emerg Med*. 2010;55(4):316–326.e1. Epub 2010 Jan 12.

25. Kucher N, Goldhaber SZ. Management of massive pulmonary embolism. *Circulation*. 2005;112:e28.

26. Kakkar VV, Hoppenstead DA, Fareed J, et al. Randomized trial of different regimens of heparins and in vivo thrombin generation in acute deep vein thrombosis. *Blood*. 2002;99:1965.

27. Buller HR, Agnelli G, Hull RD, et al. Antithrombotic therapy for venous thromboembolic disease: the Seventh ACCP Conference on Antithrombotic and Thrombolytic Therapy. *Chest*. 2004;126:401s.

28. Aklog L, Williams CS, Byrne JG, et al. Acute pulmonary embolectomy: a contemporary approach. *Circulation*. 2002;105:1416–1419.

SECTION IV

Cardiovascular Disorders

CHAPTER 12

Hemodynamic and Perfusion Monitoring

Elizabeth Lea Walters and H. Bryant Nguyen

▶ INTRODUCTION

Critically ill patients are frequently encountered in the emergency department and ICU, and practitioners in both locations are required to quickly identify and resuscitate unstable patients. Additionally, with the problems of hospital overcrowding and subsequent boarding of critical patients in the ED, hemodynamic management after the initial resuscitation is mandatory in the ED.

Hemodynamic monitoring is an integral part of the management of critically ill patients, having a diagnostic, therapeutic, and resuscitation role. The analysis of hemodynamic variables beyond traditional vital signs allows the clinician to differentiate various causes of hemodynamic instability and intervene appropriately. This chapter will discuss hemodynamic monitoring methods.

▶ ARTERIAL BLOOD PRESSURE MONITORING

Arterial blood pressure is a measure of the force exerted by circulating blood through a blood vessel. It is regulated via changes in the α-adrenergic tone of afferent vessels and varies in the different organs. Since cerebral and coronary vessels have few α-adrenergic receptors, tissue perfusion depends directly on perfusion pressure. However, tissue perfusion pressure cannot be measured directly, and arterial blood pressure has been used as a surrogate.[1]

Cardiac output (CO) and vascular tone are controlled via autoregulation, and hypotension reflects a failure of these mechanisms. Hypotension can result from severe cardiogenic or hemorrhagic shock (decreased CO), despite preserved vasomotor tone, or from a primary loss of vasomotor tone independent of CO, as in spinal cord trauma and septic shock. Normal blood pressure could occur in the setting of circulatory shock if systemic vasomotor tone proportionally increases. As a result, hypotension is always pathologic and reflects a failure of normal circulatory homeostatic mechanisms. On the other hand, normotension does not equate cardiovascular stability.

Autoregulation is determined by mean arterial pressure (MAP), and the normal range for most tissues is 65–120 mm Hg. As MAP decreases below 60 mm Hg, organ perfusion pressure is compromised and, if sustained, results in organ failure and death.[2] Thus, one target of hemodynamic monitoring is to keep the MAP higher than 65 mm Hg. However, the optimal MAP varies according to the underlying cause of hemodynamic instability. For example, in septic shock, increasing MAP greater than 65 mm Hg with fluids and vasopressors increases oxygen delivery, but does not improve indices of organ perfusion.[3] In fact, use of vasopressors to increase MAP higher than 65 mm Hg may actually result in increased mortality.[4] In cardiogenic shock, ACC/AHA guidelines recommend a systolic blood pressure (SBP) of 100 mm Hg in patients with acute myocardial infarction.[5] And in traumatic brain injury, observational studies suggested an SBP less than 90 mm Hg was an independent predictor for increased morbidity and mortality.[6] For hemorrhagic shock, delayed fluid resuscitation and tolerating an MAP of 40 mm Hg until definitive surgical intervention has been shown to improve survival.[7] Based on this evidence, the International Consensus Conference made the following recommendations: MAP >40 mm Hg in uncontrolled hemorrhage due to trauma, SBP >90 mm Hg for traumatic brain injury, and MAP >65 mm Hg for other forms of shock.[8]

SBP represents maximum pressure during ventricular ejection, diastolic pressure is the lowest pressure in the blood vessels between heart beats during ventricular filling, and pulse pressure is the difference between the two. Both SBP and diastolic pressure vary significantly throughout the vascular system. Thus, SBP can increase by up to 20 mm Hg, while the diastolic pressure similarly decreases as the pressure wave moves from the aorta to the periphery. However, MAP varies by only 1–2 mm Hg throughout the arterial system.[9] MAP can be estimated as the sum of the diastolic pressure and one third of the pulse pressure.[10]

NONINVASIVE MEASUREMENT

Palpation

SBP can be estimated by palpation of the radial, femoral, or carotid pulse in an emergency situation, with a minimum SBP of 80, 70, or 60 mm Hg, respectively. However, this method overestimates SBP when compared with invasive measurements in patients with hypovolemic shock.[11]

Sphygmomanometry

The most common method of determining arterial blood pressure is through the use of sphygmomanometry. With sphygmomanometry, blood pressure can be measured using auscultation of Korotkoff sounds or via automated oscillometric devices.[10] With oscillometric devices, the point of maximal oscillation corresponds to MAP. SBP and diastolic pressure are estimated by an empiric algorithm.[12] Oscillometric devices, in general, are more accurate than auscultation, although they may underestimate systolic blood pressure by as much as 19% and overestimate diastolic blood pressure up to 27%.[13] Variability in the auscultatory method can be due to improper cuff size, cuff placement, placement of the stethoscope bell, cuff deflation rate, dysrhythmia, observer bias, and faulty equipment.[14]

INVASIVE MEASUREMENT

Korotkoff sounds and pressure oscillations are diminished in patients with marked vasoconstriction and can underestimate SBP by more than 30 mm Hg when compared with direct measurements.[15] Invasive monitoring via intra-arterial catheterization provides instantaneous measures of MAP.

The radial artery is the most frequent site for arterial catheterization, although the femoral artery may be preferred in emergent situations and hypotensive patients.[16] Except in states of severe peripheral vasoconstriction, where radial measurements may underestimate central pressure,[9] radial and femoral artery measurements are interchangeable.[17] Other potential sites including axillary, brachial, dorsalis pedis, ulnar, tibial posterialis, and temporal arteries are rarely used.

After successful arterial catheterization, connection of the catheter to the pressure transducer should reveal an arterial waveform. The square wave flush test is applied to determine if artifact in the tubing and recording system is damping the pressure measurements (Figure 12-1). The most common source of error is due to air bubbles in the tubing system.[9] An overdamped system suggests trapped air bubbles in the tubing, resulting in falsely lowered pressure measurements, while an underdamped system will result in excessive resonance and overestimation of SBP and underestimation of diastolic pressure. Further flushing of the system to remove the air bubbles or replacement of the tubing may be required. Indications for arterial catheterization are illustrated in Table 12-1.

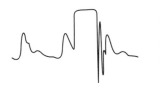

Optimally damped:
1.5 – 2 oscillations before returning to tracing. Values obtained are accurate.

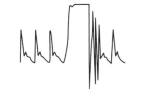

Underdamped:
> 2 oscillations. Overestimated systolic pressure, diastolic pressures may be underestimated.

Overdamped:
< 1.5 oscillations. Underestimation of systolic pressures, diastolic may not be affected.

Figure 12-1. Square wave flush test. A bolus flush of the catheter results in a square wave tracing. The number of oscillations before returning to the blood pressure tracing indicates proper damping.

► **TABLE 12-1. INDICATIONS FOR PLACEMENT OF AN ARTERIAL CATHETER**

- Continuous blood pressure monitoring of hemodynamically unstable patients
- Monitoring for optimal MAP during administration of vasoactive drugs
- Frequent blood draws for blood gases and other laboratory studies
- Calculation of pulse pressure variation (PPV) and cardiac output (CO) via pulse contour analysis

► **TABLE 12-2. FACTORS AFFECTING CENTRAL VENOUS PRESSURE**

Central venous blood volume	Venous return Cardiac output Total blood volume Regional vascular tone Vascular tone Compliance of right ventricle
Cardiovascular compliance	Myocardial disease Pericardial disease Cardiac tamponade Changes with respiration
Intrathoracic pressure	Positive end-expiratory pressure (PEEP) Intermittent positive pressure ventilation Tension pneumothorax
Tricuspid valve disease	Stenosis Regurgitation Junctional rhythm
Dysrhythmia	Atrial fibrillation Atrioventricular dissociation
Transducer reference level	Position of patient

Adapted from Polanco PM, Pinsky MR. Practical issues of hemodynamic monitoring at the bedside. *Surg Clin North Am.* 2006;86:1431–1456.

► MONITORING CENTRAL VENOUS PRESSURE

Intravenous fluids are a mainstay in the resuscitation of critical patients and are used to increase CO and arterial pressure to improve tissue oxygenation. In fact, 50% of critically ill patients will have improvement in CO and cardiac index (CI) when given a fluid challenge.[2,18]

Central venous pressure (CVP) is the pressure in the great thoracic veins proximal to the right atrium. It is measured at end expiration and is determined relative to atmospheric pressure. Using this definition, CVP may not be an accurate representation of intravascular volume as it can be affected by both anatomic and physiologic factors, such as tricuspid valve disease, cardiac compliance, abnormal right ventricular function, pulmonary vasculature disease, and arrhythmias. Other factors can also affect its measurement (Table 12-2). Thus, CVP in and of itself does not reflect blood volume status.[18,19]

While CVP monitoring is generally useful to assess global volume status, it is less useful as a guide to resuscitation. The relationship between CO and intravascular volume changes is depicted by the Starling curve. Unfortunately, a static measurement of CVP does not show where along that curve an individual patient's measurements are located. However, as an indicator of volume status, most clinicians accept that a low CVP indicates hypovolemia, while an elevated measurement suggests volume overload, with normal ranges from 0 to 10 mm Hg.[20]

Although studies have shown that measures of CVP do not necessarily correlate with circulating blood volume and even changes in CVP may not correlate with changes in blood volume, a CVP lower than 4 mm Hg in the critically ill patient should prompt fluid resuscitation with careful monitoring.[8,19] The "5–2 rule" by Weil et al to estimate a patient's volume status may be performed rapidly in the ED.[21] An initial CVP measurement is obtained, and then a 10–20 mL/min bolus of normal saline is infused for 10–15 minutes (e.g., 250 mL over 15 minutes). An increase in CVP >5 mm Hg would indicate volume overload. However, if CVP increases 2 mm Hg or less, hypovolemia should be suspected and a second fluid bolus given. Incorporated in a therapeutic protocol, CVP of 8–12 mm Hg during resuscitation of the critically ill patient in the ED is a reasonable target.[22]

NONINVASIVE MEASUREMENT

Jugular Venous Pulsation

When invasive measurement of CVP is not feasible, internal jugular venous pulsation (JVP) may be used to estimate right atrial pressure.[23] The sternal angle is approximately 5 cm above the center of the right atrium regardless of the patient's position. To obtain JVP, position the patient at a 45° angle. The vertical distance between the jugular pulsation and the sternal angle is added to that 5 cm to estimate CVP in cm H_2O. The upper limit of normal for the internal jugular vein (IJV) to pulsate is approximately 4.5 cm vertically above the sternal angle (or 9.5 cm H_2O total). Any pulsation above 4.5 cm at 45° indicates an elevated CVP. Visualization of the IJV pulsation by physical examination is not always possible in the ED, especially in trauma, obese, or uncooperative patients.

Ultrasonography

Ultrasound can be used to determine elevated jugular venous pressure in the ED. The right IJV is viewed

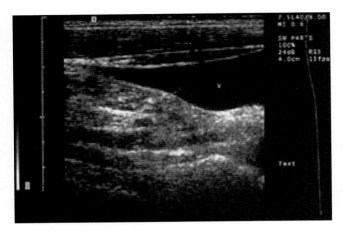

Figure 12-2. Estimating jugular venous pressure. An ultrasound longitudinal view of the internal jugular vein shows tapering at the point of jugular venous pulsation. (Reproduced with permission from Lipton B. Estimation of central venous pressure by ultrasound of the internal jugular vein. *Am J Emerg Med.* 2000;18:432–434.)

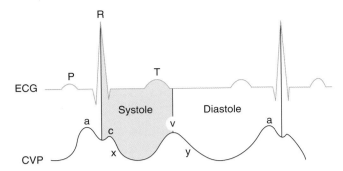

Figure 12-3. Central venous pressure waveform. Comparing the central venous waveform with the electrocardiogram waveform: (*a-wave*) atrial contraction, (*c-wave*) bulging of tricuspid valve into the right atrium at onset of systole, (*x-descent*) atrial relaxation, (*v-wave*) increase in atrial pressure due to venous return during systole, before the tricuspid valve opens, and (*y-descent*) atrial emptying into the ventricles during diastole.

with a high-frequency linear transducer (7–9 MHz). In the transverse plane with the patient in a semi-upright position, CVP is greater than 10 cm H_2O if it appears distended and larger than the adjacent common carotid artery. A near-complete collapsed IJV in the transverse view in the supine position indicates a very low CVP. In one recent study, measurement of the IJV with ultrasound showed a mean diameter in patients with CVP less than 10 cm H_2O was 7.0 mm versus 12.5 mm in patients with CVP of 10 cm H_2O and greater. Measurement of end-expiratory diameter in supine patients exhibited a high correlation to invasive measures of CVP.[24]

Another method is to visualize the right internal jugular in the longitudinal plane. With the patient in a semi-upright position, the location at which the vein tapers (collapses) is the site of the JVP (Figure 12-2). The vertical distance in centimeters between this point of vein collapse and the sternal angle is measured, and added to 5 cm, giving JVP in cm H_2O.[25]

INVASIVE MEASUREMENT

Traditionally, CVP is monitored by placing a fluid-filled catheter into the internal jugular or subclavian vein with the tip in the distal superior vena cava. The transducer should be placed at the level of the right atrium, or approximately 5 cm below the sternal angle. Because CVP measurement is affected by respirations, measurement should be taken at the end of expiration when pleural pressure has minimal effect and CVP closely approximates cardiac transmural pressure. An acceptable CVP waveform is shown in Figure 12-3. The c-wave

represents bulging of the tricuspid valve into the right atrium and occurs at the onset of systole. The base of the *c-wave* is used to determine a CVP value because it is the final pressure in the ventricle before the onset of contraction, reflecting *preload*.[20]

Occasionally, in patients with coagulopathy, patients in whom subclavian and/or IJV catheterization was unsuccessful or resulted in a complication, or those requiring immediate access, femoral vein catheterization is required to measure CVP. Studies have shown that femoral CVP may be reliable, although use of this site is often discouraged due to increased risk of infection and hematoma formation.[26] Other studies have shown that changes in venous pressure measured from a peripheral vein may correlate with similar changes in CVP.[27] Complications associated with placement of central venous lines are listed in Table 12-3. Other indications for central venous catheterization include fluid and vasopressor administration, unsuccessful or inadequate peripheral venous access, central venous oxygenation ($ScvO_2$) measurement, pulmonary artery catheterization, and transvenous pacemaker placement.

▶ CARDIAC OUTPUT MONITORING

The primary goal of resuscitation from shock is to reverse tissue hypoperfusion. Oxygen delivery is reliant on CO and the delivery of oxygenated arterial blood to the tissues. CO is in turn affected by the interaction of preload, contractility, and afterload. Vital signs and physical exam are not sufficient to estimate CO.[8] Additionally, CO does not have "normal values," but varies according to metabolic demand.

▶ **TABLE 12-3. COMPLICATIONS OF CENTRAL VENOUS LINES**

	Internal Jugular Vein (%)	Subclavian Vein (%)	Femoral Vein (%)
Arterial puncture	6.3–9.4	3.1–4.9	9.0–15.0
Hematoma	<0.1–2.2	1.2–2.1	3.8–4.4
Pneumothorax	<0.1–0.2	1.5–3.1	N/A
Hemothorax	N/A	0.4–0.6	N/A
Local infection	4.6	1.4	13.2
Blood stream infection	1.8	0.9	6.9

Data are from Merrer J, De Jonghe B, Golliot F, et al. Complications of femoral and subclavian venous catheterization in critically ill patients: a randomized controlled trial. *JAMA*. 2001; 286:700–707; Sznajder JI, Zveibil FR, Bitterman H, Weiner P, Bursztein S. Central vein catheterization:failure and complication rates bythree percutaneous approaches. *Arch Intern Med*. 1986;146:259–261; Mansfield PF, Hohn DC, Fornage BD, Gregurich MA, Ota DM. Complications and failures of subclavian-vein catheterization. *N Engl J Med*. 1994;331:1735–1738; Martin C, Eon B, Auffray JP, Saux P, Gouin F. Axillary or internal jugular central venous catheterization. *Crit Care Med*. 1990;18:400–402; Durbec O, Viviand X, Potie F, Vialet R, Albanese J, Martin C. A prospective evaluation of the use of femoral venous catheters in critically ill adults. *Crit Care Med*. 1997;25:1986–1989; Timsit JF, Bruneel F, Cheval C, et al. Use of tunneled femoral catheters to prevent catheter-related infection: a randomized, controlled trial. *Ann Intern Med*. 1999;130:729–735.

Monitoring CO helps guide treatment and response in the unstable patient. An increase in CO of >15% after a fluid challenge has been considered the gold standard reflecting fluid responsiveness.[18] Continued fluid boluses when CO does not increase can result in fluid overload and pulmonary edema. Determining the endpoint of fluid responsiveness allows optimization of CO, blood pressure, and organ perfusion. This relationship is depicted by Starling's law (Figure 12-4).[28] Thus, the focus in resuscitation should be a relative change in CO in response to therapy rather than a specific CO value.

Venous return related to respiratory changes in the intubated patient displays several predictable changes in vena caval diameters, pulmonary blood flow, and left ventricular (LV) output. In the *volume-responsive* patient, increasing intrathoracic pressure during positive-pressure inspiration decreases the pressure gradient for venous return. This results in narrowing of the venae cavae, decrease in pulmonary blood flow, and a three- to four-beat phase lag decrease in LV stroke volume and arterial pulse pressure.[2] This cyclic variation in stroke volume and arterial pulse pressure, or pulse pressure variation (PPV), reflects volume responsiveness. A PPV greater than 13% predicts a greater than 15% increase in CO after a 500-mL crystalloid bolus.[29] In high-risk surgery patients, fluid administration until

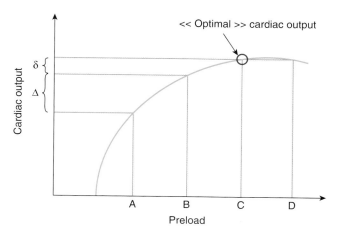

Figure 12-4. Starling's cardiac function curve. An increase in preload increases cardiac output until *optimal cardiac output* is reached (preload dependent). Initial preload increases (A to B) result in greater changes (Δ), while additional increases (B to C) have a lesser effect on cardiac output (δ). Further increases in preload beyond this point (C to D) will not result in increased cardiac output (preload independent) and may result in fluid overload and pulmonary edema.

the PPV decreased to less than 10% demonstrated improved outcome with decreased length of hospital stay.[30] However, for PPV to be accurate, the patient must be intubated and sedated so that respirations are fully synchronized with the ventilator, and without any significant dysrhythmias.[17]

In spontaneously breathing patients, postural changes such as passive leg raising (PLR) can assess volume responsiveness. The legs are raised to 30° above the chest and held for 1–2 minutes. This maneuver approximates a blood bolus similar to autotransfusion of 300 mL in a 70-kg patient that persists for approximately 2–3 minutes. Changes in heart rate, blood pressure, CVP, or CO are then observed. Studies have demonstrated that the dynamic increases in CO induced by PLR are as sensitive and specific to predicting volume responsiveness as PPV during positive-pressure mechanical ventilation.[31]

INVASIVE MEASUREMENT

CO is traditionally measured invasively with pulmonary artery catheterization. A pulmonary artery catheter (PAC; Swan–Ganz) is inserted through a large-bore introducer catheter. The PAC has a thermistor (to sense changes in temperature) located 4 cm from the tip, and a proximal port located 30 cm from the tip. CO is measured by injecting cold fluid through the proximal port, and then measuring the change in temperature of the blood over time at the thermistor. A temperature versus time curve

▶ **TABLE 12-4. HEMODYNAMIC VARIABLES OBTAINED BY THE PULMONARY ARTERY CATHETER**

- Cardiac output
- Central venous pressure
- Pulmonary artery occlusion pressure
- (Pulmonary capillary wedge pressure)
- Pulmonary vascular resistance
- Systemic vascular resistance
- Pulmonary artery pressure
- Ventricular stroke work
- Right ventricular end-systolic and end-diastolic volume
- Mixed and central venous oxygen saturation
- Systemic oxygen delivery
- Systemic oxygen consumption

is plotted and analyzed by a computer connected to the catheter, providing a *thermodilution* CO (or blood flow rate in liters per minute). Other measurements obtained by the PAC are listed in Table 12-4.

A number of studies have demonstrated PAC usage increases patient risk and utilization of resources.[32,33] However, subsequent randomized trials demonstrated no harm, but also no benefit.[34] Given the controversies and risks associated with the PAC, current expert consensus does not recommend the routine use of the PAC in the emergency department.[8] However, in patients with suspected pulmonary arterial hypertension, right ventricular dysfunction, or requiring complex fluid management, PA catheterization may still have a role in the intensive care unit.[35]

Complications from PAC insertion are similar to those of central venous catheterization. Additional complications include cardiac perforation, pulmonary artery perforation, tricuspid and pulmonary valve injury, knotting of the catheter, dysrhythmia, and heart block.

NONINVASIVE AND MINIMALLY INVASIVE MEASUREMENT

To avoid the complications associated with placement of the PAC, several noninvasive hemodynamic monitoring techniques have been devised to monitor CO.[36]

Thoracic Electrical Bioimpedance

Thoracic electrical bioimpedance (TEB) determines CO based on electrical impedance (or resistance) across the chest wall.[37] Electrodes placed on the chest measure changes in impedance, which reflect changes in blood volume within the thorax. Since the majority of flow through the thorax occurs in the aorta and vena cavae, the changes in impedance that occur in the thorax reflect changes in volume and CO within

these great vessels. Recent studies have used TEB to guide clinician assessment of ED patients with dyspnea and showed that this technology can improve the physician's differentiation of cardiac from noncardiac causes of dyspnea, and change the physician's therapeutic plan for these patients.[38] Although current studies show acceptable correlation to some invasive criterion standard measurement, TEB has some limitations, including a less reliable signal with patient movement, poor contact or placement of the skin electrodes, or any process that increases intrathoracic blood volume.[39] Additionally, cardiac dysrhythmias can affect TEB readings.

A modification to bioimpedance is *bioreactance* that uses a signal filter to analyze the relative frequency shift of the current across the thoracic cavity between the chest electrodes, rather than the changes in signal amplitude. This results in a greater signal-to-noise ratio, making it less sensitive to patient movement and external interference. Initial validation studies comparing bioreactance and PAC thermodilution CO conclude that it has acceptable accuracy.[40]

Esophageal Doppler Ultrasound

Esophageal Doppler ultrasound (EDUS) determines CO by measuring blood flow velocity in the descending aorta to determine stroke volume. A Doppler transducer probe is inserted orally or nasally into the esophagus until its tip is located at the mid-thoracic level and the characteristic signal profile is obtained. The cross-sectional area of the descending aorta is calculated via an algorithm based on the patient's age and body mass index. Using this metric, stroke volume is determined using standard transthoracic Doppler echocardiography.[41] Stroke volume is multiplied by the heart rate to give CO (CO = stroke volume × heart rate).

EDUS has high accuracy when compared with the standard PAC in measuring CO.[42] In randomized clinical trials, EDUS used in a perioperative resuscitation protocol resulted in optimal fluid resuscitation, decreased hospital length of stay, and decreased postoperative complications when compared with standard therapy.[43,44] This technology has several limitations, including operator-dependent ability to obtain and maintain the signal, need for frequent repositioning, especially with any patient movement, and discomfort in the nonventilated patient. However, the use of this technology resulted in none of the complications commonly associated with invasive central venous catherization, such as pneumothorax or arterial puncture.[45] In the ED setting, measurements of hemodynamic profile using EDUS resulted in change in shock characterization in 52% of patients, and changes in treatment plans in 68% of patients.[46]

Transcutaneous Doppler Ultrasound

Transcutaneous Doppler ultrasound (TCDUS) is similar to EDUS, except that a handheld probe is placed at the suprasternal notch with the transducer aimed downward at the aortic valve. Transaortic blood flow velocity profiles are obtained, and CO is calculated from the flow parameters. Recent validation studies comparing TCDUS with PAC measurements of CO showed that the TCDUS measurements have acceptable accuracy.[47] Interrater reliability for this technology in the ED setting is also adequate.[48] However, operator training is crucial and may require multiple patient assessments to gain proficiency.[49]

Pulse Pressure Waveform Analysis

Pulse pressure waveform analysis provides continuous monitoring of CO. Proprietary algorithms from various manufacturers analyze the arterial pressure waveform (or the pulse contour), obtained from an intra-arterial catheter. Using diastolic pressure as the baseline, the arterial pulse pressure waveform varies as a function of arterial compliance and stroke volume. Stroke volume is estimated by determining the area under the curve of the pulse waveform. Since arterial compliance varies significantly depending on blood pressure, patient condition, and any medication (e.g., vasopressor usage), the CO measured has to be regularly calibrated with some other reference standard. The two common reference standards for calibration are lithium dilution and transpulmonary thermodilution, which use changes in concentration or temperature over time, similar to the thermodilution method of the PAC.[50] A more advanced algorithm of pulse contour waveform analysis was recently introduced that does not require calibration with a CO reference standard.[51] No study has examined the accuracy of these technologies in the ED setting, but in the ICU and operating room, the arterial thermodilution calibrated pulse contour analysis method has been shown to be accurate and sensitive to small dynamic changes in CO, whereas pulse contour analysis without calibration was less validated.[52]

▶ ORGAN OXYGENATION AND PERFUSION MONITORING

The desired end result of hemodynamic monitoring is to improve tissue perfusion. However, optimal hemodynamics do not necessarily equal tissue perfusion. Recent literature has focused on microcirculation and markers of tissue hypoxia. Two methods are readily available to emergency physicians, as well as a number of promising experimental monitoring devices.

MIXED CENTRAL VENOUS SATURATION (SvO$_2$) AND CENTRAL VENOUS OXYGEN SATURATION (ScvO$_2$)

Venous oxygen saturation monitoring assesses the tissue oxygen extraction and the balance between oxygen delivery (DO$_2$) and oxygen consumption (VO$_2$). Normal oxygen extraction ratio (OER) is 25–35% and results in a venous oxygen saturation of approximately 70% of arterial DO$_2$. Venous oxygen saturation is ideally measured in the pulmonary artery as a mixed venous sample (SvO$_2$). Clinically, SvO$_2$ reflects the balance between DO$_2$ and VO$_2$, with low values reflecting inadequate DO$_2$ and/or excessive VO$_2$.

Measurement of SvO$_2$ requires placement of a PAC, while *central* venous oxygen saturation (ScvO$_2$) measurement only requires placement of a central venous catheter in the internal jugular or subclavian vein. ScvO$_2$ can be measured by drawing a standard venous blood gas from the distal port of the central venous catheter and obtaining a *measured* oxygen saturation. Continuous measurement can be performed using specialized catheters and monitors equipped with infrared oximetry and reflection spectrophotometry.

Because ScvO$_2$ reflects the oxygen balance for the upper portion of the body and does not include venous return from the coronary sinus, a large number of studies have compared ScvO$_2$ with SvO$_2$ that reflects the entire body. While ScvO$_2$ is 2–3% less than SvO$_2$ in healthy individuals, in shock states, ScvO$_2$ is typically 5–10% *higher* than SvO$_2$ as blood flow is redistributed from the abdominal vascular beds to the cerebral and coronary circulation.[53]

Clinical Use of ScvO$_2$

During initial management, despite normalization of vital signs and urine output, global tissue hypoxia may still be present.[54] ScvO$_2$ is able to detect occult inadequate DO$_2$. Regardless of the underlying cause, a low ScvO$_2$ value represents inadequate DO$_2$ relative to VO$_2$.[55] Understanding that DO$_2$ is inadequate allows the clinician to focus on the cause. DO$_2$ is dependent on CO, oxygen saturation, and hemoglobin. VO$_2$ is increased with heightened metabolic demand. Clinically, hypoxia and anemia are generally easily diagnosed and treated. Thus, a low ScvO$_2$ can be useful in suggesting that occult low CO may exist, prompting further investigation and treatment.

ScvO$_2$, as well as SvO$_2$, is a global measure of oxygen transport, and does not identify which tissues are hypoperfused. Regional areas of tissue hypoperfusion can be present even with normal ScvO$_2$ values, particularly in the lower half of the body. Additionally, certain clinical entities (e.g., terminal shock, hypothermia, cyanide poisoning) impair the ability of the tissues to extract oxygen from the blood, leading to decreased OER and high $ScvO_2$.

Targeting a normal (approximately 70%) SvO_2 as a therapeutic endpoint in the management of ICU patients has not been shown to result in improved outcome.[56] However, inclusion of $ScvO_2$ monitoring in a treatment protocol, which includes targeting CVP 8–12 mm Hg, MAP >65 mm Hg, and $ScvO_2$ >70%, for severe sepsis and septic shock patients after arrival to the ED (i.e., *early goal-directed therapy*) was shown to result in a significant mortality benefit.[22,57]

LACTATE

When DO_2 is inadequate to meet tissue oxygen demand, cellular metabolism enters an anaerobic phase. Lactate is a byproduct of anaerobic metabolism and a marker of global tissue hypoxia. Numerous studies have shown that lactate levels above 4 mmol/L (normal <2 mmol/L) are associated with worse patient outcome.[58] More important than a single lactate values is lactate clearance.[59–61] Multiple studies have demonstrated that the time to lactate clearance is critical, with times >48 hours resulting in higher morbidity and mortality.[59] Lactate clearance <24 hours is optimal for increasing survival, as lactate clearance >24 hours is associated with mortality as high as 90%.[60,61] However, lactate also increases in disease states other than shock (Table 12-5). Lactate can also have delayed clearance in patients with underlying liver disease due to impaired hepatic clearance. In the ED, the ability to decrease lactate as early as 6 hours in patients with severe sepsis or septic shock is associated with increased 60-day survival.[62]

▶ **TABLE 12-5. CONDITIONS RESULTING IN ELEVATED LACTATE**

Mechanism	Example
Tissue hypoperfusion or hypoxia	Hypotension from any cause
	Severe anemia
	Respiratory insufficiency
	Carbon monoxide poisoning
	Regional tissue hypoperfusion
Increased oxygen demand	Sepsis
	Seizure activity
	Strenuous exercise
Decreased metabolism of pyruvate	Cyanide poisoning
	Salicylate toxicity
	Thiamine deficiency
	Inborn errors of metabolism
Delayed clearance	Renal or hepatic dysfunction

EXPERIMENTAL MONITORING TECHNIQUES

Central venous oxygen saturation and lactate are measures of global hypoxia. With the current interest in assessing microcirculation, new technologies are continuously being developed and refined.[63] While these techniques remain investigational, near-infrared spectroscopy to measure peripheral tissue oxygenation has received much attention in the literature.[64–66] Other investigational modalities include orthogonal polarization spectroscopy (OPS), sublingual partial pressure of carbon dioxide ($PslCO_2$), and transcutaneous oxygen tension.[67]

▶ SUMMARY

Emergency physicians are managing greater numbers of critically ill patients, and for longer periods of time. Hemodynamic monitoring is used to identify cardiovascular instability, help determine etiology, and guide effective therapy. While no single hemodynamic variable should be used as an absolute target, understanding what modalities are available, how to optimize patient diagnosis and treatments, and understanding the overall changes in hemodynamics in response to therapies can reduce patient morbidity and mortality.

REFERENCES

1. Polanco PM, Pinsky MR. Practical issues of hemodynamic monitoring at the bedside. *Surg Clin North Am.* 2006;86:1431–1456.
2. Pinsky MR, Payen D. Functional hemodynamic monitoring. *Crit Care.* 2005;9:566–572.
3. Bourgoin A, Leone M, Delmas A, et al. Increasing mean arterial pressure in patients with septic shock: effects on oxygen variables and renal function. *Crit Care Med.* 2005;33:780–786.
4. Hayes MA, Timmins AC, Yau EH, et al. Elevation of systemic oxygen delivery in the treatment of critically ill patients. *N Engl J Med.* 1994;330:1717–1722.
5. Antman EM, Anbe DT, Armstrong PW, et al. ACC/AHA guidelines for the management of patients with ST-elevation myocardial infarction: a report of the American College of Cardiology/American Heart Association Task Force on Practice Guidelines (Committee to Revise the 1999 Guidelines for the Management of Patients with Acute Myocardial Infarction). *Circulation.* 2004;110:e82–e292.
6. Bratton SL, Chestnut RM, Ghajar J, et al. Guidelines for the management of severe traumatic brain injury. I. Blood pressure and oxygenation. *J Neurotrauma.* 2007;24(suppl 1):S7–S13.
7. Stern SA, Dronen SC, Birrer P, et al. Effect of blood pressure on hemorrhage volume and survival in a near-fatal

hemorrhage model incorporating a vascular injury. *Ann Emerg Med.* 1993;22:155–163.

8. Antonelli M, Levy M, Andrews PJ, et al. Hemodynamic monitoring in shock and implications for management. International Consensus Conference, Paris, France, 27–28 April 2006. *Intensive Care Med.* 2007;33:575–590.

9. McGhee BH, Bridges EJ. Monitoring arterial blood pressure: what you may not know. *Crit Care Nurse.* 2002;22:60–64, 66–70, 73 passim.

10. Pickering TG, Hall JE, Appel LJ, et al. Recommendations for blood pressure measurement in humans and experimental animals: part 1: blood pressure measurement in humans: a statement for professionals from the Subcommittee of Professional and Public Education of the American Heart Association Council on High Blood Pressure Research. *Circulation.* 2005;111:697–716.

11. Deakin CD, Low JL. Accuracy of the advanced trauma life support guidelines for predicting systolic blood pressure using carotid, femoral, and radial pulses: observational study. *BMJ.* 2000;321:673–674.

12. Pickering TG. Principles and techniques of blood pressure measurement. *Cardiol Clin.* 2002;20:207–223.

13. Umana E, Ahmed W, Fraley MA, Alpert MA. Comparison of oscillometric and intraarterial systolic and diastolic blood pressures in lean, overweight, and obese patients. *Angiology.* 2006;57:41–45.

14. Karnath B. Sources of error in blood pressure measurement. *Hosp Physician.* Mar 2002;38:33–37.

15. Cohn JN. Blood pressure measurement in shock. Mechanism of inaccuracy in auscultatory and palpatory methods. *JAMA.* 1967;199:118–122.

16. Scheer B, Perel A, Pfeiffer UJ. Clinical review: complications and risk factors of peripheral arterial catheters used for haemodynamic monitoring in anaesthesia and intensive care medicine. *Crit Care.* 2002;6:199–204.

17. Pinsky MR. Functional hemodynamic monitoring. *Intensive Care Med.* 2002;28:386–388.

18. Michard F, Teboul JL. Predicting fluid responsiveness in ICU patients: a critical analysis of the evidence. *Chest.* 2002;121:2000–2008.

19. Marik PE, Baram M, Vahid B. Does central venous pressure predict fluid responsiveness? A systematic review of the literature and the tale of seven mares. *Chest.* 2008;134:172–178.

20. Magder S. Central venous pressure: a useful but not so simple measurement. *Crit Care Med.* 2006;34:2224–2227.

21. Weil MH, Shubin H, Rosoff L. Fluid repletion in circulatory shock: central venous pressure and other practical guides. *JAMA.* 1965;192:668–674.

22. Rivers E, Nguyen B, Havstad S, et al. Early goal-directed therapy in the treatment of severe sepsis and septic shock. *N Engl J Med.* 2001;345:1368–1377.

23. Constant J. Using internal jugular pulsations as a manometer for right atrial pressure measurements. *Cardiology.* 2000;93:26–30.

24. Donahue SP, Wood JP, Patel BM, et al. Correlation of sonographic measurements of the internal jugular vein with central venous pressure. *Am J Emerg Med.* 2009;27:851–855.

25. Lipton B. Estimation of central venous pressure by ultrasound of the internal jugular vein. *Am J Emerg Med.* 2000;18:432–434.

26. Desmond J, Megahed M. Is the central venous pressure reading equally reliable if the central line is inserted via the femoral vein. *Emerg Med J.* 2003;20:467–469.

27. Leonard AD, Allsager CM, Parker JL, et al. Comparison of central venous and external jugular venous pressures during repair of proximal femoral fracture. *Br J Anaesth.* 2008;101:166–170.

28. Starling E. *The Linacre Lecture on the Law of the Heart given at Cambridge, 1915.* London, UK: Longmans, Green and Co; 1918.

29. Michard F, Boussat S, Chemla D, et al. Relation between respiratory changes in arterial pulse pressure and fluid responsiveness in septic patients with acute circulatory failure. *Am J Respir Crit Care Med.* 2000;162:134–138.

30. Lopes MR, Oliveira MA, Pereira VO, et al. Goal-directed fluid management based on pulse pressure variation monitoring during high-risk surgery: a pilot randomized controlled trial. *Crit Care.* 2007;11:R100.

31. Monnet X, Rienzo M, Osman D, et al. Passive leg raising predicts fluid responsiveness in the critically ill. *Crit Care Med.* 2006;34:1402–1407.

32. Connors AF Jr, Speroff T, Dawson NV, et al. The effectiveness of right heart catheterization in the initial care of critically ill patients. SUPPORT Investigators. *JAMA.* 1996;276:889–897.

33. Harvey S, Harrison DA, Singer M, et al. Assessment of the clinical effectiveness of pulmonary artery catheters in management of patients in intensive care (PAC-Man): a randomised controlled trial. *Lancet.* 2005;366:472–477.

34. Shah MR, Hasselblad V, Stevenson LW, et al. Impact of the pulmonary artery catheter in critically ill patients: meta-analysis of randomized clinical trials. *JAMA.* 2005;294:1664–1670.

35. Shure D. Pulmonary-artery catheters—peace at last? *N Engl J Med.* 2006;354:2273–2274.

36. Shoemaker WC, Belzberg H, Wo CC, et al. Multicenter study of noninvasive monitoring systems as alternatives to invasive monitoring of acutely ill emergency patients. *Chest.* 1998;114:1643–1652.

37. Marik PE, Baram M. Noninvasive hemodynamic monitoring in the intensive care unit. *Crit Care Clin.* 2007;23:383–400.

38. Lo HY, Liao SC, Ng CJ, et al. Utility of impedance cardiography for dyspneic patients in the ED. Am J Emerg Med. 2007;25:437–441.

39. Raaijmakers E, Faes TJ, Scholten RJ, et al. A meta-analysis of three decades of validating thoracic impedance cardiography. *Crit Care Med.* 1999;27:1203–1213.

40. Raval NY, Squara P, Cleman M, et al. Multicenter evaluation of noninvasive cardiac output measurement by bioreactance technique. *J Clin Monit Comput.* 2008;22:113–119.

41. Huntsman LL, Stewart DK, Barnes SR, et al. Noninvasive Doppler determination of cardiac output in man. Clinical validation. *Circulation.* 1983;67:593–602.

42. Dark PM, Singer M. The validity of trans-esophageal Doppler ultrasonography as a measure of cardiac out-

put in critically ill adults. *Intensive Care Med.* 2004;30: 2060–2066.

43. Sinclair S, James S, Singer M. Intraoperative intravascular volume optimisation and length of hospital stay after repair of proximal femoral fracture: randomised controlled trial. *BMJ.* 1997;315:909–912.

44. Noblett SE, Snowden CP, Shenton BK, et al. Randomized clinical trial assessing the effect of Doppler-optimized fluid management on outcome after elective colorectal resection. *Br J Surg.* 2006;93:1069–1076.

45. Venn R, Steele A, Richardson P, et al. Randomized controlled trial to investigate influence of the fluid challenge on duration of hospital stay and perioperative morbidity in patients with hip fractures. *Br J Anaesth.* 2002;88: 65–71.

46. Rodriguez RM, Lum-Lung M, Dixon K, et al. A prospective study on esophageal Doppler hemodynamic assessment in the ED. Am J Emerg Med. 2006;24:658–663.

47. Wong LS, Yong BH, Young KK, et al. Comparison of the USCOM ultrasound cardiac output monitor with pulmonary artery catheter thermodilution in patients undergoing liver transplantation. *Liver Transpl.* 2008; 14:1038–1043.

48. Nguyen HB, Losey T, Rasmussen J, et al. Interrater reliability of cardiac output measurements by transcutaneous Doppler ultrasound: implications for noninvasive hemodynamic monitoring in the ED. *Am J Emerg Med.* 2006;24:828–835.

49. Dey I, Sprivulis P. Emergency physicians can reliably assess emergency department patient cardiac output using the USCOM continuous wave Doppler cardiac output monitor. *Emerg Med Australas.* 2005;17:193–199.

50. Della Rocca G, Costa MG, Pompei L, et al. Continuous and intermittent cardiac output measurement: pulmonary artery catheter versus aortic transpulmonary technique. *Br J Anaesth.* 2002;88:350–356.

51. McGee WT, Horswell JL, Calderon J et al. Validation of a continuous, arterial pressure-based cardiac output measurement: a multicenter, prospective clinical trial. *Crit Care.* 2007;11:R105.

52. de Waal EE, Kalkman CJ, Rex S, et al. Validation of a new arterial pulse contour-based cardiac output device. *Crit Care Med.* 2007;35:1904–1909.

53. Scheinman MM, Brown MA, Rapaport E. Critical assessment of use of central venous oxygen saturation as a mirror of mixed venous oxygen in severely ill cardiac patients. *Circulation.* 1969;40:165–172.

54. Wo CC, Shoemaker WC, Appel PL, et al. Unreliability of blood pressure and heart rate to evaluate cardiac output in emergency resuscitation and critical illness. *Crit Care Med.* 1993;21:218–223.

55. Rady MY, Rivers EP, Nowak RM. Resuscitation of the critically ill in the ED: responses of blood pressure, heart rate, shock index, central venous oxygen saturation, and lactate. *Am J Emerg Med.* 1996;14:218–225.

56. Gattinoni L, Brazzi L, Pelosi P, et al. A trial of goal-oriented hemodynamic therapy in critically ill patients. SvO$_2$ Collaborative Group. *N Engl J Med.* 1995;333: 1025–1032.

57. Nguyen HB, Corbett SW, Steele R, et al. Implementation of a bundle of quality indicators for the early management of severe sepsis and septic shock is associated with decreased mortality. *Crit Care Med.* 2007;35: 1105–1112.

58. Perez DI, Scott HM, Duff J, et al. The significance of lacticacidemia in the shock syndrome. *Ann N Y Acad Sci.* 1965;119:1133–1141.

59. McNelis J, Marini CP, Jurkiewicz A, et al. Prolonged lactate clearance is associated with increased mortality in the surgical intensive care unit. *Am J Surg.* 2001;182: 481–485.

60. Abramson D, Scalea TM, Hitchcock R, et al. Lactate clearance and survival following injury. *J Trauma.* 1993;35:584–588. Discussion 588–589.

61. Manikis P, Jankowski S, Zhang H, et al. Correlation of serial blood lactate levels to organ failure and mortality after trauma. *Am J Emerg Med.* 1995;13:619–622.

62. Arnold RC, Shapiro NI, Jones AE, et al. Multi-center study of early lactate clearance as a determinant of survival in patients with presumed sepsis. *Shock.* 2008. Epub December 22.

63. Cohn SM, Crookes BA, Proctor KG. Near-infrared spectroscopy in resuscitation. *J Trauma.* 2003;54:S199–S202.

64. Mulier KE, Skarda DE, Taylor JH, et al. Near-infrared spectroscopy in patients with severe sepsis: correlation with invasive hemodynamic measurements. *Surg Infect.* 2008;9:515–519.

65. Mesquida J, Masip J, Gili G, et al. Thenar oxygen saturation measured by near infrared spectroscopy as a noninvasive predictor of low central venous oxygen saturation in septic patients. *Intensive Care Med.* Jun 2009;35(6):1106–1109. Epub 2009 Jan 29.

66. Rhee P, Langdale L, Mock C, et al. Near-infrared spectroscopy: continuous measurement of cytochrome oxidation during hemorrhagic shock. *Crit Care Med.* 1997;25: 166–170.

67. Lima A, Bakker J. Noninvasive monitoring of peripheral perfusion. *Intensive Care Med.* 2005;31:1316–1326.

CHAPTER 13

Acute Coronary Syndrome

John P. Marshall and Jonathan Rose

► INTRODUCTION

Acute coronary syndrome (ACS) is not a single diagnosis but a spectrum of disease. It encompasses ST-segment elevation myocardial infarction (STEMI), non-ST-segment elevation myocardial infarction (NSTEMI), and unstable angina (UA). It is a disease process that, if unrecognized, imparts upon the patient profound morbidity, if not mortality. In fact, acute myocardial infarction is the leading cause of death in the United States, if not the entire developed world.[1] For these reasons, ACS should be respected and treated expeditiously and aggressively.

► EPIDEMIOLOGY

In the United States, coronary heart disease (CHD) affected approximately 16 million people in 2005, and in 2008 an estimated 770,000 Americans had a new coronary event while 430,000 had a recurrent one.[2] CHD includes ACS as well as UA. While stable angina is an important condition, it is not a focus of this discussion because on its own, it is not directly responsible for mortality statistics (although a small number of deaths due to CHD are coded as being from angina pectoris). With respect to mortality, one in every five deaths in the United States in 2004 was due to CHD with an American suffering a coronary event once every 26 seconds and one American dying every minute as a result of a myocardial infarction.[2] The 2008 estimated cost of caring for these patients was $156.4 billion.[2] The prevalence of ACS is expected to continue to climb as increasing numbers of patients are being diagnosed with NSTEMI

and UA. This is not solely due to the aging of the population but also due to utilization of more sensitive diagnostic tests, increased availability of early invasive therapies, and treatment of comorbid conditions early and aggressively that delay the progression of disease to STEMI.[3–5]

With a heightened level of concern and recognition of these clinical entities, fewer patients have gone unrecognized. Consequently, mortality related to ACS has declined dramatically, particularly for STEMI. Unfortunately, the rate of decline has not been as great for NSTEMI and UA. This is likely due to a delay in the implementation of treatment guidelines for patients with these conditions.[6,7]

► PATHOPHYSIOLOGY

Understanding acute myocardial infarction requires understanding the pathophysiology of coronary artery thrombosis. While ACS can be caused by an embolic obstruction, this is much less common than ACS caused by atherosclerotic disease. There are two general types of atherosclerotic plaque, stable and unstable, and each produces a different presentation of ACS. The stable plaque has a thick fibrous cap that slowly thickens and produces the symptoms of classic angina such as progressively worsening exertional chest tightness. In this situation, oxygen delivery to the myocardium is gradually diminished, producing decreased tolerance of myocardial stress. Unstable plaques, however, have a thin fibrous cap suffused with inflammatory cells that make the plaques vulnerable to rupture. ACS associated with acute plaque rupture produces a spectrum of findings based on the location and degree of associated thrombosis and consequent impairment of oxygen delivery. A small thrombus can produce anginal symptoms while a higher-degree occlusion produces similar symptoms with non-ST-segment elevation myocardial infarction (NSTEMI). Complete occlusion can produce frank STEMI of differing severity depending on the amount and location of myocardium affected. Many of the treatments for ACS focus on maximizing oxygen delivery while minimizing platelet activation, aggregation, and clotting.[8]

▶ PRESENTATION

With respect to ACS, certain risk factors have been associated with the probability of developing cardiac disease over a lifetime but have been shown to be of very little utility in the acute setting.[9] Age, sex, family history, hypertension, diabetes mellitus, elevated cholesterol, obesity, smoking, and physical inactivity, while important, are not predictive of acute disease. One of the more common tools for risk stratifying patients with suspected ACS is the Thrombolysis In Myocardial Infarction (TIMI) score (Table 13-1). Associated with each score is a specific risk of poor outcome defined as death, myocardial infarction, or need for acute percutaneous coronary intervention (PCI). In a 2006 study by Pollack et al, a score of 3 or higher equates to a high risk with one study showing 5% mortality at 14 days and an 8% chance of needing PCI[10] (Table 13-2).

As with most diagnoses, an accurate history and thorough physical examination are necessary to generate a broad and appropriate differential as well as an accurate diagnosis. Unfortunately, there is no way to effectively rule out ACS by history and physical examination alone. Some patients present in a way classically referred to as "typical": poorly localized chest pain or pressure radiating to the left jaw, both shoulders, or left upper extremity; intermittent in nature; lasting

▶ **TABLE 13-1. TIMI RISK FACTORS (1 POINT EACH)**

Age 65 and above
At least three risk factors for CAD (HTN, DM, elevated cholesterol, family history, tobacco use)
Prior coronary stenosis of 50% or more
ST-segment deviation
At least two anginal events in preceding 24 h
Use of aspirin in past 7 days
Elevated serum cardiac enzymes (CK-MB; troponin)

Adapted from Pollack CV Jr, Sites FD, Shofer FS, et al. Application of the TIMI risk score for unstable angina and non-ST elevation acute coronary syndrome to an unselected emergency department chest pain population. *Acad Emerg Med.* 2006;13:13–18.

▶ **TABLE 13-2. THIRTY-DAY PROBABILITY OF POOR OUTCOME BASED ON TIMI SCORE**

TIMI Score 0	2.1%
TIMI Score 1	5%
TIMI Score 2	10.1%
TIMI Score 3	19.5%
TIMI Score 4	22.1%
TIMI Score 5	39.2%
TIMI Score 6	45%
TIMI Score 7	100%

Adapted from Pollack CV Jr, Sites FD, Shofer FS, et al. Application of the TIMI risk score for unstable angina and non-ST elevation acute coronary syndrome to an unselected emergency department chest pain population. *Acad Emerg Med.* 2006;13:13–18.

15–20 minutes at a time; exacerbated or precipitated by physical activity; relieved by rest or nitroglycerin; and associated with diaphoresis and shortness of breath. Unfortunately, most patients do not present in such a typical manner. Furthermore, certain patient populations, most notably women, the elderly, and diabetics, present with what has been termed "anginal equivalent." These symptoms may include isolated jaw, neck, shoulder, back, arm, or epigastric discomfort, as well as nausea, vomiting, dizziness, generalized fatigue, or weakness. Even more subtle, a patient may simply describe an increasing difficulty with performing his or her activities of daily living. Those with cognitive impairment, diabetics, and substance abusers may present with altered mental status. It is absolutely critical to remember that the diagnosis of UA may be based on history and physical examination alone, despite a normal electrocardiogram (ECG) or negative cardiac enzyme testing.

Physical examination for patients with ACS is most useful for evaluating other potential etiologies of the patient's complaint, although the exam has utility in predicting patients who may be at risk for a poorer outcome or who have developed a complication related to their myocardial infarction. For example, patients with unstable vital signs, jugular venous distention, pulmonary edema, and/or an S3 gallop are indicative of heart failure. A new murmur is suggestive of papillary muscle rupture. Hemiparesis can indicate aortic dissection. Each of these is associated with worse prognosis than those without these complications. Caution must be exhibited, though, when it comes to physical examination and the possibility of ascribing a patient's symptoms to a process more benign than ACS. For example, a significant proportion of ACS patients may in fact have pleuritic, positional, or reproducible chest pain on examination.[11] Simply stated, there is no single feature of physical examination that safely rules out ACS.

▶ DIAGNOSTIC APPROACH

The most crucial diagnostic study in any patient suspected of having ACS is the ECG that should be obtained within 10 minutes of the patient's arrival to the emergency department (ED) or similarly within minutes after the development of chest pain if the patient is already hospitalized. It is vital to the patient's outcome that the ECG be completed and accurately interpreted in a timely manner. Also, if not already on one, the patient should be placed on a monitor as soon as possible. For the inpatient who develops chest pain in a non-monitored setting, this may require transfer to a telemetry unit or ICU depending on the result of the ECG. If a STEMI is identified, appropriate resources should be immediately mobilized and interventions undertaken.[12,13] STEMI diagnostic criteria, as described by the American College of Cardiology (ACC) and American Heart Association (AHA), are outlined in Table 13-3.[14] Reciprocal ST-segment changes, such as depressions in opposite leads or findings on right-sided or posterior ECGs, make the diagnosis of STEMI more specific. While these criteria have been established and accepted, an ECG with these findings is still only 75% sensitive and 69% specific for STEMI.[15] Of course, there are several other conditions that may cause ST-segment elevations such as pericarditis, early repolarization, left ventricular hypertrophy, prior myocardial infarction with resultant ventricular aneurysm, etc.

As it relates to NSTEMI, the ECG is perhaps of equal importance but 1–5% of patients with a myocardial infarction will have a completely normal ECG at the time of presentation.[16] Therefore, serial ECGs are of tremendous value when considering a diagnosis of ACS and should be obtained with subsequent episodes of chest pain and with repeat cardiac enzyme testing. In fact, dynamic ECG changes associated with intermittent episodes of chest pain are most predictive of ACS. According to the ACC and AHA, ST-segment depressions greater than 0.05 mV with or without T-wave inversions are the most concerning findings associated with a poor outcome. Thirty-day mortality of patients with isolated ST-segment depressions is equivalent to those with ST-segment elevations. T-wave inversions ≥0.2 mV were next most concerning. Finally, ST-segment depressions and T-wave inversions of lesser magnitude or T waves newly upright (pseudonormalized) were found to be less concerning, but still clinically significant with regard to outcome.[16]

The necessity of accurate ECG interpretation cannot be overstated. A retrospective study of 1,684 patients with an acute myocardial infarction revealed that 12% of those patients presenting to the ED with active, ongoing ischemia, identifiable by ECG analysis, were missed.[17] While not statistically significant, there was a trend toward increased in-hospital mortality as a result.

In certain instances, the ECG may be more difficult to interpret. One such example is in the setting of a preexisting left bundle branch block (LBBB). The Sgarbossa criteria have been validated as being highly specific for a patient having an STEMI who at baseline has a LBBB (see Table 13-4).[18] The more criteria met, the more likely a STEMI is occurring. A score of 5–10 indicates an 88–99% probability of an acute STEMI. But even with 0 points, there still exists a 16% chance of an acute STEMI. Because of the low sensitivity of the Sgarbossa criteria when there are <10 points, the ECG cannot be used alone in the diagnostic evaluation of a patient with chest pain. In the right setting, however, the ECG along with the patient's history of present illness and a focused physical examination may be all that is necessary to accurately diagnose the patient and allow for swift, life-saving intervention.

In addition to electrocardiography, serum biomarker analysis is an essential tool in the setting of NSTEMI. While useful in STEMI as well, biomarkers play a less important role as treatment should be started based on the ECG alone. As mentioned earlier, UA is a diagnosis made by history, physical examination, and a consideration of alternative diagnoses by generating an appropriate differential and perhaps ruling out other

---

▶ TABLE 13-3. AHA/ACC STEMI DIAGNOSTIC CRITERIA (ANY ONE OF THE BELOW)

ST-segment elevation ≥1 mm (0.1 mV) in two or more adjacent limb leads (from AVL to III, including -aVR)

ST-segment elevation ≥1 mm (0.1 mV) in precordial leads V_4–V_6

ST-segment elevation ≥2 mm (0.2 mV) in precordial leads V_1–V_3

New left bundle branch block

Data from Myocardial infarction redefined—a consensus document of the Joint European Society of Cardiology/American College of Cardiology Committee for the Redefinition of Myocardial Infarction. *Eur Heart J*. 2000;21:1502–1513.

▶ TABLE 13-4. SGARBOSSA CRITERIA AND POINT ASSIGNMENT

ST-segment elevation ≥1 mm in a lead concordant with a QRS complex	5 points
ST-segment depression ≥1 mm in V_1, V_2, or V_3	3 points
ST-segment elevation ≥5 mm in a lead discordant with a QRS complex	2 points

Adapted from Sgarbossa EB, Pinski SL, Barbagelata A, et al. Electrocardiographic diagnosis of evolving acute myocardial infarction in the presence of left bundle-branch block. *N Engl J Med*. 1996;334:481–487.

etiologies. One may expect an unremarkable ECG and negative serum cardiac biomarker analysis in the setting of UA. Like STEMI and NSTEMI, UA is a diagnosis one cannot afford to miss. These patients still require aggressive management as they may unpredictably progress to NSTEMI or STEMI.

Serum cardiac biomarker analysis allows for diagnostic confirmation as well as risk stratification, as patients with positive results have a higher complication rate.[19,20] The most commonly used biomarkers include creatine kinase-myocardial band (CK-MB), myoglobin, and troponin T or I. The ACC and AHA guidelines no longer recommend the use of myoglobin in the evaluation of patients suspected of having NSTEMI. The marker is sensitive early in the course of the disease process, rising within 1 hour of the ischemic event, but is not at all specific. LDH, which was used as a marker for many years, is similarly not recommended due to its lack of specificity. In contrast, CK-MB and troponin are both sensitive and specific when it comes to myocardial infarction, although CK-MB is less specific than troponin as it is also found in skeletal muscle. Both enzymes rise later than myoglobin, and may reach abnormal values within 3–4 hours after an ischemic event with peak levels seen 15–20 hours after the event. CK-MB levels should decrease to a normal range within 48 hours while troponin levels remain elevated for up to 10 days. Due to their high degree of specificity, the ability of diagnostic equipment to measure even the smallest of elevated values (compared with earlier thresholds) and the current definition of acute myocardial infarction at the slightest of troponin elevations, both the prevalence and incidence of the disease have increased dramatically.[14] Of course, even small elevations identify patients at greater risk who may benefit from more aggressive intervention. There are other reasons a patient may have an elevated troponin, such as renal failure (which affects troponin I less than T), trauma, congestive heart failure (CHF), and sepsis, but each of these patients, as a consequence of his or her comorbidity, is at even greater risk and possesses a higher mortality.[21]

With all of the biomarkers, serial measurements are more useful than any one single measurement. For patients with an initially negative measurement, a second CK-MB value 2 hours later yielded a sensitivity of 93% and specificity of 94% for acute myocardial infarction.[22] Still, CK-MB is a second-line biomarker for myocardial infarction as patients with an elevated CK-MB but negative troponin have the same outcome as patients with a both a normal CK-MB and negative troponin.[19]

There have been several other novel biomarkers studied including BNP, CRP, ischemia-modified albumin, and homocysteine, but none are recommended by the AHA or ACC for the evaluation of ACS in the acute setting.

In addition to ECG and cardiac biomarker analysis, various other modalities may be utilized for evaluating the cardiac patient. In the appropriate setting, provocative testing via exercise stress testing with or without myocardial perfusion imaging and stress echocardiography is being utilized in an effort to evaluate patients for ACS with higher certainty to allow for safer discharge. Similarly, echocardiography during an acute episode of ACS can evaluate the myocardium for wall motion abnormalities. An experienced cardiac sonographer can detect changes from the normal symmetric contraction of the myocardium that may indicate cardiac stunning associated with acute ischemia.

Computed tomography (CT) has been and is still currently being investigated as an alternative to coronary angiography with the benefit of being less invasive and perhaps more readily available. Cardiac computed tomography (CCT) is a modality by which the degree of calcification of coronary arteries is measured without the need for intravenous contrast and with greater degrees of calcification indicative of a higher likelihood of a future coronary event.[23] It does not evaluate the true cardiac lumen. The greater the degree of calcification, the higher is the chance of an obstructive lesion in need of intervention being identified during coronary angiography. However, the score generated by such measurement reflects only relative or overall risk and not absolute risk or the certainty of an obstructing lesion being present.[24]

Unlike CCT, cardiac CT angiography (CCTA) evaluates the true cardiac lumen by utilizing intravenous contrast and has been shown to correlate well with findings derived from PCI. Less invasive and more readily available than PCI, CCTA is not without risk. Compared with CCT, CCTA adds the risk of exposure to intravenous contrast and involves significantly more radiation than cardiac catheterization. Furthermore, both CCTA and CCT are purely diagnostic tools. So while they may be utilized to safely discharge a certain subgroup of ED patients without need for admission and/or coronary angiography, patients who require intervention will end up receiving significantly more radiation and contrast than if they initially had a traditional cardiac angiogram. The same is true when CCTA is utilized for ED or ICU patients to determine the need for transfer to PCI-capable facilities. Furthermore, to date, published data derived from multiple, randomized, multicenter clinical trials are lacking.

Cardiac magnetic resonance imaging (CMR) with or without contrast is another novel diagnostic tool under investigation that has been shown to have a high positive predictive value and specificity for myocardial infarction.[25] Images obtained can be synchronized with the cardiac cycle and can combine both angiographic evaluation of the patient's coronary arteries and wall motion abnormalities. Like CT, CMR is also in need of additional study and validation before it can be deemed appropriate for routine clinical use.

▶ TREATMENT

The mainstay of treatment of the critical patient with ACS is focused on improving oxygen delivery to the myocardium. This is accomplished in four ways: anti-ischemic therapy, antiplatelet therapy, anticoagulation therapy, and reperfusion therapy. Anti-ischemic therapies, such as oxygen, nitroglycerin, and β-blockers, work by matching oxygen delivery and demand and therefore by increasing oxygen delivery or decreasing oxygen demand. Antiplatelet medications, such as aspirin, prevent further thrombosis by minimizing platelet activation and adhesion. Anticoagulants such as heparin inhibit clot formation via the clotting cascade or by direct thrombin inhibition. Reperfusion of ischemic myocardium is accomplished via thrombolytics or PCI, both of which are used to directly restore cardiac circulation. In some cases, these treatments will fail and the patient will require coronary artery bypass grafting (CABG) or, in the case of frank cardiogenic shock, invasive mechanical support such as intra-aortic balloon pump or left ventricular assist device placement, both of which are covered in Chapter 17.

ANTI-ISCHEMIC THERAPY

Supplemental oxygen delivery has been a standard treatment for ACS for nearly a century, although the data on its effectiveness are quite thin and inconclusive.[26,27] The recommendations from the most recent ACC/AHA guidelines strongly endorse the use of oxygen in all patients with ACS and hypoxia and less strongly endorse oxygen for all ACS patients (although they clearly indicate this is based on opinion rather than settled evidence).[28] Oxygen should be used with caution in patients with a history of COPD.

Nitrates, like oxygen, are nearly ubiquitous in the treatment of ACS, although the research on their utility is limited. The largest effect was noted in a meta-analysis of more than 80,000 patients that demonstrated that nearly 300 patients would need to be treated with nitrates to prevent one additional death.[29] Nitrates produce arterial and venous dilatation resulting in decreased cardiac preload and afterload, and subsequently decreased myocardial oxygen demand. Simultaneously, nitrate-induced coronary artery dilation can improve oxygen delivery to the myocardium. Nitrates should be administered initially via a sublingual route at doses of 0.4 mg for a total of three doses, 5 minutes apart. If anginal symptoms persist after these doses, an intravenous infusion should be started, typically at 200 mcg/min and titrated up every 3–4 minutes until the resolution of ischemia or the development of hypotension.[28] Nitrates should generally not be administered to patients who are markedly bradycardic, tachycardic, or hypotensive (systolic blood pressure below 90 mm Hg or a drop in blood pressure of greater than 30 mm Hg from their baseline).[28] Other contraindications include suspected right ventricular infarction, in which patients depend on their preload to maintain adequate blood pressure, and patients who have taken a phosphodiesterase inhibitor within 24 hours.[28] While the use of transdermal nitrates is commonplace, these preparations are of limited use in a patient with ACS due to the passive nature of administration. Active ACS in the ED or the ICU requires close monitoring and should be managed actively with periodic sublingual or continuous intravenous nitrates.

For many years, β-adrenergic blocking agents were commonly used in ACS patients to directly decrease cardiac work and oxygen demand based on early studies that showed a mortality benefit to patients who received intravenous agents on the day of their presentation.[30] Some recent studies, however, have demonstrated increased morbidity with early β-blockade. The most dramatic results came from the COMMIT study that demonstrated increased risk of cardiogenic shock in patients receiving IV β-blockers within 24 hours of myocardial infarction.[31] Based on this and similar studies, current treatment guidelines have limited their use to younger patients who do not have contraindications such as CHF, bronchospasm, cocaine abuse, low output states, heart block, and increased risk of cardiogenic shock.[28] Another recent review concluded that no evidence supports intravenous use of these agents over the oral route.[32]

Morphine has frequently been used to provide analgesia for patients with anginal pain that is refractory to nitrates. It is known to block catecholamine surge, resulting in decreased blood pressure, heart rate, and, consequently, oxygen demand.[28] It is also postulated to play a role in preventing further plaque rupture.[28] This potentially beneficial action has not been demonstrated in the literature, however. In fact, a recent observational study demonstrated an increased likelihood of death in ACS patients receiving morphine, possibly related to masking of ongoing cardiac ischemia.[33] Despite this concern, the ACC and AHA have continued to support the judicious use of morphine as the analgesic agent of choice for refractory pain associated with ACS.

ANTIPLATELET THERAPY

Aspirin is an irreversible COX-1 inhibitor that minimizes platelet activation and aggregation by blocking arachidonic acid. This prevents further clotting in ACS and was shown to reduce mortality in the ISIS-2 study that used doses of 162 mg.[34] The utility of aspirin was further confirmed in two subsequent meta-analyses.[35,36] The common practice of chewing aspirin, rather than swallowing the pills whole, has been demonstrated to deactivate platelets more quickly.[37,38] Current recommendations are for 162–325 mg of aspirin to be given immediately after the onset of symptoms, in the prehospital setting if possible, or on arrival to the hospital.[28] Aspirin should be avoided in patients with allergy or significant active bleeding or bleeding risk.[28]

Clopidogrel is a thienopyridine that also inhibits platelets irreversibly by antagonizing the adenosine diphosphate receptor. It has been shown to be equally effective for ACS in patients who cannot receive aspirin and should be given to these patients in place of aspirin for suspected ACS.[39] Some papers have recommended a 600-mg loading dose in these patients, as opposed to a 300-mg loading dose for patients who will also receive aspirin.[40] Its utility in ACS, when combined with aspirin, was demonstrated in the CRUSADE and CURE trials that both showed modest improvements in survival with dual antiplatelet therapy despite a small increase in bleeding complications.[41,42] Other studies demonstrated dual antiplatelet benefit for patients less than 75 years old with STEMI who undergo thrombolysis or for whom no revascularization treatment is planned.[43,44] Based on these findings, ACS patients who do not have PCI planned within 48 hours should receive clopidogrel 300 mg orally early in their hospital course in addition to aspirin.[28]

For patients with STEMI or planned early PCI, the use of thienopyridines is less well established. It may still be used as an aspirin substitute as described above, but there is some controversy regarding dual antiplatelet therapy in these patients. The only supporting literature on this treatment strategy demonstrated some benefit but was a somewhat flawed subgroup analysis of a larger study.[45] To date, no direct comparison exists. The use in PCI patients is further complicated by the fact that both the CURE and CRUSADE trials demonstrated additional bleeding complications for patients with dual antiplatelet therapy who underwent CABG within 5 days of administration of clopidogrel.[41,42] However, neither of these studies demonstrated an increased mortality in these patients. Since most patients do not undergo CABG within 5 days of PCI, despite the controversy, the most recent recommendation is to administer 300–600 mg of clopidogrel to all STEMI patients undergoing PCI.[46]

It should be noted that there is a newer thienopyridine, prasugrel, which is given as a 60-mg loading dose. It is also recommended for patients undergoing primary PCI but has some caveats when compared with clopidogrel: if possible, CABG should be delayed for 7 days after the last prasugrel dose and it should not be used in patients who have a history of stroke or transient ischemic attack.[46]

The final category of antiplatelet agents are glycoprotein IIb/IIIa inhibitors (GPI) that block fibrinogen cross-linking of activated platelets and consequently prevent platelet aggregation. There are two general types of GPIs: large molecule such as abciximab and small molecule such as eptifibatide and tirofiban. The largest body of data is on abciximab that has been shown to be beneficial in patients undergoing PCI for STEMI or as part of an early invasive strategy for ACS without STEMI when given in addition to aspirin with or without clopidogrel.[47,48] Similar evidence exists for small molecule GPIs for both of these categories of patients.[49,50] The evidence for abciximab in patients with ACS who undergo a conservative management strategy without planned PCI demonstrated increased complications without significant benefit.[51] No randomized studies of small molecule GPIs exist for this patient population. Therefore, the current recommendation restricts GPI use to patients at the time of catheterization as part of a double or triple antiplatelet strategy.[46] These agents are typically continued in the ICU for up to 24 hours after the time of presentation.

ANTICOAGULANT THERAPY

The commonly used anticoagulants, unfractionated heparin (UFH), low-molecular-weight heparin (LMWH), and the newer fondaparinux, function by activating the enzyme antithrombin III that in turn inactivates thrombin and factor Xa, thereby inhibiting the clotting cascade. UFH is a naturally occurring substance that contains molecules of a variety of lengths. This is relevant because the longer heparin molecules inactivate both factor Xa and thrombin, while the shorter molecules inactivate only factor Xa. LMWHs, such as enoxaparin or daltoparin, are formulations of heparin containing primarily short-chain heparin molecules and consequently inhibit factor Xa to a much greater degree than thrombin. Fondaparinux is a short-chain synthetic heparin-like molecule that functions like LMWH but only inhibits factor Xa. Because their activity is more focused, these three can be dosed subcutaneously in a more predictable manner and do not require monitoring, unlike UFH that requires a continuous infusion and monitoring of partial thromboplastin time (PTT). Because LMWH and fondaparinux do not affect thrombin, neither medication results in alteration of PTT. Similarly, LMWH is much less likely to produce heparin-induced thrombocytopenia (HIT) and fondaparinux has no risk of HIT. Consequently, both can be used for an extended period without significant risk of developing HIT, although patients with a history of HIT should preferentially receive fondaparinux.

The data on these medications in ACS are complex, with multiple competing studies producing somewhat conflicted results. Trials of UFH added to aspirin failed to show significant benefit in multiple small studies, but showed some benefit when analyzed together.[52] In contrast, the LMWHs have been shown to be directly beneficial in ACS when added to aspirin.[53] Comparisons between LMWH and UFH have been mixed with some showing benefit for LMWH and others showing no difference between LMWH or UFH.[54-56] These studies have been performed in patients receiving both conservative management and early invasive management with PCI.[57] Of note, some of these studies demonstrated an apparent increased risk of bleeding associated with LMWH, although some analysis indicates this may have been due to switching between the two medications.[58] A rational regimen should ensure that the initial anticoagulant given for ACS be continued throughout the patient's hospital stay, assuming no contraindication develops (such as HIT).

In contrast, fondaparinux has a lower rate of bleeding complications than either UFH or LMWH and has been demonstrated to be equivalent to LMWH when directly compared.[59] As a result of these data, it is currently considered a first-line option for anticoagulation in ACS patients.[28,46]

The bottom line, however, is that these medications are essentially equivalent and local culture, rather than empiric evidence, will likely play a larger role in medication selection. LMWH may carry a slightly higher bleeding risk. LMWH and fondaparinux may provide some benefit over UFH when patients are treated for longer than 48 hours due to the increased incidence of HIT after 2 days of UFH. UFH is preferred when CABG is planned within 24 hours due to its more rapid clearance.

Bivalirudin is a newer anticoagulant and functions by direct thrombin inhibition without any anti–factor Xa activity. It is derived from hirudin, a natural anticoagulant produced by leeches. It is administered as a drip, has a very rapid onset of action, and reverses very quickly when stopped. Bivalirudin also carries no risk of HIT and has produced the lowest rates of bleeding complications of any of the anticoagulants, although the literature is limited in its use for ACS. One large study demonstrated benefit in patients undergoing PCI, but was complicated by the use of other medications.[60] Bivalirudin is currently recommended as a treatment adjunct in ACS patients undergoing PCI but is best administered in consultation with the treating cardiology service.[46]

REPERFUSION THERAPY

The initial decision to reperfuse a patient with ACS should be based on the ECG. Frank STEMI indicates complete occlusion of a coronary artery and requires acute intervention. The choice of reperfusion strategies for STEMI patients is highly dependent on local

resources. The general rule is that the timeliness of reperfusion is more important than the manner in which it is achieved. Assuming equivalent availability of both approaches, PCI provides superior outcome compared with intravenous thrombolysis.[61,62] However, for patients who cannot receive PCI within 2 hours, there is no difference between the two modalities. Therefore, thrombolytics should not be delayed for PCI unless the PCI can be accomplished within 90 minutes of presentation.[46]

Thrombolytics are more widely available than PCI and have been demonstrated to produce good outcomes in STEMI patients when administered in a timely fashion. However, the quality of the outcomes worsens as time to treatment lengthens. Whenever possible, the "door to needle time," the interval between ED arrival and initiation of IV thrombolytics, should be less than 30 minutes for any STEMI patient with less than 12 hours of symptoms.[63] The currently used medications for thrombolysis are alteplase, reteplase, and tenecteplase which are all tissue plasminogen activators. While the dosing of these medications differs widely, the reperfusion and complication rates are similar and most institutions have only one of the three available. Streptokinase, which is an older thrombolytic, has generally fallen out of common use given its worse side effect profile. There are clearly defined contraindications to the administration of thrombolytics and these are listed in Table 13-5.[46]

► **TABLE 13-5. CONTRAINDICATIONS TO THE ADMINISTRATION OF FIBRINOLYTICS**

Absolute contraindications	
Prior intracranial hemorrhage	Significant head trauma within 3 months
Known structural cerebral vascular lesion	Suspected aortic dissection
Known malignant intracranial neoplasm	Active bleeding
Ischemic stroke (CVA) within 3 months	Bleeding diathesis
Relative contraindications	
Chronic severe hypertension (HTN)	Ischemic CVA greater than 3 months ago
Uncontrolled HTN (SBP >180, DBP >110)	Dementia
Prolonged CPR >10 min	Other intracranial pathology
Internal bleeding within 2–4 weeks	Active peptic ulcer
Noncompressible vascular puncture	Current anticoagulant use
Pregnancy	

Data from Antman EM, Anbe DT, Armstrong PW, et al: ACC/AHA guidelines for the management of patients with ST-elevation myocardial infarction: a report of the American College of Cardiology/American Heart Association Task Force on Practice guideline. *J Am Coll Cardiol.* 2004;44; E1–E211.

Primary PCI is the treatment of choice for STEMI if it can be accomplished in a timely fashion. The goal for PCI in the STEMI patient is to achieve a "door to balloon" time—the time between arrival and the inflation of the balloon during angioplasty—of 90 minutes or less. Systems of care in the ED should be designed to minimize the amount of time to diagnose STEMI, activate the cardiology team, and transfer the patient to the catheterization lab. For STEMI patients presenting to facilities without PCI availability, transfer to a PCI-capable institution should be initiated immediately if the patient can be transferred and treated within the 90-minute window.[64]

There are three additional, nonprimary forms of PCI that can be considered in the STEMI patient. Rescue PCI should be considered within 24 hours if a patient does not have an acceptable response to primary thrombolytic therapy as evidenced by less than 50% resolution of ST-segment elevation within 90 minutes, persistent unstable arrhythmias, persistent ischemic symptoms, or development or worsening of cardiogenic shock. Facilitated PCI is a strategy involving planned PCI after less than full-dose thrombolytics in a patient with high mortality risk when PCI is not available within 90 minutes. Follow-up PCI is common after primary fibrinolysis and considered after primary PCI if there is evidence of persistent narrowing of coronary arteries that may be amenable to further intervention.[64]

Patients with NSTEMI or ACS patients without myocardial infarction generally have only partial occlusion of the coronary vessels and the benefits of early reperfusion therapy are less clear. Classically these patients have been managed conservatively with medication followed by risk stratification, such as treadmill testing, but without reperfusion therapy. Some of these patients may also undergo diagnostic PCI, with the opportunity for stenting concerning lesions, as part of their initial hospitalization. Investigations of thrombolysis in these patients have demonstrated no benefit and a trend toward harm.[65] PCI within 48 hours, however, may confer some benefit to the ACS patient as demonstrated in a *Cochrane* systematic review of the literature and a meta-analysis, both of which were published in 2006.[66,67] A different meta-analysis showed a benefit for early PCI in patients with positive biomarkers, but no benefit in men with negative biomarkers, and a detrimental effect in women with negative biomarkers. Regardless of the initial choice of management, patients with high-risk features as described above or those with refractory or recurrent ischemia should receive early PCI and dual antiplatelet therapy assuming the patient does not have substantial comorbidities.[46]

▶ POTENTIAL COMPLICATIONS

The complications associated with ACS are clearly not just related to those of the cardiovascular system, but for the purpose of this discussion we will mention only

▶ **TABLE 13-6. KILLIP CLINICAL CLASSIFICATION**

Class	Approximate Mortality (%)
I: No congestive heart failure (CHF)	5
II: Mild CHF (bibasilar rales and an S3)	15–20
III: Frank pulmonary edema	40
IV: Cardiogenic shock	80

Reproduced with permission from Tintinalli JE, Kelen GD, Stapcyzynski JS, eds. *Emergency Medicine: A Comprehensive Study Guide.* 7th ed. McGraw-Hill Inc; 2011. Table 53-11.

those deemed most significant and related directly to the cardiovascular tree. A few of those mentioned are discussed in other sections of this book.

All types of derangements in electrical conduction may be encountered: those that have little to no effect on prognosis, such as sinus bradycardia, first-degree AV block, second-degree AV block type I, premature atrial contractions, and premature ventricular contractions, and those that have a significant impact on patient outcome, such as persistent sinus tachycardia, supraventricular tachycardia, atrial fibrillation, atrial flutter, and both right and left bundle branch blocks. With respect to ventricular tachycardia and fibrillation, the presence of either of these rhythm disturbances does not portend a poor prognosis early in the course of an acute myocardial infarction. In contrast, ventricular tachycardia or fibrillation that is delayed in its onset and encountered later in the course of disease is typically due to transmural infarction and severe ventricular dysfunction and is therefore associated with a much more grave prognosis.

As mentioned earlier, BNP as a cardiac biomarker is utilized in such a way so as to risk stratify a patient with ACS. Patients with CHF have a poorer prognosis than those without CHF. The clinical status of patients with CHF as defined by their Killip classification (Table 13-6) correlates with their percent mortality, with a higher classification indicative of a worse prognosis. For example, cardiogenic shock by itself or as a consequence of right ventricular infarction is defined as Killip Class IV and is associated with an approximate 80% likelihood of mortality, as opposed to those patients with no evidence of CHF—Killip Class I—who have an approximate 5% mortality.

A particularly lethal complication of myocardial infarction is ventricular free wall rupture that results in cardiac tamponade and death. Interventricular septum rupture may also occur, but the patient's ultimate prognosis depends on the size of the defect and the resultant degree of shunt created. Acute valvular insufficiency as a sign of papillary muscle rupture may be encountered and requires surgical correction.

Acute ascending aortic dissection, not as a consequence of but associated with acute myocardial infarction, is a rare occurrence but, when present, carries a high mortality. If unrecognized, 50% of patients will die within 48 hours. Most of these dissections involve the right coronary artery with coronary artery occlusion due to mural dissection or extravasation of blood into the pericardial space or perivascular tissues.

Other complications such as pericarditis with or without a pericardial effusion, ventricular thrombus formation with embolization, and postinfarct angina and extension are also possibilities.

▶ DISPOSITION

Ascertaining the correct disposition for patients with ACS can be difficult. The disposition of patients with definitive evidence of disease is fairly easy. Patients who have undergone PCI or thrombolysis or with evidence of ongoing cardiac ischemia should be admitted to a cardiac intensive care unit. Many ACS patients, however, present with vague symptoms without electrocardiographic or laboratory evidence of disease. The disposition of this set of patients presents a challenge and can be highly dependent on local resources. Some EDs can provide early stress testing after repeat EKG and enzyme testing that may obviate the need for admission. Other EDs offer chest pain units (CPU) with standardized pathways for monitoring and testing patients. After repeat lab testing, patients in CPUs frequently undergo risk stratification with stress testing, CT angiography, or catheterization depending on their findings and available resources.

In the ED, CPU, or on admission to the hospital, patients with suspected ACS should be observed with cardiac telemetry.[28] Given the volume of patients admitted for possible ACS and the relative paucity of telemetry beds, some researchers have attempted to develop decision rules regarding the need for telemetry monitoring. While these findings have yet to be included in the current guidelines, there have been some impressive results. One study evaluated the Goldman score, which was developed to assess perioperative cardiac risk, and found that it could reliably predict which patients could be safely admitted to an inpatient bed without telemetry monitoring.[68]

Regardless of the ultimate disposition of ACS patients, current guidelines recommend that every patient undergo an evaluation of cardiac risk. This can be accomplished via exercise or chemical stress testing, radioisotope scanning, CT angiography, or cardiac catheterization. This should be accomplished during the initial ED visit or hospitalization. Low-risk patients can have this done as an outpatient, but arrangements should be made to ensure that it is accomplished within 72 hours of discharge.[28]

REFERENCES

1. Roger VL. Epidemiology of myocardial infarction. *Med Clin North Am.* 200791:537–552.
2. Rosamond W, Flegal K, Furie K, et al. *Heart Disease and Stroke Statistics—2008 Update.* Chicago, IL: American Heart Association; 2008. Available at: http://www.americanheart.org/statistics.
3. Rogers WJ, Frederick PD, Stoehr E, et al. Trends in presenting characteristics and hospital mortality among patients with ST elevation and non-ST elevation myocardial infarction in the National Registry of Myocardial Infarction from 1990 to 2006. *Am Heart J.* 2008;156:1026–1034.
4. Giugliano RP, Braunwald E. The year in non-ST segment elevation acute coronary syndrome. *J Am Coll Cardiol.* 2008;52:1095–1103.
5. Tricoci P, Peterson ED, Roe MT. Patterns of guideline adherence and care delivery for patients with unstable angina and non-ST-segment elevation myocardial infarction (from the CRUSADE Quality Improvement Initiative). *Am J Cardiol.* 2006;98:30Q–35Q.
6. Roe MT, Halabi AR, Mehta RH, et al. Documented traditional cardiovascular risk factors and mortality in non-ST-segment elevation myocardial infarction. *Am Heart J.* 2007;153:507–514.
7. Fox KA, Goodman SG, Klein W, et al. Management of acute coronary syndromes: variations in practice and outcome; findings from the Global Registry of Acute Coronary Events (GRACE). *Eur Heart J.* 2002;23:1177–1189.
8. Yeghiazarians Y, Braunstein JB, Askari A, et al. Unstable angina pectoris. *N Engl J Med.* 2000;342:101–114.
9. Jayes RL, Beshansky JR, D'Agostino RB, et al. Do patients' coronary risk factor reports predict acute cardiac ischemia in the emergency department? A multicenter study. *J Clin Epidemiol.* 1992;45:621–626.
10. Pollack CV Jr, Sites FD, Shofer FS, et al. Application of the TIMI risk score for unstable angina and non-ST elevation acute coronary syndrome to an unselected emergency department chest pain population. *Acad Emerg Med.* 2006;13:13–18.
11. Lee TH, Cook EF, Weisberg M, et al. Acute chest pain in the emergency room: identification and examination of low-risk patients. *Arch Intern Med.* 1985;145:65–69.
12. Selker HP, Zalenski RJ, Antman EM, et al. An evaluation of technologies for identifying acute cardiac ischemia in the emergency department: a report from a National Heart Attack Alert Program Working Group. *Ann Emerg Med.* 1997;29:13–87.
13. Lau J, Ioannidis JPA, Balk E, et al. *Evaluation of Technologies for Identifying Acute Cardiac Ischemia in Emergency Departments.* Rockville, MD: Agency for Healthcare Research and Quality; May 2001. Evidence Report/Technology Assessment 26. Available at: http://www.ncbi.nlm.nih.gov/books/bv.fcgi?rid=hstat1.chapter.37233.
14. Thygesen K, Alpert JS. Myocardial infarction redefined—a consensus document of the Joint European Society of Cardiology/American College of Cardiology Committee for the Redefinition of Myocardial Infarction. *Eur Heart J.* 2000;21:1502–1513.
15. Forberg JL, Green M, Björk J, et al. In search of the best method to predict acute coronary syndrome using only

the electrocardiogram from the emergency department. *J Electrocardiol.* 2009;42:58–63.

16. Slater DK, Hlatky MA, Mark DB, et al. Outcomes in suspected acute myocardial infarction with normal or minimally abnormal admission electrocardiographic findings. *Am J Cardiol.* 1987;60:766–770.

17. Tabas JA, Rodriguez RM, Seligman HK, et al. Electrocardiographic criteria for detecting acute myocardial infarction in patients with left bundle branch block: a meta-analysis. *Ann Emerg Med.* 2008;52:329–336.

18. Sgarbossa EB, Pinski SL, Barbagelata A, et al. Electrocardiographic diagnosis of evolving acute myocardial infarction in the presence of left bundle-branch block. *N Engl J Med.* 1996;334:481–487.

19. Rao SV, Ohman EM, Granger CB, et al. Prognostic value of isolated troponin elevation across the spectrum of chest pain syndromes. *Am J Cardiol.* 2003;91;936–940.

20. Heidenreich PA, Alloggiamento T, Melsop K, et al. The prognostic value of troponin in patients with non-ST elevation acute coronary syndromes: a meta-analysis. *J Am Coll Cardiol.* 2001;38:478–485.

21. Ilva TJ, Eskola MJ, Nikus KC, et al. The etiology and prognostic significance of all-cause troponin I positivity in emergency department patients. *J Emerg Med.* 2010;38:1–5.

22. Fesmire FM, Christenson RH, Fody EP, et al. Delta creatine kinase-MB outperforms myoglobin at two hours during the emergency department identification and exclusion of troponin positive non-ST-segment elevation acute coronary syndromes. *Ann Emerg Med.* 2004;44:12–19.

23. Budoff MJ, Achenbach S, Blumenthal RS, et al. Assessment of coronary artery disease by cardiac computed tomography: a scientific statement from the American Heart Association Committee on Cardiovascular Imaging and Intervention, Council on Cardiovascular Radiology and Intervention, and Committee on Cardiac Imaging, Council on Clinical Cardiology. *Circulation.* 2006;114:1761–1791.

24. Silber S, Richartz BM. Impact of both cardiac-CT and cardiac-MR on the assessment of coronary risk. *Z Kardiol.* 2005;94(suppl 4):IV/70–IV/80.

25. Cury RC, Shash K, Nagurney JT, et al. Cardiac magnetic resonance with T2-weighted imaging improves detection of patients with acute coronary syndrome in the emergency department. *Circulation.* 2008;118:837–844.

26. Steel C. Severe angina pectoris relieved by oxygen inhalation. *BMJ.* 1900;2:1568.

27. Weijesinghe M, Perrin K, Ranchord A, et al. Routine use of oxygen in the treatment of myocardial infarction: systematic review. *BMJ.* 2009;95:198–202.

28. Anderson JL, Adams CD, Antman EM, et al. ACC/AHA 2007 guidelines for the management of patients with unstable angina/non ST-elevation myocardial infarction: a report of the American College of Cardiology/American Heart Association Task Force on Practice Guidelines. *Circulation.* 2007;116:e148–e304.

29. ISIS-4: a randomised factorial trial assessing early oral captopril, oral mononitrate, and intravenous magnesium sulphate in 58,050 patients with suspected acute myocardial infarction. *Lancet.* 1995;345:669–682.

30. Randomised trial of intravenous atenolol among 16 027 cases of suspected acute myocardial infarction: ISIS-1. First International Study of Infarct Survival Collaborative Group. *Lancet.* 1986;2:57–66.

31. Chen ZM, Pan HC, Chen YP, et al. Early intravenous then oral metoprolol in 45,852 patients with acute myocardial infarction: randomised placebo-controlled trial. *Lancet.* 2005;366:1622–1632.

32. Mattu A, Bond MC, Brady WJ. The cardiac literature 2007. *Am J Emerg Med.* 2008;26:817–833.

33. Meine TJ, Roe MT, Chen AY, et al. Association of intravenous morphine use and outcomes in acute coronary syndromes: results from the CRUSADE Quality Improvement Initiative. *Am Heart J.* 2005;149:1043–1049.

34. ISIS2 Collaborative Group. Randomised trial of intravenous streptokinase, oral aspirin, both, or neither among 17,187 cases of suspected acute myocardial infarction: ISIS2. *Lancet.* 1988;2:349–360.

35. Roux S, Christeller S, Lüdin E. Effects of aspirin on coronary re-occlusion and recurrent ischemia after thrombolysis: a meta-analysis. *J Am Coll Cardiol.* 1992;19:671–677.

36. Antithrombotic Trialists' Collaboration. Collaborative meta-analysis of randomised trials of antiplatelet therapy for prevention of death, myocardial infarction, and stroke in high risk patients. *BMJ.* 2002;324:71–86.

37. Barbash IM, Freimark D, Gottlieb S, et al. Israeli Working Group on Intensive Cardiac Care, Israel Heart Society. Outcome of myocardial infarction in patients treated with aspirin is enhanced by pre-hospital administration. *Cardiology.* 2002;98:141–147.

38. Schwertner HA, McGlasson D, Christopher M, et al. Effects of different aspirin formulations on platelet aggregation times and on plasma salicylate concentrations. *Thromb Res.* 2006;118:529–534.

39. CAPRIE Steering Committee. A randomised, blinded, trial of clopidogrel versus aspirin in patients at risk of ischaemic events. *Lancet.* 1996;348:1329–1339.

40. Harrington RA, Becker RC, Ezekowitz M, et al. Antithrombotic therapy for coronary artery disease: the Seventh ACCP Conference on Antithrombotic and Thrombolytic Therapy. *Chest.* 2004;126:513S–548S.

41. Yusuf S, Zhao F, Mehta SR, et al. Effects of clopidogrel in addition to aspirin in patients with acute coronary syndromes without ST-segment elevation. *N Engl J Med.* 2001;345:494–502.

42. Alexander D, Ou FS, Roe MT, et al. Use of and in-hospital outcomes after early clopidogrel therapy in patients not undergoing an early invasive strategy for treatment of non–ST-segment elevation myocardial infarction: results from Can Rapid risk stratification of Unstable angina patients Suppress ADverse outcomes with Early implementation of the American College of Cardiology/American Heart Association guidelines (CRUSADE). *Am Heart J.* 2008;156:606–612.

43. Chen ZM, Jiang LX, Chen YP, et al. Addition of clopidogrel to aspirin in 45,852 patients with acute myocardial infarction: randomized placebo-controlled trial. *Lancet.* 2005;366:1607–1621.

44. Sabatine MS, Cannon CP, Gibson CM, et al. Addition of clopidogrel to aspirin and fibrinolytic therapy for

myocardial infarction with ST-segment elevation. *N Engl J Med.* 2005;352:1179–1189.

45. Mehta SR, Yusuf S, Peters RJ, et al. Effects of pretreatment with clopidogrel and aspirin followed by long-term therapy in patients undergoing percutaneous coronary intervention: the PCI-CURE study. *Lancet.* 2001;358: 527–533.

46. Kushner FG, Hand M, Smith SC, et al. 2009 focused updates: ACC/AHA guidelines for the management of patients with ST-elevation myocardial infarction (updating the 2004 guideline and 2007 focused update) and ACC/AHA/SCAI guidelines on percutaneous coronary intervention (updating the 2005 guideline and 2007 focused update). *Circulation.* 2009;120;2271–2306.

47. Kastrati A, Mehilli J, Neumann FJ, et al. Abciximab in patients with acute coronary syndromes undergoing percutaneous coronary intervention after clopidogrel pretreatment: the ISAR-REACT 2 randomized trial. *JAMA.* 2006;295:1531–1538.

48. Antman EM, Giugliano RP, Gibson CM, et al. Abciximab facilitates the rate and extent of thrombolysis: results of the thrombolysis in myocardial infarction (TIMI) 14 trial. *Circulation.* 1999;99:2720–2732.

49. Gurm H, Tamhane U, Meier P, et al. A comparison of abciximab and small molecule glycoprotein IIb/IIIa inhibitors in patients undergoing primary percutaneous coronary intervention: a meta-analysis of contemporary randomized controlled trials. *Circ Cardiovasc Intervent.* 2009;2:230–236.

50. Inhibition of platelet glycoprotein IIb/IIIa with eptifibatide in patients with acute coronary syndrome. The PURSUIT Trial Investigators. *N Engl J Med.* 1998;339: 436–443.

51. Simoons ML, GUSTO IV-ACS Investigators. Effect of glycoprotein IIb/IIIa receptor blocker abciximab on outcome in patients with acute coronary syndromes without early coronary re-vascularization: the GUSTO IV-ACS randomised trial. *Lancet.* 2001;357:1915–1924.

52. Oler A, Whooley MA, Oler J, et al. Adding heparin to aspirin reduces the incidence of myocardial infarction and death in patients with unstable angina: a meta-analysis. *JAMA.* 1996;276:811–815.

53. Mikhailidis DP, Jagroop IA, Ganotakis E, et al. The FRISC Study Group. Low-molecular-weight heparin during instability in coronary artery disease. *Lancet.* 1996;347:561–568.

54. Klein W, Buchwald A, Hillis SE, et al. Comparison of low-molecular-weight heparin with unfractionated heparin acutely and with placebo for 6 weeks in the management of unstable coronary artery disease. Fragmin in unstable coronary artery disease study (FRIC). *Circulation.* 1997;96:61–68.

55. Antman EM, McCabe CH, Gurfinkel EP, et al. Enoxaparin prevents death and cardiac ischemic events in unstable angina/non-Q-wave myocardial infarction: results of the Thrombolysis In Myocardial Infarction (TIMI) 11B trial. *Circulation.* 1999;100:1593–1601.

56. Blazing MA, de Lemos JA, White HD, et al. Safety and efficacy of enoxaparin vs unfractionated heparin in patients with non-ST-segment elevation acute coronary syndromes who receive tirofiban and aspirin: a randomized controlled trial. *JAMA.* 2004;292:55–64.

57. Ferguson JJ, Califf RM, Antman EM, et al. Enoxaparin vs unfractionated heparin in high-risk patients with non-ST-segment elevation acute coronary syndromes managed with an intended early invasive strategy: primary results of the SYNERGY randomized trial. *JAMA.* 2004;292: 45–54.

58. Mahaffey KW, Ferguson JJ. Exploring the role of enoxaparin in the management of high-risk patients with non-ST-elevation acute coronary syndromes: the SYNERGY trial. *Am Heart J.* 2005;149:S81–S90.

59. Yusuf S, Mehta SR, Chrolavicius S, et al. Comparison of fondaparinux and enoxaparin in acute coronary syndromes. *N Engl J Med.* 2006;354:1464–1476.

60. Stone GW, Ware JH, Bertrand ME, et al. Antithrombotic strategies in patients with acute coronary syndromes under-going early invasive management: one-year results from the ACUITY trial. *JAMA.* 2007;298: 2497–2506.

61. Keeley EC, Boura JA, Grines CL. Primary angioplasty versus intravenous thrombolytic therapy for acute myocardial infarction: a quantitative review of 23 randomized trials. *Lancet.* 2003;361:13–20.

62. Busk M, Maeng M, Rasmussen K. The Danish multicentre randomized study of fibrinolytic therapy vs. primary angioplasty in acute myocardial infarction (the DANAMI-2 trial): outcome after 3 years follow-up. *Eur Heart J.* 2008;29:1259–1266.

63. Krumholz HM, Anderson JL, Brooks NH, et al. ACC/AHA clinical performance measures for adults with ST-elevation and non–ST-elevation myocardial infarction: a report of the ACC/AHA Task Force on Performance Measures (ST-Elevation and Non–ST-Elevation Myocardial Infarction Performance Measures Writing Committee). *J Am Coll Cardiol.* 2006;47:236–265.

64. Antman EM, Hand M, Armstrong PW, et al. 2007 focused update of the ACC/AHA 2004 guidelines for the management of patients with ST-elevation myocardial infarction: a report of the American College of Cardiology/American Heart Association Task Force on Practice Guidelines. *Circulation.* 2008;117:296–329.

65. Fibrinolytic Therapy Trialists' Collaborative Group. Indications for fibrinolytic therapy in suspected acute myocardial infarction: collaborative overview of early mortality and major morbidity results from all randomised trials of more than 1000 patients. *Lancet.* 1994;343:311–322.

66. Bavry AA, Kumbhani DJ, Rassi AN, et al. Benefit of early invasive therapy in acute coronary syndromes: a meta-analysis of contemporary randomized clinical trials. *J Am Coll Cardiol.* 2006;48:1319–1325.

67. Hoenig MR, Doust JA, Aroney CN, et al. Early invasive versus conservative strategies for unstable angina and non-ST elevation myocardial infarction in the stent era. *Cochrane Database Syst Rev.* 2006;3:CD004815.

68. Hollander JE, Sites FD, Pollack CV Jr, et al. Lack of utility of telemetry monitoring for identification of cardiac death and life threatening ventricular dysrhythmias in low-risk patients with chest pain. *Ann Emerg Med.* 2004;43;71–76.

CHAPTER 14

Hypertensive Crises

Christopher M. Perry, Qiuping Zhou, and Todd L. Slesinger

► INTRODUCTION

Hypertension is a common finding in patients presenting to the emergency department. The clinical context in which this is seen can represent a broad spectrum of disease: from asymptomatic individuals incidentally noted at triage to have elevated blood pressures to critically ill patients with hypertension-induced damage to critical organs. Determining the best management approach to such patients represents a significant challenge, as well as a frequent source of controversy, to emergency medicine and critical care clinicians.

A number of questions face the practitioner, including whether or not blood pressure reduction will be helpful or harmful, how quickly and to what level the blood pressure should be reduced, and what the appropriate agent is to use for a given situation. Additionally, the presence of preexisting conditions needs to be considered when making treatment decisions, as well as the patient's baseline blood pressure.

The diagnostic and therapeutic approach should not be algorithmic, guided strictly by numbers. Instead, clinicians should base their clinical decisions on a number of principles, most importantly the presence or absence of end-organ damage. Always treat the patient, not the number.

► EPIDEMIOLOGY

Hypertension is an increasingly important health care issue, with more than 50 million people in the United States having high blood pressure needing treatment.[1]

The prevalence increases with age, with more than half of people between the ages of 60 and 69 affected, increasing to more than three quarters of people over the age of 70.[1] Elevated blood pressures are noted in more than 25% of all patients presenting to the emergency department.[2,3] The ability to rapidly recognize and, when necessary, appropriately treat hypertension is therefore a critical skill for any practitioner in the emergency department or the intensive care unit (ICU).

► DETERMINATION OF HYPERTENSION

Essential to appropriate management is first obtaining an accurate measurement. Patients should be seated for at least 5 minutes prior to the measurement being taken, with feet on the floor and arm supported at heart level. The auscultatory method should be used, and should be performed by a trained practitioner. The cuff bladder should encircle at least 80% of the arm, and at least two measurements should be performed with the average recorded.[1]

► PATHOPHYSIOLOGY

Hypertension can be broadly divided into primary ("essential") and secondary hypertension. Essential hypertension, for which no cause is found, accounts for more than 90% of the cases of hypertension.[4] Many pathophysiologic causes have been hypothesized, but generally it is believed that the primary cause is through renal mechanisms amplified by sympathetic nervous system activity and vascular remodeling. Essential hypertension has a tendency to cluster in families, often in association with other genetically inherited syndromes.[4]

Secondary hypertension can occur through a variety of causes. Renovascular disease, such as that due to renal artery stenosis or fibromuscular dysplasia, should be suspected in any young patient with hypertension or any patient with rapidly progressive symptoms. Decreased pressures in the lower extremities or delayed femoral pulses should raise the suspicion for coarctation of the aorta. Excessive glucocorticoids, most commonly a result of iatrogenic steroid administration, are also associated with hypertension. Physical signs and symptoms such as truncal obesity, glucose intolerance, and purple striae should suggest the diagnosis. Labile blood pressures with associated paroxysmal headaches, palpitations, pallor, and diaphoresis should raise the suspicion of pheochromocytoma.

► CLASSIFICATION

The Seventh Report of the Joint National Committee on Prevention, Detection, Evaluation, and Treatment of High Blood Pressure (JNC 7), released in 2003, introduced a new classification for defining hypertension.[1] Blood pressure between 120 and 139 mm Hg systolic, and/or between 80 and 89 mm Hg diastolic, is now termed "prehypertension." Stage 1 hypertension is now defined as systolic between 140 and 159 mm Hg and/ or diastolic between 90 and 100 mm Hg. And systolic greater than 160 mm Hg and/or diastolic greater than 100 mm Hg is now classified as stage 2 hypertension.

Acute severe elevations in blood pressure can be classified in a number of ways. Most commonly, practitioners consider hypertensive "emergency" to be uncontrolled hypertension in the setting of end-organ damage, particularly damage to the renal, cerebral, or cardiovascular systems. Hypertensive "urgency," on the other hand, is generally defined as severe acutely elevated BP without evidence of acute organ damage. What constitutes "severely elevated" varies among practitioners, but is defined by JNC 7 as blood pressure greater than 180/120 mm Hg.[1]

The distinction between hypertensive emergency and urgency is critical as it dictates the timing and goals of blood pressure reduction, the need for parenteral versus oral agents, and the appropriate disposition on leaving the emergency department.

► HYPERTENSIVE URGENCIES

The majority of patients presenting to the emergency department with hypertensive urgency have previously diagnosed hypertension and most often present in the setting of various painful symptoms.[5] The level of hypertension necessitating treatment, and the choice of agent used, varies among practitioners.[5] However, most would agree that, in the absence of end-organ damage, blood pressure should not be normalized in the emergency department but instead should be controlled over a period of several days through the use of oral agents.[33]

The treatment strategy in the emergency department should begin with attempts to alleviate pain and anxiety, including providing patients with a quiet room if possible. These interventions alone may decrease the blood pressure to acceptable levels. If the patients are already being treated for hypertension, their home blood pressure medications should be given if they have not already taken them that day. If they have been compliant with their home medications, an increase in dosage can be considered or an additional agent added to their home regimen, although this should ideally be done in coordination with their primary physician.

If a decrease in blood pressure is desired over a period of hours to acceptable levels in the emergency room, oral agents such as clonidine (0.1–0.2 mg) or captopril (12.5–25 mg) may be given. However, such patients should be observed for several hours in the emergency department after drug administration.

Discharge home may be considered if the patient can be relied upon to closely follow up with his or her primary doctor within the next several days and no other compelling reason exists to admit to the hospital. All patients should be counseled on lifestyle modifications including weight loss, dietary sodium restriction, and regular aerobic activity.

It is important to note that absence of end-organ damage does not necessarily signify the absence of symptoms. Patients with hypertensive urgency may present with headache, epistaxis, anxiety, or other symptoms attributable to the elevated blood pressure. However, excessive and overly rapid correction of blood pressure elevations in such patients could precipitate ischemia to vital organs and should be avoided.

► HYPERTENSIVE EMERGENCIES

Hypertensive emergency is generally defined as uncontrolled hypertension in the setting of end-organ damage, and treatment with titratable intravenous (IV) agents should be instituted immediately. The choice of agent and the goals of therapy should be based on the specific clinical presentation and are summarized in Table 14-1. Patients with a hypertensive emergency should receive an ICU consultation.

Critical to the management of any hypertensive emergency is understanding the concept of autoregulation. Autoregulation is the ability of an organ to maintain

► TABLE 14-1. **MEDICATION OPTIONS FOR HYPERTENSIVE CRISES**

End-Organ Dysfunction	Recommended Agents
Encephalopathy	Nitroprusside, labetalol, fenoldopam, nicardipine
Stroke	Labetalol, nicardipine, nitroprusside
Acute myocardial ischemia	Nitroglycerin, esmolol, metoprolol
Acute pulmonary edema (suspected systolic dysfunction)	Nitroglycerin, ACE inhibitor, nitroprusside, fenoldopam (in combination with a loop diuretic)
Acute pulmonary edema (suspected diastolic dysfunction)	Nitroglycerin, esmolol, labetalol, metoprolol (in combination with a loop diuretic)
Aortic dissection	Labetalol, or esmolol with nitroprusside or nicardipine
Hypertension of pregnancy (preeclampsia or eclampsia)	Labetalol, nicardipine, hydralazine (consider magnesium sulfate)
Renal failure	Nitroprusside, labetalol

ACE: angiotensin-converting enzyme.

a near-constant blood flow despite variations in perfusion pressure. The autoregulatory response is intrinsic to the specific organ's vascular bed, and is independent of neural or humoral factors. Although examples of autoregulation can be seen throughout the body, it is most prominent in the cerebral, coronary, and renal vascular beds.

However, autoregulation is only maintained over a certain range of perfusion pressures. Outside of this range, changes in blood pressure are directly reflected in the microvasculature. This leads to ischemia in the setting of hypotension, and hyperperfusion injury in the setting of hypertension. Additionally, chronic hypertension can cause this autoregulatory range to be shifted to a higher range of pressures. Attempting to rapidly normalize elevated blood pressures in such patients may in fact lead to hypoperfusion and ischemia.

► PRESENTATIONS

HYPERTENSIVE ENCEPHALOPATHY

Under normal conditions, cerebral perfusion is maintained relatively stable over a wide range of blood pressures, due to the ability of the brain to autoregulate its blood flow. Hypertensive encephalopathy results from a cerebral perfusion pressure above this level of autoregulation, and represents a true medical emergency.

The precise pathophysiology of hypertensive encephalopathy is not completely understood. With sudden elevations of blood pressure, the ability of the brain to autoregulate its blood flow is lost, resulting in vasodilation, breakdown of the blood–brain barrier, and cerebral edema. It has been linked to the reversible posterior leukoencephalopathy syndrome,[7] in which acute elevations in blood pressure lead to white matter edema mostly in the posterior parietal–temporal–occipital regions of the brain. In both conditions, symptoms can be rapidly reversed with appropriate and timely lowering of blood pressure. However, if inadequately treated, these symptoms can progress to cerebral hemorrhage, coma, and death.[6]

No exact value of blood pressure is pathognomonic for hypertensive encephalopathy, although cerebral autoregulation can be overwhelmed at mean arterial pressures (MAPs) as low as 120 mm Hg in previously normotensive individuals.[6] However, individuals with chronic hypertension often have autoregulatory curves that have been shifted to higher pressures, and may not develop symptoms of hypertensive encephalopathy until MAPs have exceeded 150 mm Hg or higher.

Clinically, hypertensive encephalopathy is manifested by symptoms of headache, nausea, lethargy, altered mental status, and seizures. When associated with the reversible posterior leukoencephalopathy syndrome, symptoms may also include visual abnormalities, including cortical blindness, homonymous hemianopsia, and blurred vision.[7] On physical exam, signs of increased intracranial pressure (ICP) such as papilledema may be seen. Focal neurologic deficits are generally not found on exam, although they may occur if hemorrhage or infarction occurs. The differential diagnosis is wide and includes intracerebral hemorrhage, brain tumor, meningoencephalitis, toxidromes, and CVA.

Hypertensive encephalopathy represents a true medical emergency, and efforts at blood pressure reduction should begin immediately when this is suspected. An initial goal blood pressure reduction of 20–25% is generally advised, or a goal diastolic of 100–110 mm Hg. A titratable agent such as nitroprusside should be used, preferably with arterial line monitoring to avoid overshoot hypotension. Other agents such as fenoldopam and labetalol are acceptable alternatives.

STROKE SYNDROMES

Antihypertensive therapy in the setting of stroke remains an area of considerable controversy. In these scenarios, hypertension may represent both a contributing factor and a physiologic response to the stroke syndrome. Despite the widespread prevalence of stroke syndromes, an optimal treatment strategy regarding blood pressure management has not been established.[8,9]

Elevated blood pressures have been shown to be a prognostic indicator of stroke mortality,[9,10] but it is not clear whether this is a causal relationship or a measure of stroke severity. In the setting of ischemic stroke, there are several theoretical reasons why antihypertensive therapy would be beneficial. Lowering blood pressure could reduce edema around the damaged area, decrease the risk of hemorrhagic transformation, and lessen further vascular damage. However, aggressive treatment of hypertension in the setting of ischemic stroke could also reduce perfusion in ischemic areas. This risk of causing harm, combined with the lack of data supporting benefit, suggests that aggressive lowering of blood pressure should be avoided in the acute phase of stroke.

The Stroke Council of the American Stroke Association has offered guidelines[8] for the management of hypertension in the setting of ischemic stroke. The consensus is to withhold treatment unless the hypertension is severe, defined by this council as systolic >220 mm Hg or diastolic >120 mm Hg. The recommendation in these scenarios is treatment with labetalol 10–20 mg IV boluses every 1–2 minutes or with a nicardipine infusion of 5–15 mg/h.

These recommendations change for those patients who are candidates for thrombolytic therapy. In these patients, elevated blood pressures represent an increased danger of intracerebral hemorrhage and should thus be controlled. Blood pressure should be lowered to <185 mm Hg systolic and <110 mm Hg diastolic prior to administration of a thrombolytic agent, and should be maintained below these levels for 16 hours after therapy.[8] Again, labetalol boluses and nicardipine infusion are the recommended agents, although nitroprusside may be necessary in refractory cases.

In most cases of ischemic stroke, elevated blood pressures decrease spontaneously without treatment. Additional measures to lower ICP, such as raising the head of the bed, and measures to reduce pain and anxiety can also lower blood pressure through nonpharmacologic means.

For hemorrhagic stroke, representing approximately 15% of all strokes, the optimal treatment strategy is equally controversial.[11–13] Hypertension in the setting of intracranial hemorrhage is often severe due to increased ICPs and irritation of the autonomic nervous system. Similar concerns exist for initiating therapy including the balance between decreasing the risk of further bleeding and hemorrhagic enlargement, with the concern for decreasing cerebral perfusion pressure. As a result, no general consensus exists suggesting a compelling need to initiate antihypertensive therapy in the patient with acute intracranial hemorrhage.[11–13]

Current guidelines for patients with intracerebral hemorrhage, released in 2007 from the American Heart Association/American Stroke Association Stroke Council,[12] recommend considering aggressive therapy if the systolic is greater than 200 mm Hg or the MAP is greater than 150 mm Hg. If systolic is above 180 mm Hg or the MAP is above 130 mm Hg, and if elevated ICP is suspected, recommendations are to consider establishing ICP monitoring and maintaining a cerebral perfusion pressure between 60 and 80 mm Hg. In the absence of evidence of increased ICP, for patients with a systolic greater than 180 mm Hg or an MAP greater than 130 mm Hg, a modest reduction in blood pressure, to an MAP of 110 mm Hg or target blood pressure of 160/90 mm Hg, should be considered. However, at present, little prospective data exist to definitively recommend a specific blood pressure threshold.

In the case of aneurysmal subarachnoid hemorrhage, recommendations are to maintain the systolic blood pressure below 160 mm Hg and the MAP below 130 mm Hg.[13] However, pain control, sedation, and ICP-lowering measures, such as raising the head of the bed, should be instituted prior to administering antihypertensive agents. Additionally, the use of oral nimodipine, to prevent delayed cerebral vasospasm, will have a modest hypotensive effect, although it is not used for this purpose.

As with ischemic stroke, when the decision is made to lower blood pressure, the agents used should be rapid acting and easily titratable such as labetalol, nicardipine, or esmolol. Blood pressure monitoring should be continuous, via arterial line monitoring, or every 5 minutes.[12]

Other situations where aggressive antihypertensive therapy may be indicated in the setting of acute stroke include aortic dissection, hypertensive encephalopathy, and myocardial infarction. The systemic effects of hypertension must always be taken into account when making the decision to initiate antihypertensive therapy.

CONGESTIVE HEART FAILURE

Congestive heart failure (CHF) represents a clinical syndrome of inadequate cardiac output with a resulting cascade of events, primarily mediated through increased catecholamines, leading to increased peripheral vascular resistance, increased intravascular and interstitial volumes, and pulmonary edema. The hypertension associated with CHF can be both a cause and effect of this process and needs to be lowered rapidly, although carefully, to relieve symptoms and improve clinical outcome. Nitroglycerin is generally the first-line agent, although nitroprusside may be necessary in severe or refractory cases. Additionally, angiotensin-converting enzyme (ACE) inhibitors such as captopril or, if unable to tolerate PO, enalapril or enalaprilat may be helpful.

β-Blockers are widely used in patients with chronic CHF, but are generally avoided in acutely decompensated states due to the negative inotropic and chronotropic effects. The only exception to this would be in the case of known or suspected diastolic dysfunction. With these patients, CHF is a function of inadequacy of ventricular filling during diastole. β-Blockers may allow for additional cardiac relaxation and better filling. The ejection fraction is not typically reduced in these patients. Diastolic dysfunction is typically diagnosed with an echocardiogram, but may be suspected in a patient with decompensated heart failure without evidence of cardiomegaly.

Diuretics such as furosemide should be used to reduce fluid overload and improve work of breathing. Additional measures, including supplemental oxygen, BiPAP, and even mechanical ventilation, are often also necessary. With an improvement in respiratory status, the catecholamine surge is often relieved, subsequently lowering blood pressure and breaking the pathologic cycle.

CARDIAC ISCHEMIA

Myocardial ischemia or infarction associated with hypertension warrants immediate blood pressure–lowering therapy to minimize myocardial damage. Agents of choice include nitroglycerin and IV β-blockers such as metoprolol. ACE inhibitors are also an important part of the therapy in the setting of an acute coronary syndrome; however, care should be taken to avoid overshoot hypotension when coadministered with nitroglycerin and β-blockers.

RENAL FAILURE

Hypertension can be seen as both a consequence of and a cause of renal failure. Renal disease leads to hypertension both through increased salt retention and through the renin–angiotensin system. Additionally, uncontrolled hypertension may cause acute kidney injury and can accelerate the progression of injury in patients with chronic renal failure. Worsening kidney function in the setting of elevated blood pressures should be considered a hypertensive emergency and warrants immediate treatment.

Nitroprusside is considered a first-line agent for hypertension-induced acute renal failure, although labetalol is often preferred due to the decreased risk of overshoot hypotension. ACE inhibitors, although highly effective in controlling chronic renal disease, should be used cautiously in the setting of acute renal failure as they may worsen the process acutely.

Emergent dialysis may be indicated in patients with end-stage renal disease with acute uncontrolled hypertension in the setting of volume overload or any evidence of other end-organ dysfunction.

PREGNANCY

Hypertensive disorders complicate between 6% and 8% of all pregnancies[14] and represent a significant source of morbidity and mortality to both the mother and the fetus. Up to 15% of maternal deaths in the United States are attributable to hypertensive disorders, making it the second leading cause of maternal mortality after thromboembolic disease.[14]

Classification of pregnancy-associated hypertensive disorders is based on the level of blood pressure elevation, the presence of proteinuria, and physical signs and symptoms. Hypertension in pregnancy is defined as a systolic blood pressure ≥140 mm Hg or a diastolic pressure ≥90 mm Hg. The level of hypertension is classified as severe if the systolic blood pressure is ≥160 mm Hg or the diastolic pressure is ≥105–110 mm Hg.[15] Hypertension in pregnancy occurring prior to 20 weeks' gestation is termed chronic hypertension, most likely antedating pregnancy. Hypertension occurring after 20 weeks, but without proteinuria or any signs or symptoms, is termed gestational hypertension. Preeclampsia is defined as hypertension occurring after 20 weeks with proteinuria (>300 mg in 24 hours) or other clinical or laboratory abnormalities. Eclampsia is the occurrence of seizures or coma in the presence of preexisting preeclampsia.

Severe preeclampsia or eclampsia, or pregnancy-associated hypertension with any signs or symptoms indicative of end-organ damage, represent true hypertensive emergencies and should be treated emergently. Treatment goals in the emergency department should include blood pressure reduction, seizure prevention and control, and early obstetric consultation.

The specific goals of blood pressure reduction are not well defined. Severe, acute elevations in blood pressure can be associated with cerebral and cardiovascular complications, as well as placental abruption and uteroplacental insufficiency.[15] However, some evidence suggests a parallel between reduction in MAP and adverse effects on fetal growth.[16] Some advocate withholding treatment unless diastolic blood pressure remains persistently elevated above 105–110 mm Hg.[14]

Hydralazine has traditionally been the frontline agent of choice, although this has come into question in the recent years.[15] Nevertheless, it is still widely used and is an effective agent, although caution must be taken due to its unpredictable dose–response curve. Labetalol is now the drug of choice for pregnancy-associated hypertensive emergencies.[17] Nicardipine may also be effective, although there has been some concern about administering it in patients also receiving magnesium sulfate for seizure prophylaxis, due to the combined calcium channel–blocking activity.[15] Nitroprusside should be reserved to severe hypertension refractory to other agents, due to the potential for fetal cyanide toxicity and overshoot hypotension. ACE inhibitors are contraindicated in pregnancy.

AORTIC DISSECTION

Aortic dissection should be suspected in any patients presenting with chest and/or upper back pain, particularly pain that is sharp or "tearing" in quality and maximal at onset. However, up to 20% may present with syncope without a history of typical pain or other findings.[18] Physical exam findings pointing to a diagnosis of aortic dissection include pulse deficits, a diastolic murmur, and neurologic deficits. A high index of suspicion should always be maintained, as inappropriately treating for a presumed acute coronary syndrome or stroke could be devastating for patients with aortic dissection.

Aortic dissection represents a hypertensive emergency in which the treatment approach is two-pronged. Since propagation is dependent on both the level of hypertension and the left ventricular ejection force, therapy must be aimed at both lowering pressure and slowing the rate of pressure rise. Therefore, generally a β-blocker such as esmolol is used in combination with a vasodilator such as nitroprusside. Alternatively, labetalol, which has both α- and β-blocking effects, can be used as monotherapy.[19] Goal blood pressure should be below 120–130 mm Hg systolic.

All patients with suspected aortic dissection require prompt surgical consultation. However, aneurysms involving only the descending aorta (Stanford type B) are generally medically managed.

▶ PHARMACOLOGY

Many of the agents used to treat hypertensive urgency and emergency are described below. Parenteral agents are summarized in Table 14-2.

SODIUM NITROPRUSSIDE

Nitroprusside is an extremely powerful and effective pressure-lowering agent, acting as a potent vasodilator in both the arterial and venous systems. Due to its rapid onset of action (1–2 minutes), short half-life (3–4 minutes), and almost universal effectiveness, it is widely considered the standard drug of choice in hypertensive emergencies.

Due to its high potency, overshoot hypotension is the most common complication. Close hemodynamic monitoring, preferably with an intra-arterial line, is required. Infusion of sodium nitroprusside is generally begun at 0.3 mcg/kg/min and titrated up to goal MAP, with a maximum dose of 10 mcg/kg/min.[20]

Sodium nitroprusside is metabolized by the liver to thiocyanate that is then excreted by the kidneys. Cyanide is an intermediate metabolite in this process, although cyanide toxicity is rare. However, thiocyanate toxicity may occur in the setting of hepatic or renal failure or prolonged administration.[20] Use of this agent is also complicated by the need for special handling, as it is unstable in the presence of ultraviolet light and must be wrapped in opaque material during administration.

Caution should be used in patients in whom increased cerebral pressure is a concern, as nitroprusside acts as a cerebral vasodilator. Additionally, nitroprusside should be avoided in pregnant patients due to its ability to cross the placenta and cause toxic effects on the fetus.

FENOLDOPAM

Fenoldopam mesylate is a selective postsynaptic dopamine-1 receptor agonist that functions both as a systemic and renal vasodilator and as a natriuretic. Like nitroprusside, fenoldopam has an onset of action within minutes and a short duration of action (less than 10 minutes). Additionally, it has been demonstrated to be as effective as nitroprusside in lowering blood pressure[21] with less hypotension and no concerns of light sensitivity or thiocyanate or cyanide toxicity. For these reasons, fenoldopam is gaining favor by some as the drug of choice in treating hypertensive emergencies.

Fenoldopam is dosed initially at 0.1 mcg/kg/min and titrated in increments of 0.1 mcg/kg/min every 15 minutes until a desired pressure is reached. Side effects may include reflex tachycardia, headache, and facial flushing.

NITROGLYCERIN

Nitroglycerin is a rapidly acting vasodilator that lowers blood pressure in a dose-dependent fashion. It primarily acts on the venous system, thus decreasing preload more than afterload. It is therefore most useful in cardiac ischemia or heart failure associated with hypertension. When given intravenously, it is generally begun at 5–10 mcg/min titrating up in 5 mcg/min increments every 5 minutes until desired blood pressure is reached or the patient's symptoms have resolved.

The primary side effects of nitroglycerin are headache and tachycardia. It should be avoided in the setting of right heart failure, as a precipitous drop in cardiac output and blood pressure may result.

▶ TABLE 14-2. **DOSAGE AND EFFECTS OF COMMON PARENTERAL AGENTS IN HYPERTENSIVE EMERGENCY**

Medication	Dosage	Onset	Duration	Adverse Effects	Comments
Nitroprusside	0.3 μg/kg/min, titrate to maximum 10 μg/kg/min	Seconds	1–2 min	Cyanide toxicity, flushing, nausea, vomiting, headache, lactic acidosis	Avoid in setting of increased cerebral pressure or pregnancy Monitor for cyanide toxicity with prolonged use
Esmolol	Loading dose: 500 μg/kg over 1 min Infusion: 25 μg/kg/min, titrate to maximum 200 μg/kg/min	5–10 min	20 min	Bradycardia, nausea, flushing, bronchospasm	Avoid in acute heart failure with systolic dysfunction
Labetolol	Bolus: 20 mg initially with repeat doses of 20–80 mg Infusion: 1–2 mg/min to maximum 24 h total of 300 mg	5–10 min	6–8 h	Nausea, vomiting, bronchospasm, bradycardia, orthostatic hypotension	Avoid in acute heart failure with systolic dysfunction
Nicardipine	5 mg/h, increase by 2.5 mg/h every 5 min to maximum of 15 mg/h	5–10 min	4–6 h	Headache, nausea, flushing, reflex tachycardia	Use with caution in patients with liver failure
Nitroglycerin	5 μg/min, titrate by 5 μg/kg every 5 min to maximum 200 μg/min	Seconds	3–5 min	Headache, dizziness, tachyphylaxis	Use with caution in patients with right heart failure
Fenoldopam	0.1 μg/kg/min, titrate by 0.1 μg/kg/min every 15 min to maximum 1.6 μg/kg/min	10–15 min	30–60 min	Flushing, tachycardia, headache, nausea, vomiting	Use with caution in patients with asthma or glaucoma
Hydralazine	5–10 mg initially, repeat doses of 10 mg every 15 minutes	5–15 min	12 h	Tachycardia, headache, nausea, orthostatic hypotension	Effect may be unpredictable. Avoid in setting of myocardial ischemia or aortic dissection
Phentolamine	1–5 mg bolus 50 μg/min, titrate to maximum 500 μg/min	1–5 min	15–30 min	Flushing, reflex tachycardia, nausea, vomiting, hypotension	Used for catecholamine-induced state such as cocaine toxicity and pheochromocytoma Avoid in myocardial ischemia

HYDRALAZINE

Hydralazine is a direct arterial vasodilator, commonly used in pregnancy-induced hypertension. Onset of action is approximately 10 minutes when given intravenously with a duration of action of 4–6 hours. However, the effects can often be unpredictable, with an initial 5- to 15-minute latent period followed by an often precipitous drop in blood pressure, which may last up to 12 hours.[22,25] Doses are generally begun at 5–10 mg IV, with repeated doses of 10 mg every 10–15 minutes until goal blood pressure is reached. Reflex tachycardia is a common complication, and thus should be avoided in patients with myocardial ischemia or aortic dissection. Other adverse effects include headache, nausea, and postural hypotension. Chronic use may lead to a lupuslike syndrome.

LABETALOL

Labetalol is a combined α_1-blocker and nonselective β-blocker. The ratio of α- to β-blockade is 1:7 in the IV form.[23] As a result, labetalol is an effective blood pressure–lowering agent that has the advantage of not causing reflex tachycardia.

When given IV, onset of action is 5–10 minutes with a high volume of distribution and duration of action of approximately 6–8 hours. Dosing is usually begun at 20 mg IV for hypertensive emergencies with repeated doses of 20, 40, or 80 mg every 5–10 minutes until desired blood pressure is reached, up to a maximum of 300 mg. Alternatively, a continuous infusion of 1–2 mg/min can be begun after the initial bolus dose.

When goal blood pressure is reached, transition to oral form can be begun. Orally dosing is generally begun at 200 mg. Onset of effects with oral dosing is approximately 1–3 hours.

Labetalol has little effect on cerebral or coronary blood flow and can be used safely in patients with acute myocardial infarction. Due to its β-blockade effect, use with caution in patients with decompensated heart failure or in acute exacerbation of asthma or chronic obstructive pulmonary disease (COPD). It should also be avoided in patients with cardiac conduction system abnormalities. In low doses intravenously, due to the high ratio of β to α effects, there is a theoretical risk of paradoxical hypertension with administration to patients in high catecholamine-induced hypertension, such as that seen with pheochromocytoma or cocaine-induced hypertension.

ESMOLOL

Esmolol is a selective β_1-antagonist with an ultrashort half-life of approximately 9 minutes. It is easily titratable, due to its short duration of action of approximately 10–20 minutes. Esmolol is metabolized by red blood cell esterases, making it additionally useful in patients with hepatic and renal failure.[24]

Infusion is generally begun with a bolus of 250–500 mcg/kg over 1 minute, followed by an initial infusion of 25 mcg/kg/min. This can then be titrated up by increments of 25–50 mcg/kg/min every 4 minutes until goal blood pressure, or heart rate, is reached or to a maximum of 300 mcg/kg/min.

Adverse effects may include bradycardia, hypotension, dizziness, somnolence, nausea, and bronchospasm. As with all β-blockers, use with caution in patients with CHF, asthma, COPD, heart block, and bradycardia, or in the setting of cocaine overdose or pheochromocytoma.

NICARDIPINE

Nicardipine is a parenteral calcium channel blocker of the dihydropyridine class. It acts as a powerful vasodilator, but, unlike other calcium channel blockers such as nifedipine, it has the advantage of lacking significant negative inotropic effects.[25]

Nicardipine is generally begun at a rate of 5 mg/h and titrated every 5 minutes to a maximum of 15 mg/h or until the desired blood pressure is reached. Onset of action is within minutes, and duration of action is 4–6 hours.

Headache is a common side effect, occurring in up to 20–50% of patients.[26] Less commonly, tachycardia, nausea, and overshoot hypotension are seen. Caution should be used in patients with liver failure, as it is heavily metabolized by the liver.[27]

ENALAPRILAT

Enalaprilat is an IV ACE inhibitor that has been shown to be effective at lowering blood pressure without causing overshoot hypotension.[34] It is the active metabolite of the oral ACE inhibitor enalapril. Dosing is generally begun with a dose of between 0.625 and 1.25 mg IV. Peak effects occur within 10–15 minutes with a duration of action of 12–24 hours. Adverse effects may include renal failure, angioneurotic edema, and cough. ACE inhibitors are contraindicated in pregnancy.[28]

PHENTOLAMINE

Phentolamine is an α-adrenergic blocking agent most useful in management of catecholamine-induced hypertensive emergencies. It is generally given as 5-mg boluses, with an onset of action within 1–2 minutes and a duration of action of 10–30 minutes. It is contraindicated in the setting of myocardial ischemia, except when associated with cocaine toxicity, and may cause reflex tachycardia and tachydysrhythmias as a side effect.

CLEVIDIPINE

Clevidipine is an ultrashort-acting IV calcium channel blocker that was approved by the FDA in 2008 for the treatment of severe hypertension. It is easily titratable, with blood pressure reduction seen within 2–3 minutes of administration and a duration of action of 5–15 minutes.[29–31] Additionally, since it is cleared by plasma esterases, it requires no dosage adjustment for patients with hepatic or renal impairment. Dosing is begun at 1–2 mg/h and titrated up until desired blood pressure is reached. Titration is generally performed initially by doubling the dose every 90 seconds, although this titration should be done every 5–10 minutes if the blood pressure is near goal. A maximum of 16 mg/h is recommended; however, limited data exist for dosages up to 32 mg/h.[29–31] Adverse effects include headache, nausea, and chest discomfort.

CLONIDINE

Clonidine is a centrally acting α_2-agonist that lowers blood pressure through negative feedback on the vasomotor center of the brain, decreasing sympathetic discharge. It is an oral agent, and can be effective in cases of hypertensive urgency when blood pressure reduction is desired over a period of hours. Onset of action is between 30 minutes and 2 hours, with a duration of action of 6–8 hours. Dosing is begun at 0.1–0.2 mg orally, with additional doses 0.1 mg given hourly as necessary until goal blood pressure is reached. Side effects include sedation and dry mouth, and clonidine may sometimes cause orthostatic hypotension.[32]

CAPTOPRIL

Captopril is an oral ACE inhibitor that, like clonidine, can be useful in situations of hypertensive urgency where a more gradual blood pressure reduction is desired. Dosing is 12.5–25 mg with an onset of action between 15 and 30 minutes, and a duration of action of 4–6 hours. Side effects may include cough or skin rash. A more rare, but serious, side effect to ACE inhibitor therapy is angioedema, which may be life-threatening. ACE inhibitors are contraindicated in pregnancy.

► CONCLUSION

Hypertensive crises continue to represent a significant critical care challenge to the emergency physician. This will become increasingly more prevalent an issue as our population ages. Many factors must be considered when deciding on an appropriate treatment strategy. Therapy should always be specific to the patient and the situation, and never based on absolute values of blood pressure. The most important consideration, as always, is to remember to treat the patient, not the blood pressure.

REFERENCES

1. Chobanian A, Bakris G, Black H, et al. Seventh Report of the Joint National Committee on Prevention, Detection, Evaluation, and Treatment of High Blood Pressure. *Hypertension*. 2003;42:1206–1252.
2. Zampaglione B, Pascale P, Marchisio M, Cavallo-Perin P. Hypertensive urgencies and emergencies: prevalence and clinical presentation. *Hypertension*. 1996;27: 144–147.
3. Karras DJ, Wald DA, Harrigan RA, et al. Elevated blood pressure in an urban emergency department: prevalence and patient characteristics [abstract]. *Acad Emerg Med*. 2001;8:559.
4. Oparil S, Zaman A, Calhoun D. Pathogenesis of hypertension. *Ann Intern Med*. 2003;139:761–776.
5. Chiang W, Jamshahi B. Asymptomatic hypertension in the ED. *Am J Emerg Med*. 1998;16(7):701–704.
6. Vaughan C, Delanty N. Hypertensive emergencies. *Lancet*. 2000;356:411–417.

7. Hinchey J, Chaves C, Appignani B, et al. A reversible posterior leukoencephalopathy syndrome. *N Engl J Med*. 1996;334(8):494–500.
8. Adams H, Adams R, Brott T, et al. Guidelines for the early management of patients with ischemic stroke. A scientific statement from the Stroke Council of the American Stroke Association. *Stroke*. 2003;34:1056–1083.
9. Philips S. Pathophysiology and management of hypertension in acute ischemic stroke. *Hypertension*. 1994; 23(1):131–136.
10. Wilmot M, Leonardi-Bee J, Bath P. High blood pressure in acute stroke and subsequent outcome. A systematic review. *Hypertension*. 2004;43:18–24.
11. Adams R, Powers W. Management of hypertension in acute intracerebral hemorrhage. *Crit Care Clin*. 1997; 13(1):131–161.
12. Broderick J, Connolly S, Feldman E, et al. Guidelines for the management of spontaneous intracerebral hemorrhage in adults. 2007 update. A guideline from the American Heart Association/American Stroke Association Stroke Council, High Blood Pressure Research Council, and the Quality of Care and Outcomes in Research Interdisciplinary Working Group. *Circulation*. 2007;116:e391–e413.
13. Pancioli A. Hypertension management in neurologic emergencies. *Ann Emerg Med*. 2008;51:S24–S27.
14. Anonymous. Report of the National High Blood Pressure Education Program Working Group on High Blood Pressure in Pregnancy. *Am J Obstet Gynecol*. 2000;183(1): S1–S22.
15. Vidaeff A, Carroll M, Ramin S. Acute hypertensive emergencies in pregnancy. *Crit Care Med*. 2005;33:S307–S312.
16. von Dadelszen P, Ornstein MP, Bull SB, et al. Fall in mean arterial pressure and fetal growth in pregnancy hypertension: a meta-analysis. *Lancet*. 2000;355:87–92.
17. Sibai B. Diagnosis and management of gestational hypertension and pre-eclampsia. *Obstet Gynecol*. 2003; 102(1):181–192.
18. Neinaber A, Eagle K. Aortic dissection: new frontiers in diagnosis and management. Part I: from etiology to diagnostic strategies. *Circulation*. 2003;108:628–635.
19. Neinaber A, Eagle K. Aortic dissection: new frontiers in diagnosis and management. Part II: therapeutic management and follow-up. *Circulation*. 2003;108:772–778.
20. Friederich J, Butterworth J. Sodium nitroprusside: twenty years and counting. *Anesth Analg*. 1995;81:152–162.
21. Tumlin J, Dunbar L. Fenoldipam, a dopamine agonist, for hypertensive emergency: a multi-center randomized trial. *Acad Emerg Med*. 2000;7(6):653–662.
22. Varon J, Marik P. The diagnosis and management of hypertensive crises. *Chest*. 2000;118:214–227.
23. Lund-Johansen P. Pharmacology of combined alpha beta blockade II hemodynamic effects of labetalol. *Drugs*. 1984;28(suppl 2):35–50.
24. Gray RJ. Managing critically ill patients with esmolol: an ultra short-acting beta-adrenergic blocker. *Chest*. 1988; 93:398–403.
25. Marik P, Varon J. Hypertensive crises: challenges and management. *Chest*. 2007;131:1949–1962.
26. Wu M, Chanmugan A. Hypertension. In: Tintinalli J, Kelen G, Stapczynski JS, eds. *Emergency Medicine: A*

Comprehensive Study Guide. 6th ed. New York: McGraw-Hill; 2004:394–403.

27. Gray R. Hypertension. In: Marx JA, Hockberger RS, Walls RM, et al, eds. *Rosen's Emergency Medicine, Concepts and Clinical Practice.* 7th ed. Philadelphia, PA: Mosby Elsevier; 2009:1076–1087.

28. Strauss R, Gavras I, Vlahakos D, et al. Enalaprilat in hypertensive emergencies. *J Clin Pharmacol.* 1986;26:39–43.

29. Kenyon K. Clevidipine: an ultra short-acting calcium channel antagonist for acute hypertension. *Ann Pharmacother.* 2009;43:1258–1265.

30. Nguyen H, Ma K, Pham D. Clevidipine for the treatment of severe hypertension in adults. *Clin Ther.* 2010;32(1):11–23.

31. Erickson A, DeGrado J, Fanikos J, et al. Clevidipine: a short-acting intravenous dihydropyridine calcium channel blocker for the management of hypertension. *Pharmacotherapy.* 2010;30(5):515–528.

32. Spitalewitz S, Porush J, Oguagha C. Use of clonidine for rapid titration of blood pressure in severe hypertension. *Chest.* 1983;83:404–407.

33. Shayne P, Pitts S. Severely increased blood pressure in the emergency department. *Ann Emerg Med.* 2003;41:513–529.

34. Dipette DJ, Ferraro JC, Evans RR, et al. Enalaprilat, an intravenous angiotensin-converting enzyme inhibitor, in hypertensive crises. *Clin Pharmacol Ther.* 1985;38:199–204.

CHAPTER 15

Post-Cardiac Arrest Management

Alan C. Heffner

► INTRODUCTION

Sudden cardiac arrest is a leading cause of death in developed countries and impacts over 300,000 patients in the United States per year.[1] Despite initial resuscitation, 50% of arrest victims do not survive to discharge from the hospital. One third die from refractory cardiovascular shock or the cause of initial arrest. The remaining patients survive the initial insult only to later succumb due to organ dysfunction and neurologic injury stemming from the cardiac arrest. Among survivors, the burden of cardiac arrest persists with up to 30% of patients suffering permanent neurologic injury. These data underscore the impressive health care burden of sudden cardiac arrest.

The early post-arrest period has emerged as a critical window to impact the outcome of cardiac arrest victims. Improved morbidity and mortality achieved with therapeutic hypothermia prove the potential for treatments applied following return of spontaneous circulation (ROSC) to impact clinical outcome. As such, contemporary emergency care now emphasizes intensive support during this vulnerable and modifiable phase of illness. Priorities of the post-arrest period include stabilization of organ perfusion and oxygenation, identification and treatment of reversible causes of cardiac arrest, and initiation of neuroprotective therapy (Table 15-1). This chapter focuses on the immediate and early post-resuscitation phase of illness where timely interventions provide the greatest opportunity to achieve the goal of neurologically intact survival of cardiac arrest victims.

► THE POST-CARDIAC ARREST SYNDROME

Post-resuscitation disease is a unique multiorgan illness[2] (Table 15-2). Reperfusion following a period of whole-body ischemia and hypoxia ignites a complex systemic immunologic response. Proinflammatory cytokines, coagulation abnormalities, and endothelial dysfunction characterize a state of systemic inflammation analogous to that of severe infection.[3,4] The clinical consequence of this immune activation is macrocirculatory and microcirculatory dysfunction manifested as hemodynamic instability and early organ dysfunction.

CARDIOVASCULAR DYSFUNCTION

Low and no-flow periods of cardiac arrest are invariably associated with global ischemia. However, adequate oxygen delivery is not restored with ROSC. A brief hyperdynamic cardiovascular response is common immediately following ROSC but is typically followed by early cardiovascular deterioration.[5,6] The swiftness and degree of hemodynamic decline is inversely related to the period of cardiac arrest.[7] Persistent shock should be anticipated and represents an important target of therapy.

Post-ROSC shock is complex and multifactorial. Myocardial dysfunction stems from acute myocardial stunning, chronic disease, or the unresolved disease that incited cardiac arrest. However, primary cardiac

► TABLE 15-1. **EARLY POST-RESUSCITATION PRIORITIES**

• Provide adequate oxygenation and ventilation
• Reverse shock and stabilize hemodynamics
• Identify and treat reversible cause of cardiac arrest
• Apply neuroprotective therapies—therapeutic hypothermia
• Correct metabolic disturbances

dysfunction is rarely the sole lesion. The global cytokine storm and ischemic-reperfusion response following ROSC superimpose transcapillary leak and inappropriate vasoregulation to circulatory failure in the post-arrest period.

► HEMODYNAMIC RESUSCITATION

Hemodynamic resuscitation is a cornerstone of critical care support. Guidelines endorse an early endpoint-driven resuscitation for hemodynamic optimization following ROSC.[8,9] Early implementation of a structured hemodynamic optimization strategy improves survival in high-risk critical illness but remains untested for the post-cardiac arrest syndrome.[10-12] Standard hemodynamic manipulation focuses on preload optimization, blood pressure stabilization, and organ perfusion and oxygenation (Table 15-3). Post-resuscitation cardiovascular status is dynamic, making hemodynamic optimization an ongoing challenge. As such, invasive venous and arterial hemodynamic monitoring guidance should be strongly considered.

Systemic arterial perfusion pressure is critical to maintain adequate organ blood flow. The brain is particularly vulnerable in the post-arrest period. Impairment of cerebral autoregulation exposes the brain to hypoperfusion even in the absence of systemic hypotension.[13]

► TABLE 15-2. **POST-CARDIAC ARREST DISEASE AND PATHOPHYSIOLOGY**

Systemic ischemia–reperfusion injury	Systemic inflammatory response syndrome (SIRS) Inappropriate vasodilation Dysregulated coagulation Impaired microvascular function Early organ dysfunction
Acute myocardial dysfunction	Myocardial stunning Acute coronary syndrome
Brain injury	Anoxic brain insult Ischemic-reperfusion injury Impaired autoregulation
Persistent arrest precipitating pathology	

► TABLE 15-3. **EARLY HEMODYNAMIC RESUSCITATION GOALS FOLLOWING CARDIAC ARREST**

Resuscitation Priority	Monitor and Goal	Therapy
1. Preload optimization	Response to fluid challenge CVP 8–12 mm Hg Echo cardiac function and IVC variation Stroke volume variation	Fluid challenge
2. Perfusion pressure	MAP 65–100 mm Hg	Norepinephrine Dopamine Vasopressin
3. Perfusion optimization	Global perfusion markers ScvO$_2$ >70% Lactate clearance Clinical perfusion markers Urine output (UOP) >0.5 cm^3/kg/h Peripheral skin perfusion	Dobutamine Milrinone IABP PRBC transfusion

Early post-ROSC arterial hypotension affects more than half of patients and is associated with death and diminished functional status among survivors.[5,14-16] As such, post-ROSC blood pressure represents an important target to improve outcomes and hypotension must be scrupulously avoided.

Inappropriate vasodilation contributes to hemodynamic instability early in post-arrest shock and should be corrected with catecholamine support simultaneous with volume resuscitation. Vasopressor requirement within the first hours of care is the norm, and delaying vasopressor support risks organ hypoperfusion.[17] There is no clear single best vasoconstrictor in the post-arrest period. Norepinephrine is a preferred agent due to its potency, therapeutic dosing range, and side effect profile.[18] A minimum mean arterial pressure (MAP) goal of 65–80 mm Hg is widely recommended.

Cerebral (and likely other organ) autoregulation is impaired in the post-ROSC period with an absent or right-shifted autoregulatory range.[13] The optimal therapeutic arterial pressure and period of critical cerebral risk remain undefined. Spontaneous hypertension is associated with improved neurologic outcomes and should not be aggressively controlled in the absence of other end-organ dysfunction. MAP targets of 80–100 mm Hg may improve cerebral perfusion and have been incorporated into clinical practice.[15,19] Individual blood pressure goals should be balanced to avoid unnecessary afterload stress in patients with acute myocardial infarction or severe cardiomyopathy.

Intravascular volume depletion, stemming from capillary leak and pathologic vasodilation, contributes to post-ROSC cardiovascular insufficiency. Restoration of oxygen delivery through fluid resuscitation relies on optimizing preload to maximize stroke volume. Total volume requirements are difficult to predict at the onset of resuscitation but are often underestimated. Crystalloid resuscitation totaling 50–80 cm³/kg is typical in the first day of post-arrest support.[4,17,20] Cooled intravenous fluids serve the dual purposes of volume resuscitation and hypothermia induction.

The empiric volume challenge remains the standard means of initial fluid resuscitation. Volume expansion is achieved by infusing serial aliquots of isotonic fluid under direct observation. Crystalloid (10–20 cm³/kg) or colloid (5–10 cm³/kg) should be infused quickly (over 15–20 minutes) with serial boluses titrated to the clinical endpoint objective while monitoring for intolerance to fluid loading such as hypoxemic respiratory failure and right heart dysfunction.

A rational approach for patients who remain hypoperfused after initial empiric volume challenge incorporates selection and titration of subsequent therapy under the guidance of objective cardiovascular monitoring. In the absence of conflicting data, a target central venous pressure (CVP) of 8–12 mm Hg is frequently recommended to optimize preload. However, traditional static pressure surrogates of cardiac preload (i.e., CVP and pulmonary arterial occlusion pressure) are poor predictors of the response to fluid therapy.[21,22] Dynamic measures of volume responsiveness including respirophasic arterial and vena cava variation provide more insight and are strongly encouraged to aid in preload and hemodynamic optimization (see Chapter 47).

The ultimate goal of resuscitation is to restore oxygen delivery and tissue perfusion to meet global and regional metabolic needs. Macrocirculatory signs provide little insight into the balance of systemic oxygen delivery and utilization.[23] Resuscitation aimed to normalize traditional clinical targets of blood pressure, pulse, and CVP does not guarantee normal organ perfusion or resolution of oxygen delivery dependency and therefore risks leaving the patient in persistent compensated shock.[24,25]

Perfusion indicators are important markers of shock, and their normalization can be similarly targeted as endpoints of therapy during early resuscitation. Lactate clearance and central venous saturation (ScvO$_2$) are practical global markers of early resuscitation.[26,27] Regional perfusion estimation by clinical exam and urine output is also expected, but the role of tissue monitoring devices remains unclear. Unfortunately, no single marker of resuscitation is perfect. As such, a multimodal endpoint-driven resuscitation aiming to rapidly normalize all of several physiologic and laboratory variables is recommended (Table 15-3). Use of institutional protocolized hemodynamic order sets improves performance with resuscitation and is recommended.[17,28,29]

POST-CARDIAC ARREST MYOCARDIAL DYSFUNCTION

Acute cardiac dysfunction independent of acute coronary occlusion is common following ROSC. Global systolic and diastolic stunning can be detected within minutes of ROSC but is not clinically relevant in all patients.[30] Severity varies with cardiac function typically nadiring 6–8 hours post-ROSC.[6,20,31]

Persistent hypoperfusion despite preload optimization often signals hypodynamic shock related to cardiac dysfunction and warrants consideration of inotropic or mechanical cardiac support. Despite sometimes severe dysfunction, myocardial stunning is responsive to therapy and frequently reversible within 48–72 hours.[31,32] Inotropic support is required in up to 50% patients in some series.[17] Mechanical support in the form of intraaortic balloon counterpulsation (IABP) or extracorporeal life support (ECLS) may also be required for severe or refractory cardiogenic shock.

► PRECIPITATING PATHOLOGY

The acute precipitant of cardiac arrest must be considered as it may perpetuate shock and be amenable to specific therapy. Cardiac arrest represents the final common pathway of many lethal diseases, and prehospital data and records should be scrutinized to clarify premonitory signs and symptoms. Neurologic precipitants of cardiac arrest including subarachnoid and intracerebral hemorrhage should be considered before cooling, although neuroimaging is not mandatory for all patients.

ACUTE CORONARY SYNDROME

Heart disease remains the most common precipitant of sudden cardiac arrest in adults. The rate of acute coronary occlusion is estimated at 30–50%.[33,34] Unfortunately, acute coronary occlusion is poorly predicted by clinical history and post-ROSC electrocardiogram findings.[33] Revascularization is independently associated with survival and should be considered for all patients with strongly suspected acute coronary disease or ECG evidence of ST-elevation myocardial infarction (STEMI). Percutaneous coronary intervention (PCI) is the preferred method of revascularization and can be safely performed concurrent with therapeutic cooling.[35,36] It should not be delayed due to an uncertain neurologic prognosis.[17]

Thrombolysis is an acceptable reperfusion strategy for STEMI if PCI is not immediately available. Lysis does not carry an untoward hemorrhage risk and is associated with improved survival and neurologic outcome.[37] Coadministration with therapeutic cooling has not been well investigated. Adjunctive aspirin and heparin are recommended for suspected or confirmed acute coronary syndrome. Acute β-blocker and ACE inhibitor therapy should be withheld due to the high rate of hemodynamic instability in post-arrest patients.

DYSRHYTHMIA MANAGEMENT

Cardiac dysrhythmia, principally ventricular tachycardia or fibrillation (VT/VF), is a common precipitating cause of cardiac arrest. Reversible conditions including electrolyte disturbance and ischemia should be considered. However, the role of antidysrhythmic therapy following ROSC from VT/VF arrest remains unclear, and prophylactic administration is not supported or recommended.[9] A short course of therapy may be warranted for cases of recurrent malignant dysrhythmia or in patients who achieve ROSC in response to therapy if no alternative reversible condition is identified.

Sinus bradycardia during therapeutic cooling is common and generally well tolerated. Negative chronotropes such as β-blockers and amiodarone should be avoided unless strongly indicated. Severe bradycardia resulting in hypoperfusion during therapeutic cooling warrants mild elevation of the target temperature.

► MECHANICAL VENTILATORY SUPPORT

Even in the absence of a precipitating respiratory disease, pulmonary complications including respiratory failure, aspiration, and pneumothorax are common in cardiac arrest victims. Prehospital extraglottic airway devices should be exchanged for a cuffed endotracheal tube on patient stabilization to ensure airway protection. Adequate gas exchange and lung protection are the overriding principles of management for acute respiratory failure related to cardiac arrest (Table 15-4).

► TABLE 15-4. ACUTE RESPIRATORY MANAGEMENT

1. Lung-protective mechanical ventilation
   - Low tidal volume <7 cc/kg (ideal body weight)
   - Plateau airway pressure <30 cm H_2O
2. Avoid hyperventilation
   - Goals $PaCO_2$ 38–42 mm Hg
   - Hyperventilation ($PaCO_2$ < 35 mm Hg) should not be used to compensate for metabolic acidosis unless severe (pH < 7.0)
3. Avoid hyperoxia
   - Rapidly titrate FiO_2 to SpO_2 >95% (or PaO_2 > 70 mm Hg)

Inadvertent and purposeful hyperventilation is common with handheld resuscitation bags and contributes to auto–positive end-expiratory pressure (PEEP) with pulmonary and circulatory consequences.[38] Manual ventilation with a resuscitation bag should aim for single-handed ventilation (approximately 500 cm³) and a normal respiratory rate and minute ventilation (rate 10–14). Lung-protective, low tidal volume, ventilatory support is likewise indicated on transition to the mechanical ventilator. Goal tidal volume is less than 7 cc/kg lean body weight and may require adjustment to lower tidal volumes depending on the degree of lung injury as reflected by measured airway pressures (see Chapter 4).

The metabolic conditions of post-ischemic organ blood flow (i.e., temperature, oxygen and carbon dioxide [CO_2] tension, pH, glucose) impact the secondary reperfusion insult. Mounting evidence points to supranormal tissue oxygen in the immediate post-resuscitation period as an avoidable accelerator of reperfusion injury and neuronal damage that impacts outcome.[14,14,39] Hyperoxia can and should be avoided. Inspired oxygen concentration (FiO_2) should be rapidly titrated to physiologic levels (SpO_2 >95%) following ROSC.[40]

In contrast to cerebral autoregulation, cerebrovascular CO_2 reactivity is maintained in the post-arrest period. Hyperventilation risks cerebral vasoconstriction and hypoperfusion.[41] Normocarbia is desired (goal $PaCO_2$ 38–42 mm Hg) with minimal adjustments recommended only for profound acidemia (pH <7.0). Minute ventilation adjustments should be anticipated to maintain targeted normocapnia during the reduced metabolic rate associated with therapeutic cooling.

► POST-ARREST CEREBRAL INJURY AND RESUSCITATION

Neurologic failure is the most common cause of death and disability among patients resuscitated from cardiac arrest. The brain is uniquely vulnerable to bioenergetic failure associated with ischemia during cardiac arrest. However, reperfusion triggers a secondary cascade inciting cerebral injury that evolves over hours to days.[42,43] Historically, targeted neuroprotective drugs have not shown consistent promising results. However, therapeutic cooling trials established that therapies applied following ROSC are capable of modifying the secondary reperfusion insult and neurologic outcome.

Early prognostication of neurologic recovery among patients resuscitated from cardiac arrest is limited. Futile resuscitation efforts should not be pursued, but premature negative prognostication remains an obstacle to optimal care.[44] Signs of neurologic function immediately following ROSC are encouraging, but their absence (including posturing and absent brainstem reflexes) does not preclude recovery. Neurologic prognosis of comatose patients cannot be reliably determined by arrest events, immediate post-resuscitation neurologic exam, or neuroimaging.[45,46] Patient stabilization and initiation of neuroprotective therapies takes precedence over prognostication immediately following cardiac arrest. Accurate prediction of neurologic prognosis improves 72 hours after ROSC.

► THERAPEUTIC HYPOTHERMIA

Therapeutic cooling is an integrated neuroprotective goal of post-arrest resuscitation. The mortality of patients who achieve ROSC remains high due to the neurologic consequences rather than the cause of cardiac arrest. Therapeutic hypothermia is the only neuroprotective therapy with clear neurologic and survival benefit following cardiac arrest.[19,47,48] The landmark trials evaluated cooling in patients with a first recognized rhythm of VT/VF. Alternative rhythms were excluded to avoid experiment confounding. All other factors being equal, the brain and other organs suffer a similar injury regardless of the primary arrest rhythm or site of arrest (in-hospital vs. out-of-hospital). Observational experiences confirm the benefit of cooling for cases of non-VT/VF arrest.[49] Guidelines support application of cooling for all comatose cardiac arrest victims regardless of the initial rhythm or arrest precipitant.[9,50] Serious hemodynamic instability and the need for emergency PCI and advanced cardiorespiratory support do not contraindicate cooling.[51]

The cascade of neuronal injury is accelerated with reperfusion. Temperature modulation of reperfusion injury is greatest when implemented early, and delays negate the beneficial impact.[52] Therapeutic cooling should be initiated as soon as possible following ROSC. This has led to prehospital adoption of cooling. However, prehospital cooling does not obligate continued therapy. On arrival to the hospital, patients should be individually evaluated for candidacy of cooling based on institutional guidelines and the potential risk and benefit of continued treatment. Patients with severe or terminal illness and those unlikely to survive the intensive care unit based on their comorbid disease, irrespective of cardiac arrest, are poor candidates for cooling. Prolonged arrest intervals including >15 minutes to first resuscitation attempt or cardiac arrest longer than 40 minutes are similarly associated with poor prognosis. Intraischemic cooling during CPR is feasible and may provide benefit.[53] The therapeutic window for cooling to provide benefit is unclear, but initiation of cooling should generally occur within 6 hours of ROSC.

► **TABLE 15-5. THERAPEUTIC COOLING GUIDELINES**

1. Perform and document neurologic exam
   - Eligible patient: GCS <8 and/or no purposeful response to verbal commands
2. Hypothermia induction
   - Cooled intravenous fluids
     - 4°C 0.9% normal saline, 20–30 mL/kg bolus over 30 minutes as tolerated
   - Surface ice packs
   - Place core body temperature monitor (i.e., esophageal or bladder probe)
3. Shivering control
   - Early sedation and neuromuscular blockade
     - Midazolam 2–10 mg/h
     - Propofol 20–50 mcg/kg/min
     - Fentanyl 50–150 mcg/h
     - Vecuronium 0.1 mg/kg IV q45 min or as needed
     - Rocuronium 0.5 mg/kg IV q1 h as needed
     - Cisatracurium 0.15 mg/kg bolus followed by 3 mcg/kg/min infusion
   - Adjuncts
     - Magnesium sulfate 5 g IV over 5 h
     - Extremity skin counterwarming
4. Maintain goal 32–34°C for 12–24 h
   - Recheck serum electrolytes and ABG on reaching goal temperature
5. Rewarming
   - Slow controlled rewarming
     - 0.25–0.5°C/h to 37.5°C
   - Stop sedation once temperature reaches 36.5°C
   - Maintain normothermia (prevent hyperthermia) for 48 h

Therapeutic cooling is practically divided into induction, maintenance, and rewarming phases (Table 15-5). Induction with ice-cold (4°C) isotonic fluid is safe, inexpensive, and effective.[54,55] Application of ice packs to the neck, axilla, and groin augments induction and may be required for patients intolerant of volume loading. Core body temperature monitoring via bladder or esophageal sensor placement is recommended. Despite coma, hypnotic and opioid sedation should be employed for all patients to attenuate adrenergic response and shivering during cooling. Intermittent bolus or continuous neuromuscular blockade stops shivering and facilitates achieving rapid hypothermia. Thereafter, paralysis should only be used to combat refractory shivering that impacts maintenance temperature control. Intravenous magnesium and skin counterwarming are additional adjuncts for shivering control. External body surface or invasive cooling devices complete the induction phase and transition to maintenance temperature regulation.[56] Cooling for 12–24 hours at a goal temperature of 32–34°C is recommended. Future

► **TABLE 15-6. POTENTIAL ADVERSE PHYSIOLOGIC RESPONSES AND COMPLICATIONS ASSOCIATED WITH COOLING**

- Hypotension
  - Including vasodilation with rewarming
- Dysrhythmias
  - Sinus bradycardia during cooling is most common
- Cold diuresis
- Electrolyte abnormalities (K, Mg, Phos)
- Insulin resistance and hyperglycemia
- Coagulopathy and thrombocytopenia
- Infection (and underrecognition of signs of infection)
- Shivering
- Pancreatitis

► **TABLE 15-7. EVIDENCE-BASED CRITICAL CARE SUPPORT THERAPIES**

1. Sterile barrier precautions for all invasive procedures
2. Safe mechanical ventilation
   - Low tidal volume <7 cc/kg (ideal body weight)
   - Plateau airway pressure <30 cm H_2O
   - Endotracheal tube (ETT) cuff pressure <25 cm H_2O
3. Aspiration precautions for mechanically ventilated patients
   - Head of bed elevation >30–45° unless contraindicated
   - Orogastric or nasogastric tube decompression
4. Blood sugar control; goal BS <150 mg/dL
5. Prophylaxis
   - Gastrointestinal stress ulcer prophylaxis
   - Deep venous thrombosis prophylaxis

trials will likely explore the optimal temperature goal and treatment duration. Standard cooling blankets and ice packs are suitable for temperature maintenance, although automated servo-controlled devices prevent temperature fluctuations and facilitate slow controlled rewarming (<0.5°C/h). Although generally well tolerated, therapeutic cooling is associated with some unique physiologic changes that should be recognized (Table 15-6).

Patients ineligible for therapeutic cooling warrant active measures to avoid post-ROSC hyperthermia due to its potential to exacerbate brain injury.[57] Moderate to severe hypothermia associated with cardiac arrest warrants rewarming to the goal maintenance temperature range (32–34°C).

POST-ARREST SEIZURES

Seizures or myoclonus impact up to 30% of comatose survivors of cardiac arrest. Seizures in the post-arrest period have the potential to exacerbate cerebral injury and are associated with worse neurologic outcome. However, post-arrest seizures and status epilepticus are not associated with uniformly poor outcome. Patients should be examined for evidence of seizure activity. Routine EEG monitoring would likely reveal subclinical nonconvulsive seizures, but the timing of monitoring and impact of treatment remains unclear.[58] Standard seizure treatment with benzodiazepines, phenytoin, and barbiturates is recommended. Post-arrest myoclonus may be difficult to control, and clonazepam and levetiracetam are recommended therapies. There is no evidence to support prophylactic anticonvulsant therapy.

MISCELLANEOUS

Evidence-based supportive therapies for critical illness should be considered for all cardiac arrest patients

(Table 15-7). Post-arrest patients suffer a significant rate of serious bacterial infection. Nearly half of patients develop short-term pulmonary infection, likely a consequence of aspiration, which is associated with increased duration of mechanical ventilation and ICU stay.[59] Although therapeutic cooling is not associated with increased infection risk, temperature control obscures a principal sign of infection and may delay early respiratory sampling and treatment. Strict surveillance and early empiric antibiotics are warranted for any evidence or suspicion of aspiration given the high risk of this group.

Mixed metabolic and respiratory acidemia is common following ROSC. Cardiopulmonary support is the most important intervention to correct this condition. Extremes of blood glucose are associated with poor outcomes among post-arrest victims.[60,61] Nondiabetic patients appear more susceptible. Arrest patients are at risk for hypoglycemia and blood glucose should be serially monitored during resuscitation. Current evidence supports targeting blood glucose less than 150 mg/dL via intermittent subcutaneous insulin or insulin infusion following initial patient stabilization.[62]

Recognized complications associated with chest compressions and other resuscitation measures including rib fractures, pneumothorax, pericardial effusion, and solid and hollow abdominal organ injury should be considered.[63]

► **TABLE 15-8. AVOIDABLE PITFALLS IN THE CARE OF POST-ARREST PATIENTS**

- Failure to initiate early catecholamine support for BP stabilization
- Unnecessary hyperoxygenation
- Failure to provide revascularization therapy for patients with STEMI or strongly suspected ACS
- Delayed therapeutic cooling

► CONCLUSION

The post-cardiac arrest patient suffers a complex systemic injury cascade that continues to evolve following ROSC. Timely interventions in the immediate and early post-resuscitation phase are capable of modifying the natural trajectory of illness to achieve the goal of neurologically intact survival. Emergency care emphasizing critical care support, cardiovascular resuscitation, and neuroprotective cooling is a crucial link in the chain of survival (Table 15-8).

REFERENCES

1. Nichol G, Thomas E, Callaway CW, et al. Regional variation in out-of-hospital cardiac arrest incidence and outcome. *JAMA*. 2008;300(12):1423–1431.
2. Negovsky VA. Postresuscitation disease. *Crit Care Med*. 1988;16(10):942–946.
3. Adrie C, dib-Conquy M, Laurent I et al. Successful cardiopulmonary resuscitation after cardiac arrest as a "sepsis-like" syndrome. *Circulation*. 2002;106(5):562–568.
4. Adrie C, Laurent I, Monchi M, Cariou A, Dhainaou JF, Spaulding C. Postresuscitation disease after cardiac arrest: a sepsis-like syndrome? *Curr Opin Crit Care*. 2004;10(3):208–212.
5. Kilgannon JH, Roberts BW, Reihl LR, et al. Early arterial hypotension is common in the post-cardiac arrest syndrome and associated with increased in-hospital mortality. *Resuscitation*. 2008;79(3):410–416.
6. Chang WT, Ma MH, Chien KL, et al. Postresuscitation myocardial dysfunction: correlated factors and prognostic implications. *Intensive Care Med*. 2007;33(1):88–95.
7. Menegazzi JJ, Ramos R, Wang HE, Callaway CW. Post-resuscitation hemodynamics and relationship to the duration of ventricular fibrillation. *Resuscitation*. 2008;78(3):355–358.
8. Part 7.5: postresuscitation support. *Circulation*. 2005; 112(24 suppl):IV-84.
9. Nolan JP, Neumar RW, Adrie C, et al. Post-cardiac arrest syndrome: epidemiology, pathophysiology, treatment, and prognostication. A scientific statement from the International Liaison Committee on Resuscitation; the American Heart Association Emergency Cardiovascular Care Committee; the Council on Cardiovascular Surgery and Anesthesia; the Council on Cardiopulmonary, Perioperative, and Critical Care; the Council on Clinical Cardiology; the Council on Stroke. *Resuscitation*. 2008;79(3):350–379.
10. Kern JW, Shoemaker WC. Meta-analysis of hemodynamic optimization in high-risk patients. *Crit Care Med*. 2002;30(8):1686–1692.
11. Jones AE, Brown MD, Trzeciak S, et al. The effect of a quantitative resuscitation strategy on mortality in patients with sepsis: a meta-analysis. *Crit Care Med*. 2008;36(10):2734–2739.
12. Jones AE, Shapiro NI, Kilgannon JH, Trzeciak S. Goal-directed hemodynamic optimization in the post-cardiac arrest syndrome: a systematic review. *Resuscitation*. 2008;77(1):26–29.
13. Sundgreen C, Larsen FS, Herzog TM, Knudsen GM, Boesgaard S, Aldershvile J. Autoregulation of cerebral blood flow in patients resuscitated from cardiac arrest. *Stroke*. 2001;32(1):128–132.
14. Kilgannon JH, Jones AE, Shapiro NI, et al. Association between arterial hyperoxia following resuscitation from cardiac arrest and in-hospital mortality. *JAMA*. 2010;303(21):2165–2171.
15. Leonov Y, Sterz F, Safar P, Johnson DW, Tisherman SA, Oku K. Hypertension with hemodilution prevents multifocal cerebral hypoperfusion after cardiac arrest in dogs. *Stroke*. 1992;23(1):45–53.
16. Trzeciak S, Jones AE, Kilgannon JH, et al. Significance of arterial hypotension after resuscitation from cardiac arrest. *Crit Care Med*. 2009;37(11):2895–2903.
17. Sunde K, Pytte M, Jacobsen D, et al. Implementation of a standardised treatment protocol for post resuscitation care after out-of-hospital cardiac arrest. *Resuscitation*. 2007;73(1):29–39.
18. De BD, Biston P, Devriendt J, et al. Comparison of dopamine and norepinephrine in the treatment of shock. *N Engl J Med*. 2010;362(9):779–789.
19. Bernard SA, Gray TW, Buist MD, et al. Treatment of comatose survivors of out-of-hospital cardiac arrest with induced hypothermia. *N Engl J Med*. 2002;346(8): 557–563.
20. Laurent I, Monchi M, Chiche JD, et al. Reversible myocardial dysfunction in survivors of out-of-hospital cardiac arrest. *J Am Coll Cardiol*. 2002;40(12):2110–2116.
21. Marik PE, Baram M, Vahid B. Does central venous pressure predict fluid responsiveness? A systematic review of the literature and the tale of seven mares. *Chest*. 2008;134(1):172–178.
22. Michard F, Teboul JL. Predicting fluid responsiveness in ICU patients: a critical analysis of the evidence. *Chest*. 2002;121(6):2000–2008.
23. Rady MY, Rivers EP, Nowak RM. Resuscitation of the critically ill in the ED: responses of blood pressure, heart rate, shock index, central venous oxygen saturation, and lactate. *Am J Emerg Med*. 1996;14(2):218–225.
24. Porter JM, Ivatury RR. In search of the optimal end points of resuscitation in trauma patients: a review. *J Trauma*. 1998;44(5):908–914.
25. Rivers E, Nguyen B, Havstad S, et al. Early goal-directed therapy in the treatment of severe sepsis and septic shock. *N Engl J Med*. 2001;345(19):1368–1377.
26. Donnino MW, Miller J, Goyal N, et al. Effective lactate clearance is associated with improved outcome in post-cardiac arrest patients. *Resuscitation*. 2007;75(2): 229–234.
27. Gaieski DF, Band RA, Abella BS, et al. Early goal-directed hemodynamic optimization combined with therapeutic hypothermia in comatose survivors of out-of-hospital cardiac arrest. *Resuscitation*. 2009;80(4):418–424.
28. Kilgannon JH, Roberts BW, Stauss M, et al. Use of a standardized order set for achieving target temperature in the implementation of therapeutic hypothermia after cardiac arrest: a feasibility study. *Acad Emerg Med*. 2008;15(6):499–505.
29. Levy MM, Dellinger RP, Townsend SR, et al. The Surviving Sepsis Campaign: results of an international

guideline-based performance improvement program targeting severe sepsis. *Crit Care Med.* 2010;38(2):367–374.

30. Kern KB, Hilwig RW, Rhee KH, Berg RA. Myocardial dysfunction after resuscitation from cardiac arrest: an example of global myocardial stunning. *J Am Coll Cardiol.* 1996;28(1):232–240.

31. Kern KB, Hilwig RW, Berg RA, et al. Postresuscitation left ventricular systolic and diastolic dysfunction. Treatment with dobutamine. *Circulation.* 1997;95(12):2610–2613.

32. Ruiz-Bailen M, Aguayo de Hoyos E, Ruiz-Navarro S, et al. Reversible myocardial dysfunction after cardiopulmonary resuscitation. *Resuscitation.* 2005;66(2):175–181.

33. Spaulding CM, Joly LM, Rosenberg A, et al. Immediate coronary angiography in survivors of out-of-hospital cardiac arrest. *N Engl J Med.* 1997;336(23):1629–1633.

34. Garot P, Lefevre T, Eltchaninoff H, et al. Six-month outcome of emergency percutaneous coronary intervention in resuscitated patients after cardiac arrest complicating ST-elevation myocardial infarction. *Circulation.* 2007;115(11):1354–1362.

35. Wolfrum S, Pierau C, Radke PW, Schunkert H, Kurowski V. Mild therapeutic hypothermia in patients after out-of-hospital cardiac arrest due to acute ST-segment elevation myocardial infarction undergoing immediate percutaneous coronary intervention. *Crit Care Med.* 2008;36(6):1780–1786.

36. Knafelj R, Radsel P, Ploj T, Noc M. Primary percutaneous coronary intervention and mild induced hypothermia in comatose survivors of ventricular fibrillation with ST-elevation acute myocardial infarction. *Resuscitation.* 2007;74(2):227–234.

37. Richling N, Herkner H, Holzer M, Riedmueller E, Sterz F, Schreiber W. Thrombolytic therapy vs primary percutaneous intervention after ventricular fibrillation cardiac arrest due to acute ST-segment elevation myocardial infarction and its effect on outcome. *Am J Emerg Med.* 2007;25(5):545–550.

38. Aufderheide TP, Lurie KG. Death by hyperventilation: a common and life-threatening problem during cardiopulmonary resuscitation. *Crit Care Med.* 2004;32 (9 suppl):S345–S351.

39. Liu Y, Rosenthal RE, Haywood Y, Miljkovic-Lolic M, Vanderhoek JY, Fiskum G. Normoxic ventilation after cardiac arrest reduces oxidation of brain lipids and improves neurological outcome. *Stroke.* 1998;29(8):1679–1686.

40. Balan IS, Fiskum G, Hazelton J, Cotto-Cumba C, Rosenthal RE. Oximetry-guided reoxygenation improves neurological outcome after experimental cardiac arrest. *Stroke.* 2006;37(12):3008–3013.

41. Buunk G, van der Hoeven JG, Meinders AE. Cerebrovascular reactivity in comatose patients resuscitated from a cardiac arrest. *Stroke.* 1997;28(8):1569–1573.

42. Neumar RW. Molecular mechanisms of ischemic neuronal injury. *Ann Emerg Med.* 2000;36(5):483–506.

43. Li D, Shao Z, Vanden Hoek TL, Brorson JR. Reperfusion accelerates acute neuronal death induced by simulated ischemia. *Exp Neurol.* 2007;206(2):280–287.

44. Hemphill JC III, White DB. Clinical nihilism in neuro-emergencies. *Emerg Med Clin North Am.* 2009;27(1):27–viii.

45. Wijdicks EF, Hijdra A, Young GB, Bassetti CL, Wiebe S. Practice parameter: prediction of outcome in comatose survivors after cardiopulmonary resuscitation (an evidence-based review): report of the Quality Standards Subcommittee of the American Academy of Neurology. *Neurology.* 2006;67(2):203–210.

46. Young GB. Clinical practice. Neurologic prognosis after cardiac arrest. *N Engl J Med.* 2009;361(6):605–611.

47. Mild therapeutic hypothermia to improve the neurologic outcome after cardiac arrest. Hypothermia after Cardiac Arrest Study Group. *N Engl J Med.* 2002 Feb 21;346(8):549–556. Erratum in: *N Engl J Med.* 2002 May 30;346(22):1756. PMID:11856793.

48. Arrich J, Holzer M, Herkner H, Mullner M. Hypothermia for neuroprotection in adults after cardiopulmonary resuscitation. *Cochrane Database Syst Rev.* 2009;(4):CD004128.

49. Arrich J. Clinical application of mild therapeutic hypothermia after cardiac arrest. *Crit Care Med.* 2007;35(4):1041–1047.

50. Henry TD, Sharkey SW, Burke MN, et al. A regional system to provide timely access to percutaneous coronary intervention for ST-elevation myocardial infarction. *Circulation.* 2007;116(7):721–728.

51. Hovdenes J, Laake JH, Aaberge L, Haugaa H, Bugge JF. Therapeutic hypothermia after out-of-hospital cardiac arrest: experiences with patients treated with percutaneous coronary intervention and cardiogenic shock. *Acta Anaesthesiol Scand.* 2007;51(2):137–142.

52. Kuboyama K, Safar P, Radovsky A, Tisherman SA, Stezoski SW, Alexander H. Delay in cooling negates the beneficial effect of mild resuscitative cerebral hypothermia after cardiac arrest in dogs: a prospective, randomized study. *Crit Care Med.* 1993;21(9):1348–1358.

53. Nozari A, Safar P, Stezoski SW, et al. Critical time window for intra-arrest cooling with cold saline flush in a dog model of cardiopulmonary resuscitation. *Circulation.* 2006;113(23):2690–2696.

54. Bernard S, Buist M, Monteiro O, Smith K. Induced hypothermia using large volume, ice-cold intravenous fluid in comatose survivors of out-of-hospital cardiac arrest: a preliminary report. *Resuscitation.* 2003;56(1):9–13.

55. Polderman KH, Rijnsburger ER, Peerdeman SM, Girbes AR. Induction of hypothermia in patients with various types of neurologic injury with use of large volumes of ice-cold intravenous fluid. *Crit Care Med.* 2005;33(12):2744–2751.

56. Seder DB, Van der Kloot TE. Methods of cooling: practical aspects of therapeutic temperature management. *Crit Care Med.* 2009;37(7 suppl):S211–S222.

57. Zeiner A, Holzer M, Sterz F, et al. Hyperthermia after cardiac arrest is associated with an unfavorable neurologic outcome. *Arch Intern Med.* 2001;161(16):2007–2012.

58. Rundgren M, Westhall E, Cronberg T, Rosen I, Friberg H. Continuous amplitude-integrated electroencephalogram predicts outcome in hypothermia-treated cardiac arrest patients. *Crit Care Med.* 2010;38(9):1838–1844.

59. Gajic O, Festic E, Afessa B. Infectious complications in survivors of cardiac arrest admitted to the medical intensive care unit. *Resuscitation.* 2004;60(1):65–69.

60. Beiser DG, Carr GE, Edelson DP, Peberdy MA, Hoek TL. Derangements in blood glucose following initial resuscitation from in-hospital cardiac arrest: a report from the National Registry of Cardiopulmonary Resuscitation. *Resuscitation.* 2009;80(6):624–630.

61. Padkin A. Glucose control after cardiac arrest. *Resuscitation.* 2009;80(6):611–612.

62. Losert H, Sterz F, Roine RO, et al. Strict normoglycaemic blood glucose levels in the therapeutic management of patients within 12 h after cardiac arrest might not be necessary. *Resuscitation.* 2008;76(2):214–220.

63. Buschmann CT, Tsokos M. Frequent and rare complications of resuscitation attempts. *Intensive Care Med.* 2009;35(3):397–404.

CHAPTER 16

Vasopressors and Inotropes

Amber Rollstin, John P. Marshall, and William C. Chiu

In a shock state tissue, perfusion is compromised causing hypoperfusion to organs, cellular hypoxia, and metabolic disorder resulting in cellular injury. Injury to the organs is mainly due to the duration of the hypoperfusion and the speed with which the etiology can be treated and the shock state can be reversed. When patients are hemodynamically unstable, an important and potentially life-saving intervention is the use of vasoactive therapies to restore appropriate tissue perfusion by increasing blood flow and thereby increasing oxygenation. Vasoactive agents can be categorized by their activity and are often divided into two types: vasopressors and inotropes. The term vasopressor refers to a class of drugs that cause vasoconstriction. Typically, increasing vasoconstriction leads to an increase in systemic vascular resistance (SVR), which leads to an increase in blood pressure. The term inotrope refers to a class of drugs that increase the strength of cardiac contraction. Increasing the strength of cardiac contractions will increase the stroke volume (SV). By increasing SV, the intent is to increase the cardiac output (CO) and therefore increase blood pressure.

To review, mean arterial pressure (MAP) is the product of SVR and CO. SVR is the resistance that blood flow must overcome to reach the circulatory system; it is affected by blood viscosity, vessel length, and vessel diameter. The major determinant of SVR is the arterioles, which can manipulate blood supply by altering their diameter. Recall that keep in mind that CO is the product of SV and heart rate. SV is the quantitiy of blood that is pumped from the ventricle of the heart with each beat, which is dependent on preload (end-diastolic volume), afterload, and cardiac contractility. Vasoactive therapies are used in an attempt to manipulate these important parameters. Vasoactive drugs can also increase heart rate by increasing the sinoatrial conduction, giving them "chronotropic" properties. A

"dromotropic" effect refers to an increase in atrioventricular (AV) nodal conduction.

Prior to or concurrent with initiating vasoactive or inotropic medications, it is essential to attempt to identify the potential cause of the shock state and guide therapy based on this presumptive diagnosis.

Vasopressors and inotropic drugs are divided into two types based on their effects: adrenergic and nonadrenergic. The adrenergic agonists function at adrenergic receptors (α_1, α_2, β_1, β_2) and dopaminergic (DA) receptors. The nonadrenergic agonists exert their effect primarily via the vasopressin-specific receptor (V_1, V_2) or by inhibition of phosphodiesterase 3, which potentiates the effect of cyclic adenosine monophosphate (cAMP). It is crucial to have a good understanding of the physiologic function of these medications and their corresponding receptors and to use this understanding to guide therapy. Table 16-1 provides a summary of the physiologic responses associated with each receptor.

▶ RECPTORS

α-ADRENERGIC RECEPTORS

The main effect of α_1 stimulation is venous smooth muscle vasoconstriction. Agonism of α_2 causes vasodilation of the arteries and vasoconstriction of the veins; however, these effects are negligible and often not considered clinically significant when compared with the α_1 effect.[1]

β-ADRENERGIC RECEPTORS

Agonism at the β_1 receptor produces an increase in cardiac contraction (inotropic), increased heart rate (chronotropic), and increased atrial conduction (dromotropic). β_2 stimulation causes relaxation of the smooth

► **TABLE 16-1. PHYSIOLOGIC ACTIONS OF RECEPTORS STIMULATED BY VASOPRESSORS**

Receptor	Physiologic Response
Dopamine (DA)	Vasodilation of major vascular beds (renal, coronary, cerebral, and splanchnic) and increased renal blood flow
β_1 cardiac	Inotropy and chronotropy
β_2	Peripheral vasodilation and bronchial smooth muscle dilation
α_1	Vasoconstriction
Vasopressin 1 (V_1)	Vasoconstriction
Vasopressin 2 (V_2)	Water retention

muscle of small coronary arteries and arteries of skeletal muscle resulting in vasodilation, as well as bronchiolar dilatation. There may be a chronotropic effect at higher dosages. β_3 receptors are mainly located in adipose tissue and may have some thermogenic effect.[2]

DOPAMINERGIC RECEPTORS

There are currently five recognized subtypes of DA receptors. Their main effect is to increase contractility that results in an increased CO. Stimulation of these receptors can also result in an increased HR but this effect is dose dependent. There are also dopamine receptors in the kidney that produce diuresis and naturesis.

► SPECIFIC AGENTS

The vasopressors and inotropes that are most commonly used in the intensive care unit (ICU) are dopamine, dobutamine, epinephrine, norepinephrine, vasopressin, and phenylephrine.[3] Most vasoactive medications can cause serious complications when given through

► **TABLE 16-3. DOSAGES OF COMMON VASOPRESSORS**

Drug	Dose
Dopamine	Low dose: <5 µg/kg/min Moderate dose: 5–10 µg/kg/min High dose: >10 µg/kg/min
Dobutamine	2.0–20 µg/kg/min
Epinephrine	**For refractory hypotension** Typical dosing is 1–4 µg/min (1:10,000 solution) For anaphylaxis, the dose and route change, based on the presence of shock: **Without evidence of shock:** 0.3–0.5 mg (300–500 µg) IM q 5–10 min (1:1,000) **With evidence of shock:** 0.1 mg (100 µg) IV, which is 1.0 mL of 1:10,000 dilution IV given slowly over 3–5 min or infused at 5–15 µg/min
Norepinephrine	0.03–3.0 µg/kg/min
Vasopressin	0.04 U/min Not titrated
Phenylephrine	0.5–8 µg/kg/min 100–180 µg/min IV drip
Isoproterenol	2–10 µg/min
Milrinone	50 µg/kg bolus, and then 0.25–1 µg/kg/min

a peripheral IV (PIV), either by direct vasoconstrictive effect or via extravasation. It is recommended that these drugs be given via a central venous catheter. However, in emergent situations, these drugs can be given briefly through a PIV until a central venous catheter can be placed. Once these medications are started through a PIV, it should be a priority to obtain central venous access to minimize the time the drug is administered peripherally. A comparison of the hemodynamic effects of these agents is presented in Table 16-2, and typical dosing regimens are described in Table 16-3.

Dopamine is an immediate precursor of norepinephrine. It is an interesting drug in that it works on DA,

► **TABLE 16-2. EFFECT OF VASOPRESSORS ON HEMODYNAMIC VARIABLES**

Drug	MAP	SVR	HR	CO
Dopamine (moderate–high dose)	Increased	Increased	Increased	Increased
Dobutamine	Variable	Decreased		Increased
Epinephrine	Variable	Increased	Increased	Increased
Norepinephrine	Increased	Increased	0 → decreased	Increased
Vasopressin	Increased	Increased		Increased
Phenylephrine	Increased	Increased	0 → decreased[a]	0 → increased
Isoproterenol	Decreased	Decreased	Increased	Variable
Milrinone	Variable	Decreased		Increased

MAP, mean arterial blood pressure; SVR, systemic vascular resistance; HR, heart rate; CO, cardiac output.
[a]Phenylephrine can produce reflex bradycardia as a side effect of hypertension.

β_1, β_2, and α_1 receptors at different doses. Dopamine increases contractility and HR by direct β-adrenergic action. It also indirectly stimulates norepinephrine release from nerves, and it is this action that makes the clinical prediction of its effects difficult.[4] Dosage is based on ideal body weight. At *low dose* (1–2 μg/kg/min), dopamine acts on the DA receptors, and the effect is vasodilation of the renal, splanchnic, and mesenteric vasculatures. Some patients may become increasingly hypotensive at this dose. This is the dosage that, in the past, was termed "renal-dose dopamine" and was used to prevent acute renal failure (ARF). Several systemic reviews and one large randomized control trial concluded that dopamine did not prevent the onset of ARF. Nor did it shorten ICU or hospital length of stay, prevent the need for renal replacement therapy, or affect mortality. Low-dose dopamine is no longer recommended for the prevention or treatment of ARF.[5]

At *moderate dose* (2–5 μg/kg/min), dopamine stimulates β receptors to a greater degree than α receptors. The effect is inotropic and chronotropic but it also causes peripheral vasodilation. At *high dose* (>10 μg/kg/min), dopamine causes increased effect on the α receptors and less effect on the β receptors. Dopamine functions as more of a vasopressor at this dose.

The indications for dopamine include cardiogenic shock, particularly when peripheral vasoconstriction and cardiac stimulation are required. Dopamine is often utilized in the treatment of septic shock as well. Side effects include cardiac ectopy, tachycardia, angina, severe hypertension (HTN), dyspnea, and allergic reaction to the sulfite preservative.

Because of the varying pharmacologic effects at different doses, dopamine is unpredictable and can be difficult to titrate. Providers must remain cognizant that with increasing doses of dopamine, the activated receptor profile changes.

Dobutamine is a potent β_1 receptor agonist and weak β_2 receptor agonist. Its effects are positive inotropy and chronotropy with slight peripheral vasodilation. Dobutamine usually causes an increase in CO with or without a reduction in blood pressure.

The indications for dobutamine include low CO and decompensated heart failure without hypotension, but it is not recommended as monotherapy in markedly symptomatic cardiogenic shock. For this situation, dobutamine is typically combined with norepinephrine or dopamine to provide peripheral vasoconstriction and additional pressure support. Typical dosing of dobutamine is 2.0–20 μg/kg/min.

Side effects of dobutamine include tachycardia, HTN, hypotension, ventricular ectopy, chest pain, dyspnea, and infusion site reactions. Contraindications include hypertrophic cardiomyopathy, history of malignant ventricular tachyarrhythmias, and sulfite sensitivity. Caution should be used with this drug when treating patients with a systolic blood pressure (SBP) <100 mm Hg.

Epinephrine acts on β_1 receptors to a greater degree than α_1 and β_2 receptors, making it a chronotrope and an inotrope. Epinephrine increases SBP, but has less of an effect on diastolic blood pressure (DBP) and MAP when compared with norepinephrine. Epinephrine also causes an increase in CO. As the dosage of epinephrine increases so does SVR due to an increased effect of α_1 receptors at higher doses. Typical dosing varies depending on the clinical situation, and specific doses will be discussed under the specific indications below. It is also very important to be clear about the strength of solution—1:10,000 versus 1:1,000—when administering epinephrine for any condition. This distinction is discussed in the section "Anaphylaxis."

The indications for epinephrine include anaphylaxis and severe allergic reactions, bradycardia, refractory hypotension, and β-blocker overdose particularly for patients in whom bradycardia is the predominant abnormality.[6] For refractory hypotension, the typical dosing is 1–4 μg/min (1:10,000 solution) given intravenously. For severe allergic reactions or anaphylaxis, the dose and route is adjusted based on the presence of shock and will be discussed later in this chapter. Side effects of epinephrine include ventricular arrhythmia, HTN, and cardiac ischemia. Caution should be used in patients with cerebrovascular insufficiency, heart disease, and angina.

Norepinephrine is a strong agonist of α receptors and moderate agonist of β receptors, with greater β_1 action than β_2. The effect is vasoconstriction greater than inotropy or chronotropy. This drug's effect on α receptors is increased with increasing doses. Norepinephrine increases left ventricular afterload, SV, and both SBP and DBP.

The indications for norepinephrine include hypotensive states such as septic shock, neurogenic shock and severe hypotension secondary to pulmonary embolism. Norepinephrine may not be appropriate for single-agent use in cardiogenic shock secondary to the increased afterload it produces; however, it can be combined with dobutamine in this setting. The dose is 0.03–3.0 μg/kg/min.

Side effects of norepinephrine include reflex bradycardia, HTN, arrhythmias, and dyspnea. Norepinephrine is contraindicated in patients with sulfite allergies and may increase the risk of mesenteric or peripheral vascular thrombosis.

Vasopressin acts on V_1 receptors, which cause vasoconstriction, and V_2 receptors, which result in water retention. The primary indication for vasopressin in shock is to augment catecholamines in the treatment of septic shock, where it is used a second pressor agent. Vasopressin should not be used alone or as the first-line agent for these patients. The role of vasopressin in the treatment of other forms of vasodilatory shock has yet to be clearly defined.

The typical dosing of vasopressin is 0.04 U/min for the treatment of shock. This drug is not titrated. Side effects include cardiac ischemia, arrhythmias, mesenteric ischemia, and HTN. One advantage of vasopressin is that it maintains its effects in acidic and hypoxic environments, which are typical in shock.[2]

Phenylephrine acts on α_1 receptors, and the effect is primarily vasoconstriction at the venous and arteriolar levels causing a significant increase in MAP without significant chronotropic or inotropic effect. Because it has little direct effect on the heart rate, there is minimal chance of developing an arrhythmia, but the blood pressure elevation can lead to a reflex bradycardia. It may be used as a primary agent in hypotension after spinal anesthesia or neurologic injury. It is also very useful in patients who require a vasopressor with minimal chronotropic effect such as those with underlying atrial fibrillation or other tachydysrhythmias. Typical dosing is 0.5–8 µg/kg/min, which comes out to 100–180 µg/min via IV infusion for typically sized adults. Side effects include reflex bradycardia, HTN, and local necrosis in the event of extravasation.[7]

Contraindications to phenylephrine include hypersensitivity to sulfites. Phenylephrine should be used with caution in severe HTN, bradyarrythmia and heart block, cerebrovascular insufficiency, and coronary artery disease (CAD) as it is associated with increased oxygen demand at the coronaries.

Isoproterenol is a β_1 and β_2 agonist, and has inotropic, chronotropic, and mild vasodilatory properties. The β_2 stimulation causes decreased DBP and MAP. Indications for isoproterenol include ventricular arrhythmias secondary to AV block, symptomatic bradycardia if pacing is not immediately available, and bradycardia after heart transplantation secondary to denervation.

Isoproterenol is no longer used as an inotropic agent in clinical practice because of its tendency to cause hypotension.[8] Typical dosing is 2–10 µg/min. Side effects include ventricular arrhythmias, cardiac ischemia, and HTN or hypotension. Contraindications to isoproterenol include digoxin toxicity, angina, cardiac arrhythmia, seizure disorder, renal insufficiency or failure, and CAD, and caution should be used when considering its use in elderly patients.

Milrinone is a phosphodiesterase 3 inhibitor, which prevents the breakdown of cAMP, thereby simulating agonism at β_1 and β_2 receptors. The effects are primarily inotropic, with less chronotropy, and significant vasodilation. Indications for milrinone include severe congestive heart failure and right ventricular infract where pulmonary vasodilation serves to unload the right ventricle. Typical dosing for milrinone is a 50 µg/kg bolus, and then 0.25–1 µg/kg/min.

Side effects of milrinone include tachycardia, ischemia, hypotension, and thrombocytopenia. Contraindications include severe aortic or pulmonic obstruction and acute myocardial infarction (AMI). Use milrinone with caution in patients with atrial fibrillation or flutter, hypotension, hypertrophic subaortic stenosis, and renal impairment.

► CLINICAL INDICATIONS

The choice of vasopressor is dependent on the clinical picture and the presumed etiology of the hypotension. Specific treatments based on clinical conditions are summarized in Table 16-4. The drug is then often titrated to achieve a desired endpoint. Examples of possible endpoints include, but are not limited to, CVP 8–12 mm Hg, MAP $\geq$65 mm Hg, urine output $\geq$0.5 mL/kg/h, venous (S_vO2) or central venous ($S_{cv}O2$) oxygen saturation $\geq$70%, and improved mental status.[9] It is important to note that the optimal MAP for most conditions is unknown, but a post hoc analysis of a multicenter trial of septic shock demonstrated that elevations of the MAP >70 mm Hg by augmenting the vasopressor dosage were associated with an increase in mortality.[10] If the maximal dose of a drug is reached but not the desired endpoint, a second agent may be added. A critical care patient's hemodynamic status can change rapidly, and therefore it is important to frequently reevaluate the patient and determine if there is an ongoing need for vasopressor medication, titration, or a different agent. Excessive vasoconstriction can be detrimental, especially in the setting of inadequate CO and hypovolemia. When used in high doses without adequate volume or CO, these medications can lead to hypoperfusion of the kidneys, brain, and other organ systems.

No studies have been done to indicate that one vasopressor has improved mortality when compared with others when used for appropriate clinical conditions. The debate over dopamine and norepinephrine as the initial vasopressor of choice has been extensively studied. A recently published, large multicenter, randomized, blinded trial compared dopamine and norepinephrine as the initial vasopressor in the treatment of all patients presenting with shock regardless of etiology. This study concluded there was no mortality difference at 28 days when all forms of shock were examined.[11] In the subset of patients with cardiogenic shock, however, dopamine was significantly associated with increased mortality. It also revealed that the use of dopamine was associated with a greater number of adverse advents, such as arrhythmias, requiring medication discontinuation.[11] It seems logical that norepinephrine should be the initial vasopressor of choice, until further evidence suggests otherwise.

▶ TABLE 16-4. **TREATMENT BASED ON THE ETIOLOGY OF SHOCK**

Shock Etiology	Initial Treatment	First-Line Agent	Second-Line Agent
Hypovolemic	Intravenous fluid (2 L of crystalloid)	Blood products as indicated or further intravenous crystalloid	*Dopamine*[a] *Norepinephrine*[a] *Epinephrine*[a]
Septic	Intravenous fluid (2 L of crystalloid)	*Norepinephrine* *Dopamine*	Phenylephrine (combined with initial agent or alone if tolerated) *Vasopressin* (if catecholamine resistant) Epinephrine
Anaphylactic	Intravenous fluid (2 L of crystalloid)	*Epinephrine* (IM if no shock)	*Epinephrine* (IV if in shock)
Neurogenic	Intravenous fluid (2 L of crystalloid)	*Norepinephrine* *Dopamine* *Vasopressin*	Phenylephrine (monitor for reflex bradycardia)
Cardiogenic (right sided)	Intravenous fluid (20 mL/kg of crystalloid)	Vasopressors directed at cause of right heart failure *Norepinephrine* *Dopamine*	Additional vasopressors as needed *Milrinone* (severe CHF or RV infarct)
Cardiogenic (left sided)	Intravenous fluid as appropriate. Use caution in the setting of CHF	*Dobutamine* (without signs of shock) *Dopamine* (with signs of shock)	*Dobutamine + dopamine* *Dobutamine + norepinephrine* *Vasopressin* (added to other agents) *Milrinone* (severe CHF or RV infarct)

IM, intramuscular; IV, intravenous; CHF, congestive heart failure; RV, right ventricle.
[a]Vasopressors should only be considered as a temporizing measure in extreme cases of hypovolemic shock while fluid resuscitation continues.

Prior to initiating vasopressors, it is important to ensure that the intravascular compartment has been repleted. In the case of distributive or hypovolemic shock, an adult patient should receive 2 L of crystalloid fluid before starting vasopressors. In cardiogenic shock, the patient should receive a bolus of 20 mL/kg of crystalloid if there is right ventricular involvement. Fluid therapy is discussed at length in Chapter 47. If the blood pressure fails to respond to these measures, vasopressors should be initiated. Vasopressor activity is partially, if not significantly, reduced if the patient has not been adequately volume resuscitated.[12]

HYPOVOLEMIC SHOCK

The treatment of hypovolemic shock is initiated with crystalloid fluids, with or without colloids. Vasopressors should generally not be used since they do not address the primary problem and may lead to further hypoperfusion. If the patient is in extremis, vasopressors should be used only as a temporizing measure in the setting of hypovolemic shock while fluid resuscitation continues. The cause of hypovolemia should be identified and treated, and it is essential to distinguish between hypovolemic shock and distributive shock, which is described below. Transfusion should be considered early, particularly if the hypovolemic shock is due to blood loss. Fluid resuscitation should be continued, and

the vasopressor agent should be weaned as soon as tolerated. Consider dopamine, norepinephrine, or epinephrine as a temporizing measure in this setting.

DISTRIBUTIVE SHOCK

Distributive shock occurs when there is a fall in SVR secondary to significant peripheral vascular dilation. Causes of distributive shock include septic, anaphylactic, and neurogenic shock. Distributive shock is usually characterized by hypotension, low SVR, and normal to increased CO. Treatment will be discussed in the next subsections under the heading of each specific cause.

Septic Shock

The first-line treatments of severe sepsis and septic shock are IV fluids (IVF) and antibiotics. If the patient remains hypotensive despite adequate volume resuscitation, then vasopressors should be added to the treatment regimen. Vasopressor therapy is very important in order to improve and maintain adequate tissue perfusion in an attempt to maintain life and prevent the development of multiple organ dysfunction and failure. There has been much controversy surrounding the initial vasopressor of choice in the management of patients with septic shock. For this reason, the Surviving Sepsis Campaign guidelines recommend either dopamine or norepinephrine as the initial vasopressor for patients with septic shock.[9] Epinephrine versus norepinephrine plus dobutamine was found to have no mortality difference, in a large prospective, multicenter, randomized double-blind European study.[13] Phenylephrine can also be helpful when tachycardia or arrhythmias preclude the use of norepinephrine or dopamine.[14]

Endogenous vasopressin is released in abundance in the early stages of shock but becomes depleted with prolonged resuscitation with a resulting inappropriate vasodilation. In this setting or in the clinical setting of catecholamine-resistant shock, vasopressin can be given at a dose of 0.01–0.04 U/min.[15] However, in a randomized double-blind study of septic shock patients requiring vasopressor therapy, there was no mortality difference between the norepinephrine and norepinephrine plus vasopressin group, but the combination of norepinephrine and vasopressin allowed for more rapid weaning of norepinephrine while maintaining adequate MAP.[16]

In the patient with a persistently depressed SvO_2 or $ScvO_2$ below 70% despite adequate blood pressure response to first-line vasopressor agents and after optimizing the hematocrit to a level above 30%, dobutamine can be added. In this setting, dobutamine can significantly increase cardiac index (CI), oxygen delivery (DO_2), and oxygen consumption (VO_2), while decreasing MAP, pulmonary artery and wedge pressures, and systemic and pulmonary vascular resistances. Hypovolemic patients have a poor response to dobutamine when compared with euvolemic patients, so it is essential to ensure adequate fluid resuscitation prior to starting dobutamine.[17,18] Dobutamine should not be used as a first-line vasopressor for septic or other forms of distributive shock.

Anaphylaxis

Anaphylaxis is a hypersensitivity reaction that involves all the components of the immune system, including immunoglobulin, cytokines, leukotrienes, prostaglandins, and activation of the complement cascade. The main culprit is histamine release, which causes capillary leak resulting in hypovolemia, bronchospasm, vasospasm, and mucous gland hypersecretion.[19] The treatment of anaphylaxis should be guided by the need to prevent complications and reverse the inciting process. Special attention should be paid to securing the airway, and intubation, if indicated, should be done early. This should be followed by generous volume resuscitation, vasopressor support, and ultimately treating the histamine release.

Epinephrine is the vasopressor of choice and should be given early. Epinephrine dosage is something that is easily confused, and the literature contains a multitude of dosage variations, some in milliliters and others in milligrams or micrograms. Also, recommendations vary from country to country. First, it should be recalled that epinephrine concentrations vary. The commonly used terms, 1:1,000 and 1:10,000, are not completely obvious. Strictly speaking, these terms are structured as grams:milliliters of solution. Therefore, an epinephrine solution of 1:1,000 means 1 g of medication diluted in 1,000 mL (or 1 L) of solution. When each side of the ratio is divided by 1,000, the resulting amount is 1 mg/1 mL. This is obviously more concentrated than the 1:10,000 solution that has 1 g of medication diluted in 10,000 mL (or 10 L) of solution. In this case, dividing each side by 1,000 results in 1 mg/10 mL or 0.1 mg/1 mL. Epinephrine is packaged in a number of forms. Prefilled syringes, commonly used in cardiac arrest, come as 10 mL of 1:10,000 solution. As described above, this amounts to a total of 1 mg of epinephrine for the syringe at a concentration of 0.1 mg/mL (100 µg/mL).

The current clinical guideline recommends an initial epinephrine dose of 0.3–0.5 mg (or 300–500 µg), which is the same as 0.3–0.5 mL of a 1:1,000 solution administered intramuscularly (IM) into the anterior or lateral thigh. Also, IM injection is recommended over subcutaneous (SQ) injection due to its more rapid increase in plasma and tissue concentrations of epinephrine.[20] If shock is present or if symptoms are refractory to IM injection, then the epinephrine should be given by continuous IV infusion at a rate of 5–15 µg/min. This can easily be done by mixing 1 mg (1,000 µg) of either solution into a 100-mL bag of normal saline, which produces a concentration of 10 µg/mL. This solution can then be run at 1 mL/min, which provides the patient with 10 µg/min. In the event that the shock of anaphylaxis is refractory to epinephrine, norepinephrine or dopamine can be added.[21]

Neurogenic Shock

Neurogenic shock can be due to spinal cord injury or spinal anesthesia. The loss of sympathetic tone leads to increased venous capacitance, decreased venous return, decreased preload, decreased CO, and ultimately hypotension, often without a compensatory increased heart rate. Treatment of neurogenic shock includes careful IVF administration, and vasopressor support with α_1 stimulation for vasoconstriction with or without β_1 receptor stimulation for cardiac support. Norepinephrine and dopamine can be used for this purpose. Phenylephrine may be used as well; however, care should be taken to monitor for reflex bradycardia with this agent.

The current recommendation for blood pressure management after acute spinal injury from the American Association of Neurologic Surgeons is as follows: (1) hypotension should be avoided if possible, and if hypotension occurs, it should be corrected as soon as possible; (2) MAP goal of 85–90 mm Hg for the first 7 days following acute spinal cord injury—a MAP at this level is thought to improve spinal cord perfusion following injury. These recommendations are listed as options in the guideline as the data supporting these recommendations are limited.[22]

CARDIOGENIC SHOCK

Cardiogenic shock is the result of cardiac dysfunction and is usually associated with AMI. It is defined as hypotension not reversible with fluid therapy or hypoperfusion resulting in organ dysfunction, despite adequate left ventricular filling pressure. Cardiogenic shock is generally divided into two forms: left-sided failure, mainly due to AMI, and right-sided failure, which can have several causes. The right ventricle is thin walled, compared with the left ventricle, and can handle volume overload easier than the left side that handles much higher pressures. Similarly, right ventricular function is volume dependent, whereas left ventricular function is pressure dependent.

The treatment for cardiogenic shock is based on the side primarily involved. In the clinical setting, it is reasonable to start with the electrocardiogram (EKG) in these patients. An EKG that demonstrates a left-sided AMI indicates a left ventricular cause for cardiogenic shock. This can be followed by a bedside echocardiogram. Right ventricular dilatation indicates a right-sided cause. Echocardiography can also be used to exclude a diagnosis of cardiac tamponade in these patients.

Right ventricular failure can be caused by a wide array of clinical conditions including left-sided failure, pulmonary embolism, pulmonary HTN, sepsis, and lung disease. The treatment of cardiogenic shock from right heart failure is primarily directed at volume resuscitation to ensure adequate preload and at reversing the cause of the failure. Inotropic medication may be required as well. Right ventricular overfilling in the setting of heart failure can lead to a bulging intraventricular septum. This can diminish left ventricular function and decrease coronary perfusion resulting in myocardial ischemia or infarction.[23]

Cardiogenic shock from left-sided failure has been extensively studied, and most guidelines are directed at treating this form of cardiogenic shock. Since it is mainly due to AMI, treatment should be aimed at early revascularization and supportive care. According to the results of the SHOCK trial, which informed the American College of Cardiology/American Heart Association guidelines, emergency revascularization should be attempted immediately for patients younger than 75 years of age with cardiogenic shock from AMI.[24]

The American College of Cardiology/American Heart Association guidelines for the pharmacologic treatment of cardiogenic shock complicating AMI are as follows: (1) if SBP is 70–100 mm Hg without signs and symptoms of shock, dobutamine is the first-line agent; (2) if SBP is 70–100 mm Hg and the patient has signs and symptoms of shock, dopamine is the first-line treatment. If the response to these individual agents is inadequate, they can be used in combination or norepinephrine may be used with dobutamine. Vasopressin may also be used as a second-line agent.[15] A recent prospective randomized controlled trial in ICU patients revealed that the combination of norepinephrine–dobutamine appeared to be a more reliable and safer strategy than epinephrine alone.[25] Epinephrine was associated with a transient lactic acidosis, higher heart rate and arrhythmia, and inadequate gastric mucosa perfusion.

▶ CONCLUSION

The choice of pharmacologic treatment for shock can be very difficult. It is important to differentiate the cause of shock as quickly as possible. Initial treatment should be focused on maximizing fluid status before starting vasopressor therapy. In the undifferentiated shock patient, norepinephrine and dopamine are reasonable initial medications. As soon as the cause of shock is known, treatment should be adjusted to best address that cause. A solid understanding of the pathophysiology of the various types of shock is essential to making good decisions at the bedside.

REFERENCES

1. Tabaee A, Givertz MM. Pharmacologic management of the hypotensive patient. In: Irwin RS, Rippe JM, eds. *Irwin and Rippe's Intensive Care Medicine*. 5th ed. Philadelphia: Lippincott Williams & Wilkins; 2003:295–302.
2. Rang HP. *Pharmacology*. Edinburgh: Churchill Livingstone; 2003:163. ISBN 0-443-07145-4.
3. Gooneratne N, Manaker S. Use of vasopressors and inotropes. *UpToDate*. 2009. Available at: http://www.uptodate.com.
4. Goldberg LI. Dopamine: clinical uses of an engenous catecholamine. *N Engl J Med*. 1974 Oct 3;291(14):707–710.
5. Bellomo R, Chapman M, Finfer S, et al. Low-dose dopamine in patients with early renal dysfunction: a placebo controlled randomised trial: Australian and New Zealand Intensive Care Society (ANZICS) Clinical Trials Group. *Lancet*. 2000;356:2139–2143.
6. Anderson AC. Management of beta-adrenergic blocker poisoning. *Clin Pediatr Emerg Med*. 2008;9:4–16.
7. Gregory JS, Bonfiglio MF, Dasta JF, et al. Experience with phenylephrine as a component of the pharmaco-

logic support of septic shock. *Crit Care Med*. 1991;19: 1395–1400.

8. Vallet B, Wiel E, Lebuffe G. Resuscitation from circulatory sock. In: Fink MP, Abraham E, Vincent JL, et al. *Textbook of Critical Care*. Philadelphia, PA: Elsevier Saunders; 205–905.

9. Dellinger RP, Levey MM, Carlet JM, et al. Surviving Sepsis Campaign: international guidelines for management of severe sepsis and septic shock: 2008. *Crit Care Med*. 2008;36:296.

10. Dünser MW, Ruokonen E, Pettilä V, et al. Association of arterial blood pressure and vasopressor load with septic shock mortality: a post hoc analysis of a multicenter trial. *Crit Care*. 2009;13:6. Available at: http://ccforum.com/content/13/6/R181. Accessed on 04/01/2011.

11. De Backer D, Biston P, Devriendt J, et al. Comparison of dopamine and norepinephrine in the treatment of shock. *N Engl J Med*. 2010;362:779–789.

12. Jones AE, Kline JA. Shock. In: Marx JA, Hockberger R, Walls R. et al, eds. Rosents *Emergency Medicine*. Philadelphia, PA: Mosby Elsevier; 2006:41.

13. Annane D, Vignon P, Renault A, et al. Norepinephrine plus dobutamine versus epinephrine alone for management of septic shock: a randomised trial. *Lancet*. 2007;370:676–684.

14. Schmidt G, Mandel J. Management of severe sepsis and septic shock in adults. *UpToDate*. 2009. Available at: http://www.uptodate.com.

15. Overgaad CB, Dzavik V. Inotropes and vasopressors: review of physiology and clinical use in cardiovascular disease. *Circulation*. 2008;4(5):1043–1060.

16. Russell JA, Walley KR, Singer J, et al. Vasopressin versus norepinephrine in patients with septic shock. *N Engl J Med*. 2008;358:877–887.

17. Shoemaker WC, Appel PL, Kram HB. Hemodynamic and oxygen transport effects of dobutamine in critically ill general surgical patients. *Crit Care Med*. 1986;14: 1032–1037.

18. Rivers E, Nguyen B, Havstad S, et al. Early goal directed therapy in the treatment of sever sepsis and septic shock. *N Engl J Med*. 2001;345:1368–1377.

19. Kanji S, Chant C. Allergic and hypersensitivity reaction in the intensive care unit. *Crit Care Med*. 2010;38:S162–S168.

20. Simons F, Camargo C Jr. Anaphylaxis rapid recognition and treatment. *UpToDate*. 2009. Available at: http://www.uptodate.com.

21. Liberman P, Nicklas RA, Oppenheimer J, et al. The diagnosis and management of anaphylaxis practice parameter: 2010 update. *J Allergy Clin Immunol*. 2010;126:477–480.

22. Hadley M, Walter B. Guidelines for the management of acute cervical spine and spinal cord injuries. 2001. Available at: www.spineuniverse.com/professional/acute-cervical-spine-injury-guide, www.spineuniverse.com/pdf/traumaguide/finished1116.pdf.

23. Lahm T, McCaslin CA, Wozniak TC, et al. Medical and surgical treatment of acute right ventricular failure. *J Am Coll Cardiol*. 2010;56(18):1435–1446.

24. Sanbon TA, Sleeper LA, Bates ER, et al. Impact of thrombolysis, intra-aortic balloon pump counterpulsation, and their combination in cardiogenic shock complicating acute myocardial infarction: a report from the SHOCK Trial Registry. *J Am Coll Cardiol*. 2000;36:1123–1129.

25. Levy B, Perez P, Perny J, et al. Comparison of norepinephrine–dobutamine to epinephrine for hemodynamics, lactate metabolism, and organ function variables in cardiogenic shock. A prospective, randomized pilot study. *Crit Care Med*. 2011;39:450–455.

CHAPTER 17

Management after Cardiac Surgery

Justin T. Sambol and LaMont C. Smith

► OVERVIEW

Cardiac surgery is one of the most commonly performed major operative procedures in the United States. The indications for cardiac surgery include myocardial ischemia and infarction, heart failure, valvular dysfunction, aortic pathology, and surgery for dysrythmias. The management of patients following cardiac surgery requires a multifaceted approach and the involvement of a team of specialists. While the intensivist is often the point person for the management of the patients following open heart surgery, it is essential that the management involve the surgeon, cardiologist, and anesthesiologist, and a wide variety of other health care providers.

Successful postoperative management following cardiac surgery requires a clear understanding of the patient's preoperative conditions and the intraoperative events and management. The goal is to restore the patient's normal physiologic condition and homeostasis. As medical management and interventional cardiology procedures evolve and improve, the patients being referred for cardiac surgery are sicker and more debilitated than they were in the past. This trend is likely to continue in the years to come. Despite these increased challenges facing cardiac surgeons, patient outcomes remain very good in large part due to the postoperative management and ICU care. A systems-oriented approach is often necessary to deal with the multitude of problems facing these patients, and the cardiac system is generally the primary determinant of recovery.[1]

► HEART

HEMODYNAMIC MANAGEMENT

The goal of hemodynamic management is to maintain adequate oxygen delivery to the tissues and to minimize demands on a heart that has just undergone major surgery. Optimization of cardiac output is essential to maintain function of the brain, kidneys, gut, lungs, and other end organs necessary for optimal recovery. Postoperatively, contractility is almost always diminished, the magnitude of which is often related to the severity of chronic dysfunction, ischemia, and intraoperative events.[2]

Despite the wide array of patient disease and cardiac procedures, significant similarities exist in patient monitoring, evaluation, and management.[2] The majority of patients have continuous monitoring of EKG, pulse oximetry, blood pressure, central venous pressure (CVP) monitoring, and in most instances a pulmonary artery catheter (PAC) for monitoring mixed venous O_2 saturation (SvO_2), pulmonary artery pressures, and continuous cardiac output. Although the use of a PAC in patients undergoing cardiac surgery has been a topic of some debate,[3] it has been common practice to use PACs in almost every patient undergoing cardiac surgery. These modalities allow for measurement of oxygen consumption and mixed venous and arterial oxygen saturation, and an estimation of cardiac output. The goal is to maintain normal hemodynamic values if possible since it has been shown that normal oxygen transport and normal SvO_2 (>70%) in the immediate postoperative period can

▶ **TABLE 17-1. COMMONLY USED DRUGS FOLLOWING CARDIAC SURGERY**

Drug	Dose	Contractility	HR	MAP
Epinephrine	1–20 µg/min	4+	3+	↕ (dose dependent)
Milrinone	0.15–0.5 µg/kg/min	4+	0	↓↓↓
Dobutamine	2–20 µg/kg/min	3–4+	1–2+	↓↓
Dopamine	1–4 µg/kg/min	1+	1+	↓
	4–20 µg/kg/min	2–3+	2+	↑↑↑
Norepinephrine	2–40 µg/min	1+	1+	↑↑↑↑
Phenylephrine	20–200 µg/min	0	0	↑↑↑
Vasopressin	0.01–0.04 U/min	0	0	↑↑↑↑
Nitroglycerin	10–200 µg/min	0	1+	↓↓
Nitroprusside	0.1–10 µg/kg/min	0	2+	↓↓↓

Data modified from St. Andre and DelRossi.[2]

improve outcome.[4] Although achieving these targets can be challenging,[5-7] adjustments to volume status, afterload, heart rate and rhythm, and cardiac output can help to maximize end-organ oxygen delivery.

Blood Pressure

Mean arterial pressure (MAP) is the most dynamic physiologic variable in the first hours following cardiac surgery.[2] This can be due to a number of factors including decreased preload, vasodilatation, and cardiac contractility. Many patients' end organs are dependent on higher blood pressures; however, concerns about bleeding often lead to a struggle between maintaining a higher MAP for perfusion and keeping the pressure low to protect suture lines. Despite these concerns, the MAP should be maintained above 65 mm Hg. Volume resuscitation can be guided by CVP, and, although there is no gold standard for the type of fluid used for resuscitation, it has been our practice to use 5% albumin. There are concerns, however, about albumin extravasation,[8] and no clinical difference has been shown to suggest that there is any benefit to colloid versus crystalloid.[9] Once the patient is adequately volume resuscitated, there are a number of pharmacologic agents (Table 17-1) that can be useful for increasing vascular tone and cardiac contractility. It is essential that the intensivist have a thorough understanding of the mechanism of each of these agents and their interactions with one another.

In addition to hypotension, a small portion of patients may present with significant levels of hypertension.[2,10] This may lead to excessive bleeding and an increase in afterload that can exacerbate low cardiac output and should be treated aggressively with vasodilators.

Cardiac Contractility

Myocardial contractility following cardiac surgery can be a variable and dynamic process. Patients with low cardiac output following cardiac surgery are at significant risk for end-organ hypoperfusion if the cardiac index (CI) is below 2.2. It is essential that the source for low CI be identified and treated rapidly. Once hypovolemia, bleeding, and tamponade have been ruled out, the focus should be on instituting pharmacologic and mechanical support for the failing heart. The most useful drugs (Table 17-1) have significant inotropic and vasodilatory activity.[11] Epinephrine has both α and β effects and is very useful in the postoperative period. The $β_2$ effects are seen predominantly at lower doses, whereas the α effects predominate at higher doses. Both dobutamine and dopamine are effective β-agonists with broad dosage-dependent effects, but dobutamine has a superior effect on cardiac contractility. Milrinone, which is a cyclic phosphodiesterase inhibitor, works by increasing cAMP levels leading to increase in calcium flux and myocardial contractility. In addition to its inotropic affect, milrinone decreases vascular tone, particularly in the pulmonary bed. A randomized trial by Feneck et al[11] compared the effects of milrinone and dobutamine on low-output syndrome following cardiac surgery. They found that patients receiving dobutamine had a higher CI, heart rate, and left ventricular (LV) stroke work index than those receiving milrinone, whereas milrinone led to a greater decrease in pulmonary capillary wedge pressure. Dobutamine, however, was associated with a higher incidence of hypertension and conversion from sinus rhythm to atrial fibrillation (AF).

Mechanical Support for Low Cardiac Output

Pharmacologic support is generally effective in helping separate from cardiopulmonary bypass (CPB) and in supporting CI in the postoperative period. There are situations, however, where mechanical support is necessary such as when the CI does not increase above 2.0 despite maximum inotropic support. The intra-aortic balloon pump (IABP) is a mechanical circulatory assist device developed in 1968 by Kantrowitz et al.[12] The balloon is placed in the descending thoracic aorta just distal to the subclavian artery. The balloon inflates during diastole, increasing coronary perfusion, and deflates during systole, decreasing afterload. Its use has evolved from circulatory support of patients in cardiogenic shock to now being used as an aid to weaning patients from CPB and for postoperative low CI. It is now the most commonly used mechanical assist device with over 100,000 implanted annually.

Despite adequate volume loading, maximum inotropic support, and the use of IABP, a small percentage of patients will not be able to be weaned from CPB or will develop severe cardiogenic shock in the perioperative period. Over the last 20 years, the use of ventricular assist devices (VAD) has helped aid the failing heart after cardiac surgery. Studies have shown that patients requiring two or more high-dose inotropes to wean from CPB had better outcomes with early VAD insertion.[13] While the details of the use of VADs are beyond the scope of this chapter, it is important to understand their utility in the management of the post-cardiac surgery patient.

RATE AND RHYTHM

Following cardiac surgery, patients are prone to develop some form of dysrhythmia. Heart rate and conduction abnormalities are common following valvular and coronary surgery. Most surgeons place epicardial pacing leads on the atrium, ventricle, or both that are brought out in the subxiphoid region and can be helpful in assisting in management of bradycardia and atrial dysrhythmias. Augmentation of the heart rate, even when normal, to rates of 90–100 can be useful to increase CI. Conversely, patients may be persistently tachycardic following surgery with rates up to 120, which may be due to a variety of drugs used in the postoperative period and which often requires no intervention.

Ventricular arrhythmias such as nonsustained ventricular tachycardia (VT) are not uncommon following cardiac surgery and should prompt an examination and correction of any electrolyte disturbance. Frequent episodes or periods of sustained VT may require more aggressive therapy with antiarrhythmic drugs such as amiodarone or lidocaine and electrical cardioversion if the patient is hemodynamically compromised. These episodes should also prompt a thorough investigation of possible ischemia, particularly in coronary artery bypass graft (CABG) patients.

Atrial Fibrillation

AF occurs in 15–45% of patients undergoing cardiac surgery with the highest incidence being in patients undergoing valve and combined CABG/valve procedures. The cause for postoperative AF is not well understood but is likely due to reentry of multiple waves of excitation throughout the atria.[14] Several factors have been associated with increased risk for postoperative AF including advanced age, concomitant valve surgery, history of AF, congestive heart failure, COPD, and decreased LV function.[15] A number of strategies have been implemented to reduce the incidence of AF. β-Adrenergic blockers have been extensively studied and have shown significant efficacy in reducing AF in the postoperative setting.[15] β-Blockers should be started as early as possible in the postoperative period to reduce the incidence of AF. For patients who cannot be started on β-blockers, antiarrhythmic agents such as amiodarone and sotalol are both safe and efficacious in decreasing postoperative AF risk.

Despite the use of the preventive measures, AF remains a significant problem in the postoperative period. In most patients, AF is self-limiting and the treatment options vary based on the patient's clinical condition. One management strategy generally utilized in postoperative AF is demonstrated in Figure 17-1. For patients who are hemodynamically unstable, difficult to manage, or have a contraindication to anticoagulation, rhythm control is the preferred approach. However, in patients who are tolerating their AF, rate control and anticoagulation is the preferred approach since many of these patients will return to sinus rhythm within 3 months.

► BLEEDING

Bleeding, both intraoperatively and postoperatively, presents a significant challenge to the surgeon and intensivist in the management of the cardiac surgery patient. Excessive bleeding requires significant blood product usage that both is costly and adds significant morbidity and mortality to the patient.[16] The needs of intraoperative anticoagulation combined with the effects of platelet dysfunction by the CPB circuit lead to postoperative coagulopathy. In addition, many patients now come to the operating room with some exposure to potent antiplatelet agents such as glycoprotein IIb/IIIa inhibitors or clopidogrel (Plavix). These agents significantly disrupt platelet aggregation and may lead to increased postoperative coagulopathy.[17] In general, postoperative coagulopathy is usually due to a number of factors including thrombocytopenia, fibrinolysis, hypothermia, hemodilution, and residual or rebound heparin. This generally leads to some degree of chest tube output in the range of 50–100 cm^3/h.

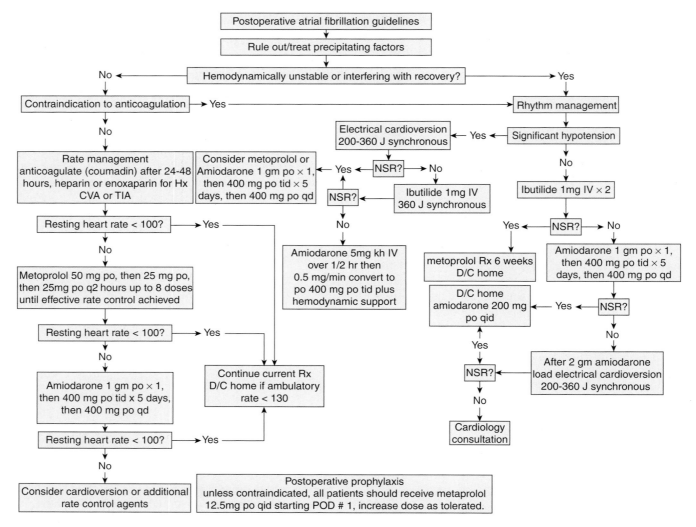

Figure 17-1. Management of postoperative atrial fibrillation. (Data from Khalpey Z, Ganim R, Rawn J. Postoperative care of cardiac surgery patients. In: Cohn LH, ed. *Cardiac Surgery in the Adult*.[82] Adapted from Maisel et al[14])

The treatment of postoperative bleeding is summarized in Table 17-2 and is dependent on the judgment of the surgeon and intensivist to determine if the patient is bleeding from surgical problems or coagulopathy. Chest tube inspection and management is essential to understand the pathophysiology of the bleeding. Generally, in coagulopathic bleeding there is no clot in the chest tubes and this can often be managed with correction of the coagulopathy and administration of blood products. Some other maneuvers that can be useful include increasing positive end-expiratory pressure (PEEP), use of epsilon aminocaproic acid, and warming. In addition, some have advocated the use of activated recombinant factor VII (rFVIIa) that has been widely reported in the management of bleeding after cardiac surgery. However, concerns about the safety, particularly in bypass patients with fresh grafts, have been raised.[18]

MEDIASTINAL RE-EXPLORATION

Patients in whom surgical bleeding is suspected often require re-exploration. This should be considered when bleeding exceeds 400 mL/h for the first hour, 300 mL/h for 2–3 hours, and 200 mL/h for 4 hours (Table 17-2). Chest tube output is not the only indicator of significant surgical bleeding since chest tubes can become clotted and blood can collect and clot in the pericardium. Hemodynamic instability not responsive to inotropic support or signs of tamponade such as elevated filling pressures or equalization of pressures should initiate a return to the operating room for re-exploration. Widening of the mediastinum on chest x-ray (CXR) or signs of tamponade on transesophageal echocardiogram can be helpful in patients where the diagnosis is questionable. On rare occasions, the

▶ TABLE 17-2. **MANAGEMENT OF POSTOPERATIVE BLEEDING**

Bleeding Scenario	Diagnosis	Treatment
<50 mL/h		
Stable BP, coagulopathy	Post-CPB	Supportive care
>100 mL/h		
Hypothermic	Hypothermia	
Acute hypotension (MAP <50 mm Hg)		
Diffuse bloody ooze	Borderline coagulopathy	
Coagulopathy		
1. High PTT, PT	Rebound heparin effect	Protamine
2. INR >1.4	Deficient clotting factors	FFP
3. Low fibrinogen	Deficient clotting factors	Cryoprecipitate
4. Platelets <10^5/μL	Thrombocytopenia	Platelets
5. Platelets >10^5/μL	Platelet dysfunction	? Platelets ± DDAVP
6. Bleeding >30 min (high D-dimers, fibrinolysis)	Fibrinolysis	FFP, cryoprecipitate
>200–300 mL/h		
>200 mL/h for 4 h	Surgical bleeding should be assumed for any of these criteria	Consider re-exploration
>300 mL/h for 2–3 h		
>400 mL/h for 1 h		

DDAVP: desmopressin (synthetic vasopressin); PTT: activated partial thromboplastin time; FFP: fresh frozen plasma; PT: prothrombin time; BP: blood pressure; CPB: cardiopulmonary bypass. Adapted and modified with permission from Khalpey Z, Ganim R, Rawn D. Postoperative care of cardiac surgery patients. In Cohn LH, ed. *Cardiac Surgery in the Adult*. 2008.[82]

patient may require re-exploration at the bedside if there is massive sudden hemorrhage or cardiac arrest is imminent. In those situations, the goal is to relieve the tamponade, restore cardiac contractile function, and temporarily control bleeding while the patient is returned to the operating room.

▶ LUNG

Postoperative pulmonary care is aimed at restoring normal pulmonary capillary permeability and interstitial lung volume, preventing or treating atelectasis, maintaining normal arterial blood gases, and preventing infection.

EARLY VERSUS DELAYED EXTUBATION

Early extubation may be defined as extubation of a patient within 3–6 hours of arrival in the ICU. The goals, as with any extubation, are to have a patient who is awake enough to protect his or her airway and adequately oxygenate and ventilate. Weaning of sedation should begin early after admission to the ICU as long as the patient is hemodynamically stable with manageable chest tube output.

There are a variety of approaches to rapid weaning including the rapid shallow breathing index (RSBI)

that is a calculated by dividing a patient's tidal volume into the observed respiratory rate during a spontaneous breathing trial of 10–30 minutes. Statistically, an RSBI of <105 is thought to be highly predictive of a successful extubation (See Chapter 5).

A T-tube trial is another way of performing a spontaneous breathing trial. The patient has supplemental oxygen administered while remaining intubated. There is no ventilatory support. Patients who tolerate a T-piece trial have a high chance of successful extubation presumably because breathing through a T-piece is more difficult than normal breathing.

Other clinicians rely on the traditional method of converting the ventilation mode to a partial support (assist control or intermittent mandatory ventilation with pressure-supported [PS] spontaneous breaths) or a total spontaneous setting when the patient is fully awake. The decision to extubate is then based on clinical observation, O$_2$ saturation, and blood gas results. Minimum settings before extubation typically are PS of 10, with a PEEP of 5. This amount of PS helps to overcome endotracheal tube resistance, and PEEP helps to maintain and recruit alveoli. No particular weaning technique has been shown to be superior to any other, and the literature does not implicate any technique as being more commonly associated with adverse outcome.

The postoperative CXR should also factor into the decision-making process. Pulmonary edema and pleural effusions are common in the early postoperative period, but are usually not large enough to be significant. Patients who do not meet the criteria for early extubation may develop larger effusions over time that may need to be drained in order to maximize the likelihood of a successful extubation. Cardiac surgery patients are also at risk for worsening pulmonary edema; therefore, diuresis may be helpful in patients who cannot be extubated early.

Definitive outcome studies are only beginning to be presented, but the data so far suggest that early extubation is not associated with any increased risk of mortality or morbidity.[19] An audit by Akhtar and Hamid of 388 postoperative CABG patients found that 196 (49.5%) patients could be extubated within 6 hours of arrival in the cardiac ICU. Of the remaining patients, reasons for prolonged intubation included deep sedation in 80 patients (46.5%), confusion in 44 (25%), excessive bleeding in 20 (11.3%), and high inotropic support in 10 (5.68%).[20]

Factors that may adversely impact successful early extubation include the effects of anesthesia on postoperative hemodynamics, stress responses and awareness, altered management in the control of pain, shivering and ischemia in the early postoperative period, and the risks of reintubation in patients who might require reoperation for bleeding. Risk factors for delayed extubation of postoperative CABG patients include increased age, female gender, postoperative use of IABP, inotrope requirement, bleeding, and atrial arrhythmia.[21]

PULMONARY MANAGEMENT FOLLOWING EXTUBATION

Once extubated, patients will need supplementary oxygen. This is usually given as a 40% face mask, and then gradually weaned to a nasal cannula. The use of bedside incentive spirometry and chest physiotherapy will help reduce atelectasis and the risk of pneumonia. In addition, short-term β-agonists help in the postextubation recovery phase, even in patients without a history of COPD or reactive airway disease.

A median sternotomy or thoracotomy incision is associated with significant pain, splinting, and decreased chest wall compliance, resulting in shallow breaths, atelectasis, and an increased risk of pneumonia.[22] Adequate pain control reduces the likelihood of postoperative splinting, atelectasis, and pneumonia. Opiates combined with rapid-acting NSAIDs such as ketorolac have been used with success.[23] Patient-controlled analgesia (PCA) may have the advantage of improved pain control as well as a reduction in the occurrence of atelectasis when compared with nurse-controlled analgesia.

▶ **TABLE 17-3. PULMONARY COMPLICATIONS AFTER CARDIAC SURGERY**

Complication	Frequency (%)
Pleural effusion	27–95
Atelectasis	17–88
Prolonged mechanical ventilation	6–58
Diaphragm dysfunction	2–54
Pneumonia	4–20
Pulmonary embolism	0.04–3.2
ARDS	0.4–2
Aspiration	2
Pneumothorax	1.5

Data adapted from Wynn and Botti.[25]

PULMONARY COMPLICATIONS

Atelectasis and pleural effusion are among the more common complications following cardiac surgery.[24] In addition, there are a number of other complications (see Table 17-3) that may complicate postoperative recovery, leading to longer stays in the ICU and hospital and increasing overall morbidity and mortality. Recognizing these potential complications and treating them early is essential to ensuring a successful postoperative outcome.

Postoperative Pulmonary Dysfunction

Postoperative pulmonary dysfunction (PPD) is a constellation of events that occurs in patients undergoing cardiac surgery. It may delay extubation, factor into extubation failure, and delay functional recovery. PPD involves alterations in pulmonary function such as increased work of breathing, shallow respiration, ineffective cough, and relative hypoxemia. All postoperative cardiac surgery patients develop some degree of PPD.

The underlying basis for PPD is the development of abnormal gas exchange, and alterations in lung mechanics. Gas exchange abnormalities include a widened alveolar–arterial oxygen gradient, increased microvascular permeability in the lung, increased pulmonary vascular resistance, increased pulmonary shunt fraction, and intrapulmonary aggregation of leukocytes and platelets.[25] Alterations in the mechanical properties of the lung lead to reductions in vital capacity, functional residual capacity, and static and dynamic lung compliance.

Premorbid conditions such as COPD and undiagnosed preoperative pneumonia can contribute to the development of pulmonary dysfunction after cardiac surgery. Postoperatively, these patients may develop pulmonary edema, atelectasis, or pneumonia. The risk of developing pneumonia increases with delayed extubation. In addition, shallow breathing, a weak cough, and splinting from inadequate pain control can also contribute to the development of PPD, leading to respiratory failure and reintubation.

CPB can contribute to pulmonary dysfunction by increasing left atrial or pulmonary venous pressure. These effects combined with reduced plasma oncotic pressure can increase extravascular lung water.[26,27] During CPB, cytotoxic and vasoactive mediators of the inflammatory response[28–32] and circulating micro-emboli[33] may reach the lung via bronchial arteries. This inflammatory response has been termed "pump lung" or "postpump syndrome." These agents increase pulmonary capillary permeability, perivascular edema, and bronchial secretions. Once CPB commences, the cessation of pulmonary ventilation results in collapsed lungs and insufficient alveolar distention to activate the production of surfactant, a situation that potentiates alveolar collapse. Abnormal pulmonary mechanics, retention of secretions, and atelectasis can also occur.[25]

The cumulative effect of premorbid conditions and CPB contributes to the development of an increased work of breathing, postoperative atelectasis, pulmonary edema, as well as an increased susceptibility to infection.

Pleural Effusions

Pleural effusions are common after cardiac surgery including CABG and can be categorized as: perioperative (within the first week), early (within 1 month), late (2–12 months), or persistent (after 6 months).[34] Among patients undergoing CABG, the prevalence of pleural effusions in the immediate postoperative period is high. In the week after CABG, the reported prevalence of pleural effusions has ranged from 40% to 75%.[35–39] Most effusions are small, unilateral, left-sided, and asymptomatic. In a study by Labidi et al, almost 7% of patients had a clinically significant pleural effusion in the 30 days postsurgery.[40] Peng et al conducted a similar study of 356 patients who were available for evaluation 1 month after undergoing CABG. The initial diagnosis of a newly developed symptomatic large pleural effusion was made in 11 patients (3.1%) within 30 days of CABG. Eight had a pleural effusion predominantly on the left side and three on the right.[41] When the presence of a pleural effusion hinders extubation or causes pulmonary dysfunction, tube thoracostomy, thoracentesis, or placement of a pig-tail catheter may be indicated.

Pulmonary Edema

CPB can cause cardiogenic pulmonary edema from hemodilution, volume overload, and reduction in oncotic pressure. It can also cause noncardiogenic pulmonary edema (NCPE) by producing a systemic inflammatory response syndrome (SIRS). This involves an increase in capillary permeability and accumulation of extravascular lung water. Surfactant production is also decreased resulting in atelectasis. Other potential causes of postoperative NCPE include blood transfusions, the administration of fresh frozen plasma to control bleeding, and preexisting lung conditions.[42] Additionally, protamine sulfate, which is often given to reverse the effects of heparin intraoperatively, has been associated with causing NCPE on rare occasions.[43]

Most cases of postoperative pulmonary edema are mild and can be treated with early diuresis. Fulminant NCPE, although rare, is associated with a high mortality. SIRS can progress to full-blown adult respiratory distress syndrome (ARDS). This syndrome is diagnosed by the presence of bilateral patchy infiltrates on CXR, normal cardiac filling pressures, relative hypoxemia, and a Pao_2/FIO_2 ratio of <200. Management of NCPE or ARDS involves mechanical ventilation with as low an FiO_2 as possible to maintain a Po_2 of 60–70. Higher settings of PEEP may be needed and must be balanced with the effect of reducing cardiac output by reducing venous return. Ventilator settings with a tidal volume of 6 mL/kg of predicted body weight have been shown to improve survival when compared with higher tidal volume.

Other maneuvers that may be useful in the management of ARDS include prone positioning that improves oxygenation but poses safety concerns in the poststernotomy patient, and high levels of PEEP (35–40 cm H_2O) that have not been shown to improve survival. High-frequency oscillatory ventilation is, in theory, the ideal "lung-protective" method, but its benefits have not been proven. No drug therapy, including corticosteroids, has been shown to improve survival in patients with ARDS. Inhaled nitric oxide, although useful in decreasing pulmonary vascular resistance and decreasing right heart failure, has no substantial impact on the duration of ventilatory support or mortality.

▶ RENAL

Patients undergoing cardiac surgery often have some degree of peripheral vascular disease, diabetes, or other predisposing factors that impact renal function. Patients at risk for developing postoperative acute kidney injury (AKI) include those of increasing age, as well as those with a history of hypertension, diabetes mellitus, and CHF. Additionally, patients who require lengthy procedures on bypass are also at risk.[44–46] AKI is a major complication of CABG surgery that is strongly associated with in-hospital mortality.[47] The incidence of AKI may be increasing despite a trend of decreasing in-hospital mortality. Some have suggested that this is

▶ **TABLE 17-4. RISK, INJURY, FAILURE, LOSS, AND END-STAGE KIDNEY (RIFLE) CLASSIFICATION**

Class	Glomerular Filtration Rate Criteria	Urine Output Criteria
Risk	Serum creatinine × 1.5	<0.5 mL/kg/h × 6 h
Injury	Serum creatinine × 2	<0.5 mL/kg/h × 12 h
Failure	Serum creatinine × 3, or serum creatinine ≥4 mg/dL with an acute rise >0.5 mg/dL	<0.3 mL/kg/h × 24 h, or anuria × 12 h
Loss	Persistent renal failure. Complete loss of kidney function >4 weeks	
End-stage kidney disease	Complete loss of kidney function >3 months	

For conversion of creatinine expressed in conventional units to SI units, multiply by 88.4. RIFLE class is determined based on the worst of either glomerular filtration criteria or urine output criteria. Glomerular filtration criteria are calculated as an increase of serum creatinine above the baseline serum creatinine level. Acute kidney injury should be both abrupt (within 1–7 days) and sustained (more than 24 hours). When the baseline serum creatinine is not known and patients are without a history of chronic kidney insufficiency, it is recommend to calculate a baseline serum creatinine using the Modification of Diet in Renal Disease equation for assessment of kidney function, assuming a glomerular filtration rate of 75 mL/min/1.73 m². When the baseline serum creatinine is elevated, an abrupt rise of at least 0.5 mg/dL to more than 4 mg/dL is all that is required to achieve class failure. From Hoste et al. *Crit Care.* 2006;10:R73.[52]

due to broader criteria for the diagnosis.[48] Some degree of renal injury almost always occurs during CPB, and postperfusion proteinuria occurs in many patients.[49] Up to 30% of patients who undergo CABG develop some degree of acute renal impairment.[50]

The Society of Thoracic Surgeons National Cardiac Surgery database defines postoperative new renal failure as a serum creatinine of >2.0 mg/dL, doubling of peak preoperative creatinine, or requirement of dialysis. The Acute Dialysis Quality Initiative formulated the Risk, Injury, Failure, Loss, and End-Stage Kidney (RIFLE) classification.[51] RIFLE defines three grades of increasing severity of AKI—risk (class R), injury (class I), and failure (class F)—and two outcome classes (loss and end-stage kidney disease). The RIFLE classification grading is based on changes in either serum creatinine or urine output from the baseline condition (see Table 17-4).

RENAL PROTECTION

AKI can be classified on the basis of the underlying pathology. The majority of postoperative AKI is due to acute tubular necrosis (ATN) or prerenal azotemia. Postobstructive uropathy and glomerulonephritis can also occur. Prerenal azotemia often develops from hypoperfusion and ischemia, but is effectively managed by restoration of normal blood flow. This may be accomplished with volume supplementation with fluid or blood, or increasing cardiac output with inotropes. ATN is thought to arise from a variety of insults to the kidney in these patients, including ischemia, general anesthesia, radiocontrast dyes, and heart failure. Blood flow decreases in the early phase of ATN, and therefore vasodilators theoretically should reduce necrosis in the kidney by restoring blood flow to the tubules. However, a prospective single-center, randomized, double-blind trial involving 80 patients undergoing cardiac surgery

studied the effects of fenoldopam at 0.05 µg/kg/min or dopamine at 2.5 µg/kg/min after the induction of anesthesia for a 24-hour period. Peak postoperative serum creatinine level, intensive care unit and hospital stay, and mortality were similar in the two groups. They concluded that there was no renal protective benefit afforded by the vasodilator fenoldopam in a high-risk population undergoing cardiac surgery.[53]

CPB and cardioplegic arrest are associated with free radical formation. These free radicals are thought to cause damage to various organs including the kidneys. Several studies have looked at free radical scavenging with agents such as *N*-acetylcysteine as a way to preserve renal function. Sisillo et al showed no difference in mortality regarding the use of *N*-acetylcysteine, although their data did suggest a decrease in the incidence of postoperative acute renal failure and ventilator days.[54] Barr and Kolodner studied 79 patients with preexisting renal disease who underwent cardiac surgery.[55] Their data suggested a protective effect of fenoldopam, *N*-acetylcysteine, or the combination when given before surgery, compared with controls. However, there was no decrease in length of ICU or hospital stay and fenoldopam was associated with perioperative hypotension.

PROGNOSIS

Ryckwaert et al, in a study of 591 patients, determined that a postoperative 20% increase in plasma creatinine after cardiac surgery was associated with an increase in mortality, especially when accompanied by multiple organ dysfunction.[56] When acute renal failure is severe enough to require renal replacement therapy (RRT), mortality rates are 50–90% compared with <3% for patients without AKI.[50,57] Possible explanations for the increased mortality associated with AKI are salt and water retention resulting in volume overload, hyperkalemia, and acid–base derangements.[58] These derangements may result in hypertension, hypotension, changes in cardiac output, as well as changes in blood flow to the liver and other organs. There is evidence that AKI may lead to insulin resistance and protein breakdown, and immunocompromise.[59] Patients with AKI also have a high incidence of infectious complications[60] and frequently develop anemia. Finally, AKI itself can lead to a noninfectious, proinflammatory response with activation of leukocytes, secretion of proinflammatory cytokines, and recruitment of neutrophils and macrophages with resultant lung injury, as has been demonstrated in animal models of ischemia–reperfusion-induced acute renal failure.[61,62]

▶ GASTROINTESTINAL TRACT

Gastrointestinal (GI) maladies are infrequent but serious complications of cardiac surgery, with high rates of morbidity and mortality. The incidence is low ranging from 0.41% to 2.0%.[63–67]; however, the mortality rate has been reported to be as high as 63%.[65–68] Patients most at risk for dying include those with New York Heart Association (NYHA) class IV and unstable symptoms, an increased need for preoperative IABP support, the need for GI surgical intervention, and patients with ischemic bowel. Zacharias et al identified eight parameters that predicted GI complications: age greater than 70 years, long duration of CPB, need for blood transfusions, reoperation, triple vessel disease, NYHA functional class IV, peripheral vascular disease, and congestive heart failure. They suggest that intra-abdominal injury is usually ischemic in nature due to low cardiac output, hypotension, blood loss, or intra-abdominal atheroemboli.[69] Other patients at risk include those with combined CABG–valve operations, prolonged ventilation time, female sex, need for vasopressors, sternal wound infection, and a history of peptic ulcer disease.[65,67,70]

The list of potential complications includes GI bleeding (most common), acute pancreatitis, perforated peptic ulcer, intestinal ischemia, cholecystitis, and small bowel obstruction.[67,71] Interestingly, Mangi et al, in their study of 8,709 patients, found the most frequent serious GI complication to be mesenteric ischemia, which developed in 67% of patients who suffered a serious GI complication.[64]

POSTOPERATIVE CARE

Postoperatively, it is important to maintain GI perfusion and an adequate CVP. The common etiological factor in developing GI complications of any kind, after cardiac surgery, seems to be postoperative splanchnic hypoperfusion with visceral ischemia.[72] CPB has been shown to decrease gastric pH, increasing the risk of erosion and bleeding. Stress ulcer prophylaxis with proton pump inhibitors reduces this risk. Other postoperative preventive measures that have had variable results in the literature include selective gut decontamination, early enteral feeding, and adjuvants to promote gut function such as glutamine, fiber, and growth hormone.[73]

Ideally, patients are extubated early in the postoperative period and are started on oral diets. For patients who are unstable or in whom complications develop that necessitate a prolonged intubation, early enteral feeding should be considered. Enteral nutritional support for critically ill patients is thought to maintain GI mucosal integrity and barrier function, and stimulate splanchnic and GI-associated lymphoid tissue blood flow. Further, when compared with parenteral nutrition, enteral nutrition improves substrate utilization, reduces the risk of sepsis, and decreases cost.[74]

▶ NEUROLOGIC COMPLICATIONS

INCIDENCE

Stroke and other neurologic impairments are among the most dreaded complications of open heart surgery for both the surgeon and the patient. The likelihood of perioperative stroke varies between 1% and 5% in most published series and is dependent on a multitude of risk factors.[75] Cognitive deterioration after cardiac surgery is far more common, although the incidence varies widely. It may affect as many as 80% of patients a few days after surgery and may persist in up to one third of patients.[76]

A retrospective report from the Society of Thoracic Surgery National Cardiac Database, of over 400,000 cardiac surgeries between 1996 and 1997, reported an overall incidence of a new neurologic event (stroke, transient ischemic attack, or unexplained coma lasting more than 24 hours) of 3.3%.[77] A prospective study evaluated 2,108 patients undergoing CABG at 24 hospitals in the United States between 1991 and 1993. Overall, 6.1% suffered a cerebral complication, roughly equally divided between stroke and encephalopathy.[78]

Neurologic injury after cardiac surgery can be classified into two types. Type I includes stroke, seizures, stupor, or coma. Type II is more common and includes intellectual deterioration and memory deficit. These complications are most often caused by microemboli and/or hypoperfusion. There may also be a contribution from the effects of general anesthesia. Some have theorized that the degree of aortic manipulation and clamping during cardiac surgery may be the predominate cause of neurologic injury later.[79,80]

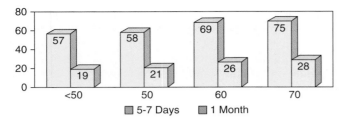

Figure 17-2. Effect of age by decade on neuropsychological outcome after coronary artery bypass graft surgery. Abnormal neuropsychological outcomes at 1 week and 1 month postoperatively are more common with advancing age. Percentages of patients with deficits on two or more tests are shown (*n* = 374). (Reproduced with permission from Hammon JW. Extracorporeal circulation: organ damage. In: Cohn LH, ed. *Cardiac Surgery in the Adult.* New York: McGraw-Hill; 2008:389–414.[82])

PATIENTS AT RISK

A study by Kolkka and Hilberman examined the characteristics of patients with neurologic complications after cardiac surgery. When compared with the 169 patients with no evidence of neurologic or neuropsychological dysfunction at discharge, the 35 patients with complications were older (65 ± 10 years vs. 55 ± 12 years), had a lower incidence of CABG as the sole surgical procedure (29% vs. 55%), a higher mortality rate (11.4% vs. 1.8%), and prolonged CPB (140 ± 45 minutes vs. 107 ± 38 minutes).[81]

Hammon identified several risk factors for neurologic damage (Figure 17-2) including proximal aortic atherosclerosis, history of neurologic disease, diabetes mellitus, use of IABP, history of hypertension, history of pulmonary disease, history of unstable angina, age (per additional decade), systolic blood pressure >180 mm Hg at admission, history of excessive alcohol consumption, history of CABG, dysrhythmia on the day of surgery, antihypertensive therapy, perioperative hypotension, ventricular venting, congestive heart failure on the day of surgery, and a history of peripheral vascular disease.[82]

POSTOPERATIVE CARE AND PREVENTION

The observation of a patient's neurologic decline after surgery is most distressing to family members. Early neurocognitive dysfunction (within 3 months of operation) is most likely related to a combination of factors that include microemboli, relative hypotension, general anesthesia, and the overall inflammatory condition initiated by CPB. Neurocognitive deficits that are present after 3 months are often permanent.[82]

There is evidence that late cognitive changes are more likely related to the presence of preoperative neurologic conditions. Patients with atherosclerotic disease that has progressed enough to require CABG often have a similar degree of cerebrovascular disease. Many have had silent cerebrovascular events. Perioperative carotid endarterectomy in patients with significant carotid artery disease helps to reduce the incidence of postoperative neurologic complications. Studies have demonstrated that neurocognitive outcomes in patients who underwent standard CABG did not differ from those in a comparable control group without surgery, at both 1 and 3 years suggesting that neurocognitive decline is not due to the surgical procedure or CPB.[83-85] On-pump versus off-pump procedures also do not seem to make a difference. The Best Bypass Surgery trial compared neurocognitive outcomes between off-pump patients and those patients who underwent on-pump CABG with CPB. They concluded that "in elderly high-risk patients, no significant difference was found in the incidence of cognitive dysfunction 3 months after either off-pump or on pump CABG."[86]

▶ ENDOCRINE

Hyperglycemia in hospitalized patients has been shown to increase both morbidity and mortality, even in nondiabetic patients.[87] Several trials have shown the benefits of intensive insulin therapy in critically ill patients, and particularly in patients undergoing cardiac surgery.[88] A trial by van den Berghe et al showed significant decreases in mortality, bloodstream infections, acute renal failure, blood transfusions, and critical care polyneuropathy in patients managed with strict glucose control.[89] Many centers have since tried to achieve strict glycemic control with a goal of blood glucose levels between 80 and 110 mg/dL.

The benefits of intensive glucose control in critically ill patients have recently come into question. Some trials have shown no benefit to intensive glucose control[90] as well as an increase in the incidence of hypoglycemia.[90,91] The Normoglycemia in Intensive Care Evaluation—Survival Using Glucose Algorithm Regulation (NICE-SUGAR) trial showed that intensive glucose control in critically ill adult patients actually increased the risk for death by 10%.[92] The investigators reported that intensive glucose control increased the absolute risk of death at 90 days by 2.6 percentage points, and that the difference in mortality was significant even after adjusting for potential confounders. Hypoglycemia was "significantly more common" in the intensive control group. The authors concluded that intensive glucose control increased mortality among adults in the ICU and that a blood glucose target of 180 mg/dL or less resulted in lower mortality than did a target of 81–108 mg/dL.

Intensively lowering blood glucose to a target of 81–108 mg/dL does not benefit critically ill patients and may well increase their risk of dying.

The risks of intensive insulin therapy may outweigh the benefits. Intensive glucose control involves insulin infusions that require close monitoring. This may also increase expenditures as well as the workload for the intensive care unit staff. At this time, a reasonable approach to hyperglycemia should have the goals of maintaining blood glucose levels as close to normal as possible with minimal fluctuations, hypoglycemia, or hypokalemia.

REFERENCES

1. Cohn L, Edmunds LH. *Cardiac Surgery in the Adult.* 2nd ed. New York: McGraw-Hill; 2003:xxiv, 1573 pp.

2. St. Andre AC, DelRossi A. Hemodynamic management of patients in the first 24 hours after cardiac surgery. *Crit Care Med.* 2005;33(9):2082–2093.

3. London MJ, Moritz T, Henderson W, et al. Standard versus fiberoptic pulmonary artery catheterization for cardiac surgery in the Department of Veterans Affairs: a prospective, observational, multicenter analysis. *Anesthesiology.* 2002;96(4):860–870.

4. Polonen P, et al. A prospective, randomized study of goal-oriented hemodynamic therapy in cardiac surgical patients. *Anesth Analg.* 2000;90(5):1052–1059.

5. Boyd O, Grounds RM, Bennett ED. A randomized clinical trial of the effect of deliberate perioperative increase of oxygen delivery on mortality in high-risk surgical patients. *JAMA.* 1993;270(22):2699–2707.

6. Yu M, et al. Effect of maximizing oxygen delivery on morbidity and mortality rates in critically ill patients: a prospective, randomized, controlled study. *Crit Care Med.* 1993;21(6):830–838.

7. Gattinoni L, et al. A trial of goal-oriented hemodynamic therapy in critically ill patients. SvO_2 Collaborative Group. *N Engl J Med.* 1995;333(16):1025–1032.

8. Ernest D, Belzberg AS, Dodek PM. Distribution of normal saline and 5% albumin infusions in septic patients. *Crit Care Med.* 1999;27(1):46–50.

9. Gallagher JD, et al. Effects of colloid or crystalloid administration on pulmonary extravascular water in the postoperative period after coronary artery bypass grafting. *Anesth Analg.* 1985;64(8):753–758.

10. Fremes SE, et al. Effects of postoperative hypertension and its treatment. *J Thorac Cardiovasc Surg.* 1983;86(1):47–56.

11. Feneck RO, et al. Comparison of the hemodynamic effects of milrinone with dobutamine in patients after cardiac surgery. *J Cardiothorac Vasc Anesth.* 2001;15(3):306–315.

12. Kantrowitz A, et al. Initial clinical experience with intraaortic balloon pumping in cardiogenic shock. *JAMA.* 1968;203(2):113–118.

13. Samuels LE, et al. Pharmacological criteria for ventricular assist device insertion following postcardiotomy shock: experience with the Abiomed BVS system. *J Card Surg.* 1999;14(4):288–293.

14. Maisel WH, Rawn JD, Stevenson WG. Atrial fibrillation after cardiac surgery. *Ann Intern Med.* 2001;135(12):1061–1073.

15. Rho RW. The management of atrial fibrillation after cardiac surgery. *Heart.* 2009;95(5):422–429.

16. Hein OV, et al. Three-year survival after four major post-cardiac operative complications. *Crit Care Med.* 2006;34(11):2729–2737.

17. Baggish AL, Sabatine MS. Clopidogrel use in coronary artery disease. *Expert Rev Cardiovasc Ther.* 2006;4(1):7–15.

18. Gill R, et al. Safety and efficacy of recombinant activated factor VII: a randomized placebo-controlled trial in the setting of bleeding after cardiac surgery. *Circulation.* 2009;120(1):21–27.

19. Higgins TL. Safety issues regarding early extubation after coronary artery bypass surgery. *J Cardiothorac Vasc Anesth.* 1995;9(5 suppl 1):24–29.

20. Akhtar MI, Hamid M. Success and failure of fast track extubation in cardiac surgery patients of tertiary care hospital: one year audit. *J Pak Med Assoc.* 2009;59(3):154–156.

21. Wong DT, et al. Risk factors of delayed extubation, prolonged length of stay in the intensive care unit, and mortality in patients undergoing coronary artery bypass graft with fast-track cardiac anesthesia: a new cardiac risk score. *Anesthesiology.* 1999;91(4):936–944.

22. Puntillo K, Weiss SJ. Pain: its mediators and associated morbidity in critically ill cardiovascular surgical patients. *Nurs Res.* 1994;43(1):31–36.

23. Gust R, et al. Effect of patient-controlled analgesia on pulmonary complications after coronary artery bypass grafting. *Crit Care Med.* 1999;27(10):2218–2223.

24. Jensen L, Yang L. Risk factors for postoperative pulmonary complications in coronary artery bypass graft surgery patients. *Eur J Cardiovasc Nurs.* 2007;6(3):241–246.

25. Wynne R, Botti M. Postoperative pulmonary dysfunction in adults after cardiac surgery with cardiopulmonary bypass: clinical significance and implications for practice. *Am J Crit Care.* 2004;13(5):384–393.

26. Maggart M, Stewart S. The mechanisms and management of noncardiogenic pulmonary edema following cardiopulmonary bypass. *Ann Thorac Surg.* 1987;43(2):231–236.

27. Boyd JE, Bewman JH, Brigham KL. Permeability pulmonary edema. Diagnosis and management. *Arch Intern Med.* 1984;144(1):143–147.

28. Tonz M, et al. Acute lung injury during cardiopulmonary bypass. Are the neutrophils responsible? *Chest.* 1995;108(6):1551–1556.

29. Chenoweth DE, et al. Complement activation during cardiopulmonary bypass: evidence for generation of C3a and C5a anaphylatoxins. *N Engl J Med.* 1981;304(9):497–503.

30. Royston D, et al. Increased production of peroxidation products associated with cardiac operations. Evidence for free radical generation. *J Thorac Cardiovasc Surg.* 1986;91(5):759–766.

31. Craddock PR, et al. Complement and leukocyte-mediated pulmonary dysfunction in hemodialysis. *N Engl J Med.* 1977;296(14):769–774.

32. Hammerschmidt DE, et al. Complement activation and neutropenia occurring during cardiopulmonary bypass. *J Thorac Cardiovasc Surg.* 1981;81(3):370–377.

33. Allardyce DB, Yoshida SH, Ashmore PG. The importance of microembolism in the pathogenesis of organ dysfunction caused by prolonged use of the pump oxygenator. *J Thorac Cardiovasc Surg.* 1966;52(5):706–715.

34. Heidecker J, Sahn SA. The spectrum of pleural effusions after coronary artery bypass grafting surgery. *Clin Chest Med.* 2006;27(2):267–283.

35. Peng MJ, et al. Postoperative pleural changes after coronary revascularization. Comparison between saphenous vein and internal mammary artery grafting. *Chest.* 1992;101(2):327–330.

36. Gale GD, et al. Pulmonary atelectasis and other respiratory complications after cardiopulmonary bypass and investigation of aetiological factors. *Can Anaesth Soc J.* 1979;26(1):15–21.

37. Daganou M, et al. Respiratory complications after coronary artery bypass surgery with unilateral or bilateral internal mammary artery grafting. *Chest.* 1998;113(5): 1285–1289.

38. Hurlbut D, et al. Pleuropulmonary morbidity: internal thoracic artery versus saphenous vein graft. Ann Thorac Surg. 1990;50(6):959–964.

39. Rolla G, et al. Effect of pleurotomy on pulmonary function after coronary artery bypass grafting with internal mammary artery. *Respir Med.* 1994;88(6):417–420.

40. Labidi M, et al. Pleural effusions following cardiac surgery. Prevalence, risk factors, and clinical features. *Chest.* 2009;136:1604–1611.

41. Peng MC, et al. Prevalence of symptomatic large pleural effusions first diagnosed more than 30 days after coronary artery bypass graft surgery. *Respirology.* 2007;12(1): 122–126.

42. Hashim SW, et al. Noncardiogenic pulmonary edema after cardiopulmonary bypass. An anaphylactic reaction to fresh frozen plasma. *Am J Surg.* 1984;147(4):560–564.

43. Brooks JC. Noncardiogenic pulmonary edema immediately following rapid protamine administration. *Ann Pharmacother.* 1999;33(9):927–930.

44. Frost L, et al. Prognosis and risk factors in acute, dialysis-requiring renal failure after open-heart surgery. *Scand J Thorac Cardiovasc Surg.* 1991;25(3):161–166.

45. MaWhinney S, et al. Identification of risk factors for increased cost, charges, and length of stay for cardiac patients. *Ann Thorac Surg.* 2000;70(3):702–710.

46. Suen WS, et al. Risk factors for development of acute renal failure (ARF) requiring dialysis in patients undergoing cardiac surgery. *Angiology.* 1998;49(10):789–800.

47. Lassnigg A, et al. Minimal changes of serum creatinine predict prognosis in patients after cardiothoracic surgery: a prospective cohort study. *J Am Soc Nephrol.* 2004;15(6):1597–1605.

48. Swaminathan M, et al. Trends in acute renal failure associated with coronary artery bypass graft surgery in the United States. *Crit Care Med.* 2007;35(10):2286–2291.

49. Feindt PR, et al. Effects of high-dose aprotinin on renal function in aortocoronary bypass grafting. *Ann Thorac Surg.* 1995;60(4):1076–1080.

50. Kuitunen A, et al. Acute renal failure after cardiac surgery: evaluation of the RIFLE classification. *Ann Thorac Surg.* 2006;81(2):542–546.

51. Bellomo R, et al. Acute renal failure—definition, outcome measures, animal models, fluid therapy and information technology needs: the Second International Consensus Conference of the Acute Dialysis Quality Initiative (ADQI) Group. *Crit Care.* 2004;8(4):R204–R212.

52. Hoste EA, et al. RIFLE criteria for acute kidney injury are associated with hospital mortality in critically ill patients: a cohort analysis. *Crit Care.* 2006;10(3):R73.

53. Bove T, et al. Renoprotective action of fenoldopam in high-risk patients undergoing cardiac surgery: a prospective, double-blind, randomized clinical trial. *Circulation.* 2005;111(24):3230–3235.

54. Sisillo E, et al. *N*-Acetylcysteine for prevention of acute renal failure in patients with chronic renal insufficiency undergoing cardiac surgery: a prospective, randomized, clinical trial. *Crit Care Med.* 2008;36(1):81–86.

55. Barr LF, Kolodner K. *N*-Acetylcysteine and fenoldopam protect the renal function of patients with chronic renal insufficiency undergoing cardiac surgery. *Crit Care Med.* 2008;36(5):1427–1435.

56. Ryckwaert F, et al. Incidence, risk factors, and prognosis of a moderate increase in plasma creatinine early after cardiac surgery. *Crit Care Med.* 2002;30(7):1495–1498.

57. Callahan M, et al. Economic consequences of renal dysfunction among cardiopulmonary bypass surgery patients: a hospital-based perspective. *Value Health.* 2003;6(2):137–143.

58. Rocktaeschel J, et al. Acid–base status of critically ill patients with acute renal failure: analysis based on Stewart–Figge methodology. *Crit Care.* 2003;7(4):R60.

59. Kellum JA, Song M, Li J. Lactic and hydrochloric acids induce different patterns of inflammatory response in LPS-stimulated RAW 264.7 cells. *Am J Physiol Regul Integr Comp Physiol.* 2004;286(4):R686–R692.

60. Thakar CV, et al. Renal dysfunction and serious infections after open-heart surgery. *Kidney Int.* 2003;64(1): 239–246.

61. Kramer AA, et al. Renal ischemia/reperfusion leads to macrophage-mediated increase in pulmonary vascular permeability. *Kidney Int.* 1999;55(6):2362–2367.

62. Donnahoo KK, et al. Review article: the role of tumor necrosis factor in renal ischemia–reperfusion injury. *J Urol.* 1999;162(1):196–203.

63. Egleston CV, et al. Gastrointestinal complications after cardiac surgery. *Ann R Coll Surg Engl.* 1993;75(1):52–56.

64. Mangi AA, et al. Gastrointestinal complications in patients undergoing heart operation: an analysis of 8709 consecutive cardiac surgical patients. *Ann Surg.* 2005;241(6):895–901. Discussion 901–904.

65. Ohri SK, et al. Intraabdominal complications after cardiopulmonary bypass. *Ann Thorac Surg.* 1991;52(4): 826–831.

66. Krasna MJ, et al. Gastrointestinal complications after cardiac surgery. *Surgery.* 1988;104(4):773–780.

67. Leitman IM, et al. Intra-abdominal complications of cardiopulmonary bypass operations. *Surg Gynecol Obstet.* 1987;165(3):251–254.

68. Lazar HL, et al. Gastrointestinal complications following cardiac surgery. *Cardiovasc Surg.* 1995;3(3):341–344.

69. Zacharias A, et al. Predictors of gastrointestinal complications in cardiac surgery. *Tex Heart Inst J.* 2000;27(2):93–99.

70. Yilmaz AT, et al. Gastrointestinal complications after cardiac surgery. *Eur J Cardiothorac Surg.* 1996;10(9):763–767.

71. Johnston G, et al. Changing perspective on gastrointestinal complications in patients undergoing cardiac surgery. *Am J Surg.* 1992;163(5):525–529.

72. Christenson JT, et al. Postoperative visceral hypotension the common cause for gastrointestinal complications after cardiac surgery. *Thorac Cardiovasc Surg.* 1994;42(3):152–157.

73. Baue AE. The role of the gut in the development of multiple organ dysfunction in cardiothoracic patients. *Ann Thorac Surg.* 1993;55(4):822–829.

74. Berger MM, et al. Intestinal absorption in patients after cardiac surgery. *Crit Care Med.* 2000;28(7):2217–2223.

75. Arrowsmith JE, Grocott HP, Newman MF. Neurologic risk assessment, monitoring and outcome in cardiac surgery. *J Cardiothorac Vasc Anesth.* 1999;13(6):736–743.

76. Svensson LG, Nadolny EM, Kimmel WA. Multimodal protocol influence on stroke and neurocognitive deficit prevention after ascending/arch aortic operations. *Ann Thorac Surg.* 2002;74(6):2040–2046.

77. Hogue CW Jr, et al. Sex differences in neurological outcomes and mortality after cardiac surgery: a Society of Thoracic Surgery National Database report. *Circulation.* 2001;103(17):2133–2137.

78. Roach GW, et al. Adverse cerebral outcomes after coronary bypass surgery. Multicenter study of Perioperative Ischemia Research Group and the Ischemia Research and Education Foundation Investigators. *N Engl J Med.* 1996;335(25):1857–1863.

79. Grega MA, Borowicz LM, Baumgartner WA. Impact of single clamp versus double clamp technique on neurologic outcome. *Ann Thorac Surg.* 2003;75(5):1387–1391.

80. Hammon JW, et al. Single crossclamp improves 6-month cognitive outcome in high-risk coronary bypass patients: the effect of reduced aortic manipulation. *J Thorac Cardiovasc Surg.* 2006;131(1):114–121.

81. Kolkka R, Hilberman M. Neurologic dysfunction following cardiac operation with low-flow, low-pressure cardiopulmonary bypass. *J Thorac Cardiovasc Surg.* 1980;79(3):432–437.

82. Cohn LH, Edmunds LH. *Cardiac Surgery in the Adult.* 3rd ed. New York: McGraw-Hill Medical; 2008:xx, 1704 pp.

83. Boeken U, et al. Neurological complications after cardiac surgery: risk factors and correlation to the surgical procedure. *Thorac Cardiovasc Surg.* 2005;53(1):33–36.

84. Selnes OA, et al. Cognitive changes with coronary artery disease: a prospective study of coronary artery bypass graft patients and nonsurgical controls. *Ann Thorac Surg.* 2003;75(5):1377–1384. Discussion 1384–1386.

85. Selnes OA, et al. Cognitive outcomes three years after coronary artery bypass surgery: a comparison of on-pump coronary artery bypass graft surgery and nonsurgical controls. *Ann Thorac Surg.* 2005;79(4):1201–1209.

86. Jensen BO, et al. Cognitive outcomes in elderly high-risk patients after off-pump versus conventional coronary artery bypass grafting: a randomized trial. *Circulation.* 2006;113(24):2790–2795.

87. Grey NJ, Perdrizet GA. Reduction of nosocomial infections in the surgical intensive-care unit by strict glycemic control. *Endocr Pract.* 2004;10 (suppl 2):46–52.

88. Goldberg PA, et al. Improving glycemic control in the cardiothoracic intensive care unit: clinical experience in two hospital settings. *J Cardiothorac Vasc Anesth.* 2004;18(6):690–697.

89. van den Berghe G, et al. Intensive insulin therapy in the critically ill patients. *N Engl J Med.* 2001;345(19):1359–1367.

90. Arabi YM, et al. Intensive versus conventional insulin therapy: a randomized controlled trial in medical and surgical critically ill patients. *Crit Care Med.* 2008;36(12):3190–3197.

91. Arabi YM, Tamim HM, Rishu AH. Hypoglycemia with intensive insulin therapy in critically ill patients: predisposing factors and association with mortality. *Crit Care Med.* 2009;37(9):2536–2544.

92. Finfer S, et al. Intensive versus conventional glucose control in critically ill patients. *N Engl J Med.* 2009;360(13):1283–1297.

CHAPTER 18

Pericardial Diseases

Joseph R. Shiber

▶ INTRODUCTION

In the 16th century, Vesalius first described the anatomy of the pericardium. In 1674, John Mayow gave the earliest account of constrictive pericarditis: "the heart was nearly covered by cartilage, adherent to its interior so that blood could scarcely enter." Richard Lower in 1689 accurately described tamponade: "a profuse effusion oppresses and inundates the heart. The walls of the heart are so compressed by the fluid circling everywhere, so that the heart cannot dilate sufficiently to receive the blood, then the pulse becomes exceedingly small, thence succeed syncope and death itself." Franz Schuh did the first successful pericadiocentesis in 1840; Churchill performed the first pericardiectomy in the United States in 1929. Claude Beck described his triad of findings in tamponade in 1935. In 1954, Edler demonstrated a pericardial effusion by ultrasound, and in 1971 Spodick described the EKG findings associated with pericarditis.[1,2]

▶ ANATOMY AND FUNCTION

The pericardial sac is formed by the visceral and parietal pericardium, which are continuous with one another at the attachment of the great vessels (Figure 18-1). The visceral component is a single mesothelial cell layer with a submesothelium that is invested directly against the myocardium. The visceral pericardium forms the pericardial fluid, an ultrafiltrate of the plasma, normally 20–50 cm^3, which is then drained via the parietal pericardium to the thoracic duct. The parietal component is approximately 1 mm thick and formed of three layers: (1) *serosa* of mesothelium; (2) *fibrosa* of dense, wavy collagen fibers and interspersed elastic fibers, also containing fibroblasts, mast cells, nerves, blood vessels, and lymphatics; (3) *epipericardium* of collagen, elastin, and adipose. It is this third layer that forms the ligaments inferiorly to the diaphragm, superiorly to the deep cervical fascia, anteriorly to the manubrium and sternum, and posteriorly to the vertebral column.[3–5]

Although there are many recognized functions of the pericardium, its removal or congenital absence is well tolerated except for partial defects that can lead to cardiac herniation. The tensile strength of the pericardium is greater than the myocardium, and it retracts when incised, suggesting that it is under tension. The pericardium maintains the heart in proper position, acts as a barrier to infection, and prevents overdilation of the chambers in response to hypervolemia. It is devoid of impulse-generating capacity, so it does not produce any EKG deflections.[5]

Intrapericardial pressure approximates pleural pressure, varying with respiration to aid in venous return and atrial filling. The tension of the pericardium evenly distributes the pericardial fluid against the heart, allowing the pericardial fluid to decrease friction, disperse gravitational and inertial forces around the heart, and distribute hydrostatic forces, giving uniform stretch of myofibrils to allow *Frank–Starling* mechanics to operate over a range of pressures.

The pericardium, circumferential myocardial fibers, and a compliant septum, together, allow for ventricular interdependence. This mechanism mostly affects diastolic interactions and balances output from both ventricles over several cycles based on the volume–pressure relationship. As the pressure in one chamber increases (due to volume filling), the compliance of the other ventricle decreases (restricting filling). The increase in right heart filling with inspiration (negative intrapericardial pressure and increased venous return, with increased pulmonary vascular capacity) is evidenced by increased tricuspid and pulmonic valve flow velocities, and simultaneous decreased left heart filling and mitral and aortic valve flow

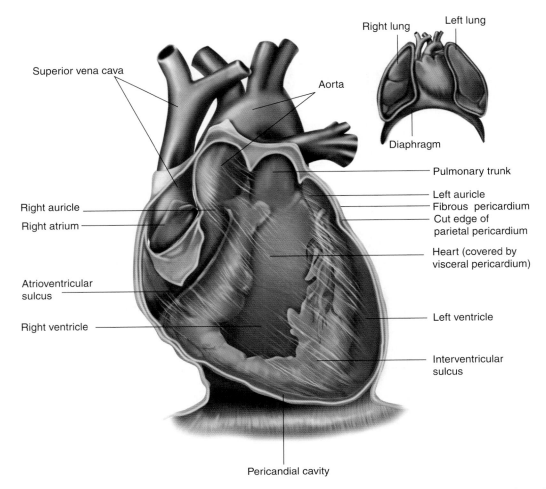

Figure 18-1. Image of the heart demonstrating the layers of pericardium making up the pericardial cavity, and covering the roots of the great vessels. (Reproduced with permission from David Shier, et al. *Hole's Human Anatomy and Physiology.* 7th ed. Copyright © 1996 TM Higher Education Group Inc. Figure 15-4.)

velocities. The opposite dynamics occur with expiration, and these volume–pressure effects are exaggerated by hypervolemia and minimized by hypovolemia.[3–5]

► PATHOPHYSIOLOGY

Pericardial diseases include pericarditis, constriction, and congenital or traumatic pericardial lesions. Although the etiologies for pericarditis are numerous (Table 18-1), the initiating factors for inflammation and effusion are shared and any of these factors, if chronic, can eventually cause pericardial constriction.[4,6]

There are three stages to pericardial inflammation: (1) vasodilation leading to transudation of a protein-poor, cell-free fluid; (2) increased vascular permeability allowing protein (fibrin) to leak; and (3) inflammatory cell migration. The presenting complaint

► **TABLE 18-1. COMMON CATEGORIES OF PERICARDIAL DISEASE**

Idiopathic
Infectious
Viral, bacterial, mycobacterial, fungal
Autoreactive
Lupus, rheumatoid arthritis, scleroderma, vasculitis, post-MI, drug induced
Neoplastic
Lung, breast, lymphoma, melanoma, mesothelioma
Metabolic
Renal failure, hemodialysis, myxedema
Traumatic
Cardiac injury (penetrating or blunt), iatrogenic (catheterization, pacer lead, venous line), radiation
Contiguous disease
Aortic dissection, ventricular aneurysm/rupture, pulmonary/ pleural disease

is usually substernal chest pain, radiating to the left scapular ridge, pleuritic, and positional (often relieved leaning forward). As an effusion develops, symptoms from compression of adjacent structures (trachea, esophagus, phrenic nerve, and recurrent laryngeal nerve) include dyspnea, cough, dysphagia, singultus, and dysphonia.[3,5,6]

Patients with pericarditis have systemic evidence of inflammation on blood testing, including a leukocytosis and elevated C-reactive protein level and erythrocyte sedimentation rate. Troponin levels are elevated in 35–50% of pericarditis cases (creatine kinase-MB fraction less often) due to epicardial inflammation, and typically return to baseline within 1–2 weeks. The magnitude of the troponin rise appears to correlate with the height of the ST-segment elevation but does not necessarily predict an adverse outcome. Serum troponin levels remaining elevated for more than 2 weeks suggest an associated myocarditis, which does predict a worse prognosis.[6,7] The initial workup and management for any patient with presumed pericarditis should be: (1) an evaluation for possible underlying or causative conditions; (2) echocardiography to determine if there is an effusion (and, if so, its size), tamponade, or other structural abnormalities; (3) alleviation of symptoms with anti-inflammatory medications; and (4) treatment for a specific condition if identified.[4,5,7]

INFECTIOUS PERICARDITIS

Viral agents are the most common cause of pericarditis, as documented by rising antibody titers, but also represent the majority of cases thought to be idiopathic (Table 18-2). Enteroviridae (Coxsackie B), Adenoviridae, Echoviridae, and Retroviridae are usually responsible, and pericardial involvement typically occurs 1–3 weeks following a URI or GI infection, although rarely pericarditis can occur with the primary infection. Viral pericarditis is typically "dry"—without a pericardial effusion—with a rub present, or may develop a small effusion that is asymptomatic and resolves spontaneously.[5,7,8] Although atrial arrhythmias can be seen, mostly with constrictive disease, patients with uncomplicated pericarditis predominantly remain in sinus rhythm and have no significant arrhythmias. When arrhythmias occur, underlying conductive disease or an associated myocarditis is usually responsible and should be sought. The classic example is Lyme pericarditis, which is really a pancarditis that can cause a bundle branch or A-V nodal block.[3,9]

Bacterial

In the pre-antibiotic era, purulent pericarditis resulted in a nearly 100% mortality rate. Unfortunately today it

▶ **TABLE 18-2. MICROBIOLOGY OF INFECTIOUS PERICARDITIS**

Viral
  HIV
  Coxsackievirus A and B
Epstein–Barr virus
  Echovirus
  Influenza
  Paramyxovirus (mumps)
  Adenovirus
  Varicella
Bacterial
  Staphylococcus
  Streptococcus
  Pneumococcus
  Gram-negative bacilli
  Meningococcus
  Gonococcus
  Haemophilus influenzae
  Bordetella pertussis
  Francisella tularensis
  Salmonella
  Campylobacter
  Listeria
  Legionella
  Mycoplasma
  Nocardia
  Actinomyces
Anaerobic
  Clostridium
  Peptostreptococcus
Rickettsial
  Typhus
  Q fever
Fungal
  Histoplasma
  Candida
  Coccidioides
  Blastomyces
  Aspergillus
Protozoal
  Toxoplasma gondii
  Entamoeba
  Trypanosoma cruzi
Parasitic
  Trichinella
  Filarioidea (microfilaria)
  Echinococcus
Mycobacterial
  Tuberculosis
  Avium-intracellulare complex

still carries a high mortality rate (30–50%) since affected patients typically have severe underlying medical disease. Bacterial pericarditis is not a primary infection but is almost exclusively a complication from an underlying one.[10,11] In one study, 13% of the cases of purulent pericarditis (confirmed by pericardial fluid analysis or at autopsy) were found in patients admitted to the ICU with a diagnosis of sepsis.[12] Risk factors include advanced age, diabetes mellitus, untreated infection (pneumonia), extensive burns, an immunosuppressed state, and a preexisting pericardial effusion (renal failure, CHF). The physician must maintain a high index of suspicion in patients with a septic presentation (fever and hypotension) to avoid missing this diagnosis since the only confirmatory test is sampling a known effusion.

The presentation is always acute, with hectic fevers and frank rigors. Tachycardia is invariably present; other findings vary, based on the underlying etiology. An evanescent three-component pericardial rub (early diastole, late diastole, and systole) is found in about one third of cases. Tamponade can develop rapidly, as an effusion of 500 cm^3 can accumulate rapidly over several days. It is important to note that after cardiac surgery, the pericardium is not typically closed, so a suppurative infection will not result in tamponade, making the diagnosis even more difficult in these patients.[10,11]

Previously, the most likely manner a patient developed suppurative pericarditis was through pneumonia with empyema development, so the most common organism was *Streptococcus pneumoniae*. The accepted etiologies of suppurative pericarditis include seeding from circulating bacteremia, contiguous intrathoracic source (empyema), penetrating trauma, surgical wounds (sternal osteomyelitis), intracardiac source, esophageal rupture with fistula formation, retropharyngeal abscess, and hepatic/subdiaphragmatic abscess. One study by Rubin demonstrated the risk of infectious endocarditis (I.E.) leading to pericardial disease; at autopsy, 13% of patients with I.E. had suppurative pericarditis, and 20% had a myocardial abscess (this figure increased to 36% if the microbe was *Staphylococcus aureus*).[10,13]

The current microbiology of pericardial infections has changed with the advent of antibiotics, as well as with the development of thoracic and cardiac surgery. Several recent studies note the trend toward more diverse microbes involved, and an important finding of anaerobes as a common cause. Since anaerobes are the leading flora of the oral cavity, where they outnumber aerobes 100:1, it reasons they would be the infectious agents if the source were esophageal, pharyngeal, GI, or pulmonic (aspiration). One large retrospective study by Brook and Frazier found primary anaerobic infections in 40% of bacterial pericarditis cases and mixed (aerobic/anaerobic) in 13%, but there were no clinical or diagnostic differences found between theses types of infections.[13,14]

Optimum therapy should include 4 weeks of a bactericidal drug, with the microbe's sensitivity known. Antibiotics penetrate well into the pericardial sac so that intrapericardial instillation is not necessary. Surgical pericardial drainage is also recommended, not only to eradicate gross pus but also to prevent constriction from occurring (a late complication with a variable time course); there has been recent evidence that supports the use of video-assisted thoracoscopic surgery (V.A.T.S.) in place of open thoracotomy.[15] If the patient were unable to tolerate these procedures, intrapericardial catheter placement would be advised. This is an old therapy that has had resurgence with multiple recent studies demonstrating its effectiveness and safety. Streptokinase and streptodornase can be instilled and the catheter clamped, and then flushed out and the procedure repeated. These substances aid in the drainage of clotted blood and thickened nucleoproteins (pus) and significantly improve resolution of loculated effusions. This procedure does not affect systemic coagulation studies and has no increased bleeding events associated, but does prevent development of constrictive disease.[16,17]

Fungal

Although there are many fungi known to cause purulent pericarditis, *Histoplasmosis* and *Candida* are the most common. These organisms usually affect immunosuppressed patients (leukemia, organ transplant, AIDS, long hospital stay on multiple antibiotics), but there are differences between these two organisms.

Histoplasmosis capsulatum spores are found in the soil of the Ohio and Mississippi river valleys, and are inhaled causing a pneumonitis. From there, hematogenous spread occurs to the mediastinal nodes and reticuloendothelial system until cellular immunity develops. In immunocompetent individuals, this process takes about 10–14 days and has a self-limited course. But in an immunosuppressed individual, pericardial disease can occur from the primary infection or at a later time from reactivation; in the latter case, the source is usually adjacent mediastinal nodes, although rarely it is disseminated disease. Ten percent of patients clinically infected will develop pericardial disease.[3,4,18]

Candida albicans and *tropicalis* are common host flora that can infect even immunocompetent individuals under certain circumstances. Intravenous drug abuse, indwelling venous catheters (particularly for parenteral nutrition with lipids), thoracic surgery, and prosthetic heart valves are risk factors for pericarditis from these entities. The route is typically hematogenous, intracardiac, or contiguous spread from a surgical site. The presentation for fungal infections is similar to bacterial, but the course is slightly slower in terms of effusion accumulation and pericardial thickening and scarring.

Therapy is similar to that of bacterial pericarditis, with systemic antifungal therapy and open drainage/pericardial resection.[3,4,19]

Tuberculous

Still the leading cause of chronic pericardial disease and constriction worldwide, tuberculosis incidence in the United States fell by 5% per year until 1985 and the increased spread of HIV. TB is now estimated to be the cause of 2–4% of all admitted pericarditis patients and 5–6% of cases with pericardial constriction. The reported incidence of pericardial involvement among patients with pulmonary tuberculosis ranges from 1% to 8%; evidence of active pulmonary disease at the time is rare, however, with only 11–50% of patients with pericarditis having positive sputum cultures.[13,20] Pericardial involvement can occur with a primary infection or reactivation of latent infection. The most common pathway is retrograde extension via lymphatics from peribronchial and mediastinal nodes; other recognized pathways include hematogenous spread from distant foci (genitourinary or skeletal) and direct extension from a contiguous source (lymph nodes, lung, pleura, spine).

Four pathologic stages have been identified: (1) *fibrinous*—fibrin deposition with many PMNs, abundant organisms, and loose granuloma formation; (2) *effusive*—serosanguineous effusion accumulation with lymphocytes and monocytes predominating; (3) *absorptive*—effusion diminishes, mycobacterium cells are now scarce, and dense caseating granulomas thicken the pericardium; (4) *constrictive*—granulomas replaced by fibrous tissue that begins to contract. Calcification may occur at any pathologic stage.[3,20,21]

Unlike bacterial pericarditis, these patients have a subacute/chronic course. The onset is insidious, with nonspecific features only, until late in the course. Diagnosis can be made by stain or culture of pericardial fluid, although this is only positive in 15% of patients clinically diagnosed with tubercular disease. These figures can be improved by doing ELISA and PCR assays on the fluid. Pericardial biopsy is thought to have the highest diagnostic yield, although still not 100%, and is dependent on the stage of disease and amount of tissue obtained. PPD testing is not helpful since patients may be anergic (low sensitivity), or may be reactive but have no pericardial involvement (low specificity). Treatment consists of four-drug therapy for at least 1 month, followed by two-drug therapy for 1–2 years. Careful follow-up is needed to evaluate for signs of constriction, and some recommend pericardiectomy as initial therapy due to the high percentage (30–50%) of appropriately treated patients that still develop constriction by 4 months. Steroids should also be given in the first month; they have been shown to significantly decrease mortality and improve patient symptoms, although they have little effect on pericardial constriction.[2,20,21]

HIV Infection

Significant cardiac morbidity due to HIV disease is estimated at 6–7%, with pericardial effusion and myocarditis the most common abnormalities. At autopsy, 40% of patients have large effusions, and several studies have found that an effusion is an independent risk factor (separate from CD4 count) for decreased survival. In a study of HIV patients, 25% had an effusion by echocardiography, of which 20% were large. The majority were asymptomatic, and at follow-up 42% of the effusions had spontaneously resolved. Still, in a series of patients requiring intervention for tamponade, the most common underlying disorders were malignancy and HIV.[22]

Pericardial disease can result from opportunistic infections, medical treatment of HIV, and the HIV itself. In these immunocompromised patients, one must consider not only viral and bacterial pathogens but also fungal, mycobacterial, and parasitic infections,[23,24] as well as noninfectious causes such as lymphoma and Kaposi's sarcoma. The risk factors for death associated with moderate–severe pericardial effusion are tuberculosis (OR 47.2), heart failure (OR 30.3), other pulmonary infection (OR 15.0), and Kaposi's sarcoma (OR 8.6). Based on this information, it would be prudent for an HIV patient symptomatic with a persistent pericardial effusion to be empirically treated for tuberculosis until that diagnosis can be excluded.[23]

Renal Failure

Uremic pericarditis occurs in 6–10% of patients with advanced renal disease before or shortly after starting dialysis and correlates with the degree of azotemia; it is unusual to occur with a BUN <60 mg/dL. Treatment is initiation or intensification of dialysis with avoidance of heparin because of concern for a hemorrhagic effusion. Dialysis-associated pericarditis occurs in 13% of patients receiving hemodialysis and, occasionally, peritoneal dialysis; the etiology and treatment are unclear.[3,6]

Myocardial Infarction

Pericarditis can occur early in the first few days post-MI due to transmural infarction that causes inflammation of the local pericardium. It is a marker of larger infarct size, but it is not associated with increased morbidity or mortality. The incidence has decreased significantly since reperfusion therapies have become the standard of care for MI.[25] Treatment is full-dose aspirin while avoiding other NSAIDs or steroids that prevent scar formation and may increase the incidence of myocardial rupture. Delayed pericarditis, also known as Dressler's syndrome, is due to a diffuse immunopathologic process involving the entire pericardium and is the same etiology of postpericardiotomy syndrome. It is best treated with ibuprofen or colchicine.[5,25,26]

Autoreactive

Pericarditis is associated with numerous autoimmune and collagen-vascular diseases. It is necessary to first evaluate for uremic, infectious, or neoplastic causes. But once these are ruled out, intensifying treatment of the underlying conditions and symptomatic analgesics are helpful. Intrapericardial steroids offer extended effectiveness without the systemic adverse effects.[27,28]

Neoplastic

Mesothelioma is the most common primary pericardial malignancy, but metastatic cancers (lung, breast, lymphoma, melanoma) are 40 times more likely to cause pericardial disease. Twenty percent of large effusions without an obvious cause have been found to be due to an undiagnosed malignancy. Neoplastic effusions are typically exudative, fibrinous, and hemorrhagic, and often require open surgical drainage. Intrapericardial chemotherapy and sclerosing agents are an option if tamponade does not exist.[3,29]

TRAUMATIC

Hemopericardium may occur secondary to penetrating or blunt chest trauma; pericardial rupture may occur following blunt injuries causing cardiac herniation that presents as tamponade. Seventeen to 45% of type A aortic dissections are complicated by hemopericardium. In these cases, unless the patient is in extremis due to tamponade, pericardiocentesis is contraindicated due to potentially extending the dissection.[30] Invasive procedures, such as endomyocardial biopsy, electrophysiology (EP) studies, permanent pacemaker insertion, and coronary angiography, can cause unintended cardiac or vascular perforation producing tamponade. EP procedures have a 1–6% risk of cardiac perforation with the risk increased by higher energy use and ablations for atrial fibrillation. Coronary perforation occurs in 0.1–0.6% of all PCI resulting in 42% mortality; its risk is increased by atheroablative procedures. The immediate treatment is to seal the coronary injury and reverse all anticoagulation while monitoring closely for tamponade.[4,30]

Tamponade

Pericardial tamponade is due to pericardial pressure exceeding cardiac chamber diastolic pressure,

▶ **TABLE 18-3. COMMON RISK FACTORS FOR PERICARDIAL TAMPONADE**

History of pericarditis
Blunt or penetrating chest trauma
Cardiac surgery
Cardiac catheterization (PCI or EP study)
Known or suspected intrathoracic neoplasm
Known or suspected aortic dissection
Renal failure or hemodialysis

therefore not allowing filling to occur. While there are several risk factors for developing pericardial tamponade (Table 18-3), only three factors determine the clinical presentation: (1) volume of fluid; (2) rate at which fluid accumulates; (3) pericardial compliance. The pressure–volume curve is nonlinear, with the initial flat section due to the pericardial reserve volume. This volume is made up of the recesses and sinuses of the pericardial sac (Figure 18-2). The gradual upslope of the curve is due to the elastic fibers stretching and the wavy collagen fibers straightening. The steep slope is due to the exhaustion of these mechanisms,

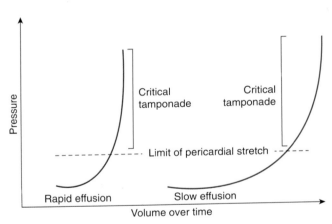

Figure 18-2. Cardiac tamponade. Pericardial pressure–volume (or strain–stress) curves are shown in which the volume increases slowly or rapidly over time. In the left-hand panel, rapidly increasing pericardial fluid first reaches the limit of the pericardial reserve volume (the initial flat segment) and then quickly exceeds the limit of parietal pericardial stretch, causing a steep rise in pressure, which becomes even steeper as smaller increments in fluid cause a disproportionate increase in the pericardial pressure. In the right-hand panel, a slower rate of pericardial filling takes longer to exceed the limit of pericardial stretch, because there is more time for the pericardium to stretch and for compensatory mechanisms to become activated. (Reproduced with permission from DH Spodick. *N Engl J Med.* 2003;349(7):684–690.)

and any increase in volume above that critical point causes severe increases in pressure that are transduced as compressive forces on the heart. If the fluid accumulates rapidly or if the pericardium is pathologically stiff, then relatively small amounts of fluid can result in marked elevations in pressure. In contrast, if the effusion grows slowly, the pericardium can gradually stretch to accommodate the volume, stretching the pressure–volume curve to the right.[2,4,31]

Symptoms of tamponade include dyspnea, tachypnea, and fatigue, while signs include tachycardia, elevated jugular venous distension, a quiet precordium, hypotension, and pulsus paradoxus. Another notable finding is dullness to percussion at the left scapular angle with bronchial breath sounds due to compressive atelectasis from the effusion. It is often commented that a pericardial rub disappears when an effusion develops, but a rub may still be present (typically on inspiration) caused by pericardial–pleural friction. The elevated pericardial pressure results in elevated right atrial and venous pressure giving a characteristic jugular venous waveform lacking the Y descent. These changes result from decreased right atrial emptying due to impaired ventricular expansion and filling.[4,31,32]

The description of *pulsus paradoxus* by Kussmaul in 1873 was of the "paradox" of not palpating a pulse despite detecting a heartbeat during inspiration. It has since been described in patients with normal physiology that during inspiration there is a consistent decrease in left ventricular stroke volume (7%) and arterial pressure (3%). These effects are due to ventricular interdependence and can be accentuated in pericardial disease, leading to the suggested renaming of the finding as *pulsus exageratus* (Figure 18-3). It is thought to be pathognomonic of tamponade when positive (inspiratory drop in SBP of 10% or 10 mm Hg), but there can be false positives as well as false negatives. A pulsus exageratus may be present without tamponade in severe COPD/asthma or with a large pulmonary embolism; exaggeration of intrathoracic pressures is believed to be responsible. Tamponade may be present without a pulsus in hypovolemia, called low-pressure tamponade; if blood volume/preload is already diminished, minimal increases in pericardial pressure limit right-sided filling without causing an effect on left-sided function. Alternatively, an atrial septal defect will shunt blood from left to right, nullifying ventricular interdependence. Finally, right ventricular hypertrophy causing a thick, noncompliant septum, aortic regurgitation, congestive heart failure, and severe left ventricular hypertrophy all increase LVEDP; these conditions also limit ventricular interdependence and therefore limit the formation of a pulsus.[4,31,32]

There are several diagnostic tests that can assist in the diagnosis of tamponade; a chest radiograph is not one of them since it gives only static anatomic data, not

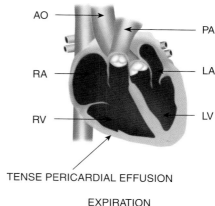

TENSE PERICARDIAL EFFUSION

EXPIRATION

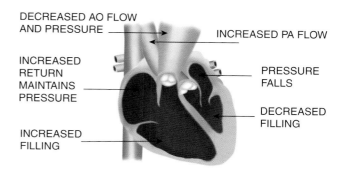

DECREASED AO FLOW AND PRESSURE

INCREASED PA FLOW

INCREASED RETURN MAINTAINS PRESSURE

PRESSURE FALLS

DECREASED FILLING

INCREASED FILLING

INSPIRATION

Figure 18-3. Schematic representation of the competitive ventricular filling that occurs during respiration with pericardial tamponade. (Reproduced with permission from Cosio FG, et al. Abnormal septal motion in cardiac tamponade with pulsus paradoxus. *Chest.* 1977;71:787.)

dynamic functional data. Acutely the pericardial silhouette will be normal, requiring approximately 250 cm³ of fluid to gather before it assumes a globular shape (Figure 18-4). *But* even if this finding is present, it still does not prove the effusion is causing any pathologic effects. Likewise, there are EKG findings suggestive of pericarditis (diffuse ST abnormalities; Figure 18-5) or an effusion (low voltages due to insulating effects, and electrical alternans; Figure 18-6), but these also are not helpful in diagnosing tamponade.[5,30]

Echocardiography is a valuable noninvasive means to evaluate a patient for tamponade, but it should be remembered that no single finding has 100% sensitivity or specificity. The presence of an effusion, graded as small (posterior only), moderate (anterior also but <1 cm), or large (>1 cm), is required, but alone does not confirm tamponade (Figure 18-7). Right atrial collapse is more sensitive but less specific for tamponade than ventricular diastolic collapse

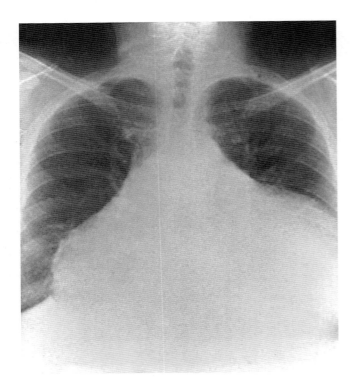

Figure 18-4. Chest radiograph of an asymptomatic patient with a large effusion due to severe CHF.

(collapse occurs when chamber pressures are lowest) (Figure 18-8). The absence of IVC plethora (suggesting normal right atrial pressure) makes the diagnosis of tamponade unlikely. Flow velocity paradoxus, the immediate marked decrease in transmitral (and increase in transtricuspid) Doppler flow with inspiration, like the pulsus, is an accentuation of normal physiology.[33,34]

On right heart catheterization, pulmonary artery wedge pressure and atrial and ventricular end-diastolic pressures are elevated and equalized (within 5 mm Hg) in tamponade. These values reflect the elevated intrapericardial pressure, but again there are other pathologic conditions that can cause diastolic equalization of pressure.

For hemodynamically stable patients (including those patients stabilized with the use of fluids and vasopressors), a controlled drainage of the effusion under guided imaging is preferable. This procedure can be done bedside with echocardiography, or in the cardiac catheterization lab under fluoroscopy while monitoring right and left heart pressures. A catheter is usually left in the pericardium for at least 72 hours to continue draining any recurrent effusion. Surgical drainage employing either a subxyphoid pericardial window or an open thoracotomy is also an option.

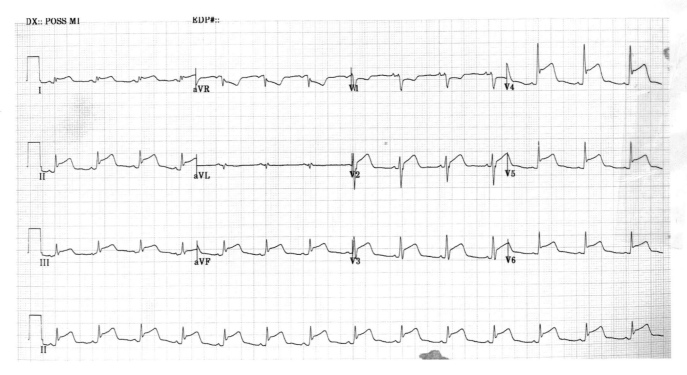

Figure 18-5. An EKG of an adolescent with fever and chest pain during an episode of diabetic ketoacidosis. Note ST-segment elevations in all leads except aVL (an isoelectric lead here so the ST segment is compressed) and aVR and V1, which have expected ST-segment depressions. PR-segment depression is best seen in lead II.

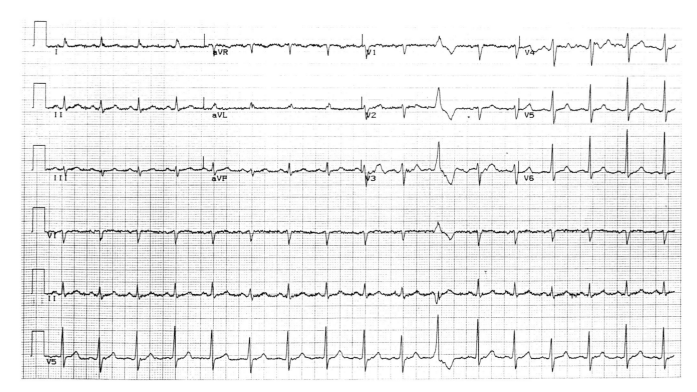

Figure 18-6. EKG of a patient with ESRD on chronic hemodialysis with a large, symptomatic effusion. Electrical alternans is present with the voltages varying over a three-beat cycle. Mild tachycardia (rate 102) and low voltages in the limb leads are also present. A pericardial window was performed.

For hemodynamically unstable patients, immediate relief of the tamponade by percutaneous subxyphoid needle aspiration is required (Figure 18-9). The patient should be positioned upright at 45° in order to have gravity assist the fluid into a dependent position

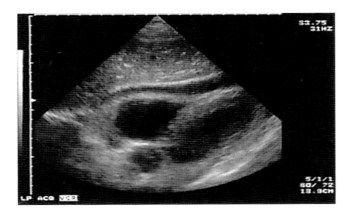

Figure 18-7. Subxiphoid pericardial ultrasound reveals a large pericardial fluid collection. (Reproduced with permission from Brunicardi FC, Andersen DK, Billiar TR, et al. *Schwartz's Principles of Surgery*. 9th ed. New York, NY: McGraw-Hill Inc; 2010. Figure 7-9.)

anteriorly. If ultrasonography is not available, a precordial lead can be clipped to the metal hub of the needle, and a continuous EKG strip is run while aspirating; epicardial contact is indicated by ST-segment elevation or PVCs indicating the needle should be withdrawn slightly. Potential serious complications include ventricular puncture, coronary artery laceration, and pneumothorax.[30,35]

CONSTRICTION

Constriction has been referred to as pseudocirrhosis because of its ability to mimic chronic liver disease. The most common etiologies include postradiation, lung and breast cancer, TB, and renal failure. The final common pathway is thickening and scarring of the pericardial layers, which, in turn, become adherent, obliterating the pericardial space. There can be focal disease, usually involving the apex and the right atrium (particularly the atrial–ventricular groove), due to increased local friction, and a minority of cases can have constriction resulting from the visceral pericardium alone.[1,3] Whatever the cause or location, the fibrotic encasement causes a fixed diastolic chamber volume with impaired expansion and an isolation of

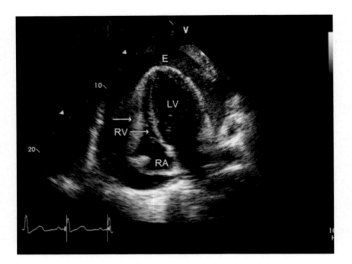

Figure 18-8. RV compression (*arrow*) in cardiac tamponade (apical four-chamber plane). RA, right atrium; RV, right ventricle; LV, left ventricle; E, effusion. (Reproduced with permission from Fuster V, O'Rourke RA, Walsh RA, Poole-Wilson P. *Hurst's the Heart*. 12th ed. New York, NY: McGraw-Hill Inc; 2008. Figure 16-135B.)

the cardiac chambers from changes in intrathoracic pressure.

Normally, the majority of ventricular filling occurs in phase 2 (rapid filling) of diastole, with up to 20% during phase 4 (atrial contraction), and increasing heart rate shortens diastole, thereby decreasing filling. With constriction, elevated atrial pressures cause increased ventricular filling (75%) in the first phase of diastole, which is then halted abruptly by mid-diastole. In this case, increasing heart rate actually improves cardiac output since very little filling occurs in the shortened late diastole.

With the abrupt cessation of filling, a "knock" is produced in 30–70% of patients; it is a loud diastolic sound 0.6–0.12 seconds after S2, but of higher frequency than an S3. Respiratory pressure variations are still transmitted to other intrathoracic structures (vena cava, pulmonary vasculature) but not to the heart. Inspiration reduces the pressure gradient between the pulmonary veins and the left heart, resulting in decreased diastolic flow and ventricular filling; based on accentuated ventricular interdependence, the septum shifts leftward allowing a simultaneous increase in right ventricular filling. The opposite effects are seen with expiration. In pure constrictive pericarditis (CP), the pulsus is usually less than 10 mm Hg and, if greater, it suggests concomitant tamponade (effusive–constrictive pericarditis).[1,3,36]

The onset of constrictive disease is typically insidious, with symptoms developing from weeks to decades after the inciting event. In one study by Ling, the average duration of symptoms prior to a diagnosis was 23.4 months. Peripheral edema, abdominal swelling (from hepatomegaly or ascites), dyspnea, and orthopnea are common initial complaints, illustrating the potential confusion with intrinsic liver disease. Physical exam will reveal elevated JVP in 96% of patients, and Kussmaul's sign (paradoxical increase in JVP with inspiration, since the right atrium cannot accommodate the increased venous return) may be present. It is not specific for constriction, however, and may be seen in any condition with elevated right heart pressures including right ventricular infarct, pulmonary hypertension, tricuspid stenosis, and restrictive cardiomyopathy (RCM). Early cessation of diastolic filling produces Fridreich's sign, a rapid *Y* descent of the JVP, seen in 94% of cases in one series. A dampened apical impulse and a pericardial knock, more prominent with squatting but attenuated by nitroglycerin, are also common findings. Pulsatile hepatomegaly with ascites was found in 70% of patients in one study, but there are differences in the liver function tests and ascitic fluid analysis of these patients with passive congestion compared with those of cirrhotic patients as seen in a study by Runyon.[36,37]

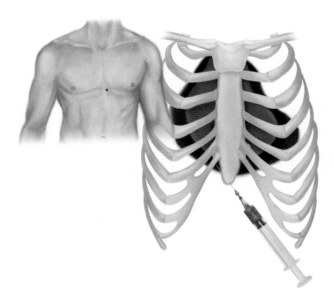

Figure 18-9. The paraxiphoid technique for *pericardiocentesis* is usually performed with the needle directed toward the left shoulder or left scapula tip. *However*, if one aims toward the tip of the right scapula, the needle tends to go parallel to the lateral border of the right heart and is less apt to penetrate the coronary artery or myocardium. (Reproduced with permission from Wilson RF. Injury to the heart and great vessels. In: Henning RS, ed. *Critical Care Cardiology*. New York, NY: Churchill Livingstone; 1989.)

EKG findings include low voltages (60%) and atrial fibrillation in the late stages (25%), although these are insensitive and nonspecific. Diagnosis can be made by CT or MRI, demonstrating a pericardial thickness of greater than 4 mm, sometimes with calcifications, but since there may be focal disease only, relying on these modalities will miss a certain percentage of cases. Echocardiography can be useful in evaluating for constriction, with transesophageal being superior to transthoracic echo in detecting pericardial thickening. Other echo findings include preserved systolic function with rapid diastolic filling causing exaggerated posterior wall and septal motion (septal bounce), early closure of the mitral valve, and premature opening of the tricuspid valve.

RCM, such as caused by amyloidosis, sarcoidosis, hemochromatosis, glycogen storage diseases, or endomyocardial elastosis, may have a similar clinical presentation and echo abnormalities to constrictive pericarditis, and it is still a challenge for cardiologists to differentiate the entities (short of sending a patient for a thoracotomy). There have been studies that have found a faster filling rate with a shorter interval to peak filling in constriction, and Garcia et al. used Doppler tissue imaging to show that left ventricular expansion peak velocity is markedly reduced in restrictive disease, but is preserved in constriction.[38]

Cardiac catheterization can also be used to help make the diagnosis, but again there is overlap of many of the findings with RCM. Right atrial pressure tracings show the typical *M* or *W* pattern formed by the prominent Y descent. Diastolic pressures are elevated and approximately equal in all four chambers, with simultaneous ventricular tracings giving a characteristic dip and plateau pattern (square root sign); RVEDP has been found to be at least one third of RVSP in 95% of constriction. If all chamber diastolic pressures are low, and there is clinical suspicion of CP, a rapid infusion of 1 L of saline may be given to identify occult disease; in a normal patient, the pressures should rise and separate, but with CP they rise and remain equally related.[4,39]

Medical therapy using diuretics may be initially attempted, but the overwhelming majority of patients will require pericardiectomy as definitive therapy. In a large series from the Mayo Clinic, preoperative risk factors were identified as severity of RVEDP elevation, renal insufficiency, and previous mediastinal radiation; intraoperative risk factors that worsen prognosis were unresectable calcifications and incomplete decortication (usually due to involvement of the epicardium). Poor postoperative response is found when the fibrosis and calcification had progressed to involve the myocardium also. Operative mortality is based on NYHA functional class status, with 1% for class I or II, 10% for class III, and 46% for class IV; these data illustrate the importance of making the diagnosis sooner rather than later.[36,37]

REFERENCES

1. Fowler NO. *The Pericardium in Health and Disease.* Mount Kisco, NY: Futura Publishing; 1985.
2. Reddy PS. *Pericardial Disease.* New York, NY: Raven Press; 1982.
3. Spodick DH. *The Pericardium: A Comprehensive Textbook.* New York, NY: Marcel Dekker; 1997.
4. Hoit BD. Pericardial disease and pericardial tamponade. *Crit Care Med.* 2007;35(8):S355–S364.
5. Ariyarajah V, Spodick DH. Acute pericarditis: diagnostic cues and common electrocardiographic manifestations. *Cardiol Rev.* 2007;15(1):24–30.
6. Little WC, Freeman GL. Pericardial disease [published erratum appears in *Circulation.* 2007;115:e406]. *Circulation.* 2006;113:1622–1632.
7. Lange RA, Hillis LD. Clinical practice: acute pericarditis [published erratum appears in *N Engl J Med.* 2005;352:1163]. *N Engl J Med.* 2004;351:2195–2202.
8. Bell EJ, McCartney RA. A study of Coxsackie B virus infections. *J Hyg.* 1984;93:197–203.
9. Nagi KS, Joshi R, Thakur RK. Cardiac manifestations of Lyme disease: a review. *Can J Cardiol.* 1996;12(5):503–506.
10. Rubin RH, Moellering RC. Clinical, microbiologic and therapeutic aspects of purulent pericarditis. *Am J Med.* 1975;59:68–77.
11. Saenz RE. Purulent pericarditis with associated cardiac tamponade caused by a highly resistant strain of *Streptococcus pneumoniae. Clin Infect Dis.* 1998;26:762–763.
12. Arsura EL, Kilgore WB, Strategos E. Purulent pericarditis misdiagnosed as septic shock. *South Med J.* 1999;92(3):285–288.
13. Brook I, Frazier EH. Microbiology of acute purulent pericarditis. *Arch Intern Med.* 1996;156:1857–1860.
14. Brook I. Pericarditis due to anaerobic bacteria. *Cardiology.* 2002;97:55–58.
15. Laisaar T. Video-assisted thoracoscopic surgery in the management of acute purulent mediastinits and empyema. *Thorac Cardiovasc Surg.* 1998;46(1):51–54.
16. Ramasamy D. Purulent pericarditis: rediscovery of an old remedy. *J Thorac Cardiovasc Surg.* 1996;111:487–488.
17. Defouilloy C, Ossart M. Intrapericardial fibrinolysis: a useful treatment in the management of purulent pericarditis. *Intensive Care Med.* 1997;23(1):117–118.
18. Kauffman CA. Histoplasmosis. *Clin Chest Med.* 2009;30:217–225.
19. Canver CC. Fungal purulent constrictive pericarditis in a heart transplant patient. *Ann Thorac Surg.* 1998;65:1792–1794.
20. Gobeil F, Dumesnil J, Cartier P. Rapidly evolving constrictive tuberculous pericarditis. *Can J Cardiol.* 1998;14(12):1467–1469.
21. Mayosi BM, Burgess LJ, Doubell AF. Tuberculous pericarditis. *Circulation.* 2005;112:3608–3616.
22. Yunis NA, Stone VE. Cardiac manifestations of HIV/AIDS: a review of disease spectrum and clinical management. *J Acquir Immune Defic Syndr Hum Retrovirol.* 1998;18:145–154.
23. Cardosa JS. Pericardial involvement in HIV infection. *Chest.* 1999;115:418–422.

24. Sudano I, Spieker LE, Noll G, et al. Cardiovascular disease in HIV infection. *Am Heart J.* 2006;151:1147–1155.

25. Imazio M, Negro A, Belli R, et al Frequency and prognostic significance of pericarditis following acute myocardial infarction treated by PCI. *Am J Cardiol.* 2009;103: 1525–1529.

26. Prince SE, Cunha BA. Postpericardiotomy syndrome. *Heart Lung.* 1997;26:165–168.

27. Pawsat D, Lee JY. Inflammatory disorders of the heart. *Emerg Med Clin North Am.* 1998;16(3):665–674.

28. Moder KG, Miller TD, Tazelaar HD. Cardiac involvement in SLE. *Mayo Clin Proc.* 1999;74:275–284.

29. DeCamp MM, Sugarbaker DJ. Malignant effusive disease of the pleura and pericardium. *Chest.* 1997;112:291s–295s.

30. Maisch B, Ristic AD. Pericardial disease. In: Fink MP, Abraham E, Vincent JL, and Kochanek PM, eds. *Textbook of Critical Care.* 5th ed. Philadelphia: Elsevier; 2005: 851–860.

31. Ariyarajah V, Sodick DH. Cardiac tamponade revisited. *Tex Heart J.* 2007;34:347–351.

32. Spodick DH. Acute cardiac tamponade. *N Engl J Med.* 2003;349:684–690.

33. Chong HH, Plotnik GD. Pericardial effusion and tamponade: evaluation, imaging modalities, and management. *Compr Ther.* 1995;21(7):378–385.

34. Tsang TS, Oh JK, Seward JB, et al. Diagnostic value of echocardiography in cardiac tamponade. *Herz.* 2000;8: 734–740.

35. Van Trigt P, Douglas J, Smith PK, et al. A prospective trial of subxiphoid pericardiotomy in the diagnosis and treatment of large pericardial effusions: follow-up report. *Ann Surg.* 1993;218:777–782.

36. Myers RB, Spodick DH. Constrictive pericarditis: clinical and pathophysiologic characteristics. *Am Heart J.* 1999;138:219–232.

37. Runyon BA. Cardiac ascites: a characterization. *J Clin Gastroenterol.* 1998;10(4):410–412.

38. Garcia MJ, Rodriguez L, Ares M, et al. Differentiation of constrictive pericarditis from restrictive cardiomyopathy: assessment of left ventricular diastolic velocities in longitudinal axis by Doppler tissue imaging. *J Am Coll Cardiol.* 1996;27:108-114.

39. Ling LH. Constrictive pericarditis in the modern era. *Circulation.* 1999;100(13):1380–1386.

SECTION V

Gastrointestinal and Renal Disorders

CHAPTER 19

Gastrointestinal Bleeding

Marie-Carmelle Elie-Turenne, Carrie A. Cregar, and Selwena Brewster

▶ INTRODUCTION

Gastrointestinal bleeding is an important cause of mortality for emergency department (ED) and critical care patients. This chapter discusses the two major types of bleeding, upper and lower, followed by detailed information on the management of these difficult patients.

▶ UPPER GASTROINTESTINAL BLEEDING

Upper gastrointestinal bleeding (UGIB) is an important cause of mortality in the ED with rates from 3% to 16%.[1-7] In the United States, UGIB represents 400,000 hospital admissions[8] and 30,000 deaths annually.[9] Hospital in-patients presenting with UGIB have a 2- to 6-fold increase of mortality compared with their ED counterparts.[1-7] Increased risk of mortality is associated with increased age, severe comorbidity, hypotension, shock, rebleeding, and the timing of the bleeding event during an in-patient hospital stay.[2,10]

CLINICAL PRESENTATION

Patients with UGIB often present with hematemesis, coffee ground vomiting, melena, or maroon stool, while hematochezia is typically associated with massive hemorrhage. The presentation of bleeding depends on the amount and location of hemorrhage. Patients may present with complications of anemia, including fatigue, chest pain, syncope, and shortness of breath. Untreated manifestations of progressive hemorrhagic shock are inevitable, including acute end-organ dysfunction and refractory hypotension.

The physical exam should include an assessment of airway, vital signs, and mentation. An abdominal exam, if tenderness is elicited, aids in localizing the source to a gastric or duodenal location. Blood on digital rectal exam may suggest both chronicity and degree of bleeding. The absence of rectal blood, however, does not exclude the existence of a gastrointestinal source. Stigmata of chronic liver disease including jaundice, telangiectasia, hemorrhoids, or caput medusae may indicate the presence of esophageal or gastric varices.

ETIOLOGY

UGIB can originate from a number of sources and are discussed below in order of frequency. A list of causes of upper GI bleeding is listed in Table 19-1.

Peptic Ulcer Disease

Despite the advent of H_2 receptor antagonists and proton pump inhibitors (PPIs), peptic ulcer disease (PUD) remains the most common etiology of UGIB accounting for 140,000 hospitalizations each year in the United States.[11] Approximately 28–59% of UGIB is represented by PUD, with the majority of duodenal, as opposed to gastric, origin.[1,12] GI bleeding from a duodenal location is fairly common owing to its abundant blood supply and the posterior location of the gastroduodenal artery to the bulb. This is the case with most massive UGIBs. The presence of large ulcers in the posterior duodenal bulb or on the lesser curvature of the stomach is associated with increased mortality.

The pathophysiology of PUD results from the overproduction of gastric acid and pepsin. These overwhelm

▶ **TABLE 19-1. CAUSES OF UPPER GASTROINTESTINAL BLEEDING**

Peptic ulcer disease	Erosive gastritis	Esophagitis
Esophageal varices	Gastric varices	Mallory–Weiss syndrome
Stress ulcers	Arteriovenous malformation	Malignancy
Nasal bleeding	Pharyngeal bleeding	Aortoenteric fistula
Leiomyoma	Telangiectasia	Angiodysplasia

the mucosal barriers and reduce mucous and bicarbonate secretion.[13] Nonsteroidal anti-inflammatory drugs (NSAIDs) cause ulcerative disease by submucosal erosion and reduction of prostaglandin production. The elevated rate of PUD witnessed in the United States parallels the high rate of NSAID use, which has been observed at 50%.[1] NSAID use is currently considered the most significant risk factor associated with UGIB. Concurrent steroid use increases the risk of ulcer formation.

Helicobacter pylori, a gram-negative bacteria residing in the mucosal layer of the stomach, is the most common causative etiology of PUD via the stimulation of gastrin production. The majority of nonbleeding duodenal (90%) and gastric (75%) ulcers are associated with *H. pylori* infections. Consequently, one large Canadian study found 45% of nonvariceal UGIB cases were *H. pylori* positive.[14] Recurrence of bleeding from *H. pylori* disease is rare when this organism is eradicated as part of ulcer treatment.[15] When present with a history of NSAID use, *H. pylori* has an additive effect and a consequent increase in UGIB risk with an odds ratio (OR) of 6.13.[16]

Less common causes of PUD are high-gastrin-secreting states such as Zollinger–Ellison tumors. Smoking, history of alcohol abuse, and acute hepatic failure may exacerbate a preexisting ulcer, decrease healing, and increase recurrence and perforation rates.

The patient with PUD classically presents with intermittent burning epigastric pain that occurs 1–3 hours after meals and is relieved by food and antacid. Constant epigastric pain suggests that there is transmucosal penetration of the ulcer. Referred back pain can be a sign of pancreatic inflammation. Diffuse peritoneal irritation and severe abdominal pain can be signs of perforation. Approximately 5% of penetrating duodenal ulcers will erode into the peritoneal cavity and cause a chemical peritonitis. Typically the patient can recall the exact time of onset of the abdominal pain, which is frequently accompanied by tachycardia and, later, dehydration, fever, and ileus. Free air underneath the diaphragm on upright chest radiograph is pathognomonic

of perforated viscous. This complication constitutes an emergency, which warrants the initiation of appropriate fluid resuscitation, pain management, and surgical consultation. In general, the elderly are at increased risk for gastric perforation. GI bleeding is the most common cause of death in PUD patients with comorbidities or over the age 65 years.[17]

The prevalence of mucosal erosive disease in UGIB ranges from 1% to 31% and is often reported as the second leading cause of UGIB. These diseases may present as esophagitis, gastritis, duodenitis, or esophageal ulcer. The pathophysiology and risk factors mimic those of PUD. The lack of standardization in reporting esophagitis and other erosive diseases across study cohorts may explain the wide spectrum of prevalence observed.[12]

Stress ulcers, a relevant subset of mucosal erosive disease, deserve particular mention in critical care patients. Uncommonly present in ED patients, stress ulcers are mucosal defects, which are induced during periods of increased physiologic demand and critical illness. Illnesses such as massive burns, trauma, elevated intracranial pressure, sepsis, and severe shock are all causes of stress ulcers. The pathophysiology of stress ulcer is unclear, but is generally thought to be caused by splanchnic hypoperfusion and poor reperfusion. The concomitant reduction in bowel motility and mucosal secretion of protective substrates are contributory. The increased acidic milieu promotes the progression of these superficial diffuse changes to ulcerative lesions. Unlike PUD, *H. pylori* plays a limited role in stress ulcers. Patients presenting with stress ulcers may be distinguished from the typical ED presentations of PUD by the following risk factors: profound persistent hypotension or shock, high-dose vasopressor use, chronic mechanical ventilation, severe burns, uremic renal failure, greater than 6 days of nasogastric tube placement, acute CNS illness, and high-dose steroid utilization.[18] Stress ulcers typically heal when the underlying clinical condition is addressed. Variants of stress ulcers include Cushing's and Curling's ulcers.

Esophageal Varices

Gastric and esophageal varices remain an important cause of UGIB accounting for 6–14% of presentations. Populations with high ethanol consumption observe higher rates secondary to liver cirrhosis. It is not uncommon for patients with no prior diagnosis of cirrhosis to present to the ED with a herald bleeding event. Varices account for 50–60% of UGIB events in the cirrhotic patient.[12] Often a consequence of cirrhosis-induced portal hypertension, varices are dilated submucosal veins in the lower esophagus or gastroesophageal junction. Varices place the patient at risk for developing a life-threatening bleeding. The sequence of events that lead to variceal rupture begins with increased hepatic resistance and increased portal blood flow. These two factors cause an increase in the portal pressure, causing dilation of preexisting vessels and the formation of varices. Repeated increases in portal pressure due to meals, ethanol, exercise, and increased abdominal pressure all cause further dilation of varices. Rupture and bleeding occur when the elastic limit of the vessel wall is exceeded.[19] Bleeding is characteristically severe and is associated with an in-patient mortality of 11–34%: the highest rates are observed in cirrhotics.[20]

Mallory–Weiss

Mallory–Weiss (MW) syndrome accounts for 2–7% of UGI bleeds.[1,5,21] The pathogenesis of MW syndrome is not completely understood, although any disease that causes retching or vomiting can induce MW. Alcoholism is the most frequently associated condition, although eating and coughing disorders, pregnancy, heavy lifting, diabetic ketoacidosis, and blunt abdominal trauma have all been described.[22,23] Linear tears, thought to occur as a result of a transient high transmural pressure gradient across the region of the gastroesophageal junction, characterize MW syndrome. Overdilation of the noncompliant lower esophagus can also produce an injury as described in postcardiopulmonary resuscitation patients.[24] There is a 0.07–0.49% incidence of MW as an iatrogenic consequence of gastroesophageal endoscopy.[25,26]

The presence of a hiatal hernia may be a predisposing factor for MW. It has been proposed that, in hiatal hernia patients, a higher pressure gradient develops in the hernia compared with the rest of the stomach during retching, thereby increasing the potential for mucosal laceration.[27] MW tears typically result in mild to moderate GI bleeding, but are rarely severe in nature. These superficial mucosal tears tend to heal rapidly and are often self-limited. Bleeding spontaneously stops in about 90% of cases, although coagulopathy or preexisting comorbidities such as thrombocytopenia and liver failure can result in refractory bleeding.[28] Low admission hematocrit (HCT), shock, or active bleeding during endoscopy is predictive of a complicated course.[29,30]

Vascular Anomalies

Vascular anomalies or angiodysplasia account for about 2–5% of acute UGIB. Upper gastrointestinal angiodysplasia occurs most commonly in the stomach, rarely in the duodenum or esophagus. Bleeding from angiodysplasia is associated with advanced age, aortic stenosis, chronic renal failure, and calcinosis, Raynaud phenomenon, esophageal dysmotility, sclerodactyly, and telangiectasia (CREST) syndrome.

Rare Causes of UGIB

Leiomyomas and gastrointestinal stromal tumors constitute about 1% of primary gastrointestinal tumors, mostly occur in the stomach, and often present with overt UGIB. Adenocarcinoma is the most common primary malignancy. It presents as a gastric mass, nonhealing ulcer, or stricture. Gastric lymphomas constitute about 5% of gastric tumors. Specifically, gastric mucosa-associated lymphoid tissues (MALTomas) are early B-cell lymphomas highly associated with chronic *H. pylori* infection. They rarely cause acute bleeding. Gastric metastases most commonly arise from lung cancer, breast cancer, and cutaneous melanoma. These malignancies frequently rebleed and have a poor long-term prognosis. Radiation and chemotherapy treatment for gastric malignancies can result in UGIB that are difficult to manage and usually require a multidisciplinary approach.[31]

Aortoenteric fistula often presents with a mild "herald bleed" followed by massive hemorrhage. This diagnosis constitutes a high mortality with delayed diagnosis. For this reason, emergency esophagogastroduodenoscopy (EGD) is indicated if this diagnosis is suspected. Aortoenteric fistula is a rare consequence of prior aortic surgery, aortic aneurysms, and severe atherosclerosis. These fistulas are typically located at the distal duodenum underscoring the role of endoscopic investigation up to this location. During EGD, if a prosthetic graft mesh is found, the scope should be withdrawn without attempting therapeutic intervention and the lesion should be treated intraoperatively due to the risk of massive bleeding.[32,33]

▶ LOWER GASTROINTESTINAL BLEEDING

Lower gastrointestinal bleeding (LGIB) accounts for about one quarter to one third of all admissions for gastrointestinal bleeding.[34] The incidence of acute LGIB is estimated at 20–27 per 100,000 adult population at risk, significantly lower compared with UGIB with 100–200 cases per 100,000 population.[35] The incidence of LGIB increases with age and is higher in men, presumably because of the increased frequency of vascular disease and diverticulosis in older men. Mortality rates of acute LGIB are consistently in the range of less than 5%.

LGIB is defined as hemorrhage that arises distal to the ligament of Treitz and encompasses a broad clinical spectrum that ranges from insignificant hematochezia to severe hemorrhage with shock.[36] Acute LGIB is defined as bleeding of less than 3 days' duration. Severe hemorrhage is defined as a decrease in HCT by 20% or a transfusion requirement of ≥2 U of blood. Other clinical data associated with severe bleeding include heart rate ≥100/min, syncope, systolic blood pressure

► **TABLE 19-2. CAUSES OF LOWER GASTROINTESTINAL BLEEDING**

Upper GI bleeding	Diverticulosis	GI carcinoma
Angiodysplasia	Arteriovenous malformation	Mesenteric ischemia
Ischemic colitis	Meckel's diverticulum	Hemorrhoids
Infectious colitis	Dieulafoy lesions	Polyps
Radiation colitis	Rectal ulcers	Trauma
Foreign bodies	Prostate biopsy	Endometriosis
Inflammatory bowel disease	Colonic varices	Portal hypertensive enteropathy

≤115 mm Hg, nontender abdominal examination, aspirin use, bleeding per rectum during the first 4 hours of evaluation, and more than two active comorbid conditions.[37]

CLINICAL PRESENTATION

Acute LGIB often presents as hematochezia, melena, or dark red blood with clots. A digital rectal exam is required. Hematochezia is the most common presentation of LGIB. However, 10–15% of hematochezia presentations are from a UGIB source.[38] Melena suggests a source of bleeding proximal to the cecum, while dark red blood with clots suggests the ascending colon.

ETIOLOGY

The most common etiologies of LGIB will be discussed in order of frequency. A list of causes of lower GI bleeding is included in Table 19-2.

Diverticular Disease

Diverticular diseases are the most common cause of significant and life-threatening LGIB, accounting for 50% of cases.[38,39] Diverticula develop where the vasa recta (intramural branches of the marginal artery supplying the colon) penetrate the colonic wall.[40] They most frequently occur in the left colon, but can exist anywhere in the colon, except the rectum. Abnormal colonic motility, defective muscular structure, increased cross-linking of collagen, and aging are all causes of diverticula. In addition, a diet low in fiber can lead to firm, small stools, which cause reduced transit time. Over time, vigorous contractions in the colon push the inner intestinal lining outwards through vulnerable points in the muscle walls.[41] High intraluminal pressure and a weak colonic wall at the sites of vessel penetration into the muscularis lead to herniation.[42] The pouches that develop are called diverticula. Diverticular hemorrhage is thought to occur when the damaged vessel ruptures at the dome or the neck of the diverticulum. The most common presentation of diverticular bleeding is massive painless rectal hemorrhage. Severe blood loss is noted in 3–5% of patients with diverticulosis. In approximately 80% of patients, diverticular bleeding resolves spontaneously.[43]

Angiodysplasia

Angiodysplasias of the intestine or arteriovenous malformations (AVMs) account for up to 30% of LGIB.[44] AVMs are found in patients older than 50 years of age and are distributed equally between the sexes. These lesions are notably associated with aortic stenosis and renal failure, especially in elderly patients. The exact mechanism of development of angiodysplasia is not fully known. Development is related to age and strain on the bowel wall.[45] Chronic venous obstruction is proposed to play an important role. When applied to the bowel lumen, the Laplace law states tension is highest in bowel segments with the greatest diameter, such as the right colon. Repeated episodes of colonic distention are associated with transient increases in lumen pressure and size. Over time, this process causes gradual dilation of the submucosal veins, the venules, and the arteriolar capillary units feeding them. Ultimately, the capillary rings dilate, the precapillary sphincters lose their competency, and a small arteriovenous communication forms.[46] A link between a deficiency of high-molecular-weight multimers of von Willebrand factor, aortic stenosis, and colonic angiodysplasia has also been proposed.[45] The hemorrhage tends to arise from the right side of the colon, with the cecum being the most common location. However, AVMs can occur anywhere in the colon, rectum, and small bowel. Most patients experience chronic bleeding, but up to 15% of patients can present with massive hemorrhage.[47]

AIDS/HIV

Patients with HIV/AIDS may have unique etiologies of gastrointestinal bleeding compared with their non-HIV cohorts. Sources of UGIB, although frequently unrelated to HIV, may include cytomegalovirus and Kaposi's sarcoma. LGIB, however, are often HIV related with etiologies including CMV colitis, hemorrhoids, and anal fissures. Because of concomitant thrombocytopenia, HIV patients may present with significant bleeding from an otherwise self-limiting source (i.e., hemorrhoid).[48]

Other Causes of LGIB

Patients with a previous history of atherosclerotic disease, vasopressor use, or shock should be assessed for ischemic colitis. Other less frequent etiologies of LGIB include malignancy, inflammatory bowel disease, NSAID use, infectious colitis, anorectal disorders, small bowel sites (i.e., Crohn's, Meckel's diverticula), and postpolypectomy bleeding.[34,36]

► MANAGEMENT OF GASTROINTESTINAL BLEEDING

Careful consideration of the management approach of gastrointestinal bleeding is needed due to the high morbidity and mortality associated with this condition. Despite advances in medical management and therapeutic interventions, the mortality from UGIB remains unchanged over the past 40 years.[49,50] For critical patients, consultation with gastroenterology and surgery should occur early in the patient's course. Several management considerations are discussed in detail below.

RESUSCITATION

The management of patients with GIBs includes initial and ongoing resuscitation. Aggressive replacement of lost volume with crystalloids and colloids is obligatory in hemodynamically unstable patients. Initial resuscitation should begin with the placement of two large-bore intravenous catheters, and administration of one to two 20 mL/kg bolus of crystalloid with the short-term goal of resolution of tachycardia and hypotension to restore tissue perfusion. Refractory hypotension or evidence of end-organ hypoperfusion should prompt the administration of packed red blood cells (PRBCs). Blood administration should not be delayed pending the results of a repeat hemoglobin (Hb) or the visualization of hematemesis, melena, or hematochezia in the setting of hemodynamic compromise.

AIRWAY CONSIDERATIONS

Massive hematemesis can result in a compromised, visibly obscured airway. Manifestations of hemorrhagic anemia may cause decline in mentation and increased aspiration risk. Moreover, endoscopic interventions in patients with frequent bouts of hematemesis, vomiting, or retching can prove challenging and may lead to further complications. Consequently, establishing a definitive airway in the anticipation of potential cardiovascular compromise and need for therapeutic endoscopic or surgical intervention may be warranted in the setting of large-volume hematemesis.

LABORATORIES

In the evaluation of the bleeding patient, blood should be immediately sent for CBC, electrolytes, calcium, renal function, glucose, prothrombin time, partial thromboplastin time, and INR, and typed for cross-matched blood. While a low Hb is the rule in cases of massive GI bleeding, slow, intermittent bleeds or early presentations can have Hb levels within normal range. In a study that identified 51% of UGIB patients who ultimately required transfusion, the mean presenting Hb was 11.3.[51] Because of the potentially dynamic nature of gastrointestinal bleeding, serial Hb and HCT should be collected to identify significant changes over time. These changes may or may not be heralded by a disruption in hemodynamics, change in clinical appearance, or symptoms such as chest pain, shortness of breath, or altered mentation. An elevated blood urea nitrogen (BUN) to creatinine ratio is suggestive of an upper GI source.[51] However, rapid transit may preclude the elevation of BUN and present with a normal ratio. The existence of thrombocytopenia or coagulopathic disturbances should prompt judicious correction with platelets, fresh frozen plasma, and/or cryoprecipitate.

GASTRIC TUBES AND LAVAGE

The placement of a gastric tube should be considered in the appropriate setting to ascertain both the existence and degree of severity of a UGIB. While nasogastric tube placement can be performed in the alert mentating patient with a gag reflex, there are multiple potential issues. Serious risks include aspiration pneumonitis, laryngospasm, and perforation of the pharyngeal and gastrointestinal structures.[52] Contraindications to placement include history of esophageal varices or strictures, recent alkaline ingestion, and a history of gastric bypass surgery. Patients with an altered level of consciousness should be intubated in order to provide airway protection prior to placement of a gastric tube. In the event of maxillofacial trauma, patients should have an orogastric tube placed to avert passing the tube through the cribriform plate. If immediate endoscopy is available, the gastric tube offers little incremental benefit and may be omitted.

Room-temperature tap water or saline lavage prior to endoscopy is considered safe and an important adjunct in management of suspected UGIB from PUD.[53]

Ice water lavage was once considered an acceptable therapeutic intervention for UGIB via gastric vessel vasoconstriction; however, this is not supported by the literature.[54] The aspiration of fresh blood indicates active bleeding, whereas an aspirate with a coffee ground appearance is associated with a subacute or chronic etiology of the UGIB. The lack of bloody aspirate does not rule out the possibility of a UGIB.[55,56]

BLOOD PRODUCT ADMINISTRATION

Blood products provide obvious benefits in repleting lost volume, replacing blood components, and correction of acidosis. However, a number of studies have demonstrated that blood product administration has been associated with immune suppression, increased nosocomial infection rates, and death.[57] Hence, it is important to properly select patients who would receive the greatest benefit from blood administration.

Patients exhibiting signs of end-organ hypoperfusion benefit from the additional oxygen-carrying capacity of PRBCs. Findings suggestive of global tissue hypoxia may include altered mental status, seizures, hypoxemia, ischemic electrocardiographic changes, or elevation of lactate, creatinine, hepatic transaminases, or troponin. In the absence of these findings, Hb should be kept at ≥ 7[57] in patients without history of coronary artery disease (CAD) and ≥ 10 in those with a history of CAD.[58]

COAGULOPATHY

GI bleeding may result from the use of anticoagulants such as warfarin, antiplatelet agents such as aspirin or clopidogrel, or NSAIDs. In addition, a history of factor deficiency or cirrhosis may indicate that a disruption in the homeostasis of the coagulation cascade exists. Therapy should be directed at correcting the underlying etiology in these cases.

Warfarin toxicity is treated with the administration of 4–6 U of FFP. Vitamin K administration will also reverse the effects of warfarin; however, its onset of action is much delayed and its effect will last 1–2 weeks. Such reversal with vitamin K should be carefully weighed against the future need to chronically anticoagulate the patient. Platelets may be administered to actively bleeding patients with a history of thrombocytopenia, salicylate, or NSAID use. Cryoprecipitate and individual clotting factors may be administered if appropriate. DDAVP or desmopressin should be considered in patients who present with chronic renal failure or uremia to increase the production of von Willebrand factor as these patients have poor platelet aggregation.

Factor VII, which is available in a recombinant formulation, complexes with tissue factor and activates factor Xa inducing the production of clot. It is approved for use in bleeding patients with hemophilia A. In cirrhosis, factor VII administration remains controversial as there are conflicting results from trials evaluating its use in the management of acute variceal bleeding.[59] Novel agents such as prothrombin complex concentrate may serve a future role in massive hemorrhage in patients with a known deficiency of Vitamin K, although they are contraindicated in patients with disseminated intravascular coagulation or liver disease.[60]

MASSIVE BLOOD TRANSFUSION

Bleeding patients who require greater than 10 U of PRBC over a 24-hour period are also at risk for the depletion of coagulation factors and platelets because of the dilutional effect. Once the first 10 U of PRBC has been administered, consideration should be made for the administration of fresh frozen plasma and platelets. The precise ratios that would render most benefit are unclear.[61,62] Patients should also be monitored for volume overload, hypothermia, hyperkalemia, hypocalcemia, and iron toxicity.[60]

PROTON PUMP INHIBITORS

PPIs act via the Na–K-ATPase channels to interrupt the production of H$^+$ ions. Increasing the gastric pH promotes platelet aggregation that is impaired in acidic environments.[63] The PPI should be administered intravenously and the patient kept NPO. When compared with placebo or H$_2$ receptor antagonist, PPI reduces the risk of rebleeding and the need for subsequent surgery in endoscopically diagnosed UGIB from peptic ulcer. PPI, however, has not been shown to reduce the overall mortality from peptic ulcer bleeding,[64] but may reduce the mortality in patients with high-risk endoscopic findings such as active bleeding or a visible vessel. PPI remains an important adjunct to endoscopy as it reduces the need for therapeutic intervention during the procedure.[65] The optimal dose and route of administration have not yet been clearly elucidated; however, suggested dosing is an initial intravenous bolus equivalent to 80 mg of omeprazole followed by an intravenous infusion of 8.0 mg/h for up to 72 hours, at which point high-dose oral PPI treatment may be initiated.[11]

OCTREOTIDE/SOMATOSTATIN

Somatostatin and its analogue, octreotide, inhibit the exocrine function of glandular tissue, which reduces both acid and pepsin secretion. Moreover, they reduce gastroduodenal mucosal blood flow that, in concert with the reduction in acid production, should theoretically prove to be of benefit in PUD. Evidence is lacking, though, in their role in the management of PUD.[66] The role of octreotide in variceal bleeding has been clearly demonstrated to facilitate hemostasis when used in conjunction with endoscopy.[67,68] The recommended regimen includes an initial bolus of 50 mcg followed by an infusion of 50 mcg/h.

VASOPRESSORS

Generally, the use of vasopressors should be discouraged in hemorrhagic shock. Hypotension should primarily be addressed by volume resuscitation with crystalloid and colloid administration. The placement of a central line in the internal jugular or subclavian veins can facilitate administration of fluids directly into the cardiac circuit as well as provide guidance in fluid administration via monitoring of the central venous pressure (CVP). A CVP reading below 8 would indicate the need for additional volume infusion.

Vasopressin, used commonly in the pre-PPI era, is an endogenous pressor normally secreted by the posterior pituitary in response to hypotensive states. It preferentially vasoconstricts sphlancnic vessels to reduce portal venous inflow and pressure. In the presomatostatin era, vasopressin was frequently utilized in cirrhotic patients who, at an advanced stage of the disease, have an impaired ability to generate systemic vascular resistance. However, vasopressin's lack of selectivity at high doses makes it a less desirable agent. Vasopressin use has been reserved for massive refractory bleeding and is administered intravenously in a dose of 0.1–1.0 U/min. Concomitant intravenous administration of nitroglycerin at 40–400 ucg/min can be used to counteract cardiac and bowel ischemic sequela of vasopressin. A synthetic analogue of vasopressin, terlipressin, is used more commonly in Europe, and may have a role in the chronic management of hepatorenal syndrome given its limited side effect profile and longer half-life.[69]

BALLOON TAMPONADE

The Sengstaken–Blakemore tube, introduced in the 1950s, is a double-balloon esophageal tamponade system used in life-threatening UGIB from esophageal or gastric varices. The gastric balloon occludes feeding vessels at the gastroesophageal junction, reducing the pressure in the esophageal varices, while the esophageal balloon provides direct compression.[70] Complications associated with its placement include esophageal or gastric rupture, pressure necrosis, and aspiration pneumonitis. An updated version, the Minnesota tube, has an added esophageal suction port to minimize aspiration. Because of the prohibitively high complication and mortality rate associated with balloon tamponade, the exhaustion of medical and endoscopic therapies prior to placement is recommended.[71] However, massive refractory hemorrhage, which precludes endoscopy or is associated with hemodynamic instability, may warrant the placement of a balloon tamponade system.

Prior to insertion of a balloon tamponade system, patients should be mechanically ventilated. The balloons and aspiration ports should be checked for integrity and patency. In the event there is no esophageal aspiration port, a nasogastric tube can be sutured onto the Sengstaken–Blakemore tube proximal to the esophageal balloon. The tube should be advanced orally approximately 50 cm into the gastric cavity. The stomach should then be aspirated of its contents. The gastric balloon can then be inflated in increments of 100 mL to a maximum of 400–500 mL. The Sengstaken–Blakemore tube should then be placed on a traction device to achieve hemostasis. If bleeding persists, the esophageal balloon may be inflated to 30–40 mm Hg. Malpositioning is not uncommon and placement should be confirmed by chest radiograph.[69,70,72,73] The Linton-Nachlas tube has a single distal balloon that may be used in patients with documented gastric varices only.[74]

SPECIAL MANAGEMENT CONSIDERATIONS IN HEPATIC CIRRHOSIS

Resuscitation and management of the hepatic cirrhosis patient deserves special attention.

Varices typically occur in the third to fourth stages of cirrhosis; these patients often preferentially pool their intravascular volume in the markedly vasodilated mesenteric circulation. Thus, persistent hypotension in these patients may be the rule. Markers of adequate resuscitation in these patients are less clear. In addition, aggressive fluid resuscitation can raise portal pressures, increasing shear stress against the already compromised varix. Moreover, dilution of coagulation factors in the cirrhotic may lead to increased or refractory bleeding.

The use of crystalloid, while appropriate initially, should be limited. The resuscitation strategy should be promptly transitioned to one that utilizes colloid in the form of PRBCs, fresh frozen plasma, platelets, or albumin as needed. Maintaining a systolic blood pressure of 80–90 mm Hg may be adequate, provided the patient is not exhibiting other signs of hypoperfusion.

Approximately 20% of UGIB cirrhotic patients are infected on admission, and 50% subsequently develop infection during hospitalization. Antibiotic administration has been shown to enhance survival in these patients.[75,76] Quinolones or cephalosporins are recommended for these patients.[77,78]

ENDOSCOPY

Esophagogastroduodenoscopy

Following adequate resuscitation, EGD is the diagnostic and therapeutic modality of choice for UGIB and may be indicated in certain cases of LGIB with unclear etiology. EGD serves the role of diagnosis, triage, and therapy.[79]

Early assessment of the etiology and severity of bleeding will dictate further therapy and need for critical care monitoring. Endoscopic management is successful in greater than 75% of patients. Despite endoscopic therapy, rebleeding occurs in about 7–29% of cases, and is most common with variceal bleeding. The benefits of EGD over other therapeutic modalities are decreased rates of further bleeding, fewer blood transfusions, lower mortality, shorter hospital stays, and lower hospital costs.[80] Treatment of UGIB with EGD depends on the etiology of the bleed.

In PUD, hemostasis can be achieved by injection therapy with epinephrine or alternative agent, mechanical clipping, or thermal treatment. Visible vessels or the presence of spurting or oozing blood predict further rebleeding and increased mortality. Almost all fatal rebleeding occurs within the first 24 hours.[63]

In MW syndrome, the occurrence of shock or active bleeding during endoscopic evaluation is predictive of recurrent bleed and warrants intensive care monitoring.[29] Sclerotherapy or injection with epinephrine may be of benefit with some MW lesions.

Endoscopic therapy of variceal bleeding may be achieved by sclerotherapy or ligation. The administration of somatostatin or octreotide early in suspected variceal bleeding facilitates achievement of hemostasis during emergent endoscopy.[81,82] The addition of antibiotic prophylaxis in cirrhotic patients appears to also reduce postendoscopic treatment failures. Endoscopy has not been shown, however, to reduce overall mortality in acute variceal bleeding, with rebleeding occurring in 10–15% of cases.[83]

Colonoscopy

Colonoscopy is the modality of choice in evaluating LGIB. Patients with hematochezia or hypotension, however, should have upper endoscopy performed first to evaluate for a brisk UGIB.[84] Although studies have demonstrated successful endoscopy can be achieved without bowel preparation, the American Society of Gastroenterology recommends thorough colon cleansing to enhance visualization of occult lesions.[85] Hemostasis is achieved by thermocoagulation, injection therapy of various agents, and mechanical methods. The incidence of complication is 1 in 1,000 with perforation occurring rarely. The diagnostic yield of urgent colonoscopy is high if performed within 12–24 hours, although may not necessarily reduce mortality, transfusion requirement, or length of stay.[86] Evidence of active bleeding, visible vessels, or adherent clot during colonoscopy is associated with a complicated course and rebleeding.[87]

DIAGNOSTIC AND INTERVENTIONAL RADIOLOGY

Angiography

Formal peripheral angiography has the capacity to identify a lesion that is actively bleeding at a rate of 0.5–1.0 mL/min. Advantages of angiography include the ability to identify the precise location of the bleed and the potential for a therapeutic intervention via embolization. Disadvantages include an inability to identify venous bleeding and a major complication rate of up to 9.1% associated with contrast administration, femoral artery thrombosis, and transient cerebral ischemic events.[88] Multidetector computed tomography angiography is equivalent to peripheral angiography in its ability to detect the site of active bleeding and is increasingly used for this purpose.[89]

Embolization can be used for UGIB lesions particularly in the case of active massive bleeding that precludes the performance of endoscopy. Embolization in this setting rarely causes ischemia and has the advantage of averting surgery but is associated with rebleeding in up to 30% of cases.[90,91]

Angiography is indicated in patients with persistent recurrent LGIB without an identified source on endoscopy or with active massive bleeding that again precludes the performance of endoscopy. If identified during angiography, most LGIB are amenable to embolization with a high success rate. In the event that hemostasis is not achieved, the interventionalist may inject methylene blue at the bleeding site to facilitate a subsequent intraoperative surgical approach.[91]

Bleeding Scan

Nuclear scintigraphy with ^{99m}Tc-labeled red blood cells or ^{99m}Tc-sulfur colloid is indicated in patients who have an occult or intermittent source of LGIB that is undetected by endoscopy or angiography. It has the advantage of increased sensitivity compared with angiography and is able to detect bleeding at a rate of 0.1 mL/min. A significant drawback to nuclear scintigraphy is that its accuracy in localizing the bleeding source rapidly declines 2 hours after study initiation.[92]

TIPS

Endoscopic treatment failures in the management of esophageal varices require transjugular intrahepatic portosystemic shunt (TIPS). The right hepatic and portal veins are accessed percutaneously via the right internal jugular vein. A cannula is then inserted to create a portosystemic communication to reduce portal pressures. When embolization of varices is performed during TIPS, the success rate is high. Complications include worsening liver function, hepatic encephalopathy, and pulmonary hypertension.[93] TIPS can be used as a bridge to liver transplantation or for palliation in advanced-stage cirrhosis. Contraindications include severe hepatic failure, hepatic encephalopathy, polycystic liver disease, right-sided congestive heart failure, malignancy, sepsis, and severe coagulopathy.[94]

SURGERY

UGIB

The advent of PPIs and therapy for *H. pylori* infection have greatly reduced the need for surgical intervention in bleeding PUD.[91] The classic indications for surgical intervention for patients with refractory bleeding despite medical or endoscopic therapy include loss of 30% of the estimated blood volume in the first 24 hours, a requirement of greater than 1,500 mL of transfused blood per 24 hours to maintain stable hemodynamics, hemorrhage to the point of hypotension or shock, and recurrent bleeding during medical therapy.[50] Patients who require surgery carry a mortality of up to 25%. Repeat endoscopic therapy, however, has been shown to reduce the need for surgical intervention without increasing mortality.[95] Moreover, when compared with surgery, angiographic embolization appears to be equally efficacious and is associated with lower morbidity.[91]

LGIB

LGIB lesions that are not amenable to endoscopic intervention or angiographic embolization should be considered for surgery. Since intraoperative identification is not feasible, preoperative localization of the bleeding lesion is necessary to prevent blind resection of bowel segments.

▶ TRIAGE AND ADMISSION

It can be difficult to predict the outcome of patients with gastrointestinal bleeding from their initial presentation; however, some literature is available on this subject. Using the Glasgow-Blatchford scoring system, UGIB patients may be safely discharged if they meet the following criteria: Hb >12.9 g/dL in men or 11.9 g/dL in women, a systolic blood pressure >109 mm Hg, pulse <100/min, BUN level <18.2 mg/dL, no melena, no history of syncope, or no past or present liver disease or heart failure. Predictors of adverse outcome and severity in LGIB include hemodynamic instability 1 hour after initial evaluation, active gross bleeding per rectum, and initial HCT ≤35%.[96]

REFERENCES

1. Longstreth GF. Epidemiology of hospitalization for acute upper gastrointestinal hemorrhage: a population-based study. *Am J Gastroenterol.* 1995;90(2):206–210.
2. Blatchford O, Davidson LA, Murray WR, Blatchford M, Pell J. Acute upper gastrointestinal haemorrhage in west of Scotland: case ascertainment study. *BMJ.* 1997;315(7107):510–514.
3. Rockall TA, Logan RF, Devlin HB, Northfield TC. Incidence of and mortality from acute upper gastrointestinal haemorrhage in the United Kingdom. Steering Committee and members of the National Audit of Acute Upper Gastrointestinal Haemorrhage. *BMJ.* 1995;311(6999):222–226.
4. Vreeburg EM, Snel P, de Bruijne JW, Bartelsman JF, Rauws EA, Tytgat GN. Acute upper gastrointestinal bleeding in the Amsterdam area: incidence, diagnosis, and clinical outcome. *Am J Gastroenterol.* 1997;92(2):236–243.
5. Czernichow P, Hochain P, Nousbaum JB, et al. Epidemiology and course of acute upper gastro-intestinal haemorrhage in four French geographical areas. *Eur J Gastroenterol Hepatol.* 2000;12(2):175–181.
6. Paspatis GA, Matrella E, Kapsoritakis A, et al. An epidemiological study of acute upper gastrointestinal bleeding in Crete, Greece. *Eur J Gastroenterol Hepatol.* 2000;12(11):1215–1220.
7. Thomopoulos KC, Vagenas KA, Vagianos CE, et al. Changes in aetiology and clinical outcome of acute upper gastrointestinal bleeding during the last 15 years. *Eur J Gastroenterol Hepatol.* 2004;16(2):177–182.
8. Gralnek IM, Barkun AN, Bardou M. Management of acute bleeding from a peptic ulcer. *N Engl J Med.* 2008;359(9):928–937.
9. Fallah MA, Prakash C, Edmundowicz S. Acute gastrointestinal bleeding. *Med Clin North Am.* 2000;84(5):1183–1208.
10. van Leerdam ME, Vreeburg EM, Rauws EA, et al. Acute upper GI bleeding: did anything change? Time trend analysis of incidence and outcome of acute upper GI bleeding between 1993/1994 and 2000. *Am J Gastroenterol.* 2003;98(7):1494–1499.
11. Leontiadis GI, Howden CW. The role of proton pump inhibitors in the management of upper gastrointestinal bleeding. *Gastroenterol Clin North Am.* 2009;38(2):199–213.

12. van Leerdam ME. Epidemiology of acute upper gastro-intestinal bleeding. *Best Pract Res Clin Gastroenterol.* 2008;22(2):209–224.

13. Suerbaum S, Michetti P. *Helicobacter pylori* infection. *N Engl J Med.* 2002;347(15):1175–1186.

14. Barkun A, Sabbah S, Enns R, et al. The Canadian Registry on Nonvariceal Upper Gastrointestinal Bleeding and Endoscopy (RUGBE): endoscopic hemostasis and proton pump inhibition are associated with improved outcomes in a real-life setting. *Am J Gastroenterol.* 2004;99(7):1238–1246.

15. Lai KC, Hui WM, Wong WM, et al. Treatment of *Helicobacter pylori* in patients with duodenal ulcer hemorrhage—a long-term randomized, controlled study. *Am J Gastroenterol.* 2000;95(9):2225–2232.

16. Huang JQ, Sridhar S, Hunt RH. Role of *Helicobacter pylori* infection and non-steroidal anti-inflammatory drugs in peptic-ulcer disease: a meta-analysis. *Lancet.* 2002;359(9300):14–22.

17. Kurata JH, Corboy ED. Current peptic ulcer time trends. An epidemiological profile. *J Clin Gastroenterol.* 1988;10(3):259–268.

18. Stollman N, Metz DC. Pathophysiology and prophylaxis of stress ulcer in intensive care unit patients. *J Crit Care.* 2005;20(1):35–45.

19. Berzigotti A, Escorsell A, Bosch J. Pathophysiology of variceal bleeding in cirrhotics. *Ann Gastroenterol.* 2001;14(3):150–157.

20. Lecleire S, Di Fiore F, Merle V, et al. Acute upper gastro-intestinal bleeding in patients with liver cirrhosis and in noncirrhotic patients: epidemiology and predictive factors of mortality in a prospective multicenter population-based study. *J Clin Gastroenterol.* 2005;39(4):321–327.

21. Katz D, Freud M, McKinnon WM. The Mallory–Weiss syndrome: evaluation by early endoscopy of its clinical picture and its incidence in upper gastrointestinal hemorrhage. *Am J Dig Dis.* 1965;10:314–323.

22. Knauer CM. Mallory–Weiss syndrome. Characterization of 75 Mallory–Weiss lacerations in 528 patients with upper gastrointestinal hemorrhage. *Gastroenterology.* 1976;71(1):5–8.

23. Yen HH, Chen YY. Diagnosing Mallory–Weiss in the ED. *Am J Emerg Med.* 2009;27(8):1010.

24. Norfleet RG, Smith GH. Mallory–Weiss syndrome after cardiopulmonary resuscitation. *J Clin Gastroenterol.* 1990;12(5):569–572.

25. Younes Z, Johnson DA. The spectrum of spontaneous and iatrogenic esophageal injury: perforations, Mallory–Weiss tears, and hematomas. *J Clin Gastroenterol.* 1999;29(4):306–317.

26. Eisen GM, Baron TH, Dominitz JA, et al. Complications of upper GI endoscopy. *Gastrointest Endosc.* 2002;55(7):784–793.

27. Fleischner FG. Hiatal hernia complex; hiatal hernia, peptic esophagitis, Mallory–Weiss syndrome, hemorrhage and anemia, and marginal esophagogastric ulcer. *JAMA.* 1956;162(3):183–191.

28. Bharucha AE, Gostout CJ, Balm RK. Clinical and endoscopic risk factors in the Mallory–Weiss syndrome. *Am J Gastroenterol.* 1997;92(5):805–808.

29. Kim JW, Kim HS, Byun JW, et al. Predictive factors of recurrent bleeding in Mallory–Weiss syndrome. *Korean J Gastroenterol.* 2005;46(6):447–454.

30. Kortas DY, Haas LS, Simpson WG, Nickl NJ 3rd, Gates LK Jr. Mallory–Weiss tear: predisposing factors and predictors of a complicated course. *Am J Gastroenterol.* 2001;96(10):2863–2865.

31. Yarris JP, Warden CR. Gastrointestinal bleeding in the cancer patient. *Emerg Med Clin North Am.* 2009;27(3):363–379.

32. Cappell MS, Friedel D. The role of esophagogastroduodenoscopy in the diagnosis and management of upper gastrointestinal disorders. *Med Clin North Am.* 2002;86(6):1165–1216.

33. Cendan JC, Thomas JB 4th, Seeger JM. Twenty-one cases of aortoenteric fistula: lessons for the general surgeon. *Am Surg.* 2004;70(7):583–587. Discussion 587.

34. Peura DA, Lanza FL, Gostout CJ, Foutch PG. The American College of Gastroenterology Bleeding Registry: preliminary findings. *Am J Gastroenterol.* 1997;92(6):924–928.

35. Longstreth GF. Epidemiology and outcome of patients hospitalized with acute lower gastrointestinal hemorrhage: a population-based study. *Am J Gastroenterol.* 1997;92(3):419–424.

36. Zuccaro G. Epidemiology of lower gastrointestinal bleeding. *Best Pract Res Clin Gastroenterol.* 2008;22(2):225–232.

37. Strate LL, Saltzman JR, Ookubo R, Mutinga ML, Syngal S. Validation of a clinical prediction rule for severe acute lower intestinal bleeding. *Am J Gastroenterol.* 2005;100(8):1821–1827.

38. Vernava AM 3rd, Moore BA, Longo WE, Johnson FE. Lower gastrointestinal bleeding. *Dis Colon Rectum.* 1997;40(7):846–858.

39. Zuckerman GR, Prakash C. Acute lower intestinal bleeding. Part II: etiology, therapy, and outcomes. *Gastrointest Endosc.* 1999;49(2):228–238.

40. Kethu SR, Rich HG. Images in clinical medicine. Bleeding colonic diverticulum. *N Engl J Med.* 2003;349(25):2423.

41. Mimura T, Emanuel A, Kamm MA. Pathophysiology of diverticular disease. *Best Pract Res Clin Gastroenterol.* 2002;16(4):563–576.

42. Stollman N, Raskin JB. Diverticular disease of the colon. *Lancet.* 2004;363(9409):631–639.

43. Lewis M. Bleeding colonic diverticula. *J Clin Gastroenterol.* 2008;42(10):1156–1158.

44. Barnert J, Messmann H. Management of lower gastrointestinal tract bleeding. *Best Pract Res Clin Gastroenterol.* 2008;22(2):295–312.

45. Warkentin TE, Moore JC, Anand SS, Lonn EM, Morgan DG. Gastrointestinal bleeding, angiodysplasia, cardiovascular disease, and acquired von Willebrand syndrome. *Transfus Med Rev.* 2003;17(4):272–286.

46. Clouse R. *Textbook of Gastroenterology.* Vol 2. 3rd ed. Philadelphia, PA: Lippincott; 1999.

47. Jensen DM, Machicado GA. Colonoscopy for diagnosis and treatment of severe lower gastrointestinal bleeding. Routine outcomes and cost analysis. *Gastrointest Endosc Clin N Am.* 1997;7(3):477–498.

48. Chalasani N, Wilcox CM. Gastrointestinal hemorrhage in patients with AIDS. *AIDS Patient Care STDS.* 1999;13(6):343–346.

49. Henrion J, Schapira M, Ghilain JM, et al. Upper gastrointestinal bleeding: what has changed during the last 20 years? *Gastroenterol Clin Biol.* September 2008.

50. Larson DE, Farnell MB. Upper gastrointestinal hemorrhage. *Mayo Clin Proc.* 1983;58(6):371–387.

51. Ernst AA, Haynes ML, Nick TG, Weiss SJ. Usefulness of the blood urea nitrogen/creatinine ratio in gastrointestinal bleeding. *Am J Emerg Med.* 1999;17(1):70–72.

52. Vale JA, Kulig K. Position paper: gastric lavage. *J Toxicol Clin Toxicol.* 2004;42(7):933–943.

53. Lee SD, Kearney DJ. A randomized controlled trial of gastric lavage prior to endoscopy for acute upper gastrointestinal bleeding. *J Clin Gastroenterol.* 2004;38(10):861–865.

54. Leather RA, Sullivan SN. Iced gastric lavage: a tradition without foundation. *CMAJ.* 1987;136(12):1245–1247.

55. Witting MD, Magder L, Heins AE, Mattu A, Granja CA, Baumgarten M. Usefulness and validity of diagnostic nasogastric aspiration in patients without hematemesis. *Ann Emerg Med.* 2004;43(4):525–532.

56. Witting MD, Magder L, Heins AE, Mattu A, Granja CA, Baumgarten M. ED predictors of upper gastrointestinal tract bleeding in patients without hematemesis. *Am J Emerg Med.* 2006;24(3):280–285.

57. Hebert PC, Wells G, Blajchman MA, et al. A multicenter, randomized, controlled clinical trial of transfusion requirements in critical care. Transfusion Requirements in Critical Care Investigators, Canadian Critical Care Trials Group. *N Engl J Med.* 1999;340(6):409–417.

58. Wu WC, Rathore SS, Wang Y, Radford MJ, Krumholz HM. Blood transfusion in elderly patients with acute myocardial infarction. *N Engl J Med.* 2001;345(17):1230–1236.

59. Dell'Era A, de Franchis R, Iannuzzi F. Acute variceal bleeding: pharmacological treatment and primary/secondary prophylaxis. *Best Pract Res Clin Gastroenterol.* 2008;22(2):279–294.

60. Hearnshaw S, Travis S, Murphy M. The role of blood transfusion in the management of upper and lower intestinal tract bleeding. *Best Pract Res Clin Gastroenterol.* 2008;22(2):355–371.

61. Malone DL, Hess JR, Fingerhut A. Massive transfusion practices around the globe and a suggestion for a common massive transfusion protocol. *J Trauma.* 2006;60(6 suppl):S91–S96.

62. Gonzalez EA, Moore FA, Holcomb JB, et al. Fresh frozen plasma should be given earlier to patients requiring massive transfusion. *J Trauma.* 2007;62(1):112–119.

63. Aabakken L. Current endoscopic and pharmacological therapy of peptic ulcer bleeding. *Best Pract Res Clin Gastroenterol.* 2008;22(2):243–259.

64. Leontiadis GI, Sharma VK, Howden CW. Systematic review and meta-analysis of proton pump inhibitor therapy in peptic ulcer bleeding. *BMJ.* 2005;330(7491):568.

65. Lau JY, Leung WK, Wu JC, et al. Omeprazole before endoscopy in patients with gastrointestinal bleeding. *N Engl J Med.* 2007;356(16):1631–1640.

66. Sgouros SN, Bergele C, Viazis N, Avgerinos A. Somatostatin and its analogues in peptic ulcer bleeding: facts and pathophysiological aspects. *Dig Liver Dis.* 2006;38(2):143–148.

67. Collins D, Worthley LI. Acute gastrointestinal bleeding: part II. *Crit Care Resusc.* 2001;3(2):117–124.

68. Arfaoui D, Elloumi H, Ajmi S. Octreotide in the treatment of acute gastrointestinal hemorrhage caused by ruptured esophageal varices. *Tunis Med.* 2004;82(10):947–950.

69. Talbot-Stern JK. Gastrointestinal bleeding. *Emerg Med Clin North Am.* 1996;14(1):173–184.

70. Bauer JJ, Kreel I, Kark AE. The use of the Sengstaken–Blakemore tube for immediate control of bleeding esophageal varices. *Ann Surg.* 1974;179(3):273–277.

71. Conn HO, Simpson JA. Excessive mortality associated with balloon tamponade of bleeding varices. A critical reappraisal. *JAMA.* 1967;202(7):587–591.

72. Chien JY, Yu CJ. Images in clinical medicine. Malposition of a Sengstaken–Blakemore tube. *N Engl J Med.* 2005;352(8):e7.

73. Roberts JR, Hedges JR, eds. *Clinical Procedures in Emergency Medicine.* 4th ed. Philadelphia: WB Saunders; 2003.

74. Chojkier M, Conn HO. Esophageal tamponade in the treatment of bleeding varices. A decadel progress report. *Dig Dis Sci.* 1980;25(4):267–272.

75. Soares-Weiser K, Brezis M, Tur-Kaspa R, Leibovici L. Antibiotic prophylaxis for cirrhotic patients with gastrointestinal bleeding. *Cochrane Database Syst Rev.* 2002;(2):CD002907.

76. Bernard B, Grange JD, Khac EN, Amiot X, Opolon P, Poynard T. Antibiotic prophylaxis for the prevention of bacterial infections in cirrhotic patients with gastrointestinal bleeding: a meta-analysis. *Hepatology.* 1999;29(6):1655–1661.

77. Rimola A, Garcia-Tsao G, Navasa M, et al. Diagnosis, treatment and prophylaxis of spontaneous bacterial peritonitis: a consensus document. International Ascites Club. *J Hepatol.* 2000;32(1):142–153.

78. de Franchis R. Evolving consensus in portal hypertension. Report of the Baveno IV consensus workshop on methodology of diagnosis and therapy in portal hypertension. *J Hepatol.* 2005;43(1):167–176.

79. Villanueva C, Colomo A, Aracil C, Guarner C. Current endoscopic therapy of variceal bleeding. *Best Pract Res Clin Gastroenterol.* 2008;22(2):261–278.

80. Lee JG, Turnipseed S, Romano PS, et al. Endoscopy-based triage significantly reduces hospitalization rates and costs of treating upper GI bleeding: a randomized controlled trial. *Gastrointest Endosc.* 1999;50(6):755–761.

81. Avgerinos A, Nevens F, Raptis S, Fevery J. Early administration of somatostatin and efficacy of sclerotherapy in acute oesophageal variceal bleeds: the European Acute Bleeding Oesophageal Variceal Episodes (ABOVE) randomised trial. *Lancet.* 1997;350(9090):1495–1499.

82. Villanueva C, Piqueras M, Aracil C, et al. A randomized controlled trial comparing ligation and sclerotherapy as emergency endoscopic treatment added to somatostatin in acute variceal bleeding. *J Hepatol.* 2006;45(4):560–567.

83. Banares R, Albillos A, Rincon D, et al. Endoscopic treatment versus endoscopic plus pharmacologic treatment

for acute variceal bleeding: a meta-analysis. *Hepatology.* 2002;35(3):609–615.

84. Jensen DM, Machicado GA. Diagnosis and treatment of severe hematochezia. The role of urgent colonoscopy after purge. *Gastroenterology.* 1988;95(6):1569–1574.

85. Davila RE, Rajan E, Adler DG, et al. ASGE guideline: the role of endoscopy in the patient with lower-GI bleeding. *Gastrointest Endosc.* 2005;62(5):656–660.

86. Green BT, Rockey DC, Portwood G, et al. Urgent colonoscopy for evaluation and management of acute lower gastrointestinal hemorrhage: a randomized controlled trial. *Am J Gastroenterol.* 2005;100(11):2395–2402.

87. Jensen DM, Machicado GA, Jutabha R, Kovacs TO. Urgent colonoscopy for the diagnosis and treatment of severe diverticular hemorrhage. *N Engl J Med.* 2000;342(2): 78–82.

88. Egglin TK, O'Moore PV, Feinstein AR, Waltman AC. Complications of peripheral arteriography: a new system to identify patients at increased risk. *J Vasc Surg.* 1995;22(6):787–794.

89. Yoon W, Jeong YY, Shin SS, et al. Acute massive gastrointestinal bleeding: detection and localization with arterial phase multi-detector row helical CT. *Radiology.* 2006;239(1):160–167.

90. Ripoll C, Banares R, Beceiro I, et al. Comparison of transcatheter arterial embolization and surgery for treatment of bleeding peptic ulcer after endoscopic treatment failure. *J Vasc Interv Radiol.* 2004;15(5):447–450.

91. Busch OR, van Delden OM, Gouma DJ. Therapeutic options for endoscopic haemostatic failures: the place of the surgeon and radiologist in gastrointestinal tract bleeding. *Best Pract Res Clin Gastroenterol.* 2008;22(2): 341–354.

92. Dusold R, Burke K, Carpentier W, Dyck WP. The accuracy of technetium-99m-labeled red cell scintigraphy in localizing gastrointestinal bleeding. *Am J Gastroenterol.* 1994;89(3):345–348.

93. Rossle M, Haag K, Ochs A, et al. The transjugular intrahepatic portosystemic stent–shunt procedure for variceal bleeding. *N Engl J Med.* 1994;330(3):165–171.

94. Colombato L. The role of transjugular intrahepatic portosystemic shunt (TIPS) in the management of portal hypertension. *J Clin Gastroenterol.* 2007;41(suppl 3):S344–S351.

95. Lau JY, Sung JJ, Lam YH, et al. Endoscopic retreatment compared with surgery in patients with recurrent bleeding after initial endoscopic control of bleeding ulcers. *N Engl J Med.* 1999;340(10):751–756.

96. Velayos FS, Williamson A, Sousa KH, et al. Early predictors of severe lower gastrointestinal bleeding and adverse outcomes: a prospective study. *Clin Gastroenterol Hepatol.* 2004;2(6):485–490.

CHAPTER 20

Acute Liver Failure: How to Orchestrate Emergency Critical Care Interventions

Thomas H. Kalb and Jennifer A. Frontera

A patient who presents emergently with acute liver failure (ALF) has an overall greater likelihood of either dying or requiring emergent transplantation than recovering without transplant.[1] Regardless of etiology, the unifying feature of ALF is a compact clinical timeline and a rapid, often precipitous natural history of disease. Whereas spontaneous recovery of liver function is possible with supportive measures, particularly with acetaminophen overdose, there remains a significant risk of spiraling decline after presentation with multiorgan failure, bleeding, and infectious complications often heralded by high-grade encephalopathy with cerebral edema.[2]

The key message for the emergency critical care practitioner is that first contact with a patient with ALF requires an orchestrated team effort to be triggered to rapidly and efficiently triage and mobilize management resources. Because of the rarity and complexity of ALF, it has been argued that ALF is best managed within the framework of a previously defined protocol, similar to the standards that have gained broad acceptance in stroke and acute coronary syndrome.[3] Such team efforts are crucial to give the patient with ALF the best opportunity for transplant-free survival. In the setting of deteriorating status, teams are required to rapidly mobilize those resources, interventions, and caregivers that are crucial to provide stabilization and life support as well as to triage rapidly and for transplantation in a crisis setting when time course may not forgive hesitation.

Recommendations and best evidence for developing this approach are substantially informed by the Acute Liver Failure Study Group (ALFSG) registry from a consortium of transplant centers that continues to prospectively collect data, report their findings, and grade level of evidence.[4] This chapter is designed as a practical guide for the emergency critical care practitioner to provide an organizational framework for key clinical interventions.

▶ FIRST CONTACT: HOW TO RECOGNIZE, DIAGNOSE, EXCLUDE MIMICS, AND PROVIDE EARLY TRANSPLANT TRIAGE

Often used interchangeably, both the terms ALF and fulminant hepatic failure are defined by the new onset of hepatocellular dysfunction as reflected by coagulopathy (INR >1.5) and encephalopathy in the absence of preexisting liver disease.[5] By convention, the further stratification of fulminant hepatic failure is based on the rapidity of encephalopathy onset in the course of illness: less than 2 weeks for acute fulminant and 8 weeks for subfulminant.[6] The ALFSG study consortium has extended that time course up to 26 weeks for entry in their multicenter data analysis, and have adopted the preferred eponymous term arguing that this captures the variable pace of illness in ALF, and better encompasses an extended range of patients who share epidemiologic, etiologic, physiologic, and management characteristics.[7] In the absence of encephalopathy or coagulopathy, population-based studies of patients at risk of ALF have defined hepatotoxicity by ALT >1,000.[8]

HOW TO SUSPECT AND MAKE THE DIAGNOSIS

As suggested by the variable terminology, the patient with ALF in the absence of prior liver disease may present with a strikingly distinct duration of symptoms, variable chief complaints, and without a clear-cut history, particularly if transaminase and INR determination are not part of initial screen. A common symptom complex of subacute fatigue, malaise, nausea, and mental status changes may be subtle and may not point overtly to ALF. Therefore, a high level of suspicion and awareness of vague or nonspecific complaints is required for an astute and rapid recognition of this disease.

EPIDEMIOLOGY, ETIOLOGY, AND OUTCOMES

The emergency critical care examiner should be aware of the common etiologic categories so as to focus attention during this key initial encounter.

A handful of categories account for the bulk of etiologies, although the complete list of possible causes is extensive. In North America, acetaminophen accounts for nearly half of the ALF caused by drug toxicity, followed distantly in etiologic prevalence by antituberculous (particularly INH and PZA), antiseizure (particularly valproic acid), and antibiotic medications.[9] Other identifiable causes of ALF include acute hepatitis B virus (HBV) infection (7%), other viral infections (3%), autoimmune hepatitis (5%), ischemic hepatitis (4%), and various other causes (5%) such as Wilson's disease, pregnancy-associated ALF, and other metabolic pathway abnormalities. Of importance, up to 15% of ALF cases remain of indeterminate etiology.[9]

As such, the first and perhaps most essential challenge is to make every attempt to obtain a complete and detailed ingestion history. To be sure, this should include all prescribed medication along with an accurate timeline. But of equal, if not more pressing, importance in the setting of ALF is that every attempt must be made to identify all nonprescription therapy, illicit drug use, and alternative/nontraditional and herbal remedy use, and to inquire about nonmedicinal ingestions (e.g., *Amanita* mushroom, nutritional or fitness supplements) that are new or noteworthy.[10] Alcohol consumption should be scrutinized, although underreporting should

be objectively ascertained by blood levels.[11] Likewise, acetaminophen overdose may be underappreciated or the result of unintentional therapeutic misadventure, and the toxicity profile may be affected by sustained or coadministration.[12] As such, it must be impressed upon the patient and family members to recall and report all recent therapies, including familiar household remedies that might be considered innocuous.

Etiology has a measurable effect on outcome. ALF from acetaminophen overdose, pregnancy, and hepatitis A has a more favorable outcome with transplant-free survival approaching 50%.[13] Spontaneous recovery is least likely with Wilson's disease, nonacetaminophen idiosyncratic drug reactions, and indeterminant causes.[14] Patients who suffer ALF due to antiepileptic medications have a significantly higher death rate after liver transplant than patients who have ALF due to other drugs.[15]

Early identification of a causal agent may be of therapeutic importance. Although treatment pathways are largely supportive and apply generically, some therapeutics may be tailored to specific etiology and may be time sensitive (see below).

INITIAL LAB TESTS: DIAGNOSIS, PROGNOSIS, AND TRANSPLANT SCREENS

In the context of history taking challenges, initial laboratory studies are crucial to sift through the diagnostic questions, and to lay the groundwork for assessment of transplant candidacy. In addition to liver function testing and INR, initial screening etiologic diagnostic studies should be sent as soon as feasible. Acetaminophen levels provide best guidance in the setting of single ingestion history, where prediction by nomogram has the greatest utility if the timing of ingestion is verifiably ascertained.[16] Liver failure is typically associated with single ingestion in excess of 10 g, and unlikely with less than 4 g.[17] However, in the setting of polypharmacy coingestion or chronic ingestion, a far lower intermittent dosage may result in hepatocellular loss. Accordingly, the receiver operating characteristic of a single acetaminophen level may have reduced negative predictive power in these settings, and thus cannot exclude acetaminophen toxicity as causal.[18] Assay for acetaminophen–protein adducts may be available in some centers, and this sensitive assay may provide clues of unappreciated acetaminophen toxicity when ALF etiology remains indeterminate.[19]

Initial evaluation should also help to discriminate among mimics that may confusingly present with a similar triad of transaminitis or hyperbilirubinemia, coagulopathy, and altered mental status. When an initial exam suggests another etiology, ultrasound examination may provide clues to biliary tract obstruction, infiltrative hepatopathy, tumor, hepatic vein obstruction, or acute exacerbation of chronic liver disease. Nonprimary hepatic disease such as sepsis, hemolytic crisis, and acute pericardial constriction may confound the first responder if coagulation abnormalities or hyperbilirubinemia are prominent. Warfarin ingestion and consumptive coagulopathy must be considered with isolated coagulopathy. Also, adverse drug reactions may occur in the context of superimposed or concomitant illness that may further cloud the distinction between hepatocellular injury and another systemic illness.

Once the diagnosis of ALF is firmly suspected or confirmed, it is essential to obtain a battery of additional laboratory studies without delay. These studies are designed to discriminate among principal ALF etiologies, further characterize the extent of hepatocellular injury, screen for metabolic derangement, and elicit nonhepatic issues that may need attention or may impact on transplant candidacy. Table 20-1 provides a comprehensive list of lab tests that are indicated. Given the magnitude and complexity of this large list, a pre-established order set that is triggered by protocol is highly recommended.

PROGNOSTICATING FROM FIRST CONTACT

Establishing a clear baseline for serial comparison and ALF trajectory is critical for subsequent decision making. Composite history, physical findings, and initial laboratory findings from first contact will form the basis of risk stratification and most importantly for comparative serial examinations that are crucial to the decision to list a patient for transplantation. The most commonly used prognostic classification scheme, the King's College Hospital criteria (see Table 20-2), uses simple measures that negatively predict transplant-free survival, originally derived from a cohort of acetaminophen-induced ALF.[20] An unambiguous baseline and a standardized plan to serially obtain and clearly document these specific components should be part of the emergency critical care team plan.

Data that support the additive value of additional serum markers of poor outcome have been debated among the transplant community.[21–23] Likewise, disease-specific prognostic indices have been evaluated in relatively small cohorts that require further validation.[24] Overall, the predictive value of any modality, including the King's College Hospital criteria, may be influenced by the interruption of the natural history of disease by transplant itself. Of course, the decision, timing, availability, and effectiveness of transplantation in any given case and in different settings compound the difficulty of comparative predictive models.

▶ **TABLE 20-1. IMMEDIATE SCREENING LABORATORY SCREEN ON SUSPICION OF ALF**

Document hepatocellular injury and initiate systemic/etiologic inquiry	Liver function panel
	PT/INR
	CBC w/ diff and platelets
	Fibrinogen
	Acetaminophen level (adduct if available)
	Toxicology screen
	Electrolytes/creatinine/uric acid
	Blood cultures
Etiology evaluation	Cytomegalovirus IgG
	Epstein–Barr virus IgG
	Hepatitis A virus IgM
	Hepatitis B virus DNA (quantitative)
	Hepatitis B surface antigen
	Hepatitis B surface antibody
	Hepatitis B core antibody
	α-Fetoprotein
	Ceruloplasmin
	Serum protein electrophoresis
	α-Smooth muscle antibody
	Antimitochondrial antibody
	Antinuclear antibody
	Liver kidney microsome antibody
	Hepatitis C virus RNA (quantitative)
Severity of hepatic and extrahepatic disturbance/ transplant triage	Urinalysis
	Arterial blood gas
	Arterial lactate
	ABO (two separate tests, 2 h apart)
	Repeat PT/INR q6 h
	Repeat transaminase level q6 h
	Repeat total and direct bilirubin q6 h

▶ **TABLE 20-2. PREDICTORS OF INCREASED MORTALITY WITHOUT EMERGENT TRANSPLANT: KING'S COLLEGE CRITERIA**

- In acetaminophen-induced ALF
  - Prothrombin time greater than 100 s (INR >6.5)
  - Arterial pH <7.30
  - Grade 3 or 4 encephalopathy
  - Serum creatinine >300 mcg/mL (3.4 mg/dL)
- In nonacetaminophen-induced ALF
  - PT greater than 100 s
  - Or three of the following five criteria:
    - Patient age less than 10 or greater than 40
    - Hepatitis due to non-A/non-B virus, halothane, or drug reaction
    - Delayed onset of encephalopathy (>1 week after onset of jaundice)
    - PT greater than 50 s (INR >3.5)
    - Serum total bilirubin >17.5 mg/dL (300 mmol/L)

Data from O'Grady JG, Alexander GJ, Hayllar KM, et al. Early indicators of prognosis in fulminant hepatic failure. *Gastroenterology.* 1989;97:439–445.

▶ SUPPORTIVE THERAPY

HOW TO MANAGE HEMODYNAMIC SUPPORT

With progressive decline in liver function, a hyperdynamic state with low systemic vascular resistance may predominate the clinical picture, and be reminiscent of, and clinically indistinguishable from, severe sepsis. This feature correlates with the Sequential Organ Failure Assessment (SOFA) score, arterial lactate, and mortality.[25] It is imperative that the mean arterial pressure (MAP) is maintained above 50–60 mm Hg to preserve organ perfusion and maintain a cerebral perfusion pressure (CPP) of >50 mm Hg. Volume resuscitation with 20–25 mL/kg isotonic crystalloid is an appropriate first maneuver, although if the patient is not responsive to an initial fluid challenge, norepinephrine is recommended.[4] There are no strict prohibitions with regard to the adverse effect of vasopressors on ALF, although experimentally, the use of vasopressin appears to have a greater predilection for cerebral vasodilation.[26]

Adrenal hyporesponsiveness has been shown to have a high incidence in ALF, and corticosteroid replacement, though controversial, may be prudent and is recommended by ALFSG in refractory hypotension.[4] Capillary permeability disturbance precipitates an increase in extravascular lung water with minimal hydrostatic pressure elevation, particularly in patients with cerebral edema, that leads to a picture of ARDS.[27] Echocardiography is indicated to exclude superimposed cardiac contractile dysfunction, pericardial disease, or undisclosed regional wall motion abnormality that may point to cardiac comorbidity and impact on surgical and anesthesia tolerance. Troponin leak is prevalent in ALF with shock, as in other forms of critical illness, and this represents a poor prognostic sign.[4]

WHEN TO INITIATE EMPIRICAL ANTIBIOTICS

With an increased duration and severity of liver dysfunction, the incidence of systemic infection rises, with bacterial and fungal sepsis reported, stemming from a blunted innate immune response coupled with catheter- and ventilator-associated barrier disruption.[4] Recommendations for empirical administration of antibiotics in the presence of systemic inflammatory response syndrome and refractory hypotension, and with progression to advanced-stage hepatic encephalopathy in the patients listed for liver transplant are based in part on the difficulty in parsing signs and symptoms that point to systemic infection in this setting.[4]

MANAGEMENT OF BLEEDING AND BLEEDING RISK

The basic guideline for the emergency critical care practitioner is to recall the central tenet of avoiding injudicious use of plasma components that might obscure the triage assessment. These products increase the risk for gas exchange disturbance due to alveolar flooding, and should be avoided unless confronted with significant bleeding or concern for hemostatic integrity in conjunction with contemplated invasive procedure.[4]

Patients in fulminant liver failure can present with abnormalities at multiple levels of the coagulation cascade. Aside from coagulation factor and fibrinogen deficiency due to synthesis disorders, patients may also present with thrombocytopenia due to splenic sequestration, disseminated intravascular coagulopathy, or platelet abnormalities because of uremia and acute renal insufficiency. It has been recommended that the use of recombinant factor VIIa (rFVIIa) be restricted to coagulopathy reversal only in the setting of severe volume overload with predicted FFP intolerance, or prior to high-risk procedures such as liver biopsy or intracranial pressure (ICP) monitor placement. Use of rFVIIa does not replete other depleted coagulation factors and carries a higher risk of DIC than other agents.[28] Additionally, the rate of arterial thrombotic events with rFVIIa is as high as 8.5%.[29]

Unactivated prothrombin complex concentrates (PCC) are marketed as Bebulin and Profilnine in the United States and Octaplex in Europe, and are sometimes referred to as factor IX concentrates. These include varying amounts of factors II, VII, IX, and X and proteins C and S. Using PCC, coagulopathy reversal of multiple factors can be achieved quickly with minimal volume and at a lower expense than rFVIIa. Since PCC does not contain factor V, some hematologists recommend additional FFP to replace this factor. All patients should receive vitamin K 10 mg intravenous (IV) once. Additionally, if the fibrinogen level is below 100 mg/dL, patients should be repleted with cryoprecipitate. Patients who have renal insufficiency should receive DDAVP 0.3 mcg/kg once for uremia-induced platelet dysfunction.

Adequate laboratory values for the placement of an ICP monitor include INR <1.5, platelets >50,000/mm^3, fibrinogen >100 mg/dL, and a normal PTT. It should be noted that multiple doses of rFVIIa or combining rFVIIa with PCC is not recommended as this can dramatically increase the risk of DIC and DIC-related complications. In patients with persistent coagulopathy, plasma exchange has been shown to be effective.[4] This may be an especially attractive option in patients who already have a dialysis catheter in place and who can tolerate an interruption from renal replacement therapy to undergo plasma exchange.

CENTRAL LINE TIMING AND SAFETY ISSUES WITH PLACEMENT

In patients with severe encephalopathy, it is most prudent to combine the acts of sedation, intubation, central line access, and blood product support, followed by an assessment for transport to computed tomography (CT) that should include a head and abdominal CT. Concern for enhanced risk of catheter-associated bloodstream infection limits the utility and may increase the hazard of femoral site placement. An internal jugular (IJ) approach is preferred over the subclavian because of improved ultrasound visualization and compressibility. Additionally, there are no contraindications to IJ line placement in patients with an elevated ICP, although maintaining the head in neutral position and avoiding bilateral IJ cannulation is preferred.

ELECTROLYTE AND FLUID MANAGEMENT

Hypoglycemia is common and needs to be expectantly screened for and managed with glucose-containing solutions as hepatic function deteriorates. Metabolic acidosis often complicates ALF, with decreased lactate flux, increased lactate production, and strong ion gap values that maintain a persistent base deficit despite the alkalinizing effects of hypoalbuminemia and hypochloremia.[30] Likewise, citrate-, acetate-, and gluconate-containing solutions may be poorly handled by the failing liver, and may represent an additional burden of unmeasured anions that can contribute to a strong ion difference and unmitigated acidosis.[31]

To avoid excess free water administration, glucose should be administered as 10% solution. Multiple aspects of ALF tend to produce hyponatremia. A deleterious effect of poorly managed water balance on patient outcomes has been observed, with both worsening encephalopathy and a significant decline in posttransplant neurologic recovery, in those recipients who had Na <130 at the time of surgery.[32] Hypophosphatemia is a notable exception to the deleterious effect of electrolyte disturbance, in that this abnormality has been attributed to recovering hepatocyte mass, and is considered to be a marker of renewed metabolic activity.[4]

WHEN TO INITIATE RENAL REPLACEMENT THERAPY

Oliguria and renal failure are common features that accompany ALF. The predilection for renal failure is highest in acetaminophen toxicity but may be precipitated in all forms of ALF.[16] The pathophysiology is likely multifactorial and may include hypovolemia, acute medullary cortical microcirculatory disturbance

with sodium avid renal failure similar to hepatorenal syndrome, or tubular damage directly from toxins including acetaminophen adducts or associated reactive oxygen species.[33] The recovery of renal function tends to mirror that of hepatic function, so that spontaneous improvement with recovery, or after transplantation, is often seen. Nonetheless, early introduction of renal replacement therapy is recommended for patients with progressive oliguria, particularly in the setting of electrolyte disturbance and volume overload, and to assist the management of plasma administration or osmotic therapies.[4] Continuous venovenous hemofiltration (CVVH) is the preferred modality by ALFSG recommendations, based on its smoother hemodynamic profile, less precipitous fluid shifts, the ability to rapidly and continuously address electrolyte disturbance, and manage osmotic therapy.[4]

SPECIFIC THERAPEUTIC INITIATIVES

Specific therapies for unique causes of ALF are few and are detailed below.

The toxic acetaminophen metabolite N-acetyl-p-benzoquinone imine (NAPQI) is normally detoxified by glutathione conjugation. N-Acetylcysteine (NAC) for acetaminophen overdose by either oral or IV route is indicated to replenish glutathione stores, and may further act by antioxidant and vasoactive mechanisms. The IV route has the advantage of improved GI tolerance and eliminates problems related to absorption.[4] Moreover, based on accumulating evidence for transplant-free survival benefit and its generally favorable safety profile, IV NAC should be strongly considered for patients with early stage nonacetaminophen ALF.[34] Treatment should be initiated immediately when ALF or hepatotoxicity is established, with a loading dose of 150 mg/kg in 500 mL dextrose 5% over 30 minutes, followed by maintenance dose 50 mg/kg over 4 hours, and then 125 mg/kg in 1,000 mL dextrose 5% over 19 hours. Most experts recommend a continuous IV infusion of NAC until the INR is less than 1.5. Because of risk of hypersensitivity reaction, IV NAC should always be administered in a monitored setting, and patients with mild allergic symptoms should have the infusion rate decreased by 50% and receive corticosteroids and antihistamine.

Other therapies in use, but of unproven benefit, include activated charcoal and high-dose IV penicillin for mushroom poisoning and corticosteroids for autoimmune hepatitis. However, corticosteroids had no demonstrated benefit in a trial of drug-induced ALF. Other emergent interventions that apply to specific etiologies include prompt delivery for pregnancy-related ALF. Consultation with the transplantation team should be conducted before initiation of etiology-specific therapy with unproven initiatives such as copper chelation, plasmapheresis, and antioxidant therapy for Wilson's disease; lamivudine or entecavir for acute hepatitis B; acyclovir for herpes simplex virus infection; and decompressive surgery or transjugular intrahepatic portosystemic shunts (TIPS) for acute Budd–Chiari syndrome.[9]

EMERGING THERAPEUTIC OPTIONS IN ALF

Hemofiltration and hemodialysis have limited capacity to remove protein-bound toxins, but newer, experimental techniques have been developed to deal with these substances. Several configurations of so-called liver support modalities have been reported in nonrandomized studies, and the results of multicenter trials are awaited. Both cell-free and bioartificial systems have been developed with the aim to remove known and unknown toxins that are released and not cleared in ALF. At present, the use of these devices has not been reported to change mortality, although endpoints such as reduced encephalopathy have raised interest in pursuing this line of research; however, their use should be considered experimental.[35]

Bridging therapies, such as auxiliary orthotopic transplant and two-stage transplantation where hepatectomy precedes transplantation by a variable interval up to days, are controversial, and have only been reported anecdotally. These extraordinary procedures are attempted only in specialized centers under dire circumstances, as in the setting of unavailable allograft in a patient with unmitigated intracranial hypertension.[36]

► ORCHESTRATING THE RESPONSE TO WORSENING ENCEPHALOPATHY

HOW TO EVALUATE MENTAL STATUS

Hepatic encephalopathy is a reversible form of neurologic dysfunction. Although its pathogenesis is not entirely understood, it is thought to be primarily due to ammonia-induced neurotoxicity. Ammonia, produced either by catabolism of nitrogenous sources or by glutamine metabolism at a mitochondrial level, has been shown to lead to astrocyte swelling and dysfunction.[37] Metabolism of glutamine into glutamate and ammonia may additionally cause stimulation of N-methyl-D-aspartic acid (NMDA) receptors triggering nitric oxide release and subsequent vasodilation. This vasodilation may lead to hyperemia and cerebral edema.[38] Additionally, cerebral autoregulation has been found to be impaired in patients with fulminant hepatic failure.[39] A variety of other mechanisms may be involved in the pathogenesis of hepatic encephalopathy including inflammation, activation of the aquaporin-4 water channel protein on astrocytes, oxindole (a tryptophan metabolite), as well as catecholamine and other neurotransmitter abnormalities.[40]

The result of this abnormal neurochemical milieu is cerebral edema, which occurs in 80% of comatose patients with acute hepatic failure and is the leading cause of death among patients suffering from fulminant ALF.[41] Hepatic encephalopathy is graded as depicted in Table 20-3.

► TABLE 20-3. HEPATIC ENCEPHALOPATHY GRADE

Grade	Level of Consciousness/ Cognitive Function	Neuromuscular Function	Psychiatric Symptoms
1	Sleep disturbance Mild confusion Impaired computations	Tremor Incoordination ±Asterixis	Euphoria/depression
2	Inattentive Moderate confusion Disorientation to time	Asterixis Slurred speech Impaired handwriting	Irritability Decreased inhibitions Personality changes
3	Marked confusion Completely disoriented Lethargic, but arousable Command following	Slurred speech Ataxia Asterixis Nystagmus Hypoactive or hyperactive reflexes	Anxiety or apathy Inappropriate or bizarre behavior Paranoia, anger, or rage
4	Noncommand following Coma	Dilated pupils Loss of cranial nerve reflexes Signs of herniation Flexor or extensor posturing Loss of reflexes	Coma

The neurologic exam should be conducted in patients who have been free of sedation for as long as possible, balancing the risks of agitation that may elevate ICP. Since neuromuscular blockade can alter brainstem reflexes and the motor exam, recently intubated patients should be tested with a train of four stimulations to ensure that neuromuscular blockade is not confounding the neurologic assessment. Table 20-4 shows an outline of neurologic domains that should be assessed in all ALF patients.

WHEN TO OBTAIN HEAD CT SCAN

Any patient with an acute deterioration in mental status or focal findings on exam should undergo a noncontrast head CT to assess for intracranial hemorrhage. Apart from this, a head CT is recommended in any patient with stage III or IV encephalopathy to evaluate for cerebral edema.[4] A normal head CT does not rule out elevated ICP and should not be used as a surrogate for ICP monitoring. In addition to a baseline CT, a head

► TABLE 20-4. **NEUROLOGIC ASSESSMENT OF THE PATIENT WITH ALF**

Neurologic Domain	Exam Features	Alarming Findings
Mental status	Orientation to self, place, time Level of attentiveness (backwards counting or months) Evaluate language (command following, fluency, naming, repeating) Evaluate higher-level cognitive functioning (calculation, praxis) Evaluate for mood disturbance	No command following Does not open eyes to voice or tactile/noxious stimulation No verbal output Does not track or saccade to voice Any change in level of attentiveness should trigger a more aggressive neurologic evaluation
Cranial nerves	Pupil reactivity, diameter, symmetry Fundoscopy to assess for papilledema, retinal hemorrhages Oculocephalic reflex (doll's eyes) Corneal reactivity (tests CN V afferent, VII efferent) Trigeminal sensation Facial symmetry Gag, palate elevation Tongue deviation	Dysarthria may indicate facial weakness or cerebellar dysfunction Loss of brainstem reflexes is an ominous sign Asymmetric pupil dilatation may indicate herniation
Motor exam	Assess upper and lower extremity motor strength Pronator drift may be an early sign of focal abnormality Noxious stimuli may be necessary to assess for posturing in grade 3 and 4 patients Assess for asterixis by having patients holding out hands as though the patient is "stopping traffic." Asterixis is negative myoclonus or loss of muscle tone and can prompt falls if lower extremity asterixis is present	Any new focal deficit should raise concern for intracranial hemorrhage Flexor or extensor posturing occurs in grade 4 encephalopathy
Sensory exam	Test to modalities of light touch, pinprick, pain, temperature, vibration, and proprioception	The sensory exam is notoriously unreliable in encephalopathic or inattentive patients
Cerebellar exam	Appendicular function: finger to nose, heel to shin Axial function: titubation, dysarthria, ataxia	Cerebellar dysfunction occurs early in hepatic encephalopathy
Gait	Evaluate normal gait, toe and heel walking and tandem gait, Romberg testing	Wide-based gait and an inability to place feet together or in tandem indicate cerebellar dysfunction
Reflexes	Deep tendon reflexes are graded as absent, 1+ (diminished), 2+ (normal), 3+ (hyperactive with spread but no clonus), 4+ (hyperactive with clonus) Babinski	Hyperactive or hypoactive reflexes can occur Upgoing toes occur with higher-grade encephalopathy

CT should be performed after insertion or removal of an ICP monitor to check positioning and for hemorrhage. Although MRI may detect cerebral edema with more sensitivity and specificity than CT, the risks of transport and the time involved in obtaining an MRI outweigh the benefits in diagnostic accuracy.

WHEN AND HOW TO INTUBATE

Encephalopathy can lead to aspiration and elevated $Paco_2$, which can exacerbate cerebral edema and elevated ICP. Noncommand following (typically grade III or IV) patients should be considered for intubation. In order to avoid spikes in ICP that can occur with laryngeal stimulation, intubation should occur in a controlled setting. Either propofol or etomidate is an appropriate induction agent. Ketamine should be avoided because it can elevate ICP. Lidocaine spray or 1 mL/kg IV bolus can be given prior to laryngoscopy to blunt increases in ICP. Succinylcholine should be avoided in patients who have been sedentary for >24 hours. Use of a video-assisted laryngoscope can facilitate intubation with fewer complications than direct laryngoscopy.

SAFE MECHANICAL VENTILATION AND PRINCIPLES OF ICP INTERACTION

Assist control volume control modes are reasonable in patients with hepatic encephalopathy. Since increasing positive end-expiratory pressure (PEEP) will increase mean intrathoracic pressure as well, elevated PEEP that exceeds central venous pressure can theoretically lead to elevations in ICP. However, studies with PEEP up to 15 cm H_2O have not shown a significant effect on ICP or CPP.[42] Permissive hypercapnia should be avoided as this will elevate ICP. Similarly, inverse ratio modes with elevated pressures for a significant duration of the respiratory cycle may inhibit jugular venous outflow and lead to increased ICP. Many fulminant liver failure patients will spontaneously hyperventilate as part of an autoregulatory response. This should not be treated. Conversely, induced hyperventilation is not recommended except in acute cases of herniation since this can lead to ischemia due to vasoconstriction.[43] Maintenance of a $Paco_2$ between 30 and 40 mm Hg is reasonable.

SEDATION PRACTICES IN THE FACE OF ENCEPHALOPATHY

Minimizing oversedation and utilizing sedation interruption are essential for continuous assessment of the neurologic exam. Adequate treatment of pain and anxiety should be addressed to minimize elevation of ICP. When selecting a sedative, renal and hepatic clearance should similarly be considered. Propofol is a typical agent with a short half-life that allows for frequent exam assessment. It does not provide any analgesia, however. Other reasonable options include fentanyl, which can minimally lower the seizure threshold, and dexmedetomidine, a centrally acting α_2-agonist that provides anxiolysis and analgesia with minimal respiratory or neurologic suppression. Midazolam is a reasonable choice in anxious patients and, like propofol, has anticonvulsant effects. It does, however, have active metabolites that can accumulate with prolonged use. All of the aforementioned agents can lower blood pressure. Paralysis is seldom necessary for adequate ventilation, but if used, it should be used judiciously and for as brief a period of time as necessary. It can substantially increase the risk for critical illness neuropathy and myopathy, mask seizure activity, and completely obscure the neurologic exam.

ICP MONITOR

Elevated ICP occurs in 86–95% of patients with grade III or IV encephalopathy.[3] Given the insensitivity of head CT to assess for cerebral edema, ICP monitoring should be considering in all noncommand following patients, typically grade III or IV encephalopathy patients. Monitoring ICP is the only way to diagnose elevated ICP and assess the efficacy of cerebral edema treatment in patients with marginal neurologic exams. Although there are no randomized trials to support the use of ICP monitoring, data suggest that monitoring can identify ICP spikes that are subclinical, lead to therapeutic changes, and provide important prognostic information. ICP monitoring is recommended by the ALFSG in grade III and IV patients who are candidates for transplantation and in some patients with advanced encephalopathy who are not liver transplant candidates, but may have survival benefit with protocolized, aggressive neurologic management.[3]

Since it is not clear that the risk of hemorrhage after adequate correction of coagulopathy is higher with intraparenchymal monitors compared with epidural ICP monitors, and since parenchymal monitors are more accurate, our practice is to place intraparenchymal monitors. Intraventricular monitor placement is not recommended due to the increased risk of bleeding.[44]

In patients who are unable to undergo ICP monitor placement, transcranial Doppler assessment of pulsatility index (peak end-diastolic flow velocity/mean flow velocity) can provide a rough assessment of whether ICP is elevated or not, but cannot quantify the ICP. Pulsatility indices >1.5 are considered abnormal. It is important to note that transcranial Doppler does not provide quantifiable or continuous ICP monitoring and in some studies has shown suboptimal sensitivity and specificity.[45]

Adequate reversal of coagulopathy is essential prior to ICP monitor placement, as described above. It is unclear if coagulation factors need to be corrected for the entire duration of time an ICP monitor is in place or if correction is only necessary during placement and removal of devices.[3] Continued aggressive coagulopathy correction can lead to volume overload, thrombosis, or DIC and may mask spontaneous liver recovery. Additionally, the expense of continued correction should be considered.

ACTIVE MANAGEMENT— PRINCIPLES OF OSMOTIC THERAPY, HYPOTHERMIA

The first steps in managing elevated ICP (defined as sustained ICP >25 cm H_2O or 20 mm Hg) involve simple measures to maximize venous outflow and avoid increases in intrathoracic or intra-abdominal pressure that can come with agitation, coughing, or ventilator dyssynchrony. All patients should have the head of the bed elevated at least 30° (unless contraindicated by hypotension), the head should be maintained midline to promote venous drainage, bilateral jugular venous catheterization should be avoided, and patients should be maintained in a comfortable pain-free state with the minimal amount of analgesics or anxiolytics required to avoid agitation or pain. Lidocaine spray can be used prior to suctioning to avoid a cough response, and an adequate bowel regimen should be prescribed to avoid straining during defecation. Generally, patients should be maintained in a euthermic, euvolemic state.

Patients should be monitored for seizures and treated appropriately since this can elevate ICP. The true incidence of seizure in fulminant liver failure patients is not clear. In small series of patients with ALF, seizure activity, including nonconvulsive status epilepticus, was identified in up to 32% of patients.[46] Additionally, paralysis should be avoided, if possible, to allow for detection of subtle clinical spells. Patients who have seized should receive antiepileptic treatment. Prophylaxis can be considered for those who have intracranial hemorrhage or very severe cerebral edema, in whom a seizure might cause herniation due to elevated ICP.[47]

Since cerebral autoregulation has been found to be impaired in patients with ALF, it is important to recognize the relationship between ICP and MAP. In patients with a global loss of autoregulation, cerebral blood flow (CBF) and cerebral blood volume (CBV) will vary passively with MAP. Since CBV is one component of intracranial volume, increases in CBV may increase ICP. Thus, MAP should not be excessively high. However,

if autoregulation is partially or regionally intact, small cerebral arterioles will dilate in an attempt to maintain CBF under circumstances of low MAP. When these arterioles dilate in the vasodilatory cascade zone, CBV increases and, as a consequence, so can ICP. Thus, at very high and very low MAPs, ICP may be elevated. For this reason, a CPP (MAP–ICP) of at least 50 mm Hg is recommended.[3]

In patients with persistently elevated ICP, osmotic therapy can be considered. Mannitol (20%, 1.0 g/kg or 100 g IV bolus) is a traditional agent that can be used for induction of a hyperosmotic state. It will cause diuresis and may cause hypotension or renal insufficiency. Alternately, hypertonic saline (3%, 30 mL over 10–20 minutes via a central line) may be used. Hypertonic saline will improve CPP to a greater extent than mannitol, but can cause flash pulmonary edema or hypotension if administered too quickly. Although hypertonic saline can also cause renal insufficiency, it is not as offensive as mannitol. Both mannitol and hypertonic saline have rheologic effects that can improve ICP. Maintenance of a hyperosmotic state can be achieved with either mannitol boluses or hypertonic saline as a bolus or continuous infusion. Mannitol is typically redosed every 6 hours for elevated ICP or serum osmolality less than 320 mOsm/L or osmolal gap greater than 50 mOsm/kg.[3] Renal insufficiency due to mannitol is typically seen with doses above 200 g per 24 hours or with a serum osmolal gap above 60–75 mOsm/kg. Hypertonic saline is typically dosed using 3% saline at 1 mg/kg/h titrated to a serum sodium of 150–155 mEq/L. Serum sodium values should be evaluated every 6 hours, and drips should be titrated accordingly. Care should be taken to avoid abrupt withdrawal of hyperosmolar treatment as this can lead to rebound cerebral edema.

Patients who are refractory to maximal osmolar therapy should be considered for induced hypothermia targeted to a core body temperature of 32–34°C, although it has not been studied in large randomized trials, and may be associated with serious complications.[48] Other options for ICP control include hyperventilation and barbiturate coma. Hyperventilation should only be used acutely during herniation. The effect of hyperventilation is short lived (1–24 hours) since the cerebral spinal fluid (CSF) will rapidly buffer the alkalotic effect. Barbiturate coma is considered the last course of action for ICP control in liver failure patients. Pentobarbital (5–20 mg/kg IV bolus followed by 1–4 mg/kg/h) is typically used and titrated to burst suppression on continuous EEG. Barbiturates cause loss of the entire neurologic exam including brainstem reflexes and, additionally, carry the complications of cardiosuppression, immunosuppression, and profound hypotension. However, barbiturates can be powerfully effective in lowering ICP by the mechanism of metabolic suppression, when patients are refractory to all other agents.

Order these lab tests:

- ❏ ABO (2 separate tests required – 2-3 hours apart)
- ❏ Liver transplant monitor
- ❏ PT/INR
- ❏ CBC w/diff and platelets
- ❏ Fibrinogen
- ❏ HCV-RNA (quant)
- ❏ AMA

- ❏ Lactate
- ❏ CMV-PCR
- ❏ HIV testing (rapid)*
- ❏ EBV IgG
- ❏ RPR
- ❏ CMV IgG
- ❏ HAV IgM
- ❏ HBV-DNA (quant)

- ❏ Uric acid
- ❏ HBsAg
- ❏ HBsAb
- ❏ HBcAb
- ❏ HCV-Ab
- ❏ Toxicology screen
- ❏ AFP
- ❏ Urinalysis

- ❏ Ceruloplasmin
- ❏ Blood cultures
- ❏ SPEP
- ❏ ASMA
- ❏ ANA
- ❏ LKM

Notify these consultants immediately:

Hepatology: Hepatology fellow on-call

Social service: Liver transplant social worker or social worker on-call

Infectious diseases: Transplant ID service

Neurology:

Cardiology:

Psychiatry (If drug overdose or psych history):

If renal dysfunction and for CVVH: Renal service

For activated factor VII: Hematology service

Transplant surgery:

Transfer service:

Neurosurgical intensivist:

Order these studies:

- ❏ Portable chest X-Ray (serial to exclude pneumonia)
- ❏ CT abdomen with liver volume or MRI abdomen with liver volume.
- ❏ If a CT or MRI cannot be done safely and in a timely manner, then bedside abdominal sonogram with doppler should be ordered to assess for portal vein patency.
- ❏ ECG
- ❏ ECHO
- ❏ CT scan of head (if stage 3-4 encephalopathy) to exclude cerebral edema

Please note that the following information is needed by the transplant coordinator to place patients upon the UNOS waiting list (whether they have fulminant liver failure or chronic liver disease)

- ❏ Full name
- ❏ Date of birth
- ❏ Social security number
- ❏ Height
- ❏ Weight
- ❏ Blood type

- ❏ Labs: creatinine, total bilirubin, albumin, INR, Na^+
- ❏ Degree of encephalopathy
- ❏ Degree of ascites
- ❏ Race and ethnicity of recipient
- ❏ HIV result

Figure 20–1. A sample MICU acute liver failure admission checklist.

▶ HOW TO PUT IT ALL TOGETHER: TRIAGE, TEAMWORK, TRANSPLANT CANDIDACY, AND EFFICIENT TRANSFER OF DATA

Clearly, an organized protocol with emergency department participation is required for the efficient care of ALF patients. The emergency critical care practitioner is most often the first responder and is best situated in the clinical arena to orchestrate the triage, diagnosis, and

teamwork for this complex, though thankfully, rare condition. Most, if not all, transplant centers have developed and implemented protocolized care with predetermined order sets and identified personnel who respond to triage triggers. Components of an organized protocol should include laboratory studies, specific consultants, and supplementary studies that are always indicated. Also, triggers for specific therapeutic interventions such as encephalopathy management should be developed with consultants. For the best practice in a given location, the

- Hepatology and transplant surgery teams will help coordinate management but MICU team is responsible for provision of all patient care

- Timely transfer of patients with acute liver failure is imperative and prioritization of such patients is essential. The hepatology team will contact the transfer service and the ICU team will discuss patient management with the transferring hospital

- Discuss with transplant ID about the need for empiric antibiotics/antifungals

- Patients should have lab tests checked no less frequently than q 4-6 hours

- Head of bed should be elevated @ 30° in intubated patients with the lights out in the room and minimalization of all stimuli (no deep suctioning)

- No lactulose should be used

- Maintain MAP with IVF; avoid pressors if at all possible. Ideal MAP should be 80 in order to provide adequate cerebral perfusion pressure

- Intubation only under controlled circumstances with attending anesthesiologist present because of coagulopathy and high risk of aspiration

- Do not correct coagulopathy unless lines need to be placed or for GI bleeding. The degree of coagulopathy is followed in serial fashion to prognosticate recovery

- Initiate gastric suppression with PPI

- Contact all necessary consultants upon admission to MICU

- Pay careful attention to acid-base and electrolytes

- Watch for hypoglycemia. Start D_{10} drip if patient unable to take p.o.

- Frequent neuro checks

- If acetaminophen is etiology, initiate and continue NAC drip until completion of protocol

- If activated factor VII is to be used, please coordinate all line placement and if applicable placement of ICP during this time

- ICP monitor placement should be considered in every patient with grade 3-4 encephalopathy.

- The mode of HD of choice is CVVH. It is to be initiated if a patient has any evidence of renal insufficiency, if the patient is mechanically ventilated or if the patient is receiving an ICP monitor. Otherwise the decision to initiate CVVH will be on a patient-by-patient basis and agreed upon by a consensus opinion of hepatology/transplant surgery.

"Every hour counts in the successful management of these complex and critically ill patients. Continuous monitoring and aggressive completion of necessary tests is essential to get these challenging patients to transplantation."

For additional recommendations, please refer to:

Raschke RA, et al. Results of a protocol for the management of patients with fulminant liver failure. Crit Care Med. 2008;36:2244-8.

Stravitz RT, et al. Intensive care of patients with acute liver failure: recommendations of the U.S. Acute Liver Failure Study Group. Crit Care Med. 2007;35:2498-508.

Figure 20–2. A sample patient management tool.

emergency critical care responder must coordinate with the local transplant center to predetermine what information will be required by the transplant team. Finally, if the diagnosis of ALF appears likely or is confirmed, the emergency critical care practitioner should be mindful of the specific demographic information that would be required of a transplant coordinator should the need arise to prepare for potential United Network of Organ Sharing (UNOS) waiting list. Ensuring the completeness of these historical components at onset may be critical to preventing transplant delay and is best accomplished by a pre-scripted protocol. As an example, a reproduction of the current protocol from our institution is offered as a template in Figures 20-1 and 20-2.

REFERENCES

1. Forde K, Reddy KR, Troxel AB, et al. Racial and ethnic differences in presentation, etiology, and outcomes of acute liver failure in the United States. *Clin Gastroenterol Hepatol.* 2009;7:1121–1126.

2. Lee WM. Acute liver failure in the United States. *Semin Liver Dis.* 2003;6:288–294.

3. Raschke RA, Curry SC, Rempe S, et al. Results of a protocol for the management of patients with fulminant liver failure. *Crit Care Med.* 2008;36:2244–2248.

4. Stravitz RT, Kramer AH, Davern T, et al. Intensive care of patients with acute liver failure: recommendations of the US Acute Liver Failure Study Group. *Crit Care Med.* 2007;35:2498–2508.

5. Trey C, Davidson C. The management of fulminant hepatic failure. *Prog Liver Dis.* 1970;3:282–298.

6. O'Grady JG, Schalm SW, Williams R. Acute liver failure: redefining the syndromes. *Lancet.* 1993 Jul 31; 342(8866):273–275.

7. Gimson AE, O'Grady J, Ede RJ, et al. Late onset hepatic failure: clinical serological and histological features. *Hepatology.* 1986;6:288–294.

8. Myers RP, Leung Y, Shaheen AA, et al. Validation of ICD-9-CM/ICD-10 coding algorithms for the identification of patients with acetaminophen overdose and hepatotoxicity using administrative data. *BMC Health Serv Res.* 2007;7:159.

9. Lee WM, Squires RH Jr, Nyberg SL, et al. Acute liver failure: summary of a workshop. *Hepatology.* 208;47:1401–1415.

10. Estes JD, Stolpman D, Olyaei A, et al. High prevalence of potentially hepatotoxic herbal supplement use in patients with fulminant hepatic failure. *Arch Surg.* 2003;138:852–858.

11. Suzuki A, Yuen N, Walsh J, et al. Co-medications that modulate liver injury and repair influence clinical outcome of acetaminophen-associated liver injury. *Clin Gastroenterol Hepatol.* 2009;7(8):882–888.

12. Fosnocht D, Taylor JR, Caravati EM. Emergency department knowledge concerning acetaminophen (paracetamol) in over-the-counter and prescription analgesics. *Emerg Med J.* 2008;25:213–216.

13. Taylor RM, Davern T, Munoz S, et al. Fulminant hepatitis A virus infection in the United States: incidence, prognosis, and outcomes. *Hepatology.* 2006;40:1589–1597.

14. Fontana R. Acute liver failure including acetaminophen overdose. *Med Clin North Am.* 2008;92:761–794.

15. Mindikoglu AL, Magder LS, Regev A. Outcome of liver transplantation for drug-induced acute liver failure in the United States: analysis of the United Network for Organ Sharing database. *Liver Transpl.* 2009;15:719–729.

16. Larson AM, Polson J, Fontana RJ, et al. Acetaminophen induced acute liver failure: results of a United States multicenter prospective study. *Hepatology.* 2005;45:1364–1372.

17. Nourjah P, Ahmad SR, Karwoski C, et al. Estimates of acetaminophen associated overdoses in the United States. *Pharmacoepidemiol Drug Saf.* 2006;15:398–405.

18. Daly FFS, O'Malley GF, Heard K, et al. Prospective evaluation of repeated supratherapeutic acetaminophen ingestion. *Ann Emerg Med.* 2004;44:393–398.

19. Davern TJ II, James LP, Hinson JA, et al. Measurement of serum acetaminophen–protein adducts in patients with acute liver failure. *Gastroenterology.* 2006;130:687–694.

20. O'Grady JG, Alexander GJ, Hayllar KM, et al. Early indicators of prognosis in fulminant hepatic failure. *Gastroenterology.* 1989;97:439–445.

21. Moller HJ, Gronbaek H, Schiodt FV, et al. Soluble CD163 from activated macrophages predicts mortality in acute liver failure. *J Hepatol.* 2007;47:671–676.

22. Bernal W, Donaldson N, Wyncoll D, et al. Blood lactate as an early predictor of outcome in paracetamol induced acute liver failure: a cohort study. *Lancet.* 2002;359: 556–562.

23. Katoonizadeh A, Decaestecker J, Wilmer A, et al. MELD score to predict outcome in adult patients with non-acetaminophen induced acute liver failure. *Liver Int.* 2007;27:329–334.

24. Taylor RM, Davern T, Santiago M, et al. Fulminant hepatitis A virus infection in the United States: incidence, prognosis, and outcomes. *Hepatology.* 2006;44:1589–1597.

25. Schmidt L, Larsen FS. Prognostic implications of hyperlactatemia, multiple organ failure, and systemic inflammatory response syndrome in patients with acetaminophen-induced acute liver failure. *Crit Care Med.* 2006;34:337–343.

26. Shawcross DL, Davies NA, Mookerjee RP, et al. Worsening cerebral hyperemia by the administration of terlipressin in acute liver failure with severe encephalopathy. *Hepatology.* 2004;39:471–475.

27. Contant CF, Valadka AB, Gopinath SP, et al. Adult respiratory distress syndrome: a complication of induced hypertension after severe head injury. *J Neurosurg.* 2001;95(4):560–568.

28. Porte RJ, Caldwell SH. The role of recombinant factor VIIa in liver transplantation. *Liver Transpl.* 2005;11(8): 872–874.

29. Mayer SA, Brun NC, Begtrup K, et al. Efficacy and safety of recombinant activated factor VII for acute intracerebral hemorrhage. *N Engl J Med.* 2008;358(20):2127–2137.

30. Funk GC, Dobeer D, Kneidinger N, et al. Acid–base disturbances in critically ill patients with cirrhosis. *Liver Int.* 2007;27:901–909.

31. Naka T, Bellomo R, Morimatsu H, et al. Acid–base balance in combined severe hepatic and renal failure: a quantitative analysis. *Int J Artif Organs.* 2008;31(4):288–294.

32. Yun BC, Kim WR, Benson JT, et al. Impact of pretransplant hyponatremia on outcome following liver transplantation. *Hepatology.* 2009;49:1610–1616.

33. Mazer M, Perrone J. Acetaminophen-induced nephrotoxicity: pathophysiology, clinical manifestations, and management. *J Med Toxicol.* 2008;4:1–6.

34. Lee WM, Hynan LS, Rossaro L, et al. Intravenous *N*-acetylcysteine improves transplant-free survival in early stage non-acetaminophen acute liver failure. *Gastroenterology.* 2009;137:856–864.

35. McKenzie TJ, Lillegard JB, Nyberg SL. Artificial and bioartificial liver support. *Semin Liver Dis.* 2008;28:210–217.

36. Ferraz-Neto BH, Moraes-Junior JM, Hidalgo R, et al. Total hepatectomy and liver transplantation as a two-stage procedure for toxic liver: case reports. *Transplant Proc.* 2008;40:814.

37. Albrecht J, Norenberg MD. Glutamine: a Trojan horse in ammonia neurotoxicity. *Hepatology.* 2006;44(4):788–794.

38. Larsen FS, Gottstein J, Blei AT. Cerebral hyperemia and nitric oxide synthase in rats with ammonia-induced brain edema. *J Hepatol.* 2001;34(4):548–554.

39. Larsen FS, Knudsen GM, Hansen BA. Pathophysiological changes in cerebral circulation, oxidative metabolism and blood–brain barrier in patients with acute liver failure. Tailored cerebral oxygen utilization. *J Hepatol.* 1997;27(1):231–238.

40. Jalan R, Olde Damink SW, Ter Steege JC, et al. Pathogenesis of intracranial hypertension in acute liver failure: inflammation, ammonia and cerebral blood flow. *J Hepatol.* 2004;41(4):613–620.

41. Ostapowicz G, Fontana RJ, Schiodt FV, et al. Results of a prospective study of acute liver failure at 17 tertiary care centers in the United States. *Ann Intern Med.* 2002;137(12):947–954.

42. McGuire G, Crossley D, Richards J, et al. Effects of varying levels of positive end-expiratory pressure on intracranial pressure and cerebral perfusion pressure. *Crit Care Med.* 1997;25(6):1059–1062.

43. Ede RJ, Gimson AE, Bihari D, et al. Controlled hyperventilation in the prevention of cerebral oedema in fulminant hepatic failure. *J Hepatol.* 1986;2(1):43–51.

44. Gray WP, Palmer JD, Gill J, et al. A clinical study of parenchymal and subdural miniature strain-gauge transducers for monitoring intracranial pressure. *Neurosurgery.* 1996;39(5):927–931. Discussion 931–932.

45. Figaji AA, Zwane E, Fieggen AG, et al. Transcranial Doppler pulsatility index is not a reliable indicator of intracranial pressure in children with severe traumatic brain injury. *Surg Neurol.* 2009;72(4):389–394.

46. Ellis AJ, Wendon JA, Williams R. Subclinical seizure activity and prophylactic phenytoin infusion in acute liver failure: a controlled clinical trial. *Hepatology.* 2000;32(3):536–541.

47. Bhatia V, Batra Y, Acharya SK. Prophylactic phenytoin does not improve cerebral edema or survival in acute liver failure—a controlled clinical trial. *J Hepatol.* 2004;41(1):89–96.

48. Stravitz RT, Larsen FS. Therapeutic hypothermia for acute liver failure. *Crit Care Med.* 2009;37(7 suppl):S258–S264.

CHAPTER 21

Acid–Base Disorders

Kevin M. Jones and William C. Chiu

The assessment of an emergency patient's acid–base status must begin with a clinical suspicion that an underlying acid–base disorder exists. That an acid–base disorder might exist in a patient presenting obtunded, hypotensive, hypoperfused, or obviously in extremis is rarely surprising. Patients with more subtle presentations or chronic, well-compensated acid–base disorders often elude clinicians in today's busy and overtasked emergency departments. One must remain diligent for clinical signs, astutely reviewing basic electrolyte panels, and remain open to the possibility that a patient may be or become more ill than he or she first appears. Knowing when to investigate for the possibility of an acid–base disorder or evaluate for complex mixed acid–base disorders requires astute clinical acumen. Unfortunately, many emergency providers today lack the ability to perform mixed acid–base assessments with facility, and many mixed or complex disorders, no doubt, go undiagnosed or undertreated.

In this chapter, we hope to review the measures of acid–base status routinely available to the emergency medicine critical care practitioner, their utility, as well as their liabilities. Using these measures, this chapter will provide a rational guide to the interpretation and initial management of a patient's acid–base status.

▶ THE HENDERSON–HASSELBALCH EQUATION

The Henderson–Hasselbalch equation in its original form IS of limited clinical utility AND is given as follows:

$$pH = pK + \log\frac{[HCO_3^-]}{[H_2CO_3]}$$

The Kassirer–Bleich equation is obtained by inserting known constants into the Henderson–Hasselbalch equation and then taking the antilog of each side.[1] The resultant equation is much more conceptually useful in understanding clinical acid–base interactions:

$$[H^+] = 24 \times \frac{P_{CO_2}}{[HCO_3^-]}$$

The Kassirer–Bleich equation makes clear the interactions between the P_{CO_2}, the bicarbonate concentration, and the free hydrogen ion concentration. If any two of these values are known, the other can be calculated.

▶ MEASURES OF ACID–BASE STATUS

SERUM BICARBONATE

The serum bicarbonate concentration is often one of the first pieces of measured laboratory data available for clinical assessment of acid–base status. Regardless of how it is labeled when reported, this value is actually a measured total CO_2 concentration.[2] The total CO_2 concentration is a combination of bicarbonate, carbonic acid, and dissolved carbon dioxide. The amount of dissolved carbon dioxide can be calculated if the measured P_{CO_2} is known by multiplying the P_{CO_2} by the solubility coefficient of CO_2 in the blood, 0.03. Hence:

$$\text{"Bicarbonate concentration"} = \text{total } CO_2$$
$$= [HCO_3^-] + [H_2CO_3] + (0.03)(P_{CO_2})$$

Most of the time, the relative contribution of the P_{CO_2} to this value is negligible, and as such is commonly ignored. It can become a significant factor in the hypercapnic patient, leading to reported total bicarbonate levels higher than would be reflected by a true assessment of the [HCO₃].

The reported serum bicarbonate can be a good initial indicator of the presence of an uncomplicated metabolic acidosis. As we can see from the Kassirer–Bleich equation, a rise in [H⁺] (decreasing pH) will necessitate an increase in the ratio of Pco₂ to [Hco₃⁻], and this will usually show up as a decreased serum bicarbonate measure. Following repeated serum bicarbonate measures is often performed to record the response to treatment for simple organic metabolic acidoses, such as ketoacidosis or lactic acidosis, when simple and relatively noninvasive measures are desired, and when complex mixed acid–base disorders have been excluded.

The serum bicarbonate is, however, not a very sensitive measure, and does not allow on its own for an analysis of the underlying disorder. In the presence of hypercapnia, as mentioned above, it can be higher than anticipated with an underlying acidemia due to the contribution of the Pco₂ and respiratory compensation. Patients with chronic lung disease or metabolic compensation can have markedly elevated serum bicarbonates at baseline, and without an appreciation for that baseline, a "normal" value can be falsely reassuring. Primary respiratory acidosis or alkalosis will produce a compensatory change in the bicarbonate levels, and can mask a mixed acid–base disorder. Reliance on the measured serum bicarbonate as a solitary measure of acid–base status should only be entertained in a simple patient without suspicion for underlying compensation and an unambiguous clinical picture.

ARTERIAL BLOOD GAS

The arterial blood gas (ABG) remains the mainstay for acid–base interpretation. While not always necessary for the identification and management of an acid–base disorder, a thorough understanding of the reported values and how to interpret them is essential. Laboratories will report values for pH, Pco₂, Po₂, [HCO₃], base excess (BE) (or deficit), and percent oxygen saturation.

The pH of the blood, normally between 7.35 and 7.45, is an assessment of the free hydrogen ion concentration in the blood. A blood pH of less than 7.35 is called *acidemia*; a blood pH of greater than 7.45 is called *alkalemia*. The pH is measured in the lab with an electrode permeable only to hydrogen ions.

The Pco₂ and Po₂ are the partial pressure of dissolved CO₂ and O₂ in the blood, respectively. They are also measured values obtained by using electrodes specific to the respective gasses.

The [HCO₃] as reported with a blood gas is calculated by using the measured pH and the measured Pco₂ using the Henderson–Hasselbalch equation. While some advocate that the measured [HCO₃] (or total CO₂ concentration) as reported in an electrolyte panel is a more reliable figure, that measured value can be flawed for the reasons discussed above. It is doubtful that either the calculated or measured [HCO₃] can uniformly be considered a more "true" assessment of the serum [HCO₃]. One should be aware of the liabilities of each approach when attempting to interpret discrepancies between the two.

The *BE* is an estimation of the amount of acid it would take to titrate 1 L of blood back to a normal pH of 7.40, assuming the Pco₂ were adjusted to a normal of 40 mm Hg. The BE is usually reported in units of milliequivalent per liter. It is calculated from the measured pH and the calculated [HCO₃⁻] according to the following equation[3]:

$$BE = 0.93 \times [HCO_3^-] + 13.77 \times pH - 124.58$$

In an acidosis, the BE is a negative value, and is often referred to as a *base deficit*. The BE is often used as a marker for metabolic acidosis, and is more reliable than the serum bicarbonate concentration as such, as it is adjusted for the effect of a concomitant respiratory disorder.

The *oxygen saturation* reported on a blood gas analysis is also a calculated value using the measured Po₂ and pH, based on the anticipated hemoglobin oxygen dissociation curve for that given pH.

▶ AN APPROACH TO THE INTERPRETATION OF ACID–BASE DISORDERS

There is an important distinction to be made between *acidemia* and *acidosis*, as well as between *alkalemia* and *alkalosis*. *Acidemia* and *alkalemia* refer to the relative abnormalities in the blood pH. *Acidosis* and *alkalosis* refer to an underlying disease process. It is possible in mixed acid–base disorders to have a low pH, hence be *acidemic*, while having a concurrent metabolic *alkalosis*. An example of this might be an *acidemic* diabetic ketoacidosis patient with a low pH and a primary metabolic *acidosis*, who also has a concurrent metabolic *alkalosis* (but not *alkalemia*) brought about by vomiting and resultant hydrogen ion depletion.

What follows is a five-step approach to the interpretation of acid–base status[2,4–8] (see Table 21-1). Whether this approach or another is used by an individual provider is not as important as is the practice that every assessment of acid–base status go through a sequenced and methodical analysis, every time.

▶ TABLE 21-1. **FIVE STEPS OF ACID–BASE ANALYSIS**

Step 1: Acidemia (pH <7.35) or alkalemia (pH >7.42)

Step 2: Primary respiratory or metabolic disturbance? (Look at P_{CO_2} on ABG or $[HCO_3]$)

Step 3: Is there appropriate compensation for the primary disorder?

Metabolic acidosis: $P_{CO_2} = (1.5 \times [HCO_3]) + 8\ (\pm 2)$

Metabolic alkalosis: $\uparrow P_{CO_2} = 0.6 \times \uparrow [HCO_3]\ (\pm 2)$

Respiratory acidosis: $\uparrow P_{CO_2}$ 10, $\uparrow [HCO_3]$ by 1 (acute) or 4 (chronic)

Respiratory alkalosis: $\downarrow P_{CO_2}$ 10, $\downarrow [HCO_3]$ by 2 (acute) or 5 (chronic)

Step 4: Is there an anion gap metabolic acidosis (AGMA)? $AG = [Na] - ([HCO_3] + [Cl])$. If AG >12, an AGMA is present

Step 5: If metabolic acidosis, is there another concomittant metabolic disturbance?

If **AGMA**, then calculate $\Delta Gap = \Delta AG - \Delta[HCO_3] = (AG - 12) - (24 - [HCO_3])$

If ΔGap is >6, there is a combined AGMA and metabolic alkalosis

If ΔGap is <−6, there is a combined AGMA and NAGMA

If **NAGMA**, for every 1 mEq/L $\uparrow[Cl]$, there should be 1 mEq/L $\downarrow[HCO_3]$

If $[HCO_3]$ decrease is less than predicted, then NAGMA and metabolic alkalosis

Reproduced with permission from Ref.[4]

▶ TABLE 21-2. **DETECTION OF PRIMARY RESPIRATORY OR METABOLIC ACID–BASE DISORDERS**

Primary Disorder	pH	P_{CO_2}	$[HCO_3]$
Metabolic acidosis	↓↓	↓	↓↓
Metabolic alkalosis	↑↑	↑	↑↑
Respiratory acidosis	↓↓	↑↑	↑
Respiratory alkalosis	↑↑	↓↓	↓

suggests a primary respiratory alkalosis, usually accompanied by a low $[HCO_3]$ representing a partial metabolic compensation. A high $[HCO_3]$ suggests a primary metabolic alkalosis, usually accompanied by a high P_{CO_2}, representing a partial respiratory compensation (see Table 21-2).

Step 3: Is there appropriate compensation for the primary disorder? In primary metabolic disorders, there should be rapid compensation for the resultant acidemia or alkalemia by the respiratory system.

Metabolic acidosis: In primary metabolic acidosis, the body will attempt to normalize the acidemia by "blowing off" CO_2. The formula of Winters and coworkers is used to calculate the predicted P_{CO_2} given the $[HCO_3]$[9]:

$$\text{Expected } P_{CO_2} = 1.5 \times [HCO_3] + 8 \pm 2$$

If the measured P_{CO_2} is less than expected, then the patient is blowing off his or her CO_2 more than would be required to compensate for the primary metabolic acidosis, and a concomitant respiratory alkalosis is present. If the measured P_{CO_2} is higher than expected, then the patient is failing to blow off enough CO_2 to compensate for the primary metabolic acidosis, and a concomitant respiratory acidosis is present.

Metabolic alkalosis: In primary metabolic alkalosis, the body will attempt to normalize the alkalemia by retaining CO_2. The expected increase in P_{CO_2} should be approximately 0.6 times the increase in the $[HCO_3]$:

$$\text{Expected increase in } P_{CO_2} = 0.6 \times ([HCO_3] - 24) \pm 2$$

If the measured P_{CO_2} is less than expected, then a concomitant respiratory alkalosis is present. If the measured P_{CO_2} is greater than expected, then a concomitant respiratory acidosis is present. A caveat to this rule is the fact that even in profound metabolic alkalosis, the P_{CO_2} will rarely rise above 50 mm Hg, which represents the upper limit of normal respiratory

Step 1: Is there a primary acidemia or alkalemia? Look at the pH as determined by the blood gas. A pH of less than 7.35 demonstrates acidemia, while a pH of greater than 7.42 demonstrates alkalemia. The direction in which the pH is deviated from normal is the effect of the primary acid–base disorder affecting the patient. While compensation for the primary disorder will decrease the effect of the primary disorder, it will never bring the pH back entirely to a normal range.

Step 2: Is the primary disorder respiratory or metabolic? Look at the P_{CO_2} from the blood gas and the serum HCO_3. Whether to use the measured total bicarbonate from an electrolyte profile or the calculated HCO_3 from a blood gas analysis remains a debate, although these authors, as a matter of routine practice, use the measured value from the electrolyte profile. In acidemia, a high P_{CO_2} suggests a primary respiratory acidosis, usually accompanied by an elevated $[HCO_3]$ representing metabolic compensation. A low $[HCO_3]$ suggests a primary metabolic acidosis, usually accompanied by a low P_{CO_2}, representing a partial respiratory compensation. In alkalemia, a low P_{CO_2}

compensation.[10] If the expected P_{CO_2} is greater than 50 mm Hg, failure to compensate fully is likely due to exceeding the limits of the respiratory compensatory mechanism rather than to a concomitant underlying respiratory alkalosis.

Respiratory alkalosis/acidosis: In primary respiratory acid–base disorders, the metabolic compensation for the primary disorder increases over time. The acute compensation occurs as a result of the bicarbonate buffering system, and occurs over the first 24–48 hours. Chronic compensation comes about as the result of the kidneys' ability to increase or decrease production of bicarbonate and to increase bicarbonate resorbtion or excretion. Chronic compensatory changes are usually seen from 72 hours and beyond. The clinician must decide, based on the history and clinical presentation, how acute the primary respiratory disorder is likely to be before being able to assess the appropriateness of the metabolic compensation. Likewise, a metabolic compensation greater or less than expected may prompt a reassessment of the acuity of the primary disorder.

In *acute* primary *respiratory acidosis*, the [HCO$_3$] should increase by 1 mEq/L for every 10 mm Hg increase in the P_{CO_2}. In a *chronic* primary *respiratory acidosis*, the [Hco$_3$] should increase by 4 mEq/L for every 10 mm Hg increase in the P_{CO_2}.

In *acute* primary *respiratory alkalosis*, the [HCO$_3$] should decrease by 2 mEq/L for every 10 mm Hg decrease in the P_{CO_2}. In a *chronic* primary *respiratory alkalosis*, the [HCO$_3$] should decrease by 5 mEq/L for every 10 mm Hg decrease in P_{CO_2}.

If the [HCO$_3$] is lower than expected, then a concomitant metabolic acidosis may be present. If the [HCO$_3$] is higher than expected, then a concomitant metabolic alkalosis may be present. It is clearly not possible for a respiratory acidosis and a respiratory alkalosis to coexist.

Step 4: Calculate the anion gap. Regardless of the primary acid–base disturbance, the anion gap (AG) should be calculated. Although the AG has limitations as a screening tool, an elevated AG should be presumed to indicate the presence of an AG acidosis. Metabolic compensation for a primary respiratory alkalosis should not elevate the AG.

Step 5: If there is a metabolic acidosis, is there another concomitant metabolic disturbance? This step is key to recognizing mixed metabolic acid–base disorders. Regardless of the primary acid–base disorder, if either step two or three identified a metabolic acidosis, proceed with the following calculations:

If there is an AG metabolic acidosis (an AG >12), then calculate the delta gap (Δgap). The Δgap is a tool that will help to reveal a concomitant metabolic alkalosis or non-AG acidosis when an AG metabolic acidosis has been found.[11] In a simple AG metabolic acidosis, the increase in the AG above normal should be matched millimolar for millimolar by a fall in the [HCO$_3$]. Let us assume the upper normal of the AG to be 12 mmol/L, and the lower normal of the [HCO$_3$] to be 22 mmol/L. If we ascribe the ΔAG to be the rise in the AG above the upper limit of normal, that is:

$$\Delta AG = AG - 12$$

and the Δ[HCO$_3$] to be the fall of the [HCO$_3$] below normal, that is:

$$\Delta[HCO_3] = 22 - [HCO_3]$$

then the Δgap can be calculated as follows:

$$\Delta Gap = \Delta AG - \Delta[HCO_3]$$

Given that in a straightforward *AG acidosis*, the rise in an AG should be perfectly matched by a fall in the [HCO$_3$], we should expect a Δgap of zero. In practice, a 2 standard deviation from the mean variation in the Δgap would give us normal values ranging from −6 to +6.[11]

If the Δgap is less than −6, it suggests a loss of [HCO$_3$] greater than should be anticipated by the *AG acidosis* known to exist. This suggests a concomitant *non-AG acidosis*. If the Δgap is greater than +6, the reduction in bicarbonate is not as great as should be expected by the known *AG acidosis*, and a concomitant *metabolic alkalosis* exists.

If there is a non-AG metabolic acidosis, then for every unit increase in the [Cl], there should be a unit decrease in the [HCO$_3$]. Remembering the discussion of electroneutrality when we looked at the AG, a decrease in the [HCO$_3$] must be accompanied by an increase in the [Cl] or in another unmeasured anion. If the increase is in an unmeasured anion, then an increase in the AG results. Since in a non-AG metabolic acidosis, we have already established a normal AG, the [Cl] *must* increase proportional to the decrease in [HCO$_3$]. If we assume a normal chloride to be 100 mmol/L, then for every 1 mmol/L increase in the chloride, we should expect a 1 mmol/L decrease in the [HCO$_3$], that is:

$$\text{Expected } \Delta[HCO_3] = \Delta[Cl]$$

If the measured [HCO$_3$] is more than 5 mmol/L greater than expected (to allow for a 2 standard

CNS depression
Chronic lung disease
Neuromuscular disorders
Acute airway obstruction
Pneumonia
Pulmonary edema
Thoracic cage injury
Hemothorax, pneumothorax
Pleural effusion
Mechanical ventilation

deviation range) based on the chloride concentration, then a concomitant metabolic alkalosis is present.

► DIFFERENTIAL DIAGNOSIS OF ACID–BASE DISORDERS

RESPIRATORY ACIDOSIS

Any etiology that limits the effective minute ventilation will result in decreased ventilation and in turn an increase in P_{CO_2}, leading to a respiratory acidosis. A list of possible causes of respiratory acidosis is shown in Table 21-3.

Treatment of a primary respiratory acidosis should be aimed at correcting the lack of respiratory drive, reducing the effective dead space, or increasing the minute ventilation. Remember that respiratory acidosis, if not the primary acid–base disorder, may be an appropriate compensation for a metabolic alkalosis! Make sure to rule out a mixed acid–base disorder before correcting it.

RESPIRATORY ALKALOSIS

Respiratory alkalosis results from excessive minute ventilation and a resultant decrease in the P_{CO_2}. Potential causes of a respiratory alkalosis are shown in Table 21-4. Hypocapnic patients are not always alkalemic, and a respiratory alkalosis is a common compensation for metabolic acidosis. As in a respiratory acidosis, respiratory

► **TABLE 21-4. CAUSES OF RESPIRATORY ALKALOSIS**

Anxiety
Hypoxia
CNS disease
Drug use—salicylates, catecholamines
Pregnancy
Sepsis/SIRS
Hepatic encephalopathy
Mechanical ventilation

alkalosis may be an appropriate compensation, and caution should be entertained in ascribing a respiratory alkalosis to psychogenic hyperventilation until an underlying mixed acid–base disorder has been ruled out. Salicylate toxicity in particular can result in severe metabolic acidosis, and any treatment that removes or inhibits respiratory compensation, which can at times seem severe, may rapidly worsen the underlying acidemia.

METABOLIC ALKALOSIS

Metabolic alkalosis is characterized by an increase in the $[HCO_3]$. It is brought about by the excess loss of hydrogen ions, the endogenous administration of bicarbonate or another anion such as lactate, acetate, or citrate, or, most commonly, the increased reabsorption of bicarbonate.

A *metabolic alkalosis* is classified as *chloride responsive* or *chloride resistant* based on the spot urine chloride concentration. A *chloride-responsive metabolic alkalosis* presents with a low urinary chloride concentration of less than 15 mEq/L, suggesting total body chloride depletion and in turn renal retention of chloride. In order to maintain electrical neutrality, low $[Cl^-]$ is accompanied by a retention of HCO_3^-, and it is this retention of HCO_3^- that brings about the resultant alkalosis. As such, chloride-responsive metabolic alkalosis is more of a problem of chloride balance than of bicarbonate balance, and restoration of chloride is what is needed to allow the kidneys to normalize the $[HCO_3^-]$ and in turn the alkalosis. Chloride-responsive metabolic alkaloses are due to gastrointestinal losses of chloride because of gastric suctioning (direct loss of hydrochloric acid [HCl]), volume depletion (reduction in space of distribution of HCO_3^-), or diuretic therapy (loss of NaCl and reduction in space of distribution of HCO_3^-).[12] Chloride-responsive metabolic alkalosis is almost always associated with a volume deficit as well, and treatment should be aimed at correcting both the volume deficit and the chloride deficit, something which is most easily accomplished with normal saline (0.9% NaCl).[13] The total deficit of chloride can be calculated according to the following equation:

$$\text{Chloride deficit (mEq)} = 0.2 \times \text{lean weight (kg)} \times (\text{normal serum } [Cl^-] - \text{measured serum } [Cl^-])$$

The volume of saline, in liters to be infused, necessary to correct the chloride deficit can then be calculated by taking the chloride deficit and dividing by 154 mEq/L (the chloride concentration of normal saline). Infusion of dilute concentrations of HCl can also be utilized to replete both hydrogen ion and chloride stores in severe cases of chloride-responsive metabolic alkalosis, although normalization of volume status with isotonic saline is recommended first.

Chloride-resistant metabolic alkalosis is characterized by a high urinary spot chloride concentration greater then 25 mEq/L. It can be brought about by either mineralocorticoid excess or profound hypokalemia.

In a state of mineralocorticoid excess, such as Cushing's syndrome or excessive mineralocorticoid administration, the kidneys inappropriately retain HCO_3^- via an aldosterone-mediated pump in the proximal tubule. The workup should be aimed at identifying and correcting the underlying cause of the mineralocorticoid excess. Acetazolamide, by blocking carbonic anhydrase, can inhibit the reabsorption mechanism in the proximal tubule and help promote appropriate renal excretion of HCO_3^-, as well as facilitate diuresis of the fluid overload that typically accompanies this state.

Hypokalemia causes an intracellular shift of hydrogen ions resulting, by means of a shift of the bicarbonate buffering equation to the left, in a relative excess of HCO_3^-. In this case, repletion of potassium along with volume repletion, if required, should correct the alkalemia.

In all cases of metabolic alkalosis, careful consideration should be made to the potential exogenous sources of alkali in the patient's medications and fluids. Acetate, citrate, or lactate in parenteral infusions, blood transfusions, or IV fluids should be considered. One of the most common causes of metabolic alkalosis, as mentioned below, is an inadvertent "overshoot" metabolic alkalosis that results from overly aggressive or inappropriate administration of alkali as treatment for metabolic acidosis.

See Table 21-5 for a review of the common causes of metabolic alkalosis.

METABOLIC ACIDOSIS

Metabolic acidosis is brought about due to the loss of extracellular bicarbonate (diarrhea, renal loss of bicarbonate, enterocuteneous fistulae), the accumulation of an endogenously produced organic acid (lactic acidosis, ketoacidosis), or the administration of an acid (salicylate, methanol, ethylene glycol, etc.).

The Anion Gap

The AG is utilized to evaluate patients with a metabolic acidosis. Metabolic acidosis can come about either due to an increase in hydrogen ion concentration or

▶ **TABLE 21-5. COMMON CAUSES OF METABOLIC ALKALOSIS**

Chloride-Responsive Urine, Cl <15 mEq/L	Chloride-Resistant Urine, Cl >25 mEq/L
Vomiting or gastric suction	Mineralocorticoid excess
Diuretics	Cushing's syndrome
Volume contraction	Licorice ingestion

▶ **TABLE 21-6. UNMEASURED IONS CONTRIBUTING TO THE NORMAL ANION GAP**

Unmeasured Anions	Unmeasured Cations
Albumin (15 mEq/L)	Calcium (5 mEq/L)
Organic acids (5 mEq/L)	Potassium (4.5 mEq/L)
Phosphate (2 mEq/L)	Magnesium (1.5 mEq/L)
Sulfate (1 mEq/L)	
Total UA (23 mEq/L)	Total UC (11 mEq/L)

due to a loss of bicarbonate. The AG helps differentiate between these two possibilities.

The concept of electroneutrality dictates that the charge of all positively charged ions in the body must be matched by an equivalent charge of negatively charged ions. The AG is the difference between the total concentration of the predominant cation (Na^+) and the total concentration of the predominant anions (Cl^-, HCO_3^-):

$$AG = [Na^+] - ([Cl^-] + [HCO_3^-])$$

The value of the AG represents the normal difference between the concentrations of cations and anions not included in the AG calculation. The cations and anions that normally contribute to the AG are shown in Table 21-6. Normal values for the AG vary slightly depending on the techniques of an individual lab. The original normal range for the AG was 8–16 mEq/L, although newer laboratory techniques have resulted in a lower normal range of 3–11 mEq/L.[14] This value represents the value of the relative charge superiority of unmeasured anions relative to unmeasured cations.

A metabolic acidosis that results in the accumulation of excess hydrogen ions will cause an increased AG. We will refer to this as an *AG metabolic acidosis*. This comes about because the excess hydrogen ions bind with free bicarbonate ions to form carbonic acid, driving the carbonic acid buffering equation to the right, resulting in a decreased concentration of bicarbonate:

$$H^+ + HCO_3^- \leftrightarrow H_2CO_3 \leftrightarrow H_2O + CO_2$$

This reduced bicarbonate concentration results in a reduced measured anion concentration, and in turn a larger AG. Caution is advised in relying too heavily on the AG as a screening measure of acidosis, especially in a clinical context where strong suspicion for organic acidosis exists. While elevated lactic acid levels should bring about a corresponding large AG, multiple studies have shown that the AG fails to predict lactate levels in both critically ill medical and trauma patients.[15–17] In the event that an organic acidosis is strongly suspected, measuring blood levels of the organic acid directly (lactate in lactic acidosis, acetate or β-hydroxybutyrate in ketoacidosis) more reliably detects or excludes the underlying disorder.

In contrast, a metabolic acidosis that comes about as a result of a loss of bicarbonate from the extracellular fluid does not result in an increase in the AG. At first, this might seem counterintuitive. When a metabolic acidosis is brought about by bicarbonate loss, however, the kidneys maintain electroneutrality by retaining chloride ions. Since both chloride and bicarbonate are measured anions, the total contribution of measured anion concentration to the AG remains unchanged, although the relative ratio of chloride to bicarbonate will increase. We will refer to this as a *non-AG metabolic* acidosis, although because of the elevated relative chloride concentration you may see *non-AG metabolic acidosis* sometimes referred to as *hyperchloremic metabolic acidosis*.[18]

Anion Gap Metabolic Acidosis

As mentioned above, an AG metabolic acidosis is brought about by the accumulation of excess hydrogen ions and the subsequent reduction in the bicarbonate concentration by means of the carbonic acid buffering system. Since the extracellular fluid must remain electrically neutral, the reduction in bicarbonate concentration must occur concurrently with an increase in another anion. The unmeasured anion that replaces bicarbonate in maintaining electrical neutrality is the conjugate base to the acid that gave off the excess hydrogen ion. In the case of lactic acidosis, lactic acid gives off its hydrogen ion, leaving behind lactate, a negatively charged ion:

$$Lactic\ acid + HCO_3^- \rightarrow Lactate^- + H^+ + HCO_3^- \rightarrow$$
$$Lactate^- + H_2CO_3 \rightarrow Lactate^- + H_2O + CO_2$$

Acids causing an AG metabolic acidosis can be inorganic (sulfate, phosphate), organic (lactate or ketoacids), or exogenous (salicylates). The most common causes of an AG metabolic acidosis can be remembered by the acronym A CAT MUDPILES (see Table 21-7).[4,19] A careful history and exam combined with confirmatory tests will help narrow the differential diagnosis.

Nonanion Gap Metabolic Acidosis

Non-AG metabolic acidosis is caused not by the addition or accumulation of an acid, but by the loss, through either renal or gastrointestinal means, of bicarbonate. Causes of non-AG metabolic acidosis are shown in Table 21-8.[19]

The urine AG can be utilized to distinguish between renal and gastrointestinal etiologies for a non-AG metabolic acidosis.[5] The urine anion gap (UAG) is calculated by obtaining the spot urine electrolyte values for Na, K, and Cl as follows:

$$UAG = (Urine[NA] + Urine[K]) - Urine[Cl]$$

▶ **TABLE 21-7. A CAT MUDPILES: COMMON CAUSES OF ANION GAP METABOLIC ACIDOSIS AND CONFIRMATORY TESTS WHERE APPROPRIATE**

Cause	Confirmatory Test(s)
Analgesics (NSAID, APAP)	Tylenol level, AST
Cyanide, carbon monoxide	CO level, cyanide level
Alcoholic ketoacidosis	Serum or urine ketones, ethanol level
Toluene	
Methanol, metformin	Osmolal gap
Uremia	Serum BUN, creatinine
Diabetic ketoacidosis	Serum or urine ketones, blood glucose
Paraldehyde, phenformin	
Iron, isoniazid	Serum iron level, abdominal radiographs
Lactic acidosis	Lactate or lactic acid level
Ethylene glycol	Osmolal gap
Salicylates	Salicylate level, urine ferric chloride

In the event of renal loss of HCO_3, the UAG would be large, as bicarbonate is not measured in the UAG and would account for a large amount of the urinary ions. In the event of gastrointestinal loss of bicarbonate, the kidneys would be retaining HCO_3, and the UAG would approximate zero.

▶ TREATMENT OF ACIDOSIS WITH EXOGENOUS BICARBONATE

Bicarbonate does not function well as a buffer, in the strictest sense of the word, at near-physiologic pH.[13] The dissociation constant or pK of the carbonic acid–bicarbonate buffering system is 6.1. If we assume that the effective range of a buffering system is within 1 pH unit of its dissociation constant (the pH level at which the acid is 50% dissociated), then the carbonic acid–bicarbonate buffering system should work effectively between a pH of 5.1 and 7.1, but would clearly not be an effective buffer at near-physiologic pH. This would be true under laboratory conditions were we simply

▶ **TABLE 21-8. HARDUP: COMMON CAUSES OF NONANION GAP METABOLIC ACIDOSIS**

Hyperalimentation
Acetazolamide
Renal tubular acidosis and renal insufficiency
Diarrhea and **D**iuretics
Ureteroenterostomy
Pancreatic fistula

titrating an acid. In the body, however, the respiratory system has the ability to remove CO_2. As H_2CO_3 is formed by the buffering of excess H^+ by HCO_3^-, the subsequent increased CO_2 can be removed via increased ventilation, pulling the buffering equation to the right, and significantly extending the effective buffering range of the system.[10]

The administration of $NaHCO_3$ solutions in an attempt to increase serum pH has been a long-standing practice and one that, on the surface, would appear to make empirical sense. The principal concern for a patient in severe acidosis (pH <7.10) is for impaired cardiac contractility.[20] Other effects of severe acidosis include centralization of blood volume, cardiac sensitization to dysrhythmias, hyperkalemia, respiratory fatigue, increased metabolic demands, insulin resistance, and obtundation or coma.[21] Clinicians often are confronted by a desire to normalize a severely acidotic pH, and the tool in our armamentarium that has been used for that purpose has been $NaHCO_3$. Arguments in favor of directly correcting an acidosis with alkali therapy hinge on two presumptions: (1) correction of the acidosis independent of addressing the underlying cause is beneficial and (2) administration of sodium bicarbonate solutions effectively corrects or improves acidosis. Neither is necessarily the case.

The administration of $NaHCO_3$ solutions has not been associated with decreased mortality, and can cause significant complications. In laboratory conditions, acidosis has been shown to be protective for ATP-deprived liver cells, delaying the onset of cell death.[22] If we presume this to be true in vivo, then correction of acidosis without normalization of the underlying causative disorder would be harmful. The exogenous administration of $NaHCO_3$ also pushes the carbonic acid buffering equation to the right:

$$H^+ + HCO_3^- \rightarrow H_2CO_3 \rightarrow H_2O + CO_2$$

This increases the P_{CO_2}, increasing the respiratory burden for clearing CO_2. In the absence of capability to increase respiratory excretion of CO_2, the net effect of $NaHCO_3$ administration may be to paradoxically lower the pH due to the increased P_{CO_2}. In an intact organism, a severe acidemia may have already brought about a maximal respiratory effort at compensation, making the lungs unable to accommodate the increased CO_2 burden. In a patient with fixed ventilation, as on a ventilator, the administration of $NaHCO_3$ often produces a paradoxical acidosis as the patient is unable to accommodate the increased CO_2 burden.

The objective when treating an organic acidosis, where an acidotic pH is almost always a marker for an underlying derangement in need of correction and not a problem itself in need of normalization, should be to correct the underlying cause of the acidosis. Restoration of tissue perfusion in lactic acidosis and of nutritional substrate in alcoholic ketoacidosis, and the administration of insulin in diabetic ketoacidosis should completely correct the underlying acidosis.[23] The administration of alkali solutions to these patients concomitant with the correction of the underlying disorder almost universally causes an overshoot alkalosis.

If a severe acidosis (pH <7.10) is present, the administration of alkali therapy may be required in bicarbonate-loosing metabolic acidosis such as profound diarrhea or renal tubular acidosis, where the body's production of HCO_3 cannot keep pace with losses. Alkali therapy can also provide a temporizing measure in the renal failure patient who develops a metabolic acidosis while hemodialysis is arranged, as such a patient will be incapable of renal compensation and increased bicarbonate production or acid excretion. Alkali therapy may also be considered in the event of massive exogenous acid ingestion that exceeds the capabilities of compensatory mechanisms, such as occurs in salicylate or toxic alcohol ingestion. In this case, the additional CO_2 transport capability supplied by sodium bicarbonate may prove a temporizing measure while arranging for hemodialysis in order to remove the exogenous acid.

If the decision is made to administer sodium bicarbonate, the goal should be to partially correct a severe acidosis to no greater a pH than 7.2, so as to prevent a reflex alkalosis after overcorrection. Inherent in the administration of sodium bicarbonate is the administration of a not insignificant amount of sodium. While commercially produced solutions are available, in practice an infusion is usually made by mixing 150 mEq (three standard 50-mEq ampoules) in 1 L of 5% dextrose in water (D5W) or 100 mEq (two standard 50-mEq ampoules) in 1 L of 0.25% sodium chloride (0.25% NaCl), yielding a near-isotonic solution.[21] The distribution of bicarbonate varies depending on the degree of acidosis, and is about 50% of lean body weight at normal pH, but increases upwards of 70% lean body weight in severe acidosis (pH <7.10).[10] If we presume to only be utilizing the administration of sodium bicarbonate in the presence of severe acidosis, and without correction upwards of a pH of 7.20, we can use 60%, or 0.6, as an estimation of the distribution of bicarbonate. Our goal should be to correct the pH to no greater than 7.20, which according to the Henderson–Hasselbalch equation should correspond to a $[HCO_3]$ of 10 mmol/L. The bicarbonate deficit can be calculated according to the following equation:

$$HCO_3^- \text{ deficit (mEq)} = 0.6 \times \text{lean body weight (kg)} \times (10 - \text{measured } [HCO_3^-])$$

The total calculated deficit should be given slowly as an infusion. The net effect of the infusion will not be manifest until upwards of 30 minutes following the infusion. It is important to stress that continuing a bicarbonate infusion until normalization of pH is observed will uniformly result in an often poorly tolerated "overshoot" alkalosis. As such, only the calculated dose should be infused, and further alkali therapy directed by subsequent blood gas and electrolyte analysis.

Alternate alkali infusions have been developed that have theoretical advantages over sodium bicarbonate including carbicarb (a 1:1 solution of sodium bicarbonate and disodium carbonate) and THAM (0.3N tromethamine). No clinical trial has demonstrated either agent to be superior to sodium bicarbonate, and their clinical use is not indicated.[10,23]

REFERENCES

1. Kassirer JP, Bleich HL. Rapid estimation of plasma carbon dioxide from pH and total carbon dioxide content. *N Engl J Med.* 1965;272:1067.

2. Narins RG, Emmett M. Simple and mixed acid–base disorders: a practical approach. *Medicine.* 1980;59:161.

3. Pon S. *Medical Calculators: Calculated Bicarbonate & Base Excess.* New York, NY; 2001. Available at: http://www-users.med.cornell.edu/~spon/picu/calc/basecalc.htm.

4. Sherman SC. *Acid–Base made Easy. Lecture Materials.* Seattle, WA; 2007.

5. Rutecki GW, Whittier FC. An approach to clinical acid–base problem solving. *Compr Ther.* 1998;24:553.

6. Morganroth M. Six steps to acid base analysis: clinical applications. *J Crit Illness.* 1990;5:460.

7. Morganroth M. An analytic approach to diagnosing acid–base disorders. *J Crit Illness.* 1990;5:138.

8. Haber RJ. A practical approach to acid base disorders. *West J Med.* 1991;155:146.

9. Albert MS, Dell RB, Winters RW. Quantitative displacement of acid–base equilibrium in metabolic acidosis. *Ann Intern Med.* 1967;66:312.

10. Rose BD, Post TW. Introduction to simple and mixed acid–base disorders. In: *Clinical Physiology of Acid–Base and Electrolyte Disorders.* 5th ed. New York: McGraw-Hill; 2001:535.

11. Wren K. The delta (delta) gap: an approach to mixed acid–base disorders. 1990;19:1310.

12. Androge HJ, Madias N. Management of life threatening acid–base disorders: part 2. *N Engl J Med.* 1998;338:107.

13. Marino PL. *Metabolic Alkalosis in the ICU Book.* 3rd ed. Lippincott Williams and Wilkins; 2007:551.

14. Winter SD, Pearson JR, Gabow PA, et al. The fall of the serum anion gap. *Medicine.* 1990;150:311.

15. Levrant J, Bounatirou T, Ichai C, et al. Reliability of the anion gap as an indicator of blood lactate in critically ill patients. *Intensive Care Med.* 1997;23:417.

16. Mikaulaschek A, Henry SM, Donovan R, et al. Serum lactate is not predicted by anion gap or base excess after trauma resuscitation. *J Trauma.* 1996;40:218.

17. Iberti TS, Lieboitz AB, Papadakos PJ, et al. Low sensitivity of the anion gap as a screen to detect hyperlactatemia in critically ill patients. *Crit Care Med.* 1990;18:275.

18. Nicolaou DD, Kelen GD. Acid–base disorders. In: Kelen GD, Stapcztnski JS, Tintinalli JE, eds. *Emergency Medicine, A Comprehensive Study Guide.* 6th ed. New York: McGraw-Hill; 2004:149.

19. Casaletto JJ. Differential diagnosis of metabolic acidosis. *Emerg Med Clin North Am.* 2005;23:771.

20. Sonnett J, Pagani FD, Baker LS, et al. Correction of intramyocardial hypercarbic acidosis with sodium bicarbonate. *Circ Shock.* 1994;42:163.

21. Androge HJ, Madias NE. Management of life-threatening acid–base disorders: the first of two parts. *N Engl J Med.* 1998;338:26.

22. Gores GJ, Nieminen AL, Fleischman KE, et al. Extracellular acidosis delays the onset of cell death in ATP-depleted hepatocytes. *Am J Physiol.* 1988;225:C315.

23. Gehlbach BK, Schmidt GA. Bench-to-bedside review: treating acid–base abnormalities in the intensive care unit—the role of buffers. *Crit Care.* 2004;8:259.

CHAPTER 22

Electrolyte Disorders

Kevin M. Jones, Samantha L. Wood, and William C. Chiu

▶ INTRODUCTION

Electrolyte disorders can be some of the most complex and subtle clinical conditions facing the critical care or emergency medicine physician. A healthy degree of suspicion coupled with vigilant electrolyte monitoring is necessary in order to avoid missing these disorders. This is particularly true as many electrolyte disorders occur secondary to other severe disease states.

▶ DISORDERS OF SODIUM

Sodium disorders are commonly encountered in clinical practice. Both hyponatremia and hypernatremia have multiple underlying causes and may develop acutely or chronically. Patients with acute or severe sodium disorders may be critically ill and require rapid, aggressive correction of their sodium abnormality, while aggressive treatment of the chronic, compensated hyponatremic or hypernatremic patient may cause dangerous fluid shifts. It is critical that the emergency physician understand how to identify, classify, and treat sodium disorders.

HYPONATREMIA

Introduction

Hyponatremia is defined as a serum sodium less than 135 mEq/L. It is commonly found in both inpatients and outpatients.[1] Even mild hyponatremia in outpatients is correlated with a poor outcome.[2] Groups at particular risk for hyponatremia include hospitalized patients, elderly patients, and patients recently started on thiazide diuretics.[3]

Presentation

The severity of symptoms due to hyponatremia depends on the rate of sodium decline as well as the absolute level. Mildly hyponatremic patients are often asymptomatic. Moderately hyponatremic patients (Na of 125–130 mEq/L) may experience nausea, headache, malaise, and myalgias and have depressed tendon reflexes. Severe hyponatremia (Na <125 mEq/L) causes mental status changes; seizure, coma, and death occur at sodium levels of below 120 mEq/L. Acute hyponatremia occurs over less than 48 hours and is likely to cause neurologic manifestations secondary to cerebral edema. In chronic hyponatremia, neurologic effects are less likely as there has been time for compensation and brain size remains normal. This compensatory response puts the patient at risk for a demyelinating syndrome if sodium is corrected too rapidly.

Evaluation

Evaluation of hyponatremia consists of a stepwise narrowing of the differential diagnosis based on history, physical exam, and laboratory testing[1,4–7] (see Figure 22-1).

Hyperosmolar or iso-osmolar hyponatremia

Hyponatremia in the absence of a hypoosmolar state is referred to as pseudohyponatremia. Hyperosmolar hyponatremia occurs when large amounts of an osmotically active substance (such as mannitol, glucose, or intravenous [IV] contrast dye) draw water into the vasculature and dilute sodium concentration. For

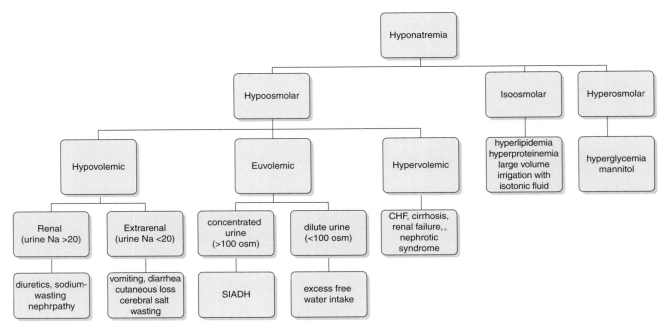

Figure 22-1. Etiologies of hyponatremia.

pseudohyponatremia secondary to hyperglycemia, a correction factor of 1.6 mEq/L sodium decrease for every 100 mg/dL rise in glucose is often used; however, experimental evidence indicates that a correction factor of 2.4 mEq/L may be more accurate.[8]

Iso-osmolar hyponatremia may be due to severe hyperlipidemia or hyperproteinemia, which causes a lab artifact in which serum water content is overestimated. Large volume irrigation with a sodium-free fluid such as sorbitol, which is frequently used in transurethral prostatic resection, can cause either an iso-osmolar or hypoosmolar hyponatremia.[9]

Hypoosmolar hyponatremia

Hypoosmolar hyponatremia is due to the net gain of free water. This may occur when water intake overwhelms the excretory capacity of the kidney or when there is an inability to suppress antidiuretic hormone (ADH) secretion secondary to true volume depletion, effective circulating volume depletion, or a primary inappropriate release of ADH.

Evaluation of the patient with hypoosmolar hyponatremia begins with an assessment of volume status based on vital signs including orthostatics, skin turgor, mucus membranes, JVD, and presence or absence of edema and ascites. Because physical exam findings can be unreliable in assessing volume status,[10] the patient's history, comorbidities, medications, and laboratory values should be incorporated into the assessment as well.

Hypovolemic hyponatremia occurs when sodium depletion exceeds free water depletion. Hypovolemia

prompts ADH release and thirst, so the patient consumes and retains free water, leading to worsened hyponatremia.

Relative sodium depletion may occur by renal or extrarenal losses of sodium and water; distinguishing between the two is based on history and measurement of urine sodium. Low urine Na (<20 mEq/L) indicates that the kidneys are appropriately reabsorbing sodium, so losses are extrarenal. Causes of extrarenal loss include vomiting, diarrhea, and cutaneous loss in burn victims. Patients presenting to the ED with hyponatremia most commonly fall into this category.[11] If urine sodium is high (>20 mEq/L), then sodium is being lost renally out of proportion to water losses. The most common cause is diuretics, and the emergency physician must be particularly alert for this condition in older patients recently started on hydrochlorothiazide. Other causes include sodium-wasting nephropathy or hypoaldosteronism.

Cerebral salt wasting syndrome (CSW) is a cause of hypovolemic hyponatremia that occurs after head injury or neurosurgical procedures. Distinguishing it from the syndrome of inappropriate antidiuretic hormone (SIADH), which may occur in the same clinical context, is critical as the treatment of CSW (administration of isotonic saline) may worsen SIADH. An assessment of the patient's volume status may help distinguish the two: patients with CSW are more likely to appear hypovolemic, whereas patients with SIADH are more likely to be euvolemic.[6] In addition, CSW patients typically produce dilute urine with a high flow rate, unlike the concentrated, low-flow urine of SIADH. Spot measurement of urinary sodium cannot distinguish between these two diseases. Additional assessment of volume status, such as degree of hemoconcentration, BUN and creatinine levels, and central venous pressure, should be considered as well.[12]

Euvolemic hyponatremia occurs when there is free water gain and/or retention with minimal sodium loss. The SIADH is diagnosed when there is a hypoosmolar hyponatremia with an inappropriately concentrated urine (>100 mOsm/kg), clinical euvolemia, absence of diuretic use, and normal renal, cardiac, adrenal, and thyroid functions. It is a frequent cause of hyponatremia in hospitalized patients and may be due to malignancy, pulmonary disease, CNS disease, or drugs[13] (see Table 22-1). Hypothyroidism and adrenal insufficiency may cause a similar clinical picture.

Euvolemic hyponatremia may also occur in the patient with normal kidney function if the amount of free water consumed is excessive (often >4 L per day). Etiologies include psychogenic polydipsia or beer potomania. An appropriately dilute urine (<100 mOsm/kg) is present as the kidney attempts to excrete free water.

Hypervolemic hyponatremia occurs in patients who are total body volume overloaded but have low effective arterial volume secondary to heart failure, cirrhosis, renal failure, or nephrotic syndrome. Hyponatremia portends a poor prognosis in heart failure patients[14] and patients with cirrhosis.[15]

Treatment

Treatment of hyponatremia depends on both the etiology and the severity of the disease. Osmotic demyelination syndrome is a dreaded complication of treatment resulting when administration of hypertonic solution causes rapid movement of water out of brain cells. The emergency physician must balance the concern for this entity with the need to treat suspected cerebral edema.

The critically ill hyponatremic patient who presents with seizure or coma should be treated aggressively to rapidly correct sodium to a safe level (>120 mEq/L). This is accomplished by administration of hypertonic saline for the first 3–4 hours after presentation or until symptoms improve. The goal rate of correction is initially 1.5–2 mEq/L/h; once symptoms improve, the rate of correction should be slowed, and should not exceed 10 mEq/L over the first 24 hours. Severe hyponatremic symptoms are likely to be due to a rapid fall in sodium without time for the brain to compensate, so rapid correction in these patients is less likely to cause a demyelinating syndrome than rapid correction in chronically hyponatremic patients.

▶ **TABLE 22-1. CAUSES OF THE SYNDROME OF INAPPROPRIATE ANTIDIURETIC HORMONE (SIADH)**

Malignancy	Lung carcinoma (small cell or mesothelioma)
	Oropharyngeal
	Gastrointestinal
	Genitourinary
	Endocrine thymoma
	Lymphoma
	Ewing's sarcoma
Pulmonary disease	Pneumonia (bacterial or viral)
	Tuberculosis
	Aspergillosis
	Asthma
	Cystic fibrosis
	Advanced chronic obstructive pulmonary disease
CNS disease	Encephalitis
	Meningitis
	Bleeding (subdural, subarachnoid, stroke)
	Intracranial mass
	Recent neurosurgical procedure
	Multiple sclerosis
	Guillain–Barré syndrome
	Cerebral sinus thrombosis
	Delirium tremens
	Acute intermittent porphyria
Drugs	Chlorpropamide
	Antidepressants
	Carbamazepine
	Nicotine
	Narcotics
	Nonsteroidal anti-inflammatory drugs (NSAIDs)
	Antineoplastic drugs
	MDMA ("ecstasy")
	AVP analogues: desmopressin, vasopressin, oxytocin
Other	Hereditary
	Idiopathic
	Transient (endurance exercise, nausea, pain, stress)

Treatment of the stable hyponatremic patient should be based on etiology. Hypovolemic patients require isotonic fluids, while euvolemic patients are treated with free water restriction. Hypervolemic patients may require diuresis in addition to free water restriction. Conivaptan, an oral V1A/V2 receptor antagonist, has been shown to increase serum sodium in patients with euvolemic or hypervolemic hyponatremia.[16]

The stable hyponatremic patient should be corrected at a rate of no more than 0.5 mEq/L/h and no more than 10–12 mEq/L/24h[6] to minimize risk of demyelination. The change in serum sodium estimated to

▶ **TABLE 22-2. SODIUM CONCENTRATIONS OF COMMON IV SOLUTIONS**

Solution	Sodium Concentration (mEq/L)
5% normal saline (NS)	855
3% NS	513
0.9% NS	154
Lactated Ringer's	130
0.45% NS	77
0.25% NS	38
5% dextrose in water	0
8.5% sodium bicarbonate (ampoule)	50 mEq/50 mL ampoule (1 mEq/mL)

result from administration of 1 L of IV fluid is calculated by the following equation:

Na change with 1L IV fluid

$$= \frac{\text{Na content IV fluid (mEq/L)} - \text{serum Na (mEq/L)}}{\text{TBW} + 1}$$

Total body water (TBW) = correction factor × weight (kg)

Correction factor:

Male	
Nonelderly	0.6
Elderly	0.5
Female	
Nonelderly	0.5
Elderly	0.45

The sodium content of common IV solutions is noted in Table 22-2. Serum sodium should be measured frequently during treatment, as calculations have limited accuracy and response to therapy is variable.[17]

HYPERNATREMIA

Introduction

Hypernatremia is defined as a serum sodium >145 mEq/L. The underlying etiology is inadequate free water intake. This condition is rare in alert people with an intact thirst mechanism; it is more prevalent in those who rely on others for their water intake. Patients over age 60 may be particularly at risk, since the protective responses of thirst and ADH release are blunted in older age. Most outpatients who present with hypernatremia are at the extremes of age, while hospitalized patients or those with altered mental status are at risk for hypernatremia regardless of age.[18]

Presentation

Hypernatremia may present with weakness, agitation, muscle twitching, hyperreflexia, ataxia, lethargy, and coma. As with hyponatremia, symptoms in hypernatremia correlate with severity and rate of sodium change. In acute or severe hypernatremia, brain shrinkage may lead to vascular rupture with cerebral bleeding. In chronic hypernatremia, the brain adapts over time by accumulation of electrolytes, so neurologic symptoms may be less pronounced; however, this adaptive response complicates management because rapid correction of hypernatremia may lead to cerebral edema.[18]

Evaluation

As with hyponatremia, an assessment of the patient's volume status will help to clarify the etiology of hypernatremia (see Figure 22-2).

Hypovolemic hypernatremia occurs when free water depletion exceeds sodium depletion. Similar to hypovolemic hyponatremia secondary to relative sodium depletion, relative free water depletion may have a renal or extrarenal cause. Renal losses are due to an osmotic diuresis caused by hyperglycemia, mannitol, or a postobstructive state. In this case, free water is lost in a dilute urine (urine osmolality <700 mOsm/kg) with concomitant renal loss of sodium (urine Na >20 mEq/L). Extrarenal losses may be due to diarrhea, NG suction, vomiting, third spacing, or skin losses as in a burn patient; urine is appropriately concentrated (>700 mOsm/kg) and renal sodium is low (<10 mEq/L).

Euvolemic hypernatremia is caused by free water loss without significant sodium loss. The cause may be renal due to diabetes insipidus (DI) or extrarenal.

DI, in which the kidney does not concentrate the urine appropriately (urine osmolality <700 mOsm/kg), will cause hypernatremia if there is insufficient access to free water. Central DI is due to decreased ADH release secondary to head trauma, neurosurgery, infiltrative disease, or an idiopathic cause. Administration of exogenous ADH will allow these patients to concentrate the urine again. In nephrogenic DI, the collecting ducts are resistant to ADH, so exogenous administration is ineffective. This condition is frequently drug related, with the most common causes being lithium, foscarnet, and clozapine. Other causes include hypercalcemia, hypokalemia, low-protein diet, and release of ureteral obstruction.[19]

Extrarenal causes include insensible losses or hypodipsia, and present with an appropriately concentrated urine (>700 mOsm/kg).

Hypervolemic hypernatremia is caused by excessive sodium gain. It is frequently iatrogenic and may

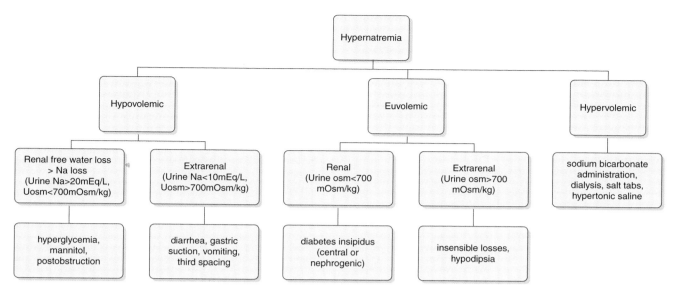

Figure 22-2. Etiologies of hypernatremia.

be due to excessive dosing of sodium bicarbonate, dialysis, salt tabs, or overcorrection with hypertonic saline.

Treatment

If the hypernatremic patient is unstable due to hypovolemia, volume resuscitation with normal saline should be aggressive until the patient is hemodynamically stable. After stabilization, fluids should be switched to 0.45% saline and correction rate monitored as described below. Although cerebral edema is a concern with rapid correction, the importance of correcting volume status outweighs the risk of this side effect. Additionally, these patients probably became hypernatremic acutely, so there has been less time for compensation and therefore lower risk of inducing cerebral edema. There should be a low threshold to get a head CT on the hypernatremic patient with neurologic deficit, as cerebral bleeding secondary to brain shrinkage and traction on cerebral vessels may occur.

As with hyponatremia, treatment of the stable hypernatremic patient will depend on the suspected etiology and volume status. The euvolemic patient may be treated with hypotonic saline; if central DI is suspected, vasopressin may be used. Hypervolemic hypernatremic patients require loop diuretics and free water replacement.

The stable hypernatremic patient should be corrected gradually to minimize the risk of cerebral edema, with a goal rate of 0.5 mEq/L/h and a maximum decrease of 10 mEq/L over a 24-hour period.[1] Expected sodium change with 1 L of fluid may be calculated by the same formula used for hyponatremia:

Na change with 1L IV fluid

$$= \frac{\text{Na content IV fluid (mEq/L)} - \text{serum Na (mEq/L)}}{\text{TBW} + 1}$$

$$\text{TBW} = \text{correction factor} \times \text{weight (kg)}$$

Correction factor:

Male	
Nonelderly	0.6
Elderly	0.5
Female	
Nonelderly	0.5
Elderly	0.45

Total free water deficit may be calculated by the following formula:

$$H_2O \text{ deficit} = \text{calculated TBW} \times \left(\frac{\text{serum Na}}{140} - 1\right)$$

The sodium content of common IV solutions is noted in Table 22-2. No more than half the free water deficit should be corrected in the first 24 hours, with the remainder corrected over the next 2–3 days. This calculation does not account for ongoing insensible losses. As in the correction of hyponatremia, predictive calculations may not be accurate, so sodium should be frequently monitored. Neurologic status should be assessed frequently, as acute changes may indicate the development of cerebral edema.

▶ DISORDERS OF POTASSIUM

Potassium disorders are the most frequently observed electrolyte disorders of hospitalized patients,[20] and probably of patients seen in the emergency department as well.[21] Given the predominantly intracellular distribution of potassium in the body, and in turn the inability to truly correct serum potassium levels acutely, treatment for disorders of potassium is by necessity a protracted endeavor.

Total body potassium stores average 50–55 mEq/kg body weight.[22] Of this, approximately 98% is contained intracellularly, and about 75% of the intracellular potassium is found in muscle tissue.[21] The remaining 2% is extracellular, and only about 0.4% of total body potassium can be found in the plasma. The concentration of potassium in the plasma is maintained in a fairly narrow range of 3.5–5.0 mmol/L. The intracellular concentration of potassium averages about 150 mmol/L. The rather steep gradient of potassium across the cell membrane is maintained by the sodium–potassium ATPase pump. It is predominantly this gradient of potassium across the cell membrane that maintains resting cell membrane potential.

Alterations in the ratio of intracellular potassium concentration to extracellular potassium concentration, $[K^+]_c \backslash [K^+]_e$, in turn alter the resting membrane potential.[22] The excitability of a membrane is defined as the difference between the resting and threshold potentials. If alterations to the $[K^+]_c \backslash [K^+]_e$ occur that increase the difference between the resting and threshold potentials, a decreased excitability is seen. Likewise, with changes in $[K^+]_c \backslash [K^+]_e$ that decrease the difference between the resting and threshold potentials, an increased excitability is seen.

The effects of hypokalemia or hyperkalemia on resting membrane potential, and in turn the degree to which symptoms or complications occur, are more directly related to the $[K^+]_c \backslash [K^+]_e$ than to the serum potassium concentration. A gradual reduction in total body potassium, where the intracellular concentration is decreased proportional to the reduction in extracellular concentration, will alter membrane excitability less than an acute change in serum potassium, where the intracellular concentration is not allowed to equilibrate. For this reason, alterations that occur due to transcellular shift of potassium into or out of cells are more likely to manifest symptoms than those that result from gradual losses or accumulations.

HYPOKALEMIA

Hypokalemia is defined as a serum potassium concentration of less than 3.5 mmol/L. Relatively mild hypokalemia, between 3.0 and 3.5 mmol/L, is often

▶ **TABLE 22-3. POTENTIAL CAUSES OF HYPOKALEMIA**

Decreased potassium intake	Medications known to cause hypokalemia
Intracellular shift of potassium	Sympathomimetics
Alkalemia	Loop and thiazide
Insulin	diuretics
Hypothermia	Osmotic diuretics
β-Adrenergic stimulation	Carbonic anhydrase
Increased potassium losses	inhibitors
Gastric suctioning/vomiting	Adrenocortical steroids
Diarrhea	Aminoglycosides
Diuretics	Amphotericin B
Hypomagnesemia	Cation-exchange resin

well tolerated by healthy people. In individuals with heart disease, particularly heart failure, even mild hypokalemia has been demonstrated to increase morbidity and mortality.[23–25] More severe hypokalemia may be associated with generalized symptoms of fatigue, weakness, and constipation. At levels under 2.5 mmol/L, muscle necrosis can occur, and at levels less than 2.0 mmol/L, an ascending paralysis, including respiratory failure, can develop. While usually not arrhythmogenic in healthy individuals, hypokalemia can induce dysrhthmias in those with underlying heart disease. Hypokalemia is well known to exacerbate the arrhythmogenic properties of digoxin.[25]

Hypokalemia can arise from deficient intake of potassium, increased excretion of potassium, or a transcellular shift of extracellular potassium into cells. See Table 22-3 for a list of potential causes of hypokalemia.

The typical American diet contains a surfeit of potassium, and, as such, hypokalemia due to decreased intake is rare. In starvation states, or more often in critically ill patients without adequate diet repletion, it is possible to elicit a potassium-deficient state in a matter of days. Adequate repletion usually prevents this.

Low serum potassium levels can be caused by total body depletion brought about by excessive potassium losses not matched by intake. Potassium losses typically occur via either renal or gastrointestinal routes. Renal potassium losses associated with diuretic use are the most common cause of hypokalemia. Nasogastric drainage can cause hypokalemia by depleting chloride levels. Concomitant magnesium depletion exacerbates renal losses, as low magnesium levels inhibit the kidney's ability to reabsorb potassium at the distal tubule. Assessment of urinary chloride levels can help to distinguish between causes of renal potassium losses: an elevated urine chloride (>25 mEq/L) is associated with magnesium depletion or diuretic-induced losses, while a low urine chloride (<15 mEq/L) is associated with nasogastric drainage or alkalosis-induced potassium losses.

Gastrointestinal losses of potassium arise due to diarrhea. The potassium concentration of stool is about 75 mEq/L. In states of excessive stool volume loss, potassium losses can quickly add up.

Several factors can promote a transcellular shift of potassium from the extracellular space into the cells, leading to a low serum potassium level despite normal total body potassium stores, including hypothermia, alkalosis, and multiple medications—such as insulin and any of the sympathomimetics. Profound hypothermia may also present with immediate or delayed hyperkalemia as the result of tissue death.

Many medications induce hypokalemia. In the ED or ICU, β-agonists are the most common culprit, although their effect at therapeutic doses is minimal, typically resulting in reductions in serum potassium levels of less than 0.5 mEq/L.[26] Other medications known to cause hypokalemia include loop and thiazide diuretics, osmotic diuretics, carbonic anhydrase inhibitors, adrenocortical steroids, natural penicillins, aminoglycosides, and amphotericin B.[27] See Table 22-3 for a list of potential causes of hypokalemia.

Treatment of the Hypokalemic Patient

Treatment of the hypokalemic patient should begin with identification and correction of any causes for intracellular shifts of potassium. Magnesium levels should be checked and hypomagnesemia corrected prior to attempts at potassium repletion, as hypomagnesemia will preclude effective potassium repletion. If true potassium depletion is thought to exist, potential causes should be identified, beginning with a thorough review of the patient's medication profile. If causes of ongoing potassium loss can be mitigated, do so. It is often the case that treatments iatrogenically causing potassium depletion are required due to the patient's underlying disease processes. In these cases, attempts should be made to establish adequate ongoing potassium supplementation in order to prevent repeat episodes of hypokalemia. Repletion of potassium must be done relatively slowly allowing for stable equilibration between the intracellular and extracellular compartments. Too rapid repletion of potassium will cause rapid rises in serum potassium concentrations, and in turn acutely increase the $[K^+]_c \backslash [K^+]_e$. IV repletion of potassium is routinely performed using potassium chloride solutions at a rate not in excess of 20 mEq/h. In cases of severe symptomatic potassium depletion, rates as high as 100 mEq/h have been reported as being used without ill effect.[28] Due to the irritating properties of the hyperosmotic potassium chloride solutions, infusion via a large central vein is preferred.

Oral potassium supplementation is better suited to ongoing supplementation than to rapid repletion.

Oral administration has the advantage that the rate of GI absorption inherently limits rapid changes in serum potassium concentrations. Oral potassium chloride salts can be used, or, in the context of concomitant hypophosphatemia, potassium phosphate salts.

Given the difficulty in estimating total body potassium deficit from the serum potassium level, it should come as no surprise that estimating the total amount of repletion required is difficult at best. In addition, the serum concentration to total body potassium stores relationship is not a linear one. Ongoing losses of potassium during attempts at repletion make calculating total repletion doses required more difficult. Due to the large intracellular distribution of potassium and the necessity of slow repletion, several days of repletion are often necessary in order to normalize serum concentrations safely, and the best way to track the amount of repletion required is to monitor repeated serum potassium concentrations. Due to the nonlinear nature of the serum potassium concentration to total body potassium levels, early repletion is likely to have minimal effects on serum concentration while smaller amounts of repletion will have more dramatic effects on serum concentration as the patient's total body potassium concentrations approach normal. As a general rule, however, a total of 175 mEq of potassium, given over several doses, should be needed for every 0.5 mEq/L decrease in the serum potassium level.[29]

HYPERKALEMIA

Elevated serum potassium levels are potentially arrhythmogenic due to their destabilizing effect on the myocardial cell membrane. See Table 22-4 for a list of potential causes of hyperkalemia.

▶ **TABLE 22-4. POTENTIAL CAUSES OF HYPERKALEMIA**

Decreased potassium excretion	Medications known to cause hyperkalemia
Renal failure	Citrate
Type IV renal tubular acidosis	Penicillin G
Hypoaldosteronism	Spironolactone/amelioride
Extracellular shift of potassium	Triamterene
Acidemia	Trimethoprim
β-Adrenergic blockade	β-Blockers
Hyperkalemic periodic paralysis	Digoxin
Drug induced	Angiotensin-converting enzyme inhibitors
Loss of cellular integrity	Angiotensin receptor blockers
Hemolysis	Succinylcholine
Ischemia	Heparin
Necrosis	

Hyperkalemia may be due to inability to excrete excess potassium, as occurs in renal failure, or due to a release of intracellular potassium into the extracellular space. Release of intracellular potassium stores can occur either as a result of a transcellular shift, as mentioned above, or as a result of cell ischemia and necrosis. Acutely ischemic skeletal muscle or gut, given the high concentration of potassium in muscle cells, can cause dramatic releases of potassium. Complications due to the rapid development of hyperkalemia following reperfusion of ischemic tissue are often cited as a proximate cause of death following crush injury. Hyperkalemia is rarely caused by excessive intake, except when associated with renal failure. The effects of hyperkalemia can be seen transiently if too rapid repletion of potassium is undertaken, without allowing time for the extracellular and intracellular compartments to equilibrate. Multiple medications can induce hyperkalemia, including cation-exchange resins, citrate, spironolactone/amelioride, triamterene, trimethoprim, digoxin, angiotensin-converting enzyme inhibitors, angiotensin receptor blockers, heparin, and succinylcholine.[27] See Table 22-4 for a list of potential causes of hyperkalemia.

The immediate concern following the identification of hyperkalemia is the need to stabilize myocardial cell membranes in order to prevent arrhythmic complications. A 12-lead EKG should be obtained, and examined for evidence of cell membrane instability. EKG abnormalities associated with mild hyperkalemia include large-amplitude T waves, and "peaked" or "tented" T waves. Moderate hyperkalemia can result in PR interval prolongation, decreased P-wave amplitude or disappearance, QRS complex widening, and conduction blocks with escape beats. Severe hyperkalemia can result in a sine-wave pattern, ventricular fibrillation, and eventually asystole[30] (see Figure 22-3).

If hyperkalemia has produced electrocardiographic evidence of myocardial instability, administration of calcium-containing salt solution should be undertaken immediately, as calcium will help stabilize the myocardial membrane, while subsequent efforts are made to normalize the serum potassium concentrations. Calcium is commonly available in calcium chloride and calcium gluconate solutions. Calcium chloride should only be infused via a large central line, as it is very hyperosmolar. Administration of 10 mL of 10% calcium chloride or

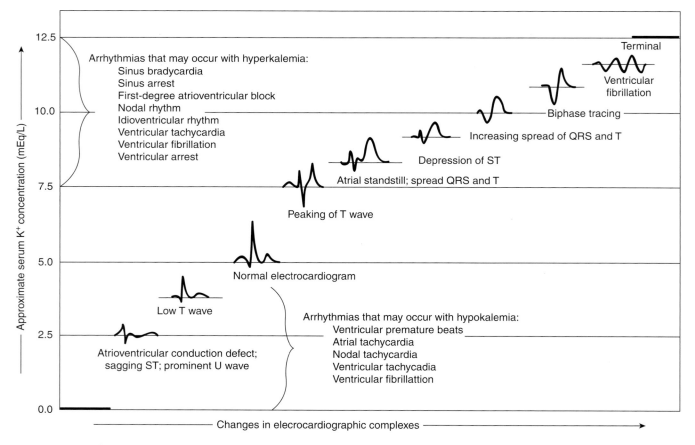

Figure 22-3. Correlation between serum potassium concentration and EKG findings. (Reproduced with permission from Stone CK, Humphries RL. *Current Diagnosis and Treatment: Emergency Medicine.* 6th ed. McGraw-Hill, Inc; 2008. Figure 42-2.)

30 mL of 10% calcium gluconate will have effects within minutes, but those effects will only last 30–60 minutes, requiring that other acute interventions be undertaken in that interval.

Treatments for hyperkalemia can be divided into those that temporize the hyperkalemia by inducing an intracellular shift of potassium and those that remove total body potassium. The former may be more appropriate if the hyperkalemia is suspected to be due to transcellular shifts of potassium as opposed to a total body excess of potassium.

Aggressive hydration with isotonic normal saline IV solution will help dilute the serum potassium, as well as promote diuresis and renal excretion of potassium if the patient is not oliguric. In the context of ischemia, aggressive resuscitation will help minimize ongoing potassium release by restoring perfusion.

Sodium bicarbonate induces an intracellular shift of potassium by inducing relative alkalemia. Because sodium bicarbonate and calcium salt solutions can precipitate when coadministered, some authors have advocated not using sodium bicarbonate if calcium salt administration is being performed. The risks of coadministration of sodium bicarbonate and calcium salts can be minimized by administering them through separate IV lines and/or temporally spacing their respective administration if the advantages of sodium bicarbonate administration are felt to be warranted.

β-Agonists cause an intracellular shift of potassium. Because β-agonists have arrhythmogenic properties of their own, some caution may be advised in their utilization, particularly in the presence of hyperkalemic EKG changes. The use of β_2-specific agonists, and albuterol in particular, can lower the serum potassium concentration acutely.

Insulin causes an intracellular shift of potassium. Because of insulin's obvious effect on serum blood sugars, it usually requires the coadministration of a dextrose-containing solution to prevent hypoglycemia. Typical dosing is 10 U of regular insulin administered with one or two ampoules of 50% dextrose in water (25–50 g D50).

Sodium polystyrene sulfonate (SPS) is a gastrointestinal-binding resin that exchanges sodium cations for potassium cations in the intestinal lumen, resulting in the fecal excretion of potassium. It does not work acutely as it requires the progressive equilibration of potassium across the intestinal mucosa. Effects are usually seen within 4–6 hours. Faster onset may be seen with the use of a retention enema of SPS. It is used more typically in the chronic renal failure patient in order to help prevent hyperkalemia. When initiated early in the acutely hyperkalemic patient, SPS may help prevent later rebound hyperkalemia after the effect of other acute interventions has begun to wane.

Diuretics are a frequent cause of hypokalemia, so it should be no surprise that they are employed to counter hyperkalemia. Non–potassium-sparing diuretics, most commonly furosemide, induce renal excretion of potassium. When using diuretics to remove excess potassium, replace urinary fluid output with isotonic IV fluid.

Hemodialysis will acutely clear elevated serum potassium levels as well as normalize hyperkalemia-inducing metabolic acidosis, and is the treatment of choice for acute severe hyperkalemia. The rate of clearance will vary depending on the dosing of dialysis and the diasylate chosen. Patient's electrolytes should be monitored closely following hemodialysis, as rebound hyperkalemia often occurs as the intracellular and extracellular compartments reequilibrate. Repeat runs of hemodialysis or a steady state of continuous renal replacement therapy may be required. As the initiation of hemodialysis often requires a significant amount of time, even in the well-resourced facilities, its availability should not preclude the early application of other more immediately available interventions.

▶ DISORDERS OF MAGNESIUM

Magnesium is the second most prevalent intracellular cation, next to potassium. It serves as a cofactor for enzymatic reactions involving adenosine triphosphate (ATP), including the sodium–potassium ATPase pump responsible for maintaining cell membrane potential. Magnesium also regulates the transport of calcium into smooth muscle cells.

Total body magnesium stores are approximately 24 g in the adult. Only about 1% of this is located in the extracellular fluid compartment, making imputation of the total body magnesium status from serum measures very difficult.[31]

MAGNESIUM DEFICIENCY

Effects of Magnesium Deficiency

There are no characteristic clinical findings specific for magnesium deficiency. Hypokalemia and/or hypocalcemia suggest the possibility of magnesium depletion, as low magnesium levels will impair renal absorption of potassium and the secretion of parathyroid hormone (PTH), respectively.

Cardiac dysrhythmias are associated with magnesium depletion, as magnesium is a cofactor in the sodium–potassium ATPase pump. Depletion of magnesium can result in depolarized myocytes and predispose to tachydysrhythmias. Magnesium depletion will accentuate the effects of digitalis toxicity, as both agents have their effect on the sodium–potassium ATPase membrane pump.[32] This is of particular concern as patients on digitalis are often also prescribed diuretics. Magnesium deficiency is associated classically with torsades de pointes, where the rapid administration of magnesium is a first-line therapy.

Magnesium's effect on smooth muscle has led to its use as an adjunctive therapy in severe asthma, although to what degree magnesium depletion might be contributory to the exacerbation of that disease state is unclear.

Causes of Magnesium Deficiency

Like potassium, low magnesium levels may be due to intracellular shifts of magnesium, or due to renal or gastrointestinal losses. Non–potassium-sparing diuretics, and in particular the loop diuretics, impair magnesium reabsorption and result in renal losses. Lower GI losses due to diarrhea result in loss of magnesium in the stool. Unlike potassium, however, upper GI losses due to vomiting or gastric drainage rarely lead to significant magnesium losses. Drug-induced causes of renal magnesium loss other than diuretics include use of aminoglycosides, amphotericin, pentamidine, cisplatin, and cyclosporine.[27] Digitalis, insulin, and epinephrine can all cause intracellular shifts in magnesium. Absent excessive losses, low magnesium levels are not frequently due to poor dietary intake in developed countries. An exception to this has been in the alcoholic population, where magnesium deficiency due to poor diet may impair attempts at thiamine repletion, as magnesium is a cofactor in the metabolism of thiamine into thiamine pyrophosphate.[33] See Table 22-5 for a list of potential causes of magnesium deficiency.

Diagnosis of Magnesium Deficiency

To even a greater degree than with potassium, the serum magnesium level is a poor measure of total body magnesium stores. The majority of magnesium is intracellular or within bone, and of the extracellular magnesium, much is protein bound and inert. Serum magnesium levels do not distinguish between ionized and bound forms of magnesium, and unlike calcium, specific ionized magnesium assays are not routinely available in most labs.[34]

Low serum levels of magnesium almost always reflect deficiency and warrant repletion, but many patients with deficiencies of magnesium have normal levels of serum magnesium. In the absence of renal disease or of renal losses of magnesium, the urine magnesium level may be a useful measure.

Often the only indication that magnesium may need repletion is the clinical suspicion brought about by identifying a predisposing condition. Patients on loop diuretics, those with refractory hypokalemia or hypocalcemia, anyone with an osmotic diuresis, those with lower GI losses due to diarrhea, and alcoholics undergoing thiamine repletion may all warrant repletion of magnesium based on clinical suspicion alone, regardless of otherwise normal serum magnesium levels.

Treatment of Magnesium Deficiency

Repletion of magnesium, as with potassium, must be done over time, although for different reasons. Once magnesium is infused, the shift from extracellular to intracellular fluid compartment is gradual, and renal excretion of perceived excess magnesium begins almost immediately after infusion. As such, a single dose of IV magnesium is likely to only have an effect on serum concentrations for about 30 minutes unless followed up by a steady-state administration over time while intracellular stores are repleted. Oral magnesium agents are useful in the outpatient environment to supplement diet and prevent deficits due to diuretic use, but are rarely adequate to replete deficits in the acute setting.

The IV solution of 50% magnesium sulfate ($MgSO_4$) is the agent most commonly available. This solution contains 4 mEq/mL of elemental magnesium. The 50% $MgSO_4$ solution is very hyperosmolar (4,000 mOsm/L), and should be diluted 5:1 to a 10% solution in normal saline before infusing.

Magnesium-depleted patients should be treated differently based on the severity of their depletion.[34,35] For mild asymptomatic hypomagnesemics, assume a total magnesium deficit of 1–2 mEq/kg. Because approximately 50% of the repleted magnesium will be lost in urine before intracellular equilibration, replete twice the anticipated deficit. Administer 1 mEq/kg over the first 24 hours, and then 0.5 mEq/kg per day over the next 3–4 days. If enteral access exists, oral repletion may be appropriate.

▶ **TABLE 22-5. POTENTIAL CAUSES OF MAGNESIUM DEFICIENCY**

Gastrointestinal losses	Medications known to cause magnesium deficiency
Diarrhea	
Renal losses	Aminoglycosides
Medication induced	Amphotericin B
Alcoholism	Cisplatin
Hypercalcemia	Cyclosporine
	Digoxin
	Diuretics
	Ticarcillin
	Foscarnet
	Methotrexate

For moderate hypomagnesemia (<1 mEq/L), add 6 g of $MgSO_4$ to 250 mL of normal saline and infuse over 3 hours, and then 5 g of $MgSO_4$ in 250 mL of normal saline over the next 6 hours, and finally 5 g of $MgSO_4$ every 12 hours for the next 5 days.

For severe life-threatening hypomagnesemia, or repletion in the context of torsades de points or seizure activity, infuse 2 g of $MgSO_4$ IV over 2–5 minutes. This dose may be repeated. Follow this with 5 g $MgSO_4$ in 250 mL of normal saline over the next 6 hours, and then an additional 5 g of $MgSO_4$ every 12 hours for 5 days.

MAGNESIUM EXCESS

Elevated magnesium levels are rarely a problem outside the context of renal failure, as excess magnesium is excreted renally with great facility. Symptomatically, hyporeflexia is seen at serum levels around 4 mEq/L, first-degree AV block at levels around 5 mEq/L, complete heart block at levels around 10 mEq/L, and cardiac arrest at levels around 13 mEq/L.[36] It would be rare to achieve clinically problematic elevated levels of magnesium in the context of renal failure without first encountering clinically significant hyperkalemia, unless an untoward level of magnesium intake were being undertaken. Hemodialysis is the treatment of choice for malignant hypermagnesemia. The administration of calcium salts, either calcium chloride or gluconate, can be used to temporize the conduction delays due to excess magnesium while hemodialysis is arranged.

▶ DISORDERS OF CALCIUM

Calcium is the most abundant electrolyte in the human body, but the vast majority of it (99%) is found in bone. The portion of calcium in the serum, which is measured on routine calcium concentration assays, exists partially as albumin or other protein-bound calcium, partially as chelated calcium, and partially as ionized calcium. Only the ionized calcium is metabolically active and of interest clinically. Unfortunately, routine lab values fail to distinguish between the different forms of serum calcium. Since variations in albumin concentration, as well as variations in the degree of calcium binding to albumin, directly affect the ionized calcium proportion, attempts at imputing the ionized calcium level from the total serum level of calcium are difficult at best. A number of calculations have been proposed to adjust the serum calcium concentration based on the serum albumin concentration; none of them reliably work in the acutely ill patient.[37] The only way to meaningfully appreciate the concentration of active ionized calcium is to directly measure the ionized calcium with an ion-specific probe. Fortunately, direct serum measurement of ionized calcium levels can now be routinely performed in most labs in a timely fashion. Normal values for serum ionized calcium are between 1.1 and 1.3 mmol/L (4.5–5.0 mg/dL).

HYPOCALCEMIA

Effects of Hypocalcemia

Hypocalcemia induces increased excitability of muscle tissue, leading to cardiac irritability and muscle twitching (evidenced by the oft-referenced but not sensitive Chvostek's and Trousseau's signs). Ionized hypocalcemia also impairs strength in muscle contractions, due to calcium's role in actin/myosin chain interactions. The result is progressive twitching leading eventually to tetany of skeletal muscles and hyperreflexia. Tetany of the laryngeal muscles may occur, creating an airway emergency. Cardiovascular effects include increased excitability and ectopy along with decreased myocardial function.

Causes of Hypocalcemia

Hypocalcemia is often seen in the acutely ill patient. While disorders of parathyroid function are the most common causes of hypocalcemia in the outpatient, they are rarely the culprit in the critically ill patient. Hypocalcemia in the critically ill patient is often multifactorial. See Table 22-6 for a list of potential causes of ionized hypocalcemia.

▶ TABLE 22-6. POTENTIAL CAUSES OF IONIZED HYPOCALCEMIA

Nonmedication induced	Medication induced	
Hypoparathyroidism	Fluoride poisoning	Primidone
Vitamin D deficiency	Bisphosphonates	Aminoglycosides
Chronic renal failure	Calcitonin	Phenobarbitol
Pancreatitis	Amphotericin B	Heparin
Citrate excess	Cimetidine	Chemotherapeutic agents
Tumor lysis syndrome	Phenytoin	Loop diuretics
Hyperphosphatemia	Ketoconazole	Isoniazid
Hypomagnesemia		
Sepsis/systemic inflammatory response syndrome		

Medications that can induce hypocalcemia include fluoride poisoning, bisphosphonates, calcitonin, amphotericin B, cimetidine, ethanol, foscarnet, citrate, albumin, heparin, phenytoin, rifampin, aminoglycosides, loop diuretics, isoniazid, and propothiouracil.[27]

Hypomagnesemia can blunt calcitriol production as well as blunt the end-organ response to calcitriol. For this reason, repletion of magnesium in the case of low magnesium levels or refractory ionized hypocalcemia is recommended. Hyperphosphatemia can lead to chelation of ionized calcium in renal failure. Chelation of ionized calcium also occurs during massive blood transfusions, where large cumulative infused amounts of citrate (used as anticoagulant in stored blood products) can drop the ionized calcium levels. For this reason, monitoring and repletion of ionized calcium should be performed as necessary during massive transfusions, particularly in the context of refractory hypotension.[38]

Sepsis and the systemic inflammatory response syndrome (SIRS) are associated with hypocalcemia, probably due to decreased PTH and calcitriol production.[39] No clinical benefit has been seen to ionized calcium repletion in sepsis if patients are asymptomatic, and it is not clear if sepsis-related ionized hypocalcemia is protective or deleterious.

Treatment of Hypocalcemia

Treatment of ionized hypocalcemia is 2-fold: (1) identify and treat the underlying disorder that gave rise to the ionized hypocalcemia; (2) replete symptomatic or severe (<0.8 mmol/L) ionized hypocalcemia emergently. Calcium only requires urgent repletion if symptomatic or if approaching critically low levels. Previous studies have suggested no advantage to repletion of asymptomatic ionized hypocalcemia above levels of 0.65 mmol/L,[40] while one recent study indicated increased adverse outcomes only in patients with ionized calcium levels below 0.8 mmol/L.[41] Calcium administration is not benign, particularly in the context of tissue hypoxia, where calcium administration can aggravate cellular injury.[42] Rapid infusion of calcium solutions can cause bradycardia, hypotension, and vasodilatation. When indicated, IV repletion should be undertaken with either calcium gluconate or calcium chloride. Calcium gluconate and calcium chloride each comes in 10-mL vials, each containing 100 mg of its respective compound. Calcium chloride, however, has three times the elemental calcium of calcium gluconate (27 mg/mL [1.36 mEq/mL] vs. 9 mg/mL [0.46 mEq/mL], respectively). Calcium chloride is significantly more hyperosmolar than calcium gluconate (2,000 mOsm/L vs. 680 mOsm/L), and so should only be infused through a large central line.

Both solutions should be diluted in normal saline or dextrose 5% in water prior to administration. Calcium will equilibrate between the extracellular and intracellular space following infusion, and the immediate results seen following infusion will wane within 30 minutes of administration unless a follow-up infusion is started.[40] A total of 200 mg of elemental calcium (corresponding to approximately 8 mL of 10% calcium chloride, or 22 mL of 10% calcium gluconate) may be required to increase the ionized calcium 0.1 mmol/L.

HYPERCALCEMIA

Hypercalcemia, defined as an increase in ionized calcium greater than 2.6 mmol/L, is rare in critically ill patients. The most common cause of hypercalcemia in the ED, as in outpatients, is primary hyperparathyroidism, which can be diagnosed with a PTH level. When present in critically ill patients, hypercalcemia is most often associated with underlying malignancy, although it may also be seen in other disorders that result in increased bone resorption such as sarcoidosis or with prolonged immobilization. A few medications can cause hypercalcemia, including thiazide diuretics, lithium, and vitamin D or A supplementation.[27]

Effects of Hypercalcemia

Mild hypercalcemia is often asymptomatic. Gastrointestinal symptoms include ileus, constipation, nausea, and vomiting due to smooth muscle relaxation. Patients often suffer from severe lethargy, dehydration due to polyuria, and stupor. Cardiac features include shortened QTc, broadened T waves, and first-degree AV block. There is very poor correlation between serum calcium levels and the severity of symptoms.[43]

Treatment of Hypercalcemia

IV fluid hydration and diuresis to promote renal excretion are indicated if the patient is symptomatic, or in the case of ionized calcium levels greater than 3.5 mmol/L.[44] If underlying malignancy is suspected to exist, use of salmon calcitonin or bisphosphanates may be useful. Hydrocortisone may be useful in the case of multiple myeloma.[45]

▶ DISORDERS OF PHOSPHORUS

Phosphorus (PO_4) exists predominantly in bone, and as free ionic PO_4 intracellularly. PO_4 is critical in all ATP-related energy-requiring cellular activities such as glycolysis and high-energy phosphate bond formation. Normal serum levels of PO_4 are 2.5–5.0 mg/dL, or 0.8–1.6 mmol/L.

HYPOPHOSPHATEMIA

Hypophosphatemia can be the result of an intracellular shift of PO_4, an excess of PO_4 secretion, or a deficiency in PO_4 intake.

Effects of Hypophosphatemia

Hypophosphatemia is usually clinically silent unless very profound. The effects of hypophosphatemia are all related to cellular energy production, including a decrease in cardiac output observed in heart failure patients, a theoretical decrease in skeletal muscle strength, and reports of difficulty weaning from ventilators due to respiratory muscle weakness.[46,47] Multiple reports of cardiac arrest, cardiovascular collapse, or profound encephalopathy associated with profound hypophosphatemia exist in the emergency medicine literature, many associated with intracellular shifts of PO_4 during high-dose insulin therapy for DKA.[48–50]

Causes of Hypophosphatemia

The transit of glucose into cells is an active process in which PO_4 is cotransported into the cell. As such, both the feeding of a patient who has been nutritionally deprived and the aggressive use of insulin for tight euglycemic control can cause dramatic intracellular shifts of glucose, and in turn PO_4. Any time nutritional support is started on a patient after a period of deprivation, gradual increases in caloric intake along with frequent assessment of serum PO_4 levels should be undertaken.

Alkalosis can cause intracellular shift of PO_4, presumably due to increased glycolysis that accompanies increased intracellular pH. This is seen to a far greater degree in respiratory alkalosis than in metabolic alkalosis, and accounts for the increased incidence of hypophosphatemia seen in chronic obstructive pulmonary disease (COPD) patients.[51]

The use of β-receptor sympathomimetics is associated with a transient intracellular shift of PO_4, although the clinical significance of this is not clear.[52] The same response to sympathetic tone may account for the hypophosphatemia seen in sepsis or SIRS.

The use of antacid compounds, such as sucralfate or aluminum hydroxide, can bind phosphate in the upper gastrointestinal tract and impair its absorption.

Other medications that can cause hypophosphatemia include glucocorticoids, insulin, and, when in overdose, acetaminophen, aspirin, and theophylline.[27]

▶ **TABLE 22-7. POTENTIAL CAUSES OF HYPOPHOSPHATEMIA**

Internal redistribution	Medications known to cause hypophosphatemia
Refeeding syndrome	Antacids
Respiratory alkalosis	Sucralfate
Sepsis/systemic inflammatory response syndrome	Phosphate binders
	Aspirin (in overdose)
Decreased intestinal absorption	Catecholamines
Inadequate dietary intake	Acetaminophen (in overdose)
Chronic diarrhea	Glucocorticoids
Increased urinary losses	Diuretics
Hyperglycemia	Theophylline (in overdose)
Osmotic diuresis	

Osmotic dieresis, as a result of either hyperglycemia or administration of an osmotic diuretic, can impair renal reabsorption, and lead to urinary wasting of phosphate.

See Table 22-7 for a list of potential causes of hypophosphatemia.

Treatment of Hypophosphatemia

PO_4 can be repleted in IV formulation with either sodium phosphate (93 mg/mL [3 mmol/mL] PO_4, 4.0 mEq/mL sodium) or potassium phosphate (93 mg/mL [3 mmol/mL] PO_4, 4.4 mEq/mL potassium). Patients presenting with a serum PO_4 of less than 2.0 mg/dL should receive 15 mmol of sodium phosphate in 100 mL of sodium chloride, infused over 2 hours. If a concomitant hypokalemia exists, potassium phosphate can be substituted at an equal dose. If follow-up serum PO_4 levels at 6 hours remain less than 2 mg/dL, identical repeat doses can be administered up to 45 mmol of PO_4 in a 24-hour period.[53] If no central venous access is available, the above doses should be diluted in a total of 250 mL of normal saline in order to prevent phlebitic complications of infusing a hyperosmolar solution. Oral PO_4-containing solutions, such as K-Phos or Neutra-Phos, cannot be used effectively for the large doses of PO_4 required to replete severe hypophosphatemia (<1.0 mg/dL), as they tend to promote diarrhea, but can be used to maintain PO_4 levels once repletion via IV is complete, or to replete mild asymptomatic phosphate deficits.[54] Repletion of mild to moderate hypophosphatemia in the ED may be accomplished with the administration of 2–3 g of sodium phosphate or potassium phosphate, most formulations of which contain 8 mmol of PO_4 per packet or capsule. Daily PO_4 intake requirements, absent excessive losses, are about 1,200 mg (38 mmol) per day orally or about 800 mg (25 mmol) per day IV for a 70-kg adult.

HYPERPHOSPHATEMIA

Hyperphosphatemia occurs as the result of renal failure or the widespread necrosis of cells, as in ischemia/reperfusion, rhabdomyolysis, or tumor lysis. The principal concern is for the formation of calcium–PO_4 insoluble complexes and subsequent profound hypocalcemia. Treatment is with IV hydration, and the administration of PO_4-binding agents via the gastrointestinal tract, such as sucralfate, aluminum-containing antacids, or calcium acetate. Hemodialysis, while rarely necessary, may be employed to promote PO_4 clearance in the renal failure patient.[55]

REFERENCES

1. Lin M, Liu SJ, Lim IT. Disorders of water imbalance. *Emerg Med Clin North Am.* 2005;23:749.
2. Sajadieh A, Binici Z, Maridsen MK, et al. Mild hyponatremia carries a poor prognosis in community subjects. *Am J Med.* 2009;122:679.
3. Palmer BF, Gates JR, Lader M. Causes and management of hyponatremia. *Ann Pharmacother.* 2003;37:1694.
4. Yeong-Hau HL, Shapiro JI. Hyponatremia: clinical diagnosis and management. *Am J Med.* 2007;120:653.
5. Biswas M, Davies JS. Hyponatremia in clinical practice. *Postgrad Med J.* 2007;83:373.
6. Verbalis JG, Goldsmith SR, Greenberg A, et al. Hyponatremia treatment guidelines 2007: expert panel recommendations. *Am J Med.* 2007;120:S1.
7. Reynolds RM, Padfield PL, Seckl JR. Disorders of sodium balance. *BMJ.* 2006;332:702.
8. Hillier TA, Abbott RD, Barrett EJ. Hyponatremia: evaluating the correction factor for hyperglycemia. *Am J Med.* 1999;106:399.
9. Hahn RG. Fluid absorption in endoscopic surgery. *Br J Anaesth.* 2006;96:8.
10. McGee S, Abernathy WB, Simel DL. The rational clinical exam: is this patient hypovolemic? *JAMA.* 1999;281:1022.
11. Lee C, Guo H, Chen J. Hyponatremia in the emergency department. *Am J Emerg Med.* 2000;18:264.
12. Rahman M, Friedman WA. Hyponatremia in neurosurgical patients: clinical guidelines development. *Neurosurgery.* 2009;65:925.
13. Ellison DH, Berl T. The syndrome of inappropriate antidiuretic hormone. *N Engl J Med.* 2007;356:2064.
14. DeLuca L, Klein L, Udelson JE, et al. Hyponatremia in patients with heart failure. *Am J Cardiol.* 2005;96:19L.
15. Kim WR, Biggins SW, Kremers WK, et al. Hyponatremia and mortality among patients on the liver transplant waiting list. *N Engl J Med.* 2008;359:1018.
16. Annane D, Decaux G, Smith N. Efficacy and safety of oral conivaptan, a vasopressin-receptor antagonist, evaluated in a randomized, controlled trial in patients with euvolemic or hypervolemic hyponatremia. *Am J Med Sci.* 2009;337:28.
17. Nguyen MK, Kurtz I. Analysis of current formulas used for treatment of the dysnatremias. *Clin Exp Nephrol.* 2004;8:12.
18. Adrogue HJ, Madias NE. Hypernatremia. *N Engl J Med.* 2000;342:1493.
19. Sands JM, Bichet DG. Nephrogenic diabetes insipidus. *Ann Int Med.* 2006;144:186.
20. Acker CG, Johnson JP, Palevsky PM, et al. Hyperkalemia in hospitalized patients: cause, adequacy of treatment, and results of an attempt to improve physician compliance with published therapy guidelines. *Arch Intern Med.* 1998;158:917.
21. Schaefer TJ, Wolford RW. Disorders of potassium. *Emerg Med Clin North Am.* 2005;23:723.
22. Rose DB, Post TW. Introduction to disorders of potassium balance. In: *Clinical Physiology of Acid–Base and Electrolyte Disorders.* 5th ed. New York: McGraw-Hill; 2001:822.
23. Gennari FJ. Hypokalemia. *N Engl J Med.* 1998;339:451.
24. Bowling CB, Pitt B, Ahmed MI. Hypokelemia and outcomes in patients with chronic heart failure and chronic kidney disease: findings from propensity matches studies. *Circ Heart Fail.* 2010;3:253.
25. Kjeldsen K. Hypokalemia and sudden cardiac death. *Exp Clin Cardiol.* 2010;15:e96.
26. Allon M, Copkney C. Albuterol and insulin for treatment of hyperkalemia in hemodialysis patients. *Kidney Int.* 1990;38:869.
27. Buckley MS, LeBlanc JM, Cawley MJ. Electrolyte disturbances associated with commonly prescribed medications in the intensive care unit. *Crit Care Med.* 2010;38:S253.
28. Kim GH, Han JS. Therapeutic approach to hypokalemia. *Nephron.* 2002;92 (suppl 1):28.
29. Marino PL. *Potassium. The ICU Book.* 3rd ed. Philadelphia, PA: Lippincott Williams and Wilkins; 2007.
30. Diercks DM, Shumaik GM, Harrigan RA, et al. Electrocardiographic manifestations: electrolyte abnormalitis. *J Emerg Med.* 2004;27:153.
31. Elin RJ. Assessment of magnesium status. *Clin Chem.* 1987;33:1965.
32. Cohen L, Kitzes R. Magnesium sulfate and digitalis-toxic arrhythmias. *JAMA.* 1983;249:2808.
33. Dyckner T, Ek B, Nyhlin H, et al. Aggravation of thiamine deficiency by magnesium depletion: a case report. *Acta Med Scand.* 1985;218:129.
34. Mareno P. *Magnesium. The ICU Book.* 3rd ed. Philadelphia, PA: Lippincott Williams and Wilkins; 2007:611.
35. Oster JR, Epstein M. Management of magnesium depletion. *Am J Nephrol.* 1988;8:349.
36. Van Hook JW. Hypermagnesemia. *Crit Care Clin.* 1991;7:215.
37. Slomp J, van der Voort PH, Gerritsen RT, et al. Albumin adjusted calcium is not suitable for diagnosis of hyper- and hypocalcemia in the critically ill. *Crit Care Med.* 2003;31:1389.
38. Lier H, Bottger BW, Hinkelbein J, et al. Coagulation management in multiple trauma: a systematic review. *Intensive Care Med.* 2011. Epub ahead of print.
39. Jankowski S, Vincent JL. Calcium administration for cardiovascular support in critically ill patients: when is it indicated? *J Intensive Care Med.* 1995;10:91.
40. Zaloge GP. Hypocalcemia in critically ill patients. *Crit Care Med.* 1992;20:251.

41. Moritoki E, Inbyung K, Nichol A, et al. Ionized calcium concentration and outcome in critical illness. *Crit Care Med.* 2011;39:314.

42. Vincent J-L, Bredas P, Jankowski S, Kahn RJ. Correction of hypocalcaemia in the critically ill: what is the haemodynamic benefit? *Intensive Care Med.* 1995;21:838.

43. Kacprowicz RF, Lloyd JD. Electrolyte complications of malignancy. *Emerg Med Clin North Am.* 2009;27:257.

44. Forster J, Querusio L, Burchard KW, Gann DS. Hypercalcemia in critically ill surgical patients. *Ann Surg.* 1985;202:512.

45. Stewart AF. Clinical practice: hypercalcemia associated with cancer. *N Engl J Med.* 2005;352:373.

46. Aubier M, Murciano D, Lecocguic Y. Effect of hypophosphatemia on diaphragmatic contractility in patients with acute respiratory failure. *N Engl J Med.* 1985; 313:420.

47. Knochel JP. The pathophysiology and clinical characteristics of severe hypophosphatemia. *Arch Intern Med.* 1977;137:203.

48. Osuka A, Matsuoka T, Idoguchi K. Is this the worst outcome of metabolic syndrome? Hypophosphatemia and resulting cardiac arrest during the treatment of diabetic ketoacidosis with hypertriglyceridemia. *Intern Med.* 2009; 48:1391.

49. Megarbane B, Guerrier G, Blancher A, et al. A possible hypophosphatemia-induced, life threatening encephalopathy in diabetic ketoacidosis: a case report. *Am J Med Sci.* 2007;333:384.

50. Bohannon NJ. Large phosphate shifts with treatment for hyperglycemia. *Arch Intern Med.* 1989;149:1423.

51. Shiber JR, Mauut A. Serum phosphate abnormalities in the emergency department. *J Emerg Med.* 2002;23:395.

52. Bodenhamer J, Bergstrom R, Brown D, et al. Frequently nebulized beta-agonists for asthma: effects on serum electrolytes. *Ann Emerg Med.* 1992;21:1337.

53. Rosen GH, Boullata JI, O'Rangers EA, et al. Intravenous phosphate repletion regimen for critically ill patients with moderate hypophosphatemia. *Crit Care Med.* 1995;24:1204.

54. Miller DW, Slovis CM. Hypophosphatemia in the emergency department therapeutics. *Am J Emerg Med.* 2000;18:457.

55. Rutecki GW, Whittier FC. Life-threatening phosphate imbalance: when to suspect, how to treat. *J Crit Illness.* 1997;12:699.

CHAPTER 23

Acute Renal Failure and Renal Replacement Therapy

Alex Flaxman and Deborah Stein

► INTRODUCTION

In keeping with the role of providing organ support, such as managing a ventilator for pulmonary support, or pressors for cardiovascular support, it is often the intensivist's role to provide support for failing kidneys. This chapter will focus on when and how to provide that support.

Normally functioning kidneys are important in several homeostatic mechanisms:

1. The production of hormones such as erythropoietin and renin
2. Partial conjugation required to activate vitamin D that is necessary to absorb enteral calcium
3. The regulation of acid–base status along with the lungs
4. The filtration of the blood and regulation of concentrations of solutes such as sodium and potassium
5. The elimination of fluid and waste products such as urea

It is assisting or replacing these last three functions—solute clearance and volume regulation—that will be the focus of this chapter.

► RENAL FAILURE

Depending on the population studied, the incidence of renal failure (RF) in ICU patients has been reported to be as high as 25%.[1,2] There is disparity, however, in how RF is defined in clinical practice as well as in the literature. This has led to initiation of renal support at different levels of renal function, which makes it difficult to compare studies, construct studies, or extrapolate findings to one's own patient population.

The Acute Dialysis Quality Initiative Group (ADQI), a group formed in 2000 "to provide an objective, dispassionate distillation of the literature description of the current state of practice of dialysis and related therapies,"[3] recently proposed a classification scheme for diagnosing acute renal failure (ARF).[4] Commonly referred to as the RIFLE criteria, the acronym itself describes the level of renal dysfunction:

R—Risk of renal dysfunction
I—Injury to the kidney
F—Failure of kidney function
L—Loss of kidney function
E—End-stage kidney disease

Each level (R-I-F-L-E) of renal dysfunction can be classified or diagnosed by either the glomerular filtration rate (GFR) or urine output (UO).

The GFR is generally considered a better measure of renal function/failure, although it is typically only measured via surrogates such as creatinine clearance. Interpreting a change in GFR requires knowledge of the baseline creatinine that is not always available. For instance, a previously healthy trauma patient who is now acutely ill may have never had his or her baseline serum creatinine measured, while a patient whose primary doctor sends a basic metabolic panel including blood urea nitrogen (BUN) and creatinine every year, or an elective surgery candidate who had preoperative labs drawn, will have a known baseline creatinine.

In the event that a baseline creatinine is not known, or for providers who are more comfortable, UO can also be used. The advantage of UO is that it can be used on all patients except for patients anuric prior to their acute illness (e.g., end-stage renal patients already on dialysis) or in whom UO cannot be measured (e.g., patients with ureteral diversions such as ureterosigmoidostomy). Furthermore, UO is recorded on ICU flow sheets and is a noninvasive or minimally invasive parameter that is easy to measure and follow.

The ADQI group released a graphical representation of the criteria, as shown in Figure 23-1.

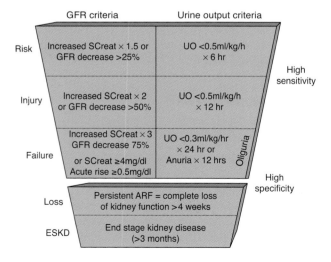

Figure 23-1. The RIFLE criteria. (Reproduced with permission from Acute Dialysis Quality Initiative [ADQI], http://www.adqi.net.)

The shape of the diagram (wider at the top) is meant to indicate a higher sensitivity (S_n). Therefore, more patients will meet these criteria, while patients who do not meet the criteria are unlikely to have RF (i.e., low risk of false negatives). As might be expected, these same criteria have a lower specificity (S_p), so many patients who meet these criteria will not have ARF (i.e., higher risk of false positives).

Similarly, the criteria at the bottom of the diagram have a lower S_n and may miss patients who do have RF (i.e., higher risk of false negatives). However, these criteria have a high S_p, so as patients progressively meet the criteria toward the bottom of the picture, they are more likely to have true RF (i.e., low risk of false positives).

As more studies use the ADQI Group's RIFLE criteria, it will likely become easier to compare studies with each other, and to identify studies whose populations are similar to one's own population, leading to better evidence-based approaches.

▶ WHEN TO INITIATE RENAL SUPPORT

The indications for initiating renal support can be remembered by the mnemonic AEIOU RSI:

A—**A**cidosis
E—**E**lectrolyte abnormality
I—**I**ntoxication, **I**ngestion, and **I**mmune modulation (still controversial)
O—Fluid **O**verload
U—**U**remia
R—**R**habdomyolysis
S—**S**epsis (especially in multiorgan failure) (still controversial)
I—after **I**V contrast (for patients with renal insufficiency [RI] or ARF)[5–7]

Renal support should be initiated if the patient has any of the above indications. In the case of patients who will receive IV contrast, this is particularly true if the patient has baseline RI that is resistant to treatment.

▶ BACKGROUND FOR RENAL SUPPORT

Renal replacement therapy (RRT) is a therapy designed to clear the blood of substances and volume that functioning kidneys would normally remove. The most commonly thought of substances that RRT clears are volume, potassium, and urea.

There are two broad categories of RRT: intermittent renal replacement therapy (IRRT) and continuous renal replacement therapy (CRRT). IRRT is the more familiar of these two. The most common modality used in IRRT is hemodialysis (HD), and the abbreviation often seen is intermittent hemodialysis (IHD).

In its most common form, an outpatient with chronic renal failure (CRF) goes to a dialysis center and receives HD for 3 hours, three times per week; usually Monday–Wednesday–Friday or Tuesday–Thursday–Saturday. By following a specific lifestyle, such as a renal diet and limiting fluid intake, these sessions are enough to remove solutes and fluid and thereby approximate what normal human kidneys accomplish with continuous normal blood flow. When such patients are admitted to a hospital (for renal or unrelated issues), they should receive their normal HD sessions, with adjustments made for their acute illness. Either such sessions can be run at the patient's bedside or, if the patient is stable for transport, the patient may be moved to the hospital's dialysis center.

The advantage of IHD is cost, in terms of both time and resources. IHD requires a specialized nurse, but only for 9 hours per week. The general disadvantages of IHD are the requirement of large vascular access (usually initially done with a long-term indwelling dual-lumen vascular catheter, and later via a surgically constructed arteriovenous fistula or graft, aka a "shunt"), and the need to attend a dialysis center three times per week for 3 hours. Another major disadvantage is the buildup of substances (potassium, urea) and body fluid (blood volume, edema) over 2–3 days with rapid resolution over 3 hours. These shifts are not as gentle on a patient as the continuous clearance performed by the patient's own kidneys.

Emergency physicians are acutely aware of this issue since patients with dialysis disequilibrium often present to the emergency department (ED). In addition to lesser symptoms such as headache, vertigo, and weakness, dialysis disequilibrium can cause seizure, intracerebral hemorrhage, cerebral edema, and even death.[8]

Among outpatients, however, not everyone is a candidate for traditional IHD. For outpatients in whom sufficient vascular access cannot be obtained (either with a long-term indwelling catheter or with construction of an arteriovenous graft), peritoneal dialysis is an option for IRRT. However, patients must be otherwise hemodynamically stable, and still urinate in sufficient quantity.

In peritoneal dialysis, a surgeon implants a port into the patient's peritoneal space. The patient, a visiting nurse, or an automated machine (at night, while the patient sleeps) adds fluid via the access port. The dialysis fluid remains in the abdomen, equilibrating with the patient's interstitial fluid. The fluid along with solutes and electrolytes (such as urea and potassium) is then drained and discarded, and new fluid is added. This must be done manually several times per day or,

if at night, automatically several times overnight. The primary advantages of PD are 2-fold. First, it avoids the huge chemical and fluid shifts associated with a 2- to 3-day buildup between traditional HD sessions and removal over 3 hours. Second, it is convenient since a reliable patient can administer this therapy himself or herself, at home. The main disadvantages of PD are complications related to the catheter—specifically local infection (cellulitis) and peritonitis, which can be fatal—and cardiac and pulmonary dysfunction related to negative effects on diaphragmatic excursion secondary to the excess intra-abdominal fluid.[9]

For outpatients who have poor vascular access and are also not PD candidates, alternative vascular access must be sought. One approach is to place an access port to dialyze using a plexus such as the lumbar plexus.

Outpatient modalities, however, are often not appropriate for use in the ICU. Since, as previously discussed, up to 25% of ICU patients will develop ARF at some point during their illness, intensivists must be able to support the kidneys as they would support any other organ.

Whether the RF is transient and will resolve with the patient's illness or will become permanent, a patient in ARF will require some renal support. If permanent, patients may eventually require outpatient IHD as described above. But while in the acute phase of his or her illness, it is difficult to determine if a patient's renal function will recover. Furthermore, even for patients who were already on IHD, a critical illness may prevent the performance of IHD.

One reason is that during a critical illness, patients become nutritionally deficient. To maintain a patient on every other day renal dialysis, it is necessary to restrict fluid and, more importantly, protein intake. But it is precisely the protein intake that will help the patient recover. When on CRRT, patients can be fed, enterally or parenterally, without concern of urea accumulation over 2–3 days. In other words, there is no need to limit feeding for patients on CRRT while there is such a limitation for patients receiving IHD.

Due to the high blood flow volumes (remember, IHD accomplishes in 9 hours what normal kidneys do in 168 hours), there is a significant blood pressure drop when IHD is initiated. This blood pressure drop is not benign. This hemodynamic instability, however temporary, has been reported to cause loss of consciousness and myocardial infarction, and has even caused patients with partial RF (sometimes called RI) to go into complete RF.[10] Furthermore, for patients with hemodynamic instability, IHD may be contraindicated. In the past, some of these patients were treated with PD, but the clearances were generally not sufficient, and in many of those cases (such as abdominal injury or infection) PD was contraindicated.[11] For these patients, CRRT is the answer.

▶ THE FINAL ARGUMENT

Despite the number of critical care patients who have contraindications to IHD, many feel that if a patient can tolerate it, IHD should be the preferred modality, mainly due to cost. This is false. Countless studies have shown a reduction in mortality and morbidity when patients go on CRRT.

As previously mentioned, differences in when renal replacement therapies are initiated, which modalities are used, which settings are used, and when they are halted make reviewing the literature a challenge. However, several key concepts have been proven over and over.

Kellum et al performed a meta-analysis and found that, after pooling studies that enrolled patients with similar APACHE II scores, mortality was lower in patients treated with CRRT.[12] Furthermore, when adjusted for study quality and severity of illness, mortality was still noted to be lower in patients treated with CRRT. The only negative conclusion was that it was not possible to determine the optimum timing, modality, and dose of CRRT.

Perhaps the most convincing evidence was an unexpected conclusion from Jacka et al. In their study, they found that among patients who survived their critical illness, those who received continuous venovenous renal replacement therapy (CVVRRT), as opposed to IHD, were more likely to recover their renal function and not require IHD on a long-term or permanent basis.[13] This conclusion was also suggested by Waldrop et al,[14] though not proven since their study was not powered to detect this outcome. This study drew two conclusions: (1) that patients who suffer ARF secondary to a critical illness have such a high mortality from their inciting event that the massive mortality risk obscures any small benefit CVV might incur and (2) that perhaps studies have been evaluating the wrong endpoint and should instead be powered to study recovery of renal function after CVV versus IHD, rather than mortality benefit.

Finally, one common theme stands out among all the studies. One absolute indication for CVV over IHD is hemodynamic instability (i.e., hypotension) too severe to withstand IHD. Such a degree of hypotension is an indicator of sicker patients. It is difficult to randomize patients to IHD or CVV due to this difference and the fact that these patients are, by necessity, typically placed in the CVV groups. These studies then fail to show a difference between IHD and CVV. One interpretation of this outcome is that CVV may be demonstrating itself to be a superior modality, by achieving survival rates with sicker patients comparable to that achieved by IHD with healthier patients.

▶ THE SIMPLEST CIRCUIT-SCUF

At its core, CRRT is the same as IHD. In each modality, blood is removed from the patient, "bad" substances and excess fluid are removed, and the "cleaned" blood is then returned to the patient.

In the most basic of RRT setups Figure 23-2, blood is removed from the patient at a rate called the blood flow rate, or Q_B. It is put through a hydrostatic pump that contains a filter with holes in it. Any solute dissolved or suspended in the fluid that is smaller than the size of the holes (such as potassium and urea) will go through. Different filters have different size holes, but generally the holes are 500–50,000 d—large enough to allow passage of fluid and solutes, but small enough to prevent loss of plasma proteins such as albumin (80,000 d). This allows fluid and small solutes to be removed without also removing plasma proteins or RBCs. The remainder of the fluid is then returned to the patient.

The fluid extracted is an ultrafiltrate (UF) of plasma. As expected, it has a mild yellow color and resembles urine. The amount of UF generated is expressed in terms of milliliters per minute. Solutes are removed via "solute drag," that is, the solutes are dragged along with the fluid forced out of the system.

The setup in Figure 23-2 is called slow continuous ultrafiltrate (SCUF), and is the most basic of CRRT modalities. It is not used often because solute clearance is limited to the concentration in the fluid removed. All other CRRT setups, however, build on the foundation of SCUF.

When blood is returned to the patient, it is returned into a central vein. However, the blood draw line can be placed in an artery or a vein.

- If blood is drawn from an artery, this is called continuous arteriovenous renal replacement therapy (CAVRRT, usually shortened to CAVRT or CAVH where the H stands for hemofiltration [HF]).
- If blood is drawn from a vein, this is called CVVRRT (usually shortened to CVVRT, CVVH, or, more commonly, CVV).

When RRT was first developed, blood was taken from an artery. This allowed for a simpler mechanism

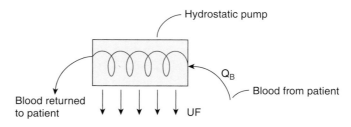

Figure 23-2. Slow continuous ultrafiltration (SCUF). UF: ultrafiltrate; Q_B: blood flow.

because no pump was required. The system used the patient's blood pressure (and therefore the patient's heart) as the driving force to keep blood moving through the system. However, CAVRT had many complications, mostly due to the arterial cannulation. Tominaga et al reported arteriovenous fistulas (when an adjacent artery and vein—such as the femoral vessels—were cannulated), pseudoaneurysms, DVTs, ischemia in limbs distal to the arterial cannulation secondary to clot embolization, and persistent bleeding requiring surgical intervention.[15] They noted that the rates of vascular complications with CAVRT are similar to those of the arterial access for angiograms—something not reported in CVVRT, at all—suggesting that the complication is related to the arterial cannulation itself, rather than the dwell length of the catheter. In addition to the complications reported by Tominaga et al, Bellomo et al reported shunt failures requiring revisions, infections, bleeding from the shunt itself, recurrent clotting requiring invasive intervention, and hematomas from failed arterial cannulations.[16]

Even more importantly, patients receiving CAVRT have shown a higher mortality compared with those receiving CVVRT.[17] It is postulated that this mortality is a result of the lower clearance rates achievable with CAVRT as opposed to CVVRT. In fact, many patients placed on CAVRT required IHD for additional solute clearance.[11,16–18] Finally, CAVRT requires the patient's heart to do all the work. For patients already hypotensive (one of the major reasons to put a patient on CRRT instead of IHD), this places more demand on a heart already strained, results in lower blood flow, and is a contributing factor to the lesser clearance obtainable with CAVRT.[11,17]

The main hindrance to CVVRT instead of CAVRT was the pump and circuit technology. Specifically, CVV setups require air detectors and bubble traps, to prevent air emboli to the lungs, and closer monitoring.[15] Once technology evolved to safely include a pump, CVV became the preferred modality. In this setup, blood is drawn from a central vein, "cleaned" by the CRRT setup, and then returned to a central vein.

▶ VASCULAR ACCESS

For CVV vascular access, a large-bore, dual-lumen catheter placed into a central vessel provides a "take blood" line and a "return blood" line with one stick. If such a catheter is not available, RRT can be administered with two independent large-bore, single-lumen, central lines. However, this doubles the risk of cannulation since two vessels would need to be cannulated instead of one.[16]

For patients who are dependent on other technology, it may be possible, though generally not preferred, to pull blood from that other technology. For patients

on extracorporeal membrane oxygenation (ECMO), cardiac bypass, or cardiopulmonary bypass, it is possible to have the "take blood" line come off the other pump.[9] This is, however, not recommended due to infectious risks, and is only to be used as a method of last resort. The blood is still returned directly to the patient, not back to the other pump.

CRRT catheters should be placed as far away as possible from other medication infusion lines. Of course, when hooking up the CRRT circuit to the central venous catheter, the intake line should be upstream from the return line, or the circuit will yield a vastly reduced efficiency.

▶ A BASIC RRT CIRCUIT—CVVHF

SCUF as shown in Figure 23-2 limits solute clearance to the concentration in the patient's plasma and the volume of fluid that can be removed. However, consider Figure 23-3. In this setup, blood is removed from the patient at rate Q_B, just as in SCUF (Figure 23-2). However, the blood is then mixed with "good fluid" called the "substitution fluid" (SF).

This mix is then put through the same hydrostatic pump and the fluid not extracted as UF is then returned to the patient. The advantage here is that by adding the SF, the circuit can filter more volume than if relying on the Q_B alone.

For example, consider renal support in two identical patients. The first will be supported using SCUF as in Figure 23-2, with the Q_B set to be 100 mL/min. Using SCUF alone, the amount of solute removed is limited by how much fluid we can remove from the patient. If the patient is hypotensive and cannot suffer to have any plasma volume removed, no solute can be cleared at all.

For the second patient, supported as in Figure 23-3, the same Q_B of 100 mL/min is set, but also with SF at 2 L/h. If the UF rate is set at 2 L/h, the patient's blood can be filtered, yet the patient left isovolemic. In other words, the renal support is no longer limited by the patient's volume and hemodynamic status.

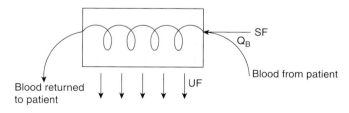

Figure 23-3. Continuous venovenous hemofiltration (CVVHF). Substitution fluid (SF) running "prefilter." UF: ultrafiltrate; Q_B: blood flow.

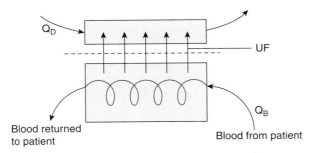

Figure 23-4. Continuous venovenous hemodialysis (CVVHD). Q_D: dialysate fluid flow; UF: ultrafiltrate; Q_B: blood flow.

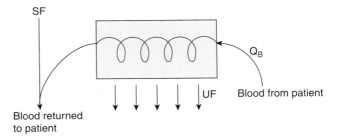

Figure 23-5. Continuous venovenous hemofiltration (CVVHF). Substitution fluid (SF) running "postfilter." UF: ultrafiltrate; Q_B: blood flow.

This setup is called hemofiltration, or HF. Since it is a CVV setup, it may also be referred to as CVVH or CVVHF. This chapter will use the CCVH**F** abbreviation to contrast it with continuous venovenous hemodialysis (CVVH**D**), described below.

Remember, in CVVHF, the SF mixes with the blood.

► CVVHD

Another way to configure a CVV circuit is to use a membrane instead of a filter (see Figure 23-4).

In this case, blood is still withdrawn from the patient at rate Q_B. However, instead of using the pump to push the blood against a filter and to obtain a UF, the blood is pumped along a membrane, forcing some plasma across the membrane. On the other side of the membrane is a fluid that may be the same as the SF in the CVVHF setup above (Figure 23-3). However, in this setup, it is called the dialysis fluid, or dialysate, run at rate Q_D. The dialysate runs along its side of the membrane in a direction opposite, or countercurrent, to the blood. In addition to the small amount of solute cleared in the UF via solute drag (as in SCUF, Figure 23-2), diffusable substances such as potassium and urea flow across the membrane down their concentration gradients into the dialysate, which is then discarded.

Set up in this manner, the CVV circuit is called hemodialysis, or HD and so the full abbreviation is CVVHD.

► REMOVING FLUID

Many critical care patients on RRT will require volume removal in addition to solute removal in order to avoid volume overload. Taking the example of the CVVHF circuit (Figure 23-3), the Q_B can be set to be 100 mL/min and the SF is set to normal saline running at 2 L/h. If the UF is set to be 2 L/h, solute will be removed without the removal of volume. If the UF is set to be 2.5 L/h, however, solute will still be removed but now also a net of 0.5 L/h of fluid will be removed, creating a negative fluid balance of 0.5 L/h.

► A MORE EFFICIENT RRT SETUP

Above, SF was added to the blood before the combined fluid went through the filter (called "prefilter"). The problem with this is that this method dilutes out the "bad substances" and then tries to filter the combined fluid. Consider the setup shown in Figure 23-5 instead.

In this case, Q_B is still 100 mL/min. But now, as opposed to the setup above, solute is filtered at full concentration. Setting UF rate equal to the SF rate clears solute while maintaining an even fluid balance. Similarly, setting UF higher than the SF clears solute and fluid.

The advantage of this setup is more HF (i.e., higher solute clearance). The disadvantage of this setup is that as more concentrated solute is pushed through the filter, the filter clogs faster. While it seems a straightforward solution to "simply change the filter," the technical realities entail halting the system (during which time the patient is receiving no RRT), removing the old filter, and recycling and restarting the system. Error—including infection, air emboli, etc.—can be introduced in any one of these steps. An increased number of system halts increases the number of times a complication may develop and thereby increases the complication risk as the access ports and other parts of the system are manipulated.

► THE BEST OF BOTH WORLDS: PREFILTER AND POSTFILTER

The setup shown in Figure 23-6 is simply a combination of the previous two modalities (Figures 23-3 and 23-5). In this case, some SF is run prefilter and some is run postfilter. By running some SF prefilter, the solute is diluted, reducing the efficiency of solute clearance but prolonging the life of the filter. As discussed above, this reduces the number of times the filter must be changed and therefore reduces the number of times complications such as DVT or air emboli could occur. Conversely, running some SF postfilter allows for more efficient removal of solutes at the expense of filter life.

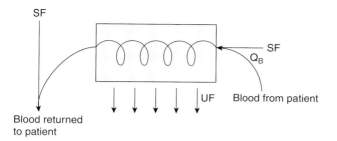

Figure 23-6. Continuous venovenous hemofiltration (CVVHF). Substitution fluid (SF) running "prefilter" and "postfilter." UF: ultrafiltrate; Q_B: blood flow.

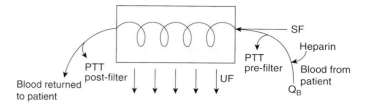

Figure 23-7. CVVHF—showing anticoagulation with heparin and location of blood draws for partial thromboplastin time (PTT). SF: substitution fluid; UF: ultrafiltrate; Q_B: blood flow.

This combination of running the SF both prefilter and postfilter may provide the best compromise of solute clearance and filter uptime. However, this has not been well studied and there are no studies demonstrating the optimal combination of fluids (e.g., 30% prefilter and 70% postfilter). In addition, this combined approach adds another layer of complexity to an already complex setup.

▶ THE FINAL STEP: ANTICOAGULATION

As in any extracorporal circuit (cardiac bypass, ECMO), blood will clot in a CVV setup. CVV circuits, therefore, require anticoagulation. The interesting quirk of such systems is that unlike systemic anticoagulation for myocardial infarction or pulmonary embolus, the goal in this case is to anticoagulate only the circuit while not affecting the patient. In practice, the patient is always affected to a degree, but it is the goal to minimize anticoagulation of blood in the patient.

To anticoagulate the circuit, but not the patient, anticoagulant is infused after blood is removed from the patient but before entering the CRRT pump, that is, it is given prefilter. Prefilter measurements must be taken to ensure adequate anticoagulation of the CVV circuit, and postfilter measurements must be taken to ensure minimal effect on the patient or, in the case of some anticoagulants, to counteract their effects once back in the patient.

The most common anticoagulant used is heparin. To measure the effectiveness of heparin and for dosing guidance, a prefilter and postfilter partial thromboplastin time (PTT) should be checked. Figure 23-7 shows a complete CVV circuit with prefilter SF using heparin as the anticoagulant.

In reality, a postfilter PTT can be drawn from the patient rather than from the CVV return line. In fact, it may be more prudent to draw a PTT directly from the patient in order to minimize the infectious risks of the CVV circuit. Protocols should be instituted to allow the nurse running the CRRT to adjust the heparin independently based on the PTT.

There are, however, several contraindications to heparin. If a patient has or develops heparin-induced thrombocytopenia (HIT) or an allergy to heparin (including low-molecular-weight heparin), heparin can no longer be used. Similarly, if a patient is bleeding or has a risk of bleeding, such as trauma or recent surgery, other anticoagulants should be considered.

The next most common anticoagulant is trisodium citrate (TSC). Like the citrate added to stored blood to prevent clotting, the citrate in TSC chelates calcium, preventing activation of platelet adenosine diphosphate (ADP) and thereby inhibiting platelet aggregation and initiation of the clotting cascade.[19]

As with all anticoagulants in CRRT, the TSC should be added to the blood draw line (i.e., as it comes out of the patient) in order to ensure anticoagulation of the CRRT circuit. But the calcium level must be restored within the patient to prevent systemic anticoagulation. Systemic anticoagulation of the patient will be prevented if the patient's ionized calcium (iCa^{2+}) level is maintained at normal levels.[19] Therefore, a calcium drip must also be running.

A postfilter iCa^{2+} should be checked and the calcium drip adjusted accordingly. Protocols should be instituted to allow the nurse to adjust the calcium drip independently. Note that a calcium drip (usually calcium chloride) requires another central venous access line. Furthermore, calcium drips are compatible with few other medications or drips and therefore require their own, dedicated, central venous port. It is theoretically possible to infuse the calcium in the blood return line; however, since the calcium drip will be changed more often than the CRRT circuit and the indwelling catheter, this puts the patient at additional risk for complications. There are large-bore, dual-lumen catheters that contain a third smaller port. If such a catheter provides adequate blood flow for CRRT, the third port provides a convenient site for the calcium drip. Note that the third port must be sufficiently far from the blood draw port to prevent drawing the calcium drip into the CRRT circuit (which would cause clots in the circuit and fail to restore the patient's coagulation status to normal).

There are two additional disadvantages to TSC. First, for every molecule of citrate, there are three molecules of sodium, which risks hypernatremia. Utilizing a low-sodium SF can compensate to some degree, but many patients will still become hypernatremic requiring a different anticoagulant.

Second, the liver will metabolize the citrate in TSC to bicarbonate. Unchecked, this can lead to a metabolic alkalosis. While in certain situations providing an alkalinizing fluid may be beneficial, most historic indications for administering bicarbonate have been debunked and patients who develop a metabolic alkalosis from the TSC should have the TSC drip altered, the SF changed to compensate, or be switched to another anticoagulant.

There are other less commonly used anticoagulants. These include hirudin (originally isolated from leeches), argatroban, bivalirudin, and others. In fact, if a patient is not able to tolerate any anticoagulant, the circuit can even be run with high blood flows and frequent saline flushes to attempt to minimize clotting.

SPECIAL SITUATIONS WHERE ANTICOAGULATION IS NOT REQUIRED

There are a few instances where patients do not require separate anticoagulation for the CRRT circuit. Note that, in both of these instances, the patients are still receiving anticoagulation of some type. The only difference is they are already systemically anticoagulated and so dedicated anticoagulation of the CRRT circuit is not necessary.

Drotrecogin alfa (recombinant human activated protein C [rhAPC]) is the drug that has shown a measurable decrease in the mortality of patients with severe sepsis. Given as a 96-hour continuous IV infusion, its main risk is that of bleeding that can be significant and even terminal.[20] It stands to reason that patients receiving rhAPC who also are receiving CVV do not require additional anticoagulation. Although formal studies are lacking, there is one case series of three patients receiving rhAPC and CVV who were not given any additional anticoagulation.[21] Although the filters clotted earlier in patients on rhAPC versus patients on heparin, the difference was not statistically significant. Therefore, given the significant risk of bleeding during rhAPC infusion, it seems reasonable to withhold extra anticoagulation such as heparin or TSC until and unless the filter clots earlier than expected.

Once the rhAPC infusion is ended (either for rhAPC-related complications such as allergy or bleeding or at completion of the 96-hour infusion), patients must be placed back on traditional anticoagulation. If rhAPC is readministered, the anticoagulation should again be held during this second infusion, and restarted when it is complete.

There have been no dedicated studies on the topic of patients who require anticoagulation for reasons other than the CVV circuit (e.g., thromboembolism, atrial fibrillation, mechanical heart valve), but in these patients it is probably not necessary to run separate anticoagulation for the CRRT circuit. Although there have been no studies on this topic, it seems reasonable to only administer anticoagulation prefilter with the goal of achieving postfilter anticoagulation sufficient for the patient's condition. In the case of heparin, administer sufficient heparin prefilter such that the postfilter PTT is at the level required for the patient's condition. If the patient has bleeding complications from this approach and it becomes necessary to stop systemic anticoagulation, one must revert to anticoagulating the circuit in such a way as to not affect the patient.

▶ SUBSTITUTION FLUIDS

The selection of an SF starts with some basic principles and then moves into the "art" of medicine. It is also strongly influenced by the fluids available at a particular institution.

Theoretically, as Q_B and SF infusion rates are raised higher and higher, in either HF or dialysis, the plasma will start to approximate those fluids. Therefore, it might seem that certain fluids should not be used. However, the patient's current condition should be taken into account when choosing an SF. For instance, if a patient is hyperkalemic, it would be prudent to start with a fluid that has no potassium in it, and then change once the patient's potassium level normalizes in order to prevent an equally dangerous hypokalemic state. Furthermore, it is known from other sources that most patients in diabetic ketoacidosis do not benefit from exogenous bicarbonate administration in the absence of cardiac effects. However, a patient with cardiac instability from a low pH secondary to a toxic ingestion might benefit from an SF with significant amounts of bicarbonate. Some commonly available SFs are listed in Table 23-1.

Three other issues are worth mentioning here:

1. A hospital pharmacist should be able to make an SF or dialysate with almost any concentration of ions such as sodium, potassium, bicarbonate, etc. That having been said, it is rather time intensive to do this for a fluid used at a rate of 2–6 L/h. It also introduces another source of possible error since it is something nonstandard that must be mixed ad hoc. It is also significantly more expensive than using fluids that are "off-the-shelf." Custom fluids are generally used only for the rarest of circumstances where an extra degree of control is required. For instance, it might be useful in pediatrics where the smaller

► TABLE 23-1. **COMMONLY USED SUBSTITUTION FLUIDS**

	Human Plasma	0.9% NaCl	NaHCO$_3$ 150 mEq (Three Ampoules) in 1 L Sterile Water	Prismasate 0 K$^+$	Prismasate 4 K$^+$
Na$^+$ (mEq/L)	135–145	154	150	140	140
Cl$^-$ (mEq/L)	95–105	154	0	109.5	113
K$^+$ (mEq/L)	3.5–5	0	0	0	4
Mg$^+$ (mEq/L)	1.5–2	0	0	1	1.5
Lactate (mEq/L)	0.5–2	0	0	3	3
HCO$_3^-$ (mEq/L)	22–26	0	150	32	32
Glucose (mEq/L)	70–110	0	0	0	110
Acetate (mEq/L)	0	0	0	0	0
Ca^{2+} (mEq/L)	8.5–10.5	0	0	3.5	2.5
Osmolarity (mOsm/L)	275–295	308	300	287	300

body weights limit the amount of fluid one can administer, regardless of the content of that fluid.

2. Consider fluids that make it easier to run the machine. For instance, Prismasate is often available in 5-L bags, while normal saline is available in only 1-L bags. Therefore, if the patient's condition will allow Prismasate, it is an easier fluid for the nurse to administer as it only requires a bag change every 5 L, rather than every 1 L. This also reduces the number of manipulations to the system's lines and therefore reduces the risk of infection.

3. Finally, fluids can be combined. So, for someone who is dangerously hyperkalemic, it might be prudent to start with Prismasate 0K in order to lower the potassium into a safer range as quickly as possible. As the potassium approaches a normal level, but is still elevated, a bag of Prismasate 0K and a bag of Prismasate 4K can be connected together with a "Y" connector, effectively giving a new fluid, Prismasate 2K. This will still lower the patient's potassium but minimize the risk of dangerous hypokalemia. When the patient's potassium normalizes, a switch to Prismasate 4K alone will maintain the potassium in the normal range. Similarly, a mixture of 0.45% NaCl with 75 mEq of NaHCO$_3$ will yield a fluid with a sodium concentration of 152 mEq/L, chloride concentration of 77 mEq/L, and HCO$_3$ concentration of 75 mEq/L, for a total osmolarity of 304 mOsm/L.

► FILTER

Although there are different filter configurations for CVV, because of cost considerations, generally an institution will have only one or two filters available. In the case that a different filter is desired, or even being considered, a renal consultation can be very helpful with some of the less common configurations. One example might be the use of a charcoal filter for patients with an ingestion or overdose.

► LABS

Although there are no studies examining minimum required labs for patients while on CVV, it seems prudent to send blood every 6 hours for sodium, potassium, chloride, bicarbonate, urea, creatinine, glucose, calcium, magnesium, and phosphorous. Appropriate anticoagulation labs should also be obtained (prefilter and postfilter PTTs for patients receiving heparin and prefilter and postfilter iCa^{2+} levels for patients receiving TSC). Arterial blood gases should be sent at regular intervals, or more often as the patient's status or other treatments dictates. Furthermore, bleeding times, activated clotting time, and thromboelastograms may be useful in specific circumstances.

► ALL TOGETHER NOW

For maximum clearance, CVVHF and CVVHD can be run simultaneously. As a combination of CVVHF and CVVHD, this setup is termed continuous venovenous hemodiafiltration (CVVHDF). This setup combines the advantages of convective clearance with diffusive clearance, giving clearance rates superior to either modality alone. Such a setup, complete with prefilter and postfilter SF, anticoagulation with heparin, and prefilter and postfilter PTTs, is pictured in Figure 23-8.

Note that covering everything above the dotted line leaves a CVVHF circuit as pictured in Figure 23-7. Eliminating the prefilter and postfilter SFs and additional UF leaves the CVVHD circuit pictured in Figure 23-4.

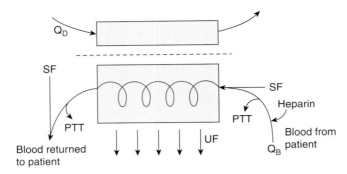

Figure 23-8. Continuous venovenous hemodiafiltration (CVVHDF). Q_D: dialysate fluid flow; PTT: partial thromboplastin time; SF: substitution fluid; UF: ultrafiltrate; Q_B: blood flow.

▶ **TABLE 23-2. CLEARANCE OF DIFFERENT MODALITIES OF CRRT**

Modality	Urea Clearance (g/day)	Middle Molecule Clearance
SCUF	1–4	+
CVVHF	22–24	++
CVVHD	24–30	−
CVVHDF	36–38	+++

Table 23-2 shows the relative clearances of CVVHF versus CVVHD versus CVVHDF. As you can see, CVVHDF results in higher clearance rates, but not exponentially so.

▶ TERMINATING RENAL SUPPORT

Just as there is a relative lack of strong evidence-based support for when and how to initiate CRRT, there is a lack of evidence guiding when to withdraw renal support. Uchino et al reported on current practices of 54 ICUs across 23 countries. While not a prospectively derived treatment rule, they found that, by far, UO was the best predictor of successfully weaning renal support, that is, the best indicator of recovery of renal function.[22,23] The next best indicator was creatinine clearance, but its predictive power was far inferior to that of UO.

▶ DIFFERENT MACHINES

Note that some machines have different terminology for the various settings. Some machines use the terms Q_B, SF, and UF as described above. But one manufacturer has set the machine such that UF will automatically equal the SF. That means if the machine is set to add SF at 2 L/h, the UF will automatically be 2 L/h. This may seem confusing but it is actually a safety measure. If you do not set the UF (or if you leave it at UF = 0), the machine will automatically keep the patient isovolemic. If you want to make the patient negative, you would then set a UF >0. However, the same machine will not account for any volume from the anticoagulation fluid. Depending on the fluid used and the concentration, especially for TSC, the volume of that fluid may be significant.

The take home point is that familiarity with the machine, or machines, in use is of vital importance. This includes knowing which settings are in milliliters per minute, and which are in liters per hour. Standardized forms greatly aid this effort.

There needs to be a strong working relationship between the physicians and nurses so everyone is using the same vocabulary. All physicians who will be evaluating or writing recommendations for the therapy must be using the same terminology. This should include the intensivist, the renal consulting service, and even consulting cardiologists who will need to know the details of the patient's fluid management.

In-services should be run to educate staff on which machines are in use, how to set them up, and how to troubleshoot them. This should be required for all nurses and doctors directly involved in the running of the therapy (intensivist, nephrologist) and should be made available to all others who may need to understand the therapy (e.g., cardiologist). Online modules greatly aid in this effort and, in fact, may completely suffice for the latter group.

▶ MEDICATION DOSING

Medication dosing for patients on CVV is beyond the scope of this text. The calculations are complex, and not always completely studied. To calculate appropriate dosing, one must take into consideration the clearance of the substance that is a function of the following items:[24]

- Volume of distribution of the medication, and whether a loading dose is required
- Whether a certain medicine is cleared more by diffusion (dialysis) or convection (HF)
- What modality the patient is on: CVVHF, CVVHD, and CVVHDF
- If on CVVHF, whether SF is prefilter, postfilter, or both
- Filtration fraction (how much plasma is filtered across the membrane given a certain Q_B)
- The sieving coefficient (how easily the medicine crosses the membrane)

Given these factors, medication dosing for these patients should involve close consultation with the pharmacology service.

▶ FEVER

The evaluation of fever in patients requiring RRT is complicated by the fact that all of the CVV modalities involve an extracorporal circuit. The CVV machine itself has a heater to keep the blood warm, but the blood must still pass through tubing exposed to the environment. This means that the blood tubing "bleeds" heat from the patient. This heat loss may make a normothermic patient hypothermic. More importantly, by clearing middle molecules, such as the cytokines that produce fever, CVVHF and CVVHDF (but not CVVHD) may mask a normothermic patient developing a fever. It would seem prudent, then, to lower the threshold for considering a temperature elevation as a true fever, for instance, 100°F (37.8°C) instead of the more traditional 100.4°F (38°C). It would also seem prudent to send routine blood cultures at some predefined interval based on the patient's condition or local practice. There are currently no studies that define the optimal interval for routine blood cultures.

▶ SEPSIS

For patients with severe sepsis, CVVHF holds promise as a therapy to modulate the immune response. Specifically, HF, in clearing middle molecules, also clears the cytokines that have been implicated in the harmful immune response of sepsis. In contradistinction to solutes and fluid volume that are cleared by convection, cytokines are cleared by adsorbing to the CVVHF filter. It can be shown that CVVHF clears cytokines because when weighing a filter after being used for CVVHF in a patient with sepsis, the filter weighs more. However, since cytokines exert their influence at the tissue level, and since the filter does not remove all cytokines, it remains to be shown if clearing the cytokines truly modulates the septic response.[25,26] Some also argue that in clearing such cytokines, CVVHF also clears the downregulating or beneficial cytokines. While true, the balance in a septic patient seems to be more toward the more harmful cytokines. Until filters can selectively remove the harmful cytokines, nonselective removal of cytokines seems a reasonable therapy. To achieve the clearance rates necessary to clear cytokines in septic shock, CVVHF must be run with high SF rates, and the filter must be changed every 6 hours, which is when the adsorption capability of the filter declines. At that point, the filter will still clear solute, but will not remove additional cytokines. This remains one of the most promising therapies for the future treatment of septic shock.

▶ THE FUTURE

CRRT, as "the kindler, gentler" RRT, will continue to evolve. Unlike traditional dialysis, CVV does not require a water source, and so can be implemented not only in patients not candidates for IHD but also in locations not set up to handle IHD.

As critical care moves closer to the front lines of medical care, there may be instances where it would be beneficial to start this therapy in the ED. For emergency physicians to run this therapy, they must be familiar with its requirements in order to facilitate its initiation in the ED. This may include placing a large-bore, dual-lumen central line, ordering the CVV machine, ordering the necessary fluids (SF, anticoagulation, etc.), and rearranging staff (or calling in additional staff) to free up a nurse capable of running the CVV machine.

Furthermore, "liver dialysis" is starting to become a technically feasible therapy. While not likely to be an ED therapy, it holds out great promise for hepatic support for any of a number of diseases, including overdoses, "liver help" during a critical illness, and as a bridge to a liver transplant. Its development will naturally draw heavily from the RRT world, and those already equipped to manage RRT will be in the best position to manage hepatic replacement therapy.

REFERENCES

1. De Mendonça A, Vincent JL, Suter PM, et al. Acute renal failure in the ICU: risk factors and outcome evaluated by the SOFA score. *Intensive Care Med.* 2000;26:915.
2. Schwilk B, Wiedeck H, Stein B, et al. Epidemiology of acute renal failure and outcome of haemodiafiltration in intensive Care. *Intensive Care Med.* 1997;23:1204.
3. Acute Dialysis Quality Initiative (ADQI). Available at: http://www.adqi.net.
4. Bellomo R. Defining, quantifying, and classifying acute renal failure. *Crit Care Clin.* 2005;21:223.
5. Marenzi G, Bartorelli AL. Recent advances in the prevention of radiocontrast-induced nephropathy. *Curr Opin Crit Care.* 2004;10(6):505.
6. Stacul F, Adam A, Becker CR. Strategies to reduce the risk of contrast-induced nephropathy. *Am J Cardiol.* 2006;98(6A):59K.
7. Meschi M, Detrenis S, Musini S. Facts and fallacies concerning the prevention of contrast medium-induced nephropathy. *Crit Care Med.* 2006;34(8):2060.
8. Meiera P, Vogtb P, Blanca E. Ventricular arrhythmias and sudden cardiac death in end-stage renal disease patients on chronic hemodialysis. *Nephron.* 2001;87:199.
9. Ronco C, Bellomo R, Ricci Z. Continuous arteriovenous hemofiltration in critically ill patients. *Nephrol Dial Transplant.* 2001;16(suppl 5):67.
10. Manns M, Sigler MH, Teehan BP. Intradialytic renal haemodynamics—potential consequences for the management of the patient with acute renal failure. *Nephrol Dial Transplant.* 1997;12:865.
11. Lauer A, Saccaggi A, Ronco C. Continuous arteriovenous hemofiltration in the critically ill patient. Clinical use and operational characteristics. *Ann Intern Med.* 1983;99(4):455.

12. Kellum JA, Angus DC, Johnson JP. Continuous versus intermittent renal replacement therapy: a meta-analysis. *Intensive Care Med.* 2002;28(1):29.

13. Jacka MJ, Ivancinova X, Gibney RT. Continuous renal replacement therapy improves renal recovery from acute renal failure. *Can J Anaesth.* 2005;52(3):327.

14. Waldrop J, Ciraulo DL, Milner TP. A comparison of continuous renal replacement therapy to intermittent dialysis in the management of renal insufficiency in the acutely ill surgical patient. *Am Surg.* 2005;71(1):36.

15. Tominaga GT, Ingegno M, Ceraldi C, et al. Vascular complications of continuous arteriovenous hemofiltration in trauma patients. *J Trauma.* 1993;35(2):285.

16. Bellomo R, Parkin G, Love J. A prospective comparative study of continuous arteriovenous hemodiafiltration and continuous venovenous hemodiafiltration in critically ill patients. *Am J Kidney Dis.* 1993;21(4):400.

17. Storck M, Hartl WH, Zimmerer E. Comparison of pump-driven and spontaneous continuous haemofiltration in postoperative acute renal failure. *Lancet.* 1991; 337(8739):452.

18. Kierdorf H. Continuous versus intermittent treatment: clinical results in acute renal failure. *Contrib Nephrol.* 1991;93:1.

19. Monchi M, Berghmans D, Ledoux D. Citrate vs. heparin for anticoagulation in continuous venovenous hemofiltration: a prospective randomized study. *Intensive Care Med.* 2004;30:260.

20. Bernard G, Vincent JL, Laterre PF. Efficacy and safety of recombinant human activated protein C for severe sepsis. *N Engl J Med.* 2001;344(10):699.

21. de Pont AC, Bouman CS, de Jonge E. Treatment with recombinant human activated protein C obviates additional anticoagulation during continuous venovenous hemofiltration in patients with severe sepsis. *Intensive Care Med.* 2003;29:1205.

22. Uchino S, Bellomo R, Morimatsu H. Discontinuation of continuous renal replacement therapy: a post hoc analysis of a prospective multicenter observational study. *Crit Care Med.* 2009;37(9):2576.

23. Finkel K, Podoll W, Amber S. Comment: discontinuation of continuous renal replacement therapy: when is enough enough? *Crit Care Med.* 2009;37(9):2664.

24. Choi G, Gomersall C, Tian Q. Principles of antibacterial dosing in continuous renal replacement therapy. *Crit Care Med.* 2009;37(7):2268.

25. De Vriese AS, Colardyn FA, Philippe JJ. Cytokine removal during continuous hemofiltration in septic patients. *J Am Soc Nephrol.* 1999;10(4):846.

26. Piccinni P, Dan M, Barbacini S. Early isovolaemic haemofiltration in oliguric patients with septic shock. *Intensive Care Med.* 2006;32(1):80.

SECTION VI

Neurologic and Neurosurgical Disorders

CHAPTER 24

Alterations in Mental Status

Nestor D. Tomycz and David W. Crippen

The human brain, then, is the most complicated organization of matter that we know.

Isaac Asimov

► INTRODUCTION

The complexity of the brain renders its normal functioning—especially the production of consciousness—uniquely vulnerable to acute metabolic derangements and structural deformation. As a perpetual glucose and oxygen glutton, the brain is extremely intolerant of sudden changes in energy homeostasis and in vivo neurons begin to die after only minutes of fuel deprivation. Likewise, the diffuse circuitry responsible for consciousness in the brain makes anatomic insults involving both cerebral hemispheres and the brainstem reticular activating system necessary and sufficient to perturb mental status. Regardless of etiology, altered mental status (AMS) or brain failure frequently prolongs hospital length of stay and worsens the prognosis of patients in the critical care setting. Rapid diagnosis is necessary to differentiate imminently life-threatening brain failure from more benign, reversible forms. As an amalgam of evidence-based practice and our clinical experience, this chapter will focus on the diagnostic and management challenges of AMS in the intensive care unit (ICU).

► CONSCIOUSNESS AND THE EXAMINATION OF MENTAL STATUS

AMS is an impairment of consciousness, which is comprised of arousal and awareness.[1] Arousal refers to general brain wakefulness, while awareness defines whether the individual has knowledge of his or her own existence and surroundings. Awareness demands a certain degree of arousal but it may be dissociated as is best exemplified by the persistent vegetative state (PVS)—awake patients without clinically demonstrable self-awareness.[2]

Mental status forms the core of any neurologic examination. Caregivers at all levels should be trained to abandon labeling a patient "unresponsive" in favor of more descriptive categories based on the physical examination: lethargy, obtundation, stupor, and coma (Table 24-1).[3,4] Lethargic patients manifest decreased alertness but retain awareness of their environment. Obtunded patients require a stimulus to rouse and follow simple commands but have lost awareness of their immediate surroundings. Stuporous patients do not follow commands and require a continuous painful stimulus to exhibit signs of arousal. Finally, comatose patients exhibit no awareness and no significant arousal response to even painful stimuli. Coma results from bilateral cerebral hemisphere impairment or dysfunction of the reticular activating system in the brainstem;

▶ **TABLE 24-1. DESCRIPTIVE CATEGORIES OF ALTERED MENTAL STATUS**

Cloudy consciousness	A mild deficit in the speed of information processing by the brain, resulting from mechanical disruption of cerebral substance; can be seen after mild to moderate head trauma and may persist for several months. Recent memory may be diminished, but long-term memory remains intact
Lethargy	A decrease in alertness, resulting in impaired ability to perform tasks normally accomplished without effort. Patients rouse briefly in response to stimuli and then settle back to inactivity when left alone. They retain awareness of their immediate environment
Obtundation	A decrease in awareness and alertness when stimulated. Patients rouse briefly and follow simple commands but are unaware of their immediate surroundings. Following arousal, they settle back to inactivity
Stupor	A state in which the patient cannot communicate clearly but can be aroused by continued painful stimulation. Arousal may manifest only as withdrawal from painful stimuli. As soon as the stimulus is removed, the patient settles back to inactivity
Coma	A state in which the patient does not respond to the most vigorous stimuli

▶ **TABLE 24-2. GLASGOW COMA SCALE**

Eye opening	
Spontaneous	4
To voice	3
To pain	2
None	1
Verbal response	
Oriented	5
Confused	4
Inappropriate	3
Incomprehensible	2
None	1
Motor response	
Follows commands	6
Localizes to pain	5
Withdraws to pain	4
Flexion to pain	3
Extension to pain	2
None	1

The GCS is composed of a motor, verbal, and eye opening score; however, some studies have suggested that the most useful (because it can be performed on intubated patients) and predictive component of the GCS is the motor score.[14,15] Moreover, besides its limited utility in intubated patients (in which the verbal score is replaced by "T"), the GCS has often been criticized for failing to include brainstem reflexes.[16] Nevertheless, the GCS remains the reigning worldwide consciousness scale and continues to facilitate both clinical research and decision making.

The motor component of the GCS deserves particular attention because it contains the most information and typically requires the most practice and effort to confidently extract from the physical examination. To meet the criteria of following commands, we recommend that the patient must show two fingers or wiggle his or her thumb to a verbal command. A common pitfall occurs in aphasic patients, who may mimic the examiner and therefore make it seem as though commands are being followed. Similarly, we recommend strict criteria for determining localizing, wherein the patient exhibits both cranial and caudal localization of the stimulus. Finally, withdrawal should be recognized as being a fairly complex and nonstereotypical movement of an extremity away from a painful stimulus; it must be distinguished from the more simple, posturing flexion and extension movements.

unilateral hemispheric disease (such as a middle cerebral artery stroke) does not typically lead to coma unless there is associated midline shift and resultant contralateral hemispheric dysfunction. Although these categories are useful to help qualitatively describe the level of depressed consciousness in a patient, the lack of standardized definitions for these terms makes them prone to misuse and variable interpretation.

The Glasgow Coma Scale (GCS) remains one of the most important quantitative barometers for mental status (Table 24-2). Although originally designed by neurosurgeons in 1974 to classify patients with traumatic brain injury (TBI), the GCS has become a common language among acute care providers and has stood the test of time due to its ease of use, minimal interobserver variability, and prognostic capability.[5–7] GCS is no longer solely a TBI tool, and its predictive value has been demonstrated in other diagnoses such as intracerebral hemorrhage, subarachnoid hemorrhage, intracranial subdural hematoma, ischemic stroke, Alzheimer's dementia, and poisoning.[8–13]

▶ **DIFFERENTIAL DIAGNOSIS OF ALTERED MENTAL STATUS**

Although there are myriad causes of AMS in the ICU, the basic dichotomy in brain failure is whether it has been anatomically or metabolically engendered. Clinical acumen gives the physician a general gestalt as to what type of cognitive reserve one can expect in a patient. Cognitive reserve is a function of patient age, baseline brain function, brain volume, comorbidities, and perhaps duration of stay in an ICU. For example, one may expect that a urinary tract infection might cause obtundation in an 82-year-old woman in the ICU but would be reluctant to attribute such a cause to obtundation in a 30-year-old patient. History provided by the patient's family can aid in the diagnosis of AMS by both helping gauge cognitive reserve (e.g., by identifying baseline brain function and whether there are signs of an underlying dementia) and identifying substance abuse disorders, most notably alcohol dependence. As a good rule of thumb, anatomic causes of AMS (intracerebral hemorrhage, ischemic stroke, subarachnoid hemorrhage, cerebral venous sinus thrombosis, vasospasm, hydrocephalus) tend to have a more rapid onset, tend to cause a greater decrement in GCS, and are usually more immediately life-threatening than many of the "bad humor" encephalopathies such as fever, hyponatremia, or septic encephalopathy.

Pupil size and light reactivity and motor exam symmetry are typically preserved in metabolic encephalopathy. Even in the presence of nondepolarizing neuromuscular blockade when motor exam has been lost, pupil reactivity is typically preserved.[17] Dilation of a pupil with loss of light reactivity heralds third cranial nerve compression with very few exceptions; rarely seizure may cause this same response.[18] Prospective studies have confirmed that both anisocoria and light reflex loss have high positive predictive values for structural coma.[19] Extremely small symmetric and reactive pupils may be caused by a pontine lesion. Moreover, metabolic encephalopathy may amplify or accentuate a baseline motor asymmetry (e.g., an old hemiparesis from stroke may become more pronounced in the presence of hyponatremia) but rarely manifests with a motor exam asymmetry. Recalling the brain's appetite for glucose, hypoglycemia is one cause of metabolic encephalopathy and rapid-onset coma that may cause a focal neurologic deficit along with AMS; glucose determination must accompany any acute evaluation of AMS since hypoglycemic episodes in diabetics have not uncommonly been misdiagnosed as strokes.[20,21]

The prevalence of etiologies for AMS in the ICU undoubtedly depends on the type of unit. Multiple studies have shown that AMS prolongs hospital stay and is an independent risk factor for mortality in the ICU.[22–26] In one study of 1,758 patients admitted to a medical ICU for a non-neurologic reason, metabolic encephalopathy was found to be the primary cause of AMS followed by seizures; among the metabolic encephalopathies, septic encephalopathy was the leading culprit followed by hepatic and renal encephalopathies.[27]

In another study involving patients in a medical ICU, Isensee et al reported that metabolic encephalopathy was the most frequent cause of AMS and those patients with AMS had more than double the mortality rate than was seen in patients without AMS.[28]

▶ SEPTIC ENCEPHALOPATHY

Septic encephalopathy is a leading cause of AMS in the critical care setting; however, the pathogenesis for brain failure in sepsis remains unknown. As a neurophysiologic indicator of brain failure, abnormal evoked potentials were found in 84% of septic ICU patients in one study.[29] Recent studies using mouse models of lipopolysaccharide-induced encephalopathy have suggested that the cytokine tumor necrosis factor (TNF) plays an important role in initiating and maintaining an inflammatory state in the brain.[30] Brain microabscesses, abnormal amino acid metabolism, changes in brain neurotransmitter concentrations, reduced cerebral blood flow and oxygen utilization, and weakening of the blood–brain barrier with resultant cerebral edema have all been implicated in the pathogenesis of septic encephalopathy.[31–34] Cerebrospinal fluid analysis is normal or with mild protein elevation, and electroencephalogram (EEG), the most sensitive test for septic encephalopathy, usually demonstrates a pattern consistent with metabolic encephalopathy with diffuse slow waves (predominantly delta waves) often with a triphasic pattern. Rarely, septic encephalopathy may manifest with focal neurologic deficits in addition to AMS.[35] Regardless of the causes, sepsis in the ICU causes acute AMS and may often leave patients with long-term cognitive morbidity. Animal models are helping to pave the way toward therapies that might counter the pathophysiologic mechanisms behind brain failure in sepsis; however, at the present time, our only defense is early identification and treatment of infection.

▶ NONCONVULSIVE STATUS EPILEPTICUS

There are little epidemiologic data on seizures in critical care; however, even one seizure in an adult ICU patient may double mortality.[25] While the management of isolated partial or generalized seizures and status epilepticus is generally well known among intensivists, much less attention has been granted to subclinical seizures and nonconvulsive status epilepticus (NCSE). There is no current international EEG-based definition or classification scheme for NCSE. NCSE has been defined as AMS associated with continuous epileptiform changes on EEG in the absence of motor signs.[36] Unfortunately, the diagnosis of NCSE is further hampered by a lack of a pathognomonic EEG pattern. NCSE may be focal or

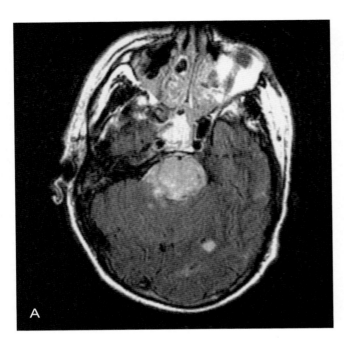
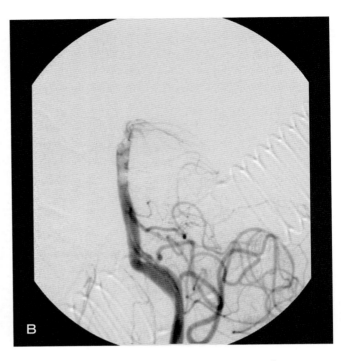

Figure 24-1. Locked-in syndrome. Axial FLAIR sequence MRI of the brain demonstrating a massive pontine infarction in a 46-year-old man with locked-in syndrome secondary to basilar artery thrombosis (A). Cerebral angiography demonstrating thrombus in the distal basilar artery (B).

generalized based on EEG that most commonly shows spike-and-wave or polyspike-and-wave discharges (usually with frequency <2–3 Hz); some have divided the EEG patterns in NCSE into five categories: continuous focal spike and wave, continuous generalized spike and wave, continuous generalized sharp and wave, continuous focal sharp and wave, and continuous periodic lateralized epileptiform discharges.[37] The prevalence of NCSE in patients with coma has been estimated to be as high as 3–8%; this is likely underestimated because the more commonly utilized routine EEG (20–30 minutes) is less sensitive for convulsive and nonconvulsive epileptic activity than continuous EEG.[38] The diagnosis of NSCE is therefore often missed, and this has been a frequent argument among proponents of continuous EEG monitoring in the ICU; NCSE, independent of etiology, worsens patient morbidity and mortality.[39,40] Current treatment for NCSE involves prescribing benzodiazepines (especially lorazepam and midazolam), antiepileptics (phenytoin, fosphenytoin, valproate, and phenobarbital), and intravenous anesthetics such as propofol with a goal of suppressing EEG abnormalities.[41]

► LOCKED-IN SYNDROME

Locked-in syndrome (LIS) is the constellation of anarthria, quadriplegia, and horizontal gaze paresis caused most commonly by an ischemic insult to the ventral pons[42] (Figure 24-1). Patients with LIS can communicate solely with blinking and vertical eye movements. LIS is not a disorder of consciousness but can easily be misconstrued as coma since there is a near complete deprivation of voluntary activity. Especially in patients with brainstem pathology, physicians must remember to assess for vertical eye motion prior to declaring a patient comatose. While still a grave diagnosis, LIS needs to be identified and distinguished from coma because there may be a counterintuitive potential for good recovery with supportive care and aggressive rehabilitation.[43]

► PERSISTENT VEGETATIVE STATE AND MINIMALLY CONSCIOUS STATE

Brought to the public eye by the case of Terry Schiavo, the PVS is a form of AMS in which there is preserved alertness, sleep–wake cycles, and autonomic control but absent awareness and only reflexive movements.[44] If such patients exhibit some nonreflexive movements as well, they are classified as being in a minimally conscious state (MCS). The PVS and MCS may develop as patients recover from coma. Head trauma with diffuse axonal injury and anoxia are the major brain insults that engender the PVS. Neuroimaging tools such as functional magnetic resonance imaging (MRI) have reinvigorated ethical debates concerning the PVS by demonstrating that these patients may retain some component of conscious awareness.[45] Nevertheless, the PVS remains a devastating diagnosis and reversibility is rare. Emerging technologies such as deep brain stimulation offer the potential of augmenting consciousness in these patients.[46]

▶ BRAIN FAILURE

In vitro studies have shown that central nervous system neurons can tolerate between 20 and 60 minutes of complete ischemic anoxia without irreversible injury.[47] However, the injury in vivo is much more severe and occurs in much less time. Immediately after cessation of circulation to the brain, the cerebral vessels dilate in response to the local environmental factors and increased $Paco_2$. Because the brain has no stores of glucose, cellular metabolism quickly ceases. Loss of nutrients and hypoxia cause the most sensitive structures to lose cellular integrity. This results in leakage from capillaries, edema, and disruption of cells and leads to release of lysosomes, proteases, and other damaging compounds into the surrounding tissues.[48] This in turn results in clogged microcirculation, stasis, and a vicious circle of increasing damage backing up into the macrocirculation. If this process is allowed to continue for a variable length of time and blood flow is then reestablished, the increased pressure gradient in the damaged area tends to disrupt the architecture, much like the sudden bursting of the Hoover Dam might do to downstream communities. The result is a progressive postresuscitative hypoperfusion state, in which blood flow is decreased to below the 20% level within 90 minutes postreperfusion and remains at this low level for up to 18 hours.[49,50]

Two theories have been offered to explain these phenomena: (1) Massive calcium (Ca^{2+}) overloading of the cells may be the initial stage of irreversible damage.[51] Normally, the extracellular Ca^{2+} level is high and the intracellular level is low. The damage of the cell membrane from hypoxia and loss of nutrient flow allows the gradient to shift and Ca^{2+} to enter the cell, causing interference with enzymes, DNA, RNA, mitochondria, and energy production cycles. Infusion of high levels of Ca^{2+} into precapillary arterioles causes vasospasm and a vicious cycle of decreased flow, more depletion of oxygen and nutrients, and so on. (2) During ischemia, oxygen-free radicals may be created by abnormal metabolism. These free radicals attack DNA, RNA, and mitochondria, resulting in irreversible damage.[52]

▶ BRAIN DEATH

As it pertains to brain death in the United States, philosophical ruminations on the meaning of life and death are fortuitously muffled by state law.[53] Brain death is a legal death that is relatively resistant to interpretation.[54]

The brain death exam basically interrogates the brainstem at a body temperature greater than 32°C and in the absence of drugs that can suppress the central nervous system or the neuromuscular junction. It is a diagnosis of what is, not what might be.[55] Simply put, brain death equals legal death. Once objective criteria are met on physical examination, a physician can pronounce a patient brain dead; some states require more than one physician to make this pronouncement. The family is informed that the patient has died, life support is withdrawn, and a death certificate is completed. Overall, the criteria behind brain death are similar worldwide.

A brief summary of a typical brain death protocol is presented here:[56]

> The cause of injury must be known. There must be clear evidence of an acute, catastrophic, irreversible brain injury. This is extremely important. There must be clear, objective evidence of brain injury on computed tomography (CT) or MRI of the brain that is compatible with the physical exam. A physical exam compatible with brain death is by itself insufficient, as numerous tabloid media sources routinely proclaim when supposed brain dead patients unexpectedly awaken.

Reversible conditions that may confuse the clinical diagnosis of brain death must be excluded, including:

> Hypothermia; body temperature must be greater than 32°C
>
> Drug intoxication or inadvertent neuromuscular blockade
>
> Hypoperfusion and shock

The physical examination:

> No response to verbal or visual command
>
> No spontaneous ventilation
>
> No spontaneous musculoskeletal movements to pain
>
> Pupils fixed and nonreactive
>
> No oculocephalic reflex
>
> Negative oculovestibular reflex
>
> No corneal reflex
>
> No gag or cough reflex

The apnea test: This test should be the last test and should be conducted after two clinical exams (separated by the mandatory observation period) have confirmed the absence of brainstem function. The patient is disconnected from the ventilator while oxygenation of the lungs continues passively. By calculation ($Paco_2$ rises 4 Torr in the first minute and 3 Torr every minute thereafter), the patient is allowed to build up to a $Paco_2$ of 60 Torr or more without becoming hypoxic. If there is no respiratory effort, the test is considered confirmatory.[57]

The EEG: An EEG is not necessary for confirmation of brain death, as small artifacts may confuse the issue. If ordered, the EEG should show electrocerebral silence for at least 30 minutes and must conform to established criteria for brain death.[58]

When the cause of death cannot be determined without absolute accuracy, consider cerebral angiography. The absence of intracranial arterial circulation as demonstrated by four-vessel angiography confirms brain death.[59]

Normally, two separate examinations are done, one by a neurologist or neurosurgeon and the other by a critical care specialist or anesthesiologist with critical care experience. If, after this extensive clinical examination, the patient shows no sign of neurologic function and the cause of the injury is known, the patient can be pronounced dead (by neurologic criteria) and a death certificate is completed with the time of death noted as the time the protocol was completed.

REFERENCES

1. Plum F, Posner JB. *The Diagnosis of Stupor and Coma.* 3rd ed. Philadelphia, PA: FA Davis Company; 1982:1–86.

2. Kinney HC, Samuels MA. Neuropathology of the persistent vegetative state. A review. *J Neuropathol Exp Neurol.* 1994;53(6):548–558.

3. Crippen D. Brain failure and brain death. In: *ACS Surgery: Principles and Practice.* WebMD Inc.: New York; 2005.

4. Crippen D. Neurologic monitoring in the intensive care unit. *New Horiz.* 1994;2:107.

5. Gabbe BJ, Cameron PA, Finch CF. The status of the Glasgow Coma Scale. *Emerg Med (Fremantle).* 2003;15(4):353–360.

6. Matis G, Birbilis T. The Glasgow Coma Scale—a brief review. Past, present, future. *Acta Neurol Belg.* 2008;108(3):75–89.

7. Bastos PG, Sun X, Wagner DP, et al. Glasgow Coma Scale score in the evaluation of outcome in the intensive care unit: findings from the acute physiology and chronic health evaluation III study. *Crit Care Med.* 1993;21(10):1459–1465.

8. Davies JO, Eddleston M, Buckley NA. Predicting outcome in acute organophosphorus poisoning with a poison severity score or the Glasgow Coma Scale. *QJM.* 2008;101(5):371–379.

9. Amirjamshidi A, Abouzari M, Rashidi A. Glasgow Coma Scale on admission is correlated with postoperative Glasgow outcome scale in chronic subdural hematoma. *J Clin Neurosci.* 2007;14(12):1240–1241.

10. Cho DY, Chen CC, Lee HC, et al. Glasgow Coma Scale and hematoma volume as criteria for treatment of putaminal and thalamic intracerebral hemorrhage. *Surg Neurol.* 2008;70(6):628–633.

11. Weingarten S, Bolus R, Riedinger MS, et al. The principle of parsimony: Glasgow Coma Scale score predicts mortality as well as the APACHE II score for stroke patients. *Stroke.* 1990;21(9):1280–1282.

12. Benesch CG, McDaniel KD, Cox C, et al. End-stage Alzheimer's disease. Glasgow Coma Scale and the neurologic examination. *Arch Neurol.* 1993;50(12):1309–1315.

13. Oshiro EM, Walter KA, Piantadosi S, et al. A new subarachnoid hemorrhage grading system based on the Glasgow Coma Scale: a comparison with the Hunt and Hess and World Federation of Neurological Surgeons Scales in a clinical series. *Neurosurgery.* 1997;41(1):140–148.

14. Healey O, Osler TM, Rogers FB, et al. Improving the Glasgow Coma Scale score: motor score alone is a better predictor. *J Trauma.* 2003;54(4):671–678.

15. Ross SE, Leipold C, Terregino C, et al. Efficacy of the motor component of the Glasgow Coma Scale in trauma triage. *J Trauma.* 1998;45(1):42–44.

16. Sternback GL. The Glasgow Coma Scale. *J Emerg Med.* 2000;19(1):67–71.

17. Schmidt JE, Tamburro RF, Hoffman GM. Dilated nonreactive pupils secondary to neuromuscular blockade. *Anesthesiology.* 2000;92(5):1476.

18. Gadoth N, Margalith D, Bechar M. Unilateral pupillary dilation during focal seizures. *J Neurol.* 1981;225(3):1432–1459.

19. Tokuda Y, Nakazato N, Stein GH. Pupillary evaluation for differential diagnosis of coma. *Postgrad Med J.* 2003;79:49–51.

20. Carter F, Taylor C. Transient hypoglycemia hemiparesis. *J Natl Med Assoc.* 2002;94(11):999–1001.

21. Boylan-Starks L. Hypoglycemia hemiplegia: a case study. *Heart Lung.* 1995;24(4):330–332.

22. Stevens RD, Pronovost PJ. The spectrum of encephalopathy in critical illness. *Semin Neurol.* 2006;26(4):440–451.

23. Ely EW, Shintani A, Truman B, et al. Delirium as a predictor of mortality in mechanically ventilated patients in the intensive care unit. *JAMA.* 2004;291(14):1753–1762.

24. Ely EW, Gautam S, Margolin R, et al. The impact of delirium in the intensive care unit on hospital length of stay. *Intensive Care Med.* 2001;27(12):1892–1900.

25. Ropper AH, Green DR, Diringer MN, Green DM, Mayer SA, Bleck TP. *Neurological Complications of Critical Medical Illness in Neurological and Neurosurgical Intensive Care.* 4th ed. Philadelphia, PA: Lippincott Williams and Wilkins; 2004:190.

26. Consales G, De Gaudio AR. Sepsis associated encephalopathy. *Minerva Anestesiol.* 2005;71:39–52.

27. Bleck TP, Smith MC, Pierre-Louis SJ, et al. Neurologic complications of critical medical illness. *Crit Care Med.* 1993;21:98–103.

28. Isensee LM, Weiner LJ, Hart RG. Neurological disorders in a medical intensive care unit: a prospective survey. *J Crit Care.* 1989;4:208–210.

29. Zauner C, Gendo A, Kramer L, et al. Impaired subcortical and cortical sensory evoked potential pathways in septic patients. *Crit Care Med.* 1992;30:1136–1139.

30. Alexander JJ, Jacob A, Cunningham P, et al. TNF is a key mediator of septic encephalopathy acting through its receptor, TNF receptor-1. *Neurochem Int.* 2008;52(3):447–456.

31. Davies DC. Blood–brain barrier breakdown in septic encephalopathy and brain tumours. *J Anat.* 2002;200(6):639–646.

32. Papadopoulos MC, Davies DC, Moss RF, et al. Pathophysiology of septic encephalopathy: a review. *Crit Care Med.* 2000;28(8):3019–3024.

33. Hamed SA, Hamed EA, Abdella MM. Septic encephalopathy: relationship to serum and cerebrospinal fluid levels of adhesion molecules, lipid peroxidases and S-100B protein. *Neuropediatrics.* 2009;40(2):66–72.

34. Bowton DL. CNS effects of sepsis. *Crit Care Clin.* 1989;5(4):785–792.

35. Bello JHSM, Park M. Sepsis-associated encephalopathy as a differential diagnosis with motor deficit plus altered mental status. *Clinics.* 2007;62(2):199–202.

36. Epstein D, Diu E, Abeysekera T. Review of non-convulsive status epilepticus and an illustrative case history manifesting as delirium. *Aust J Ageing.* 2009;28(3):110–115.

37. Siddiqui M, Jamil N, Malik A. Frequency of non-convulsive status epilepticus in patients with impaired level of consciousness. *J Pak Med Assoc.* 2009;59(5):296–298.

38. Alroughani R, Javidan M, Qasem A, et al. Non-convulsive status epilepticus: the rate of occurrence in a general hospital. *Seizure.* 2009;18(1):38–42.

39. Hirsch LJ. Continuous EEG monitoring in the intensive care unit: an overview. *J Clin Neurophys.* 2004;21(5):332–340.

40. DeLorenzo RJ, Waterhouse EJ, Towne AR, et al. Persistent nonconvulsive status epilepticus after the control of convulsive status epilepticus. *Epilepsia.* 1998;39:833–840.

41. Murthy JM. Nonconvulsive status epilepticus: an under diagnosed and potentially treatable condition. *Neurol India.* 2003;51(4):453–454.

42. Patterson JR, Grabois M. Locked-in syndrome: a review of 139 cases. *Stroke.* 1986;17(4):758–764.

43. Tomycz ND, Holm M, Horowitz M, et al. Extensive brainstem ischemia on neuroimaging does not preclude meaningful recovery from locked-in syndrome: two cases of endovascularly managed basilar thrombosis. *J Neuroimaging.* 2003;17:1–3.

44. The Multi-Society Task Force on PVS. Medical aspects of the persistent vegetative state. *N Engl J Med.* 1994;330:1499–1508.

45. Owen AM, Coleman MR, Boly M, et al. Detecting awareness in the vegetative state. *Science.* 2006;313(5792):1402.

46. Yamamoto T, Katayama Y, Kobayashi K, et al. DBS therapy for a persistent vegetative state: ten years follow-up results. *Acta Neurochir Suppl.* 2003;87:15–18.

47. Safar P, Bircher N. *Cardiopulmonary Cerebral Resuscitation.* 3rd ed. Philadelphia, PA: WB Saunders Co; 1988.

48. Steen PA, Milde JH, Michenfelder JD. No barbiturate protection in a dog model of complete cerebral ischemia. *Ann Neurol.* 1979;5:343.

49. Nozari A, Rubertsson S, Wiklund L. Improved cerebral blood supply and oxygenation by aortic balloon occlusion combined with intra-aortic vasopressin administration during experimental cardiopulmonary resuscitation. *Acta Anaesthesiol Scand.* 2000;44:1209.

50. Shaffner DH, Eleff SM, Koehler RC, et al. Effect of the no-flow interval and hypothermia on cerebral blood flow and metabolism during cardiopulmonary resuscitation in dogs. *Stroke.* 1998;29:2607.

51. Bowersox SS, Singh T, Luther RR. Selective blockade of N-type voltage-sensitive calcium channels protects against brain injury after transient focal cerebral ischemia in rats. *Brain Res.* 1997;747:343.

52. Maragos WF, Korde AS. Mitochondrial uncoupling as a potential therapeutic target in acute central nervous system injury. *J Neurochem.* 2004;91:257.

53. Searle J, Collins C. A brain-death protocol. *Lancet.* 1980;1:641.

54. Kaste M, Palo J. Criteria of brain death and removal of cadaveric organs. *Ann Clin Res.* 1981;13:313.

55. Jastremski M, Powner D, Snyder J, et al. Problems in brain death determination. *Forensic Sci.* 1978;11(3):201.

56. Bernat JL, Culver CM, Gert B. On the definition and criteria of death. *Ann Intern Med.* 1981;94(3):389–394.

57. Jeret JS, Wijdicks EF. Pronouncing brain death: contemporary practice and safety of the apnea test. *Neurology.* 2009;73(2):159–160.

58. Guérit JM, Amantini A, Amodio P, et al. Consensus on the use of neurophysiological tests in the intensive care unit (ICU): electroencephalogram (EEG), evoked potentials (EP), and electroneuromyography (ENMG). *Neurophysiol Clin.* 2009;39(2):71–83.

59. Escudero D, Otero J, Marqués L, et al. Diagnosing brain death by CT perfusion and multislice CT angiography. *Neurocrit Care.* 2009;11(2):261–271. Epub June 30, 2009.

CHAPTER 25

Management of Acute Intracranial Hypertension

Asma Zakaria and Imoigele P. Aisiku

The cranial vault is a rigid structure containing brain, blood, and cerebrospinal fluid (CSF). According to the Monro–Kellie doctrine, the volume of this chamber is unchangeable, and any addition of contents must be matched by a displacement of volume elsewhere. The goal of this chapter is to briefly outline the pathophysiologic processes that result in volume shifts in the cranium and measures that can be taken to identify and treat these conditions.

► WHAT IS INTRACRANIAL PRESSURE?

Intracranial pressure (ICP) is defined as the pressure exerted on the dura mater by the intracranial contents.[1] It comprises the sum of three partial pressures:

$$ICP = P_{Cerebrum} + P_{Blood} + P_{CSF}$$

Any increase in the partial pressure of one compartment will cause a decrease in the pressure of another to maintain a constant ICP. The change in volume divided by a change in ICP is defined as intracranial compliance. Initially, the addition of volume is easily accommodated in the vault without a corresponding increase in pressure. Once this "compensatory reserve"[2] is exhausted, the pressure rises rapidly in response to an increase in volume (Figure 25-1).

Normal ICP ranges between 5 and 15 mm Hg or 7.5 and 20 cm H_2O.[3]

An increase in ICP can jeopardize the cerebral perfusion pressure (CPP) that is defined as follows:

$$CPP = MAP - ICP$$

where MAP is the mean arterial pressure, and hence the cerebral blood flow (CBF) = CPP/cerebral vascular resistance (CVR).

Although transient ICP elevations of up to 100 cm H_2O have been tolerated by the human brain under experimental conditions,[4] sustained ICP values above 20 mm Hg are associated with worse outcomes in brain trauma patients. CPP is less predictive of neurologic outcome as long as it is maintained above 60 mm Hg.[5]

► CEREBRAL AUTOREGULATION

In normal physiologic states, CBF remains stable or "autoregulated" over a wide range of CPP through cerebral arteriolar vasodilation and vasoconstriction.[6] CPP and ICP are clinical surrogates for CBF and therefore are utilized as clinical diagnostic and therapeutic indices. CVR is increased or decreased based on alterations in CPP when autoregulation is intact. As CBF decreases beyond the limits of autoregulation, the brain increases its oxygen extraction fraction (OEF) to compensate

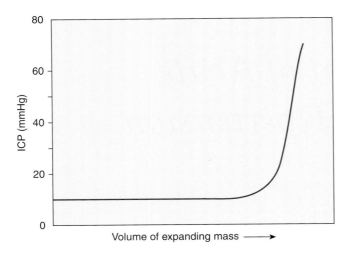

Figure 25-1. The pressure–volume curve: Until a certain point, the skull can accommodate volume without a significant change in pressure. Beyond this, any increase in volume is associated with a disproportional increase in intracranial pressure.

for reduced blood flow. In the neurologically injured brain, the concept of autoregulation may be disrupted and therefore the normal compensatory measures may not exist. Any therapeutic measures directed toward improving the injured brain or other organ systems should consider this pathophysiologic process/concept prior to instituting therapy.

▶ CLINICAL SIGNS OF INTRACRANIAL HYPERTENSION

The clinical presentation of elevated ICP depends on the etiology and varies in reliability. Signs include somnolence, papilledema, a symptom complex of headache, nausea/vomiting, and blurry/double vision, or a complex of bradycardia, irregular respirations, and widened pulse pressure (Cushing's triad).[7] Cushing proposed that these findings in the presence of profound intracranial hypertension were a sign of medullary ischemia. However, this constellation can be seen anytime there is distortion of the brainstem even in the setting of normal ICP[8] and should be considered an ominous trend without a specific clinical correlation to intracranial hypertension.

Acute increases in ICP such as those due to epidural hematomas, subarachnoid hemorrhage (SAH), or severe brain trauma usually present with a more global impairment in cerebral function such as low Glasgow Coma Scale (GCS) score, headache, nausea, and vomiting. Venous bleeds, subdural hematomas, brain tumors, and malignant strokes are more likely to present as focal neurologic deficits progressing to one of the herniation

syndromes and elevated ICP. In these patients, it is important to monitor for worsening paresis, cranial nerve palsies (especially third and sixth nerves), and pupillary changes.

▶ RADIOGRAPHIC SIGNS OF INTRACRANIAL HYPERTENSION

Any patient with suspected intracranial hypertension should undergo emergent neuroimaging. Concerning findings include:

1. Presence of acute intraventricular, subarachnoid, epidural, or subdural blood
2. Obliteration of the third ventricle or basal cisterns[9]
3. Dilation of the contralateral temporal horn[10]
4. Obstructive hydrocephalus with enlarged lateral ventricles and transependymal flow[3]
5. Midline shift
6. Diffuse or focal cerebral edema—loss of gray–white junction, large-vessel ischemia, or large areas of vasogenic edema resulting in sulcal effacement

▶ HERNIATION SYNDROMES

The shifting of intracranial contents from one intracranial compartment to the next because of mass effect is called herniation.[11] There are different types of herniation syndromes: (1) transtentorial herniation; (2) central herniation; (3) tonsillar herniation; and (4) subfalcine herniation (Figure 25-2).

▶ INDICATIONS FOR ICP MONITORING

ICP should be measured whenever elevation of ICP is suspected in patients who will benefit from the procedure. There is insufficient level 1 evidence to support a standard for ICP monitoring or to confirm that it improves outcomes. According to the most recent traumatic brain injury (TBI) guidelines,[12] there is level II evidence that all salvageable patients with a GCS score of 3–8 and an abnormal computed tomography (CT) scan should have some form of ICP monitoring. Level III evidence supports ICP monitoring in all patients with severe TBI and a normal CT who have two of the following: age >40 years, unilateral or bilateral motor posturing, or a systolic blood pressure <90 mm Hg. Beyond these guidelines, indications are less well defined, although ICP monitoring is used in poor-grade SAH, intraventricular hemorrhage, intraparenchymal hemorrhage, meningitis, acute liver failure, hydrocephalus, etc.

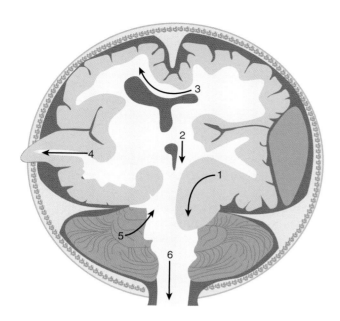

Figure 25–2. Herniation syndromes: (1) uncal herniation can result in third cranial nerve, posterior cerebral artery, and midbrain compression; (2) central herniation can cause downward displacement of the entire brainstem with lateral gaze palsy; (3) subfalcine herniation can result in strangulation of the anterior cerebral artery under the falx; (4) extracranial herniation can occur through a traumatic skull defect or therapeutic craniectomy; (5) upward tentorial herniation can occur due to posterior fossa masses; (6) tonsillar herniation can result in brainstem compression, pupillary dilation, and cardiorespiratory arrest.

▶ MEASUREMENT OF INTRACRANIAL PRESSURE

The gold standard for ICP monitoring is direct measurement in the lateral ventricle (Figure 25-3). This allows for continuous monitoring of the ICP and CSF drainage for ICP control. External ventricular drains (EVDs) are inserted into the ventricle through a burr hole. They are connected to a transducer and a drainage bag, which is positioned at a set level above the tragus to maintain the desired ICP. It is important to remember that the height of the collecting bag relative to the tragus is often measured in cm H_2O, while ICP is measured in millimeters of mercury. The biggest complications of EVDs are malfunction and infection. Infection rates from 5% to 20% have been documented in the literature[13] and are related to surgical technique, duration of EVD placement, frequency of manipulation, and catheter flushing. In general, more than three placement attempts and flushing more than twice for malfunction should be avoided.[1] Neither routine catheter exchange nor the use of prophylactic antibiotics is recommended to reduce infections.[14]

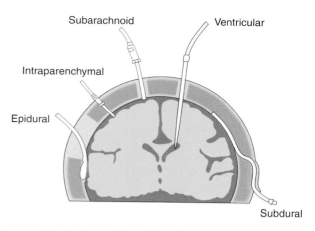

Figure 25–3. Location of various intracranial pressure monitors.

Intraparenchymal monitors are less invasive and independent of head position. They cannot be rezeroed once inserted, although the newer models have less drift, making this less of an issue.[15] These devices measure pressure in the anatomic compartment that they are placed in, which may not be an accurate assessment of global (ventricular) ICP.

Subarachnoid bolts are hollow saline-filled bolts that are screwed into the burr hole. The fluid in the lumen is continuous with the CSF in the subarachnoid space and the transmitted pressure is considered the ICP. The main advantages of this device are the ease of insertion and the low risk of infection and bleeding. However, they do not allow for CSF drainage, are less accurate than EVDs, and tend to get occluded by swollen brain.[16]

Epidural devices are fiberoptic catheters that are placed in the space between the skull and dura. Although they have a low risk of infection and bleeding, they are often inaccurate.

▶ MANAGEMENT OF INTRACRANIAL HYPERTENSION

Once the diagnosis of intracranial hypertension has been established, the treatment can be directed to the cause: CSF drainage for hydrocephalus, steroids, and resection for intracranial tumors and craniectomy for strokes. General principles of ICP management continue until definitive treatment can be implemented, or if the patient is not a candidate for any of the above. As with all emergencies, the airway, breathing, and circulation must be stabilized before any further steps are taken.

POSITION

A change in head position from 0° to 60° is associated with a significant decrease in ICP[17] as it improves venous return and decreases CSF hydrostatic pressure. Unfortunately, this is coupled with a drop in MAP and CPP[18] that may adversely affect patients with impaired cerebral autoregulation. A midline head position ensures that both jugular veins are open and draining. Special attention should be given to collars and endotracheal tube (ETT) holders, which may be constrictive and impair venous return.

HYPERVENTILATION

A decrease in P_{CO_2} effectively decreases the ICP[19] by causing cerebral arteriolar constriction and reducing cerebral blood volume. The effect generally lasts for less than 24 hours, and prolonged hyperventilation should be avoided. Level II evidence discourages maintaining P_{CO_2} levels below 25 mm Hg in TBI patients given the risk for global ischemia.[20] In general, eucapnia should be maintained and hyperventilation should be avoided or only used as a temporizing measure.

HEMODYNAMICS

As the ICP rises, the MAP reflexively increases to maintain CPP. More protocols are now incorporating CPP-targeted therapies with a lower limit ≥ 60 mm Hg. This allows for less use of vasopressors and fewer pulmonary complications than ICP-driven management of brain injury.[21]

HYPEROSMOLAR THERAPY

Mannitol is the most commonly used osmotic agent in the treatment of intracranial hypertension. It is usually dosed as a bolus infusion at 0.25–1.0 g/kg body weight. It does not cross the blood–brain barrier (BBB) in uninjured brain tissue but can in areas where the BBB is compromised, creating a reverse osmotic effect. Mannitol acutely expands the intravascular volume, increasing CBF. This in turn enhances oxygen delivery to the brain and causes vasoconstriction in areas of the brain where autoregulation is intact, resulting in a decrease in ICP. Mannitol also creates an osmotic gradient between the cells and plasma, resulting in reduction of intracerebral volume and a drop in ICP. There is subsequent urinary osmotic diuresis, which should be replaced by intravenous fluids to avoid dehydration, hypotension, and renal failure. These side effects are more common when the drug is dosed frequently, continuously, or in large volumes, especially at serum osmolarities greater than 320 mOsm.[22] Renal toxicity is one of the primary concerns with usage of mannitol especially when given in scheduled dosing regimens or in continuous intravenous formats. It is related to

mannitol accumulation, and therefore osmolar gap should be calculated in multiple-dose formats:

$$\text{Osmolar gap} = \text{measured POsm} - \text{calculated POsm}$$

$$\text{Plasma osmolarity (POsm)} = 2[\text{Na}] + \frac{[\text{glucose}]}{18} + \frac{[\text{BUN}]}{2.8}$$

There have been no randomized controlled trials to prove mannitol's superiority over other agents or an improvement in outcomes with its use.

Hypertonic saline (HS) reduces ICP by creating a hyperosmolar gradient across the BBB. ICP reduction has been noted to last for ≤ 2 hours but may be maintained for longer with a continuous infusion.[23] Side effects include electrolyte abnormalities, heart failure, and phlebitis. In a recent comparison of equiosmolar mannitol and 7.5% HS, both equally reduced ICP but mannitol had the added benefit of improving CPP. Since then, a series of patients refractory to mannitol were treated with 7.5% HS with marked reduction in ICP and improvement in brain tissue oxygen tension ($PbtO_2$) and cerebral and systemic hemodynamics.[24] Thirty- and 60-mL boluses over 15 minutes of 23.4% saline as a single osmotic agent have also been found to be safe and effective in reducing ICP and improving CPP and $PbtO_2$.[25]

TEMPERATURE

Fever has been associated with adverse outcomes in all forms of brain injury, most likely secondary to an increase in brain metabolic demands. Induced moderate hypothermia (32–34°C) has been used to reduce cerebral edema but no definite benefit has been seen with the exception of postcardiac arrest anoxic injury. Outcomes are influenced by the depth and duration of hypothermia, as well as the rate of rewarming.[26] Passive rewarming of patients who were hypothermic on arrival to the hospital was associated with worse outcomes than patients who were maintained at hypothermic temperatures.[27] Shivering, a common side effect, elevates ICP and may require higher does of sedation or neuromuscular blockade. Other side effects include coagulopathy, arrhythmias, and suppressed immune responses. At this time, the advantages of hypothermia as a neuroprotective agent have not been proven to be greater than the risks, and treatment should be guided toward maintenance of normothermia. Questions that need to be answered include what patient populations may benefit, if any, what degree of hypothermia, and for how long hypothermia should be maintained.

BARBITURATES, ANALGESIA, & PARALYTICS

Barbiturates reduce ICP by reducing brain metabolism and therefore CBF and volume. Pentobarbital is more commonly used given its intermediate half-life (approximately 20 hours) and is usually administered as a bolus of 10–30 mg/kg followed by an infusion of 0.5–3 mg/kg/h with the goal of achieving burst suppression. Barbiturates alone are seldom sufficient for the control of ICP when compared with mannitol.[28] Their use is fraught with multiple side effects including profound cardiac suppression, vasodilation, and immunosuppression. The hypotension and associated drop in CPP often negates any advantages of ICP control and patients often need to be hemodynamically supported on vasopressors. The use of barbiturates should therefore be limited to patients who have elevated ICP that are refractory to standard medical and surgical management.[29] Propofol has been used as an alternative to barbiturates because of its very short half-life, reduction in cerebral metabolism, and anti-seizure properties.[30] Its use is limited by hypotension as well as by the fact that it is lipid solvent, which can cause severe hypertriglyceridemia and increased CO_2 production. The risk of propofol infusion syndrome, although rare, discourages many practitioners from long-term usage.

Pain, agitation, and shivering can increase cerebral metabolic demand and ICP. Patients should be on adequate doses of opioid analgesics to avoid this. When shivering or motor posturing is intractable, neuromuscular blockade with nondepolarizing aminosteroidal agents can be used. The pharmocokinetics of these agents may be altered in the setting of hypothermia and they should be dosed accordingly.

DECOMPRESSIVE CRANIECTOMY

Removal of part of the skull for ICP control aims to negate the Monro–Kellie doctrine of fixed volume by allowing the brain to swell out of the cranial defect.[31] Craniectomy has been used to treat intractable intracranial hypertension due to strokes, SAH, TBI, and intracranial hemorrhage. Although there is level 1 evidence supporting the use of decompression in malignant strokes,[32] the data for TBI are restricted to case series. Two randomized control trials are underway to determine the benefit of decompression in TBI patients.[33] If surgical decompression is considered, it should be done expeditiously and generously, ideally after the first-tier treatments have failed.

REFERENCES

1. Jantzen JP. Prevention and treatment of intracranial hypertension. *Best Pract Res Clin Anaesthesiol.* 2007;21: 517–538.
2. Czosnyka M, Smielewski P, Timofeev I, et al. Intracranial pressure: more than a number. *Neurosurg Focus.* 2007;22:E10.
3. Eccher M, Suarez JI. Cerebral edema and intracranial dynamics—monitoring and management of intracranial pressure. In: Suarez JI, ed. *Critical Care Neurology and Neurosurgery.* Totowa, New Jersey: Humana Press; 2004.
4. Ryder HW, Espey FF, Kimbell FD, et al. The mechanism of the change in cerebrospinal fluid pressure following an induced change in the volume of the fluid space. *J Lab Clin Med.* 1953;41:428–435.
5. Juuls N, Morris GF, Marshall SB, et al. Intracranial hypertension and cerebral perfusion pressure: influence on neurological deterioration and outcome in severe head injury. *J Neurosurg.* 2000;92:1–6.
6. Diringer MN, Axelrod Y. Hemodynamic manipulation in the neuro-intensive care unit: cerebral perfusion pressure therapy in head injury and hemodynamic augmentation for cerebral vasospasm. *Curr Opin Crit Care.* 2007;13:156–162.
7. Stern WE. Intracranial fluid dynamics: the relationship of intracranial pressure to the Monro–Kellie doctrine and the reliability of pressure assessment. *J R Coll Surg Edinb.* 1963;9:18–36.
8. Stern WE. Studies in experimental brain swelling and brain compression. *J Neurosurg.* 1959;16:676–704.
9. Teasdale E, Cardoso E, Galbraith, et al. CT scan in severe diffuse brain injury: physiological and clinical correlations. *J Neurol Neurosurg Psychiatry.* 1984;47: 600–603.
10. Sadhu VK, Sampson J, Haar FL, et al. Correlation between computed tomography and intracranial pressure monitoring in acute head trauma patients. *Radiology.* 1979;133:507–509.
11. Blumenfeld H. Brain and environs: cranium, ventricles and meninges. In: Blumenfeld H, ed. *Neuroanatomy through Clinical Cases.* Sunderland, MA: Sinauer Associates Inc; 2002.
12. Brain Trauma Foundation, American Association of Neurological Surgeons, Congress of Neurological Surgeons, et al. Guidelines for the management of severe traumatic brain injury. VI. Indications for intracranial pressure monitoring. *J Neurotrauma.* 2007;24:S37–S44.
13. Beer R, Lackner P, Pfausler, et al. Nosocomial ventriculitis and meningitis in neurocritical care patients. *J Neurol.* 2008;255:1617–1624.
14. Lozier AP, Sciacca RR, Romagnoli MF, et al. Ventriculostomy-related infections: a critical review of the literature. *Neurosurgery.* 2002;51:170–181.
15. Czosnyka M, Pickard JD. Monitoring and interpretation of intracranial pressure. *J Neurol Neurosurg Psychiatry.* 2004;75:813–821.
16. North B, Reilly P. Comparison among three methods of intracranial pressure recording. *Neurosurgery.* 1986;18:730–732.
17. Schwarz S, Georgiadia D, Aschoff A, et al. Effects of body position on intracranial pressure and cerebral perfusion in patients with large hemispheric stroke. *Stroke.* 2002;33:497–501.
18. Oertel M, Kelly DF, Lee JH, et al. Efficacy of hyperventilation, blood pressure elevation, and metabolic suppression therapy in controlling intracranial pressure after head injury. *J Neurosurg.* 2002;97:1045–1053.
19. Brain Trauma Foundation, American Association of Neurological Surgeons, Congress of Neurological

Surgeons, et al. Guidelines for the management of severe traumatic brain injury. XIV. Hyperventilation. *J Neurotrauma.* 2007;24:S87–S90.

20. Huang SJ, Hong WC, Han YY, et al. Clinical outcome of severe head injury using three different ICP and CPP protocol-driven therapies. *J Clin Neurosci.* 2006;13:818–822.

21. Allen CH, Ward JD. An evidence-based approach to management of increased intracranial pressure. *Crit Care Clin.* 1998;14:485–495.

22. Qureshi AI, Suarez JI. Use of hypertonic saline solutions in treatment of cerebral edema and intracranial hypertension. *Crit Care Med.* 2000;28:3301–3313.

23. Francony G, Fauvage B, Falcon D, et al. Equimolar doses of mannitol and hypertonic saline in the treatment of increased intracranial pressure. *Crit Care Med.* 2008;36:795–800.

24. Oddo M, Levine JM, Frangos S, et al. Effect of mannitol and hypertonic saline on cerebral oxygenation in patients with severe traumatic brain injury and refractory intracranial hypertension. *J Neurol Neurosurg Psychiatry.* 2009;80:916–920.

25. Rockswold GL, Solid CA, Paredes-Andrade E, et al. Hypertonic saline and its effect on intracranial pressure, cerebral perfusion pressure, and brain tissue oxygen. *Neurosurgery.* 2009;65:1035–1042.

26. McIntyre LA, Fergusson DA, Hébert PC, et al. Prolonged therapeutic hypothermia after traumatic brain injury in adults: a systematic review. *JAMA.* 2003;289:2992–2999.

27. Clifton GL, Miller ER, Choi SC, et al. Hypothermia on admission in patients with severe brain injury. *J Neurotrauma.* 2002;19:293–301.

28. Roberts I. Barbiturates for acute traumatic brain injury. *Cochrane Database Syst Rev.* 2000:CD000033.

29. Brain Trauma Foundation, American Association of Neurological Surgeons, Joint Section on Neurotrauma and Critical Care, et al. Guidelines for the management of severe traumatic brain injury. XI. Anesthetics, analgesics and sedatives. *J Neurotrauma.* 2007;24:S71–S76.

30. Raslan A. Bhardwaj A. Medical management of cerebral edema. *Neurosurg Focus.* 2007;22:E12.

31. Rangel-Castilla L, Gopinath S, Robertson CS. Management of intracranial hypertension. *Neurol Clin.* 2008;26:521–541.

32. Kakar V, Nagaria J, John Kirkpatrick P. The current status of decompressive craniectomy. *Br J Neurosurg.* 2009;23:147–157.

33. Sahuquillo J, Arikan F. Decompressive craniectomy for the treatment of refractory high intracranial pressure in traumatic brain injury. *Cochrane Database Syst Rev.* 2006;25:CD003983.

CHAPTER 26

Stroke

Alex M. Barrocas and Beth A. Longenecker

▶ INTRODUCTION

Stroke continues to be a major cause of morbidity and mortality in adult populations worldwide. Over 750,000 patients are newly diagnosed with stroke each year in the United States alone, and this entity remains the third most frequent cause of death among adults.[1] This disease is a leading cause of disability in the adult population. More than 50% of stroke sufferers will be left with permanent disability, 25% will require some assistance with activities of daily living, and 25% of patients will remain in an institutional setting 6 months poststroke.[2]

The management of acute stroke had been strictly supportive until 1995 when the National Institute of Neurological Disorders and Stroke (NINDS) rt-PA Stroke Study Group published their trial of recombinant tissue plasminogen activator (rt-PA) in the treatment of acute ischemic stroke.[3] The availability of an effective therapy triggered a renewed interest in treatment of acute ischemic infarction as well as the development of specialized "stroke centers" in an attempt to improve outcome in patients with cerebral ischemic infarction. These interventions have improved the outcomes in acute ischemic infarction; however, the 30-day mortality following acute stroke is still unacceptably high at 15–30%.[4] Clearly, more interventions are needed in this devastating disease. New hope has been instilled with the advent of interventional neuroradiology.

It is now even more important for the emergency physician to be able to recognize acute ischemic infarction, order appropriate imaging studies, initiate intravenous (IV) thrombolytic therapy and rapidly consult neurologists and interventional neuroradiologists. This paradigm is akin to the treatment of

ST-elevation myocardial infarction (STEMI). This chapter will review (1) basic neurologic syndromes as localized by their arterial distributions (i.e., anterior cerebral artery [ACA], middle cerebral artery [MCA], posterior cerebral artery [PCA], basilar artery, etc.) as an effort to simplify recognition of large-vessel infarctions, (2) new imaging modalities, (3) initial medical management, and (4) interventional management.

▶ RECOGNIZING ACUTE ISCHEMIC INFARCTION

Computed tomography (CT) scans do not "rule out" acute ischemic infarctions. This is an unfortunate reality that forces the non-neurologist to perform a detailed neurologic examination. Identifying these patterns can assist in the identification of stroke syndromes that can be treated with thrombolytic therapy, as opposed to stroke syndromes that do not follow vascular territories such as hemorrhages, venous infarctions (extremely rare), or stroke mimics such as extreme ranges of blood sugar, seizures, or tumors. The history of a sudden onset of neurologic deficit and the time of onset are paramount to making the diagnosis and treatment decisions.

The presentation of acute stroke follows distinctive anatomic patterns that are predictive of the involved arterial territory. Here are anatomic structures and associated syndromes as supplied by each major vessel:

ACA: The first segment (A1) of the ACA gives rise to the recurrent artery of Huebner that supplies the caudate head, anterior limb of the internal capsule, and anterior aspect of the putamen and globus pallidus (there is some variability). Infarcts to these structures can result in confusion, and arm and face weakness. The remainder of the ACA supplies the medial surface of the cerebral hemisphere and the superior aspect of the frontal and parietal lobes. Infarcts in these territories may result in lack of initiative, abulia, paratonia ("gegenhalten") (anterior frontal lobes), contralateral leg paralysis (superior aspect of the motor cortex—the precentral gyrus), and to a lesser extent arm paralysis (in particular, the shoulder). In bilateral frontal infarction, akinetic mutism, paraplegia, incontinence, and apathy with amnesia may result. Lower extremity contralateral sensory loss may be present if the postcentral gyrus is affected. Other nuances may occur in ACA territory strokes, but these are out of the scope of this review.

MCA: The MCA is the most common site of ischemic stroke and the largest branch of the internal carotid artery (ICA). It supplies the majority of the lateral surface of the cerebral hemisphere and the deep structures of the frontal, insular, and parietal lobes. The lenticular striate arteries arise off the M1 segment and supply the corona radiata, external capsule, claustrum, putamen, part of the globus pallidus, body of the caudate nucleus, and superior aspect of the anterior and posterior limbs of the internal capsule. The clinical picture of the MCA territory infarction depends on the site of occlusion. Contralateral face, arm, and leg weakness manifests when the precentral gyrus (primary motor cortex) is affected. Contralateral face, arm, and leg sensory loss occurs when the postcentral gyrus (primary sensory cortex) is affected. Gaze preference to the affected side may occur when the frontal eye fields are affected. In the dominant hemisphere, the various aphasias occur when Wernicke's, Broca's, or communicating fibers are affected. Complicated sensory syndromes such as alexia with agraphia (left angular gyrus), and combinations of finger agnosia, acalculia, right–left disorientation, and agraphia (Gerstmann syndrome) may also be encountered in posterior MCA territory infarctions. Neglect, denial (agnosagnosia), apraxias, sudden confusional states, and agitated delirium may also occur with parietal lobe infarctions. Contralateral visual field cuts (homonymous hemianopsia, or homonymous inferior quadrantanopsia) may occur if the parietal radiations are affected. Clinical manifestations of infarcts to the lenticulostriate territory include hemiplegia and less often dysarthria alone or upper limb clumsiness. Of course, other nuances to MCA territory ischemic infarctions exist that are out of the scope of this review.

PCA: The PCAs are the terminal branches of the basilar artery; however, 25% of the time they have an embryonic origin off the ICA (aka fetal PCA). The PCA supplies the occipital lobes and the inferomedial portions of the temporal lobes. Numerous small branches off the P1 segments and sometimes the top of the basilar artery supply the mesencephalon, thalamus, and adjacent structures. Proximal PCA occlusion may simulate MCA occlusion when it causes hemiparesis, hemianopsia, hemispatial neglect aphasia, and sensory loss. Cortical signs may be pseudolocalizers in the event of thalamic involvement. The PCA gives a splenial branch (splenium of the corpus callosum) that makes anastamosis with the ACA. Infarction of the splenium can result in alexia without agraphia, "pure word blindness," and sometimes color anomia and/or object/photograph anomia. The cortical branches of the PCA are the anterior temporal, posterior temporal, parieto-occipital, and calcarine arteries. These supply the inferior aspect of the temporal lobe and the parietal radiations, and terminate with the calcarine branch that supplies the visual cortex. Cortical PCA branch occlusion almost always presents with a contralateral visual field cut. Involvement of the calcarine artery may be associated with ipsilateral eye pain. Involvement of bilateral PCAs may result in cortical blindness. Patients are often unaware of their "cortical blindness" (Anton's syndrome).

Vertebral and basilar arteries: The vertebral arteries give rise to the posterior inferior cerebellar arteries (PICAs) that supply the inferior cerebellum and inferior vermis. Infarcts here result in ataxia. The vertebral arteries then merge in what is referred to as the vertebral–basilar junction (VBJ) to give rise to the basilar artery. The basilar artery gives rise to the anterior inferior cerebellar arteries (AICAs), which when infarcted result in ataxia and possible hearing loss if the labyrinthine artery arises off the AICA. The superior cerebellar artery (SCA) is near the top of the basilar artery and supplies the superior vermis and the superior aspect of the cerebellar hemispheres. Infarcts here can vary from limb ataxia to truncal ataxia or both. The mid and the top segments of the basilar artery give off perforating branches into the brainstem (medulla and pons) and thalamus/midbrain, respectively. The top of the basilar branches has overlap with the perforating branches that arise off the P1 segments of the PCAs. These perforating vessels allow for the plethora of "posterior circulation syndromes" (Table 26-1).

▶ TABLE 26-1. POSTERIOR CIRCULATION SYNDROMES

1. Ipsilateral oculomotor palsy with contralateral cerebellar ataxia (Nothnagel syndrome)
2. Ipsilateral oculomotor palsy with contralateral hemiplegia (Weber syndrome)
3. Ipsilateral oculomotor palsy with contralateral ataxia and hemichoreoathetosis (Benedikt syndrome)
4. Nuclear oculomotor palsy (rare), characterized by:
   a. Unilateral oculomotor weakness with contralateral superior rectus weakness
   b. Bilateral oculomotor weakness with sparing of the levator palpebra
5. Unilateral internuclear ophthalmoplegia (INO): inability of the affected eye to cross the midline medially
6. Wall-eyed bilateral internuclear ophthalmoplegia (WEBINO syndrome): neither eye can cross the midline medially
7. Dorsal rostral midbrain (Parinaud syndrome) characterized by:
   a. Supranuclear upward gaze palsy
   b. Defect of convergence
   c. Convergence-retraction nystagmus
   d. Light-near dissociation
   e. Collier's sign (lid retraction)
   f. Skewed deviation
8. Pseudoabducens palsy: no lateral eye movement on the affected side
9. Midbrain corectopia
10. Peduncular hallucinosis, primarily visual lesions of mobile objects, often animated, colorful, and frequently pleasant: no hallucinations occur with mid and cephalic lesions involving the cerebral peduncles or the medial substantia nigra pars reticulata bilaterally
11. Decerebrate rigidity
12. Locked-in syndrome
13. Disturbances of consciousness

▶ IMAGING IN ACUTE STROKE

Differentiating an acute ischemic stroke from a hemorrhage is nearly impossible by history and physical exam alone. This is the reason why a CT scan must be done. Acute ischemic stroke cannot be "ruled out" by CT scan. It is hemorrhage that can be ruled out. Once hemorrhage has been excluded and the remainder of the inclusion/exclusion criteria satisfied, thrombolytic therapy may be administered. It is important to note that acute ischemic stroke is usually not visible on a CT scan in its early stages (typically less than 6 hours).

Imaging has progressed in several fronts. Magnetic resonance imaging (MRI) has the diffusion-weighted imaging (DWI) sequence where acute ischemic stroke can be seen within minutes of infarction. CT scanning remains more commonly available and has the advantage of being quick. To this end, progress in CT scanning includes CT angiography (CTA) and CT perfusion (CTP). MRI advances also include the perfusion sequences.

With CTA, it is now possible to identify large-vessel occlusions in the brain within seconds. In addition, part of the etiologic workup of the stroke can be attained simultaneously by performing a CTA of the neck. Now, carotid stenosis and intracranial vessel integrity (occlusion, vasculopathy, dissection, or stenosis) can be determined within minutes of performing the initial head CT.

Perfusion studies have been referred to as "physiologic imaging." In simple terms, perfusion imaging can determine a delay in the arrival of contrast (blood) to the vascular bed in question. If there is a delay to a certain territory, say the right MCA, for example, one can spend more time analyzing the vasculature leading to and including the right MCA in the hopes of identifying (1) a treatable source, for example, carotid stenosis and (2) the actual clot/occlusion causing the stroke (Figure 26-1).

Physiologic imaging has further progressed with analysis of the concept of "mismatch." Infarcted or otherwise dead tissue can be demonstrated on MRI DWI. Perfusion defects may be equal to the amount of tissue already dead, or they can be greater giving rise to a new definition of penumbra: underperfused territory that is at risk of dying (Figures 26-2 and 26-3).

▶ MEDICAL MANAGEMENT OF ACUTE ISCHEMIC STROKE

The NINDS trial in 1995 provided evidence that intervention is possible in the setting of ischemic stroke. By administering IV rt-PA within 3 hours, 30% of patients improved to near-normal exams at 3 months with a 6% risk of intracranial hemorrhage (ICH). However, only a small percentage of patients are candidates for IV rt-PA. Even in the subgroup receiving thrombolytic therapy, appropriate supportive care can significantly reduce morbidity.

THE ABC'S

While the majority of patients with acute ischemic stroke will not require intubation or ventilatory support, endotracheal intubation should be considered in those patients who are obtunded or those who have lost airway protective reflexes. Also, many patients will have impaired mobility of their oropharynx, placing them at risk for aspiration. As pneumonia has been shown to be an important cause of death after cerebrovascular events,[5] it is prudent to keep these patients NPO until their swallowing ability has been evaluated.

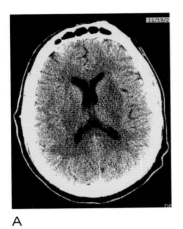

A

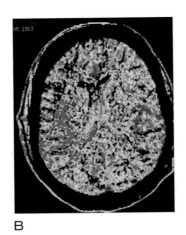

B

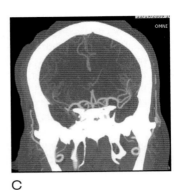

C

Figure 26-1. (A–D) A 46-year-old man presented with left face, arm, and leg hemiplegia (NIHSS 20). CT demonstrates no hemorrhage. CT perfusion demonstrates elevated mean transit time (MTT) in the right MCA territory. CTA demonstrates occlusion of the right distal M1/proximal M2 segment. Angiography confirms the occlusion despite intravenous t-PA. The occlusion was recanalized successfully with 11 mg intra-arterial t-PA and wire disruption of the clot. Postprocedure, the patient's residual deficit was mild nasolabial flattening.

D

Blood pressure (BP) management immediately following acute ischemic stroke remains somewhat controversial. Hypertension is common in the immediate poststroke period and is felt to be a protective response—an attempt to provide adequate perfusion to the ischemic penumbra that surrounds the area of acute infarct. There is some evidence demonstrating a correlation between hypertension in the first 24 hours after stroke and increased mortality.[6,7] There is also evidence that rapid reduction of BP may contribute to morbidity after acute stroke.[8] It is generally believed that extreme hypertension contributes to poor outcome in the setting of stroke, but there is no evidence that clearly defines the upper limits of BP that should be considered a trigger for therapy. This is not the case in those patients receiving thrombolytic therapy, where there are clearly defined limits (systolic BP [SBP] <185 mm Hg and diastolic BP [DBP] <110 mm Hg) beyond which the risk of ICH is increased.[9]

The current American Heart Association/American Stroke Association (AHA/ASA) guidelines for management of hypertension in acute stroke are as follows:

1. Aggressive management of BP should be considered in all patients who demonstrate evidence of severe end-organ damage from hypertension in addition to acute stroke. This includes patients with hypertensive encephalopathy, acute renal failure, aortic dissection, acute myocardial infarction (MI), or acute congestive heart failure.

2. If a patient will be undergoing thrombolytic therapy or other reperfusion intervention, BP should be lowered to an SBP of less than 185 mm Hg and a DBP of less than 110 mm Hg.

3. In those who are not candidates for intervention, a less aggressive approach is recommended. Antihypertensive agents should be held until SBP remains above 220 mm Hg or DBP remains above 120 mm Hg.

In all instances, it is recommended that the agent of choice be easily titratable to prevent rapid sustained declines in BP. The current guidelines recommend labetalol 10 mg IV repeated every 10–20 minutes to a maximum dose of 200 mg, labetalol 10 mg IV followed by a 2–8 mg/min infusion, or nicardipine infusion starting at 5 mg/h and titrated to desired BP or a maximum dose of 15 mg/h.[10] Hypotension is uncommon in patients with acute stroke. If it develops, the cause should be actively sought—aortic dissection, acute MI, etc. Cardiac dysrhythmias, blood loss, or volume depletion should all be considered. Therapy should be directed at the underlying cause and may include volume replacement and pressors if hypotension persists. Certainly patients

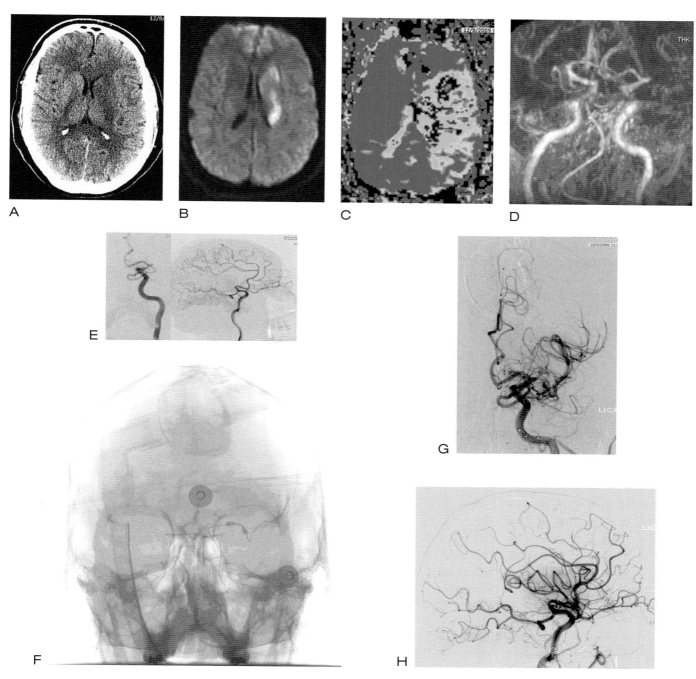

Figure 26-2. (A–H) A 45-year-old man presents with sudden onset of global aphasia and 2/5 hemiparesis at 3.5 hours onset time. The patient was not given IV t-PA, although now given ECASS III, he would have been a candidate. CT demonstrates no hemorrhage. Early findings in the caudate are more obvious on MRI/DWI. MRI perfusion demonstrates a full MCA territory perfusion defect. This case demonstrates well the concept of diffusion–perfusion mismatch. Clearly there is brain to save (penumbra). The MRA demonstrates an occlusion of the left MCA M1 segment. Angiography confirms the left M1 occlusion. Intra-arterial t-PA and the MERCI device were used unsuccessfully in efforts to recanalize the vessel. Angioplasty was performed successfully leaving a mild residual stenosis. This correlates to the pathophysiology, as the patient was using cocaine the previous night. Recall cocaine induces transient platelet aggregability, vasospasm, and cardiac arrhythmias secondary to sympathomimetic effects. The patient's residual deficit correlates to the original MRI/DWI: deficits that localize to the caudate. A clear demonstration of perfusion defect correlating to deficits that were reversible—proof of concept of the penumbra saved.

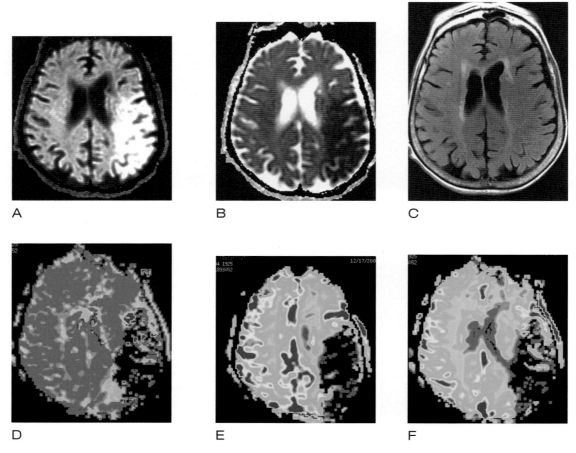

Figure 26-3. (A–F) Matched diffusion–perfusion defect. This patient is not a candidate for interventional or arguably intravenous thrombolysis because the area of infarction (hyperintense on DWI) matches the area of perfusion defect, making this a "completed infarction" in this 84-year-old woman with sudden-onset aphasia, right hemiplegia, right hemisensory loss, and right homonymous hemianopsia in the context of atrial fibrillation.

may sustain ischemic infarction in the setting of arterial stenosis and hypotension. Neurovascular imaging is warranted (CTA or MRA of the head and neck).

MANAGEMENT OF GLUCOSE

Hyperglycemia is a common phenomenon immediately poststroke and has been shown to be associated with worsened outcome. The correlation is strongest in the population without diabetes mellitus. Hyperglycemia in the critically ill is often referred to as stress hyperglycemia and is characterized by elevation in catecholamines, cortisol, growth hormone, glucagon, gluconeogenesis, insulin levels, insulin resistance, and insulin-like growth factor-1 (IGF-1) protein. There is evidence that hyperglycemia worsens outcome and increases the risk of ICH in patients receiving rt-PA.[11] While current evidence demonstrates worsened outcome in the setting of hyperglycemia poststroke, there is no solid evidence to guide the means of therapy or the level to which

glucose control should be maintained. The majority of randomized controlled trials (RCTs) available that deal with glucose control are studies that looked at insulin therapy in patients in the intensive care unit (ICU) setting for illnesses other than stroke. These studies indicate variable benefit from tight glycemic control and demonstrated a significant risk of hypoglycemia with worsened outcome in patients in the treatment arm.[12] The largest RCT looking specifically at tight glucose control in stroke patients is the GIST-UK trial. The methods for maintaining infusion and monitoring glucose were highly labor intensive, and the results were neutral with effect on morbidity and mortality.[13] The current AHA/ASA guidelines are to begin intervention for serum glucose levels of >140–185 mg/dL and to try to maintain levels between 80 and 140 mg/dL. Therapy can involve repeated boluses of insulin or IV infusion.[10] In all instances, careful monitoring is needed and hypoglycemia should be avoided as this also has been shown to have a negative effect on patient outcome.

► THROMBOLYSIS IN ACUTE STROKE

The goal of the treatment of acute ischemia is rapid reperfusion in patients who present within the therapeutic window. Every ischemic stroke patient must be evaluated quickly. Time is brain. Early stroke treatment is associated with better outcome.[14] Treatment of the symptoms of ischemic infarction begins as soon as the diagnosis is made, in other words, once the CT scan excludes the hemorrhage. Give aspirin. Aspirin has been shown in numerous trials to reduce the frequency of subsequent ischemic events.[15] Per rectum aspirin may be safely administered in patients with swallowing or face weakness.

With the publication of the NINDS trial in 1995, thrombolytic therapy entered the spotlight. The study demonstrated significant benefit of therapy, but also demonstrated a 6% risk of ICH in the treatment arm. Significant controversy ensued among the emergency medicine community. Did the benefit of lytics outweigh the risk? Could rt-PA be safely used in the community setting? Can thrombolytic therapy safely be initiated in the absence of a neurologist? A plethora of research ensued.

As of 2010, thrombolytic therapy is widely accepted and is widely used throughout the United States and Europe. However, not all hospitals have initiated protocols for the use of rt-PA in this setting. This may be due to a lack of neurology coverage in many areas of the country—it is estimated that 20% of the population is served by emergency departments that lack immediate access to a neurologist. The literature supports the use of thrombolytics even in the absence of an onsite neurologist. Teleneurology is becoming increasingly popular and has been shown to be safe and efficacious.[16,17] Also, in spite of subtleties in stroke presentation, accuracy of diagnosis by emergency physicians has been demonstrated[18] and thrombolytic treatment can be safely initiated using a standard protocol, even in the absence of a neurologist.[19] Current evidence-based medicine indicates that rt-PA can be safely used in the community setting, so long as strict adherence to protocols is maintained. The rate of ICH remains at 6% in most studies, but has been noted to be lower (1.7%) in the SITS-MOST observational study.[20] The current AHA/ASA guidelines[10] for the use of rt-PA in the setting of acute ischemic stroke recommend treatment for patients who fit the following profile: Patients must have a measurable neurologic deficit that is not clearing spontaneously and is not minor and isolated. In those with more severe deficits—National Institutes of Health Stroke Scale (NIHSS) >22—caution is advised, because while there may be some benefit to therapy, there is a significant increase in the incidence of ICH. Contraindications to rt-PA therapy are listed in Table 26-2.

► **TABLE 26-2. CONTRAINDICATIONS TO RECOMBINANT TISSUE PLASMINOGEN ACTIVATOR (rt-PA) THERAPY**

1. Head trauma in the preceding 3 months
2. Myocardial infarction in the preceding 3 months
3. GI or urinary tract hemorrhage in the preceding 21 days
4. Major surgery in the preceding 14 days
5. Any history of prior intracranial hemorrhage
6. Arterial puncture at a noncompressible site in the past 7 days
7. Active bleeding or acute trauma/fracture on current physical examination
8. Elevated aPTT or INR >1.7
9. Platelet count below 100,000/mm³
10. Hypoglycemia (<50 mg/dL)
11. Seizure with postictal neurologic deficits
12. CT with multilobar infarction (>1/3 the cerebral hemisphere)
13. Hypertension (SBP >185 mm Hg and/or DBP >110 mm Hg)

Older age is not in and of itself a contraindication to thrombolytic therapy. Prior suggestions that rt-PA should be withheld in patients older than 80 years have been questioned, and data analysis has shown that there is some benefit to treatment in this age group. Overall, these patients still have poorer outcomes than younger patients when suffering an acute stroke, but the incidence of ICH among this population is not higher than in younger patients treated with thrombolytics.[21,22]

The recommended dose of rt-PA in the setting of acute stroke is 0.9 mg/kg with a maximum dose of 90 mg. The initial 10% of the dose is administered as an IV bolus given over 1 minute and the remaining is infused over 60 minutes. It is markedly important to obtain a weight on all patients in whom thrombolysis is considered. Overestimation of weight and subsequent overdosing of rt-PA is one of the more common violations of protocol and is thought to contribute significantly to the incidence of ICH in this patient population.[23] Another frequently noted protocol violation is failure to adequately control BP. Frequent monitoring of BP should be initiated in these patients, and antihypertensives should be administered if the SBP is 180 mm Hg or higher and the DBP is 105 mm Hg or higher.

The decision to treat patients with thrombolytics is time dependent. In the initial NINDS trial, there was a significant increase in the incidence of ICH in patients receiving rt-PA more than 3 hours after symptom onset. For years, the "3-hour window" has been the gold standard. Over the past 5 years, multiple studies have asked the following question: Is it possibly safe to expand this therapeutic window? The most definitive is the European Cooperative Acute Stroke Study (ECASS) III trial, published in September 2008. The trial was multicentered, randomized, and placebo controlled and enrolled patients with stroke onset 3–4.5 hours prior to receiving therapy. There was a significant improvement in neurologic outcome at 90 days in the treatment group. The incidence of ICH was also larger in the treatment arm, with symptomatic ICH occurring in 2.7% of those receiving lytics. There was no significant difference in mortality between the groups.[24] As a result of this trial, the AHA/ASA guidelines for the use of thrombolytics in acute stroke have been revised. It is now a Class IB recommendation for lytics to be used in patients for up to 4.5 hours after the onset of symptoms.[25] As failure to present within the 3-hour window is one of the most common reasons why thrombolytic therapy is not provided to stroke patients, the new time window is likely to increase the number of patients receiving therapy, and will contribute to improved outcome among patients with acute ischemic stroke.

Even so, there will be patients who are not candidates for IV thrombolysis or those who present with a greater delay after symptom onset. These patients need no longer all fall into the category of "supportive care only." Over the past 15 years, an entire specialty, interventional neuroradiology, has developed, and now there are a multitude of techniques that have been added to the therapeutic armamentarium.

▶ INTERVENTIONAL MANAGEMENT OF STROKE

Indications for the interventional management of acute ischemic infarction parallel those for IV thrombolysis with a few important variations: (1) time window is increased to 6 hours; (2) inclusion criteria now include the presence of an occluded vessel by CTA; and (3) anticoagulation is not a contraindication. Absolute contraindications are hemorrhage and hypoattenuation of the region in question on CT (in other words, the region of brain where the deficits localize is already infracted). Patients may receive IV rt-PA and then undergo intra-arterial (IA) thrombolysis safely[26] or receive IA thrombolysis in the 3- to 6-hour window safely.[27] In patients who are anticoagulated or have recently received surgery, mechanical thrombectomy is an option employing devices such as Mechanical Embolus Removal in Cerebral Ischemia (MERCI) thrombectomy device[28] and Penumbra Aspiration System.[29] The aforementioned studies have demonstrated efficacy and safety in interventional thrombolysis and thrombectomy in patients with acute cerebral ischemia. This is different from demonstration of efficacy in the medical treatment of acute cerebral ischemia. Although level 1 evidence for the interventional treatment of stroke is pending, there are numerous reports of success in the literature.

REFERENCES

1. Lloyd-Jones D, Adams R, Carnethon M, et al. Heart disease and stroke statistics 2009 update: a report from the American Heart Association Statistics Committee and Stroke Statistics Subcommittee. *Circulation.* 2009;119:e72.
2. Petrea RE, Biser AS, Sashadri S, et al. Gender differences in stroke incidence and poststroke disability in the Framingham Heart Study. *Stroke.* 2009;40:4.
3. The National Institute of Neurological Disorders and Stroke rt-PA Stroke Study Group. Tissue plasminogen activator for acute ischemic stroke. *N Engl J Med.* 1995;333:1581–1587.
4. Carandang R, Seshadri S, Beiser A, et al. Trends in incidence, lifetime risk, severity, and 30-day mortality of stroke over the past 50 years. *JAMA.* 2006;296:2944.
5. Katzan IL, Cebul RD, Husak SH, et al. The effect of pneumonia on mortality among patients hospitalized for acute stroke. *Neurology.* 2003;60:620–625.
6. Vemmos KN, Spengos K, Tsivgoulis G, et al. Factors influencing acute blood pressure values in stroke subtypes. *J Hum Hypertens.* 2004;18:253–259.
7. Aslanyan S, Fazekas F, Weir CJ, et al, GAIN International Steering Committee and Investigators. Elevated pulse pressure during the acute period of ischemic stroke is associated with poor stroke outcome. *Stroke.* 2004;35:e153–e155.
8. Castillo J, Leira R, Garcia MM, et al. Blood pressure decrease during the acute phase of ischemic stroke is associated with brain injury and poor stroke outcome. *Stroke.* 2004;35:520–526.
9. Brott T, Lu M, Kothari R, et al. Hypertension and its treatment in the NINDS rt-PA Stroke Trial. *Stroke.* 198;29:1504–1509.
10. Adams HP, del Zoppo G, Alberts MJ, et al. Guidelines for the early management of adults with ischemic stroke: a guideline from the American Heart Association/American Stroke Association, Stroke Council, Clinical Cardiology Council, Cardiovascular Radiology and Intervention Council, and the Atherosclerotic Peripheral Vascular Disease and Quality of Care Outcomes in Research and Interdisciplinary Working Groups: the American Academy of Neurology affirms the value of this guideline as an educational tool for neurologists. *Stroke.* 2007;38;1655–1711.
11. Bruno A, Levine SR, Frankel MR, et al, NINDS rt-PA Stroke Study Group. Admission glucose level and clinical outcomes in the NINDS rt-PA Stroke Trial. *Neurology.* 2002;59:669–674.
12. Brunkhorst FM. Intensive insulin therapy in patients with severe sepsis and septic shock is associated with an increased rate of hypoglycemia—results from a multicenter randomized controlled study (VISEP). *Infection.* 2005;33:19.
13. Gray CS, Hildreth AJ, Sandercock PA, et al. GIST Trialists Collaboration. Glucose–potassium–insulin infusions in the management of post-stroke hyperglycemia: the UK Glucose Insulin in Stroke Trial (GIST-UK). *Lancet Neurol.* 2007;6:397–406.

14. Marler JR, Tilley BC, Lu M, et al. Early stroke treatment associated with better outcome: the NINDS rt-PA Stroke Study. *Neurology*. 2000;55(11):1649–1655.

15. Mohr JP, Choi DW, Grotta JC, Weir B, Wolf PA, eds. Stroke: Pathophysiology, Diagnosis, and Management; 4th ed. Churchill Livingston. 2004.

16. Shafquat S, Kvedar JC, Guanci MM, et al. Role for telemedicine in acute stroke: feasibility and reliability of remote administration of the NIH stroke scale. *Stroke*. 1999;30;2141–2145.

17. Wiborg A, Widder B. Teleneurology to improve stroke care in rural areas: the Telemedicine in Stroke in Swabia (TESS) project. *Stroke*. 2003;34;2951–2956.

18. Hemmen TM, Meyer BC, McClean TL et al. Identification of nonischemic stroke mimics among 411 code strokes at the University of California, San Diego, Stroke Center. *J Stroke Cerebrovasc Dis*. 2008;17(1):23–25.

19. Batmanian JJ, Lam M, Matthews C, et al. A protocol-driven model for the rapid initiation of stroke thrombolysis in the emergency department. *Med J Aust*. 2007;187(10):567–570.

20. Wahlgren N, Davalos A, Ford GA, et al. Thrombolysis with alteplase for acute ischaemic stroke in the Safe Implementation of Thrombolysis in Stroke-Monitoring Study (SITS-MOST): an observational study. *Lancet*. 2007;369;275–282.

21. DeKeyser JD, Gdovinova Z, Uyttenboogaart M, et al. Intravenous alteplase for stroke: beyond the guidelines and in particular clinical situations. *Stroke*. 2007;38; 2612–2618.

22. Engelter ST, Bonati LH, Lyrer PA. Intravenous thrombolysis of stroke patients in ≥ 80 versus < 80 years of age—a systematic review across cohort studies. *Age Ageing*. 2006;35:572–580.

23. Lopez-Yunez AM, Runo A, Williams LS, et al. Protocol violations in community based rTPA stroke treatment are associated with symptomatic intracranial hemorrhage. *Stroke*. 2001;32;12–16.

24. Hacke W, Kaste M, Bluhmki E, et al. Thrombolysis with alteplase 3 to 4.5 hours after acute ischemic stroke. *N Engl J Med*. 2008;359(13):1317–1329.

25. del Zoppo GJ, Saver JL, Jauch EC, et al, on behalf of the American Heart Association Stroke Council. Expansion of the time window for treatment of acute ischemic stroke with intravenous tissue plasminogen activator: a science advisory from the American Heart Association/American Stroke Association. *Stroke*. 2009;40:2945–2948.

26. Lewandowski CA, Frankel M, Tomsick TA, et al. Combined intravenous and intra-arterial rt-PA versus intra-arterial therapy of acute ischemic stroke: Emergency Management of Stroke (EMS) Bridging Trial. *Stroke*. 1999;30;2598–2605.

27. Furlan A, Higashida R, Wechsle L, e al. Intra-arterial prourokinase for acute ischemic stroke. The PROACT II study: a randomized controlled trial: prolyse in acute cerebral thromboembolism. *JAMA*. 1999;282;2003–2011.

28. Smith WS, Sung G, Starkman S, et al. Safety and efficacy of mechanical embolectomy in acute ischemic stroke: results of the MERCI trial. *Stroke*. 2005;36:1432–1438.

29. Penumbra Pivotal Stroke Trial Investigators. The penumbra pivotal stroke trial: safety and effectiveness of a new generation of mechanical devices for clot removal in intracranial large vessel occlusive disease. *Stroke*. 2009;40(8):2761–2768.

CHAPTER 27

Intracranial Hemorrhage

Alex M. Barrocas and Beth A. Longenecker

▶ SPONTANEOUS INTRACRANIAL HEMORRHAGE

Intracranial hemorrhage (ICH) accounts for 15% of all strokes, and there are approximately 37,000 cases in the United States per year. These patients have the highest mortality of all stroke subsets (>30%) and 50% of deaths occur in the first 48 hours after the event. Survivors of ICH often have profound neurologic deficits and only the minority will regain functional independence at 6 months.[1]

The incidence of ICH increases exponentially with age and is higher in men than in women. Independent risk factors for ICH include arterial hypertension (the most significant risk factor, present in 75%), alcohol abuse, thrombolytic therapy, cocaine or amphetamine use, cigarette smoking, and diabetes mellitus.[2–4]

Anticoagulant therapy and daily aspirin use are also independent risk factors for ICH. In a meta-analysis of the literature, for every 1,000 patients treated with aspirin for 5 years, there will be one excess ICH caused by this therapeutic intervention. On the other hand, 14 acute myocardial infarctions will be avoided in this same population, so benefits of therapy far outweigh risk.[5] Patients on anticoagulant therapy have a 7- to 10-fold higher incidence of ICH. The mortality in this population is 60%, almost double that of the general population. ICH occurs in 2–9 per 100,000 patients receiving anticoagulant therapy per year. A strong association between overanticoagulation and ICH exists; however, the majority of bleeds occur in patients with a therapeutic international normalized ratio (INR).[6]

This chapter will discuss the diagnosis and management of spontaneous intracerebral hemorrhage and will then separately address diagnostic and management strategies for subarachnoid hemorrhage (SAH).

PRESENTATION AND DIAGNOSIS

Patients with an ICH generally present with sudden onset of neurologic deficits (Figure 27-1). These are often rapidly progressive. A full neurologic examination including mental status, cranial nerves, motor strength, sensory, reflexes, and cerebellar coordination should be documented on presentation to the emergency room and followed sequentially (hourly neuro checks). Exam findings can help localize the lesion, but more importantly, form the baseline to evaluate for signs of deterioration. Cerebral hemispheric subcortical white matter or putamenal hemorrhages can present with gaze deviation (involvement of eye fields—gaze toward the lesion) and/or contralateral hemiparesis/plegia, aphasia (dominant side—perisylvian subcortical white matter), neglect or agnosias (parietal subcortical white matter), and contralateral hemianopsia (occipital lobe subcortical white matter). Thalamic hemorrhages can present with aphasia (dominant side), neglect (nondominant side), contralateral sensory or motor deficits (if adjacent internal capsule motor fibers are involved), oculomotor derangements, visual field cuts, and/or small reactive pupils. Brainstem lesions can present with coma, quadriparesis, locked-in syndrome, horizontal gaze paresis, ocular bobbing, pinpoint pupils, nystagmus, hyperthermia, and abnormal breathing patterns. Fixed midposition pupils and hippus are suggestive of midbrain involvement. Cerebellar hemorrhages can present with limb or truncal ataxia, nystagmus, skewed gaze, brainstem findings secondary to mass effect on the brainstem, and signs of elevated intracranial pressure (ICP)/hydrocephalus from complete effacement of the fourth ventricle or cerebral aqueduct.

The diagnostic test of choice at this time remains noncontrast computed tomography (CT). CT angiography (CTA) is useful in identifying aneurysms or vascular malformations. Active bleeding can be seen as contrast

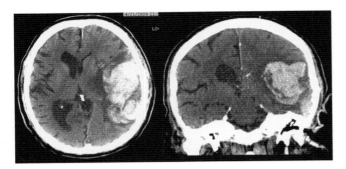

Figure 27–1. CT lobar hemorrhage. The patient presented with sudden-onset right face, arm, and leg weakness with alteration of consciousness. Coronal sequence is particularly useful at demonstrating uncal herniation.

extravasation into the hematoma "spot sign" on these studies. Increase in ICH is seen in 38% of patients within the first 3 hours of ictus and two thirds of those are within the first hour. Hemorrhages from chronic hypertension commonly occur in the basal ganglia, thalamus, pons, and cerebellum, among other sites (Figure 27-2). These sites are supplied by perforating vessels that are susceptible to lipohyalinosis, fibrinoid necrosis, and Charcot–Bouchard microaneurysms in the setting of chronic hypertension. Hemorrhages from amyloid angiopathy usually occur in a lobar distribution. This disease is characterized by β-amyloid deposition in small- and medium-sized vessels, history of Alzheimer's disease, recurrent hemorrhages (of various sorts—subdural, subarachnoid, etc.), and Apo E2 and E4 alleles.

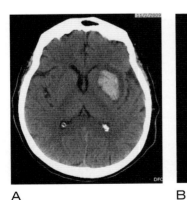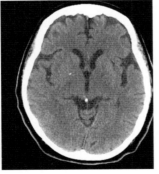

A   **B**

Figure 27–2. (A and B) CT hypertensive hemorrhage. Note the left basal ganglia hemorrhage encompassing the left putamen and globus pallidus. Six-month follow-up CT reveals small linear cystic encephalomalacia in the site of prior hemorrhage consistent with the form of healing in the brain by cavitation. The site of hypertensive hemorrhages is most commonly in the territory of perforating vessels (basal ganglia—lenticular striate arteries; pons—basilar perforators; thalamus—thalamoperforators).

Hemorrhages from vasculopathy usually result from rupture of small- or medium-sized vessels. History is critical in making this diagnosis as typically the hemorrhage is preceded by months of headache, and neurologic deficits such as cognitive decline and psychiatric symptoms from multiple small strokes. Vasculopathy can be seen with infectious diseases such as herpes, tuberculosis, bacterial/fungal/viral vasculitis, syphilis, systemic diseases such as polyarteritis nodosa, Wegener's granulomatosis, Churg–Strauss syndrome, systemic lupus erythematosis, rheumatoid arthritis, Sjögren's disease, hepatitis, Behçet's disease, sarcoidosis, drug induced (cocaine), etc.

MEDICAL MANAGEMENT OF PATIENTS WITH ICH

Airway Management

Patients with ICH often deteriorate rapidly and require careful monitoring of their airway. Endotracheal intubation should be performed in patient with Glasgow Coma Scale (GCS) score of 8 or lower, or those unable to manage secretions. If patients require transfer from a carefully monitored setting or to an outside facility, realize that there is the potential for these patients to suffer airway compromise and consider intubation in patients who are obtunded. Rapid sequence induction should be performed prior to intubation. The use of lidocaine prior to intubation has not been proven to prevent increases in ICP and is of questionable benefit.[7] The preferred induction agents should be short acting and should not increase ICP. Current recommendations are for the use of etomidate or propofol in the setting of acute ICH. Propofol can cause a rapid decrease in blood pressure (BP), but this generally is responsive to boluses of isotonic fluids. Midazolam should be avoided as it may adversely affect ICP. A short-acting nondepolarizing agent such as rocuronium is preferred to the shorter-acting succinylcholine in patients at risk for increased ICP.[8] The evidence is incomplete, but it does suggest that succinylcholine may increase ICP in those with a space-occupying lesion in the cranium. If a decision is made to use succinylcholine, pretreatment with a "defasciculating" dose of a nondepolarizing agent such as vecuronium or pancuronium should be employed as this has been demonstrated to protect against such increases in ICP.[9]

There are no unique aspects to ventilator management in patients following acute ICH. Hyperoxygenation is not necessary, and hyperventilation should be reserved as a temporizing measure for patients with elevations in ICP. Positive end-expiratory pressure (PEEP) of up to 12 mm Hg may safely be used and will not increase ICP so long as mean arterial pressure (MAP) is maintained.[10]

Blood Pressure Management

There is still some controversy over definite limits at which to begin therapy for hypertension in patients following spontaneous ICH. Prior literature showed possible increases in morbidity and mortality accompanying aggressive management of hypertension. However, two recent trials, the INTERACT and the ATACH trials,[11,12] demonstrated that it is safe to aggressively lower BP in patients with ICH. The studies are not sufficient to establish parameters for BP control, nor do they provide sufficient evidence to demonstrate improved outcome in patients receiving aggressive early lowering of BP. As such, the American Heart Association/ American Stroke Association (AHA/ASA) continues to support the 2007 recommendations[1] as follows:

1. If systolic BP (SBP) is >200 mm Hg or MAP is >150 mm Hg, consider aggressively lowering pressure using an agent given by intravenous (IV) infusion.
2. For SBP >180 mm Hg or MAP >130 mm Hg in the setting of possible increased ICP, consider lowering BP via either continuous infusion or intermittent administration of IV medications while monitoring the ICP.
3. Consider lowering BP to 160/90 mm Hg if SBP >180 mm Hg or MAP is >130 mm Hg in patients with no evidence of increased ICP. Again, continuous IV infusion or intermittent dosing of medication is appropriate. The guidelines were modified to include the following in the 2009 update by the AHA/ASA: If a patient presents with an SBP of 150–220 mm Hg, it is probably safe to acutely lower the SBP to 140 mm Hg.[13] In general, agents chosen for BP control in this setting should be easy to titrate and have a relatively short duration of action. The most frequently recommended agents include IV nicardipine, labetalol, or esmolol.

Minimizing Hematoma Expansion

It is widely recognized that hematoma expansion during the first 6 hours after an ICH is predictive of poor outcome. Patients with coagulopathy, be it inherent or iatrogenic, should receive agents that attempt to correct the abnormality and therefore limit hematoma size. Patients who have a severe coagulation factor deficiency or severe thrombocytopenia should receive appropriate factor replacement or platelets.[13]

In patients who have received recombinant tissue plasminogen activator (rt-PA) and suffer symptomatic ICH, there are no solid guidelines available. Current recommendations are to infuse 6–8 U of platelets as well as cryoprecipitate that contains factor VIII.[14]

In patients suffering ICH who have been on heparin, reversal with protamine sulfate, 1 mg for every 100 U of heparin given (within the first 30 minutes of heparin administration), is indicated; 0.75 mg/100 U heparin of protamine within 31–60 minutes, 0.5 mg/ 100 U heparin of protamine within 61–120 minutes, and 0.4 mg/100 U heparin of protamine at greater than 2 hours of heparin administration, keeping in mind the half-life of heparin is 2 hours. The total dose should not exceed 50 mg, and protamine should be injected slowly by IV as rapid infusion may trigger hypotension.[1]

People receiving oral anticoagulants, such as warfarin, account for 12–14% of all ICH patients. The current AHA/ASA guidelines for patients with elevated INR are to (1) withhold warfarin; (2) give IV vitamin K (dose: 2 mg, slow IV)—be prepared for a possible anaphylactic response when administering IV vitamin K; (3) use either fresh frozen plasma (FFP) 15 mL/kg or prothrombin complex concentrates (PCC) 50–150 mL to provide vitamin K–dependent clotting factors. PCC may hold some benefit over FFP as there is less volume loading and PCC has been shown to more rapidly improve INR. However, no current studies have demonstrated improved outcome with their use and the product is far more costly. Current AHA/ASA recommendations are for either product.[1]

There has been a great deal of interest in the use of recombinant factor VIIa in acute hemorrhage; however, in phase III trials, there was no improvement in outcome in patients with ICH receiving rVIIa and there was some increase in arterial thrombus in the treatment arm.[15] Current AHA/ASA guidelines state that there is no indication for rVIIa in unselected patients, but many still contend that its use should be considered in those patients with ICH who were receiving oral anticoagulant therapy if neurosurgical intervention is a possibility.

Other Management Considerations

It is critical to attempt to minimize secondary brain injury following ICH. Studies have shown an improved outcome in these patients when managed in a specialized neuroscience intensive care unit (NICU); as such, this is the most appropriate setting for these patients whenever possible.[16]

Management of Increased Intracranial Pressure

Patients with large intracerebral hematomas or with intraventricular involvement are at increased risk of developing increased ICP. There are no techniques specific to management in the subset of patients with ICH. The standard medical therapies remain unchanged: (1) the head of the bed should be maintained at 30°; (2) 20% mannitol should be infused in a dose of 1–1.5 g/kg; (3) hyperventilation may provide a temporary decrease in ICP and should be initiated with a goal toward maintaining the patient's Pco_2 at 25–30 mm Hg; (4) barbiturates, such as pentobarbital, given in 5-mg boluses every 10–15 minutes may improve ICP in intractable cases; (5) intracranial monitoring of ICP or ventriculostomy with drainage of cerebrospinal fluid (CSF) should also be considered on an individual basis.[1,8] Intraventricular administration of rt-PA has been explored in patients with ICH but is still considered investigational by the AHA/ASA.[1]

Rigid control of glucose has been shown to be beneficial in surgical intensive care unit (SICU) patients; however, hypoglycemia must also be avoided. Several studies in patients with closed head injury have demonstrated episodes of hypoglycemia and possible increased risk of mortality.[17] The current AHA/ASA guidelines are for less aggressive management than the recommended tight glucose control of 80–110 mg/dL and instead call for maintenance of euglycemia and avoidance of hypoglycemia.[1]

Fever has been shown to worsen outcome in patients with ICH; conversely, there is no evidence demonstrating that temperature control improves outcome in these patients. It is recommended that antipyretics and cooling blankets be employed to maintain euthermia.[1,8]

Patients with lobar ICH are at increased risk for seizure. Prophylactic antiepileptic medications are not currently recommended by the AHA/ASA. Treatment should begin if the patient has clinical seizures or in patients with changes in mental status who demonstrate seizure on electroencephalography (EEG). Continuous EEG monitoring should be considered in patients with mental status depression that is out of proportion to the degree of demonstrated brain injury.[1] Initial management of seizures should begin with benzodiazepines such as lorazepam 0.1 mg/kg, followed by a loading dose of phenytoin or fosphenytoin (20 mg/kg).[8]

Patients are at increased risk for thromboembolic events while under care in the NICU. It is recommended that all patients be placed in compression stockings with intermittent compression devices to the lower extremities. Once bleeding has been documented to have stopped, low-dose subcutaneous low-molecular-weight heparin or unfractionated heparin may be considered for deep vein thrombosis (DVT) prevention.[1]

The current recommendations for surgical intervention are based largely on the STICH trial[18] that did not confirm benefit for surgery in patients with superficial lobar hemorrhage. The trial did demonstrate worsened outcome in patients with deeper hemorrhages undergoing surgery. The current AHA/ASA guidelines are for early surgical intervention in patients with cerebellar

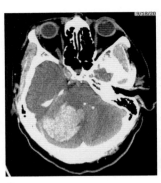 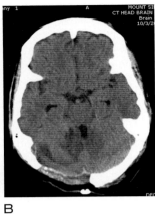

A   B

Figure 27–3. (A and B) Cerebellar hemorrhage and 2 weeks postoperative CT. Note the mass effect that the hematoma causes on the fourth ventricle (fully compressed), and complete effacement of the quadrigeminal plate cistern and brainstem. On the 2-week postdecompressive craniectomy follow-up CT, the fourth ventricle is again visible and the mass effect on the brainstem relieved with residual encephalomalacia in the area of hemorrhage. Immediate relief of the compressive effect of the hematoma is the objective of the surgical intervention.

hemorrhage with rapid deterioration, brainstem compression, or hydrocephalus (Figure 27-3). Craniotomy may be considered in patients with large hemorrhages >30 mL within 1 cm of the surface of the brain. Finally, the use of minimally invasive techniques for clot evacuation is still considered investigational.[1]

Finally, the current AHA/ASA guidelines address the issue of mortality in patients with ICH. It is well published that the majority of patients who die from ICH will do so during their initial acute hospitalization. Newer studies that have looked at lack of intervention (do not resuscitate [DNR] orders) in the initial phase of treatment in patients with ICH have demonstrated that "early care limitations" may be an independent risk factor for mortality in this population.[19,20] The AHA/ASA now recommends that implementation of DNR orders in patients who do not currently have them in place should not be initiated until the second hospital day.[1]

▶ SUBARACHNOID HEMORRHAGE

SAH accounts for approximately 5% of all strokes and about 1% of all patients presenting to the emergency department with the complaint of headache. While the incidence of SAH has remained relatively unchanged, mortality has significantly improved, remaining anywhere from 33% to 45%.[21,22] The most common cause of nontraumatic SAH is rupture of an intracranial aneurysm and will be the focus of this discussion. Numerous other causes of SAH exist, including intracranial arterial dissection, arteriovenous malformation (AVM), dural arteriovenous fistula (AVF), infectious aneurysms, infectious endocarditis, trauma, coagulation disorders, cocaine abuse, cervical origin (from a spinal AVM or AVF), cavernous malformations, vasculitis, vasculopathy, intracranial tumor, sickle cell anemia, pituitary apoplexy, and intracranial venous sinus thrombosis to list a few for which cerebral angiography is indicated in the diagnostic evaluation.

Independent risk factors for the development of SAH include cigarette smoking, hypertension, cocaine, and heavy use of alcohol.[23] Certain genetic syndromes are also linked to formation of aneurysm and SAH. These include α_1-antitrypsin deficiency, autosomal dominant polycystic kidney disease,[24] type IV Ehlers–Danlos syndrome,[25] and familial intracranial aneurysm syndrome (defined as first-degree relatives with $\geq$2 affected members). Patients with this disorder tend to have multiple aneurysms and a 10% risk of having an aneurysm compared with 2% in general population, and tend to suffer aneurysmal rupture at an early age. Patients with a history of ruptured aneurysm have an annual rate of new aneurysm formation of 1–2%.[26]

The diagnosis of spontaneous SAH requires a high index of suspicion. It is estimated that approximately between 5% and 12% of patients with this type of bleed remain undiagnosed.[27,28] This is a dismal statistic, as failure to diagnose SAH considerably increases morbidity and mortality.

The most common presenting symptom of SAH is sudden onset of severe headache. Patients may describe the headache as the "worst headache of my life." Severe headache is present in up to 80% of patients with subarachnoid bleeding. Patients may also present with nausea, vomiting, neck pain, or alterations in mental status or focal neurologic deficits, frequently cranial nerve palsies.[21] It should be remembered that improvement of pain in response to conventional therapies used for headache control does *not* rule out SAH, and this thought process is a trap to be avoided. Initial neurologic examination is predictive of outcome in SAH as shown by the Hunt and Hess scale where grade 1 is asymptomatic to mild headache and nuchal rigidity; grade 2 is moderate–severe headache, nuchal rigidity, but no neurologic deficit other than cranial neuropathy; grade 3 is drowsiness, altered sensorium, and/or mild focal neurologic deficit; grade 4 is stupor and/or moderate–severe hemiparesis; grade 5 is coma/decerebrate posturing.[29] The 30-day survival is 70% for grades 1–3, and 20% for grades 4 and 5.[30] Modern advancements in treatment of SAH (in 1995) including the advent of interventional neuroradiology for endovascular treatment of vasospasm have improved these figures at least

in good grades (1–3) that demonstrate 86% return to independent functioning.[31] Further improvement in outcomes is expected as the technological advancements in endovascular treatments continue.

The diagnosis of SAH should begin with radiographic analysis. Noncontrast CT remains the initial test of choice, with a sensitivity of 98–100% in the first 12 hours following SAH. Sensitivity declines with time, and falls to 93% at 24 hours and to as low as 57% at 6 days after the event.[21] CTA may be helpful in identification of aneurysm and is highly sensitive for aneurysms larger than 5 mm; however, sensitivity is low in detecting smaller aneurysms. Magnetic resonance angiography (MRA) is also a helpful tool in identifying cerebral aneurysm, but again sensitivity is limited and is highest for aneurysms of >5 mm in diameter.

For these reasons, the gold standard used to rule out SAH in patients with suspected SAH and a nondiagnostic, noncontrast CT remains the lumbar puncture. The sensitivity of this test, when properly performed and interpreted, approaches 100% with a 99% negative predictive value. Tubes 1 and 4 should be sent for a cell count, and >400 red blood cells (RBC) (which does not decrease from tube 1 to tube 4) and an elevated opening pressure are suggestive of SAH. Finding xanthochromia is diagnostic of this disorder; however, it may take up to 12 hours for RBCs to lyse sufficiently to produce this finding. There is evidence to support the use of visual inspection to make this diagnosis and suggests that spectrophotometry is not necessary to safely exclude SAH.[32]

TREATMENT OF ANEURYSMAL SUBARACHNOID HEMORRHAGE

The object of aneurysmal SAH treatment is to prevent rerupture of the aneurysm. Early treatment (within 48 hours) is recommended to prevent the 67% mortality rate associated with rebleeding.[21] There is a 3–4% risk of rebleeding in the first 24 hours and 2% risk in the second day. Each subsequent day carries a 0.3% risk and 15–20% risk in the first weeks. If left untreated, there is a 50% risk of rerupture in the first 6 months.[33] Securing an aneurysm may be performed either by open microsurgical technique (clipping) or via endovascular technique (coiling) (Figure 27-4). The international subarachnoid aneurysm trial (ISAT) randomized 2,143 spontaneous SAH patients to clipping versus coiling within 28 days of SAH ictus. Although the randomization process is heavily criticized, at 1 year there was a 24% major disability or death in the endovascular group versus 31% in the surgical group ($P = .0019$). At the 7-year follow-up, the mortality was significantly higher in the surgically treated group ($P = .03$), and seizure rates were higher as well. The early rebleeding risk was higher with the

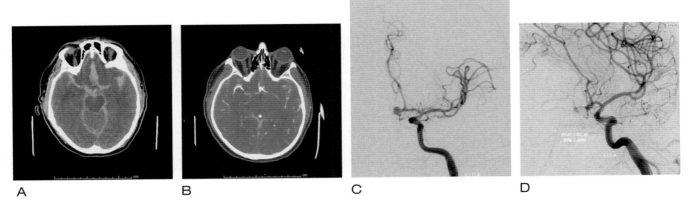

A   B   C   D

Figure 27–4. (A–D) CT scan demonstrates diffuse subarachnoid hemorrhage. CTA demonstrates a left anterior communicating artery aneurysm pointing right and upward. This is confirmed on cerebral angiography. Postaneurysm coil embolization angiogram is demonstrated. Note the lack of filling within the aneurysm.

endovascular group at the 30-day follow-up, but at 7 years it was similar in both groups.[33,34] The optimal method of treatment remains individualized for each patient depending on aneurysm morphology, location, and patient characteristics.

MEDICAL MANAGEMENT OF SUBARACHNOID HEMORRHAGE

Patients requiring airway or ventilatory support should be managed as in the prior discussion of patients with ICH. All patients with SAH are best served by admission to an NICU preferably in a facility with access to experts in neurovascular interventional care. Management of patients with SAH should be set with the goals to prevent rebleeding and to limit vasospasm in the cerebral circulation.

BP should be maintained at normal levels in these patients until the ruptured aneurysm is secured (coiled or clipped). Appropriate analgesia may assist in this endeavor. Antiemetics are indicated to prevent vomiting and subsequent increases in ICP. As in ICH, hyperglycemia and hyperthermia may worsen outcome and should be avoided.[21,36]

The second arm of medical treatment is an attempt to prevent vasospasm and subsequent decreased cerebral blood flow. Patients with vasospasm will present with new onset of focal neurologic deficits that may either resolve or continue on to permanent ischemic infarction. Up to 15% of patients with episodes of vasospasm post-SAH will either suffer a stroke or die from this process in spite of maximal therapy.[21] Oral nimodipine (60 mg every 4 hours) should be started as soon as possible once the diagnosis is obtained in an effort to prevent the development of this complication, and continued for 21 days. Early intervention is the key to preventing rebleeding and allowing for hypertensive/hypervolemic therapy in the setting of arterial vasospasm. Symptomatic vasospasm occurs in 20–40% of patients with aneurysmal SAH within days 5–21. Cerebral ischemia or infarction results from symptomatic vasospasm. Risk factors include poor grade, thick blood on CT, sentinel bleed, fever, early angiographic spasm, volume depletion, low cardiac output, and smoking. Endovascular treatment of vasospasm can reverse symptoms of delayed ischemia. Treatment may consist of intra-arterial medication delivery (verapamil, milrinone, among others) and/or angioplasty, and treatment within 2 hours of symptom onset is ideal.

Finally, patients with SAH are at risk for other complications, including seizure, DVT, hydrocephalus, and hyponatremia. Compression stockings and intermittent compression devices should be used to prevent the development of DVT. Subcutaneous administration of anticoagulants may be used once the aneurysm is safely secured (clipped or coiled). Prophylactic use of anticonvulsants remains controversial but may be considered.[21] Seizures should be managed as with seizures from any cause, first with lorazepam or another benzodiazepine followed by anticonvulsants such as phenytoin or fosphenytoin.[36] External ventricular drains should be placed in patients with hydrocephalus or evidence of increased ICP (i.e., Cushing's triad or decreased sensorium with hydrocephalus seen on CT). Prior to securing the aneurysm, the ICP should be kept at the high end of normal (20 mm Hg CSF). The theory is to reduce the transdome pressure in an effort to reduce the rerupture rate. Once the aneurysm is secured, the drain may be kept open to a level of 10 mm Hg CSF. Finally, hyponatremia occurs in between 10% and 30% of all patients with SAH. It was originally suggested that this is a form of syndrome of inappropriate antidiuretic hormone (SIADH); however, fluid restriction and volume contraction have been shown to worsen outcome in this population. Cerebral salt wasting syndrome (CSW) is most often the cause and has been postulated to be related to alterations in brain natriuretic peptide (BNP) levels. CSW is differentiated from SIADH in that in CSW there is volume depletion with the loss of sodium as opposed to SIADH where there is normovolemia or hypervolemia. When urine output exceeds fluid input, the diagnosis of CSW should be considered. Current AHA/ASA guidelines are to maintain euvolemia, use isotonic fluids to maintain a normal fluid balance, use fludrocortisone acetate, and consider the use of 3% hypertonic saline to correct hyponatremia in these patients.[21] Caution is advised not to correct hyponatremia too quickly as to cause central pontine myelinolysis; however, this is rare in patients with hyponatremia less than 24 hours' duration. This is avoided by not exceeding 8 mEq/24 hours in the chronically hyponatremic patient.

REFERENCES

1. Broderick J, Connolly S, Feldmann E, et al. Guidelines for the management of spontaneous intracerebral hemorrhage in adults: 2007 update: a guideline from the American Heart Association/American Stroke Association Stroke Council, High Blood Pressure Research Council, and the Quality of Care and Outcomes in Research Interdisciplinary Working Group. *Stroke.* 2007;38:2001–2023.

2. Ariesen MJ, Claus SP, Rinkel JGE et al. Risk factors for intracerebral hemorrhage in the general population: a systematic review. *Stroke.* 2003;34:2060–2065.

3. Wojak JC, Flamm ES. Intracranial hemorrhage and cocaine use. *Stroke.* 1987;18:712–715.

4. Buxton N, McConachie NS. Amphetamine abuse and intracranial haemorrhage. *J R Soc Med.* 2000;93:472–477.

5. Gorelick PB, Weisman SM. Risk of hemorrhagic stroke with aspirin use: an update. *Stroke.* 2005;36;1801–1807.

6. Steiner T, Rosand J, Diringer M. Intracerebral hemorrhage associated with oral anticoagulant therapy: current practices and unresolved questions. *Stroke.* 2006;37;256–262.

7. Robinson M, Clancy N. In patients with head injury undergoing rapid sequence intubation, does pretreatment with intravenous lingocaine/lidocaine lead to an improved neurological outcome? A review of the literature. *Emerg Med J.* 2001;18:453–457.

8. Rincon F, Mayer SA. Clinical review: critical care management of spontaneous intracerebral hemorrhage. *Crit Care.* 2008;12:237–251.

9. Clancy M, Halford S, Walls R, et al. In patients with head injuries undergoing rapid sequence intubation using succinylcholine, does pretreatment with a competitive neuromuscular blocking agent improve outcome? A literature review. *Emerg Med J.* 2001;18:373–375.

10. Georgiadis D, Schwarz S, Baumgartner RW, et al. Influence of positive end-expiratory pressure on intracranial pressure and cerebral perfusion pressure in patients with acute stroke. *Stroke.* 2001;32;2088–2092.

11. Anderson CS, Huang Y, Wang JG, et al. Intensive blood pressure reduction in acute cerebral haemorrhage trial (INTERACT): a randomized pilot trial. *Lancet Neurol.* 2008;7:391–399.

12. Quereshi AI. Antihypertensive treatment of acute cerebral haemorrhage (ATACH): rationale and design. *Neurocrit Care.* 2007;6:56–66. Results presented at International Stroke Conference, New Orleans, February 2008.

13. Morgenstern LB, Hemphill JC III, Anderson C, et al. Guidelines for the management of spontaneous intracerebral hemorrhage: a guideline for healthcare professionals from the American Heart Association/American Stroke Association. *Stroke.* 2010;41:2108–2129.

14. Adams HP Jr, Adams RJ, Brott T, et al. Guidelines for the early management of patients with ischaemic stroke: A scientific statement from the Stroke Council of the American Stroke Association. *Stroke.* 2003;34:1056–1083.

15. Mayer SA, Brun NC, Begtrup K, et al. Recombinant activated factor VII for acute intracerebral hemorrhage. *N Engl J Med.* 2005;352:777–785.

16. Diringer MN, Edwards DF. Admission to a neurologic/neurosurgical intensive care unit is associated with reduced mortality rate after intracerebral hemorrhage. *Crit Care Med.* 2001;29:635–640.

17. Oddo M, Schmidt JM, Carrera E, et al. Impact of tight glycemic control on cerebral glucose metabolism after severe brain injury: a microdialysis study. *Crit Care Med.* 2008;36:3233–3238.

18. Mendelow AD, Gregson BA, Fernandes HM, et al. Early surgery versus initial conservative treatment in patients with spontaneous supratentorial intracerebral haematomas in the International Surgical Trial in Intracerebral Haemorrhage (STICH): a randomised trial. *Lancet.* 2005;365:387–396.

19. Zahuranec DB, Brown DL, Lisabeth LD, et al. Early care limitations independently predict mortality after intracerebral hemorrhage. *Neurology.* 2007;68:1651–1657.

20. Zurasky JA, Aiyagari V, Zazulia AV, et al. Early mortality following spontaneous intracerebral hemorrhage. *Neurology.* 2005;64:725–727.

21. Bederson JB, Connolly ES Jr, Batjer HH, et al. Guidelines for the management of aneurysmal subarachnoid hemorrhage: a statement for healthcare professionals from a special writing group of the Stroke Council, American Heart Association. *Stroke.* 209;40:994–1025.

22. Edlow JE. Diagnosis of subarachnoid hemorrhage. Are we doing better? *Stroke.* 2007;38:1129–1131.

23. Feigin VL, Rinkel GJE, Lawes CM, et al. Risk factors for subarachnoid hemorrhage: an updated systematic review of epidemiological studies. *Stroke.* 2005;36:2773–2780.

24. Schievink WI, Torres VE, Piepgras DG, et al. Saccular intracranial aneurysms in autosomal dominant polycystic kidney disease. *J Am Soc Nephrol.* 1992;3:88–95.

25. Schievink WI, Limburg M, Oorthuis JW, et al. Cerebrovascular disease in Ehlers–Danlos syndrome type IV. *Stroke.* 1990;21:626–632.

26. Bederson JB, Awad IA, Wiebers DO, et al. Recommendations for the management of patients with unruptured intracranial aneurysms: a statement for healthcare professionals from the Stroke Council of the American Heart Association. *Stroke*. 2000;31:2742–2750.

27. Vermeulen MJ, Schull MJ. Missed diagnosis of subarachnoid hemorrhage in the emergency department. *Stroke*. 2007;38:1216–1221.

28. Kowalski RG, Claassen J, Kreiter KT, et al. Initial misdiagnosis and outcome after subarachnoid hemorrhage. *JAMA*. 2004;291:866–869.

29. Hunt WE, Hess RM. Surgical risk as related to time of intervention in the repair of intracranial aneurysms. *J Neurosurg*. 1968;28:14–20.

30. Longstreth WT Jr, Nelson LM, Koepsell TD, et al. Clinical course of spontaneous subarachnoid hemorrhage: a population-based study in King County, Washington. *Neurology*. 1993;43:712–718.

31. Le Roux PD, Elliot JP, Downey L, et al. Improved outcome after rupture of anterior circulation aneurysms: a retrospective 10-year review of 224 good-grade patients. *J Neurosurg*. 1995;83:394–402.

32. Dupont SA, Wijdicks EF, Manno EM, et al. Thunderclap headache and normal computed tomographic results: value of cerebrospinal fluid analysis. *Mayo Clin Proc*. 2008;83(12):1326–1331.

33. Naidech AM, Janjua N, Kreiter KT, et al. Predictors and impact of aneurysm rebleeding after subarachnoid hemorrhage. *Arch Neurol*. 2005;62:410–416.

34. Molyneux AJ, Kerr RS, Stratton I, et al. International subarachnoid aneurysm trial (ISAT) of neurosurgical clipping versus endovascular coiling in 2143 patients with ruptured intracranial aneurysms: a randomized trial. *Lancet*. 2002;360(9342):1267–1274.

35. Molyneux AJ, Kerr RS, Stratton I, et al. International subarachnoid aneurysm trial (ISAT) of neurosurgical clipping versus endovascular coiling in 2143 patients with ruptured intracranial aneurysms: a randomized comparison of effects on survival, dependency, seizures, rebleeding, subgroups, and aneurysm occlusion. *Lancet*. 2005;366(9488):809–817.

36. Suarez JI, Tarr RW, Selman WR, et al. Aneurysmal subarachnoid hemorrhage. *N Engl J Med*. 2006;354:387–396.

CHAPTER 28

Traumatic Brain Injury and Spinal Cord Injury

Jason A. Ellis, Kiwon Lee, and Dorothea Altschul

▶ INTRODUCTION

Traumatic brain injury (TBI) and traumatic spinal cord injury (TSI) represent pathologies that result from a diverse spectrum of primary insults to the central nervous system (CNS). Nearly 2 million cases of neurotrauma, including both TBI and TSI, occur annually in the United States making it an important public health issue.[1-3] In addition to the long-term physical disabilities and the psychosocial impairments seen in neurotrauma survivors, the economic burden of TBI and TSI is significant. The cost of TBI in the United States is estimated to be somewhere between $40 and $200 billion.[3-6] For TSI, it is estimated that the lifetime total cost directly attributable to spinal cord injury in a 25-year-old patient may exceed $3 million.[2]

Advancements in our understanding of the pathophysiology of CNS injury post-trauma have led to improvements in the critical care of patients with TBI and TSI. Indeed, the development of standardized guidelines for aggressive medical and surgical management of these patients has been credited for helping to improve outcomes.[7,8] For severely brain- and/ or spinal cord–injured patients, it is crucial that a multidisciplinary approach be taken from the outset. The foremost principle guiding the management of TBI and TSI patients is to minimize the secondary neural injury that inevitably follows a primary CNS insult. Appropriate and timely emergency stabilization, critical care management, and surgical interventions are essential for delaying the progression of secondary CNS injury. Toward this end, the clinician treating TBI and TSI patients must be able to assess, monitor, and treat the multitude of physiologic derangements that result from and also facilitate CNS injury. In this chapter, we review the epidemiology, pathophysiology, and critical care management of TBI and TSI patients. As neurosurgical intervention—whether at the bedside or in the operating room—is generally necessary for TBI and TSI patients, the surgical indications for pathology encountered in the emergency and critical care setting will also be reviewed.

▶ EPIDEMIOLOGY

TRAUMATIC BRAIN INJURY

The Centers for Disease Control and Prevention (CDC) estimates that 1.7 million people sustain TBI annually.[1] Of this total, approximately 52,000 die, 275,000 are hospitalized, and 1.365 million are treated and released from an emergency department. However, the actual number of TBI cases is uncertain as many patients either receive care in the field or do not seek medical attention at all. The causes of TBI in all age groups combined are: falls in 35.2%, motor vehicle accident in 17.3%, being struck in 16.5%, assault in 10%, and other or unknown causes in 21%. Among all age groups, males have higher incidences of TBI and on average present with TBI about 1.4 times more frequently than females. The CDC identified three age groups—children aged 0–4 years, adolescents aged 15–19 years, and adults aged 65 years and older—as most likely to sustain TBI. Children aged 0–4 years had the highest rate of TBI-related emergency department visits (1,256 per 100,000 population) while hospitalization (339 per 100,000 population) and death (57 per 100,000 population) rates were highest among those 75 years and older. TBI-related death rates have substantially declined in the past 30 years and can mostly be attributed to primary prevention. Motor vehicle–related TBI deaths declined 22% and firearm-related TBI deaths declined 14% between 1989 and 1998.[9] Recent data indicate more modest declines or relative stability in TBI mortality trends.[1,10]

TRAUMATIC SPINAL CORD INJURY

The National Spinal Cord Injury Statistical Center (NSCISC) collects and dispenses the most comprehensive epidemiologic data on spinal cord injury in the United States. They estimate the annual incidence of spinal cord injury at 40 cases per million population, representing about 12,000 new cases each year in the United States.[2,11] About 80% of these injuries occur in males. The most common causes of spinal cord injury include motor vehicle accident in 41.3%, fall in 27.3%, and violence in 15%. Cervical spinal cord injuries are the most common comprising over 50% of lesions within the NSCISC database, followed by thoracic, lumbar, and sacral lesions. Among all levels of injury, cervical lesions confer the worst prognosis with ventilator dependency having a strong negative association with survival. Death in spinal cord–injured patients most commonly results from respiratory infections and septicemia associated with urinary infections and decubitus ulcers.

▶ PATHOPHYSIOLOGY

An appreciation for the pathophysiologic mechanisms at work after TBI and TSI is important for the development and implementation of effective clinical therapeutic strategies. Although typically treated separately, the pathophysiologies of both TBI and TSI have a number of similarities. Most notably, the injury due to both TBI and TSI can be understood in terms of primary and secondary insults to neural tissue. Primary injury denotes the initial mechanical damage secondary to energy transmission during impact while secondary injury results from the destructive tissue-intrinsic and body systemic response to primary injury. The critical care of TBI and TSI patients is directed at minimizing secondary injury. Detailed accounts of the molecular and cellular mechanisms of TBI and TSI have been given.[12–15] Here we present a concise review of the pathophysiology of TBI and TSI with emphasis on delineating pathologic processes that are routinely targeted clinically.

BLOOD FLOW

Both TBI and TSI are associated with focal and/or global hypoperfusion to the brain and spinal cord, respectively.[13,14,16,17] Hypoperfusion can result from a number of mechanisms including microvascular or macrovascular damage, vasospasm, neurogenic/spinal shock, loss of autoregulation, or mechanical tissue disruption. Decreased blood flow to neural tissue results in ischemia and ultimately infarction as cellular metabolic demands exhaust available resources. For these reasons, it is unsurprising that reductions in cerebral blood flow (CBF) and hypotension portend a worse prognosis for TBI patients.[18–23] The evidence suggests this may be true in TSI patients as well; however, further studies are warranted.[24,25]

Paradoxically, focally increased blood flow resulting in hyperemia may also result from acute injury to neural tissue. Hyperemia is similarly as deleterious to the injured brain and spinal cord as is hypoperfusion. Mechanistically, both processes result in a mismatch between blood flow and cellular metabolism. Additionally, by facilitating oxidative damage to cells, promoting tissue edema, and increasing intracranial pressure (ICP), hyperemia further promotes secondary injury in the acute setting.[12–14]

METABOLISM

Metabolic dysfunction results after TBI and TSI due to impaired delivery and/or utilization of oxygen and glucose within the injured brain and spinal cord.[12–14] As neural cells depend on the production of high-energy molecules from aerobic metabolism to meet their energy requirements, even modest reductions in oxygen and glucose are poorly tolerated.[12,26] The ionic fluxes associated with primary cellular injury result in the initiation of energy-dependent processes such as membrane transport in an attempt to restore homeostasis. As energy stores become depleted, especially within the ischemic penumbra, cell death occurs.[12]

INFLAMMATION

The robust inflammatory reaction seen within the damaged brain and spinal cord is a major component of both negative secondary injury processes and positive, reparative processes.[12–14,26] At the site of injury, leukocyte recruitment and concurrent expression of inflammatory mediators such as TNF-α, interleukins, and complement molecules promote vascular permeability, edema, and progressive tissue damage. Inhibition of this cytotoxic inflammatory milieu is a major target for the development of neuroprotective therapies.

EXCITOTOXICITY

TBI and TSI are associated with excessive release of excitatory neurotransmitters such as glutamate in response to hypoxia.[12–14,26] This in turn results in major ionic flux involving sodium, potassium, and calcium across cell membranes. The accumulation of intracellular calcium in particular is associated with many toxic processes such as lipase and peroxidase activation as well as free radical generation.

▶ ETIOLOGIES OF INJURY

TBI can be caused by a number of mechanisms that involve deforming brain tissue at various strain rates. This may range from the relatively low strain rates imparted during simple collision to the higher rates associated with ballistic and blast mechanisms. Injuries can be divided into two main categories—open (including penetrating) and closed head injuries. Open head injuries involve violation of the skull and can result from foreign body (i.e., bullet, arrow, knife) entry or direct blunt force (i.e., blow from baseball bat). Closed head injury is most often caused by direct blunt force; however, primary blast– or shock wave–induced injuries are becoming increasingly prevalent in the military theater.

▶ INITIAL ASSESSMENT AND CLASSIFICATION

The initial assessment of neurotrauma patients should begin with the familiar ABCs: evaluate the airway, confirm breathing with effective ventilation, and assess the circulatory status. Cervical hard collar placement and body immobilization on a rigid backboard is warranted for all trauma patients.[27] Clinically deteriorating patients and those with a Glasgow Coma Scale (GCS) score of 8 or less should be intubated as they are unable to adequately protect their airway. Precautions such as logrolling and inline stabilization during intubation are prudent until spinal stability is verified.[27] Cardiac, hemodynamic, respiratory, and pulse oximetry monitoring is necessary for all patients with moderate and severe TBI (see below) as well as in all TSI patients.[16,17,28] Hypoxemia (SaO_2 <90%) and hypotension (systolic blood pressure <90 mm Hg) should be avoided in both TBI and TSI patients. TBI outcomes have clearly been shown to be worse if hypoxia or hypotension is present, and the available evidence suggests that the same holds true for TSI.[16,17,24,28] Intubation, volume resuscitation with intravenous fluids or transfusion, and the use of vasopressor medications may be necessary to achieve these initial goals.

Visual inspection of the general physical condition of the patient should be carried out. Evidence of basal skull fracture (periorbital or postauricular ecchymoses, cerebrospinal fluid [CSF] rhinorrhea/otorrhea), facial fracture, or spine deformity should be noted. At a minimum, the initial neurologic examination should encompass assessment of the following: (1) level of consciousness with a determination of the GCS (Table 28-1), (2) cranial nerve (CN) function with particular attention to the size, symmetry, and reactivity of pupils, and (3) gross motor and sensory examination of the extremities. In cases of suspected spinal cord injury, a more detailed motor exam and determination of a specific sensory level is appropriate. Additionally, a digital rectal exam checking for voluntary anal sphincter contraction should be performed and an American Spinal Injury Association (ASIA) impairment scale grade (see below) should be assigned.[29]

While in the acute period, all patients with TBI should be neurologically examined on a regular basis—at least every hour for the first 24 hours (hyperacute period) and then less often as clinically indicated. In general, cerebral edema is greatest from 48 to 96 hours following injury. Thereafter, edema resolution ensues with most patients showing some measure of clinical improvement.

▶ **TABLE 28-1. GLASGOW COMA SCALE**

Points	Eye Opening	Verbal Response	Motor Response
6	—	—	Obeys commands
5	—	Oriented	Localizes to pain
4	Spontaneous	Confused	Withdraws to pain
3	To speech	Inappropriate	Flexor posturing
2	To pain	Incomprehensible	Extensor posturing
1	None	None	None

CLINICAL SEVERITY OF BRAIN INJURY

Patients with a GCS of 8 or less are considered to have severe TBI and will require advanced medical care in the prehospital setting as well as neurocritical care management. Severe TBI is associated with significant neurologic injury often with structural lesions revealed by neuroimaging (e.g., head computed tomography [CT] scan revealing skull fracture, intracranial hemorrhage, and early diffuse cerebral edema). After initial resuscitation and stabilization in the field, patients with severe TBI should be evacuated to the nearest Level 1 trauma center with neurosurgical capability. Patients presenting with moderate TBI (GCS 9–12) should also be treated in the critical care setting while those with mild TBI (GCS 13–15) may or may not require hospital admission.[30–33]

It should be noted that in addition to the GCS parameter, mild TBI is formally defined as the presence of loss of consciousness for 30 minutes or less, post-traumatic amnesia not greater than 24 hours, any alteration in mental status at the time of injury, or focal neurologic deficit.[34] In clinical practice, concussion and mild TBI are often used interchangeably; however, the terms are subtly distinct if only because they were independently defined by different expert panels. The American Academy of Neurology (AAN) defines concussion as a trauma-induced alteration in mental status with confusion and amnesia being the hallmarks.[35] As the GCS does not provide enough detail to give a useful clinical picture in cases of mild TBI or concussion, a variety of scales have been developed (Table 28-2).[35,36]

A great deal of clinicopathologic heterogeneity exists in head injury classifications and so physician judgment taking into account the entire clinical picture as well as neuroimaging findings is paramount.[37] While the classifications and grading scales developed by expert consensus are clinically useful, their use is typically not supported by class I evidence.[32]

▶ **TABLE 28-2. CANTU AND AMERICAN ACADEMY OF NEUROLOGY (AAN) CONCUSSION GRADING SCALES**

Grade	Cantu	AAN
1	a. No LOC b. PTA <30 min	a. No LOC b. Transient confusion c. Symptom resolution in <15 min
2	a. LOC <5 min b. PTA >30 min (<24 h)	a. No LOC b. Transient confusion c. Persistent symptoms >15 min
3	a. LOC >5 min b. PTA >24 h	a. Any LOC

LOC, loss of consciousness; PTA, post-traumatic amnesia.

▶ **TABLE 28-3. AMERICAN SPINAL INJURY ASSOCIATION (ASIA) IMPAIRMENT SCALE**

Grade	Features
A	Complete injury. No motor or sensory function below lesion level
B	Incomplete injury. Sensory but not motor function preserved below lesion level
C	Incomplete injury. Muscle grade less than 3 in more than half of key muscles below lesion level
D	Incomplete injury. Muscle grade 3 or more in more than half of key muscles below lesion level
E	Normal function

SPINAL CORD INJURY SYNDROMES

Spinal cord injuries may be categorized as either complete or incomplete (Table 28-3). Both categories of acute spinal cord injury require patients to be monitored and treated in a critical care setting.[17]

A complete spinal cord injury (ASIA A) results in loss of all motor and sensory function at or just caudal to the cord lesion level. Acutely, spinal shock with flaccid paralysis, areflexia, and autonomic dysfunction is seen below the lesion level.[38,39] For cervical lesions, this may result in bradyarrhythmias, conduction block, and hypotension due to disrupted sympathetic outflow. Although this clinical picture represents a spinal cord transection syndrome, an actual anatomic transection is rare.[38]

In contrast to complete injury, incomplete spinal cord injuries (ASIA B–D) are associated with varying levels of motor and sensory preservation. Several incomplete spinal cord injury syndromes have been described and include the following:

1. Central cord syndrome: This syndrome presents with upper greater than lower extremity weakness, urinary dysfunction, and varying degrees of sensory disturbance. It is thought to result from a cervical hyperextension injury in the setting of cervical spondylosis.

2. Brown-Séquard syndrome: Penetrating trauma resulting in spinal cord hemisection is the usual cause of this syndrome. The clinical findings of Brown-Séquard syndrome include: (1) ipsilateral motor paralysis and loss of posterior column function (proprioception and vibratory sense) below the lesion and (2) contralateral dissociated sensory loss with loss of pain and temperature but preserved light touch sensation.

3. Anterior cord syndrome: Cord infarction in the territory of the anterior spinal artery causes this syndrome. Traumatic etiologies such as disc

herniation or retropulsion of a vertebral body fragment may result in occlusion of the anterior spinal artery causing paralysis below the lesion level and bilateral dissociated sensory loss (pain and temperature sensation) with sparing of position sense.

4. Conus medullaris syndrome: This syndrome affects the most caudal region of the spinal cord and presents with bladder and anal sphincter dysfunction, impotence, and saddle anesthesia. Lower extremity motor weakness may be limited. Conus medullaris syndrome must be distinguished from cauda equina syndrome, which affects lumbosacral nerve roots rather than the spinal cord. Pain and lower extremity weakness are more prominent in cauda equina syndrome.

5. Posterior cord syndrome: This syndrome is poorly defined and uncommonly seen in TSI. Lesions causing this syndrome damage the dorsal columns causing reduced proprioception, paresthesias, and dysesthetic (burning) pain. Alternate descriptions include additional corticospinal tract involvement producing weakness below the lesion.

▶ RADIOGRAPHIC EVALUATION

HEAD INJURY IMAGING

A noncontrast head CT should be the initial imaging modality used to evaluate TBI patients. Although criteria have been developed to help identify TBI patients who require head CT,[40,41] its liberal use appears justifiable in even mild cases to rule out pathology requiring immediate surgical intervention.[32,42] The Marshall CT classification that segregates diffuse brain injury into several categories is often a helpful prognostic guide (Table 28-4).[43] Conventional catheter cerebral and cervical angiography should be performed in cases of penetrating brain injury when breach of a major vessel is suspected. Brain magnetic resonance imaging (MRI) is generally not indicated in the acute setting.

SPINAL CORD INJURY IMAGING

In patients with evidence of spinal cord injury, a CT scan of the entire spine should be performed to evaluate known spinal lesions and to rule out additional, noncontiguous vertebral injuries.[24] An MRI of the known or suspected area of spinal cord injury should also be performed. MRI is superior to CT for the detection of traumatic intervertebral disc herniation, spinal ligament disruption, and epidural hematoma (EDH).

CERVICAL SPINE CLEARANCE

Cervical spine injury is found in association with TBI in 2–6% of patients. Thus, cervical spine immobilization with a hard collar should be continued in all trauma patients until either clinical or radiographic clearance can be accomplished.[44,45] Initial spine imaging in both obtunded and awake symptomatic patients should include cervical spine x-rays in three views (anteroposterior [AP], lateral, odontoid) with clear visualization from the craniocervical junction to the C7–T1 junction. Any x-ray abnormalities should be followed up with cervical spine CT. If cervical radiographs and CT are unrevealing, either dynamic flexion–extension x-ray (fluoroscopy for obtunded patients) or cervical spine MRI within 48 hours of injury is required for clearance.

▶ SURGICAL INDICATIONS

The initial management of TBI and TSI patients aims to both stabilize and identify pathology requiring emergent surgical intervention. A working knowledge of the surgical indications for the most commonly seen neurosurgical pathology in this population is therefore

---

▶ TABLE 28-4. **MARSHALL CLASSIFICATION OF DIFFUSE BRAIN INJURY**

Category	Features on Noncontrast Head CT	Outcome at Discharge[a]
Diffuse injury I	a. No pathology	27% good 34.6% moderate
Diffuse injury II	a. Midline shift 0–5 mm with visible basal cisterns b. No high or mixed density lesion >25 cm³	8.5% good 26% moderate
Diffuse injury III	a. Midline shift 0–5 mm with cisterns compressed or absent b. No high or mixed density lesion >25 cm³	3.3% good 3.1% moderate
Diffuse injury IV	a. Midline shift >5 mm b. No high or mixed density lesion >25 cm³	3.1% good 3.1% moderate

[a]Data from Marshall L, Marshall S, Klauber M, et al. A new classification of head injury based on computerized tomography. *J Neurosurg.* 1991;75(suppl):S14–S20.

essential for any physician caring for TBI and TSI patients. Through the combined efforts of the Brain Trauma Foundation and the Congress of Neurological Surgeons, evidence-based recommendations were codified in the *Guidelines for the Surgical Management of Traumatic Brain Injury*.[46] The specific intracranial traumatic lesions and the indications for surgery are outlined below. As the indications for emergency surgery in TSI patients are not well defined, only a brief discussion will be given. It is important to keep in mind that guidelines only provide recommendations for patients meeting specific criteria. Thus, clinical judgment must also guide management in each unique scenario.

EPIDURAL HEMATOMA

An acute EDH with a volume greater than 30 mL should be evacuated regardless of the patient's GCS score. In patients with GCS less than 9, pupillary abnormalities, or other focal neurologic deficits, a craniotomy for evacuation should occur as soon as possible. An EDH with volume less than 30 mL, thickness less than 15 mm, and midline shift less than 5 mm in a patient with GCS greater than 8 and no focal deficits may be managed nonoperatively with serial head CT and close observation.[47]

SUBDURAL HEMATOMA

An acute subdural hematoma (SDH) with thickness greater than 10 mm or midline shift greater than 5 mm should be evacuated regardless of the patient's GCS score. If the patient is comatose (GCS <9) and has pupillary abnormality or ICP >20 mm Hg or had a clinical decline by 2 or more GCS points, hematoma evacuation as soon as possible is also indicated.[48]

PARENCHYMAL LESIONS

Traumatic parenchymal lesions include both focal and nonfocal lesions. The focal lesions occur at the site of impact (coup) or opposite the site of impact (contrecoup) and include intracerebral hematoma (ICH), contusion, and infarction. Nonfocal lesions include diffuse injury typically resulting in hemispheric or global cerebral edema. Patients with traumatic parenchymal mass lesions causing neurologic deterioration, refractory intracranial hypertension, or evidence of mass effect on CT should be treated surgically. Similarly, any lesion greater than 50 mL should be evacuated. In patients with GCS 6–8, a lesion greater than 20 mL should be evacuated if it is frontal or temporal in location and causing more than 5 mm of midline shift and/or cisternal compression.[49] Contusions commonly affecting the orbitofrontal and anterior temporal lobes must be observed with particular vigilance. Delayed hematomas that can manifest or "blossom" within hours to days may require urgent craniectomy (Figure 28-1).

POSTERIOR FOSSA MASS LESIONS

A traumatic posterior fossa mass lesion should be evacuated by suboccipital craniectomy if there is radiographic evidence of mass effect or if neurologic dysfunction is referable to the lesion. As neurologic decline can be precipitous in patients with these lesions, surgery should be performed as soon as possible.[50]

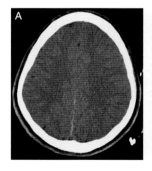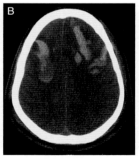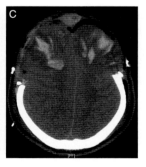

Figure 28–1. Intracerebral hematoma expansion within bifrontal contusions. This 27-year-old male patient presented with a GCS score of 3 after being ejected head first from a motorcycle during a collision. Initial noncontrast head CT was significant for bilateral frontal lobe contusions with early evidence of sulcal effacement (A). A follow-up noncontrast head CT performed 9 hours after initial presentation showed the interval development of large bilateral intraparenchymal hemorrhages (B). The patient subsequently developed refractory intracranial hypertension necessitating performance of a bilateral frontotemporal craniectomy with duraplasty for ICP control (C).

DEPRESSED CRANIAL FRACTURES

Closed (simple) nondepressed, typically linear, cranial fractures are not surgical lesions unless associated with an intracranial mass. On the other hand, depressed cranial fractures may be managed either surgically or nonsurgically depending on the particular case. Patients with open (compound) cranial fractures depressed greater than the thickness of the cranium should undergo early elevation of the bone fragments and debridement of the wound. Open cranial fractures with depression less than 1 cm and no dural penetration, significant intracranial hematoma, frontal sinus involvement, gross deformity, wound infection, pneumocephalus, or gross wound contamination may be treated nonoperatively. Although not rigorously supported in the literature, closed depressed cranial fractures are often surgically treated if the extent of depression is greater than the thickness of the adjacent calvarium to effect better cosmesis and lower rates of post-traumatic seizure (PTS) and neurologic deficit. Nonoperative management, however, is a treatment option in these cases.[51]

PENETRATING BRAIN INJURY

Penetrating brain injury involves both missile and nonmissile trauma to the brain. No strict guidelines dictate when surgical debridement, hematoma evacuation, and/or removal of protruding foreign body are warranted. In one study of gunshot wounds to the head, it was suggested that all patients with GCS 9–15 should have aggressive surgical therapy; patients with GCS 6–8 should have surgical therapy if no transventricular, multilobar, or dominant hemisphere injury is present; and patients with GCS 3–5 should have surgical therapy only if a large extra-axial hematoma is present.[52]

SPINAL DECOMPRESSION AND STABILIZATION

There are no well-defined indications for emergency decompression and stabilization in TSI patients.[53,54] While animal studies suggest that early decompression is beneficial, the available human studies do not consistently indicate improved neurologic outcomes. A recent systematic review concluded that urgent decompression in patients experiencing neurologic deterioration, with bilateral locked facets in the setting of incomplete tetraplegia, or cervical cord injury may be appropriate.[55] However, further studies are warranted to clarify the role of emergent surgical intervention in TSI patients.

▶ INTENSIVE CARE MEASURES

No discrete segregation exists between the emergency care, the surgical care, and the critical care of neurotrauma patients. The intensive care management of TBI and TSI patients begins in the field with first responders and continues until the patient is stable for intensive care unit (ICU) discharge. At all phases of care, the goal is to prevent additional primary injuries and to minimize the extent of secondary injury to the CNS. The recommendations set forth in the Brain Trauma Foundation's *Guidelines for the Management of Severe Traumatic Brain Injury*[7] and in the American Association of Neurological Surgeons/Congress of Neurological Surgeons Joint Section on Disorders of the Spine and Peripheral Nerves' *Guidelines for the Management of Acute Cervical Spine and Spinal Cord Injuries*[56] are invaluable resources detailing medical management. Additional guidelines have been released in an attempt to optimize prehospital, combat-related, and neurosurgical care. These include the *Guidelines for Prehospital Management of Traumatic Brain Injury*,[57] the *Guidelines for the Field Management of Combat-Related Head Trauma*,[58] and the previously mentioned *Guidelines for the Surgical Management of Traumatic Brain Injury*.[46]

BLOOD PRESSURE AND OXYGENATION

As already emphasized in the section "Initial Assessment and Classification," both hypotension (systolic blood pressure <90 mm Hg) and hypoxia (SaO_2 <90% or PaO_2 <60 mm Hg) should be avoided.[28] As an additional measure to improve spinal cord perfusion in TSI patients, it is recommended that a mean arterial pressure (MAP) of 85–90 mm Hg be maintained for 7 days after the injury.[16] At a minimum arterial and central venous pressure (CVP), line placement is usually done in neurotrauma patients. Swan–Ganz catheter placement or use of arterial catheter device monitors is also helpful for hemodynamic optimization.

INTRACRANIAL PRESSURE MONITORING

A number of devices are available for ICP monitoring. Intraventricular devices provide the most accurate and reliable measurements of ICP and also allow for therapeutic drainage of CSF. However, in the setting of global cerebral edema with collapse of the lateral ventricles, ventriculostomy may not be possible. Parenchymal ICP monitors are also accurate and useful when ventriculostomy is not possible but their inability to effect CSF diversion makes them less ideal. Subarachnoid, subdural, and epidural ICP monitors are the least favored devices.[59]

ICP monitoring is often initiated in all salvageable severe TBI (GCS 3–8) patients and in select patients with GCS >8 whose neurologic exam cannot be followed. The guidelines recommend ICP monitoring in salvageable severe TBI patients with: (1) an abnormal head CT or (2) a normal head CT and two or more of the following—age over 40 years, motor posturing, and systolic blood pressure less than 90 mm Hg.[60]

CEREBRAL PERFUSION PRESSURE

Cerebral perfusion pressure (CPP) is defined as the difference between the MAP and the ICP. CPP maintenance is an important clinical parameter that can be used to prevent the reductions in CBF that are associated with poor outcome. While the literature points to no clear optimal CPP target, multiple studies suggest maintenance within the range of 50–70 mm Hg with a goal of 60 mm Hg for the severe TBI population.[61] Addressing CPP begins with placing an arterial line and providing fluid resuscitation to euvolemia. In order to increase the osmolar gradient between the systemic vasculature and the brain, hyperosmolar intravenous solutions should be used. Normal saline—which is hyperosmolar relative to blood—is commonly used. Another option is hypertonic saline, which is a useful adjunctive therapy in managing cerebral edema and intracranial hypertension (see below).

CONTROLLING INTRACRANIAL PRESSURE

Consensus recommendations based on class II evidence suggest that treatment for ICP should be initiated for values above 20 mm Hg.[62] Nonetheless, it is important to remember that herniation may occur at pressures below this value and so the entire clinical picture must be assessed. The methods below detail a fairly stepwise approach to the treatment of intracranial hypertension in neurotrauma patients. At all stages during the escalation of ICP-lowering therapy, a high suspicion for enlarging mass lesion must be entertained with a low threshold for obtaining a head CT.

1. General measures: The general measures used for decreasing ICP include ensuring neutral head position, elevating the head of bed (HOB), providing adequate sedation and analgesia, and avoiding fever. A neutral head position allows for unimpeded venous drainage out of the intracranial compartment, thus decreasing cerebral blood volume and ICP. Keeping the HOB elevated at 30–45° also enhances venous outflow. Agitation, discomfort, endotracheal tube–induced coughing, tensing the abdominal musculature, and elevated sympathetic tone all increase ICP. The use of adequate sedation and analgesia with agents such as propofol or midazolam is helpful with these issues.

   As fever is known to increase both the cerebral metabolic rate and ICP, maintenance of normothermia along with the prevention of shivering is important. Although TBI alone can induce a fever, this should be a diagnosis of exclusion. Febrile patients must be appropriately assessed for underlying infection with tests including complete blood count, chest x-ray, urinalysis, and cultures of blood and urine. Fever reduction can be achieved with acetaminophen, cooling blankets or vests, or intravascular devices. If a patient develops severe shivering, one should consider administering meperidine, buspirone, magnesium, or increasing sedation with or without pharmacologic paralysis.

2. CSF drainage: One of the major benefits to ICP monitoring with an intraventricular device is that it allows for CSF diversion. Unclamping the intraventricular catheter and draining 3–5 mL of CSF is one of the fastest and most effective methods of lowering ICP.

3. Hyperventilation: Hyperventilation reduces ICP by causing cerebral vasoconstriction. As CBF is also reduced by cerebral vasoconstriction, one must necessarily question the safety of hyperventilation in the setting of TBI. The only randomized controlled trial addressing this question found significantly worse outcomes at 6 months in a subgroup of patients hyperventilated to a $Paco_2$ of 25 mm Hg as compared with the control group ventilated to a $Paco_2$ of 35 mm Hg.[63] Based on this along with additional class III data, prophylactic hyperventilation is not recommended in TBI patients.[64] However, hyperventilation may be briefly used as a temporizing measure in an acute setting such as active or imminent herniation. The clinical response is very fast and lasts anywhere from a few minutes to hours. Efficacy subsequently wanes due to metabolic compensation within the CSF and brain tissue. When employed, efforts should be made to wean the patient from this type of therapy as soon as other interventions become effective.[65]

4. Osmotherapy: Mannitol is the most commonly used ICP-reducing osmotic agent in the setting of TBI. It is an osmotic diuretic that lowers ICP through both rheologic and osmotic

effects. Mannitol administration immediately expands plasma volume reducing blood viscosity, increasing CBF, and increasing cerebral oxygen delivery. More delayed osmotic effects dehydrate the intracellular and interstitial brain compartments pulling water intravascularly. Bolus administration at doses of 0.25–1 g/kg is effective.[66] In an effort to prevent renal toxicity, a cutoff serum osmolarity of 320 mOsm is often used. This value is somewhat arbitrary and so in the setting of ICP crisis a higher osmolarity may be tolerated. Avoiding severe hypernatremia (Na >160 mEq/L) is also prudent as this has been associated with increased mortality.[67]

Hypertonic saline is also an osmotic agent that effectively lowers ICP. Hypertonic saline concentrations up to 23.4% are frequently used in clinical practice, and it may represent an important alternative to mannitol for controlling ICP.[68] However, it is less well studied in the TBI population and recommendations regarding the use of hypertonic saline have been deferred.

5. Surgical decompression: Approximately 10–15% of severe TBI patients experience intracranial hypertension refractory to maximal medical therapy.[69] At present, decompressive surgery is one of the last strategies save high-dose barbiturate therapy employed in the management of such patient. It remains to be seen whether the promising results obtained from retrospective cohort studies[69] will be reflected in ongoing randomized controlled trials.

6. Barbiturate therapy: TBI patients with intracranial hypertension refractory to maximal medical and surgical therapy may be treated with high-dose barbiturates.[70] The beneficial effects of barbiturates are attributed to their ability to induce cerebral vasoconstriction, decrease cerebral metabolism and CBF, and act as a free radical scavenger. Given the plethora of complications associated with the use of high-dose barbiturates, one must consider this a "last ditch" effort as their prophylactic use has no benefit. If barbiturate coma is to be used, pentobarbital may be administered with an intravenous loading dose of 10 mg/kg over 30 minutes followed by an infusion at 1–3 mg/kg/h titrated to burst suppression on electroencephalogram (EEG). Barbiturates are myocardial depressants and thus aggressive cardiovascular management is necessary to maintain systemic blood pressure. ICP unresponsive to this therapy is an ominous sign and consideration for further neurosurgical decompression is warranted.

HYPOTHERMIA

Systemic hypothermia with target temperatures between 33°C and 35°C has been used in neurotrauma patients. Although there are known benefits in terms of ICP control to avoiding fever, the data are less clear regarding the neuroprotective effects of prophylactic hypothermia. No mortality benefit to prophylactic hypothermia has been demonstrated in TBI patients. However, benefit by other measures such as the Glasgow Outcome Score is supported by the available literature.[71]

In the TSI population as well, the evidence for therapeutic benefit from systemic hypothermia is not yet available and awaits the results of ongoing clinical trials.[72] A committee from the Joint Section of the AANS and the CNS concluded that there is insufficient evidence to recommend either for or against the practice of local or systemic hypothermia in the treatment of acute spinal cord injury.[73]

BRAIN OXYGEN MONITORING

Low brain oxygenation as measured globally by jugular venous oxygen saturation ($S_{jv}O_2$) or locally by brain tissue oxygen tension ($P_{bt}O_2$) is associated with poor outcomes.[74] Desaturations of $S_{jv}O_2$ to values less than 50% have been shown to indicate various ischemia inducing pathologies such as elevated ICP, hypocarbia, arterial hypoxia, systemic hypotension, and cerebral vasospasm. Sheinberg et al showed a trend toward increasing death rates in TBI patients who had multiple $S_{jv}O_2$ desaturations.[75] Similarly the length of time $P_{bt}O_2$ levels were less than 15 mm Hg is also associated with increased death rates.[76] In a recent retrospective series, TBI patients managed with $P_{bt}O_2$-directed therapy had better outcomes than patients managed with standard ICP/CPP-directed therapy.[77] Interestingly elevated $S_{jv}O_2$ levels (>75%) are associated with poor outcomes and may be an indication of hyperemia or infarction.[78] Therefore, brain oxygen monitoring not only gives information on brain state but also provides another parameter that can be clinically optimized.

STEROIDS

1. Steroids in TBI: Corticosteroids have no role in the management of severe TBI. Class I data from large randomized controlled studies indicate that they neither improve outcome nor lower ICP in this setting.[79,80] Indeed, the data suggest that the use of steroids is harmful in TBI patients.

2. Steroids in TSI: Findings from the second National Acute Spinal Cord Injury Study (NASCIS II) form much of the basis for using corticosteroids after TSI.[81] This multicenter randomized

controlled study concluded that the administration of methylprednisolone within the first 8 hours after spinal cord injury improves neurologic recovery. The dosage protocol used was an initial intravenous bolus of 30 mg/kg/h followed by infusion at 5.4 mg/kg/h for 23 hours. In a follow-up study—NASCIS III—improved motor recovery was seen if the methylprednisolone infusion continued for 47 hours in the subgroup of patients who began steroid therapy between 3 and 8 hours after injury.[82] While this protocol is often implemented in clinical practice, it cannot be considered standard of care given the numerous criticisms leveled at the NASCIS studies. The current guidelines suggest methylprednisolone therapy as an option with the proviso that harmful side effects are more consistent than evidence of clinical benefit.[83]

SEIZURE PROPHYLAXIS

Seizures may be seen in up to 25% of TBI patients within the first 7 days of injury and in up to 42% after this.[84] The literature currently supports the use of seizure prophylaxis to decrease the occurrence of early (within 7 days of injury) PTS but not for late PTS. Therefore, continuation of anticonvulsant therapy for more than 1 week following TBI is not recommended.[84] While phenytoin has been the historical drug of choice in the setting of TBI, use of levetiracetam or newer agents such as lacosamide may be similarly beneficial with a better side effect profile, no known significant drug–drug interactions, and no need for serum level monitoring.[85–87]

REFERENCES

1. Faul M, Xu L, Wald M, Coronado V. *Traumatic Brain Injury in the United States: Emergency Department Visits, Hospitalizations and Deaths 2002–2006*. Atlanta, GA: Centers for Disease Control and Prevention, National Center for Injury Prevention and Control; 2010.
2. Spinal cord injury facts and figures at a glance. National Spinal Cord Injury Statistical Center (NSCISC); February 2010. Available at: https://www.nscisc.uab.edu.
3. Coronado V, Thurman D, Greenspan A, Weissman B. Epidemiology. In: Jallo J, Loftus C, eds. *Neurotrauma and Critical Care of the Brain*. New York: Thieme; 2009.
4. Max W, MacKenzie E, Rice D. Head injuries: costs and consequences. *J Head Trauma Rehabil*. 1991;6(2):76–91.
5. Miller T, Zaloshnja E, Hendrie D. Cost of traumatic brain injury and return on helmet investment in the United States. In: Jallo J, Loftus C, eds. *Neurotrauma and Critical Care of the Brain*. New York: Thieme; 2009.
6. Traumatic brain injury. Centers for Disease Control and Prevention; 2010. Available at: http://www.cdc.gov/TraumaticBrainInjury.
7. Bullock MR, Povlishock JT. Guidelines for the management of severe traumatic brain injury. Editor's commentary. *J Neurotrauma*. 2007;24(suppl 1):2 p preceding S1.
8. Carney NA, Ghajar J. Guidelines for the management of severe traumatic brain injury. Introduction. *J Neurotrauma*. 2007;24(suppl 1):S1–S2.
9. Adekoya N, Thurman DJ, White DD, Webb KW. Surveillance for traumatic brain injury deaths—United States, 1989–1998. *MMWR Surveill Summ*. 2002;51(10):1–14.
10. Rutland-Brown W, Langlois JA, Thomas KE, Xi YL. Incidence of traumatic brain injury in the United States, 2003. *J Head Trauma Rehabil*. 2006;21(6):544–548.
11. *Annual Report for the Spinal Cord Injury Model Systems*. National Spinal Cord Injury Statistical Center (NSCISC); Birmingham, AL; 2009.
12. Bullock M, Gugliotta M. Pathophysiology. In: Jallo J, Loftus C, eds. *Neurotrauma and Critical Care of the Brain*. New York: Thieme; 2009.
13. Kwon BK, Tetzlaff W, Grauer JN, Beiner J, Vaccaro AR. Pathophysiology and pharmacologic treatment of acute spinal cord injury. *Spine J*. 2004;4(4):451–464.
14. Werner C, Engelhard K. Pathophysiology of traumatic brain injury. *Br J Anaesth*. 2007;99(1):4–9.
15. Ropper A, Gress D, Diringer M, Green D, Mayer S, Bleck T. *Neurological and Neurosurgical Intensive Care*. Philadelphia: Lippincott Williams & Wilkins; 2004.
16. American Association of Neurological Surgeons/Congress of Neurological Surgeons Joint Section on Disorders of the Spine and Peripheral Nerves. Blood pressure management after acute spinal cord injury. *Neurosurgery*. 2002;50(3 suppl):S58–S62.
17. American Association of Neurological Surgeons/Congress of Neurological Surgeons Joint Section on Disorders of the Spine and Peripheral Nerves. Management of acute spinal cord injuries in an intensive care unit or other monitored setting. *Neurosurgery*. 2002;50(3 suppl):S51–S57.
18. Dunn I, Frerichs K, Day A, Kim D. Perioperative management of severe traumatic brain injury in adults. In: Schmidek H, Roberts D, eds. *Operative Neurosurgical Techniques*. Philadelphia: Saunders Elsevier; 2006.
19. Fieschi C, Battistini N, Beduschi A, Boselli L, Rossanda M. Regional cerebral blood flow and intraventricular pressure in acute head injuries. *J Neurol Neurosurg Psychiatry*. 1974;37(12):1378–1388.
20. Jaggi JL, Obrist WD, Gennarelli TA, Langfitt TW. Relationship of early cerebral blood flow and metabolism to outcome in acute head injury. *J Neurosurg*. 1990;72(2):176–182.
21. Robertson CS, Contant CF, Gokaslan ZL, Narayan RK, Grossman RG. Cerebral blood flow, arteriovenous oxygen difference, and outcome in head injured patients. *J Neurol Neurosurg Psychiatry*. 1992;55(7):594–603.
22. Chesnut RM, Marshall LF, Klauber MR, et al. The role of secondary brain injury in determining outcome from severe head injury. *J Trauma*. 1993;34(2):216–222.
23. Marmarou A, Anderson R, Ward J, et al. Impact of ICP instability and hypotension on outcome in patients with severe head trauma. *J Neurosurg*. 1991;75:S59–S66.

24. Consortium for Spinal Cord Medicine. Early acute management in adults with spinal cord injury: a clinical practice guideline for health-care professionals. *J Spinal Cord Med.* 208;31(4):403–479.

25. Ploumis A, Yadlapalli N, Fehlings MG, Kwon BK, Vaccaro AR. A systematic review of the evidence supporting a role for vasopressor support in acute SCI. *Spinal Cord.* 2010;48(5):356–362.

26. Kuniyoshi S, Suarez J. Traumatic head injury. In: Suarez J, ed. *Critical Care Neurology and Neurosurgery.* Totowa, N.J.: Humana Press; 2004.

27. American Association of Neurological Surgeons/Congress of Neurological Surgeons Joint Section on Disorders of the Spine and Peripheral Nerves. Cervical spine immobilization before admission to the hospital. *Neurosurgery.* 2002;50(3 suppl):S7–S17.

28. Bratton SL, Chestnut RM, Ghajar J, et al. Guidelines for the management of severe traumatic brain injury. I. Blood pressure and oxygenation. *J Neurotrauma.* 2007;24(suppl 1):S7–S13.

29. American Association of Neurological Surgeons/Congress of Neurological Surgeons Joint Section on Disorders of the Spine and Peripheral Nerves. Clinical assessment after acute cervical spinal cord injury. *Neurosurgery.* 2002;50(3 suppl):S21–S29.

30. Jagoda AS, Bazarian JJ, Bruns JJ Jr, et al. Clinical policy: neuroimaging and decisionmaking in adult mild traumatic brain injury in the acute setting. *Ann Emerg Med.* 2008;52(6):714–748.

31. Heller J, Maas A. Severe brain injury. In: Jallo J, Loftus C, eds. *Neurotrauma and Critical Care of the Brain.* New York: Thieme; 2009.

32. Miele V, Bailes J. Mild brain injury. In: Jallo J, Loftus C, eds. *Neurotrauma and Critical Care of the Brain.* New York: Thieme; 2009.

33. Timmons S, Winestone J. Moderate brain injury. In: Jallo J, Loftus C, eds. *Neurotrauma and Critical Care of the Brain.* New York: Thieme; 2009.

34. Kay T, Harrington D, Adams R, et al. Definition of mild traumatic brain injury. *J Head Trauma Rehabil.* 1993;8(8):86–87.

35. Practice parameter: the management of concussion in sports (summary statement). Report of the Quality Standards Subcommittee. *Neurology.* 1997;48(3):581–585.

36. Cantu RC. Head injuries in sport. *Br J Sports Med.* 1996;30(4):289–296.

37. Culotta VP, Sementilli ME, Gerold K, Watts CC. Clinicopathological heterogeneity in the classification of mild head injury. *Neurosurgery.* 1996;38(2):245–250.

38. Atkinson PP, Atkinson JL. Spinal shock. *Mayo Clin Proc.* 1996;71(4):384–389.

39. Ditunno JF, Little JW, Tessler A, Burns AS. Spinal shock revisited: a four-phase model. *Spinal Cord.* 2004;42(7):383–395.

40. Haydel MJ, Preston CA, Mills TJ, Luber S, Blaudeau E, DeBlieux PM. Indications for computed tomography in patients with minor head injury. *N Engl J Med.* 2000;343(2):100–105.

41. Stiell IG, Wells GA, Vandemheen K, et al. The Canadian CT Head Rule for patients with minor head injury. *Lancet.* 2001;357(9266):1391–1396.

42. Stein SC, Burnett MG, Glick HA. Indications for CT scanning in mild traumatic brain injury: a cost-effectiveness study. *J Trauma.* 2006;61(3):558–566.

43. Marshall L, Marshall S, Klauber M, et al. A new classification of head injury based on computerized tomography. *J Neurosurg.* 1991;75(suppl):S14–S20.

44. American Association of Neurological Surgeons/Congress of Neurological Surgeons Joint Section on Disorders of the Spine and Peripheral Nerves. Radiographic assessment of the cervical spine in symptomatic trauma patients. *Neurosurgery.* 2002;50(3 suppl):S36–S43.

45. American Association of Neurological Surgeons/Congress of Neurological Surgeons Joint Section on Disorders of the Spine and Peripheral Nerves. Radiographic assessment of the cervical spine in asymptomatic trauma patients. *Neurosurgery.* 2002;50(3 suppl):S30–S35.

46. Bullock M, Chesnut R, Ghajar J, et al. Guidelines for the surgical management of traumatic brain injury. *Neurosurgery.* 2006;58(3 suppl):S1–S62.

47. Bullock MR, Chesnut R, Ghajar J, et al. Surgical management of acute epidural hematomas. *Neurosurgery.* 2006;58(3 suppl):S7–S15. Discussion Si–Siv.

48. Bullock MR, Chesnut R, Ghajar J, et al. Surgical management of acute subdural hematomas. *Neurosurgery.* 2006;58(3 suppl):S16–S24. Discussion Si–Siv.

49. Bullock MR, Chesnut R, Ghajar J, et al. Surgical management of traumatic parenchymal lesions. *Neurosurgery.* 2006;58(3 suppl):S25–S46. Discussion Si–Siv.

50. Bullock MR, Chesnut R, Ghajar J, et al. Surgical management of posterior fossa mass lesions. *Neurosurgery.* 2006;58(3 suppl):S47–S55. Discussion Si–Siv.

51. Bullock MR, Chesnut R, Ghajar J, et al. Surgical management of depressed cranial fractures. *Neurosurgery.* 2006;58(3 suppl):S56–S60. Discussion Si–Siv.

52. Grahm TW, Williams FC Jr, Harrington T, Spetzler RF. Civilian gunshot wounds to the head: a prospective study. *Neurosurgery.* 1990;27(5):696–700. Discussion 700.

53. Fehlings MG, Tator CH. An evidence-based review of decompressive surgery in acute spinal cord injury: rationale, indications, and timing based on experimental and clinical studies. *J Neurosurg.* 1999;91(1 suppl):1–11.

54. Baisden J, Maiman D, Ducker T. Timing of spinal surgery: argument for elective surgery. In: Benzel E, ed. *Spine Surgery: Techniques, Complication Avoidance, and Management.* Philadelphia: Elsevier; 2005.

55. Fehlings MG, Perrin RG. The timing of surgical intervention in the treatment of spinal cord injury: a systematic review of recent clinical evidence. *Spine (Phila Pa 1976).* 2006;31(11 suppl):S28–S35. Discussion S36.

56. American Association of Neurological Surgeons/Congress of Neurological Surgeons Joint Section on Disorders of the Spine and Peripheral Nerves. Guidelines for the management of acute cervical spine and spinal cord injuries. *Neurosurgery.* 2002;50(3 suppl):S1–S124.

57. Badjatia N, Carney N, Crocco TJ, et al. Guidelines for prehospital management of traumatic brain injury 2nd edition. *Prehosp Emerg Care.* 2008;12(suppl 1):S1–S52.

58. Knuth T, Letarte PB, Ling G, et al. *Guidelines for the Field Management of Combat-Related Head Trauma.* New York: Brain Trauma Foundation, 2005.

59. Bratton SL, Chestnut RM, Ghajar J, et al. Guidelines for the management of severe traumatic brain injury. VII. Intracranial pressure monitoring technology. *J Neurotrauma*. 2007;24(suppl 1):S45–S54.

60. Bratton SL, Chestnut RM, Ghajar J, et al. Guidelines for the management of severe traumatic brain injury. VI. Indications for intracranial pressure monitoring. *J Neurotrauma*. 2007;24(suppl 1):S37–S44.

61. Bratton SL, Chestnut RM, Ghajar J, et al. Guidelines for the management of severe traumatic brain injury. IX. Cerebral perfusion thresholds. *J Neurotrauma*. 2007;24(suppl 1):S59–S64.

62. Bratton SL, Chestnut RM, Ghajar J, et al. Guidelines for the management of severe traumatic brain injury. VIII. Intracranial pressure thresholds. *J Neurotrauma*. 2007;24(suppl 1):S55–S58.

63. Muizelaar JP, Marmarou A, Ward JD, et al. Adverse effects of prolonged hyperventilation in patients with severe head injury: a randomized clinical trial. *J Neurosurg*. 1991;75(5):731–739.

64. Bratton SL, Chestnut RM, Ghajar J, et al. Guidelines for the management of severe traumatic brain injury. XIV. Hyperventilation. *J Neurotrauma*. 207;24(suppl 1):S87–S90.

65. Bratton SL, Chestnut RM, Ghajar J, et al. Guidelines for the management of severe traumatic brain injury. *J Neurotrauma*. 2007;24(suppl 1):S1–S106.

66. Bratton SL, Chestnut RM, Ghajar J, et al. Guidelines for the management of severe traumatic brain injury. II. Hyperosmolar therapy. *J Neurotrauma*. 2007;24(suppl 1):S14–S20.

67. Aiyagari V, Deibert E, Diringer MN. Hypernatremia in the neurologic intensive care unit: how high is too high? *J Crit Care*. 2006;21(2):163–172.

68. Ogden AT, Mayer SA, Connolly ES Jr. Hyperosmolar agents in neurosurgical practice: the evolving role of hypertonic saline. *Neurosurgery*. 2005;57(2):207–215. Discussion 207–215.

69. Aarabi B, Hesdorffer DC, Ahn ES, Aresco C, Scalea TM, Eisenberg HM. Outcome following decompressive craniectomy for malignant swelling due to severe head injury. *J Neurosurg*. 2006;104(4):469–479.

70. Bratton SL, Chestnut RM, Ghajar J, et al. Guidelines for the management of severe traumatic brain injury. XI. Anesthetics, analgesics, and sedatives. *J Neurotrauma*. 2007;24(suppl 1):S71–S76.

71. Bratton SL, Chestnut RM, Ghajar J, et al. Guidelines for the management of severe traumatic brain injury. III. Prophylactic hypothermia. *J Neurotrauma*. 2007;24(suppl 1):S21–S25.

72. Levi AD, Casella G, Green BA, et al. Clinical outcomes using modest intravascular hypothermia after acute cervical spinal cord injury. *Neurosurgery*. 2010;66(4):670–677.

73. Resnick D, Kaiser M, Fehlings M, McCormick P. Hypothermia and human spinal cord injury: position statement and evidence based recommendations from the AANS/CNS Joint Sections on Disorders of the Spine and the AANS/CNS Joint Section on Trauma; 2007. Available at: http://www.spinesection.org/hypothermia.php.

74. Bratton SL, Chestnut RM, Ghajar J, et al. Guidelines for the management of severe traumatic brain injury. X. Brain oxygen monitoring and thresholds. *J Neurotrauma*. 2007;24(suppl 1):S65–S70.

75. Sheinberg M, Kanter MJ, Robertson CS, Contant CF, Narayan RK, Grossman RG. Continuous monitoring of jugular venous oxygen saturation in head-injured patients. *J Neurosurg*. 1992;76(2):212–217.

76. Valadka AB, Gopinath SP, Contant CF, Uzura M, Robertson CS. Relationship of brain tissue PO_2 to outcome after severe head injury. *Crit Care Med*. 1998;26(9):1576–1581.

77. Spiotta AM, Stiefel MF, Gracias VH, et al. Brain tissue oxygen-directed management and outcome in patients with severe traumatic brain injury. *J Neurosurg*. 2010;113(3):571–580.

78. Cormio M, Valadka AB, Robertson CS. Elevated jugular venous oxygen saturation after severe head injury. *J Neurosurg*. 1999;90(1):9–15.

79. Bratton SL, Chestnut RM, Ghajar J, et al. Guidelines for the management of severe traumatic brain injury. XV. Steroids. *J Neurotrauma*. 2007;24(suppl 1):S91–S95.

80. Edwards P, Arango M, Balica L, et al. Final results of MRC CRASH, a randomised placebo-controlled trial of intravenous corticosteroid in adults with head injury—outcomes at 6 months. *Lancet*. 2005;365(9475):1957–1959.

81. Bracken MB, Shepard MJ, Collins WF, et al. A randomized, controlled trial of methylprednisolone or naloxone in the treatment of acute spinal-cord injury. Results of the Second National Acute Spinal Cord Injury Study. *N Engl J Med*. 1990;322(20):1405–1411.

82. Bracken MB, Shepard MJ, Holford TR, et al. Administration of methylprednisolone for 24 or 48 hours or tirilazad mesylate for 48 hours in the treatment of acute spinal cord injury. Results of the Third National Acute Spinal Cord Injury Randomized Controlled Trial. National Acute Spinal Cord Injury Study. *JAMA*. 1997;277(20):1597–1604.

83. American Association of Neurological Surgeons/Congress of Neurological Surgeons Joint Section on Disorders of the Spine and Peripheral Nerves. Pharmacological therapy after acute cervical spinal cord injury. *Neurosurgery*. 2002;50(3 suppl):S63–S72.

84. Bratton SL, Chestnut RM, Ghajar J, et al. Guidelines for the management of severe traumatic brain injury. XIII. Antiseizure prophylaxis. *J Neurotrauma*. 2007;24(suppl 1):S83–S86.

85. Jones KE, Puccio AM, Harshman KJ, et al. Levetiracetam versus phenytoin for seizure prophylaxis in severe traumatic brain injury. *Neurosurg Focus*. 2008;25(4):E3.

86. Szaflarski JP, Sangha KS, Lindsell CJ, Shutter LA. Prospective, randomized, single-blinded comparative trial of intravenous levetiracetam versus phenytoin for seizure prophylaxis. *Neurocrit Care*. 2010;12(2):165–172.

87. Parkerson KA, Reinsberger C, Chou SH, Dworetzky BA, Lee JW. Lacosamide in the treatment of acute recurrent seizures and periodic epileptiform patterns in critically ill patients. *Epilepsy Behav*. 2011;20(1):48–51.

SECTION VII

Hematologic and Endocrine Disorders

CHAPTER 29

Transfusion in Critical Care

Julie A. Mayglothling and Therese M. Duane

▶ INTRODUCTION

Fresh, warm whole blood most effectively restores red cell mass, plasma volume, clotting factors, and platelets. However, given shortages of blood products, the use of whole blood transfusions is not realistic. The use of component product transfusion is the mainstay of blood banking and transfusion practice, effectively utilizing a scare resource while matching the components transfused to the specific needs of the patient. Whole blood is usually separated into packed red blood cells (PRBC), fresh frozen plasma (FFP), and platelet concentrate soon after donation. The plasma can be further separated into cryoprecipitate and cryopoor plasma, or undergo further fractionation to individual plasma proteins.

Indications for blood component therapy can be divided into two main categories: (1) enhancement of oxygen-carrying capacity by increasing red blood cell (RBC) mass and (2) replacement of coagulation components due to loss, dysfunction, or consumption.

▶ ANEMIA AND PACKED RED BLOOD CELL TRANSFUSION

Anemia is one of the most common abnormal laboratory findings among critically ill patients. The effect of anemia on outcome and the determination of transfusion triggers has been the subject of much debate in recent literature.

Historically, the decision to transfuse has been guided by the hemoglobin (Hb) concentration, usually 10 mg/dL. However, given the risks associated with PRBC transfusion and recent literature supporting better or similar outcomes with lower transfusion triggers, the optimal Hb level at which to transfuse patients remains unclear.

BENEFITS OF RBC TRANSFUSION

The main function of RBCs is to transport oxygen from the lungs to the peripheral tissues. Oxygen delivery (DO_2) is calculated by multiplying the cardiac output (CO) times the arterial oxygen content (CaO_2):

$$DO_2 = CO \times CaO_2$$

where DO_2 is in milliliters per minute, CO in deciliters per minute, and CaO_2 in milliliters per deciliter.

And CaO_2 is calculated by the following equation:

$$CaO_2 = (SaO_2 \times 1.34 \times [Hb]) + (0.0031 \times PaO_2)$$

where SaO_2 is the arterial oxygen saturation (%), 1.34 the oxygen-carrying capacity of Hb (mL/g), [Hb] the Hb concentration (g/dL), 0.0031 the solubility of oxygen in plasma at 37°C, and Pao_2 is measured in millimeters of mercury.

Under normal conditions, DO_2 exceeds oxygen consumption (VO_2) by three to five times. However, in situations where the VO_2 of the peripheral tissues is greatly increased, or DO_2 is decreased by anemia or decreased CO, VO_2 can exceed DO_2 and result in tissue hypoxia. Increasing the [Hb] is one of the ways to increase the blood's oxygen-carrying capacity, and therefore increase DO_2. Additionally, transfusion can increase blood volume for patients following acute blood loss or hemorrhage and alleviate symptoms of anemia such as dyspnea, weakness, and fatigue.

DRAWBACKS OF RBC TRANSFUSION

Despite the theoretical benefits of transfusion described above, it is associated with multiple risks. There is risk of human error resulting in a transfusion reaction, most commonly an acute hemolytic reaction, from receiving incorrectly matched blood. Febrile reactions, namely, nonhemolytic/noninfectious reactions secondary to antileukocyte antibodies, are also possible in up to 7% of blood product recipients. There is risk of allergic reaction ranging from urticaria to frank anaphylaxis that is usually a result of the passive transfer of sensitizing antibodies. Additionally, transmission of communicable diseases such as human immunodeficiency virus (HIV) and viral hepatitis is possible, although this risk, with modern blood banking techniques, is now exceedingly remote.[1] Finally, metabolic derangements can occur with transfusion, such as hypocalcemia and hyperkalemia.

More commonly, especially in the critically ill population, transfusion of PRBCs is associated with increased risk of infection, including wound infections, sepsis and pneumonia,[2,3] increased incidence of multiple organ failure (MOF),[4] and increased risk of acute lung injury (ALI) and acute respiratory distress syndrome (ARDS).[5] In addition, transfusions are associated with longer intensive care unit (ICU) and hospital length of stay (LOS), more complications, and increased mortality.[6] These effects are dose-dependent, meaning the more units of blood that are transfused, the higher the risk of complications.

The reason for the increased morbidity and mortality in patients receiving PRBCs is not completely clear, although recent interest has focused on immunomodulating effects of transfused RBCs and RBC storage lesions (age of transfused RBCs) as possible mechanisms. It has been suggested that leukodepleted blood may have less immunomodulating properties and, hence, reduce the complications associated with the transfusion of nonleukodepleted blood,[7–9] but there is still considerable debate about the benefit of leukoreduction and which patients will benefit most from receiving leukoreduced blood.[10] Similarly, age of transfused RBCs has also been suggested as a possible explanation for the adverse effects associated with RBC transfusion. Well-documented changes occur to the RBC product during ex vivo storage, including a reduction in RBC deformability, altered RBC adhesiveness and aggregability, and a reduction in 2,3-diphosphoglycerate and adenosine triphosphate (ATP). These changes reduce posttransfusion viability of RBCs and limit DO_2.[11] The clinical effect of these changes is uncertain; however, some studies have suggested that transfusion of "older" RBCs may be associated with adverse effects.[12–14] But a 2009 review of 27 studies of postsurgical, ICU, and trauma patients could not establish definitive relationship between the age of transfused RBCs and outcome in adult patients, except possibly for trauma patients receiving massive transfusion.[15]

TRANSFUSION THRESHOLD

There have been multiple retrospective and observational studies that demonstrate that the use of blood transfusions for the treatment of anemia in hemodynamically stable critically ill patients is not associated with improved outcome. The CRIT Study, performed in the United States and published in 2004, documented that 44% of all patients received blood transfusions and the number of units transfused was independently associated with worse outcomes.[16] Similarly, a European study by Vincent et al showed an ICU transfusion rate of 37%. In this study, the group of patients who received a transfusion had a higher mortality rate compared with the nontransfused group despite similar degrees of organ dysfunction.[17]

The Transfusion Requirements in Critical Care (TRICC) trial conducted in Canada is the only prospective, adequately powered study that randomized patients to either a restrictive transfusion strategy (patients transfused if Hb dropped below 7 mg/dL and maintained between 7 and 9 mg/dL) or a liberal strategy (patients transfused when Hb fell below 10 mg/dL and maintained at 10–12 mg/dL). The overall hospital mortality was significantly lower in the restrictive transfusion group (22.2% vs. 28.1%, $P = .05$), and although 30-day mortality was similar in the two groups (18.7% vs. 23.3%, $P = .11$), mortality rates were significantly lower in patients randomized to the restrictive transfusion group who were <55 years of age and less acutely ill. The authors concluded that a restrictive strategy of red cell transfusion is at least as effective as, and possibly superior to, a liberal transfusion threshold for hemodynamically stable critically ill adults.[18] Despite these recommendations, multiple studies demonstrate that transfusion practices have not changed significantly.

One patient population that may be an exception to the restrictive transfusion threshold is elderly patients with evidence of myocardial ischemia. A group of 79,000 patients >65 years of age admitted to the hospital with myocardial infarction was retrospectively reviewed. Those patients with lower hematocrit (HCT) levels on admission had higher 30-day mortality. In addition, blood transfusion was associated with a lower 30-day mortality among those patients with an HCT <24%. The patients who had an HCT above 30% did not have improved mortality from transfusion.[19] It is important to remember that this study was performed in patients with evidence of myocardial ischemia. A history of coronary artery disease (CAD) or patients at risk for ischemia do not fall into this category.[20]

SEPSIS

The Surviving Sepsis Campaign recommends that during the first 6 hours of resuscitation of severe sepsis or septic shock, if central venous oxygen saturation of 70% is not achieved with fluid resuscitation to a central venous pressure (CVP) of 8–12 mm Hg, then transfuse PRBCs to an HCT >30% and/or initiate dobutamine infusion.[21] This recommendation is based on the study of Rivers et al regarding early goal-directed therapy for sepsis.[22] Once initial resuscitation of tissue hypoxia is achieved, and in the absence of myocardial ischemia, the restrictive transfusion threshold should then be targeted.

TRAUMA

The trauma patient with hemorrhagic shock should be transfused regardless of Hb levels. However, in the absence of ongoing blood loss or hemorrhagic shock, there is no benefit of a "liberal" transfusion threshold in hemodynamically stable trauma patients.[23] In a prospective study of over 15,000 trauma patients, blood transfusion was shown to be an independent predictor of mortality, ICU admission, ICU LOS, and hospital LOS. Those patients who received blood transfusion in the first 24 hours were more than three times as likely to die.[24]

TRAUMATIC BRAIN INJURY

One area that remains unclear is transfusion criteria for those patients with traumatic brain injury (TBI). One retrospective review showed that more days with an HCT <30% were associated with improved neurologic outcome, but the lowest measured HCT was associated with lower Glasgow Coma Scale (GCS) score on hospital discharge. The authors concluded that patients with TBI should not have different transfusion thresholds than other critical care patients, but prospective studies need to be done to support this recommendation.[25]

RECOMMENDATIONS

A number of guidelines regarding the indications for RBC transfusion have been published between 1997 and 2007. Most recently, a joint task force of the Eastern Association for the Surgery of Trauma (EAST) and the American College of Critical Care Medicine (ACCM) of the Society of Critical Care Medicine (SCCM) performed a comprehensive literature review of the topic and graded the evidence using scientific assessment methods. Table 29-1 includes an abridged summary of their 2009 evidence-based recommendations

regarding the use of RBC transfusion in adult trauma and critical care.[26]

Anemia in critical illness is extremely common, and up to 40% of ICU patients will be transfused during their hospital stay. Physicians must weigh the risks and benefits of transfusion. PRBC transfusions are associated with increased incidence of infection, MOF, ALI, and ARDS across heterogeneous patient groups. Based on existing literature, no one transfusion trigger should be used in all patients. However, the evidence is sufficient to state that transfusions are rarely beneficial when Hb level exceeds 10 g/dL (HCT >30%) in the absence of acute blood loss, and using a restrictive strategy for transfusion (transfusing PRBC when Hb levels fall below 7 mg/dL) is just as effective, and likely superior to, a liberal strategy in hemodynamically stable critically ill patients.

▶ FRESH FROZEN PLASMA

FFP is plasma separated from the RBCs and platelets of whole blood and placed at −18°C or below within 8 hours after collection. By definition, "1 U" of FFP has the equivalent plasma coagulation factors as 1 U of whole blood and one bag contains approximately 200–250 mL. Once thawed, FFP must be used within 24 hours or the amount of factors V and III begins to decline. FFP is not a concentrate and must be ABO compatible.

INDICATIONS

Transfusion of FFP is indicated in the presence of active bleeding or prior to major invasive procedures with known or suspected coagulation abnormalities due to inadequate production, malfunction, loss, or consumption of multiple clotting factors.[27–30] Liver failure, warfarin overdose, vitamin K deficiency, and dilutional coagulopathy are some indications for plasma transfusion. Patients with a deficiency of a single clotting factor are more appropriately treated with factor concentrates or cryoprecipitate.

Coagulopathy is supported by prothrombin time (PT) or international normalized ratio (INR) greater than 1.5 times normal, or activated partial thromboplastin time (aPTT) greater than 1.5 times the top of the normal range.[31] Even in the setting of excessive warfarin effects, transfusion of plasma products should not be used to reverse elevated INR in the absence of bleeding, unless urgent invasive or surgical procedures are required.[32]

MILD TO MODERATE COAGULOPATHY

The ability of FFP to reverse mild to moderate coagulopathy (INR 1.1–2) has been shown to be poor.[33,34]

▶ **TABLE 29-1. ABRIDGED SUMMARY OF 2009 CLINICAL PRACTICE GUIDELINE FOR RED BLOOD CELL TRANSFUSION IN ADULT TRAUMA AND CRITICAL CARE FROM THE ACCM/SCCM AND EAST PRACTICE MANAGEMENT WORKGROUP "DATA FROM"[26]**

A. Indications for RBC transfusion in the general critically ill patient
  • RBC transfusion is indicated for patients with evidence of hemorrhagic shock (Level 1)
  • RBC transfusion may be indicated for patients with evidence of acute hemorrhage and hemodynamic instability or inadequate oxygen delivery (Level 1)
  • A "restrictive" strategy of RBC transfusion (transfuse when Hb <7 g/dL) is as effective as a "liberal" strategy (transfusion when Hb <10 g/dL) in critically ill patients with hemodynamically stable anemia, except possibly in patients with acute myocardial ischemia (Level 1)
  • The use of only Hb level as a "trigger" for transfusion should be avoided (Level 2)
  • In the absence of acute hemorrhage, RBC transfusion should be given as single units (Level 2)
  • RBC transfusion should not be considered as an absolute method to improve tissue oxygen consumption in critically ill patients (Level 2)
B. RBC transfusion in sepsis
  • The transfusion needs for each septic patient must be assessed individually (Level 2)
C. RBC transfusion in patients at risk for or with ALI and ARDS
  • All efforts should be initiated to avoid RBC transfusion in patients at risk for ALI and ARDS after completion of resuscitation (Level 2)
D. RBC transfusion in patients with neurologic injury and diseases
  • There is no benefit of a "liberal" transfusion strategy in patients with moderate-to-severe traumatic brain injury (Level 2)
E. RBC transfusion risks
  • RBC transfusion is associated with increased nosocomial infection (Level 2)
  • RBC transfusion is an independent risk factor for MOF and SIRS (Level 2)
  • There is no definitive evidence that prestorage leukocyte depletion of RBC transfusion reduces complication rates (Level 2)
  • RBC transfusions are independently associated with longer ICU and hospital LOS, increased complications, and increased mortality (Level 2)
  • There is a relationship between transfusion and ALI and ARDS (Level 2)
F. Alternatives to RBC transfusion
  • Recombinant human erythropoietin (rHuEpo) administration improves reticulocytosis and hematocrit and may decrease overall transfusion requirements (Level 2)
  • Hemoglobin-based oxygen carriers (HBOCs) are undergoing investigation for use in critically ill and injured patients but are not yet approved for use in the United States (Level 2)
G. Strategies to reduce RBC transfusion
  • The use of low-volume adult or pediatric blood sampling tubes is associated with a reduction in phlebotomy volumes and a reduction in blood transfusion (Level 2)
  • Reduction in diagnostic laboratory testing is associated with a reduction in phlebotomy volumes and a reduction in blood transfusion (Level 2)

Regardless of the number of units of FFP transfused, there is a low likelihood that the INR will be corrected to normal levels.[35] Specifically, current evidence does not support the use of prophylactic plasma transfusion for minimally invasive procedures in the setting of mildly abnormal coagulation tests such as paracentesis, thoracentesis,[28] or central venous catheter insertion.[36]

Approximately 25% of clotting activity is required for hemostasis. Given that the plasma volume of humans is usually 40 mL/kg, the amount required is approximately 10–15 mL/kg, or 2–3 U of FFP, in the absence of ongoing losses or consumption. This is a general guideline, and clinicians should follow clinical course and coagulation parameters to guide transfusion, remembering that mild to moderate coagulopathy may not be corrected with FFP.

MASSIVE TRANSFUSION

Prophylactic transfusion of FFP is indicated in patients receiving massive transfusion (defined as greater than 10 U of PRBC in a 24-hour period). The exact ratio of FFP to PRBC transfusion has been a debate for many years. Historically, the FFP:PRBC ratio ranged from 1:4 to 1:10 and the initiation of almost any massive transfusion protocol using multiple different ratios had been shown to improve mortality.[37] Recent literature in both military and civilian trauma patients supports using higher ratios of FFP. The optimal ratio appears to be between 1:1 and 1:3 FFP to PRBC[38–40] and is a source of continued study.

► CRYOPRECIPITATE

Cryoprecipitate is obtained from the precipitate of frozen plasma once it is thawed. It has high concentrates of factor VIII, fibrinogen, factor XIII, and von Willebrand factor but the volume of cryoprecipitate is smaller, approximately 10 mL, and multiple units are often combined for transfusion. Despite the small volume of cryoprecipitate, it carries the same infectious risk as 1 U of FFP. Indications for transfusion of cryoprecipitate include fibrinogen deficiency with levels less than 100 mg/dL, mostly encountered during massive bleeding or consumptive coagulopathy; von Willebrand disease; and hemophilia A when factor VIII concentrates are not available.[31]

► PLATELETS

Platelets are required for primary hemostasis and circulate normally at a count of 150–400 × 10⁹/L. Each concentrate of platelets contains approximately 5.5×10^{10} platelets and is derived from 1 U of whole blood or from plateletpheresis donations. Once collected, platelets can be stored for up to 5 days, and they are pooled with concentrates from multiple donors before transfusion. ABO compatibility is not required, but is preferred because small amounts of donor leukocytes and plasma are transfused along with the platelets. Each unit of platelets is expected to increase the platelet count by $5–10 \times 10^{9}$/L in the absence of consumption or ongoing loss, and the usual dose is 1 U per 10 kg of body weight.

There is no single target platelet count under which transfusion is recommended for all patients. When platelet counts fall below 5×10^{9}/L, there is a possibility of spontaneous hemorrhage and a high risk of hemorrhage with trauma or an invasive procedure.[41] Given these risks, platelets should be administered regardless of apparent bleeding, when platelets drop below this level.[42] At counts greater than 50×10^{9}/L, bleeding due to platelet deficiency is unlikely and prophylactic transfusion is normally not indicated. For patients with active bleeding and those undergoing invasive or surgical procedures, the current recommendation is that platelet counts should be maintained above 50×10^{9}/L.[31] Some recommend targets of 100×10^{9}/L in the setting of intracranial hemorrhage or multisystem trauma.[43]

Platelet counts between 5×10^{9} and 50×10^{9}/L have variable risks of hemorrhage due to thrombocytopenia, and the issue of prophylactic platelet transfusion is controversial between these levels. Clinical observation and evaluation of the patient's other risk factors for bleeding must guide transfusion practices. Prior recommendations were to transfuse platelets whenever the platelet count was less than 20×10^{9}/L, but recent literature recommends lowering that trigger to 10×10^{9}/L.[44,45]

Patients suffering from a destructive cause for thrombocytopenia rarely benefit from platelet transfusion because the transfused platelets are rapidly destroyed. Patients with such conditions as idiopathic thrombocytopenia purpura (ITP), hypersplenism, disseminated intravascular coagulation (DIC), sepsis, platelet antibodies, or those after cardiac surgery with extracorporeal bypass fall under this category. In the presence of a life-threatening hemorrhage or surgery, transfusion may be beneficial for its short-term effect. Platelet transfusion is contraindicated in such conditions as thrombotic thrombocytopenic purpura (TTP)[46] and hemolytic uremic syndrome (HUS) because of worse outcomes, and is therefore reserved for life-threatening hemorrhage with these conditions. Heparin-induced thrombocytopenia (HIT) was also thought to be a contraindication for platelet transfusion; however, recent guidelines conclude that platelet transfusion can be considered in patients with HIT and overt bleeding, or those thought to be at high risk of bleeding.[47]

► ERYTHROPOIETIN

The use of recombinant erythropoietin (EPO) has been shown to reduce the need for RBC transfusions in patients with chronic renal failure, as well as those with anemia of chronic disease, such as cancer and acquired immune deficiency syndrome (AIDS).[48] Despite the decrease in production of endogenous EPO that accompanies critical illness,[49] the use of recombinant EPO in critically ill patients has been controversial. Multiple studies using recombinant EPO have shown conflicting results.[50,51] The use of recombinant EPO may result in a small decrease in RBC transfusion for some patients, but it does not show an overall mortality benefit and appears that the risk of thrombotic events likely outweighs the benefits in most critically ill patients.[51] The one subset of patients that may benefit from recombinant EPO is patients with multiple trauma,[52] but the reason for this is unclear and the practice continues to be controversial.

► CONCLUSIONS

Transfusion of blood components can be an essential part of the management of critically ill patients. However, despite the growing body of evidence recommending specific transfusion thresholds and more judicious use of blood products, many transfusion practices continue to be rooted in tradition. Transfusion carries with it multiple risks, including an increased risk of infection, MOF, ALI, and mortality for every unit of component administered. Practitioners must have a clear understanding of these risks in order to use blood component therapy safely and effectively.

REFERENCES

1. Busch MP, Kleinman SH, Nemo GJ. Current and emerging infectious risks of blood transfusions. *JAMA*. 2003;289:959–962.

2. Edna TH, Bjerkeset T. Association between blood transfusion and infection in injured patients. *J Trauma*. 1992;33(5):659–661.

3. Hill GE, Frawley WH, Griffith KE, Forestner JE, Minei JP. Allogenic blood transfusion increases the risk of postoperative bacterial infections: a meta analysis. *J Trauma*. 2003;53(5):908–914.

4. Moore FA, Moore EE, Sauaia A. Blood transfusion. An independent risk factor for postinjury multiple organ failure. *Arch Surg*. 1997;132(6):620–624.

5. Looney MR, Gropper MA, Matthey MA. Transfusion related acute lung injury: a review. *Chest*. 2004;126(1):249–258.

6. Blumberg N. Allogenic transfusion and infection: economic and clinical implications. *Semin Hematol*. 1997;34(3 suppl 2):34–40.

7. Raghavan M, Marik PE. Anemia, allogenic blood transfusion, and immunomodulation in the critically ill. *Chest*. 2005;127:295–307.

8. Fergusson D, Khanna MP, Tinmouth A, et al. Transfusion of leukoreduced red blood cells may decrease postoperative infections: two meta-analyses of randomized controlled trials. *Can J Anaesth*. 2004;51:417–424.

9. Hebert PC, Tinmouth A, Corwin HL. Controversies in RBC transfusion in the critically ill. *Chest*. 2007;131:1583–1590.

10. Corwin HL, AuBuchon JP. Is leukoreduction of blood components for everyone? *JAMA*. 2003;289:1993–1995.

11. Ho J, Sibbald WJ, Chin-Yee IH. Effects of storage on efficacy of red cell transfusion: when is it not safe? *Crit Care Med*. 2003;31:S687–S697.

12. Marik PE, Sibbald WJ. Effect of stored-blood transfusion on oxygen delivery in patients with sepsis. *JAMA*. 1993;269:3024–3029.

13. Fitzgerald RD, Martin CM, Dietz GE, et al. Transfusion red blood cells stored in citrate phosphate dextrose adenine-1 for 28 days fails to improve tissue oxygenation in rats. *Crit Care Med*. 1997;25:726–732.

14. Tinmouth A, Chin-Yee I. The clinical consequences of the red cell storage lesion. *Transfus Med Rev*. 2001;15:91–107.

15. Lelubre C, Piagnerelli, M, Vincent JL. Association between duration of storage of transfused red blood cells and morbidity and mortality in adult patients: myth or reality? *Transfusion*. 2009;49:1384–1394.

16. Corwin HL, Gettinger A, Pearl RG, et al. The CRIT Study: anemia and blood transfusion in the critically ill—current clinical practice in the United States. *Crit Care Med*. 2004;32:39–52.

17. Vincent JL, Baron JF, Reinhart K, et al. Anemia and blood transfusion in critically ill patients. *JAMA*. 2002;288:1499–1507.

18 Hebert PC, Wells G, Blajchman MA, et al. A multicenter, randomized, controlled clinical trial of transfusion requirements in critical care. Transfusion Requirements in Critical Care Investigators, Canadian Critical Care Trials Group. *N Engl J Med*. 1999;340(6):409–417.

19. Wen-Chih W, Saif SR, Yongfei W, et al. Blood transfusion in elderly patients with acute myocardial infarction. *N Engl J Med*. 2001;345(17):1230–1236.

20. Hebert PC, Tinmouth A, Corwin H. Anemia and red cell transfusion in critically ill patients. *Crit Care Med*. 2003;31(12 suppl):S672–S677.

21. Dellinger RP, Carlet JM, Masur H, et al. Surviving Sepsis Campaign guidelines for management of severe sepsis and septic shock. *Crit Care Med*. 2004;32(3):858–873.

22. Rivers E, Nguyen B, Havstad S, et al, Early Goal-Directed Therapy Collaborative Group. Early goal-directed therapy in the treatment of severe sepsis and septic shock. *N Engl J Med*. 2001;345(19):1368–1377.

23. McIntyre L, Hebert PC, Wells G, et al, Canadian Critical Care Trials Group. Is a restrictive transfusion strategy safe for resuscitated and critically ill trauma patients? *J Trauma*. 2004;57(3):563–568.

24. Malone DL, Dunne J, Tracey JK, et al. Blood transfusion, independent of shock severity is associated with worse outcome in trauma. *J Trauma*. 2003;54(5):898–905.

25. Carlson AP, Schermer CR, Lu SW. Retrospective evaluation of anemia and transfusion in traumatic brain injury. *J Trauma*. 2006;61:567–571.

26. Napolitano LM, Kurek S, Luchette FA, et al, American College of Critical Care Medicine of the Society of Critical Care Medicine, Eastern Association for the Surgery of Trauma Practice Management Workgroup. Clinical practice guideline: red blood cell transfusion in adult trauma and critical care. *Crit Care Med*. 2009;37:3124–3157.

27. Consensus conference. Fresh-frozen plasma. Indications and risks. *JAMA*. 1985;253:551–553.

28. McVay PA, Toy PTCY. Lack of increased bleeding after paracentesis and thoracentesis in patients with mild coagulation abnormalities. *Transfusion*. 1991;21:164–171.

29. Shanberge JN, Quattrochiocchi-Longe T. Analysis of fresh frozen plasma administration with suggestions for ways to reduce usage. *Transfus Med*. 1992;2:189–194.

30. Gajic O, Dzik WH, Toy P. Fresh frozen plasma and platelet transfusion for nonbleeding patients in the intensive care unit: benefit or harm? *Crit Care Med*. 2006;34(5 suppl):S170–S173.

31. Practice parameter for the use of fresh-frozen plasma, cryoprecipitate, and platelets. Fresh-Frozen Plasma, Cryoprecipitate, and Platelets Administration Practice Guidelines Development Task Force of the College of American Pathologists. *JAMA*. 1994;271:777–781.

32. Ansell, J, Hirsh, J, Hylek, E, et al. Pharmacology and management of the vitamin K antagonists: American

College of Chest Physicians Evidence-Based Clinical Practice Guidelines (8th Edition). *Chest.* 2008;133:160S.

33. Stanworth SJ, Brunskill SJ, Hyde CJ, et al. Is fresh frozen plasma clinically effective? A systematic review of randomized controlled trials. *Br J Haematol.* 2004;126(1):139–152.

34. Holland LL, Brooks JP. Toward rational fresh frozen plasma transfusion: the effect of plasma transfusion on coagulation test results. *Am J Clin Pathol.* 2006;126(1):133–139.

35. Abdel-Wahab OI, Healy B, Dzik WH. Effect of fresh-frozen plasma transfusion on prothrombin time and bleeding in patients with mild coagulation abnormalities. *Transfusion.* 2006;46(8):1279–1285.

36. Doerfler ME, Kaufman B, Goldenberg AS. Central venous catheter placement in patients with disorders of hemostasis. *Chest.* 1996;110:185–188.

37. Cotton BA, Au BK, Nunez TC, et al. Predefined massive transfusion protocols are associated with a reduction in organ failure and postinjury complications. *J Trauma.* 2009;66(1):41–48.

38. Holcomb JB, Wade CE, Michalek JE, et al. Increased plasma and platelet to red blood cell ratios improves outcomes in 466 massively transfused civilian trauma patients. *Ann Surg.* 2008;248(3):447–458.

39. Zink KA, Sambasivan CN, Holcomb JB, et al. A high ratio of plasma and platelets to packed red blood cells in the first 6 hours of massive transfusion improves outcomes in a large multicenter study. *Am J Surg.* 2009;197(5):565–570.

40. Snyder CW, Weinberg JA, McGwin G, et al. The relationship of blood product ratio to mortality: survival benefit or bias? *J Trauma.* 2009;66:358–364.

41. Slichter SJ. Controversies in platelet transfusion therapy. *Annu Rev Med.* 1980;31:509–540.

42. NIH Consensus Conference. Platelet transfusion therapy. *JAMA.* 1987;257:1777–1780.

43. British Committee for Standards in Haematology, Blood Transfusion Task Force. Guidelines for the use of platelet transfusions. *Br J Haematol.* 2003;122:10.

44. Beutler E. Platelet transfusion: the 20,000/ul trigger. *Blood.* 1993;81:1411–1413.

45. Heckman K, Weiner GJ, Strauss RG, et al. Randomized evaluation of the optimal platelet count for prophylactic platelet transfusion in patients undergoing induction therapy for acute leukemia. *Blood.* 1993;82(S1):192a.

46. Harkness DR, Byrnes JJ, Lian EC-Y, et al. Hazard of platelet transfusion in thrombotic thrombocytopenic purpura. *JAMA.* 1981;246:1931.

47. Warkentin TE, Greinacher A, Koster A, et al. Treatment and prevention of heparin-induced thrombocytopenia: American College of Chest Physicians Evidence-Based Clinical Practice Guidelines (8th Edition). *Chest.* 2008;133:340S.

48. Eschbach JW, Egrie IC, Downing MR, et al. Correction of the anemia of end-stage renal disease with recombinant human erythropoietin. *N Engl J Med.* 1987;316:73–79.

49. Rogiers P, Zhang H, Leeman M, et al. Erythropoietin response is blunted in critically ill patients. *Intensive Care Med.* 1997;23(2):159–162.

50. Corwin HL, Gettinger A, Pearl RG, et al. Efficacy of recombinant human erythropoietin in critically ill patients: a randomized controlled trial. *JAMA.* 2002;288(22):2827–2835.

51. Corwin HL, Gettinger A, Fabian TC, et al. Efficacy and safety of epoetin alfa in critically ill patients. *N Engl J Med.* 2007 6;357(10):965–976.

52. Napolitano LM, Fabian TC, Kelly KM, et al. Improved survival of critically ill trauma patients treated with recombinant human erythropoietin. *J Trauma.* 2008;65(2):285–297.

CHAPTER 30

Deep Venous Thrombosis

Amy Tortorich and David R. Gens

▶ INTRODUCTION

In the United States, it is estimated that roughly 100 per 100,000 people per year experience a first-time venous thromboembolism (VTE). Of these cases, two thirds are caused by deep venous thrombosis (DVT).[1] Much literature has been devoted to the occurrence of VTE in hospitalized patients who are ill or recovering from a surgical procedure. However, many patients present as outpatients to the emergency room with symptoms related to their VTE. This chapter focuses on the current practices for evaluation and diagnosis of DVT and hopes to help guide the emergency physician through the current evidence-based clinical practice guidelines for antithrombotic and thrombolytic therapy.[2]

▶ ANATOMY AND PATHOPHYSIOLOGY

Lower extremity DVT is subdivided into proximal (thigh) and distal (calf) vein thrombosis. Proximal DVT is considered of more clinical importance since it is more commonly associated with serious disease and potentially fatal outcomes.

Venous thrombi are composed mainly of fibrin and red blood cells, with the number of platelets and leukocytes being variable. The development, progression, and breakdown of venous thromboemboli reflect a balance between thrombogenic stimuli and protective mechanisms. In the 19th century, Virchow identified and described thrombogenic stimuli. Virchow is credited with outlining the now classic triad of hypercoagulability, endothelial injury, and stasis in association with VTE.[3] The presence of the above factors alters the balance between endogenous fibrinolysis and fibrin formation that contributes to the formation and proliferation of a thrombus.[1] The protective mechanisms against thromboembolic formation are inactivation of activated coagulation factors by circulating inhibitors such as antithrombin and activated protein C, clearance of activated coagulation factors and soluble fibrin polymer complexes by mononuclear phagocytes and the liver, and plasma and endothelial cell–derived fibrinolytic enzyme lysis of fibrin.[4]

Using Virchow's triad as a framework, one can better understand the factors that predispose the development of venous thrombosis and the protective mechanisms that counter thrombogenic stimuli. This allows for a better understanding of the various risk factors and treatments for venous thrombi.

HYPERCOAGULABILITY

The activated clotting factors in blood are regulated by inhibitors on the surface of endothelial cells and circulating antiproteinase. Hypercoagulable states offset the balance and tip the natural clotting cascade in the direction of fibrin production and clot formation. This can be seen as a result of reduced levels of inhibitors or an increase in activated clotting factors. Activation of coagulation may result from the contact of factor XII with collagen on the damaged vessels' exposed subendothelium.[5] Malignant cells contain a cysteine protease that can directly activate factor X. This may be one mechanism by which malignancy can induce thrombosis.[6] Fibrin formation is enhanced by acquired states of hypercoagulability. Genetic thrombophilias and neoplastic abnormalities increase fibrin formation or decrease fibrinolysis.

VASCULAR INJURY

The processes that initiate a venous thrombosis are less certain and felt to be much different from those that initiate an arterial thrombosis. In arterial thrombosis, a clear relationship between blood vessel injury and thrombus formation has been demonstrated. Following the rupture of an atherosclerotic plaque, the endothelial layer of the vessel is lost, exposing subendothelial ligands such as von Willebrand factor (VWF) and collagen. Platelets have specific receptors for these ligands and therefore bind, signaling additional cofactors and initiating thrombin formation.[7,8]

The mechanisms by which damage to the venous vessel wall initiates a thrombus formation are less understood. Gross vessel wall injury does not appear to be a prerequisite for venous thrombi formation. A study of 41 autopsies failed to identify any gross vessel wall injury in 49 of 50 lower extremity thrombi.[9] However, vascular endothelium can be damaged in other ways: endotoxins, inflammatory cytokines, and hypoxia.

Inflammation results in the activation of the endothelium, which leads to the release of granules that contain VWF and membrane-bound P-selectin. The proteins can attach to the endothelial surface as well as bind leukocytes.[7] Leukocytes, in particular monocytes, are able to synthesize tissue factor (TF).[10]

Additionally there are animal data suggesting that TF-bearing microvesicles may participate in DVT formation. In a mouse model, elevated levels of leukocyte-derived microvesicles were shown to be associated with greater thrombus mass.[11] Other studies have demonstrated elevated TF antigen levels and TF–VIIa activity in cancer patients.[12] The increased numbers of TF-bearing microvesicles may play a role in the associated hypercoagulability. This theory is supported by autopsy studies that demonstrated DVT not associated with vessel trauma is frequently bilateral.[23]

Additionally, arterial thrombi cellular composition is different from that of venous thrombi. Platelets compile the core of arterial thrombi and are the cellular components attaching to the vessel wall.[13] Venous thrombi are composed predominantly of fibrin, and they are the fibrin-rich regions of the thrombi found at the sight of attachment to the vessel wall.[9] The lack of platelets found at the site of attachment of a venous thrombus could explain why antiplatelet drugs have had limited efficacy for venous thrombosis.[8]

VENOUS STASIS

Venous stasis leads to an increase in fibrin cross-linking.[14] Contraction of the calf muscles enhances venous return from the lower extremities. Blood is propelled upward, preventing pooling in the legs. Stasis, conversely, leads to a reduction in venous blood flow. Diminished blood flow allows the accumulation of prothrombotic substances (such as thrombin) that otherwise would be washed downstream where they are inactivated. In general, thrombin from the lower extremities is washed into the capillary bed of the lung, which has a large surface area coated with antithrombotic substances.[7]

Venous stasis may also lead to local hypoxia. By allowing stagnation of blood, the hemoglobin in the erythrocytes is desaturated, stimulating hypoxia responses in leukocytes, platelets, and endothelial cells.[15] Hypoxia can lead to local ischemia that has been shown to activate the expression of P-selectin on endothelial cells.[16] It has been proposed that the expression of P-selectin enables the TF-bearing microvesicles to initiate coagulation and thrombosis.[8]

▶ RISK FACTORS

There are numerous risk factors that promote the formation of VTE. The major ones are listed in Table 30-1.[1,17,18] Ethnicity has also been shown to influence the prevalence of VTE. Hispanics and Asians have a lower adjusted risk of VTE than Caucasians and African Americans.[19,20] Advancing age correlates with an increased rate of thromboembolism. An increased occurrence of VTE is observed with each decade over the age of 60.[4] Persons under the age of 15 have an incidence of VTE of less than 5 cases per 100,000. After the age of 80, however, the incidence increases to 500 cases per 100,000.[21,22]

Factor V Leiden is currently recognized as the most common hereditary abnormality predisposing to venous thrombosis. The substitution of glutamine for arginine at residue 506 in the factor V molecule makes factor V resistant to proteolysis by activated protein C.[4] The gene mutation follows autosomal dominant inheritance and is more prevalent in Caucasians.[23] A patient who is homozygous for the factor V Leiden mutation has a marked increase risk of thromboembolism (estimated 80-fold increase risk) and presents at an earlier age than those who are heterozygous.[24] Figure 30-1 shows the coagulation pathway and where circulating inhibitors function to protect against thromboembolic formation. Deficiency in circulating inhibitors leads to increased thrombus formation.

▶ **TABLE 30-1. RISK FACTORS FOR VENOUS THROMBOEMBOLISM**

Patient-specific factors
Prior episode of venous thromboembolism
Increasing age
Obesity
Increased estrogen states (pregnancy or puerperium, oral contraceptive pills, hormonal therapy)
Immobility (paralysis, travel, hospital or nursing home resident)
Inherited thrombophilia
Factor V Leiden mutation
Prothrombin gene mutation
Protein S deficiency
Protein C deficiency
Antithrombin (AT) deficiency
Hyperhomocysteinemia
Medical conditions
Stroke
Congestive heart failure
Chronic obstructive pulmonary disease
Neuromuscular weakness syndromes (e.g., Guillain–Barré)
Myocardial infarction
Burns
Malignancy (higher risk during chemotherapy and radiotherapy)
Medications: tamoxifen, bevacizumab, thalidomide, lenalidomide
Lupus anticoagulants/antiphospholipid antibody syndrome
Surgery
Major surgery: abdominal, gynecologic, urologic, orthopedic, neurosurgery
Cancer-related surgery
Trauma
Multisystem trauma
Fractures of the hip and pelvis
Major fracture
Spinal cord injury
Spinal fracture
Other
Indwelling central venous catheter
Prolonged mechanical ventilation
Consumptive coagulopathy
Heparin-induced thrombocytopenia

▶ DIAGNOSIS

CLINICAL PRESENTATION

The initial symptoms of a DVT are variable and largely nonspecific: cramping, a sense of fullness, paresthesia, or pain in the thigh or calf. A physical examination may reveal unilateral swelling, erythema or discoloration, and warmth of the affected extremity; tenderness to palpation; dilation of superficial collateral veins; and a palpable venous cord. The classic Homan's sign (sharp pain in the calf or posterior aspect of the knee on passive dorsiflexion of the foot) is insensitive and nonspecific.[25] A patient with minor signs and symptoms may have extensive DVT, while someone with severe leg pain and swelling may not have a DVT demonstrated by objective testing. Clinical examination is correct only about 50% of the time.

The subtle and nonspecific presentation of a DVT can make it difficult to clinically differentiate the diagnosis from a broad differential diagnosis. Thus, objective testing is needed to confirm or exclude the diagnosis of DVT. Several objective tests are available for establishing the diagnosis of DVT.

▶ OBJECTIVE TESTING

D-DIMER

D-dimer (DD) units are produced as the fibrinolytic system degrades cross-linked fibrin. They are generated by the action of factor XIIIa on fibrin monomers and polymers. Monoclonal antibodies in DD assays recognize the fragments from cross-linked fibrin. A small percentage of plasma fibrinogen is physiologically converted to fibrin and then degraded. Thus, small amounts of DD are present in healthy individuals. However, increased concentrations are seen in conditions in which fibrin formation is enhanced and subsequently degraded by plasmin. On average, the plasma level is increased 8-fold in VTE and, moreover, the level falls in parallel with symptom duration and the start of anticoagulant treatment.[26] The plasma half-life is approximately 8 hours and DD fragments are cleared by the kidney and reticuloendothelial system.[27]

The detection of the monoclonal antibody–DD fragment complexes is performed by various techniques: enzyme-linked immunosorbent assay (ELISA), immunofiltration, and sandwich-type or agglutination techniques. Describing the various commercial DD assays is beyond the scope of this text. Each diagnostic system has its own cutoff levels. Clinicians should be knowledgeable of the specific test their facility uses and, furthermore, should only use DD assays that have been appropriately validated in prospective outcome studies.[27]

A number of clinical conditions increase DD levels: infection, inflammation, cancer, surgery, trauma, extensive burns or bruises, ischemic heart disease, stroke, peripheral artery disease, ruptured aneurysm or aortic dissection, pregnancy, and cerebral sinus thrombosis.[26] The diagnostic yield of DD is lower in the elderly as the concentrations of DD rise in the normal aging population. In a cost-effectiveness analysis of a single study of 1,029 patients, one group of investigators demonstrated using DD was cost-saving until the age of 79.[28]

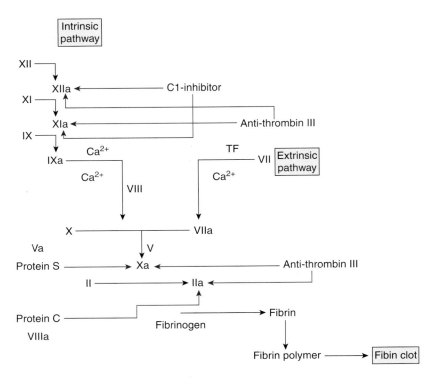

Figure 30–1. Blood coagulation cascade. Black arrows indicate procoagulant property of a substance. Red arrows indicate coagulation-inhibiting property of a substance. Deficiency in coagulation-inhibiting factors enhances coagulation. Ca^{2+}, calcium; TF, tissue factor; a, activated.

The objective diagnostic imaging tests currently most useful in diagnosing patients with clinically suspected DVT are ultrasound (US) imaging and venography. Both have been validated through clinical trials that include prospective studies with long-term follow-up establishing the safety of withholding anticoagulation treatment in patients with negative results.

ULTRASOUND

Venous US has become the standard diagnostic test in patients with a suspected DVT. The two common methods of US used in assessing the presence of DVT are compression US and duplex.

A 2005 meta-analysis examined the diagnostic accuracy of US for DVT as well as performed a separate analysis of different US techniques: (1) compression US only; (2) color Doppler only; (3) continuous wave Doppler only; (4) duplex (combined compression and color Doppler US); (5) triplex (combined compression, color Doppler, and continuous wave Doppler US).[29] This study determined diagnostic accuracy varies according to the technique used. Optimal sensitivity was demonstrated by using duplex or triplex US. Optimal specificity was seen by using compression

US alone. The authors conclude that compression US alone is probably the appropriate technique for patients with a low probability of DVT, whereas duplex or triplex US would be the appropriate technique when evaluating patients at high risk for DVT or to identify distal DVT.

In compression US, evaluating for a venous thrombosis consists of determining vein patency or the lack thereof (Figure 30-2). To determine venous patency, the gold standard is to determine if the vein collapses completely under pressure, which is directly visualized with US when the lumen disappears entirely (Figures 30-3 and 30-4). Continuous wave Doppler also evaluates blood flow and direction, but as a graphic depiction.[31]

A duplex US combines color Doppler with compression US. The color Doppler represents flow within a vein. The specific color maps are assigned to a variety of speeds and one of two directions (toward or away from the US transducer).[31]

Augmentation is a technique to confirm blood flow through a section of an extremity. It utilizes either pulsed wave or color Doppler. While evaluating the proximal portion of a venous segment (e.g., the common femoral vein), the sonographer squeezes the calf that sends a rush of venous blood past the transducer. The increased

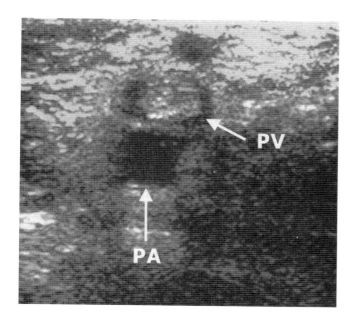

Figure 30–2. An echogenic thrombus can be seen within the popliteal vein. PV, popliteal vein; PA, popliteal artery. (Reproduced with permission from Ref.[30], second edition, Chapter 15, p. 390, Figure 15-33.)

blood flow is seen on Doppler that is thought to indicate the absence of a completely occlusive thrombus. Patients with venous disease and other comorbidities may lack positive augmentation. Additionally, a partially occluding thrombus or previously established collaterals may still show augmentation.[32]

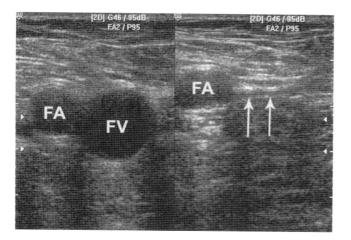

Figure 30–3. A split screen showing the common femoral artery (FA) and common femoral vein (FV). The left is without compression. The right is the view after pressure has been applied with the transducer causing the femoral vein to collapse with its wall barely visible (arrows). (Reproduced with permission from Ref.[30], second edition, Chapter 15, p. 382, Figure 15-13.)

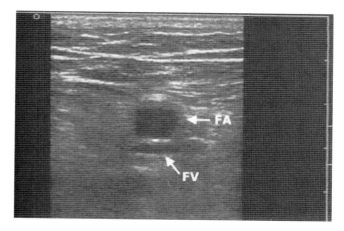

Figure 30–4. Incomplete collapse of the femoral vein. If adequate pressure has been applied, this view indicates a thrombus is likely present within the femoral vein. FV, femoral vein; FA, femoral artery. (Reproduced with permission from Ref.[30], second edition, Chapter 15, p. 383, Figure 15-17.)

EMERGENCY PHYSICIANS' ROLE IN US DIAGNOSIS OF DVT

The utilization of the bedside US examination by emergency physicians has evolved from a clinical need to improve efficiency of patient care. Many hospitals do not have vascular laboratory services available during off-hours. This limited availability has resulted in some emergency physicians developing the practice of administering empirical treatment to those patients who are suspected of having a DVT. The patient is then discharged home to return the next day for a formal study. Empirical treatment with anticoagulation involves risk, particularly for patients in whom anticoagulation is problematic. Studies have shown that emergency physicians performing US examinations of the lower extremities themselves decrease time to patient disposition.[33] Extensive training is not required. Emergency medicine residents have been shown to be able to perform a limited duplex examination with good accuracy after very limited instruction (90 minutes).[34] The increased ability of emergency physicians to perform a bedside US examination will hopefully decrease the practice of empirical treatment with anticoagulation and serve to help discharge patients more quickly who can then obtain a follow-up study as an outpatient.

CT VENOGRAPHY

Using computed tomography (CT) to diagnosis DVT is an area under active investigation. One such example is the PIOPED II study. This prospective multicenter study of 711 patients compared the clinical value of

CT venography (CTV) after multidetector CT (MDCT) angiography (CTA) with venous compression sonography for the diagnosis of VTE.[35] The investigators demonstrated a 95.5% concordance between CTV and sonography for the diagnosis or exclusion of DVT. They conclude both studies yield equivalent diagnostic results and the choice of imaging techniques should be made on the basis of safety, expense, and time constraints.

Protocols to image the pulmonary arteries and the subdiaphragmatic deep veins (including the legs) should ideally require no additional contrast medium beyond that which is already required for a CT pulmonary angiogram. Yet, not all patients being evaluated for a DVT require a CT pulmonary angiogram. Utilizing CT solely to evaluate for DVT exposes the patient to a radiation dose, potential nephrotoxic intravenous (IV) contrast, and the expense of CT.

MR VENOGRAPHY

The diagnostic accuracy of magnetic resonance (MR) venography is comparable to that of contrast venography (CV), yet outcome data are lacking. Additionally, the high cost of MR venography is a limitation for widespread use. Unlike US, MR imaging (MRI) is able to image the pelvic vasculature and vena cava. MRI does not require the use of ionizing radiation, which makes it an attractive option for certain patient populations such as pregnant patients with suspected VTE.

A prospective single-center study of 24 randomly selected patients compared true fast imaging with steady-state precession (FISP) MR venography for suspected DVT with contrast agent–enhanced venography.[36] The authors conclude that MR venography for DVT is sensitive and specific in the pelvis and thigh, but has poor sensitivity below the popliteal vein. Additionally, 11 of the 14 patients without DVT had an alternative diagnosis suggested by MR venography: muscle tear, chronic venous insufficiency secondary to previous DVT, edema, and subcutaneous (SC) fat/fluid artifact related to clinically confirmed congestive cardiac failure or cellulitis. The ability of MR to provide an alternative diagnosis is an added benefit. MR has some disadvantages: transport of a very sick critical care patient to MR can be difficult, some ventilators are not compatible with MR, and an awake patient may suffer from claustrophobia.

CONTRAST VENOGRAPHY

CV had long been considered the diagnostic test of choice for DVT. However, due to patient discomfort and difficulty in obtaining an adequate study, venography is not recommended as the initial screening test. Noninvasive tests demonstrating equivalent diagnostic accuracy have significantly reduced venography use. Venography is currently reserved for situations in which noninvasive testing is nondiagnostic or impossible to perform. For a CV study to be adequate, complete visualization of the deep venous system (from the calf to the pelvic veins and the inferior vena cava [IVC]) must be obtained[37]: the internal iliac venous system (hypogastric veins) will not be visualized unless a catheter is directed up into this system. A constant intraluminal filling defect present in two or more views is the most reliable criterion in diagnosing an acute DVT.[38]

▶ ADDITIONAL SOURCES OF VENOTHROMBOEMBOLISM

UPPER EXTREMITY DVT

Although the majority of DVTs occur in the lower extremities, upper extremity (UE) thrombi are becoming more common than previously thought. There are two forms of UE DVT: (1) effort thrombosis and (2) secondary thrombosis.

Effort thrombosis (Paget–von Schrötter syndrome) is due to an underlying chronic venous compression caused by musculoskeletal variations of the thoracic outlet. The subclavian vein can be compressed by a cervical rib or hypertrophied cervical muscles in the athlete (especially in the weight lifter) during Valsalva maneuver (hence "effort" thrombosis): the sudden stasis of blood leads to thrombosis.

In secondary thrombosis, the increased incidence of UE DVT is most likely a result of increased utilization of central venous catheters, pacemaker wires, and an increase in treated malignancy.[31] UE DVTs involve the subclavian, axillary, or brachial veins. Clinical manifestations are similar to those seen in lower extremity DVT and include edema; dilated collateral veins over the arm, neck, or chest; limb pain and discoloration. Pulmonary embolism (PE), recurrent UE DVT, and rarely postthrombotic (phlebitic) syndrome (PTS) of the arms are all potential complications of UE DVTs.[2]

MAY–THURNER SYNDROME

May–Thurner syndrome is an anatomic pattern in which hemodynamically significant compression of the left common iliac vein occurs between the overlying right common iliac artery and the underlying vertebral body. Most commonly it is seen in women, between the ages of 20 and 50. Typically it presents as either chronic venous insufficiency or a large iliofemoral DVT. The diagnosis should be considered in patients with recurrent left lower extremity DVT or chronic, refractory DVT of the left lower extremity. DVT episodes associated with May–Thurner syndrome can be recurrent and/or not respond to treatment with anticoagulation by itself. Treatment can require catheter-directed thrombolysis (CDT), venous angioplasty, and/or intravascular stenting.[39]

PHLEGMASIA CERULEA DOLENS

Phlegmasia cerulea dolens is an uncommon form of massive proximal (iliofemoral) venous thrombosis of the lower extremities. Venous obstruction results leading to a sharp rise in venous pressure, massive interstitial fluid shifts, decreased arterial perfusion due to vasospasm from inflammation, compartment syndrome, and gangrene.[1] This results in a lower extremity that is tense, cool, swollen, painful, and cyanotic (Figure 30-5).[40] The resulting gangrene, compartment syndrome, and arterial compromise can lead to circulatory collapse and

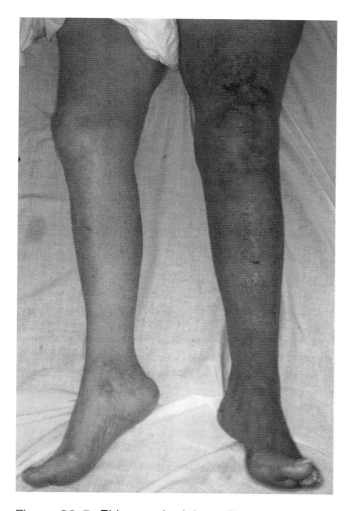

Figure 30–5. Phlegmasia dolens. The left leg is noted to have a bluish discoloration and swelling. (Reproduced with permission from Ref.[40], second edition, Chapter 12, p. 370, Figure 12-29.)

shock. Systemic anticoagulation should not be delayed as death or loss of the limb may result. IV thrombolytic therapy's role in treatment is controversial. Emergency thrombectomy should be considered.

▶ TREATMENT

The American College of Chest Physicians (ACCP) published their first consensus statement on antithrombotic therapy in 1986. The most recent ACCP guidelines were released in 2008. This section aims to summarize the 2008 ACCP guidelines on therapy for VTE with regards to their application to patients seen by the emergency medicine physician. Unless otherwise referenced, all recommendations are from the 8th Edition *ACCP Evidence-Based Clinical Practice Guidelines.*[2]

Briefly, before considering the use of anticoagulant therapy, one must consider if the patient has any contraindications to anticoagulation. The absolute contraindications to anticoagulation treatment include severe active bleeding; intracranial bleeding; recent brain, eye, or spinal cord surgery; and malignant hypertension. Relative contraindications include recent cerebrovascular accident, active gastrointestinal tract bleeding, recent major surgery, severe hypertension, severe renal or hepatic failure, and severe thrombocytopenia (platelets less than 50,000/μL).[4]

INITIAL ANTICOAGULATION OF ACUTE DVT OF THE LEG

The main therapy of acute DVT of the leg is anticoagulation. Initial treatment of this disease aims to prevent thrombus extension as well as early and late recurrences of VTE. As patients treated with vitamin K antagonist (VKA) alone have a high rate of recurrence/extension, it is recommended that heparin (or low-molecular-weight heparin [LMWH] or fondaparinux) is started along with VKA at the time of diagnosis.[41] For patients with objectively confirmed DVT, the guidelines recommend five options for the initial treatment of DVT: (1) SC LMWH without monitoring; (2) IV unfractionated heparin (UFH) with monitoring; (3) SC UFH with monitoring; (4) weight-based SC UFH without monitoring; and (5) SC fondaparinux without monitoring. All options were given a Grade 1A recommendation. Additionally, if there is a high clinical suspicion for DVT or a delay before diagnostic testing can be performed, the guidelines recommend treatment with anticoagulants should begin before testing (Grade 1C). The initial treatment with LMWH, UFH, or fondaparinux should continue for at least 5 days and until the international normalized ratio (INR) is ≥2.0 for 24 hours (Grade 1C). This recommendation is based on the observation that, regardless of the INR, factor II activity is not significantly reduced earlier than 5 days after starting warfarin. The combination of a relatively long half-life of factor II and the short half-life of protein C and protein S is thought to provoke a paradoxical hypercoagulable state if heparin/LMWH/fondaparinux is stopped prematurely.[41]. The initiation of VKA should not be delayed but instead initiated together with LMWH, UFH, or fondaparinux on the first treatment day (Grade 1A). Warfarin can typically be started at a dose of 10 mg in young (less than 60 years), healthy patients and at a dose of 5 mg in older patients and those being hospitalized. The dose of VKA is adjusted to maintain a target INR of 2.5 (range 2.0–3.0) (Grade 1A).

Low-Molecular-Weight Heparin

The guidelines prefer SC LMWH to treatment with IV UFH. They recommend initial treatment with SC LMWH once or twice daily, as an outpatient if possible (Grade 1C), or as an inpatient if necessary (Grade 1A) over treatment with IV UFH. They recommend against routine monitoring with anti–factor Xa level measurements (Grade 1A). However, as LMWH is cleared by the kidneys, in patients with severe renal failure, UFH over LMWH is suggested (Grade 2C).

IV Unfractionated Heparin

The guidelines recommend an initial IV bolus (80 U/kg or 5,000 U), followed by a continuous infusion (initially at a dose of 18 U/kg/h or 1,300 U/h). The dose is then adjusted to achieve and maintain an APPT prolongation that corresponds to therapeutic heparin levels.

SC Unfractionated Heparin

If monitored SC UFH is chosen, the guidelines recommend an initial dose of 17,500 U, or a weight-adjusted dose of approximately 250U/kg bid. The dose is then adjusted to achieve and maintain an activated partial thromboplastin time (APTT) prolongation corresponding to therapeutic heparin levels (Grade 1C).

If fixed-dose unmonitored SC UFH is selected, the guidelines recommend an initial dose of 333 U/kg followed by a twice-daily dose of 250 U/kg instead of nonweight-based dosing (Grade 1C).

Fondaparinux

Fondaparinux is a synthetic pentasaccharide. Like LMWH, it can be administered SC without monitoring and has been shown to be effective in the treatment of acute DVT (Grade 1A). The disadvantage of fondaparinux is a prolonged half-life (17 hours) and the absence of an antidote.

TREATMENT STRATEGIES OF THROMBUS REMOVAL FOR ACUTE DVT

Actively removing the thrombi has the potential to decrease acute symptoms and the risk for PTS, and can be limb-saving in phlegmasia cerulea dolens. By removing the thrombus, venous obstruction is reversed and valvular function is restored that may prevent late development of venous valvular incompetence. The guidelines further speculate that thrombus removal and subsequent relief of venous obstruction may reduce the risk of recurrent VTE.

Catheter-Directed Thrombolysis

The guidelines state CDT may be beneficial in select patients: those with symptoms present for less than 14 days, iliofemoral DVT, life expectancy ≥1 year, and good functional status demonstrate a low risk of bleeding. They suggest CT can be utilized to reduce acute symptoms and postthrombotic morbidity at institutions with the appropriate expertise and resources available (Grade 2B). Following successful CDT, the guidelines suggest utilizing balloon angioplasty and stents to correct underlying venous lesions (Grade 2C). If expertise and resources are available, pharmacomechanical thrombolysis (e.g., with inclusion of thrombus fragmentation and/or aspiration) is preferred to CDT alone as it shortens treatment time (Grade 2C). Patients who have undergone successful CDT are still recommended the same intensity and duration of anticoagulant therapy as recommended for those patients who do not receive CDT (Grade 1C).

Systemic Thrombolytic Therapy

For patients with a low risk of bleeding, extensive proximal DVT, symptoms present for less than 14 days, life expectancy ≥1 year, and a good functional status, the guidelines suggest if CDT is not available, systemic thrombolytic therapy may be used to reduce acute symptoms and postthrombotic morbidity (Grade 2C).

Operative Venous Thrombectomy

Operative venous thrombectomy is typically reserved for iliofemoral DVT. For patients with acute iliofemoral DVT, good functional status, life expectancy ≥1 year, and symptoms present for less than 7 days, the guidelines suggest operative venous thrombectomy to decrease acute symptoms as well as postthrombotic morbidity at institutions with appropriate expertise and resources (Grade 2B). However, if patients do not have a high risk of bleeding, the guidelines suggest that CDT is generally preferable to operative venous thrombectomy (Grade 2C). After undergoing operative venous thrombectomy, the guidelines recommend the same intensity and duration of anticoagulant therapy as for those not undergoing venous thrombectomy (Grade 1C).

VENA CAVAL FILTERS FOR THE PATIENT WITH A DVT

The placement of an IVC filter is not without risk. IVC thrombosis can occur in up to 5% of patients after placement of the filter.[40] Currently, no randomized trial has evaluated the efficacy of IVC filters alone (without concurrent anticoagulation) in preventing PE in those with an acute DVT. The guidelines differentiate their recommendations for vena cava filter placement based on the ability to utilize anticoagulation. They recommend against the routine use of a vena cava filter in addition to anticoagulants (Grade 1A). For patients with VTE who cannot receive anticoagulation due to a risk of bleeding, the placement of an IVC filter is recommended (Grade 1C). In addition, for those patients in whom an IVC filter was inserted as an alternative to anticoagulation, the guidelines recommend that that they should subsequently be given a standard course of anticoagulant therapy if their risk of bleeding resolved (Grade 1C).

DURATION OF ANTICOAGULANT THERAPY

In determining the duration of anticoagulant therapy, the ACCP guidelines differentiate acute episode of VTE provoked by a reversible risk factor from those episodes of VTE that are unprovoked (idiopathic VTE). Reversible provoking risk factors include major factors such as surgery, hospitalization, or plaster case immobilization, all within 1 month; and minor factors such as estrogen therapy, pregnancy, prolonged travel (>8 hours), or the previously noted major factors if their occurrence was 1–3 months prior to the diagnosis of VTE. Additional factors considered were if the DVT was confined to the distal veins (isolated calf DVT) and whether the DVT was a first episode of VTE.

- For patients with a DVT secondary to a transient (reversible) risk factor, the recommended treatment is with a VKA for 3 months over treatment for shorter periods (Grade 1A).
- For patients with an unprovoked DVT, the recommended treatment is with a VKA for at least

3 months (Grade 1A). The guidelines further recommend that all patients with unprovoked DVT be evaluated for the risk-to-benefit ratio of long-term therapy (Grade 1C). Long-term treatment is recommended for those patients who have a first unprovoked VTE that is a proximal DVT, do not have risk factors for bleeding, and can adhere to good anticoagulant monitoring (Grade 1A). Long-term treatment is also recommended for patients with a second episode of unprovoked DVT (Grade 2B).

- For patients with DVT and cancer, LMWH is recommended for the first 3–6 months of long-term anticoagulation (Grade 1A). Subsequent anticoagulant therapy with VKA or LMWH is recommended indefinitely or until the cancer has resolved (Grade 1C).
- In those patients who are receiving long-term anticoagulation therapy, the risk-to-benefit ratio of continuing treatment for the individual patient should be reassessed at periodic intervals (Grade 1C).
- In patients who are unexpectedly found to have an asymptomatic DVT, the same initial and long-term anticoagulation is recommended as that for comparable patients with a symptomatic DVT (Grade 1C).

INTENSITY OF ANTICOAGULANT EFFECT

- The guidelines recommend that the dose of VKA should be adjusted to maintain a target INR of 2.5 (range 2.0–3.0) for all durations of treatment (Grade 1A).
- The guidelines recommend against high-intensity VKA therapy (INR range 3.1–4.0) in comparison to an INR range of 2.0–3.0 (Grade 1A).

TREATMENT OF ACUTE UE DVT

Patients with acute UE DVT are recommended the same initial treatment with therapeutic doses of LMWH, UFH, or fondaparinux as described for lower extremity DVT. The recommendation is against the routine use of systemic or catheter-directed thrombolytic therapy for the majority of patients with acute UE DVT (Grade 1C). In select patients with acute UE DVT (recent onset of severe symptoms and a low risk of bleeding), the recommendations do suggest that CDT may be used for initial treatment if available expertise and resources are present (Grade 2C). The majority of patients with acute UE DVT are recommended against the routine use of surgical thrombectomy, transluminal angioplasty, catheter extraction, stent placement, staged approach to lysis followed by interventional or surgical procedure, or superior vena cava (SVC) filter placement (Grade 1C).

However, in select patients (having a primary UE DVT, failing anticoagulant or thrombolytic treatment, and having severe persistent symptoms), the above interventions are recommended if available (Grade 2C). In patients with acute UE DVT, the placement of an SVC filter is suggested when anticoagulant treatment is contraindicated and clear evidence of DVT progression or clinically significant PE is present (Grade 2C). The recommended treatment for an acute UE DVT is VKA for ≥3 months (Grade 1C). For a UE DVT that is associated with an indwelling central venous catheter, the guidelines recommend against catheter removal if it is functional and an ongoing need for the catheter is present (Grade 2C). If a UE DVT is associated with an indwelling catheter that has been removed, the guidelines recommend against shortening the duration of long-term anticoagulant treatment to less than 3 months (Grade 2C).

HOME VERSUS IN-PATIENT TREATMENT FOR DVT

A recent *Cochrane* review concluded home management is both cost-effective and preferred by patients.[42] Six randomized controlled trials (RCTs) involving 1,708 patients compared home (LMWH) with hospital (LMWH or UFH) treatment for DVT. Patients treated at home with LMWH were less likely to have recurrence of VTE, and had lower mortality and fewer major bleeds. However, the home treatment patients were more likely to have minor bleeding than those treated in the hospital.

► POSTTHROMBOTIC SYNDROME

The PTS is a frequent complication of DVT. Patients complain of pain, swelling, heaviness, cramps, and itching or tingling of the affected leg. Ulcerations can occur. Standing and walking usually aggravate symptoms, whereas rest and elevation of the leg improve symptoms. Ipsilateral recurrent venous thrombosis is strongly associated with subsequent development of moderate or severe postthrombotic symptoms.[43] Therefore, prevention of recurrent thrombi likely reduces PTS. Utilization of a properly fitted compression stocking at the time of diagnosis and continued for at least 2 years can be effective in the reduction of postthrombotic symptoms.[44] Stockings that are fitted to the patient with a specific pressure gradient may be prescribed.

► APPENDIX

The grading system used in the *ACCP Evidence-Based Clinical Practice Guidelines* (8th Edition) are as follows: Grade 1 recommendations are strong, indicating the benefits do or do not outweigh risks, burden,

and cost. Grade 2 recommendations are weaker and made when there is less certainty regarding the magnitude of the benefits, risks, burden, and cost. With a Grade 2 recommendation, individual patient values and preferences may become more important. An A, B, or C label is also given to all recommendations signifying the quality of evidence on which a given recommendation is based: A is the highest quality (e.g., multiple, well-designed RCTs with concordant results); B is of intermediate quality (e.g., one RCT or multiple trials without concordant results); and C is the lowest quality (e.g., small, observational study with significant potential for selection or reporting bias).[45]

REFERENCES

1. Fields JM, Goyal M. Venothromboembolism. *Emerg Med Clin North Am.* 2008;26:649–683, viii.
2. Kearon C, Kahn SR, Agnelli G, et al. Antithrombotic therapy for venous thromboembolic disease: American College of Chest Physicians Evidence-Based Clinical Practice Guidelines (8th Edition). *Chest.* 2008;133:454S–545S.
3. Virchow R. *Gesammalte abhandlungen zur wissenschaftlichen medtzin.* Frankfurt: Medinger Sohn & Company; 1856.
4. Lichtman MA, Williams WJ, Beutler E, et al. *Williams Hematology.* New York: McGraw-Hill Professional; 2005.
5. Merli GJ. Pathophysiology of venous thrombosis, thrombophilia, and the diagnosis of deep vein thrombosis-pulmonary embolism in the elderly. *Clin Geriatr Med.* 2006;22:75–92, viii–ix.
6. Gordon SG, Franks JJ, Lewis B. Cancer procoagulant A: a factor X activating procoagulant from malignant tissue. *Thromb Res.* 1975;6:127–137.
7. Lopez JA, Chen J. Pathophysiology of venous thrombosis. *Thromb Res.* 2009;123(suppl 4):S30–S34.
8. Lopez JA, Kearon C, Lee AY. Deep venous thrombosis. *Hematology (Am Soc Hematol Educ Program).* 2004: 439–456.
9. Sevitt S. The structure and growth of valve-pocket thrombi in femoral veins. *J Clin Pathol.* 1974;27:517–528.
10. Osterud B, Bjorklid E. The tissue factor pathway in disseminated intravascular coagulation. *Semin Thromb Hemost.* 2001;27:605–617.
11. Myers DD, Hawley AE, Farris DM, et al. P-selectin and leukocyte microparticles are associated with venous thrombogenesis. *J Vasc Surg.* 2003;38:1075–1089.
12. Rao LV. Tissue factor as a tumor procoagulant. *Cancer Metastasis Rev.* 1992;11:249–266.
13. Friedman MH, Brinkman AM, Qin JJ, et al. Relation between coronary artery geometry and the distribution of early sudanophilic lesions. *Atherosclerosis.* 1993;98: 193–199.
14. Bockenstedt P. D-dimer in venous thromboembolism. *N Engl J Med.* 2003;349:1203–1204.
15. Ogawa S, Gerlach H, Esposito C, et al. Hypoxia modulates the barrier and coagulant function of cultured

bovine endothelium. Increased monolayer permeability and induction of procoagulant properties. *J Clin Invest.* 1990;85:1090–1098.

16. Closse C, Seigneur M, Renard M, et al. Influence of hypoxia and hypoxia–reoxygenation on endothelial P-selectin expression. *Thromb Res.* 1997;85:159–164.

17. Bongard FS, Sue DY, Vintch JRE. *Current Diagnosis & Treatment: Critical Care.* New York: 3rd ed. McGraw-Hill; 2008:640.

18. Marino PL, Sutin KM. *The ICU Book.* Philadelphia: Williams & Wilkins; 2006:82.

19. White RH. The epidemiology of venous thromboembolism. *Circulation.* 2003;107:I4–I8.

20. Klatsky AL, Armstrong MA, Poggi J. Risk of pulmonary embolism and/or deep venous thrombosis in Asian-Americans. *Am J Cardiol.* 2000;85:1334–1337.

21. Anderson FA Jr, Wheeler HB, Goldberg RJ, et al. A population-based perspective of the hospital incidence and case-fatality rates of deep vein thrombosis and pulmonary embolism. The Worcester DVT Study. *Arch Intern Med.* 1991;151:933–938.

22. Silverstein MD, Heit JA, Mohr DN, et al. Trends in the incidence of deep vein thrombosis and pulmonary embolism: a 25-year population-based study. *Arch Intern Med.* 1998;158:585–593.

23. Mazza JJ. Hypercoagulability and venous thromboembolism: a review. *WMJ.* 2004;103:41–49.

24. Rosendaal FR, Koster T, Vandenbroucke JP, et al. High risk of thrombosis in patients homozygous for factor V Leiden (activated protein C resistance). *Blood.* 1995; 85:1504–1508.

25. Vaccaro P, Van Aman M, Miller S, et al. Shortcomings of physical examination and impedance plethysmography in the diagnosis of lower extremity deep venous thrombosis. *Angiology.* 1987;38:232–235.

26. Righini M, Perrier A, De Moerloose P, et al. D-dimer for venous thromboembolism diagnosis: 20 years later. *J Thromb Haemost.* 2008;6:1059–1071.

27. Hager K, Platt D. Fibrin degeneration product concentrations (D-dimers) in the course of ageing. *Gerontology.* 1995;41:159–165.

28. Righini M, Nendaz M, Le Gal G, et al. Influence of age on the cost-effectiveness of diagnostic strategies for suspected pulmonary embolism. *J Thromb Haemost.* 2007;5:1869–1877.

29. Goodacre S, Sampson F, Thomas S, et al. Systematic review and meta-analysis of the diagnostic accuracy of ultrasonography for deep vein thrombosis. *BMC Med Imaging.* 2005;5:6.

30. Blaivas M. Deep venous thrombosis. In: Ma OJ, Mateer JR, Blaivas M, eds. *Emergency Ultrasound.* 2nd ed, New York: McGraw-Hill Publishing; 2007:373–391.

31. Blaivas M. Ultrasound in the detection of venous thromboembolism. *Crit Care Med.* 2007;35:S224–S234.

32. Blaivas M, Lambert MJ, Harwood RA, et al. Lower-extremity Doppler for deep venous thrombosis—can emergency physicians be accurate and fast? *Acad Emerg Med.* 2000;7:120–126.

33. Theodoro D, Blaivas M, Duggal S, et al. Real-time B-mode ultrasound in the ED saves time in the diagnosis of deep vein thrombosis (DVT). *Am J Emerg Med.* 2004;22:197–200.

34. Jacoby J, Cesta M, Axelband J, et al. Can emergency medicine residents detect acute deep venous thrombosis with a limited, two-site ultrasound examination? *J Emerg Med.* 2007;32:197–200.

35. Goodman LR, Stein PD, Matta F, et al. CT venography and compression sonography are diagnostically equivalent: data from PIOPED II. *AJR Am J Roentgenol.* 2007;189:1071–1076.

36. Cantwell CP, Cradock A, Bruzzi J, et al. MR venography with true fast imaging with steady-state precession for suspected lower-limb deep vein thrombosis. *J Vasc Interv Radiol.* 2006;17:1763–1769.

37. Tapson VF, Carroll BA, Davidson BL, et al. The diagnostic approach to acute venous thromboembolism. Clinical practice guideline. American Thoracic Society. *Am J Respir Crit Care Med.* 1999;160:1043–1066.

38. Rabinov K, Paulin S. Roentgen diagnosis of venous thrombosis in the leg. *Arch Surg.* 1972;104:134–144.

39. Fazel R, Froehlich JB, Williams DM, et al. Clinical problem-solving. A sinister development—a 35-year-old woman presented to the emergency department with a 2-day history of progressive swelling and pain in her left leg, without antecedent trauma. *N Engl J Med.* 2007;357:53–59.

40. Suner S, Savitt D. Extremity conditions. In: Knoop KJ, Stack LB, Storrow AB, eds. *Atlas of Emergency Medicine.* 2nd ed. New York: McGraw-Hill Professional; 2002:370.

41. Houman Fekrazad M, Lopes RD, Stashenko GJ, et al. Treatment of venous thromboembolism: guidelines translated for the clinician. *J Thromb Thrombolysis.* 2009;28:270–275.

42. Othieno R, Abu Affan M, Okpo E. Home versus inpatient treatment for deep vein thrombosis. *Cochrane Database Syst Rev.* 2007;(3):CD003076.

43. Prandoni P, Lensing AW, Cogo A, et al. The long-term clinical course of acute deep venous thrombosis. *Ann Intern Med.* 1996;125:1–7.

44. Brandjes DP, Buller HR, Heijboer H, et al. Randomised trial of effect of compression stockings in patients with symptomatic proximal-vein thrombosis. *Lancet.* 1997;349:759–762.

45. Schunemann HJ, Cook D, Guyatt G. Methodology for antithrombotic and thrombolytic therapy guideline development: American College of Chest Physicians Evidence-Based Clinical Practice Guidelines (8th Edition). *Chest.* 2008;133:113S–122S.

CHAPTER 31

Hyperglycemic Emergency

Grace S. Lee and Shyoko Honiden

► INTRODUCTION

Diabetic ketoacidosis (DKA) and hyperosmolar hyperglycemic state (HHS) encompass two severe complications of diabetes mellitus (DM). The incidence is increasing in the United States, with 120,000 hospitalizations for DKA in 2005, which was a 20% increase compared with 2000.[1] Of the hospitalizations for DKA in 2005, 72% were 44 years old or younger, 21% were between 45 and 64 years old, and <1% were 65 years old or older.[1] Although the rate of hospitalizations for DKA continues to rise, mortality from DKA has been declining, and in 2005 mortality was 0.8 deaths per 100,000.[1] HHS, on the other hand, has a lower rate of hospitalization but a higher mortality at a rate of 5–20%.[2,3] The cost of DKA is profound and the aggregate cost of its hospitalizations is approximately $850 million.[4]

► DEFINITION OF DKA AND HHS

DKA is defined by the following criteria (Table 31-1): plasma glucose >250 mg/dL, arterial pH ≤7.30, serum bicarbonate ≤18 mEq/L, presence of urinary and serum ketones, and an anion gap >10 mEq/L.[2] It is further divided into mild, moderate, and severe based on the degree of acidemia that corresponds to an arterial pH of 7.25–7.30, 7.00 to <7.24, and <7.00, respectively, or a serum bicarbonate level of 15–18, 10 to <15, and <10 mEq/L, respectively.[2] HHS is defined by the following criteria: plasma glucose >600 mg/dL, an arterial pH >7.30, serum bicarbonate >18 mEq/L, an effective serum osmolality >320 mOsm/kg (where effective serum osmolality = 2[measured Na$^+$ (mEq/L)] + glucose [mg/dL]/18).[2,5] Although HHS was previously called hyperglycemic hyperosmolar nonketotic state (HHNKS), small urinary and serum ketones may be seen in this condition and thus their presence does not exclude the diagnosis of HHS.[2] DKA and HHS in reality lie along a continuum, and up to 33% of patients may have a clinical presentation in which features of both are present in varying degrees.[3]

Traditionally, DKA was thought to occur only in type 1 DM and HHS in type 2 DM. There is a newly recognized entity, however, of ketosis-prone type 2 DM.[6] These patients present with DKA resulting from decreased insulin secretion and action but they characteristically recover β-islet cell function within a few months.[5,6] In long-term follow-up, up to 40% of these patients remain without exogenous insulin requirements 10 years after their initial presentation with DKA.[5-7] Patients with ketosis-prone type 2 DM as a group tend to have obesity, family history of DM, lack of genetic HLA association, and low prevalence of autoimmune markers.[6] There is a predilection for African, African American, and Hispanic patients—somewhere between 20% and 50% of patients with new-onset DKA in this demographic may fit this description—but cases have also been reported in other populations (Native American, Japanese, Chinese, Caucasian).[6]

► PATHOPHYSIOLOGY OF DKA AND HHS

DKA is characterized by a state of relative insulin deficiency and concurrent increase in counterregulatory hormones (such as glucagon, cortisol, catecholamines, and growth hormone).[2,5] Hyperglycemia occurs due to increased gluconeogenesis and glycogenolysis, and

▶ **TABLE 31–1. DIAGNOSTIC CRITERIA FOR DKA AND HHS**

	DKA			HHS
	Mild (Plasma Glucose >250 mg/dL)	Moderate (Plasma Glucose >250 mg/dL)	Severe (Plasma Glucose >250 mg/dL)	Plasma Glucose >600 mg/dL
Arterial pH	7.25–7.30	7.00 to <7.24	<7.00	>7.30
Serum bicarbonate (mEq/L)	15–18	10 to <15	<10	>18
Urine ketone[a]	Positive	Positive	Positive	Small
Serum ketone[a]	Positive	Positive	Positive	Small
Effective serum osmolality[b]	Variable	Variable	Variable	>320 mOsm/kg
Anion gap[c]	>10	>12	>12	Variable
Mental status	Alert	Alert/drowsy	Stupor/coma	Stupor/coma

[a]Nitroprusside reaction method.
[b]Effective serum osmolality: 2(measured Na^+ [mEq/L]) + glucose (mg/dL)/18.
[c]Anion gap: $(Na^+) - (Cl^- + HCO_3^-$ [mEq/L]).
Copyright 2009 American Diabetes Association, *Diabetes Care*. 2009;32:1335–1343. Reprinted with permission from The American Diabetes Association.

decreased peripheral glucose utilization in the liver, muscle, and adipocytes.[5] Insulin deficiency and elevated cortisol levels lead to: (a) increased proteolysis, which creates amino acid substrates that further fuel gluconeogenesis, and (b) increased lipolysis, which creates glycerol and free fatty acids (FFA).[5] The latter undergo β-oxidation in the liver, which in turn generates ketone bodies, such as β-hydroxybutyrate and acetoacetate.[5] Generation of these weakly acidic ketone bodies leads to the characteristic anion gap metabolic acidosis.[5] Glycerol is used for further gluconeogenesis.[5] Excess glucagon relative to insulin causes a decrease in malonyl CoA leading to the disinhibition of carnitine palmitoyl acyltransferase I (CPT I).[8] CPT I facilitates ketogenesis by transporting FFA into the mitochondria for oxidation.[8] Finally, as volume depletion causes prerenal azotemia, the ability to excrete glucose and ketoanions declines.[9]

In addition to the well-described metabolic disturbances outlined above, patients in states of hyperglycemic emergency also exhibit evidence of hypercoagulability and inflammation.[8,10,11] Markers of coagulation, fibrinolysis, and platelet activity rise during DKA and may clinically manifest as thromboses, myocardial infarction (MI), and disseminated intravascular coagulation.[8,10] In both DKA and HHS, a proinflammatory milieu develops as cytokines and other markers of cardiovascular risk and oxidative stress rise.[11]

The pathophysiology of HHS, on the other hand, is not completely understood but just as in DKA, osmotic diuresis leads to a loss of electrolytes and a free water deficit.[3] The magnitude of total body water deficit is much greater in HHS and may exceed 9 L, whereas in DKA it typically ranges around 6 L.[3] This leads to marked hyperosmolarity, hypovolemia, and intravascular and extravascular dehydration triggering an increase in counterregulatory hormones, which further worsens hyperglycemia and insulin resistance.[5,8] In HHS, ketone production is minimal if not absent because enough insulin is present to suppress lipolysis.[5,12]

▶ **DIAGNOSIS AND EVALUATION**

Patients typically present with fatigue, weakness, polyuria, polydipsia, weight loss, and possibly altered mental status depending on the severity of presentation.[2] Additional history often present in DKA (but not HHS) includes generalized abdominal pain, nausea, and vomiting that tends to track the severity of acidemia.[2,13] The pain may be of such severity that an acute abdomen is considered during the evaluation in 50–75%.[5,13] The tempo of illness differs: DKA develops rather quickly within 24 hours, whereas HHS develops over a course of a few days to weeks.[2] In DKA, the physical exam may reveal tachycardia, hypotension, lethargy, dry mucous membranes, poor skin turgor, breath with fruity odor (due to ketones), Kussmaul respirations, and abdominal tenderness.[2] Altered mental status, lethargy, and even coma are possible in both conditions, although they are more common in HHS due to the degree of hyperosmolarity.[3,14] In particular, obtundation and coma are typically seen when the effective osmolality is greater than 330 mOsm/kg.[5] If the patient's osmolality is less than 320 mOsm/kg and obtundation is present, one must consider other etiologies for the altered mental status.[2,5] In HHS, physical exam findings may include signs of dehydration as well as additional neurologic changes such as seizures or hemiparesis, making a thorough neurologic evaluation paramount.[2]

Initial evaluation should include an investigation for a precipitating factor. The most common precipitant for both DKA and HHS is infection.[2] Others include intentional or accidental insulin noncompliance, pancreatitis, cerebrovascular accident, MI, and medications (e.g., corticosteroids, diuretics, β-blockers, calcium channel blockers, cimetidine, diazoxide, phenytoin, sympathomimetic agents, pentamidine, typical or atypical antipsychotics).[2,3,15] Elderly patients in particular have a greater risk of developing HHS due to poor thirst response and their dependence on others for free water access.[2,3] Other risk factors for DKA include psychological illness, eating disorders, and cocaine use.[2,16] There are also some endocrine disorders that are associated with hyperglycemia: acromegaly, glucocorticoid excess, pheochromocytoma, thyrotoxicosis, and hyperaldosteronism.[15] Some patients with Cushing's syndrome and DM may even develop HHS.[15]

Initial objective data should include an assessment of glycemia, readily obtained via fingerstick glucose, and a urinalysis to evaluate for ketones. A detailed initial laboratory evaluation is outlined in Table 31-2. Of note, leukocytosis is typically seen in DKA with or without the presence of infection.[2] If the patient's white blood cell count is greater than $25 \times 10^3/mm^3$ or bandemia is 10% or greater, however, one should suspect a true infection.[2,17] Nonspecific elevations in lipase and amylase, up to greater than three times normal values, may also be seen in up to 25% of patients with DKA and thus one cannot diagnose acute pancreatitis by this laboratory value alone.[18] An arterial blood gas (ABG) should be performed to determine the degree of acidemia.[2] In general, admission to the intensive care unit (ICU) is warranted if there is evidence of airway compromise, hemodynamic instability, severe acidemia, or any other finding that would suggest impending decompensation (e.g., suspected gastric dilation, acute abdomen).

Pseudohyponatremia may be present in the setting of hyperglycemia due to the shift of water to the extracellular space. For each 100 mg/dL of glucose greater than 100, 1.6 mEq/L must be added to the measured serum sodium level to arrive at the corrected sodium value.[3] Although this is the traditional teaching, reevaluation of this correction factor showed that for serum glucose greater than 400 mg/dL, a factor of 2.4 mEq/L was more appropriate and thus may be helpful in HHS.[3,8]

The patient's serum potassium level may initially be elevated or near normal, which is falsely reassuring as total body potassium levels are typically quite depleted.[3] Insulin normally drives potassium into the intracellular space—as such, in the setting of absolute or relative insulin deficiency, potassium shifts to the extracellular space.[9] Once treatment with insulin is initiated, the astute clinician must be prepared for a rapid decrease in the serum potassium level. Patients are at risk of developing cardiac arrhythmias and should be kept on telemetry.[9]

▶ TABLE 31–2. **INITIAL EVALUATION IN DKA AND HHS**

Metabolic Evaluation	Infectious Evaluation	Imaging, Miscellaneous
Glucose	CBC with differential	Chest x–ray (CXR)
Urinalysis (for ketones)	Urinalysis	Electrocardiogram (ECG)
ABG	Urine culture	Abdominal plain film[c]
Electrolytes	Blood cultures	
• Sodium[a]	Viral nasal swab	
• Potassium		
• Chloride[a]		
• Bicarbonate[a]		
• Calcium		
• Magnesium		
• Phosphate		
Serum ketones		
Blood urea nitrogen (BUN)		
Creatinine		
Lactic acid		
Osmolarity		
Overdose panel[b]		
Urine toxicology panel[b]		
Liver function tests[c]		
Lipase[c]		

[a]Use to calculate the anion gap: AG = sodium − (chloride + bicarbonate).
[b]Tests to be considered if patient presents with recurrent DKA.[14,16]
[c]Tests to be considered if abdominal pathology is suspected.

▶ TREATMENT

The goals in the treatment of DKA and HHS are to treat the hypovolemia, free water deficit, hyperglycemia, electrolyte abnormalities, and the precipitating factor if one is present. A recent consensus statement proposed a revised treatment algorithm for DKA and HHS (Figure 31-1).[2] Both conditions require frequent monitoring of mental status, vital signs, and urine output. Laboratory monitoring may need to occur at 2- to 4-hour intervals until resolution.[2]

Initial treatment with intravenous fluids (IVF) is necessary in both DKA and HHS to replete the intravascular and interstitial spaces. Correction of hyperosmolarity has the added benefit of improving the patient's response to insulin.[19] First, normal saline (0.9% NaCl) should be given at a rate of 15–20 mL/kg body weight/h or 1–1.5 L over the first hour. At this point, based on the patient's hemodynamics, hydration status, serum sodium level, and urine output, the next composition of IVF is determined as outlined in Figure 31-1. If the patient remains hypotensive, isotonic fluids are continued. Insulin infusion is held until hemodynamic stability is achieved because when insulin is given, water moves from the extracellular to the intracellular space and thus can worsen hypotension.[8] Once the patient is normotensive, insulin infusion should begin at 0.1 U/kg/h. When determining the resuscitation rate, the patient's cardiac and renal functions are also taken

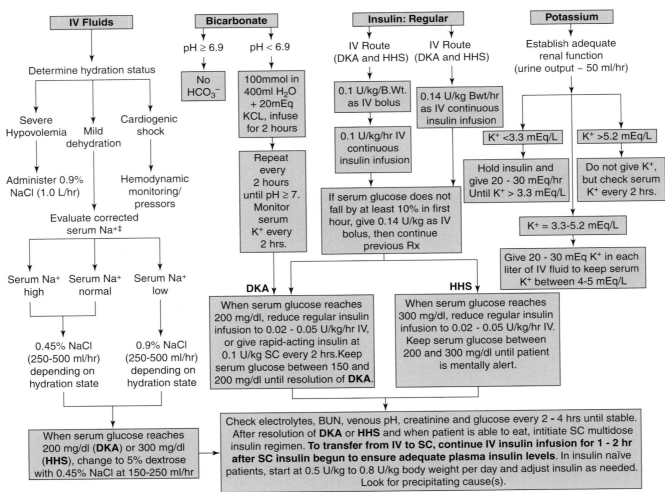

†15-20 ml/kg/h. ‡Serum Na+ refers to the corrected Na+ = measured serum Na+ + 1.6 mEq for every 100mg/dl of glucose over 100 mg/dl. B.Wt = body weight. IV = intravenous. SC = subcutaneous. (Copyright 2009 American Diabetes Association, *Diabetes Care*, Vol. 32, 2009; 1335-1343. Reprinted with permission from The American Diabetes Association.)

Figure 31–1. Management of adult patients with DKA or HHS.

into consideration. When the plasma glucose reaches 200–250 mg/dL in DKA (300 mg/dL in HHS), dextrose is added to the IVF to prevent hypoglycemia and insulin is continued at a lower rate, as ketoacidosis persists longer than hyperglycemia. It is important to continue insulin treatment well after resolution of hyperglycemia in order to suppress lipolysis and subsequent ketoacid production.

Regular intravenous (IV) insulin is typically used due to its relatively short half-life (5–17 minutes) and ease of administration. Studies have shown, however, that insulin therapy may be administered intravenously, subcutaneously, or intramuscularly with good effect.[20] In particular, treatment of mild and moderate DKA with rapid-acting insulin every 1–2 hours outside of the ICU has been demonstrated to be as effective as regular IV insulin therapy in the ICU.[2,21] As for the use of bolus insulin, the traditional treatment protocol involves giving a 0.1-U/kg body weight bolus followed by a continuous infusion of 0.1 U/kg/h.[2] A recent study, however, demonstrated that an initial bolus of insulin is unnecessary if patients are given 0.14 U/kg body weight/h.[22] Thus, at this time it appears that either method may be used to initiate treatment. In general, blood glucose should decline at a steady rate of 50–75 mg/dL/h. Until this is achieved, the rate of the insulin infusion may be doubled every hour.[23]

Given the expected decline in serum potassium level with the initiation of insulin therapy, insulin should be held if the patient's potassium is less than 3.3 mEq/L as the intracellular shift of potassium triggered by insulin may further worsen hypokalemia and place the patient at risk for cardiac arrhythmias. The goal of potassium repletion is to maintain a level around 4–5 mEq/L. Repletion should begin when the level is at the upper limit of normal (5 mEq/L). Typically, adding 20–30 mEq/L of potassium to each liter of IVF will help prevent hypokalemia.[2]

Patients with DKA also have total body phosphate depletion but studies have not convincingly shown benefit in aggressively repleting phosphate in these patients and doing so may carry the risk of hypocalcemia.[2,23,24] However, if serum phosphate levels are less than 1 mEq/L or if the patient has comorbid conditions including respiratory depression, cardiac or respiratory compromise, or anemia, then repletion is warranted.[2,23]

Resolution of DKA occurs when the blood glucose is less than 200 mg/dL and two of the following occur: serum bicarbonate level ≥15 mEq/L, venous pH >7.3, and/or anion gap ≤12 mEq/L. Resolution of HHS occurs when the osmolality and mental status have normalized. At this time, subcutaneous insulin may be initiated with at least 1–2 hours of overlap with the insulin infusion to prevent relapse. Regarding the dose of subcutaneous insulin, the patient's home insulin regimen may be used if it had been working well for the patient prior to the episode. In newly diagnosed diabetic patients, dosing should start at 0.5–0.8 U/kg per day. The total daily dose should be divided into a basal and bolus regimen. One approach is to allocate 50% of the total daily dose as long-acting insulin such as glargine and to divide the remainder into three equal mealtime boluses of rapid-acting insulin (e.g., aspart or lispro).[2]

Bicarbonate therapy is controversial in the treatment of DKA. As DKA is treated, ketoacidosis should improve because ketone bodies are metabolized in the citric acid cycle.[8] This leads to the production of carbon dioxide and water, which leads to regeneration of bicarbonate.[8] Studies have failed to demonstrate that bicarbonate therapy has any benefit in improving morbidity or mortality in patients with severe DKA (pH 6.9–7.1).[2,25] There are no randomized controlled trials, however, that have examined the role of bicarbonate therapy in DKA patients with a pH <6.9.[9] In severe acidemia, patients are at risk for developing cerebral vasodilatation, coma, decreased myocardial contractility, and gastrointestinal (GI) complications.[2,26] Given these risks, the current recommendation is to give bicarbonate therapy to DKA patients with a pH <6.9. It is important to note that bicarbonate therapy carries the risks of worsening hypokalemia, worsened intracellular acidosis, cerebral edema, and paradoxical central nervous system acidosis.[2] See Figure 31-1 for dosing.

► COMPLICATIONS

Potential complications during treatment of DKA and HHS include cerebral edema, hypoglycemia, hypokalemia, hyperchloremic metabolic acidosis, fluid overload, acute respiratory distress syndrome (ARDS), thromboembolism, and acute gastric dilation due to gastroparesis.[2,3,8,27]

Cerebral edema is rarely seen in adult patients with DKA, and the exact mechanism of cerebral edema is not entirely clear. Most of the literature is in the pediatric population. There is evidence to support the following theories: inflammatory mediators, cerebral ischemia, hypoxia, and rapid decline in serum osmolality due to aggressive IVF.[2] If present, patients may develop a headache, altered level of consciousness, papilledema, bradycardia, hypertension, seizures, incontinence, or even respiratory arrest.[2,3,27] Treatment includes giving mannitol and mechanically ventilating the patient.[27]

A more common complication is development of hyperchloremic non-anion gap metabolic acidosis resulting from large amounts of normal saline given during treatment and the decrease in ketoanions as DKA resolves.[9] In addition, fluid overload or ARDS could also occur and thus frequent cardiopulmonary assessment is vital.[9] Given the possibility of gastroparesis and resulting gastric dilation, serial abdominal exams and an abdominal plain film should take place if there are sufficient clinical concerns.[8]

▶ SUMMARY

DKA and HHS lie along a continual spectrum, and are frequently encountered diabetic complications in the acute care setting with significant economic burden and morbidity for the patient. With prompt diagnosis and careful management, DKA and HHS can be successfully managed with improved patient outcomes.

REFERENCES

1. Centers for Disease Control. National Diabetes Surveillance System. Available at: http://www.cdc.gov/diabetes/statistics/complications_national.htm. Accessed December 19, 2009.
2. Kitabchi AE, Umpierrez GE, Miles JM, et al. Hyperglycemic crises in adult patients with diabetes. *Diabetes Care.* 2009;32:1335.
3. Ennis ED, Kreisberg RA. Diabetic ketoacidosis and the hyperglycemic hyperosmolar syndrome. In: LeRoith D, Taylor SI, Olefsky JM, eds. *Diabetes Mellitus.* 3rd ed. Philadelphia: Lippincott Williams & Wilkins; 2004:627.
4. Agency for Healthcare Research and Quality. Healthcare Cost & Utilization Project (HCUP). Available at: http://hcupnet.ahrq.gov/HCUP.net.jsp. Accessed December 18, 2009.
5. Kitabchi AE, Nyenwe EA. Hyperglycemic crises in diabetes mellitus: diabetic ketoacidosis and hyperglycemic hyperosmolar state. *Endocrinol Metab Clin North Am.* 2006;35:725.
6. Umpierrez GE, Smiley D, Kitabchi AE. Narrative review: ketosis-prone type 2 diabetes mellitus. *Ann Intern Med.* 2006;144:350.
7. Mauvais-Jarvis F, Sobngwi E, Porcher R, et al. Ketosis-prone type 2 diabetes in patients of sub-Saharan African origin: clinical pathophysiology and natural history of beta-cell dysfunction and insulin resistance. *Diabetes.* 2004;53:645.
8. Magee MF, Bhatt BA. Management of decompensated diabetes. Diabetic ketoacidosis and hyperglycemic hyperosmolar syndrome. *Crit Care Clin.* 2001;17:75.
9. Kitabchi AE, Umpierrez GE, Murphy MB, et al. Management of hyperglycemic crises in patients with diabetes. *Diabetes Care.* 2001;24:131.
10. Büyükaşik Y, Ileri NS, Haznedaroğlu IC, et al. Enhanced subclinical coagulation activation during diabetic ketoacidosis. *Diabetes Care.* 1998;21:868.
11. Stentz FB, Umpierrez GE, Cuervo R, et al. Proinflammatory cytokines, markers of cardiovascular risks, oxidative stress, and lipid peroxidation in patients with hyperglycemic crises. *Diabetes.* 2004;53:2079.
12. Kitabchi AE, Fisher JN, Murphy MB, et al. Diabetic ketoacidosis and the hyperglycemic, hyperosmolar nonketotic state. In: Kahn CR, Weir GC, eds. *Joslin's Diabetes Mellitus.* 13th ed. Philadelphia: Lea & Febiger; 1994:738.
13. Umpierrez G, Freire AX. Abdominal pain in patients with hyperglycemic crises. *J Crit Care.* 2002;17:63.
14. Umpierrez GE, Kelly JP, Navarrete JE, et al. Hyperglycemic crises in urban blacks. *Arch Intern Med.* 1997;157:669.
15. Trence DL, Hirsch IB. Hyperglycemic crises in diabetes mellitus type 2. *Endocrinol Metab Clin North Am.* 2001;30:817.
16. Nyenwe EA, Loganathan RS, Blum S, et al. Active use of cocaine: an independent risk factor for recurrent diabetic ketoacidosis in a city hospital. *Endocr Pract.* 2007;13:22.
17. Slovis CM, Mork VGC, Slovis RJ, et al. Diabetic ketoacidosis and infection: leukocyte count and differential as early predictors of serious infection. *Am J Emerg Med.* 1987;5:1.
18. Yadav D, Nair S, Norkus EP, et al. Nonspecific hyperamylasemia and hyperlipasemia in diabetic ketoacidosis: incidence and correlation with biochemical abnormalities. *Am J Gastroenterol.* 2000;95:3123.
19. Bratusch-Marrain PR, DeFronzo RA. Impairment of insulin-mediated glucose metabolism by hyperosmolality in man. *Diabetes.* 1983;32:1028.
20. Fisher JN, Shahshahani MN, Kitabchi AE. Diabetic ketoacidosis: low-dose insulin therapy by various routes. *N Engl J Med.* 1977;297:238.
21. Umpierrez GE, Latif K, Stoever J, et al. Efficacy of subcutaneous insulin lispro versus continuous intravenous regular insulin for the treatment of patients with diabetic ketoacidosis. *Am J Med.* 2004;117:291.
22. Kitabchi AE, Murphy MB, Spencer J, et al. Is a priming dose of insulin necessary in a low-dose insulin protocol for the treatment of diabetic ketoacidosis? *Diabetes Care.* 2008;31:2081.
23. Kitabchi AE, Umpierrez GE, Murphy MB, et al. Hyperglycemic crises in adult patients with diabetes: a consensus statement from the American Diabetes Association. *Diabetes Care.* 2006;29:2739.
24. Fisher JN, Kitabchi AE. A randomized study of phosphate therapy in the treatment of diabetic ketoacidosis. *J Clin Endocrinol Metab.* 1983;57:177.
25. Morris LR, Murphy MB, Kitabchi AE. Bicarbonate therapy in severe diabetic ketoacidosis. *Ann Intern Med.* 1986;105:836.
26. Mitchell JH, Wildenthal K, Johnson RL. The effects of acid–base disturbances on cardiovascular and pulmonary function. *Kidney Int.* 1972;1:375.
27. Roberts MD, Slover RH, Chase HP. Diabetic ketoacidosis with intracerebral complications. *Pediatr Diabetes.* 2001;2:109.

CHAPTER 32

Glucose Management in Critical Care

Ari J. Ciment and Joseph Romero

► INTRODUCTION

The American Diabetes Association (ADA) defines inpatient hyperglycemia as a fasting blood glucose (BG) >126 mg/dL or a random BG >200 mg/dL that reverts to normal after discharge.[1] The prevalence of hyperglycemia in the acutely ill patient in the intensive care unit (ICU) has been shown to be as high as 83%.[2] Hyperglycemia in critical illness may occur due to stress-related surges in counterregulatory hormones, preexisting diabetes, impaired glucose tolerance, and insulin resistance. Whether it is a condition necessitating intervention or a marker of disease severity, hyperglycemia has been shown to be an independent risk factor for increased mortality in the ICU.[3] Despite this association, tight glycemic control (TGC) has not been shown to consistently improve patient outcomes and surprisingly may, in some subgroups, cause more harm than good. This chapter examines the historical background, essential pathophysiology, associations, key clinical studies, current protocols, and recommendations regarding hyperglycemia in the critically ill.

► HISTORICAL BACKGROUND

Hyperglycemia was first detected as glucosuria in ether-anesthetized patients 150 years ago, and in 1877, Bernard described hyperglycemia in a canine model of hemorrhagic shock.[4] For many years, hyperglycemia in the critically ill was considered an adaptation to stress and was not treated. In fact, some early ICU practitioners recognized insulin resistance and believed that elevated glucose levels (160–200 mg/dL) would promote cellular glucose uptake. In 2001, Van den Berghe demonstrated a statistically significant mortality benefit with TGC in surgical ICU patients. Subsequently, many professional societies including the Surviving Sepsis Campaign (SSC) in 2004 endorsed TGC.[5] The Leuven (Van den Berghe et al) medical trial in 2006, Efficacy of Volume Substitution and Insulin Therapy in Severe Sepsis (VISEP, Brunkhorst et al) trial in 2008, and Normoglycemia in Intensive Care Evaluation—Survival Using Glucose Algorithm Regulation (NICE-SUGAR, Finfer et al) and Glucontrol (Preiser et al) trials published in 2009 have contributed most to the continuously evolving issue of glucose management in the critically ill patient.

► PATHOPHYSIOLOGY OF HYPERGLYCEMIA IN ICU SETTING

Risk factors for the development of hyperglycemia include preexisting diabetes mellitus, advanced age, infusion of catecholamine pressors, glucocorticoids, obesity, excessive dextrose resuscitation, sepsis, hypothermia, hypoxia, uremia, and cirrhosis.[6] These proven risk factors highlight the multifactorial pathophysiologic mechanisms underlying ICU hyperglycemia.

In the critically ill patient, hyperglycemia can be explained by increased glucose production (glycogenolysis and gluconeogenesis) and decreased peripheral uptake (insulin resistance) (Figure 32-1):

Increased glucose production: Counterregulatory hormones and catecholamines such as glucagon, growth hormone, cortisol, and epinephrine increase adipose tissue lipolysis and skeletal muscle proteolysis. The end products from this process (glycerol, alanine, and lactate) then fuel hepatic gluconeogenesis. By directly enhancing hepatic glycogenolysis, the above hormones simultaneously further raise glucose levels. Impairment of cellular glycogen synthesis is another important pathway leading to increased glucose levels.

Decreased peripheral uptake: In a healthy subject, insulin binds to its receptor triggering a signaling pathway that ultimately leads to the translocation of the intracellular Glut4 protein to the plasma membrane where it is responsible for glucose uptake. Although not well understood, it has been postulated that critical illness inhibits Glut4 translocation resulting in hyperglycemia. Counterregulatory hormones and cytokines are believed to play an important role in this process.

Insulin resistance, defined as ongoing gluconeogenesis, glycogenolysis, lipolysis, and proteolysis despite normal or elevated insulin levels, is directly or indirectly (via counterregulatory hormones) modulated

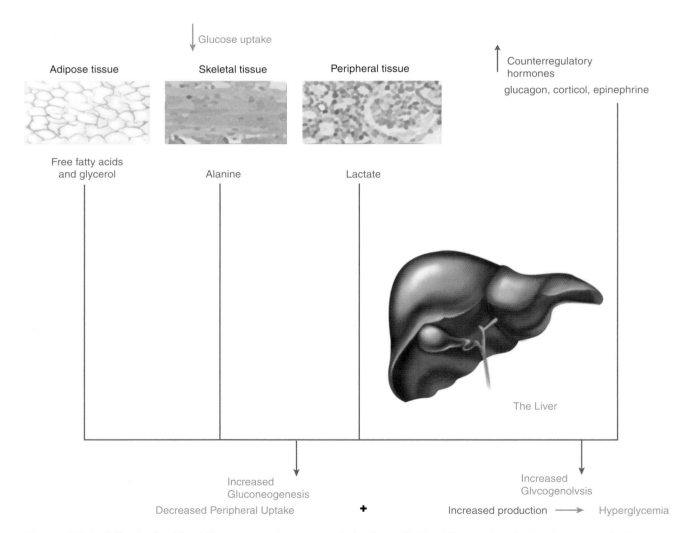

Figure 32-1. Effect of critical illness on glucose metabolism. Critical illness leads to decreased glucose uptake in adipose, skeletal, and peripheral tissues despite normal or high insulin levels, so-called insulin resistance. Counterregulatory hormones stimulate lipolysis, proteolysis, and glycolysis. The end products glycerol, alanine, and lactate are then used in the liver for gluconeogenesis. The simultaneous hormone-induced glycogenolysis further contributes to the ensuing hyperglycemic state.

by proinflammatory cytokines such as tumor necrosis factor (TNF)-α, interleukin (IL)-1, and IL-6.

► ASSOCIATION OF HYPERGLYCEMIA AND POOR OUTCOME

Even prior to the seminal randomized control trial (RCT) by Van den Berghe et al in 2001 that showed a statistically significant 30% excess mortality, there have been numerous retrospective studies showing a strong association between poor ICU-related outcomes in hyperglycemic patients.[7] For instance, Sung et al demonstrated that admission hyperglycemia in trauma patients was an independent risk factor for increased mortality, ICU length of stay, and infection.[8] In traumatic brain injury patients, Young et al showed significantly worse 3-month and 1-year outcomes if the BG levels were >200 mg/dL.[9] In patients with ischemic and hemorrhagic stroke, Weir et al demonstrated that a plasma glucose concentration above 144 mg/dL predicted poorer chances of survival and functional independence, even after adjusting for age and stroke severity.[10]

Similar results have been found in retrospective studies, which focused on a heterogeneous population of ICU patients. Most notably, Krinsley studied 1,826 consecutive ICU patients (roughly 80% medical and 20% surgical) and found that hospital mortality increased progressively as glucose values increased, reaching 43% among patients with mean glucose values exceeding 300 mg/dL.[3]

Among surgical patients, one of the key mechanisms by which insulin may improve outcomes is through reduction in infections. Studies supporting such a connection have demonstrated a 3-fold increased risk of postoperative wound infections and a 4-fold increased incidence of intravascular infections in hyperglycemic surgical ICU patients.[5,6]

► KEY TRIALS OF HYPERGLYCEMIC CONTROL IN ICU POPULATION

Initial enthusiasm for intensive insulin therapy (IIT) stimulated by the initial Leuven surgical trial was dampened by the subsequent four RCTs that not only failed to show clear mortality benefits but also highlighted the possible dangerous consequences of IIT.

Subgroup analysis of the initial Leuven surgical trial showed that the greatest mortality benefit was achieved in patients who had a prolonged ICU stay of >5 days.[11] Consequently, the Leuven medical trial specifically targeted patients with prolonged (>3 days) ICU stay. Although demonstrating a mortality benefit in that subgroup once again, the intention-to-treat design failed to demonstrate a mortality benefit of IIT in overall patients

and is widely considered a negative trial despite the listed morbidity benefits in all subgroups.[12]

The purpose of the VISEP trial was to determine if the benefit of strict glucose control applied to patients with severe sepsis and septic shock. Due to unacceptably high hypoglycemia rates, the VISEP trial was prematurely terminated and did not reach the recruitment goal. The trial's subsequent lack of power coupled with potential confounding agents inherent in the four-arm design may explain why this trial also failed to show an IIT benefit for both mortality and morbidity.[13]

A noteworthy point of the negative Glucontrol trial was the lower BG target levels (140–180 mg/dL vs. 180–200 mg/dL) in the conventional arm. Although terminated early for protocol violations and failure to reach target BG levels, those IIT patients who did reach target levels still did not have a mortality benefit when compared with the conventional arm.[14]

Finally, the largest and most definitive trial to date, NICE-SUGAR, showed a significantly *increased* mortality rate in the IIT group at 90 days and no positive effect on morbidity as well. For reasons that are not yet clear, excess deaths were predominantly due to cardiovascular causes. Interestingly, despite worse mortality, there were no observable differences in ICU or hospital length of stay, new organ failure rates, ventilator days, bacteremia, or transfusion requirements between the two groups. Also noteworthy is that roughly 33% of the NICE-SUGAR patients were surgical and, unlike the original Leuven surgical trial, there was no mortality benefit in this subgroup.[15]

A concise summary of the key trials highlighting the study population, endpoints, adverse effects, and criticisms can be found in Table 32-1.

► SELECTED SUBGROUP POPULATIONS

In addition to the aforementioned key RCTs, TGC has also been studied in patients with acute myocardial infarctions (MI), coronary artery bypass grafts (CABG), and cerebral vascular accidents (CVA).

MI AND POST-CABG PATIENTS

Hyperglycemia has been shown to be a risk factor for mortality in patients with acute MI. In a study of 16,781 patients with acute MI, the mortality rate increased incrementally with each 10 mg/dL rise in glucose over 120 mg/dL.[16] Studies have shown that hyperglycemia in the presence of ischemia is associated with decreased collateral circulation, increased infarct size, and prolonged QT interval.[17] Since hyperglycemia has been clearly linked to less "Thrombolysis in Myocardial

▶ **TABLE 32-1. REVIEW OF PROSPECTIVE RANDOMIZED TRIALS OF GLYCEMIC CONTROL AMONG CRITICALLY ILL PATIENTS[11-15]**

Study/Year	Population; No. of Pts; Centers	Goal Glucose Level	Primary Outcome and Endpoints	Adverse Effects	Key Findings and Comments	Key Criticisms
Leuven Surgical/2001	Surgical ICU; 1,548; single site	TGC, 80–110 mg/dL; conventional, 180–200 mg/dL	ICU mortality: TGC, 4.6%; Conv, 8%; $P < .04$	Hypoglycemia: TGC, 5%; Conv, 0.7%	TGC reduced mortality during ICU/hospital stay, morbidity, renal failure, hyperbilirubinemia, bloodstream infection, duration of mechanical ventilation, and ICU/hospital stay	Use of parenteral nutrition to achieve caloric goals in both groups. High mortality rates in the control group (8%)
Leuven Medical/2006	Medical ICU; 1,200; single site	TGC, 80–110 mg/dL; conventional, 180–215 mg/dL	In-hospital mortality: TGC, 37.3%; Conv, 40.0%; $P = .33$	Hypoglycemia: TGC, 18.7%; Conv, 3.1%	<3-Day ICU stay: TGC-no significant difference in mortality. Decreased duration of mechanical ventilation, ICU and hospital length of stay. >3-Day ICU stay: TGC-decreased mortality in hospital and at 90 days, duration of mechanical ventilation, ICU and hospital length of stay	Subjective inclusion criteria (ICU length of stay >3 days). Unusually high rates of hypoglycemia in TGC group
VISEP/2008	Medical and surgical ICU (only with pts. with severe sepsis/shock); 537; 18 sites	TGC, 80–110 mg/dL; conventional, 180–200 mg/dL	28-Day mortality: TGC, 24.7%; Conv, 26%; $P = .74$	Hypoglycemia: TGC, 17%; Conv, 4.1%	Stopped early for safety concerns due to large number of hypoglycemic episodes in TGC. Before trial was stopped, there was no difference in mortality at 28 and 90 days	Large number of hypoglycemic episodes in TGC group
Glucontrol/2006	Medical and surgical ICU; 1,101; 21 sites	TGC, 110–140 mg/dL; conventional, 140–180 mg/dL	ICU mortality: TGC, 17.2%; Conv, 15.3%; $P = .41$	Hypoglycemia: TGC, 8.7%; Conv, 2.7%	Trial was terminated early after the first interim analysis due to failure to achieve targeted blood glucose levels and high rates of hypoglycemia	Failure to achieve targeted blood glucose levels. High rates of hypoglycemia
NICE-SUGAR/2009	Medical and surgical ICU; 6,104; 42 sites	TGC, 81–108 mg/dL; conventional, <180 mg/dL	90-Day mortality: TGC, 27.5%; Conv, 24.9%; $P = .02$	Hypoglycemia: TGC, 6.8%; Conv, 0.5%	TGC: increased mortality at 90 days. No difference between groups in need for dialysis, duration of mechanical ventilation, or days in ICU/hospital	Subjective inclusion criteria (ICU length of stay >3 days). Achievement of glucose levels modestly above target range in large portion of TGC group

TGC, tight glucose control; Conv, conventional control.

Infarction (TIMI)" flow before primary percutaneous coronary intervention (PCI), it has been hypothesized to be a strong prothrombotic stimulus initiating procoagulant factors and inhibiting thrombolysis.[18] In addition to counteracting these deleterious procoagulant effects, insulin blocks the accumulation of free fatty acids generated from ischemia-induced myocardial anaerobic metabolism that otherwise would promote further oxygen debt and arrhythmias.[19]

Initial enthusiasm was sparked by the Diabetes and Insulin–Glucose Infusion in Acute Myocardial Infarction (DIGAMI) trial, an RCT which studied diabetics with acute MI. An impressive 30% mortality reduction was shown in the glucose, insulin, and potassium (GIK) infusion group.[20] However, the larger and more recent 2005 follow-up study, DIGAMI-2, did not replicate such findings.[21] Similarly, the CREATE-ECLA trial showed no difference in mortality, cardiac arrest, or cardiogenic shock in ST-elevation MI (STEMI) patients randomized to a GIK infusion.[22] Although the subsequent HI-5 study in 2006 also did not show a mortality benefit in diabetic acute MI patients randomized to GIK, there was a significantly lower incidence of heart failure and reinfarction in that group that has revived the pro-IIT debate.[23]

It is worth noting that unlike the TGC studies such as NICE-SUGAR and the Leuven trials, the GIK infusion acute MI studies such as the aforementioned CREATE-ECLA and DIGAMI trials did not really achieve TGC. Ostensibly these trials focused more on insulin therapy than on the control of hyperglycemia.

Hyperglycemia is a known risk factor for mortality, deep sternal wound infections, and increased length of stay in patients undergoing CABG. The ongoing large Portland Diabetic Project that is a prospective, nonrandomized, observational study including 5,510 diabetic patients has shown a dramatic and significant 60–77% decrease in mortality and infection risk when employing a continuous insulin infusion.[24]

CVA PATIENTS

Patients with acute stroke (CVA) have been shown to have worse outcomes when hyperglycemic. The detrimental effects of hyperglycemia may include increasing tissue acidosis secondary to anaerobic glycolysis, lactic acidosis, and free radical production along with a possible contribution to cerebral edema via an effect on the blood-brain barrier.[25] There is a recognized 3-fold increase in hemorrhagic transformation in tissue plasminogen activator (tPA)-treated hyperglycemic post-CVA patients as well. A 2001 comprehensive cohort review demonstrated a 3-fold increase in 30-day mortality among hyperglycemic post-CVA patients.[26] While admission BG >140 mg/dL has significant long-term mortality

association, Baird et al found that persistent hyperglycemia (BG > 200 mg/dL) during the first 24 hours after stroke independently predicted expansion of the volume of ischemic stroke and poor neurologic outcomes.[27] A 2009 large observational Glycemia in Acute Stroke (GLIAS) study showed that a BG >155 mg/dL or higher at any time within the first 48 hours from stroke onset was associated with poor outcome independently of stroke severity, infarct volume, diabetes, or age.[28]

To date, few RCTs studying BG control in the post–CVA patient have been published. One such RCT, the GIST-UK trial in 2008, did not show a mortality or morbidity effect of IIT in acute CVA patients, but was underpowered and the length of treatment (24 hours) was minimal.[29] Additionally, the IIT group in the GIST-UK trial only had a mean BG level of 10.3 mg/dL lower than the control group. Since it was suggested that greater reductions in BG levels might be needed to show a clinical benefit, two recent RCTs focused on the clinical feasibility and safety of more aggressive intensive insulin protocols. These studies, which focused on patients with preexisting diabetes, suggested clinical benefit, but were unable to demonstrate definitive improvement.[30,31] Of importance, the aforementioned prospective RCTs excluded nondiabetics because they tend to self-correct and enter the target range without intervention.

Given the paucity of RCTs, the guidelines for BG control in CVA patients vary and are constantly evolving. The European Stroke Organization guidelines recommend starting insulin therapy when the BG is >10 mmol/L (181 mg/dL).[32] The Stroke Council of the American Stroke Association, which in 2003 initially recommended BG control only when the BG is >300 mg/dL, has recently changed the BG target to 140–185 mg/dL (7.7–10.2 mmol/L).[33]

For a detailed summary of the MI and CVA studies, see Table 32-2.

▶ RISKS OF HYPOGLYCEMIA IN THE ICU

The Leuven surgical and medical, NICE-SUGAR, VISEP, and Glucontrol trials, as well as the aforementioned RCTs in selected subgroup populations, have all shown a risk of hypoglycemia in the intensive glucose control groups. Symptoms of hypoglycemia such as headache, fatigue, confusion, and dysarthria are often masked in an ICU patient and may not become evident until the BG is <40 mg/dL. Complications of such severe hypoglycemia include coma, seizures, and even cardiac arrest. In 2007, Krinsley and Grover identified severe hypoglycemia in ICU patients as an independent risk factor for mortality. In fact, a single episode of severe hypoglycemia was shown to significantly increase the risk of mortality over 2-fold. The populations at greatest

▶ TABLE 32-2. REVIEW OF PROSPECTIVE RANDOMIZED TRIALS OF GLYCEMIC CONTROL AMONG MI AND CVA PATIENTS[20-23,29]

Study/Year	Population; No. of Patients; Centers	Goal Glucose Level	Intervention	Primary Outcome and Endpoints	Key Findings and Comments	Key Criticisms
DIGAMI/1999	MI patients with admission glucose >198 mg/ dL; 620; 19 sites	TGC: 126–180 mg/ dL Conv: physician discretion	TGC: insulin and glucose infusion for >24 h, and then SQ insulin for 3 months Conv: glucose control at the discretion of treating physician	Mortality during an average follow-up of 1.6–5.6 years: TGC, 33%; Conv, 44%; $P = .011$	Improved mortality in the TGC group	Inconsistent glucose control in the Conv group due to physician discretion and no goal glucose level
DIGAMI 2/2005	MI patients with admission glucose >198 mg/ dL; 1,253; 48 sites	TGC (1 and 2): fasting (126–180 mg/dL) Conv: physician discretion	TGC (1): 24-h insulin and glucose infusion followed by long-term SQ insulin TGC (2): 24-h insulin and glucose infusion followed by glucose control at the discretion of treating physician Conv: glucose control at the discretion of treating physician	2-Year mortality: TGC (1), 23.4%; TGC (2), 21.2%; Conv (3), 17.9% P-value: 1:2 = .832; 1:3 = .157; 2:3 = .203	No difference in mortality or morbidity between the three groups	Inconsistent glucose control in the Conv group due to physician discretion and no goal glucose level; 14% of the Conv group received insulin and glucose infusion as per the treating physician Significant differences in the patient characteristics of the three groups Study was stopped early due to slow recruitment rates
CREATE-ECLA/2005	STEMI patients; 20,201; 470 sites	No set glucose goals	Test group: glucose, insulin, and potassium (GIK) infusion-infused over 24 hours after admission along with 7 days of low-molecular-weight heparin, reviparin Control: usual care	30–Day mortality: GIK, 10%; Cont, 9.7%; $P = .45$	No difference in mortality, cardiogenic shock, or cardiac arrest in patients s/p STEMI	No correlation with previous, smaller studies involving GIK infusion Test group had glucose infusion as part of insulin drip that may have led to negative results

Study/Year	Population	Glucose goal	Intervention	Mortality	Outcome	Comments
HI-5/2006	MI patients with admission blood glucose >140 mg/dL; 240; 6 sites	TGC: 72–180 mg/dL. Conv: no set glucose goals	TGC: insulin and dextrose infusion for at least 24 h after admission. Conv: patients remained on their usual diabetes therapy, including SQ insulin. Metformin was discontinued on admission. If blood glucose >288 mg/dL, SQ insulin was permitted	Inpatient mortality: TGC, 4.8%; Conv, 3.5%; $P = .75$. 3-Month mortality: TGC, 7.1%; Conv, 4.4%; $P = .42$. 6-Month mortality: TGC, 7.9%; Conv, 6.1%; $P = .62$	No difference in mortality. TGC: lower incidence of cardiac failure and evidence of reinfarction at 3 months	Significant difference in blood glucose between TGC and Conv groups was not achieved. Mean duration of time from symptoms to infusion initiation in TGC group was 13 h
GIST-UK/2007	Acute stroke patients: excluding pts with h/o IDDM and hyperglycemia on presentation >17 mmol/dL (306 mg/dL); 933; multicenter	GIK infusion: 72–126 mg/dL. Control: no set glucose goals. If glucose >306 mg/dL, insulin infusion could be started based on physician discretion	GIK: glucose, insulin, and potassium infusion for at least 24 h after admission. Control: 0.9% saline infusion at 100 mL/h	90-Day mortality: GIK, 30%; control, 27.3%; $P = .37$	No difference in mortality. GIK: reduced mean serum glucose levels by 10 mg/dL and blood pressure by 9 mm Hg	Trial was stopped early due to slow enrollment. Most patients had only moderate elevations in plasma glucose on admission, and patients with severely high serum glucose (>306 mg/dL) were excluded from the study. GIK infusion was labor intensive and had a 15.7% incidence of hypoglycemia requiring rescue treatment

TGC, tight glucose control; Conv, conventional treatment; Cont, control; MI, myocardial infarction; STEMI, ST-elevation myocardial infarction; IDDM, insulin-dependent diabetes mellitus.

risk of mortality secondary to hypoglycemia were the patients with preexisting diabetes, on mechanical ventilation, with an admitting diagnosis of septic shock, and with a very high Acute Physiology and Chronic Health Evaluation (APACHE) score.[34] It has been suggested that the mortality benefit provided with IIT can perhaps be offset if IIT is too intense and thus finding the right balance is of utmost importance.

▶ TREATMENT AND RECOMMENDATIONS

In review, although it is clear that severe hyperglycemia is associated with poor outcomes, there are no convincing data to suggest that the tightest glucose control (80–110 mg/dL) provides mortality benefits. An early single-center surgical study showing morbidity and mortality improvements rushed in an era of intensive insulin protocols around the world, but subsequent studies including medical patients and a more heterogeneous group of ICU patients have failed to replicate this finding.

The updated SSC guidelines recommended that patients with severe sepsis and hyperglycemia should be placed on intravenous (IV) insulin infusion to reduce BG levels with a goal of <150 mg/dL.[35] In June 2009, an addendum published by the SSC glucose control subgroup in response to the NICE-SUGAR publication recommended against IIT aimed at BG 80–110 mg/dL in patients with severe sepsis. They did however recommend considering glucose control when levels exceed 180 mg/dL, with a goal BG approximating 150 mg/dL.[36] In 2009 the ADA and American Association of Clinical Endocrinologists (AACE) guidelines recently advocated a BG target of 140–180 mg/dL with initiation of insulin therapy when BG is >180 mg/dL.[37]

Glycemic control in the ICU can be obtained by either IV or subcutaneous (SQ) insulin. In a systematic literature review by Meijering et al in 2005, the IV route achieved a target BG level in a higher number of patients than the SQ route alone.[38] The standard of care in the ICU is to use IV infusions when feasible and not SQ and IV together.

There are at least 18 current insulin protocols available, but the concept is the same: achieve the best BG control while minimizing the risk of hypoglycemia.[39] A typical "sliding" protocol, as seen in the Leuven surgical trial, sets a predetermined amount of insulin according to the range in which the last BG value fell. On the other hand, "dynamic" protocols, such as Goldberg's Yale protocol, make adjustments based on glycemic levels, as well as the rate of change and the degree of insulin resistance.

In transitioning from the ICU to general or intermediate care within the hospital, BG control is still targeted, albeit less tightly. The use of a basal–bolus regimen (i.e.,

adding basal coverage in addition to the sliding scale dose) has been shown to be almost two times more effective at achieving target BG levels in non-ICU patients than the traditional sliding scale protocols alone.[40]

▶ THE FUTURE OF ICU HYPERGLYCEMIC CONTROL

Current and future studies focus on incorporating some new approaches evaluating metrics of hyperglycemia beyond average values, such as glycemic variability. Interesting ongoing studies with the goal of avoiding or reducing insulin use focus on utilizing insulin-like growth factor-1 (IGF-1, a signal in the insulin pathway) and glucagon-like peptide-1 (GLP-1, a glucose-lowering incretin) or even simply restricting carbohydrates.[41] Providing better and safer target BG levels, improving protocol adherence via online and computerized tools, and incorporating advanced glucose monitoring devices (such as continuous glucose sensors) are also exciting subjects for future investigation, and are likely to contribute to the evolution of glycemic control in the ICU population.

REFERENCES

1. American Diabetes Association. Standards of medical care in diabetes—2009. *Diabetes Care.* 2009;32(suppl 1):S13–S61.
2. Saberi F, Heyland D, Lam L, et al. Prevalence, incidence, and clinical resolution of insulin resistance in critically ill patients: an observational study. *J Parenter Enteral Nutr.* 2008;32:227–235.
3. Krinsley JS. Association between hyperglycemia and increased hospital mortality in a heterogeneous population of critically ill patients. *Mayo Clinic Proc.* 2003;78:1471–1478.
4. Van den Berghe G. How does blood glucose control with insulin save lives in intensive care? *J Clin Invest.* 114:1187–1195, 2004.
5. Dellinger RP, Carlet JM, Masur H, et al. Surviving Sepsis Campaign guidelines for management of severe sepsis and septic shock. *Crit Care Med.* 2004;32:858–873.
6. McCowen KC, Malhotra A, Bistrian BR. Stress-induced hyperglycemia. *Crit Care Clin.* 2001;17:107–124.
7. Van den Berghe G, Wouters PJ, Bouillon R, et al. Outcome benefit of intensive insulin therapy in the critically ill: insulin dose versus glycemic control. *Crit Care Med.* 2003;31:359–366.
8. Sung J, Bochicchio GV, Joshi M, et al. Admission hyperglycemia is predictive of outcome in critically ill trauma patients. *J Trauma Inj Infect Crit Care.* 2005;59:80–83.
9. Young B, Ott L, Dempsy R, et al. Relationship between admission hyperglycemia and neurologic outcome of severely brain-injured patients. *Ann Surg.* 1989;210:466–472.

10. Weir CJ, Murray GD, Dyker AG, et al. Is hyperglycemia an independent risk predictor of poor outcome after acute stroke? Results of a long-term follow up study. *BMJ.* 1997;314:1303–1306.

11. Van den Berghe G, Wouters P, Weekers F, et al. Intensive insulin therapy in the critically ill patients. *N Engl J Med.* 2001;345:1359–1367.

12. Van den Berghe G, Wilmer A, Hermans G, et al. Intensive insulin therapy in the medical ICU. *N Engl J Med.* 2006;354:449–461.

13. Brunkhorst FM, Engel C, Bloos F, et al. Intensive insulin therapy and pentastarch resuscitation in severe sepsis. *N Engl J Med.* 2008;358:125–139.

14. Preiser JC, Devos P, Ruiz-Santana S, et al. A prospective randomised multi-centre controlled trial on tight glucose control by intensive insulin therapy in adult intensive care units: the Glucontrol study. *Intensive Care.* 2009;35:1738–1748.

15. NICE-SUGAR Study Investigators, Finfer S, Chittock DR, Su SY, et al. Intensive versus conventional glucose control in critically ill patients. *N Engl J Med.* 2009;360:1283–1297.

16. Kosiborod M, Inzucchi SE, Krumholz HM, et al. Glucometrics in patients with acute myocardial infarction. Defining the optimal outcome-based measure of risk. *Circulation.* 2008;117:1018–1027.

17. Deedwania P, Kosiborod M, Barret E, et al. Hyperglycemia and acute coronary syndrome. *Circulation.* 2008;117:1610–1619.

18. Timmer JR, Ottervanger JP, de Boer MJ, et al. Hyperglycemia is an important predictor of impaired coronary flow before reperfusion therapy in ST-segment elevation myocardial infarction. *J Am Coll Cardiol.* 2005;45:999–1002.

19. Oliver MF, Opie LH. Effects of glucose and fatty acids on myocardial ischemia and arrhythmias. *Lancet.* 1994;343:155–158.

20. Malmberg K, Norhammar A, Wedel H, et al. Glycometabolic state at admission: important risk marker of mortality in conventionally treated patients with diabetes mellitus and acute myocardial infarction: long–term results from the Diabetes and Insulin-Glucose Infusion in Acute Myocardial Infarction (DIGAMI) study. *Circulation.* 1999;99:2626–2632.

21. Maimberg K, Ryden L, Wedel H, et al. Intense metabolic control by means of insulin in patients with diabetes mellitus and acute myocardial infarction (DIGAMI 2): effects on mortality and morbidity. *Eur Heart J.* 2005;26:650–661.

22. Mehta SR, Yusuf S, Diaz R, et al. Effect of glucose-insulin-potassium infusion on mortality in patients with acute ST-segment elevation myocardial infarction: the CREATE-ECLA randomized controlled trial. *JAMA.* 2005;293:437–446.

23. Cheung, NW, Wong, VW, McLean M. The hyperglycemia: Intensive Insulin Infusion in Infarction (HI-5) study. A randomized controlled trial of insulin infusion therapy for myocardial infarction. *Diabetes Care.* 2006;29:765–770.

24. Furnary AP. Rationale for glycemic control in cardiac surgical patients: the Portland Diabetic Project. *Insulin.* 2006;1(suppl A):S24–S29.

25. Lindsberg PJ, Roine RO. Hyperglycemia in acute stroke. *Stroke.* 2004;35:363–364.

26. Capes SE, Hunt D, Malmberg K, et al. Stress hyperglycemia and prognosis of stroke in nondiabetic and diabetic patients: a systematic overview. *Stroke.* 2001;32:2426–2432.

27. Baird TA, Parsons MW, Phanh T, et al. Persistent post-stroke hyperglycemia is independently associated with infarct expansion and worse clinical outcome. *Stroke.* 2003;34:2208–2214.

28. Fuentes B, Castillo J, San Jose B, et al. The prognostic value of capillary glucose levels in acute stroke. The Glycemia in Acute Stroke (GLIAS) study. *Stroke.* 2009;40:562–568.

29. Gray CS, Hildreth AJ, Sandercock PA, et al. Glucose-potassium-insulin infusions in the management of post-stroke hyperglycaemia: the UK Glucose Insulin in Stroke Trial (GIST-UK). *Lancet Neurol.* 2007;6:397–406.

30. Bruno A, Kent TA, Coull BM, et al. Treatment of Hyperglycemia in Ischemic Stroke (THIS): a randomized pilot trial. *Stroke.* 2008;39:384–389.

31. Johnston KC, Hall CE, Kissela BM, et al. Glucose Regulation in Acute Stroke Patients (GRASP) trial: a randomized pilot trial. *Stroke.* 2009;40:3804–3809.

32. European Stroke Organization (ESO) Executive Committee, ESO Writing Committee. Guidelines for management of ischaemic stroke and transient ischaemic attack 2008. Available at: http://www.eso-stroke.org.

33. Adams HP Jr, del Zoppo G, Alberts MJ, et al. Guidelines for the early management of adults with ischemic stroke. *Stroke.* 2007;38:1655–1711.

34. Krinsley JS, Grover A. Severe hypoglycemia in critically ill patients: risk factors and outcomes. *Crit Care Med.* 2007;35:2262–2267.

35. Dellinger RP, Levy MM, Carlet JM, et al. Surviving Sepsis Campaign: international guidelines for management of severe sepsis and septic shock. *Crit Care Med.* 208;36:296–327.

36. Surviving sepsis guidelines. Surviving Sepsis Campaign statement on glucose control in severe sepsis. Available at: http://www.survivingsepsis.org.

37. Moghissi ES, Korytkowski MT, DiNardo M, et al. American Association of Clinical Endocrinologists and American Diabetes Association consensus statement on inpatient glycemic control. *Diabetes Care.* 2009;32:1119–1131.

38. Meijering S, Corstjens AM, Tulleken JE, et al. Towards a feasible algorithm for tight glycaemic control in critically ill patients: a systematic review of the literature. *Crit Care.* 2006;10:R19. Published online.

39. Nazer LH, Chow SL, Moghissi ES. Infusion protocols for critically ill patients: a highlight of differences and similarities. *Endocr Pract.* 2007;13:137–146.

40. Umpierrez, GE, Smiley, D, Zisman, A, et al. Randomized study of basal-bolus insulin therapy in the inpatient management of patients with type 2 diabetes (RABBIT 2 trial). *Diabetes Care.* 2007;30:2181–2186.

41. Clinical trials. Comparison of two strategies for glycemic control in acute ischemic stroke. Available at: http://www.clinicaltrial.gov/NCT00747279.

CHAPTER 33

Adrenal Insufficiency

Evie G. Marcolini and William C. Chiu

► BACKGROUND

Adrenal gland function has provided great academic material for investigation and controversy. It was not until 1937 that 17-hydroxy-11-dehydrocorticosterone, or cortisone, was isolated by Reichstein from the adrenal cortex. By 1947, synthetic cortisone was developed. At the same time, in addition to the use of cortisone for Addison's disease, this compound was found to have a therapeutic effect in patients with rheumatoid pain through its ability to inhibit stress and inflammation.

Adrenal insufficiency presents as chronic primary (about 5 per million incidence) or secondary (about 200 per million incidence). Both of these entities are more common in women, and diagnosis peaks anywhere from the fourth to the sixth decade. Historically, the most common cause of adrenal insufficiency was tuberculous adrenalitis. In developed countries, autoimmune adrenalitis has become a much more common cause of adrenal insufficiency, as tuberculous adrenalitis still plays a major role in the disease in developing countries.[1]

The adrenal gland has two anatomic divisions. The medulla secretes the catecholamines epinephrine and norepinephrine, and the cortex produces mineralocorticoids (via the renin–angiotensin system) and glucocorticoids. Critical illness and stress activate the hypothalamic–pituitary–adrenal (HPA) axis and stimulate the release of hypothalamic corticotropin-releasing hormone (CRH) and pituitary adrenocorticotropic hormone (ACTH).[2] ACTH secretion reaches its effector organ, the adrenal cortex, where it stimulates the synthesis and secretion of glucocorticoids, mineralocorticoids, and adrenal androgens. The mechanisms regulating ACTH secretion during stress are multifactorial, with the stimulatory effect of CRH and the inhibitory influence of cortisol. The "closed-loop" negative feedback of cortisol to the HPA axis acts to suppress the secretion of CRH, ACTH, and cortisol itself (Figure 33-1).

Physiologic ACTH and cortisol secretion have a diurnal pattern with nadirs at 10 PM and 2 AM, and peak at 8 AM. During infection and inflammatory states, cortisol levels are increased through stimulation of the hypothalamus and pituitary by cytokines and a reduction in the negative feedback loop. The diurnal variation of cortisol secretion is lost, and resources are shifted away from mineralocorticoid and androgen production toward corticosteroid production. ACTH release can also be increased by the influence of endorphinergic pathways and from the acute (but not chronic) administration of morphine. Even with the negative feedback loop in place, during periods of high stress (after major surgery, septic shock), the adrenal cortex is also influenced directly by paracrine pathways, endothelin, atrial natriuretic peptide, or cytokines.

The adrenocortical response to stress has several mechanisms. Cortisol is 90% bound to cortisol-binding globulin, with less than 10% in the free bioavailable form. This cortisol-binding globulin is downregulated by as much as 50% during acute illness, particularly sepsis, making more cortisol available in the free form. Cortisol has been shown to upregulate intracellular glucocorticoid receptors through a positive feedback mechanism. Glucocorticoid receptors have also shown to increase their level of binding activity in skeletal muscle.

All of the above mechanisms allow for glucocorticoid production to enable physiologic compensation in periods of acute stress. Glucocorticoids increase blood glucose levels via hepatic gluconeogenesis, and inhibit adipose tissue glucose uptake. They stimulate free fatty acid and amino acid release as well as increase proteolysis to supply energy and substrate for stress response.

Glucocorticoids contribute toward the synthesis of catecholamines, allowing for maintenance of cardiac

Hypothalamic-pituitary-adrenal axis
closed-loop negative feedback inhibition

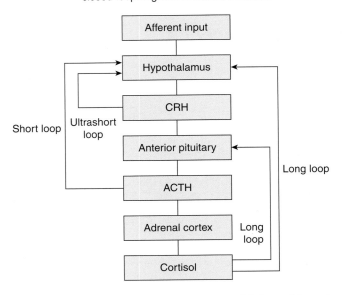

Figure 33-1. There are three types of "closed-loop" negative feedback systems in the hypothalamic-pituitary-adrenal (HPA) axis. Corticotropin-releasing hormone (CRH) acts directly on the hypothalamus to control its own secretion in the ultrashort-loop system. Adrenocorticotropic hormone (ACTH) feeds back on the hypothalamus in the short–loop system. Glucocorticoids exert a negative feedback on the anterior pituitary and hypothalamus in the long-loop system.

contractility, vascular tone, and blood pressure. They also decrease nitric oxide and prostaglandin production, with the result of maintaining hemodynamic stability. Glucocorticoids also have anti-inflammatory and immunosuppressive qualities through their downregulating influence on lymphocytes, natural killer cells, monocytes, macrophages, eosinophils, neutrophils, mast cells, and basophils.

In spite of the beneficial actions of cytokines and cellular mediators in an acute stress response, there is evidence that these cytokines and mediators can also have the opposite effect, resulting in decreased ACTH production, impaired corticosteroid production, and an increase in cortisol half-life, which may represent decreases in the number, expression, and function of glucocorticoid receptors. In short, mediators released in the septic patient can have a positive or negative effect on adrenal response and the net effect may depend on timing, severity of illness, and/or extent of mediator production.

In primary adrenal insufficiency, the adrenal gland fails to produce cortisol. In addition to autoimmune and infectious etiologies, this can be caused by bilateral adrenal hemorrhage, metastases, sarcoidosis, amyloidosis, adrenalectomy (such as in the case of resistant Cushing's syndrome), acquired immune defi-

ciency syndrome (AIDS), antiphospholipid syndrome, or medication-induced effects (such as antineoplastics, etomidate, ketoconazole, and mifepristone).[3] Secondary adrenal insufficiency, in which the pituitary gland produces insufficient ACTH, is typically caused by a regional tumor, autoimmune causes, genetic mutations, pituitary apoplexy postpartum (Sheehan's syndrome), head trauma, or chronic exogenous glucocorticoid administration.

A life-threatening episode of acute adrenal insufficiency typically manifests in severe hypotension, acute abdominal pain, vomiting, and fever. Hypoglycemic seizures may present in pediatrics or recurrent hypoglycemia in patients with type I diabetes. The common clinical signs of chronic adrenal insufficiency include fatigue, energy loss, reduced muscle strength, increased irritability, weight loss, nausea, and anorexia. Primary adrenal failure will likely result in hyperpigmentation, due to the stimulation of melanocytes by ACTH, whereas secondary adrenal failure will manifest with pale skin color. Mineralocorticoid deficiency may also be present, resulting in hyponatremia, hyperkalemia, dehydration, hypovolemia, hypotension, and prerenal failure.

► CRITICAL ILLNESS–RELATED CORTICOSTEROID INSUFFICIENCY

The holy grail of adrenal insufficiency in critically ill patients is the question of how to assess adrenal function. Notwithstanding the myriad of effects that can be affected by cytokines and mediators on the HPA axis, we are so far unable to test end-organ effects of cortisol, so the diagnosis is commonly based on serum cortisol levels. This has resulted in a variety of studies and beliefs about the most accurate method to assess the serum cortisol level and its subsequent clinical implications.[4] Many centers utilize the cosyntropin stimulation test, by administering 250 mcg of synthetic corticotropin and checking the serum level of cortisol before, and 30 and 60 minutes after injection. A level below 18–20 mcg/dL, or increase less than 9 mcg/dL, is considered diagnostic of adrenal insufficiency. Some centers believe that a lower dose (1 mcg) of cosyntropin is more sensitive and specific.

It is important to recognize that the increase in cortisol following a stimulation test is indicative of reserve levels of cortisol, as opposed to adrenal function. The best way to determine whether or not the HPA axis is functioning adequately is to test the entire axis, which, in the case of severely stressed critically ill patients, is already taking place via the stressors of hypotension, hypoxemia, fever, and hypoglycemia. Therefore, a random cortisol level in the face of critical illness should provide adequate information on adrenal insufficiency. A random cortisol level greater than 25 mcg/dL is considered to indicate adequate HPA axis functioning, based on the fact that patients with trauma, surgery, and critical illness have been found to have cortisol levels in the 30–50 mcg/dL range that can last for a week. It is also worth noting that critically ill patients lose the diurnal nature of cortisol secretion, so timing of a random level should not be an issue.

Adrenal insufficiency can manifest in critically ill patients up to an incidence of 77%, depending on the criteria. Previous steroid use, depending on the dose and duration of use, may contribute to suppression of the HPA axis, especially if used for more than 30 days. Immunosuppression and other infections, while not necessarily causing primary adrenal insufficiency in the outpatient setting, have become the most significant etiology of such in the critically ill patient. It is also noteworthy that patients with sepsis and systemic inflammatory response syndrome (SIRS) criteria commonly manifest primary adrenal failure, consisting of suppression of the HPA axis as well as glucocorticoid receptor expression. This has been shown to be reversible on resolution of the septic episode.

There is general agreement that adrenal insufficiency in the critically ill patient portends a higher mortality, and that some level of steroid treatment improves outcome. The difficult questions to clarify become how to assess for adrenal insufficiency, at what cutoff level does the patient require steroids, and what dosing should be used. The current recommendations by the Surviving Sepsis Campaign are to administer intravenous corticosteroids (hydrocortisone 200–300 mg per day, for 7 days in three or four divided doses or by continuous infusion) for adult septic shock patients after blood pressure is identified to be poorly responsive to fluid resuscitation and vasopressor therapy.[5] It is also recommended that each intensive care unit (ICU) have a standardized protocol for deciding when it is appropriate to start steroids and how to administer them.

It is also worth noting that there are many drug–drug interactions that may occur with steroid administration. Glucocorticoids can decrease the drug blood levels of aspirin, warfarin, insulin, isoniazid, and oral hypoglycemic agents, but they can increase the levels of cyclophosphamide and cyclosporine. Drugs that can increase the level of glucocorticoid blood concentration include antacids, carbamazepine, cholestyramine, colestipol, ephedrine, mitotane, phenobarbital, phenytoin, and rifampin, while cyclosporine, erythromycin, oral contraceptives, and troleandomycin increase them.

Steroid administration should be tapered as the critically ill patient's clinical picture improves, so as to avoid hemodynamic and immunologic rebound. Hydrocortisone is the corticosteroid of choice, since most studies were performed using this formulation, and it is the closest in physiologic characteristics to cortisone. Hydrocortisone also has mineralocorticoid activity, which must be considered and replaced if other glucocorticoids are utilized.

In summary, critical illness–related corticosteroid insufficiency (CIRCI) can be a significant factor in the progress of the critically ill patient, but many questions remain unanswered at this time. Table 33-1 lists

▶ **TABLE 33-1. TWELVE RECOMMENDATIONS OF THE AMERICAN COLLEGE OF CRITICAL CARE MEDICINE INTERNATIONAL TASK FORCE. "DATA FROM"[6]**

Critical illness-related corticosteroid insufficiency
1. Dysfunction of the HPA axis in critical illness is best described by the term *critical illness-related corticosteroid insufficiency* (CIRCI)
2. The terms *absolute* and *relative* adrenal insufficiency are best avoided in the context of critical illness

Diagnosis of adrenal insufficiency
3. At this time, adrenal insufficiency in critical illness is best diagnosed by a delta cortisol (after 250 μg cosyntropin) of <9 μg/dL or a random total cortisol of <10 μg/dL
4. The use of free cortisol measurements cannot be recommended for routine use at this time
5. The ACTH stimulation test should not be used to identify those patients with septic shock or ARDS who should receive GCs

Who to treat with glucocorticoids?
6. Hydrocortisone should be considered in the management strategy of patients with septic shock, particularly those patients who have responded poorly to fluid resuscitation and vasopressor agents
7. Moderate-dose GC should be considered in the management strategy of patients with early severe ARDS (PaO_2/FiO_2 of <200) and before day 14 in patients with unresolving ARDS

How to treat
8. In patients with septic shock, intravenous hydrocortisone should be given in a dose of 200 mg/day in four divided doses or as a bolus of 100 mg followed by a continuous infusion at 10 mg/h (240 mg/day)
9. The optimal duration of GC treatment in patients with septic shock and early ARDS is unclear
10. GC treatment should be tapered slowly and not stopped abruptly
11. Treatment with fludrocortisone (50 μg orally once daily) is considered optional
12. Dexamethasone is not recommended for the treatment of septic shock or ARDS

the 12 recommendations from the American College of Critical Care Medicine.[6] It is important to have a protocolized practice in the care of these patients and to participate in and follow in the research advances in this very important topic.

REFERENCES

1. Oelkers W. Adrenal insufficiency. *N Engl J Med.* 1996; 335:1206–1212.
2. Marik PE, Zaloga GP. Adrenal insufficiency in the critically ill: a new look at an old problem. *Chest.* 2002;122: 1784–1796.
3. Arlt W, Allolio B. Adrenal insufficiency. *Lancet.* 2003;361: 1881–1893.
4. Jacobi J. Corticosteroid replacement in critically ill patients. *Crit Care Clin.* 2006;22: 245–253.
5. Dellinger RP, Levy MM, Carlet JM, et al. Surviving Sepsis Campaign: international guidelines for management of severe sepsis and septic shock: 2008. *Crit Care Med.* 2008;36: 296–327.
6. Marik PE, Pastores SM, Annane D, et al. Recommendations for the diagnosis and management of corticosteroid insufficiency in critically ill adult patients: consensus statements from an international task force by the American College of Critical Care Medicine. *Crit Care Med.* 2008;36:1937–1949.

SECTION VIII

Infectious Disorders

CHAPTER 34

Approach to Fever in Critical Care

Marnie E. Rosenthal

▶ PART I: FEVER IN THE ICU: BACKGROUND AND PATHOPHYSIOLOGY

INTRODUCTION

Fever is an adaptation mechanism of the body in response to internal and external environmental stressors, and is a key indicator of immune system activation. Normal body temperature is maintained by peripheral nerves that transmit signals back to the hypothalamus. Fever occurs when cytokines cause an increase in body temperature in association with a rise in hypothalamic set point, and consists of three clinical phases: chill, fever, and flush. Elevated body temperatures can broadly be classified as hyperthermia syndromes and infectious and noninfectious fever (see Table 34-1). Hyperthermia occurs when thermoregulatory mechanisms fail and when heat production exceeds heat loss through either overproduction of heat or decrease in heat loss. Such examples of heat overproduction include thyrotoxicosis, pheochromocytoma, adrenal crisis, or salicylate toxicity via interruption of the citric acid cycle and uncoupled oxidative phosphorylation. Heatstroke or anticholinergic toxicity is mediated by a deficiency in mechanisms of heat dissipation. Some hyperthermia syndromes fall into both categories, such as postanesthesia neuroleptic malignant syndrome (NMS), and may cause profound hyperpyrexia. It is important to differentiate fever from hyperthermia because hyperthermia due to thermoregulatory failure is treated by a lowering of the body temperature by physical mechanisms (conduction, convection, evaporation); antipyretics are not effective. Both noninfectious and infectious causes of elevated body temperatures in the intensive care unit (ICU) will be discussed in detail in following sections.

DEFINITION

The average body temperature set point is 37.0°C (98.6°F) and may vary by 0.5–1.0°C according to time of day or hormonal milieu: it is highest at 6:00 AM and for women at the time of ovulation. Fever is defined in multiple ways. It is an isolated core body temperature >38.0°C (100.4°F) or two consecutive elevations of greater than 38.3°C. In neutropenic patients, fever may be defined as a single temperature greater than 38.3°F (101.0°F) or greater than 38.0°C (100.4°F) for 60 minutes. The American College of Critical Care Medicine and the Infectious Diseases Society of America (ACCM/IDSA) define a fever as a rise in body temperature greater than 38.3°C (101°F) and recommend any new fever be investigated.[1] However, in immunocompromised or elderly individuals, a lower cutoff may be appropriate, as these patients may not be able to mount substantial febrile responses. Additionally, the fever response may be attenuated in patients with azotemia or congestive heart failure, or in patients receiving antipyretics or pain control with an antipyretic combination.

EPIDEMIOLOGY

Fever is common in critically ill patients and warrants clinical attention. Infections are the leading cause of temperature elevation in hospitalized patients, whereas hypothalamic disorders are less common. In patients

▶ **TABLE 34-1. CAUSES OF FEVER IN THE ICU**

Excessive heat production	Delirium tremens, exercise, heatstroke, malignant hyperthermia, neuroleptic malignant syndrome, pheochromocytoma, recreational drugs (cocaine, phencyclidine, methylenedioxymethamphetamine [ecstasy], lysergic acid diethylamide [LSD]), salicylates, serotonin syndrome, seizure, tetanus, toxicity
Disordered heat dissemination	Anticholinergics, dehydration, heatstroke, neuroleptic malignant syndrome
Hypothalamic	Encephalitis, granulomatous disease (sarcoid and tuberculosis [TB]), neuroleptic malignant syndrome, thrombotic disease, trauma, tumors
Infections	Bacteremia, catheter-related infections, central nervous system infections, *Clostridium difficile*–associated diarrhea, fungal infections, parasitic infections, pneumonia, postoperative fever, septic thrombophlebitis, sinusitis, surgical site infections, urinary tract infection, viremia

admitted to an ICU with severe sepsis, the incidence of fever approached 90%.[2] Prospective and retrospective studies have described wide ranges of fever prevalence in the ICU, ranging from 30% to 70%, with the highest incidence seen in noncardiac surgical patients in one study.[3,4] In the neuro-ICU, the incidence of fever may approach 70%, only half of the fevers being due to infection, mainly nosocomial pulmonary infection.[5] The incidence of hyperpyrexia due to anesthesia-induced malignant hyperthermia (MH) estimates ranges from 1:250 to 1:250,000, with a recent study evaluating 2001–2005 New York state discharge data establishing local incidence as 1 in 100,000.[6]

PATHOPHYSIOLOGY

Basal metabolic activity in the liver and heart accounts for the majority of the body's heat production, while the skin accounts for the majority of heat dissipation. The lungs add a minor amount to basal metabolic heat dissipation through conduction and evaporation. Temperature is regulated not by one single neural area, but by feedback loops involving the hypothalamus, brainstem, and spinal cord that interact with the autonomic, somatic, and endocrine systems (see Figure 34-1). The earliest published observations regarding temperature

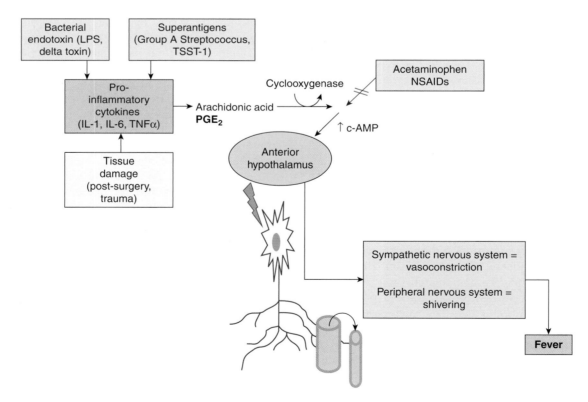

Figure 34-1. Pathogenesis of fever.

regulation appeared in 1912 and described thermal sensitivity of the hypothalamic region.[7] Further understanding was provided in the 1960s with three influential papers describing the role of the preoptic area of the anterior hypothalamus in thermoregulation.[8–10] Stimulation by the anterior hypothalamus causes vasoconstriction and sweating, while posterior hypothalamic activation induces shivering. Vasoconstriction in response to an increased hypothalamic set point begins in the hands and feet as blood is shunted centrally. Shivering develops as a heat conservation mechanism to increase heat production from skeletal muscle. The nature of the response depends on ambient temperature; animal models injected with exogenous substances that raise temperature set point will increase heat production in a cold environment or decrease heat loss in a warm environment.

Fever is regulated at the level of the hypothalamus through pyrogen release by activated immune cells. Exogenous pyrogens, such as lipopolysaccharide (LPS) endotoxin in gram-negative bacteria or exotoxins such as toxic shock syndrome toxin (TSST) in *Staphylococcus aureus*, trigger febrile responses in the host. LPS complexes with a binding protein and attaches to the CD14 receptor of a macrophage resulting in cytokine release.[11] Cytokines are soluble intracellular signal proteins that regulate local and systemic immune processes. Formulated as large-molecular-weight polypeptides, they are produced by monocytes, macrophages, and glial cells in response to inflammation, infection, or injury.[12,13] Interleukin (IL) 1 and tumor necrosis factor (TNF) are structurally unrelated cytokines with a strikingly similar biologic function; both are secreted by antigen-presenting cells that augment binding and activation of T cells and promote growth and differentiation of B cells. TNF-α is produced by activated macrophages in response to LPS of gram-negative organisms, whereas TNF-β is a product of T lymphocytes. Together, IL-1, IL-6, and TNF are collectively referred to as proinflammatory cytokines (see Table 34-2).

Endogenous pyrogen, later reclassified as lymphocyte-activating factor and eventually found to be part of the IL-1 family, was the earliest isolated cellular product implicated in fever induction.[14] Animal models of endogenous pyrogens indicate the febrile response is mediated by activation of calcium channels and can be attenuated by calcium channel blockers such as nifedipine or verapamil.[15] The IL-1 gene family composed of IL-1α, IL-1β, and IL-1 receptor antagonist (IL-1ra) is encoded on the long arm of chromosome 2. Variable number tandem repeat polymorphisms in this receptor antagonist region are linked to autoimmune dysregulation syndromes such as psoriasis and inflammatory bowel disease.[16] IL-1β is a potent inducer of IL-6 that is critical in the fever response as evidenced by the absence of fever production in IL-6-deficient knockout mice.[17,18] Cytokines bind to and activate their own receptor, activating phospholipase A_2 resulting in release of arachidonic acid, which is the substrate of cyclooxygenase and the rate-limiting enzyme in prostaglandin biosynthesis.[19]

Increased levels of IL-1, IL-6, interferon-γ, and TNF-α act on the hypothalamus to raise its inherent set point through the catecholamine cells of the medulla oblongata and the circumventricular organs.[20] The organum vasculosum of the lamina terminalis (OVLT) is a vascular sensory organ of the brain that is unique in that it is composed of a capillary bed that lacks a blood–brain barrier and can therefore monitor the osmotic, ionic, and hormonal environment of the blood.[21] When pyrogens are detected by the OVLT, prostaglandin E_2 (PGE_2) is released that triggers the PGE_2 receptor on glial cells to release cyclic adenosine monophosphate (C-AMP). This activates the febrile response via the hypothalamic feedback loops involving vasoactive substances and neurotransmitters such as norepinepherine, dopamine, and serotonin.[22] Additionally, these cytokines are also released during tissue trauma, especially IL-6.[23]

Endogenous antipyretics such as IL-10, a protein product of T-helper cells, have been shown in mouse models to inhibit the production of endogenous IL-1β, IL-6, and TNF during LPS-induced fevers.[18,24] Additionally, arginine vasopressin, α-melanocyte-stimulating hormone, and glucocorticoids counter and limit the duration of fever.[25]

TEMPERATURE MEASUREMENT

In the ICU, body temperature may be measured peripherally or centrally. Temperature is most accurate when measured by thermistors on pulmonary artery catheters (the gold standard), bladder catheters, or esophageal probes. Rectal probes provide a close approximation of core temperature. Generally readings from rectal thermometers are a few tenths of a degree higher than core temperatures. Rectal thermometers are somewhat invasive for the awake and alert patients and are contraindicated in neutropenic

► **TABLE 34-2. CYTOKINES INVOLVED IN TEMPERATURE REGULATION**

Proinflammatory Cytokines	Antipyretic Cytokines
IL-1	IL-4
IL-6	IL-10
IFN-α	Arginine vasopressin
TNF-α	Melanocyte-stimulating hormone
	Glucocorticoids

IL, interleukin; IFN, interferon; TNF, tumor necrosis factor.

patients. Oral temperature measurements are convenient, safe, and minimally invasive, although readings may be confounded by ingestion of hot or cold fluids, or mouth breathing. Additionally patients with decreased level of consciousness, arousal states, or altered mental status may not be able to comply with placement of a thermometer under the tongue. Readings may vary depending on the location of sublingual thermometer placement, and are generally 0.4°C (0.7°F) lower than rectal temperatures.[26] Infrared tympanic membrane thermometers are less accurate than intravascular probes and rectal or oral thermometers. Temporal artery thermometers and axillary or femoral skinfold temperatures should not be used to record temperatures in an ICU.[27]

EFFECTS ON THE HOST

Conflicting evidence exists as to outcome associations with elevated temperature in ICU patients. One study suggested that crude mortality was higher in febrile patients (34.5% vs. 18.7%); however, when adjusted for patient severity, fever was no longer associated with mortality ($P = 0.384$).[28] Low-grade fever was common in the ICU, and outcome varied by admission criteria.[4] High fever was associated with an increased risk of death (20% vs. 12%) in a large literature review.

Numerous studies have found that after controlling for baseline predictors of poor outcome, fever in acute subarachnoid hemorrhage is independently associated with increased morbidity, including cognitive impairment, and mortality.[29,30] In stroke patients, the earlier the fever onset, the greater the amount of cognitive dysfunction; hyperthermia appearing after 24 hours was not associated with poorer outcome.[31]

Controversy exists as to whether treating a fever is beneficial for the host. Elevated temperatures result in tachycardia, increased minute ventilation, resting energy expenditure, oxygen consumption, and sympathetic tone. Hyperthermia has been associated with rhabdomyolysis, disseminated intravascular coagulation, and multisystem organ failure.[32] In animal models, fever has been shown to decrease the serum level of iron, which is a growth factor for many microbes.[33] It may reduce the expression of virulence factors, enhance antibiotic susceptibility by lowering minimum inhibitory concentrations, and augment host responses.[34,35] A recent study in a trauma ICU that randomized patients to permissive or aggressive treatment (650 mg acetaminophen q 6 hours) for fevers >38.5°C was stopped after the first interim analysis due to a statistically significant increase in deaths in the aggressively treated group ($P = 0.06$).[36] Despite the lack of evidence-based outcomes data, pharmacologic and physical means of fever reduction are commonly employed.

▶ PART II: ETIOLOGY OF FEVER IN THE ICU

NONINFECTIOUS CAUSES OF FEVER

Drug Fever

Drug fever is often a diagnosis of exclusion based on the background of administration of a new medication. A hallmark sign of drug fever is the disappearance of fever after the medication is stopped and reappearance after it is restarted. This is most often the result of a hypersensitivity reaction, and commonly occurs 7–10 days after the administration of an agent; it may be accompanied by rash, urticaria, or serum sickness. Although any medication can cause hypersensitivity reaction, antimicrobials (especially β-lactams), antimycobacterials, antiepileptics, antiarrhythmics (such as quinidine and procainamide), and antihypertensives (methyldopa and phenytoin) are common causes of fever.[37] Certain classes of pharmacologic agents are associated with hyperthermia through disordered thermoregulatory mechanism. Sympathomimetics, anticholinergics, neurotransmitter active drugs, such as dopamine antagonists, serotonergic agents, and monoamine oxidase inhibitors, as well as inhaled anesthetics can disrupt the balance between heat production and dissipation. MH occurs in genetically predisposed individuals after exposure to certain pharmacologic agents. It is the result of a large efflux of calcium triggered by inhalation anesthetics or succinylcholine on a background of a genetic defect in the ryanodine, or calcium release channel in the sarcoplasmic reticulum of skeletal muscle.[38] NMS can be seen with antipsychotic agents such as haloperidol, prochlorperazine, and metoclopramide or with the withdrawal of dopaminergic agents. It is characterized by muscular rigidity, autonomic dysregulation, extrapyramidal side effects, and hyperthermia, and is thought to be due to dopamine antagonism within the hypothalamus.[39] Serotonin syndrome has similar clinical features, but also involves diarrhea, tremor, and myoclonus. It is related to excessive 5HT1A receptor stimulation, and may be exacerbated with the use of linezolid.[40] Illicit drugs such as phencyclidine (PCP), ecstasy (methylenedioxymethamphetamine [MDMA]), lysergic acid diamide (LSD), and cocaine have been implicated in hyperthermia syndromes. MDMA ingestion leads to central deregulation of thermogenesis via activation of the sympathetic nervous system and an excessive release of norepinepherine with an uncoupling of adrenoreceptors and loss of heat dissipation.[41]

Head Injury

Elevated core temperature is common after many types of neurologic injury (ischemic, hemorrhagic, or traumatic) and is associated with increased risk of adverse outcome, even after controlling for confounders or modifiers, such severity of illness, diagnosis, age, and infection. Human and animal models have shown that fever exacerbates ischemic neuronal damage and is proportional to the degree of pyrexia.[42] Hyperthermia postcardiac resuscitation was associated with an unfavorable neurologic recovery after cardiac pulmonary resuscitation.[43] Fever was found to be strongly associated with an increased intensive care and overall length of stay, and higher overall mortality.[44,45]

Heatstroke

Heatstroke occurring in warm environments may be exertional or nonexertional in origin, and may be exacerbated by dehydration or antihistamines. Defined as a core temperature 40°C (>104°F), individuals at the extremes of age are at risk for nonexertional heatstroke during hot weather and heat waves. It is associated with upregulation of heat shock proteins in the brain that function as molecular chaperons and cellular repair proteins with cytoprotective effects.[46]

Neurologic Causes of Fever

Although fever may occur in up to one quarter of neuro-ICU patients, almost half are noninfectious.[47] Stroke or subarachnoid hemorrhage can trigger febrile responses in noninfected patients, as can head trauma and neurosurgery involving the floor of the third ventricle.[48]

Miscellaneous

Vasculitis, hyperthyroidism, or mesenteric ischemia can trigger febrile responses in noninfected patients. A low-grade fever can also be seen in the cardiac care unit post–myocardial infarction, resulting from epicardial inflammation after a transmural infarct. Dressler's syndrome, likely mediated by antimyocardial antibodies, can also present with fever and a friction rub up to 2–3 months post–myocardial infarction.

Blood is an irritant, and when it accumulates or stagnates, it may induce fever. Hematomas and pulmonary embolism have been associated with fever.[49] However, contrary to common dictum, deep vein thrombosis is not a common cause of isolated fevers as evidenced by a number of recent studies evaluating the rate of fever in patients with lower extremity deep venous thrombosis.[50,51] Transfusion reactions are possible during or after receipt of blood products.

Noninfectious intra-abdominal processes such as pancreatitis, acalculous cholecystitis, and mesenteric ischemia are causes of fever in critically ill patients, and these entities frequently present with associated clinical signs and symptoms. Rheumatologic disorders such as systemic lupus erythematosus, and adult Still's disease, as well as occult malignancy, are uncommon, albeit possible, causes of fever in ICU patients.[52]

INFECTIOUS CAUSES OF FEVER

Central Nervous System Infection

Focal neurologic abnormalities generally occur with central nervous system (CNS) infection; however, in critically ill patients, a high index of suspicion is warranted even in the absence of focal findings, and appropriate imaging studies and culture data should be obtained.[53] Fever is the most common acute presentation of bacterial meningitis in children; in adults and the elderly, confusion, nuchal rigidity, and headache are more common.[48] Bacterial meningitis may occur after any neurosurgical procedure, but is most common with procedures related to open head trauma.[54]

Diarrhea

For evaluation of fever in the ICU, ACCM/IDSA defines diarrhea as more than two stools per day that conform to the container in which they are placed.[53] Enteral feedings and medications are common causes of loose stool or diarrhea in the ICU patient. The most common enteric cause of fever in the ICU is *Clostridium difficile* and should be suspected in any patient with fever, elevated white blood cell count, and antimicrobial therapy or chemotherapy administration within 60 days of diarrhea onset. Other organisms that cause fever and diarrhea are generally community associated and rarely acquired after a patient is admitted to an ICU. Therefore, sending stools for routine culture or ova and parasites should be avoided unless the patient was admitted to the hospital with diarrhea or is human immunodeficiency virus (HIV) positive, or as part of an outbreak investigation.[53] In patients with negative *C. difficile* toxin assays, it is important to consider increased gastrointestinal (GI) motility as a side effect of medications, enteral feedings, or hemorrhagic enterocolitis due to *Klebsiella oxytoca*.[55,56]

Intravascular Devices

Patients should be examined daily for signs of catheter entry site infections and phlebitis, and any expressed purulence should be sent for Gram stain and culture. Short-term peripheral and noncuffed central catheters should be removed if infection is suspected; with evidence of a tunnel infection or septic physiology, the catheter should be removed, cultured, and reinserted at a different site.[53] It is not necessary to routinely culture all catheters removed from ICU patients, as catheters are frequently colonized within the lumen and this may not correlate with infection.[53]

Pneumonia

Pneumonia is a common cause of infection acquired in the ICU and a predominant cause of fever, especially in mechanically ventilated patients. For initial fever evaluation, a portable chest radiograph is sufficient. In the nonintubated patient, expectorated sputum or nasal/endotracheal aspirate is adequate to evaluate airway colonization or infection.[53] Aspirates from the inner channel of the bronchoscope in intubated patients reflect upper airway colonization and may lead to overtreatment of colonizing organisms. Mini-bronchoalveolar lavage (BAL) or blind bronchoscopy, with a protected brush, is a reliable sampling method to obtain lower respiratory secretions.[57] Respiratory cultures should be processed within 2 hours of collection.

Postoperative Fever

Fever is a common phenomenon in the first 48 hours after surgery. Initially, the etiology is noninfectious, but after 96 hours fevers can often be attributed to infectious processes.[58] Wound infections are rare immediately postop, with the exception of *S. pyogenes* or clostridial infections that may present in the first 3 postoperative days. In the febrile postoperative patient, surgical sites should be examined daily for erythema, purulence, or tenderness, and incisions should be opened and cultured if infection is expected.[53] New or persistent fevers after 96 hours warrant careful surgical site inspection as well as investigation into other etiologies of fever, including thromboembolic disease, drug reaction, MH, or catheter-related infection.

Sinusitis

Nosocomial maxillary sinusitis is a common entity in intubated patients and should be included in the differential diagnosis of fever in an ICU patient.[59] Either two major criteria (cough, purulent nasal discharge) or one major plus two minor criteria (headache, earache, facial or tooth pain, malodorous breath, sore throat, or wheezing) suggest acute bacterial sinusitis in the outpatient setting; however, in critically ill patients, these signs may not be evident.[60] Additionally, sinus films may be of limited value and sinus computed tomography (CT) or magnetic resonance imaging (MRI) scans may be difficult to obtain. For a definitive diagnosis, puncture and sampling of the involved sinus under aseptic technique should be performed.[53] A prospective study of new-onset fever in surgical ICU patients after excluding bacteremia, catheter-related infections, or pneumonia found sinusitis diagnosed by three-view sinus films accounted for 24% of fevers, and the predominant microbiology was *Klebsiella* and *Pseudomonas*.[61] Another study found the common pathogens by maxillary sinus aspirates were *Acinetobacter* (32%) and anaerobes (21%) and a combination of a nasal decongestant and topical nasal steroid was effective in decreasing the incidence of sinusitis in mechanically ventilated trauma patients.[62]

Urinary Tract Infection

Urinary tract infection is among the most frequent nosocomial infection in the ICU, and a common cause of fevers due to frequent bladder instrumentation. Not surprisingly, increased duration of catheter days is correlated with the risk of cystitis and pyelonephritis.[63] The predominant pathogens involved in urinary tract infections in ICU patients include multidrug-resistant gram-negative rods. Cultures should be collected from the sampling port of the catheter and not the drainage bag, and processed by the microbiology laboratory within 1 hour. A colony count from a catheterized patient of $>10^3$ cfu/mL represents true infection.[53]

Immunocompromised Patients

Immunocompromised patients (i.e., HIV/acquired immune deficiency syndrome [AIDS], induced immune suppression from solid organ or bone marrow transplants, chemotherapy, or immune modulation therapy) are at risk for opportunistic bacterial, viral, and fungal infections. Special consideration must be given to immunodeficient patients with fevers. A broad range of infectious organisms can be seen, including cytomegalovirus, *Pneumocystis jerovicii*, *Aspergillus*, and endemic mycoses such as *Histoplasma* and *Coccidioides*.

► PART III: DIAGNOSIS AND MANAGEMENT OF FEVER IN THE ICU

DIAGNOSTIC APPROACH

Approach to the febrile patient begins with a proper diagnosis and management of the underlying disorder. Pseudosepsis, characterized by fever, elevated leukocyte counts with a left shift, and sepsis physiology with elevated heart rate and hypotension, can closely mimic infectious fevers, but may be attributed to rheumatologic, endocrine, or neurologic disturbances. Adrenal insufficiency and thyroid storm have been mistaken for sepsis.[64] The magnitude of temperature elevation does not provide clues to the etiology, as fevers greater than 102°F may be present with both infectious and noninfectious causes.

Accurate history and physical exam, along with careful review of the hospital course, including previous in-patient or outpatient workup, is the first step in diagnosis and management of the febrile patient in the ICU. The 2008 ACCM/IDSA guidelines recommend that a new onset of temperature <36.0°C or >38.3°C warrants a clinical assessment.[53] A thorough physical exam should be performed, including conjunctival and fundoscopic ocular exam, detailed oropharyngeal inspection, careful auscultative cardiopulmonary exam, and full skin exam including catheter insertion sites and dependent or posterior body surfaces when possible. Radiographic imaging should be employed if clinical signs warrant further investigation. Laboratory investigation based on results of a clinical assessment may include a complete blood count with a differential, complete metabolic panel, urine and sputum microscopy and culture, and additional Gram stain and culture specimens from any concerning site. Blood cultures are the only mandatory evaluation and should follow certain guidelines. According to the 2008 ACCM/IDSA guidelines for evaluation of new fever in critically ill adult patients, within the first 24 hours of a fever, and prior to initiation of antibiotics, three to four blood cultures from separate puncture sites should be drawn after decontamination with 2% chlorohexidine gluconate, preferentially, or 1–2% tincture of iodine.[53] Patients with intravascular access should have one set drawn through the line and one set drawn peripherally. Access to intravascular device and stopper on the blood culture bottle should be swabbed with 70% alcohol and allowed to dry for 30 seconds prior to drawing 20–30 mL of blood for inoculation. Additional blood cultures should be drawn only for a suspicion of continuation or recurrent bacteremia or for a test of cure 48–96 hours after appropriate antimicrobial or antifungal therapy.

ANTIPYRESIS

Despite a lack of compelling evidence-based medicine, fever is commonly treated by pharmacologic and physical mechanisms to establish euthermia in the ICU. Rationale for treating hyperthermia includes therapeutic effect on metabolic consumption and patient comfort. In one study, external cooling was shown to decrease oxygen consumption by 20% in febrile critically ill patients if treated with paralytics to prevent shivering; however, if shivering was not inhibited, external cooling was shown to increase oxygen consumption.[65] In a large clinical trial, treatment with intravenous ibuprofen

reduced core temperature, heart rate, oxygen consumption, and lactic acid blood levels but did not decrease organ failure or 30-day mortality.[66]

The goal of treating fever is to reduce the hypothalamic set point and restore the balance of heat production and dissipation. Pharmacologic therapy includes nonsteroidal anti-inflammatory drugs (NSAIDs) and steroids, while physical mechanisms range from externally applied cooling blankets, fans, or ice packs to chilled intravenous fluids, gastric lavage, or intravascular catheter-based techniques. NSAIDs and acetaminophen/paracetamol inhibit the cyclooxegenase pathway and formation of $PGEE_2$, and foster a return to a normothermic hypothalamic set point.[67] Aspirin and NSAIDs effectively reduce fever, but can have an anticoagulant effect on platelets. Acetaminophen is the preferred antipyretic in adults, but increases the risk of Reye's syndrome in children and should be avoided. If bacteremia or infection is suspected, targeted antimicrobial therapy should be initiated and de-escalated as appropriate microbiologic information becomes available.

Drug hypersensitivity reactions should be treated with medication withdrawal. MH should be treated with immediate withdrawal of the anesthetic agent in conjunction with intravenous dantrolene and procainamide to prevent ventricular arrhythmia.

▶ CONCLUSION

Fever is a well-preserved adaptive mechanism that may provide a survival benefit to the host. It is a common, nonspecific physical exam finding in the ICU, which warrants attention. An automatic and protocol drive toward normothermia should be avoided, as the etiology differs depending on underlying medical or surgical factors. Appropriate interventions range from careful observation to immediate and aggressive action, and should be decided on a case-by-case basis; no single "fever workup" should be implemented across all patient populations.

▶ ACKNOWLEDGEMENT

The author would like to thank Kathleen Casey, MD, for critical review of this manuscript.

REFERENCES

1. O'Grady NP, Barie PS, Bartlett JG, et al. Practice guidelines for evaluating new fever in critically ill adult patients. Task Force of the Society of Critical Care Medicine and the Infectious Diseases Society of America. *Clin Infect Dis*. 1998;26(5):1042–1059.

2. Arons MM, Wheeler AP, Bernard GR, et al. Effects of ibuprofen on the physiology and survival of hypothermic sepsis. Ibuprofen in Sepsis Study Group. *Crit Care Med.* 1999;27(4):699–707.

3. Circiumaru B, Baldock G, Cohen J. A prospective study of fever in the intensive care unit. *Intensive Care Med.* 1999;25(7):668–673.

4. Laupland KB, Shahpori R, Kirkpatrick AW, Ross T, Gregson DB, Stelfox HT. Occurrence and outcome of fever in critically ill adults. *Crit Care Med.* 2008;36(5):1531–1535.

5. Badjatia N. Fever control in the neuro-ICU: why, who, and when? *Curr Opin Crit Care.* 2009;15(2):79–82.

6. Brady JE, Sun LS, Rosenberg H, Li G. Prevalence of malignant hyperthermia due to anesthesia in New York State, 2001–2005. *Anesth Analg.* 2009;109(4):1162–1166.

7. Barbour HG. Die Wirkung unmittelbärer Erwärmung und Abkülung der Wärmezentra auf die Körpertemperature. *Arch Exp Pathol Pharmakol.* 1912;70(1):1–36.

8. Hammel HT, Hardy JD, Fusco MM. Thermoregulatory responses to hypothalamic cooling in unanesthetized dogs. *Am J Physiol.* 1960;198:481–486.

9. Hammel HT, Jackson DC, Stolwijk JA, Hardy JD, Stromme SB. Temperature regulation by hypothalamic proportional control with an adjustable set point. *J Appl Physiol.* 1963;18:1146–1154.

10. Hellstrom B, Hammel HT. Some characteristics of temperature regulation in the unanesthetized dog. *Am J Physiol.* 1967;213(2):547–556.

11. Dentener MA, Bazil V, Von Asmuth EJ, Ceska M, Buurman WA. Involvement of CD14 in lipopolysaccharide-induced tumor necrosis factor-alpha, IL-6 and IL-8 release by human monocytes and alveolar macrophages. *J Immunol.* 1993 1;150(7):2885–2891.

12. Dinarello CA, Cannon JG, Wolff SM. New concepts on the pathogenesis of fever. *Rev Infect Dis.* 1988;10(1):168–189.

13. Dinarello CA. The interleukin-1 family: 10 years of discovery. *FASEB J.* 1994;8(15):1314–1325.

14. Murphy PA, Simon PL, Willoughby WF. Endogenous pyrogens made by rabbit peritoneal exudate cells are identical with lymphocyte-activating factors made by rabbit alveolar macrophages. *J Immunol.* 1980;124(5):2498–2501.

15. Stitt JT, Shimada SG. Calcium channel blockers inhibit endogenous pyrogen fever in rats and rabbits. *J Appl Physiol.* 1991;71(3):951–955.

16. Tarlow JK, Blakemore AI, Lennard A, et al. Polymorphism in human IL-1 receptor antagonist gene intron 2 is caused by variable numbers of an 86-bp tandem repeat. *Hum Genet.* 1993;91(4):403–404.

17. Chai Z, Gatti S, Toniatti C, Poli V, Bartfai T. Interleukin (IL)-6 gene expression in the central nervous system is necessary for fever response to lipopolysaccharide or IL-1 beta: a study on IL-6-deficient mice. *J Exp Med.* 1996 1;183(1):311–316.

18. Kozak W, Kluger MJ, Soszynski D, et al. IL-6 and IL-1 beta in fever. Studies using cytokine-deficient (knockout) mice. *Ann N Y Acad Sci.* 1998;856:33–47.

19. Cao C, Matsumura K, Ozaki M, Watanabe Y. Lipopolysaccharide injected into the cerebral ventricle evokes fever through induction of cyclooxygenase-2 in brain endothelial cells. *J Neurosci.* 1999;19(2):716–725.

20. Buller KM. Role of circumventricular organs in pro-inflammatory cytokine-induced activation of the hypothalamic–pituitary–adrenal axis. *Clin Exp Pharmacol Physiol.* 2001;28(7):581–589.

21. Saper CB, Breder CD. Endogenous pyrogens in the CNS: role in the febrile response. *Prog Brain Res.* 1992;93:419–428. Discussion 28–29.

22. Mallick BN, Jha SK, Islam F. Presence of alpha-1 adrenoreceptors on thermosensitive neurons in the medial preoptico-anterior hypothalamic area in rats. *Neuropharmacology.* 2002;42(5):697–705.

23. Mitchell JD, Grocott HP, Phillips-Bute B, Mathew JP, Newman MF, Bar-Yosef S. Cytokine secretion after cardiac surgery and its relationship to postoperative fever. *Cytokine.* 2007;38(1):37–42.

24. Fiorentino DF, Zlotnik A, Mosmann TR, Howard M, O'Garra A. IL-10 inhibits cytokine production by activated macrophages. *J Immunol.* 1991;147(11):3815–3822.

25. Leon LR. Invited review: cytokine regulation of fever: studies using gene knockout mice. *J Appl Physiol.* 2002;92(6):2648–2655.

26. Rabinowitz RP, Cookson ST, Wasserman SS, Mackowiak PA. Effects of anatomic site, oral stimulation, and body position on estimates of body temperature. *Arch Intern Med.* 1996;156(7):777–780.

27. Kistemaker JA, Den Hartog EA, Daanen HA. Reliability of an infrared forehead skin thermometer for core temperature measurements. *J Med Eng Technol.* 2006;30(4):252–261.

28. Kiekkas P, Filos KS, Karanikolas M, Aretha D, Baltopoulos GI. Relationships between fever and outcome in intensive care unit patients. *Crit Care Med.* 2008;36(11):3127–3128.

29. Oliveira-Filho J, Ezzeddine MA, Segal AZ, et al. Fever in subarachnoid hemorrhage: relationship to vasospasm and outcome. *Neurology.* 2001;56(10):1299–1304.

30. Fernandez A, Schmidt JM, Claassen J, et al. Fever after subarachnoid hemorrhage: risk factors and impact on outcome. *Neurology.* 2007;68(13):1013–1019.

31. Castillo J, Davalos A, Marrugat J, Noya M. Timing for fever-related brain damage in acute ischemic stroke. *Stroke.* 1998;29(12):2455–2460.

32. Henry JA, Jeffreys KJ, Dawling S. Toxicity and deaths from 3,4-methylenedioxymethamphetamine ("ecstasy"). *Lancet.* 1992;340(8816):384–387.

33. Grieger TA, Kluger MJ. Fever and survival: the role of serum iron. *J Physiol.* 1978;279:187–196.

34. Kluger MJ, Kozak W, Conn CA, Leon LR, Soszynski D. The adaptive value of fever. *Infect Dis Clin North Am.* 1996;10(1):1–20.

35. Mackowiak PA, Marling-Cason M, Cohen RL. Effects of temperature on antimicrobial susceptibility of bacteria. *J Infect Dis.* 1982;145(4):550–553.

36. Schulman CI, Namias N, Doherty J, et al. The effect of antipyretic therapy upon outcomes in critically ill patients: a randomized, prospective study. *Surg Infect (Larchmt).* 2005;6(4):369–375.

37. Mackowiak PA, LeMaistre CF. Drug fever: a critical appraisal of conventional concepts. An analysis of 51 episodes in two Dallas hospitals and 97 episodes

reported in the English literature. *Ann Intern Med.* 1987;106(5):728–733.

38. Roth J, Rummel C, Barth SW, Gerstberger R, Hubschle T. Molecular aspects of fever and hyperthermia. *Immunol Allergy Clin North Am.* 2009;29(2):229–245.

39. Henderson VW, Wooten GF. Neuroleptic malignant syndrome: a pathogenetic role for dopamine receptor blockade? *Neurology.* 1981;31(2):132–137.

40. Lawrence KR, Adra M, Gillman PK. Serotonin toxicity associated with the use of linezolid: a review of postmarketing data. *Clin Infect Dis.* 2006;42(11):1578–1583.

41. Mills EM, Banks ML, Sprague JE, Finkel T. Pharmacology: uncoupling the agony from ecstasy. *Nature.* 2003;426(6965):403–404.

42. Stocchetti N, Rossi S, Zanier ER, Colombo A, Beretta L, Citerio G. Pyrexia in head-injured patients admitted to intensive care. *Intensive Care Med.* 2002;28(11):1555–1562.

43. Zeiner A, Holzer M, Sterz F, et al. Hyperthermia after cardiac arrest is associated with an unfavorable neurologic outcome. *Arch Intern Med.* 2001;161(16):2007–2012.

44. Diringer MN, Reaven NL, Funk SE, Uman GC. Elevated body temperature independently contributes to increased length of stay in neurologic intensive care unit patients. *Crit Care Med.* 2004;32(7):1489–1495.

45. Greer DM, Funk SE, Reaven NL, Ouzounelli M, Uman GC. Impact of fever on outcome in patients with stroke and neurologic injury: a comprehensive meta-analysis. *Stroke.* 2008;39(11):3029–3035.

46. Horowitz M, Robinson SD. Heat shock proteins and the heat shock response during hyperthermia and its modulation by altered physiological conditions. *Prog Brain Res.* 2007;162:433–446.

47. Commichau C, Scarmeas N, Mayer SA. Risk factors for fever in the neurologic intensive care unit. *Neurology.* 2003;60(5):837–841.

48. Powers JH, Scheld WM. Fever in neurologic diseases. *Infect Dis Clin North Am.* 1996;10(1):45–66.

49. Murray HW, Ellis GC, Blumenthal DS, Sos TA. Fever and pulmonary thromboembolism. *Am J Med.* 1979;67(2):232–235.

50. Diamond PT, Macciocchi SN. Predictive power of clinical symptoms in patients with presumptive deep venous thrombosis. *Am J Phys Med Rehabil.* 1997;76(1):49–51.

51. Kazmers A, Groehn H, Meeker C. Do patients with acute deep vein thrombosis have fever? *Am Surg.* 2000;66(6):598–601.

52. Laupland KB. Fever in the critically ill medical patient. *Crit Care Med.* 2009;37(7 suppl):S273–S278.

53. O'Grady NP, Barie PS, Bartlett JG, et al. Guidelines for evaluation of new fever in critically ill adult patients: 2008 update from the American College of Critical Care Medicine and the Infectious Diseases Society of America. *Crit Care Med.* 2008;36(4):1330–1349.

54. Cunha BA, Shea KW. Fever in the intensive care unit. *Infect Dis Clin North Am.* 1996;10(1):185–209.

55. Ringel AF, Jameson GL, Foster ES. Diarrhea in the intensive care patient. *Crit Care Clin.* 1995;11(2):465–477.

56. Zollner-Schwetz I, Hogenauer C, Joainig M, et al. Role of *Klebsiella oxytoca* in antibiotic-associated diarrhea. *Clin Infect Dis.* 2008 1;47(9):e74–e78.

57. Campbell GD Jr. Blinded invasive diagnostic procedures in ventilator-associated pneumonia. *Chest.* 2000;117(4 suppl 2):207S–211S.

58. Garibaldi RA, Brodine S, Matsumiya S, Coleman M. Evidence for the non-infectious etiology of early postoperative fever. *Infect Control.* 1985;6(7):273–277.

59. Bert F, Lambert-Zechovsky N. Microbiology of nosocomial sinusitis in intensive care unit patients. *J Infect.* 1995;31(1):5–8.

60. Shapiro GG, Rachelefsky GS. Introduction and definition of sinusitis. *J Allergy Clin Immunol.* 1992;90(3 pt 2):417–418.

61. van Zanten AR, Dixon JM, Nipshagen MD, de Bree R, Girbes AR, Polderman KH. Hospital-acquired sinusitis is a common cause of fever of unknown origin in orotracheally intubated critically ill patients. *Crit Care.* 2005;9(5):R583–R590.

62. Pneumatikos I, Konstantonis D, Tsagaris I, et al. Prevention of nosocomial maxillary sinusitis in the ICU: the effects of topically applied alpha-adrenergic agonists and corticosteroids. *Intensive Care Med.* 2006;32(4):532–537.

63. Cheadle WG. Current perspectives on antibiotic use in the treatment of surgical infections. *Am J Surg.* 1992;164(4A suppl):44S–47S.

64. Marik PE, Zaloga GP. Adrenal insufficiency in the critically ill: a new look at an old problem. *Chest.* 2002;122(5):1784–1796.

65. Manthous CA, Hall JB, Olson D, et al. Effect of cooling on oxygen consumption in febrile critically ill patients. *Am J Respir Crit Care Med.* 1995;151(1):10–14.

66. Bernard GR, Wheeler AP, Russell JA, et al. The effects of ibuprofen on the physiology and survival of patients with sepsis. The Ibuprofen in Sepsis Study Group. *N Engl J Med.* 1997;336(13):912–918.

67. Plaisance KI, Mackowiak PA. Antipyretic therapy: physiologic rationale, diagnostic implications, and clinical consequences. *Arch Intern Med.* 2000;160(4):449–456.

CHAPTER 35

Principles of Antimicrobial Use in Critical Care

Anu Osinusi and Manjari Joshi

Critically ill patients are at very high risk of developing severe infections, with incidence rates typically about 5- to 10-fold higher than general wards. Estimates from the National Nosocomial Infections Surveillance (NNIS, now the National Healthcare Safety Network [NHSN]) system demonstrated that approximately 1.7 million nosocomial infections occurred in US hospitals in 2002. Twenty-four percent of these infections occurred in the intensive care unit (ICU), a rate of 13 per 1,000 patient days,[1] while other studies have demonstrated incidence rates between 9% and 37%.[2,3] Critically ill patients have numerous insults to normal host mechanisms. Skin integrity is usually compromised by peripheral and central access devices or wounds. Certain immunosuppressive medications decrease the ability of the immunologic defenses to function properly. Furthermore, other underlying medical conditions, such as diabetes, malnutrition, and renal disease, may predispose patients to infectious complications.

Antimicrobials are consistently among one of the most important and commonly prescribed drugs, and appropriate policies for their use must exist in the ICU. The success of these drugs is dependent on many factors, and it is therefore imperative for health care providers to have a clear understanding of antimicrobial use in the critically ill patient.

General principles of antimicrobial use in critical care should include the following[4–6]:

- *Health care providers need to have a clear understanding that all fevers and leukocytosis are not always caused by infections.* Systemic inflammatory response syndrome (SIRS) can be due to many noninfectious causes; thus, empirical antimicrobials are not always indicated.
  - Pursue diagnostic studies for both infectious and noninfectious causes until a diagnosis is reached.
- Always attempt to arrive at a diagnosis for the syndrome encountered.
  - Clinical outcomes are improved when a diagnosis is reached and targeted therapy is provided.
- Develop an empirical antimicrobial therapy based on differential diagnosis and predicted mortality.
  - Treat patients with sepsis with broad-spectrum antibiotics empirically.
  - Modify therapy to the most narrow-spectrum antibiotic when site and microbiology of the infection is defined.
  - Source control is essential for optimal care.
- Appropriately dose antimicrobials to achieve adequate dosing and minimize toxicity.
  - In cases of sepsis, early and appropriate administration is essential to improve survival.
  - Modification of doses in patients with renal or hepatic dysfunction.
  - Awareness of drug interactions with other medications.
- Define and continually address duration of antimicrobial therapy.
  - Tailor therapy based on microbiologic results and clinical response.
  - Discontinue antimicrobials if a noninfectious etiology is documented.
  - Base duration of therapy on clearly established standards.

- Address antibiotic resistance.
  - Antimicrobial stewardship.
  - Antimicrobial resistance surveillance.

► CHOICE OF THE PROPER ANTIMICROBIAL AGENT

A number of factors must be considered in choosing the appropriate antimicrobial for a given infection. These can be grouped into three major categories, namely, microbial, host, and drug factors.

MICROBIAL FACTORS

It is important for health care professionals to have some knowledge about the identity of the infecting organism or at least make a reasonable guess of its identity on available information. It is useful to know what organisms cause infections in that particular ICU. For example, it is a known fact that *Staphylococcus aureus* and *Pseudomonas aeruginosa* are the most common infecting agents in special units such as burn units. Second, information about the susceptibility of the infecting/likely organism should be as current as possible. An antibiogram, updated regularly by the local microbiology lab, can be an important tool for appropriate antimicrobial selection. It is also imperative for health care professionals to be well informed about important characteristics of certain microbes such as toxin-producing strains of staphylococci, streptococci, or clostridia. In many instances, antibiotics are started without the exact knowledge of the infecting organisms. In such cases, familiarity with the specific characteristics of the organisms could help with selection of appropriate antimicrobial therapy. For instance, a healthy person with a rapid onset of cellulitis most likely has an infection caused by toxin-producing strains of streptococci or staphylococci. Management should include aggressive surgical debridement and antimicrobial therapy such as clindamycin targeted toward the toxin production.

HOST FACTORS

A number of host factors influence antimicrobial efficacy, toxicity, and the selection of antibiotic therapy:

1. History of allergies to previous antimicrobial agents.
2. Age: Many physiologic functions such as renal capacity decline with age. Absorption of certain antibiotics, for example, penicillin G varies with age. Several adverse effects have also been noted to occur with increased incidence in older adults. In some cases, this may be due to specific disease states or impairment of physiologic processes, but in certain cases, the only identified factor is age. An example is the increased hepatotoxicity of isoniazid observed with age.[7]
3. Renal or hepatic abnormalities: The kidneys and liver serve as the major routes of excretion of antimicrobials. In patients with impaired renal and/or hepatic function, toxic levels of antibiotics can cause severe side effects.
4. Pregnancy: All antibiotics cross the placenta to a varying degree, and many antibiotics are also secreted in breast milk. Therefore, the fetus or infant can be exposed to adverse effects of a drug.[8,9]
5. Genetic or metabolic abnormalities: In certain individuals, the presence of genetic or metabolic abnormalities may also have a significant effect on the toxicity of a given antimicrobial agent.[10] Examples include acetylation of certain drugs in Asians and potentiation of hypoglycemic effects of sulfonylureas by sulfonamides in diabetics.
6. Site of infection: For antimicrobial therapy to be effective, an adequate concentration of the drug must be delivered to the site of infection usually at least equal to the minimum inhibitory concentration (MIC) of the organism. Other considerations include[11–13]:
   i. Protein binding of the drug.
   ii. Antibiotic penetration to various sites, for example, blood–brain barrier in meningitis.
   iii. Local factors such as the presence of pus and devitalized tissue can lead to inactivation of certain antibiotics. Foreign bodies can serve as a nidus for microbes to adhere and produce biofilms as seen in prosthetic joint infections. In addition, changes in oxygen tension and pH especially in the urinary tract can serve to enhance the effect of certain antibiotics such as aminoglycosides or nitrofurantoin at either alkaline or acidic environments, respectively.

DRUG FACTORS

Antibacterial drugs are usually divided into two groups: those that are primarily bacteriostatic (inhibit growth of the organism) and those that are primarily bactericidal (kill the organism). Bacteriostatic drugs require the aid of host defenses to clear tissues of the infecting organism. In cases where the host defenses are deficient or impaired at the site of infection, for example, meningitis and endocarditis, the organism will resume growth on stopping the bacteriostatic drug. These circumstances therefore require the use of bactericidal drugs, while in most other infections bacteriostatic drugs are sufficient. In more recent decades, it has become apparent that pharmacokinetic (PK) and pharmacodynamic (PD) properties are the major determinants of in vivo efficacy of antimicrobial agents.[14]

Pharmacodynamic Properties

Antimicrobial PD seeks to measure drug exposure with microbiologic or clinical effects.[15] For certain antibiotics, the rate of killing is closely related to the length of time the concentration of the drug is sustained above breakpoint MIC (time-dependent activity), while for others, killing rates are more related to the peak concentration above breakpoint (concentration-dependent activity).[16] Many antibiotics also demonstrate suppressive effects on bacterial growth even after their concentrations have fallen below the MIC. This is described as the post-antibiotic effect (PAE). Based on the above, there are three largely recognized patterns defining the PK/PD properties of the major classes of antibiotics[17–19]:

1. Time-dependent killing and minimal to moderate PAE. The amount of time that free antimicrobial concentrations remain above the MIC (T >MIC) for the organism is the PK/PD index correlating with efficacy. Different classes of β-lactams exhibit this pattern of activity.
2. Time-dependent killing and prolonged PAE. This goal of dosing is to optimize the amount of drug, and the area under the concentration–time curve at 24 hours/MIC ($AUC_{0–24}$/MIC) ratio. This is the index most closely associated with efficacy. Antimicrobials such as linezolid, vancomycin, tigecycline, and quinupristin/dalfopristin represent this class of drugs.
3. Concentration-dependent killing and a prolonged PAE. The peak concentration/MIC (C_{max}/MIC) ratio and/or $AUC_{0–24}$/MIC ratio are the best PK/PD parameters correlating with efficacy. This is predictive of activity of aminoglycosides, fluoroquinolones, metronidazole, and daptomycin.

Pharmacokinetic Properties and Critical Illness

PK describes the time course of drug levels in the body as a result of absorption, distribution, and elimination. Critically ill patients are subject to several pathophysiologic conditions that may substantially alter the PK of antimicrobials that in turn can influence the efficacy of the drug. Most often, variations in the volume of distribution and renal or hepatic function are the most common pathophysiologic conditions affecting drug disposition in critically ill individuals.

Volume of distribution and drug concentrations

In many instances in critical illness, the volume of distribution is usually greater than in noncritically ill patients. This is usually as a result of increased capillary permeability resulting from endothelial damage as well as reductions in oncotic pressure from hypoalbuminemia all leading to fluid extravasation. This is very particularly important when dealing with hydrophilic antibiotics such as β-lactams, aminoglycosides, and vancomycin. These antibiotics are distributed primarily in the extracellular fluid (ECF), and in cases of significant interstitial extravasation, the plasma levels may drop substantially resulting in clinical failure. This has been well described with aminoglycosides that are concentration-dependent bactericidal drugs.[20,21] It is therefore important to monitor drug concentrations and consider higher doses for most hydrophilic antibiotics when an edematous state is present.[22,23] On the other hand, with lipophilic antibiotics such as quinolones that have a large volume of distribution, changes in interstitial fluid volume are not as relevant.

Renal dysfunction and drug concentrations

Most antibiotics are cleared from the body largely through the kidneys. In critical illness, many patients develop renal impairment that may easily lead to drug accumulation. Furthermore, many patients are supported by renal replacement therapies (RRT) such as hemodialysis or continuous RRT that clear drugs from the system similar to a kidney functioning with a glomerular filtration rate (GFR) ≤35 mL/min. While some antibiotics such as vancomycin and aminoglycosides have easily measurable drug levels used as surrogates for toxic levels, many other drugs do not have measurable levels and toxic levels are difficult to ascertain.[24]

Conversely, the use of hemodynamically active drugs (dopamine) and the hyperdynamic phase of extensive burns or early sepsis can modify renal blood flow with an increase in GFR leading to increased renal clearance of most hydrophilic and lipophilic antimicrobials.[25] Finally in many instances, serum creatinine and estimated clearance often fail to estimate renal function appropriately and the adjustments may cause an overdosage.[26] Table 35-1 lists the antimicrobials that do not require dosage adjustment in renal disease.

Hepatic dysfunction and drug concentrations

Several antimicrobials have well-documented effects on hepatic function. These are usually categorized into inducers or inhibitors that can have huge impacts on concomitantly administered drugs. Inhibitors of certain

▶ TABLE 35-1. **SELECTED ANTIMICROBIALS THAT DO NOT REQUIRE DOSAGE ADJUSTMENTS IN RENAL DISEASES AND ANTIMICROBIALS THAT REQUIRE ADJUSTMENTS IN LIVER DISEASE**

Antibacterials		Antifungals	Antivirals
Azithromycin	Linezolid	Anidulafungin	Ribavirin
Ceftriaxone[a]	Minocycline	Caspofungin[a]	Many HIV medications
Chloramphenicol[a]	Nafcillin[a]	Itraconazole (solution)[a]	
Clindamycin[a]	Pyrimethamine	Ketoconazole	
Doxycycline	Rifaximin	Micafungin	
Metronidazole	Tigecycline[a]	Voriconazole (oral)[a]	

[a]Drugs that require adjustment with hepatic failure.

hepatic enzymes such as erythromycin and ciprofloxacin that inhibit CYPA12 can interfere with theophylline metabolism leading to toxicity. Others such as rifampin that induces Cy P450 can result in lowering the levels of other drugs such as Coumadin. The effect of hepatic metabolism on the majority of antimicrobials is very limited and protein binding is also low enough to make no difference in efficacy. Therefore, there is rarely any need to make dose adjustments to many antimicrobials in critical illness with hepatic dysfunction.[27]

▶ INITIAL SELECTION OF ANTIMICROBIAL THERAPY

Prompt, effective, and targeted antimicrobial therapy is crucial for treating a critically ill patient with suspected infection. Higher mortality is associated with both delay in therapy and inappropriate treatment.[4,5] Often, critically ill patients present with a nonspecific SIRS syndrome that stems from either infectious or noninfectious causes. To define the etiology of the SIRS syndrome, a thorough investigation should be undertaken. If the patient is critically ill, and an infectious etiology is suspected, antimicrobials should be empirically initiated based on a number of factors. Figure 35-1 provides an overview of the variables used in the decision-making process for the selection of antimicrobial agents.

After selection of initial therapy, it is important to evaluate each patient on a daily basis. The evaluation should be comprehensive and include the following assessments:

1. Is the cause of SIRS syndrome infectious or noninfectious?
2. If it is infectious, what is the site of the infection and what organisms (type and susceptibility) are associated with it?
3. Is there adequate source control?
4. Assessment of clinical response to therapy.
5. Modification of therapy based on the clinical data and patient response.
6. Defining the duration of antimicrobial therapy.
7. Stopping antimicrobial therapy if the patient is stable, but is not improving and no infectious etiology of the SIRS syndrome is apparent. This is one of the hardest concepts to accept in a critically ill patient. In this setting, most health

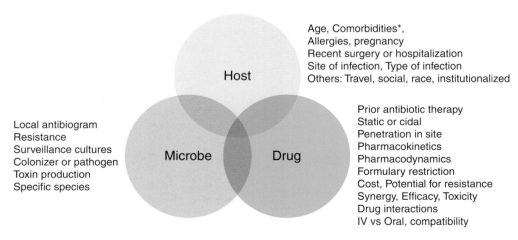

*Comorbidities: diabetes, smoking, obesity, immunosuppression, dialysis, and organ dysfunction.

Figure 35-1. Variables for decision making for antibiotic choices.

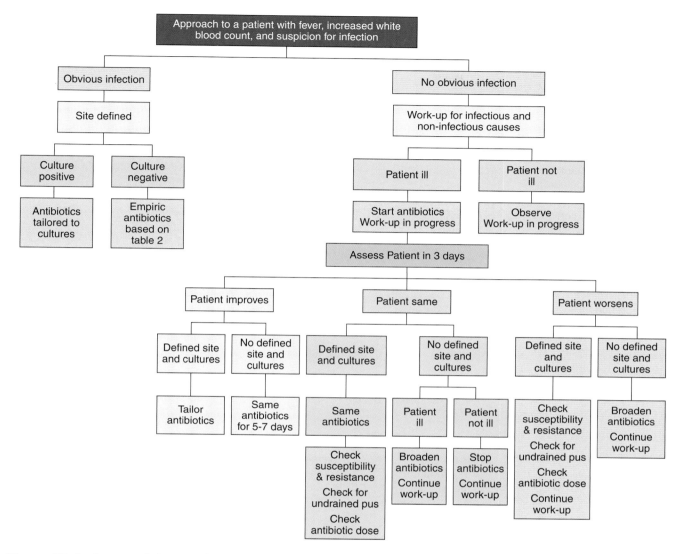

Figure 35-2. Approach to a patient with suspected infection.

care providers change antimicrobial therapy or add more potent antibiotics to the existing regimen. This practice masks the underlying SIRS syndrome that contributes to a delay in the correct diagnosis. Additionally, it is associated with antimicrobial-related side effects and the emergence of antimicrobial resistance. During the time period of antimicrobial withdrawal, the patient needs to be closely observed for any signs of clinical decompensation. It is also important to keep evaluating the patient for the etiology of SIRS syndrome.

Figure 35-2 provides an approach to the management of patients with suspected infection.

Once the site of infection and the causative organisms are identified, antimicrobial therapy needs to be optimized. Table 35-2 provides a summary of the spe-

cific organisms and the antimicrobial agents with the most activity against them. Additionally, alternative therapy, secondary options, as well as selected therapy for multidrug-resistant (MDR) organisms is included.

ANTIMICROBIAL COMBINATION

Many infections can be treated by single agents. However, in certain circumstances, antimicrobial combinations can be considered. When antimicrobial agents are combined, the interactions exhibited against an organism in vitro can be indifference, synergism, or antagonism.

Certain circumstances in critical care where combination antimicrobials might be appropriate include:

- Initial therapy in immunocompromised/critically ill patients, for example, neutropenic fevers when the initial nature of the infection is unclear.

► **TABLE 35-2. RECOMMENDED ANTIMICROBIAL THERAPY FOR SELECTED PATHOGENS[28]**

Pathogen	Recommended	Alternative	Other Options
Gram-positive cocci			
Staphylococcus aureus (methicillin-sensitive)	Oxacillin Nafcillin	CEPH 1 (cefazolin) Clindamycin Vancomycin	Carbapenems BL/BLI; FQ Macrolides, linezolid Quin-Dalfo, daptomycin Tigecycline
S. aureus (methicillin-resistant) (health care associated)[a]	Vancomycin	Daptomycin Linezolid Quin-Dalfo	Tigecycline TMP/SMX (some strains resistant)
S. aureus (methicillin-resistant) (community acquired)[a] • Mild-moderate	TMP/SMX or doxycycline ± rifampin	Clindamycin (if D test is negative)	Vancomycin Daptomycin Linezolid Tigecycline
S. aureus (methicillin-resistant) (community acquired)[a] • Severe infection	Vancomycin	Daptomycin Linezolid	
Coagulase-negative staphylococci	Vancomycin ± rifampin	TMP/SMX ± rifampin	Daptomycin[b] Linezolid[b] Tigecycline[b]
S. pneumoniae (penicillin-sensitive)	Penicillin G	Multiple agents	–
S. pneumoniae (penicillin-resistant, MIC ≥2)	Vancomycin ± rifampin or gatifloxacin/ levofloxacin/moxifloxacin		For nonmeningeal infections: CEPH 3/4 Linezolid Tigecycline[b] Quin–Dalfo
S. pyogenes (A, B, C, F, G)	Penicillin G or V + clinda for serious group A strep infections + gent for group B strep infections	All β–lactams All macrolides CEPH 1/2	Macrolide resistance increasing
Listeria monocytogenes	Ampicillin	TMP/SMX	Penicillin G (high dose) Erythromycin APAG (synergy with β-lactams)
Enterococcus (penicillin-sensitive)	Penicillin or ampicillin ± gentamicin	Vancomycin ± gentamicin	–
Enterococcus (penicillin-resistant/ vancomycin-sensitive)	Vancomycin ± gentamicin	Linezolid	Daptomycin Tigecycline
Enterococcus (penicillin-sensitive, vancomycin + streptococci/ gent resistant)[a]	Penicillin G Ampicillin Nitrofurantoin or fosfomycin (UTIs only)	Linezolid[a]	Daptomycin Tigecycline
Enterococcus faecium (PCN, AMP, vancomycin + streptococci/gent resistant)[a]	Linezolid Quin-Dalfo ± FQ, rifaximin, doxycycline, chloramphenicol		Daptomycin Tigecycline

▶ **TABLE 35-2. RECOMMENDED ANTIMICROBIAL THERAPY FOR SELECTED PATHOGENS**[28] **(CONTINUED)**

Pathogen	Recommended	Alternative	Other Options
Gram-negative rods			
Escherichia coli *Klebsiella* spp. *Enterobacter* spp.	Recommended agents vary with the clinical setting		
Klebsiella pneumonia (ESBL producer)[a]	Imipenem Meropenem	CEPH 4	PIP-TZ[a] TC-CL[a]
Klebsiella pneumoniae (carbapenemase producer)[a]	Colistin		Tigecycline[a]
Serratia marcescens	FQ Carbapenems CEPH 3	Aztreonam Gentamicin	TC-CL PIP-TZ
MDR *Acinetobacter* (resistant to IMP, FQ, APAG, CEPH 3, AP Pen)[a]	AMP–SB–colistin Amikacin	Polymyxin B Tigecycline[b]	
Pseudomonas aeruginosa	PIP-TZ Ceftazidime/cefepime IMP/MERO Aminoglycosides	FQ (↑ resistance) Aztreonam	Combination therapy for serious infections
Anaerobes			
Bacteroides fragilis	Metronidazole	Cefoxitin Carbapenems, BL/BLI Tigecycline	Clindamycin[a] Cefotetan[a]
Clostridium perfringens	Penicillin G ± clindamycin	Doxycycline	Cefoxitin, cefazolin Erythromycin BL/BLI
Clostridium difficile	Metronidazole	Vancomycin (oral)	Nitazoxanide, rifaximin

AP Pen, antipseudomonal penicillin; APAG, antipseudomonal aminoglycoside (amikacin, tobramycin, gentamicin); BL/BLI, β-lactam/β-lactamase inhibitors (ampicillin–sulbactam [AMP-SB], piperacillin–tazobactam [PIP-TZ], ticarcillin–clavulanate [TC-CL]); CEPH 1/2, first- and second-generation cephalosporins; CEPH 3/4, third- and fourth-generation cephalosporins; clinda, clindamycin; FQ, fluoroquinolones (moxifloxacin, levofloxacin, gatifloxacin, ciprofloxacin); gent, gentamicin; IMP, imipenem; MERO, meropenem; TMP/SMX, trimethoprim/sulfamethoxazole.
[a]Select organisms with published increasing resistance.
[b]Activity demonstrated in a few published studies; *not* FDA-approved for this indication.

- Critically ill patients with suspected sepsis of an unknown source need to be empirically covered with broad-spectrum drugs to cover methicillin-resistant *Staphylococcus aureus* (MRSA), resistant gram-negative rods (GNR), and possible anaerobes.
- Polymicrobial infections: Intra-abdominal, pelvic, and diabetic foot infections are often caused by a mix of aerobic and anaerobic organisms requiring broad coverage. Antibiotics such as carbapenems, β-lactamases, and β-lactamase inhibitors provide broad coverage that can be utilized as monotherapy.[29,30]
- Synergism: Use of combination antimicrobials has proven synergistic only in limited clinical settings.[31,32] An example is the use of the combination of penicillin and aminoglycosides for the treatment of enterococcal endocarditis

that results in cure rates comparable to those achieved for endocarditis caused by less resistant streptococci. Similarly, synergistic combination therapy may be useful in the treatment of infections with *S. viridans, S. aureus,* and *P. aeruginosa.*

Although the use of antimicrobial combinations may be beneficial, inappropriate use can result in adverse events that include antagonism, increased cost, side effects, and the emergence of resistant organisms.

ANTIMICROBIAL RESISTANCE IN CRITICAL CARE

In current times, antimicrobial resistance is becoming more prevalent while antimicrobial development is relatively stagnant. This phenomenon has been shown to lead to increased morbidity and mortality, higher risk of severe infections, longer hospital stay, and increased costs.[33,34] It is therefore important that health care providers learn how to achieve clinical efficacy, without further compromising the existing antibiotic armamentarium.

Bacterial resistance of antimicrobials occurs mainly through four mechanisms, namely, altered uptake due to decreased permeability, increased efflux, target modification, and hydrolysis or modification of the antibacterial agent (most predominant mechanism).

The emergence of resistance and spread of resistant microorganisms in critical care units are dependent on several factors, including the propensity of the microorganism to acquire resistance, the presence of human and inanimate reservoirs in which resistant organisms can survive, and existing institutional strategies for use of antimicrobial agents. The emergent nature of care, prolonged hospital stay, use of invasive devices, prior antibiotic use, and the increasing presence of chronically ill patients in critical care units have also played a significant role. Additionally, transmission of resistant organisms often occurs among the debilitated and elderly inmates of the long-term care facilities. When these colonized patients fall ill, they are often admitted to ICUs, where they are responsible for further spreading antimicrobial resistance.

Several strategies have been utilized to prevent the spread of resistant organisms and they include:

- Hand washing, protective barriers, and educational programs for health care workers;
- Patient isolation and use of dedicated equipment in patients with resistant organisms;
- Use of surveillance cultures and antimicrobial resistance surveillance in critical care;
- Early and prompt diagnosis of infections;
- Appropriate antibiotic use with targeted empirical therapy and knowledge of local antibiograms;
- Antimicrobial stewardship to curtail emergence of resistance.

The features of antimicrobial stewardship[7,35,36] are described as follows:

- Prospective audits with intervention and feedback
- Formulary restriction and preauthorization
- Clinical pathways and guidelines
- Dose optimization
- Combination therapy guidelines
- Streamlining and de-escalating/tailoring therapy
- Antimicrobial cycling and switching
- Parenteral to oral conversion as soon as possible

ANTIMICROBIAL PROPHYLAXIS FOR SURGICAL PROCEDURES

For surgical prophylaxis to be maximally effective, knowledge of the risks of the procedure, likely infecting organism, antimicrobial dosing, and premorbid history of resistant organisms are crucial. It has been recommended that antibiotics must be started usually 2 hours before surgical incision or even closer to incision time.[37] For most surgical procedures, the duration is not defined but most often a single dose is employed. In procedures lasting more than 3 hours, additional doses of rapidly excreted antibiotics should be given. A recent consensus statement by the National Surgical Infection Project advises that antibiotic prophylaxis be started within 1 hour of the incision (except vancomycin and quinolones). They should be supplemented intraoperatively if the procedure lasts for more than two half-lives, and in most cases not be extended beyond 24 hours.[38] There are also PK considerations that may render the standard prophylaxis dose with suboptimal concentrations in patients with high body mass index (BMI).[39]

Key points in selecting appropriate prophylactic therapy include:

- Type of procedure (Table 35-3)
- Coverage against expected flora (Table 35-3)
- Local resistance patterns
- Allergies
- Penetration of antibiotic into the required site
- Risk factors for acquisition of resistant pathogens

ANTIVIRALS IN CRITICAL CARE

Viral infections are more commonly seen in patients with acquired immune deficiency syndrome (AIDS) and neutropenia, and in patients in immunocompromised states. However, during winter months, severe episodes of influenza can result in respiratory failure and may require admission to a critical care unit. In the last few decades, there have been remarkable advances in antiviral therapy. Prior to the 1970s, a diagnosis of a severe viral infection was treated largely with supportive care. Today, there are several treatment alternatives for some viral infections as shown in Table 35-4.

ANTIFUNGAL THERAPY IN CRITICAL CARE

In the last two decades, fungal diseases have become progressively more important in critically ill patients. Immunocompromised patients with serious fungal

▶ **TABLE 35-3. ANTIMICROBIAL PROPHYLAXIS BY PROCEDURE AND LIKELY INFECTING ORGANISMS[40,41]**

Type of Procedure	Typical Microbiologic Flora at the Site	Recommended	Alternate
Cardiovascular/thoracic	S. aureus, CoNS	Cefazolin or cefuroxime	Vancomycin
Gastroduodenal/biliary	GNR, streptococci, oropharyngeal anaerobes	Cefazolin, cefoxitin, cefuroxime, or cefotetan	Ampicillin-sulbactam TC-CL
Colonic	GNR, anaerobes	Oral: neomycin + erythromycin or metronidazole	
		Intravenous: cefoxitin or cefazolin + metronidazole	Clindamycin or metronidazole + ciprofloxacin or aztreonam
Head and neck	S. aureus, streptococci, oropharyngeal anaerobes	Cefazolin or clindamycin	Addition of gentamicin controversial
Neurosurgical	S. aureus, CoNS	Cefazolin or clindamycin	Vancomycin
Obstetrics/gynecologic • Hysterectomy • C-section • Abortion	GNR, enterococci, group B streptococci, anaerobes	Cefazolin, cefoxitin, cefotetan, or cefuroxime PCN G or cefazolin	Ampicillin–sulbactam Doxycycline
Orthopedic	S. aureus, CoNS, streptococci, GNR	Cefazolin or ceftriaxone	Vancomycin
Urologic (preoperative bacteriuria)	GNR	Cefazolin followed by nitrofurantoin or TMP/SMX	

infections often require critical care, and patients in critical care settings are often susceptible to these infections.

In the past decade, the rate of hospital-acquired fungal infection has nearly doubled with the greatest increase in critically ill surgical patients.[42]

Several factors have been identified as independent predictors for invasive fungal complications during critical illness.[43–46] They include:

- Duration of ICU care and invasive mechanical ventilation
- Diabetes mellitus
- Neutropenia
- Organ transplantation and immunosuppression
- Solid and hematologic malignant tumors

- Long-term use of central venous catheters and urinary catheters
- Candida colonization
- Use of broad-spectrum antibiotics
- Use of corticosteroids
- Total parenteral nutrition (TPN)
- Burns
- Gastrointestinal surgery

The major pathogenic fungal organisms encountered in critical care are Candida albicans (59% of candidal isolates), Candida glabrata, other non-albicans Candida spp., Aspergillus, and other emerging fungal organisms such as zycomycetes.[43,46]

Fungal therapy is usually used in four different settings in the ICU, namely, prophylactic, preemptive,

▶ **TABLE 35-4. SPECTRUM OF SELECTED ANTIVIRALS IN CRITICAL CARE WITH PERMISSION[28]**

	HSV-1	HSV-2	CMV	VZV	EBV	Flu A	Flu B	RSV	Adenovirus
Acyclovir/famciclovir/valacyclovir	+++[a]	+++[a]	+/−[a]	+++[a]	+	0	0	0	0
Ganciclovir/valganciclovir	++	++	+++[a]	+	++	0	0	0	+/−
Cidofovir	++	++	+++	+	++	0	0	0	+
Foscarnet	++	++	+++	++	++	0	0	0	0
Ribavirin	0	0	0	0	0	0	0	+	0
Amantadine/rimantadine	0	0	0	0	0	++[a]	0	0	0
Oseltamivir/zanamivir	0	0	0	0	0	++[a]	++[a]	0	0

Flu, influenza; 0, no activity; +/−, possible activity; +++, first-line activity; ++, second-line activity; +, third-line (least active).
[a]Resistant strains reported.

▶ TABLE 35-5. SELECTED ANTIFUNGALS IN CRITICAL CARE WITH PERMISSION[28]

Antifungal Agent	Indications for Use	Special Comments
Fluconazole	+++: *C. albicans, C. tropicalis, C. parapsilosis, C. guillermondi* +: *C. lusitaniae* ±: *C. glabrata* Fungistatic to *Aspergillus,* coccidiomycosis, cryptococcus, blastomycosis, histoplasmosis, *Sporothrix*	No activity against *C. krusei, Aspergillus,* fusarium, *Scedosporium*
Voriconazole	+++: *C. albicans, C. parapsilosis, C. tropicalis, C. guillermondi* ++: *C. krusei, C. lusitaniae* +: *C. glabrata* *Aspergillus,* fusarium, *Scedosporium,* dermaticeous molds, coccidiomycosis, cryptococcus, blastomycosis, histoplasmosis, *Sporothrix*	No activity against zycomycetes (mucor, rhizopus, etc.)
Posaconazole	+++: *C. albicans, C. parapsilosis, C. tropicalis, C. guillermondi* ++: *C. krusei, C. lusitaniae* +: *C. glabrata* *Aspergillus,* fusarium, *Scedosporium,* dermaticeous molds, zycomycetes, coccidiomycosis, cryptococcus, blastomycosis, histoplasmosis, *Sporothrix*	*Liquid formulation that has to be taken with fatty meals*
Caspofungin Micafungin Anidulafungin	*C. albicans, C. parapsilosis,*[a] *C. glabrata, C. tropicalis, C. krusei, C. lusitaniae, C. guillermondi*[a]	Case reports of combination therapy with polyenes against mold infections
Amphotericin B • Standard • Lipid complex • Liposomal	*C. albicans, C. parapsilosis, C. glabrata, C. tropicalis, C. krusei, C. lusitaniae, C. guillermondi* *Aspergillus,* fusarium, zycomycetes, coccidiomycosis, cryptococcus, blastomycosis, histoplasmosis, *Sporothrix*	More nephrotoxicity with standard formulation No activity against *Aspergillus terreus* spp.

+++, higher activity; ++, active (second line); +, least active (third line); ±, possible activity.
[a]Higher MIC.

empiric, and definitive. Prophylactic therapy is hardly employed in critical care except in high-risk patients such as neutropenic patients, bone marrow patients, or solid organ transplant patients.[46,47] Preemptive therapy is used rarely and involves the treatment of patients at high risk of developing deep candidiasis identified by clinical or laboratory markers. These could include patients with severe burns, patients on extracorporeal membrane oxygenation systems or left ventricular assist devices, or patients with pancreatitis.[48]

Empirical therapy is used in the treatment of patients suspected to have deep candidiasis without microbiologic, histologic, or serologic confirmation, while definitive therapy is the treatment of established deep candidiasis. Table 35-5 is a list of available antifungal agents.

In summary, antimicrobials remain a crucial part of the armamentarium of drugs in critically ill patients. The judicious use of these drugs is essential not only for good patient outcomes but also for prevention of antimicrobial resistance.

REFERENCES

1. Klevens RM, Edwards JR, Richards CL, et al. Estimating health care-associated infections and deaths in U.S. hospitals, 2002. *Public Health Rep.* 2007;122:160.
2. Osmon S, Warren D, Seiler NM, et al. The influence of infection on hospital mortality for patients requiring > 48 h of intensive care. *Chest.* 2003;124:1021.
3. Vincent JL. Nosocomial infections in adult intensive-care units. *Lancet.* 2003;361:2068.
4. Rello J. Importance of appropriate initial antibiotic therapy and de-escalation in the treatment of nosocomial pneumonia. *Eur Respir Rev.* 2003;16:33.
5. Kollef MH, Sherman G, Ward S, Fraser VJ. Inadequate antimicrobial treatment of infections: a risk factor for hospital mortality among critically ill patients. *Chest.* 1999;115:462.

6. Dellit TH, Owens RC, McGowan JE, et al. Infectious Diseases Society of America and the Society for Healthcare Epidemiology of America guidelines for developing an institutional program to enhance antimicrobial stewardship. *Clin Infect Dis.* 2007;44:159.

7. Nolan CM, Goldberg SV, Buskin SE. Hepatotoxicity associated with isoniazid preventative therapy. *JAMA.* 1999;281:1014.

8. Nahum GG, Uhl K, Kennedy DL. Antibiotic use in pregnancy and lactation: what is and is not known about teratogenic and toxic risks. *Obstet Gynecol.* 2006;107:1120.

9. Meyer JM, Rodvold KA. Antimicrobials during pregnancy. *Infect Med.* 1995;12:420.

10. Roy PD, Majumder M, Roy B. Pharmacogenomics of anti-TB drugs-related hepatotoxicity. *Pharmacogenomics.* 2008;9:311.

11. Merrikin DJ, Briant J, Rolinson GN. Effect of protein binding on antibiotic activity in vivo. *J Antimicrob Chemother.* 1983;11:233.

12. Dickinson GM, Bisno AL. Infections associated with indwelling medical devices. *Antimicrob Agents Chemother.* 1989;33:597.

13. Pillai SK Eliopoulos G, Moellering RS. Principles of anti-infective therapy. In: Mandell GL, Bennett JE, Dolin R, eds. *Mandell, Douglas, and Bennett's Principles and Practice of Infectious Diseases.* 7th ed. Philadelphia, Churchill Livingstone; 2009:247.

14. Scaglione F, Paraboni L. The influence of pharmacokinetics/pharmacodynamics of antibacterials in their dosing regimen selection. *Expert Rev Anti Infect Ther.* 2006;4:479.

15. Thomas JK, Forrest A, Bhavnani SM, et al. Pharmacodynamic evaluation of factors associated with the development of bacterial resistance in acutely ill patients during therapy. *Antimicrob Agents Chemother.* 1998;42:521.

16. Drusano GL. Antimicrobial pharmacodynamics—critical interactions of 'bug and drug'. *Nat Rev Microbiol.* 2004;2:289.

17. Craig WA. Pharmacokinetic/pharmacodynamic indices: rationale for antibacterial dosing of mice and men. *Clin Infect Dis.* 1998;26:1.

18. Craig WA. Basic pharmacodynamics of antibacterials with clinical applications to the use of β-lactams, glycopeptides and linezolid. *Infect Dis Clin North Am.* 2003;17:479.

19. Godke J, Karam G. Principles governing antimicrobial therapy in the intensive care unit. In: Parrillo J, Dellinger PR, eds. *Critical Care Medicine—Principles of Diagnosis and Management in the Adult.* 3rd ed. St. Louis, Mosby; 2008:1074.

20. Vrhovac B, Sarapa N, Bakran I, et al. Pharmacokinetic changes in patients with edema. *Clin Pharmacokinet.* 1995;28:405.

21. Dasta JF, Armstrong DK. Variability in aminoglycoside pharmacokinetics in critically ill surgical patients. *Crit Care Med.* 1988;16:327.

22. De Paepe P, Belpaire FM, Buylaert WA. Pharmacokinetic and pharmacodynamic considerations when treating patients with sepsis and septic shock. *Clin Pharmacokinet.* 2002;41:1135.

23. Joukhadar C, Frossard M, Mayer BX, et al. Impaired target site penetration of beta-lactams may account for therapeutic failure in patients with septic shock. *Crit Care Med.* 2001;29:385.

24. Bugge JF. Pharmacokinetics and drug dosing adjustments during continuous venovenous hemofiltration or hemodiafiltration in critically ill patients. *Acta Anaesthesiol Scand.* 2001;45:929.

25. Weinbren MJ. Pharmacokinetics of antibiotics in burn patients. *J Antimicrob Chemother.* 1999;44:319.

26. Roberts JA, Lipman J. Antibacterial dosing in intensive care: pharmacokinetics, degree of disease and pharmacodynamics of sepsis. *Clin Pharmacokinet.* 2006; 45:755.

27. Mehrotra R, DeGaudio R, Palazzo M. Antibiotic pharmacokinetic and pharmacodynamic considerations in critical illness. *Intensive Care Med.* 2004;30:2145.

28. Gilbert DN, Moellering RC, Eliopoulos GM, et al. *The Sanford Guide to Antimicrobial Therapy.* 39th ed. Antimicrobial Therapy, Inc., Sperryville, VA. 2009.

29. Babinchak T, Ellis-Grosse E, Dartois N, et al, Tigecycline 301 Study Group. The efficacy and safety of tigecycline for the treatment of complicated intra-abdominal infections: analysis of pooled clinical trial data. *Clin Infect Dis.* 2005;41:S354.

30. Lipsky BA, Armstrong DG, Citron DM, et al. Ertapenem versus piperacillin/tazobactam for diabetic foot infections (SIDESTEP): prospective, randomised, controlled, double-blinded, multicentre trial. *Lancet.* 2005; 366:1695.

31. Sexton DJ, Tenenbaum MJ, Wilson WR, et al. Ceftriaxone once daily for four weeks compared with ceftriaxone plus gentamicin once daily for two weeks for treatment of endocarditis due to penicillin-susceptible streptococci. Endocarditis Treatment Consortium Group. *Clin Infect Dis.* 1998;27:1470.

32. Falagas ME, Matthaiou DK, Bliziotis IA. The role of aminoglycosides in combination with a beta-lactam for the treatment of bacterial endocarditis: a meta-analysis of comparative trials. *J Antimicrob Chemother.* 2006;57:639.

33. McGowan JE Jr. Resistance in nonfermenting gram-negative bacteria: multidrug resistance to the maximum. *Am J Infect Control.* 2006;34:S29.

34. Asche C, McAdam-Marx C, Seal B, et al. Treatment costs associated with community-acquired pneumonia by community level of antimicrobial resistance. *J Antimicrob Chemother.* 2008;61:1162.

35. MacDougall C, Polk RE. Antimicrobial stewardship programs in health care systems. *Clin Microbiol Rev.* 2005;18:638.

36. Martin C, Ofotokun I, Rapp R, et al. Results of an antimicrobial control program at a university hospital. *Am J Health Syst Pharm.* 205;62:732.

37. Garey KW, Dao T, Chen H, et al. Timing of vancomycin prophylaxis for cardiac surgery patients and the risk of surgical site infections. *J Antimicrob Chemother.* 2006;58:645.

38. Bratzler DW, Houck PM. Antimicrobial prophylaxis for surgery: an advisory statement from the National Surgical Infection Prevention Project. *Clin Infect Dis.* 2004;38:1706.

39. Edminston CE, Krepel C, Kelly H, et al. Perioperative antibiotic prophylaxis in the gastric bypass patient: do we achieve therapeutic levels? *Surgery.* 2004; 136:738.

40. American Society of Health-System Pharmacists. ASHP therapeutic guidelines on antimicrobial prophylaxis in surgery. *Am J Health Syst Pharm.* 1999;56:1839.

41. Korinek AM, Golmard JL, Elcheick A, et al. Risk factors for neurosurgical site infections after craniotomy: a critical reappraisal of antibiotics prophylaxis on 4,578 patients. *Br J Neurosurg.* 2005;19:155.

42. Vincent JL, Anaissie E, Bruining H, et al. Epidemiology, diagnosis and treatment of systemic *Candida* infection in surgical patients under intensive care. *Intensive Care Med.* 1998;24:206.

43. Cornwell EE, Belzberg H, Berne TV, et al. The pattern of fungal infections in critically ill surgical patients. *Am Surg.* 1995;61:847.

44. Blumberg HM, Jarvis WR, Soucie JM, et al. Risk factors for candidal bloodstream infections in surgical intensive care unit patients: the NEMIS prospective multicenter study. *Clin Infect Dis.* 2001;33:177.

45. Paphitou NI, Ostrosky-Zeichner L, Rex JH. Rules for identifying patients at increased risk for candidal infections in the surgical intensive care unit: approach to developing practical criteria for systematic use in antifungal prophylaxis trials. *Med Mycol.* 2005;43:235.

46. Goodman JL, Winston DJ, Greenfield RA, et al. A controlled trial of fluconazole to prevent fungal infections in patients undergoing bone marrow transplantation. *N Engl J Med.* 1992;326:845.

47. Marr KA, Seidel K, Slavin MA, et al. Prolonged fluconazole prophylaxis is associated with persistent protection against candidiasis-related death in allogeneic marrow transplant recipients: long-term follow-up of a randomized, placebo-controlled trial. *Blood.* 2000;96:2055.

48. Edwards JE Jr, Bodey GP, Bowden RA, et al. International conference for the development of a consensus on the management and prevention of severe candidal infections. *Clin Infect Dis.* 1997;25:43.

CHAPTER 36

Sepsis and Septic Shock

David A. Farcy, John Yashou, and Emanuel Rivers

▶ INTRODUCTION

Of the 120 million patients presenting to the emergency department (ED) in the United States per year, 2.9% or over 600,000 carry a diagnosis of severe sepsis and septic shock in the United States. The overall hospital mortality for sepsis, severe sepsis, and septic shock is 15%, 20%, and 45%, respectively. Sepsis is responsible for 9% of the deaths or 210,000 deaths per year in the United States. By comparison, 180,000 persons die of acute myocardial infarction and 200,000 die of lung or breast cancer annually. Many patients with severe sepsis and septic shock present to the ED where there are often long delays before transfer to an intensive care unit (ICU) bed. Sepsis is the most expensive diagnosis admitted to hospitals accounting for over $50 billion in health care costs each year. It is because of these aforementioned factors that the ED has become a logical focal point for sepsis diagnosis and treatment. It is during the first 6 hours that sepsis management can improve outcomes in one of every six patients who present with the disease.[1]

Risk factors and comorbidities that increase the incidence and mortality include age, gender, race, multidrug-resistant organisms, severity of chronic illnesses, and overcrowding of the EDs.[2] Because ED visits increase with age, a higher proportion of patients will come from this population. The incidence of sepsis in adult patients over age 85 is 26.2/1,000 versus 0.2/1,000 in children.[3] Over 115 million patients present to the ED per year and 2.9% of these patients have sepsis that accounts for over 600,000 annually, with a mean stay of 4.7 hours. Approximately 20.4% of the patients stay longer than 6 hours.[4] The ED accounts for 50% of all hospital admissions for sepsis. Because of ED overcrowding and long lengths of stay, the ED becomes a significant portal of entry to realize improved outcomes.[5]

▶ THE PATHOGENESIS OF SEPSIS

A series of pathogenic events are responsible for the transition from simple infection or sepsis to severe sepsis and septic shock. When an organism enters the body, the reaction is a systemic response that creates a systemic inflammatory response syndrome (SIRS). This reaction may be self-limited or may create a generalized systemic response. SIRS is the result of a release of proinflammatory and anti-inflammatory mediators. There is also a release of apoptotic proteins and an activation of the coagulation cascade. These processes can lead to malignant microvascular injury, thrombosis, and diffuse endothelial disruption, resulting in impaired tissue oxygenation. Furthermore, there is an imbalance between oxygen delivery and oxygen consumption. When organ dysfunction accompanies this response, this marks the onset of severe sepsis. Global tissue hypoxia and cytopathic (cellular) hypoxia develops, leading to multiple organ dysfunction and irreversible shock.

▶ THE DEFINITION OF SEPSIS

The American College of Chest Physicians (ACCP), the Society of Critical Care Medicine (SCCM), and International Sepsis Definitions Conference (ISDC) provided

▶ TABLE 36-1. SUMMARY OF DEFINITIONS

Infection

Defined as a pathologic process caused by the invasion of normally sterile tissue, fluid, or body cavity by pathogenic microorganisms.

Systemic inflammatory response syndrome (SIRS)

Defined as a physiologic response to an inflammatory process to a variety of severe clinical insults, manifested by at least two or more of the following:

1. Temperature >38°C or <36°C
2. Heart rate >90 beat/min
3. Respiratory rate >20 breaths/min or $Paco_2$ <32 mm Hg
4. WBC count >12,000 or < 4,000/mm^3 or >10% immature (band) forms

Sepsis

Sepsis is a systemic inflammatory response to an infection, defined as at least two SIRS conditions as a result of infection

Severe sepsis

Defined as acute sepsis-induced organ dysfunction, hypoperfusion (lactic acidosis, oliguria, or mental status alteration), or hypotension

Septic shock

Defined as sepsis-induced persistent hypotension, despite adequate fluid resuscitation along with the presence of perfusion abnormalities, which may include but are not limited to lactic acidosis, oliguria, and mental status alteration

▶ TABLE 36-2. DIAGNOSTIC CRITERIA FOR SEPSIS

Infection,[a] documented or suspected, and some of the following:

General variables

Fever (core temperature >38.3°C)
Hypothermia (core temperature <36°C)
Heart rate >90/min or >2 SD above the normal value for age
Tachypnea
Altered mental status
Significant edema or positive fluid balance (>20 mL/kg over 24 h)
Hyperglycemia (plasma glucose >120 mg/dL or 7.7 mmol/L) in the absence of diabetes

Inflammatory and hematologic variables

Leukocytosis (WBC count >12,000/μL)
Leukopenia (WBC count <4,000/μL)
Normal WBC count with >10% immature forms
Döhle's bodies, toxic granulation, and vacuoles
Plasma C-reactive protein >2 SD above the normal value
Plasma procalcitonin >2 SD above the normal value
Hemoconcentration (dehydration)
Thrombocytopenia
Fibrin degradation products

Hemodynamic variables

Arterial hypotension (SBP <90 mm Hg, MAP <70 mm Hg, or an SBP decrease >40 mm Hg in adults or >2 SD below normal for age)
Mixed venous oxygen saturation (SvO_2 >70%)
Cardiac index >3.5 L/min/m

Organ dysfunction variables

Arterial hypoxemia (Pao_2/FiO_2 <300)
Acute oliguria (urine output <0.5 mL/kg//h or 45 mmol/L for at least 2 h)
Creatinine increase >0.5 mg/dL
Coagulation abnormalities (INR >1.5 or aPTT >60 s)
Ileus (absent bowel sounds)
Thrombocytopenia (platelet count <100,000/μL)
Hyperbilirubinemia (plasma total bilirubin >4 mg/dL or 70 mmol/L)

Tissue perfusion variables

Hyperlactatemia (>2 mmol/L)
Decreased capillary refill or mottling

SD, standard deviation; WBC, white blood cell; SBP, systolic blood pressure; MAP, mean arterial blood pressure; SvO_2, mixed venous oxygen saturation; INR, international normalized ratio; aPTT, activated partial thromboplastin time.
[a]Infection defined as a pathologic process induced by a microorganism.

the definition of SIRS. SIRS is the systemic inflammatory response that is seen in a variety of infectious or non-infectious insults. The conference saw SIRS as a continuum, worsening and evolving to sepsis, severe sepsis, and septic shock (Table 36-1).[6] The definitions were still vague and not specific; for the 2001 International Sepsis Definition Conference definitions, the SIRS definition was expanded in the attempt to increase early diagnosis (Table 36-2).[7]

▶ BIOMARKERS AND DIAGNOSTICS IN SEPSIS

Biomarkers as diagnostic, therapeutic, and prognostic tools in sepsis continue to evolve. C-reactive protein (CRP) and lactate were the first to be used in risk stratification. A more sensitive and specific marker is procalcitonin (PCT); it has higher sensitivity and specificity.[8,9] PCT is currently being used in European countries to risk-stratify septic patients. In addition, PCT has been incorporated in recent guidelines as a first choice in management of sepsis. Recently, other markers have shown similar sensitivity and specificity as PCT. These markers include interleukin (IL)-1 receptor antagonist, protein C, and neutrophil gelatinase–associated lipocalin, which are key components of sepsis pathophysiology including inflammation, activation of coagulation, and renal/organ dysfunction, respectively.[10] This multimarker approach may offer an advantage for identifying patients likely to develop severe sepsis and earlier implementation of sepsis bundles.

▶ SURVIVING SEPSIS CAMPAIGN

The Surviving Sepsis Campaign (SSC)[11] was initiated in 2002 to improve the diagnosis, survival, and management of patients with sepsis by addressing the challenges associated with it. It developed three phases to carry its mission statement. Phase I started in October 2002 at the Barcelona Declaration at the 15th Annual Congress of the European Society for Intensive Care Medicine. It called for a 25% global reduction of mortality by 2009. The first-phase agenda includes the following points: public awareness, provider education, international standardization of care, improving early diagnosis and treatment, and providing access to post-ICU patient care.[12]

The second phase of the campaign was released as a set of guidelines for sepsis management in March 2004 and April 2004. The biggest achievement of this phase was the availability of unrestricted educational grants. The updated sepsis guidelines were released in 2008 and used the GRADE system. The GRADE system is a system developed to evaluate literature that includes grade of recommendation, assessment, development, and evaluation.

▶ IDENTIFICATION OF HIGH-RISK PATIENTS

The early detection of high-risk patients facilitates the rapid implementation of the sepsis bundles. High-risk patients are defined as patients who remain hypotensive (systolic blood pressure <90 mm Hg) after a 20–40 mL/kg fluid challenge or who have a lactate greater than 4 mmol/L.[13] Base deficit may be useful when present. However, up to 20% of patients may have a normal base deficit but elevated lactate.[14] While single lactate levels are helpful, serial lactates (every 3–6 hours) carry significant prognostic implications for morbidity and mortality.[15]

▶ ANTIBIOTICS AND SOURCE CONTROL

In multivariate studies, inadequate antibiotic therapy was shown to be a significant risk factor for sepsis. There is a 10% increase in hospital mortality among patients who receive inadequate therapy.[16] In addition, the failure to initiate antibiotics prior to or within the first hour of onset of hypotension is associated with an increased mortality of 7.6% for each hour antibiotic was delayed.[17] The recommendation for early administration of intravenous (IV) broad-spectrum antibiotics should be within 3 hours of arrival to the ED and 1 hour for non-ED ICU admissions.[18]

Prior to initiating any antibiotic treatment, appropriate cultures should be obtained, and, if needed, lumbar puncture or stool cultures should be collected. The goal is to start the appropriate antibiotics that will most likely attack the offending organism. Another consideration is the local antibiotic resistance patterns. Drug cost, pharmacokinetics, and interaction should also be considered when selecting the appropriate antibiotic.[19] The selection of the appropriate antibiotics also has significant outcome implications (Table 36-3).

The most common cause of sepsis is pneumonia (47%), intra-abdominal processes (18%), urinary tract infection (UTI) (18%), and bloodstream infection (12%). Other sites of infection include skin infections (rarely), nosocomial meningitis, and indwelling catheters.[16,18]

There are two different divisions of pneumonia: either nosocomial pneumonia or pneumonia without risk factors of multidrug-resistant pathogens. In nosocomial pneumonia, the most common organism is Enterobacteriaceae (30–40%), *Pseudomonas aeruginosa* (17–30%), and *Staphylococcus aureus* (7–15%). Treat this type of infection with a β-lactam active against *P. aeruginosa* ± aminoglycoside ± glycopeptide or linezolid if methicillin-resistant *S. aureus* (MRSA) is suspected. For pneumonia without risk factors for multidrug-resistant pathogens, the most common organism is *S. aureus* (45%), *Haemophilus influenzae* (20%), gram-negative bacilli (20%), and *Streptococcus pneumoniae* (9%). The recommended empirical antibiotic for this group is third-generation cephalosporin ± macrolide if intracellular bacteria are suspected.[19]

Another leading cause of sepsis includes UTI (60–70%), most commonly from Enterobacteriaceae including *Escherichia coli* (40%). This infection is usually treated with ciprofloxacin or if *P. aeruginosa* is suspected, ceftriaxone or ceftazidime ± aminoglycoside.[19] A bloodstream infection related to a catheter caused by *Staphylococcus* sp. (50%) and Enterobacteriaceae (30%) should be treated with a glycopeptide or linezolid with β-lactam that has activity against *P. aeruginosa*.[21]

Other causes of sepsis include intra-abdominal sepsis (usually gram-negative bacilli [60%] that include *E. coli* [40%], *P. aeruginosa* [30%]); gram-positive cocci (30%) include *Enterococcus* species.[22] Anaerobes and fungi can also cause sepsis. Treatment for gram-negative includes piperacillin–tazobactam or third/fourth-generation cephalosporin + metronidazole, or impenem ± fluconazole ± aminoglycoside.

Skin infection and nosocomial meningitides are rare causes of sepsis. Skin infection organisms include *Streptococcus* sp. and *Staphylococcus* sp.[23] While nosocomial meningitides may be caused by gram-negative bacilli, more commonly, *Acinetobacter* sp., *Staphylococcus* sp., and *Streptococcus* sp. can be the causative organism.[24]

▶ TABLE 36-3. ANTIBIOTIC CHOICE[16-25]

Site	Organism	Antibiotic
Pneumonia: nosocomial	1. Enterobacter 2. *Pseudomonas aeruginosa* 3. *Staphylococcus aureus*	1. β-Lactam 2. Add aminoglycoside 3. Add linezolid if suspect MRSA
Pneumonia: community acquired	1. *S. aureus* 2. *Streptococcus pneumoniae* 3. Gram-negative	Third-generation cephalosporin or macrolide
Urinary tract infection	1. Enterobacteriaceae (*Escherichia coli*) 2. *P. aeruginosa* 3. *Enterococcus* sp.	1. Ciprofloxacin 2. Ceftriaxone or ceftazidime 3. May add aminoglycoside
Abdominal source	1. Gram-negative bacilli (*E. coli*, *P. aeruginosa*) 2. Gram-positive cocci (*Enterococcus* sp.) 3. Anaerobes (*Bacteroides* sp.)	1. Piperacillin–tazobactam 2. Ceftriaxone, ceftazidine, or cefepime plus metronidazole 3. Imipenem, with fluconazole and aminoglycoside
Skin source	1. *Streptococcus* sp. 2. *Staphylococcus* sp. 3. Anaerobes	1. β-Lactam/lactamase inhibitor 2. Pipercillin/tazobactam 3. Cefoxitin
Indwelling catheter septicemia	1. *Staphylococcus* sp. 2. Enterobacteriaceae 3. *P. aeruginosa*	Linezolid with β-lactam
Meningitis	1. Gram-negative bacilli (*Acinetobacter* sp.) 2. *Staphylococcus* sp. 3. *Streptococcus* sp.	1. Meropenem with glycopeptide 2. Cefotaxime with fosfomycin

Selection depends on each region pattern. The most common causes are given in the table.

Source control is strategic in the early management of sepsis. It includes drainage of infected fluids, debridement of infected soft tissues, removal of infected devices or foreign bodies, and, finally, definite measures to correct anatomic derangement resulting in ongoing microbial contamination and to restore optimal function. A clear diagnostic approach to source identification and eradication should be determined within the first 6 hours of sepsis presentation.[25]

▶ EARLY GOAL-DIRECTED THERAPY

A goal-directed hemodynamic resuscitation within the first 6 hours of severe sepsis/septic shock includes a systematic approach to restoration of systemic oxygen delivery through a manipulation of preload (volume), afterload (blood pressure), and contractility (stroke volume) in order to preserve effective tissue perfusion while avoiding excessive increases in myocardial oxygen consumption (i.e., avoiding tachycardia and maintaining coronary perfusion pressure). There have been multiple studies that have shown when early goal-directed therapy (EGDT) is performed within the first 6 hours of disease presentation, outcomes are improved (Table 36-4). Specifically, patients are managed by (Table 36-5): (1) fluid resuscitation with either crystalloid or colloid to achieve a central venous pressure (CVP) goal of 8–12 mm Hg, (2) vasoactive agents to achieve a mean arterial pressure (MAP) goal of 65–90 mm Hg, (3) blood transfusion to a hematocrit ≥30%, (4) inotrope therapy, and (5) intubation, sedation, and paralysis as necessary to achieve a central venous oxygen saturation ($ScvO_2$)

▶ TABLE 36-4. SEPSIS RESUSCITATION BUNDLE BY THE INSTITUTE FOR HEALTHCARE IMPROVEMENT AND THE SURVIVING SEPSIS CAMPAIGN

Sepsis resuscitation bundle (should be accomplished as soon as possible and scored over the first 6 h of treatment):
- Serum lactate measured
- Blood cultures obtained prior to antibiotic administration
- Broad-spectrum antibiotics administered within 3 h for ED presentation and 1 h for non-ED ICU presentation
- In the event of hypotension (MAP <65 mm Hg or SBP <90 mm Hg) and/or lactate ≥4 mmol/L (36 mg/dL):
  - Initiate fluid resuscitation with 20 mL/kg of crystalloid (or colloid equivalent)
  - Start vasopressor for hypotension not responding to initial fluid to maintain MAP ≥65 mm Hg or SBP ≥90 mm Hg
- In the event of persistent hypotension or lactate ≥4 mmol/L (36 mg/dL):
  - Achieve central venous pressure (CVP) of ≥8 mm Hg
  - Achieve central venous oxygen saturation ($ScvO_2$) of ≥70%

► **TABLE 36-5. SURVIVING SEPSIS CAMPAIGN GUIDELINES FOR MANAGEMENT OF SEVERE SEPSIS AND SEPTIC SHOCK**

Initial resuscitation goals for sepsis-induced tissue hypoperfusion
- Central venous pressure: 8–12 mm Hg
- Mean arterial pressure: ≥65 mm Hg
- Urine output: ≥0.5 mL/kg/h
- Central venous oxygenation (superior vena cava oxygen saturation [$ScvO_2$]): ≥70%

≥70% as measured by intermittent or continuous central venous monitoring (Figure 36-1). EGDT should be employed as the first means of resuscitation with simultaneous prioritization of appropriate empirical antimicrobials and source control.[19]

Fluid Therapy

Decreased oral intake, increased insensible losses, arterial and venous dilation, and transudation of fluid into the extravascular fluid compartment lead to volume depletion. Because of these factors, initial fluid resuscitation should consist of rapid delivery of at least 20 mL/kg of crystalloid or colloid equivalent. If the patient needs further fluid resuscitation, it should be guided by CVP measurement. If CVP <8 mm Hg, the patient should receive 500-mL bolus every 30 minutes until the CVP >8 mm Hg.[26,27] The type of fluid has not been shown to have outcome benefit. See Table 36-6 for fluid choices.

Early fluid administration should not be confused with the adverse effects of late or liberal fluid administration in acute lung injury. The Fluids and Catheters Treatment Trial (FACTT) followed patients for 43 hours after being admitted to the ICU and 24 hours after developing a lung injury. The study showed no difference in the 60-day mortality rate.[33] Conservative fluid management showed significantly improved lung function, decreased need for mechanical ventilation, and improvement of central nervous system function secondary to decreased need for sedation.[34] It must be remembered that this is after the initial resuscitation.

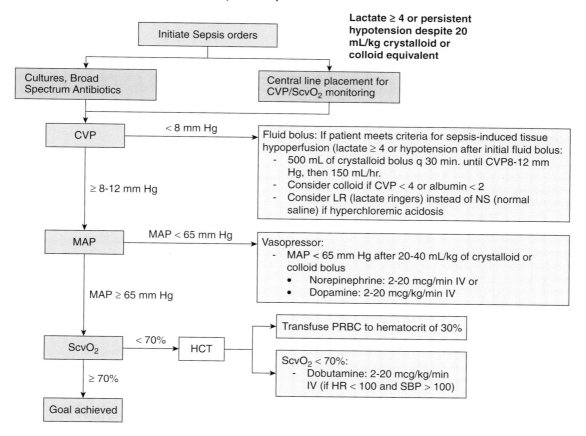

If patients meet entry criteria of severe sepsis or septic shock:

Figure 36–1. Diagram derived from early goal-directed therapy in the treatment of severe sepsis and septic shock.

► TABLE 36-6. **FLUID THERAPY**

Normal saline	Normal saline is a slightly hyperosmolar solution containing 154 mEq/L of both sodium and chloride. Due to the relatively high chloride concentration, normal saline carries a risk of inducing hyperchloremic metabolic acidosis when given in large amounts[27]
Lactated Ringer's	Lactate can accept a proton and subsequently be metabolized to CO_2 and water by the liver, leading to release of CO_2 in the lungs and excretion of water by the kidneys. LR results in a buffering of the acidemia that is advantageous over normal saline. Due to the fact that LR contains potassium, albeit a very small amount, there is a small risk of inducing hyperkalemia in patients with renal insufficiency or renal failure. There is a theoretical issue of using LR because of the significant immune activation and induction of cellular injury caused by the D-isomer of lactated Ringer's. Replacement of the lactate with ethyl pyruvate or β-hydroxybutyrate or using only the L-isomer of lactate in Ringer's solution decreases this adverse effect[27]
Albumin	Albumin is a protein derived from human plasma. It is available in varying strengths from 4% to 25%. The Saline versus Albumin Fluid Evaluation (SAFE) study compared fluid resuscitation with albumin or saline on mortality and found similar 28-day mortalities and secondary outcomes in each arm.[28] However, a subset analysis of patients with sepsis and acute lung injury resuscitated with albumin showed a decrease in mortality, although statistically it was insignificant. There was a significant increase in mortality in trauma patients particularly with head injury[27]
Hydroxyethyl starch	Hydroxyethyl starch (HES) is a synthetic colloid derived from hydrolyzed amylopectin, and has been found to be harmful, causing renal impairment at recommended doses and impairing long-term survival at high doses.[29] It can also cause coagulopathy and bleeding complications from reduced factor VIII and von Willebrand factor levels, as well as impaired platelet function. Hydroxyethyl starch increases the risk of acute renal failure among patients with sepsis and reduces the probability of survival. It should be avoided in sepsis[29-31]
Dextrans	Dextrans, another of the artificial colloids, are glucose polymers synthesized by *Leuconostoc mesenteroides* bacteria grown in sucrose media. They are not frequently used for rapid plasma expansion, but rather to lower blood viscosity. This class can cause renal dysfunction, as well as anaphylactoid reactions. The final group of artificial colloids is the gelatins. Gelatins are produced from bovine collagen. Because they have a much smaller molecular weight, they are not as effective expanding plasma volume; however, they cost less.[32] They too have been reported to cause renal impairment, as well as allergic reactions ranging from pruritus to anaphylaxis. Gelatins are not currently available in North America

Vasopressor Use

The homeostatic balance between vasodilatation and vasoconstriction is altered in severe sepsis and septic shock.[35] In sepsis, the predominant feature is systemic vasodilatation. Nitric oxide synthesis production increases in sepsis; the vascular smooth muscle relaxes. The endogenous vasoconstriction is less studied. In septic shock, smooth muscle is poorly responsive to norepinephrine. When the blood pressure decreases, endogenous arginine vasopressin (AVP) increases. AVP is released by the neurohypophysis to induce water conservation by the kidneys; thus, it helps to regulate osmotic pressures and cardiovascular homeostasis.[36]

Exogenous vasopressors

If a patient continues to be hypotensive with vasopressor dependency after adequate volume resuscitation, central venous and arterial access should be obtained. In EGDT, if CVP <8 mm Hg, the patient should be given boluses of 500-mL aliquots every 30 minutes until CVP >8 mm Hg. In a severe hypotensive patient,

vasopressors should be started sooner. Vasopressors should be started if MAP <65 mm Hg and CVP >8 mm Hg, or prior to fluid resuscitation in the presence of very low MAP.[19,37] Table 36-7 shows some exogenous vasopressors with their side effects.

Inotropic Therapy

Prior to EGDT, ICU-based studies using inotropic therapy targeting supranormal goals of oxygen delivery were associated with an increased mortality rate.[53] In EGDT, the timing, patient selection, and physiologic goals were different. Dobutamine was started at a lower dose and titrated up to achieve $ScvO_2$ ≥70% (Figure 36-1). For an initial resuscitation in a busy ED, $ScvO_2$ can be used as a convenient surrogate for mixed venous oxygen saturation (SvO_2).[26,54] A resuscitation endpoint of SvO_2 of 65% and $ScvO_2$ of 70% is recommended by the SSC.

Blood Product Administration

The rationale for transfusing a severely septic or a septic shock patient due to impaired marrow response and

► TABLE 36-7. **EXOGENOUS VASOPRESSORS**

Drug	Side Effects and Comments
Norepinephrine	Norepinephrine has the physiologic properties of a vasoconstrictor and an inotrope.[38] Martin et al found favorable outcomes in 7- and 28-day mortality while the other vasopressors did not extrapolate to be having either a negative or positive association in mortality with multivariant analysis.[39] Marik et al. compared norepinephrine with dopamine showing improved splanchnic oxygen utilization by norepinephrine[40]
Dopamine	The majority of the effects of dopamine <5 μg/kg/min are seen in the renal, mesenteric, and coronary dopaminergic receptors. At doses 5–10 μg/kg/min, β-adrenergic effects are seen that increase cardiac contractility. At higher doses >10 μg/kg/min, β-adrenergic effects predominate with arterial vasoconstriction.[41] A randomized clinical trial of low-dose dopamine in septic shock patients showed no protective effects from renal insufficiency.[42] Jakob showed increased splanchnic oxygen consumption even in the face of increased splanchnic blood flow.[38,43] One observational study suggests that dopamine administration may be associated with increased mortality rates in shock[44]
Phenylephrine	Phenylephrine has primary selectivity for α_1-receptors in increasing peripheral resistance.[38] It is most ideal in patients who present with tachycardia. Phenylephrine lacks significant inotropic or chronotropic effects and is recommended to be used in caution with those in cardiac dysfunction in sepsis. One concern is the increase in oxygen consumption, decrease in splanchnic blood flow, and decrease in cardiac output for septic shock patients[45]
Ephedrine	Causes palpitations, hypertension, and cardiac arrhythmias; an indirect-acting CNS stimulant; limited long-term value as therapy for shock
Epinephrine	De Backer et al investigated the splanchnic circulation in septic shock patients with epinephrine compared with the other vasopressors and found a dose-dependent redistribution phenomenon away from hepatosplanchnic system, lowering splanchnic blood flow despite a higher cardiac output.[46] Hyperlactatemia has been described as a detrimental effect of epinephrine; however, Levy describes this effect as being transient with a 24-hour recovery independent of hypoxemia and likely is an adaptive physiologic response to maintain carbohydrate metabolism under an aggressive circulatory insult.[47] Epinephrine may attenuate excessive activity of inflammatory cytokines during infections and may have antithrombotic properties.[47] In persistent hypotension while on dopamine, the addition of epinephrine was not a significant factor for prediction of mortality.[39] Martin et al investigated the management of septic shock with either epinephrine or norepinephrine plus dobutamine and found no difference in mortality[39,47,48]
Vasopressin	Landry et al observed that septic shock patients have reduced vasopressin levels and were responsive to exogenous vasopressin infusion.[49] Ertmer et al were also able to show how the addition of dobutamine dosed at 5–10 μg/kg/min reversed the vasopressin impairment in CI, DO_2I, and SvO_2 and even increased the MAP.[50] The VASST multicenter trial investigated vasopressin as an adjunctive and alternative therapy to norepinephrine and showed no statistical 28- or 90-day mortality difference[45,51]

erythropoietin levels may be to improve low hemoglobin levels in the presence of global tissue hypoxia.[55] When septic shock or global tissue hypoxia is combined with anemia, transfusion is recommended. When resuscitating patients with large volumes of fluid, a dilutional anemia is common. In the presence of an elevated or low $ScvO_2$, transfusion to a hematocrit of 30% is recommended.

When should packed red blood cells, fresh frozen plasma, antithrombin, and platelets be transfused? As per guidelines, red blood cells should be transfused when hemoglobin is <7 g/dL to a target of 7–9 g/dL except in patients with significant coronary artery disease or acute hemorrhage where hemoglobin >10 g/dL is maintained.[19] Fresh frozen plasma should not be transfused to correct coagulopathy unless there is bleeding or a planned invasive procedure. Antithrombin therapy

should not be used. Transfuse platelets when the count is <5,000/mm³ regardless of bleeding, or if count is 5,000–30,000/mm³ with significant bleeding risk.

Corticosteroids and the Septic Patient

In the stress of sepsis, the adrenal response may not be sufficient; thus, a relative adrenal insufficiency results. This has given rise to the existence of adrenal dysfunction. While early studies have shown that steroid replacement has no benefit and may cause harm,[56–58] Annane et al in 2002 showed that replacement of hydrocortisone at 50 mg every 6 hours showed improved outcomes and decreased vasopressor use.[59] More recently, the Corticosteroid Therapy of Septic Shock (CORTICUS) study enrolled a wider population range.[60] Specifically, patients with systolic blood pressure less than

90 mm Hg for 1 hour regardless of vasopressor use, septic shock patients from the ICU up to the first 72 hours, and patients where etomidate was used were enrolled. By comparison, Annane et al only enrolled persistent hypotensive patients for 1 hour or greater and septic shock patients for the first 8 hours, and excluded any person where etomidate was used within 6 hours.[59] CORTICUS showed no significant difference in 28-day mortality between corticosteroid and placebo.[60] However, in a subset analysis of patients similar to the first trial, the mortality benefit was significant.

A clinical caveat is to withhold the use of steroid for 6–8 hours until the patient reaches the endpoints of EGDT. There is a 14% reduction in vasopressor use during the first 6 hours by giving fluids alone. By delaying steroid use in this setting, there will be a decreased use. In the latest 2008 guidelines of the SSC, the use of IV hydrocortisone is recommended for adult patients with persistent hypotensive septic shock where the blood pressure does not respond to fluid therapy and vasopressors. The guidelines went one step further by making the cosyntropin stimulation test elective and recommending against the use of dexamethasone as a substitute to hydrocortisone.[19]

In an ED rapid sequence intubation (RSI), etomidate is commonly used.[61] In ICU studies, continuous infusion of etomidate in septic patients led to adrenal insufficiency; this in turn led to an increase in mortality.[62] Another study in surgical patients showed that prolonged use of etomidate lowered plasma cortisol level.[63] The use of a single dose of etomidate during RSI is currently under debate. Recently, ketamine is being used as an alternative RSI agent with a favorable hemodynamic profile. Further studies are needed in this area.

Activated Protein C

During sepsis, the inflammatory complexes (cytokines and coagulation mediators) in the body start to damage endothelial cells and coagulation in the microcirculation leading to end-organ dysfunction and finally death.[64] The body inhibits coagulation by tissue factor pathway inhibitor, antithrombin, and the protein C system.[65] Endogenous activated protein C inhibits thrombosis, inflammation, and apoptosis. Severe sepsis patients with low activated protein C are associated with increased mortality.[66] The Recombinant Human Activated Protein C Worldwide Evaluation in Severe Sepsis (PROWESS) study demonstrated reduction of mortality rate from 30.9% in the placebo to 24.7% in the treatment group; the study was stopped early after these findings.[64] The increased survival was confirmed only in higher severities of illness, as reflected by a higher APACHE II score ≥25 or multiple organ

▶ **TABLE 36-8. ABSOLUTE AND RELATIVE CONTRAINDICATIONS OF RECOMBINANT HUMAN ACTIVATED PROTEIN C**

Absolute contraindications to the use of recombinant human activated protein C (rhAPC):
- Active internal bleeding
- Recent (within 90 days) hemorrhagic stroke
- Recent (within 60 days) intracranial/intraspinal surgery, or severe head trauma
- Trauma with risk of life-threatening bleeding
- Presence of epidural catheter
- Intracranial neoplasm or mass lesion (known or suspected)
- Hypersensitivity to rhAPC

Relative contraindications to the use of recombinant human activated protein C (rhAPC):
- Heparin use (>15 U/kg/h)
- Platelet count <30,000/mm²
- Thrombolytic therapy within 3 days
- Oral anticoagulant or glycoprotein IIb/IIIa inhibitors within 7 days
- Ischemic stroke within 90 days
- Intracranial AV malformation or aneurysm
- Known bleeding diathesis
- Chronic severe hepatic disease
- HIV infection with CD4 count <50/mm³
- Recent surgery within 30 days
- Single organ dysfunction due to sepsis
- Pediatric patients

dysfunction. The Extended Evaluation of Recombinant Human Activated Protein C (ENHANCE) study showed similar mortality benefit as PROWESS with increase of bleeding; if recombinant human activated protein C (rhAPC) is started within the first 24 hours, then the mortality was 22.9% versus 27.4% if rhAPC is started >24 hours.[67]

In the ED, the use of rhAPC is limited only to instances where admission to the ICU is delayed.[19] Pursuant to the current guidelines, rhAPC is recommended in the presence of sepsis-induced acute organ dysfunction associated with a clinical assessment of high risk of death (APACHE II scores ≥25) and with no absolute contraindications or relative contraindications that outweigh benefit (Table 36-8).

Ventilation with Low Tidal Volume

As mentioned previously, the lung is the most common site of infection. The inflammatory cascade in the lung leads to pulmonary parenchymal damage. This damage causes dysfunction in the respiratory system that may lead to acute respiratory distress syndrome (ARDS). ARDS is defined as an acute onset of respiratory failure with a ratio of arterial partial pressure of oxygen and fractional inspired concentration of oxygen (Pao_2/FiO_2) <200 regardless of positive end-expiratory pressure (PEEP), bilateral infiltrates, and pulmonary capillary wedge pressure (PCWP).[68] A study was performed using lung-protective ventilation (LPV) (6 mL/kg tidal volumes and a plateau pressure <30 cm H_2O) versus conventional volumes (ARDSNET study).[69] This study showed that in patients with lung injury, LPV was associated with 9% absolute reduction in mortality. The ARDSNET study also showed that permissive hypercapnea (hypoventilation and mild respiratory acidosis [pH 7.3–7.45]) was tolerated.

Guidelines recommend in severe sepsis or septic shock to avoid high tidal volume coupled with high plateau pressures by decreasing tidal volumes to 6 mL/kg (based on predicted body weight) with the goal of maintaining end-inspiratory plateau pressure <30 cm H_2O. Set PEEP based on severity of oxygenation deficit. Consider intermittent prone positioning treatment for patients who require potentially injurious FiO_2 levels or plateau pressure >30 cm H_2O.[19] To prevent ventilator-associated pneumonia, raise head of bed 45° unless contraindicated.

Glycemic Control

Hyperglycemia is noted to be prevalent in critically ill patients. Intensive glucose control between 80 and 110 mg/dL showed to be more beneficial in surgical intensive care unit (SICU) versus medical intensive care unit (MICU) patients.[70,71] In the MICU population, there was not any benefit to intensive glucose control. In fact, there were patients who developed hypoglycemia.[71]

The 2008 SSC recommends that after the first 6 hours, blood glucose <150 mg/dL and greater than lower limit of laboratory normal be maintained.[19] In addition, continuous insulin and glucose infusion should be used and the blood glucose levels should be monitored every 30–60 minutes until the levels are stabilized; once stabilized, the levels should be monitored every 4 hours. The Campaign also recommends a longer ICU stay when patients receive IV insulin. All patients on IV insulin therapy should receive a glucose calorie source; caution should be observed when using point-of-care glucose to make sure that the plasma values are not overestimated.

Prophylaxis

Prophylactic unfractionated heparin or low-molecular-weight heparin should be administered as soon as the patient is admitted. A mechanical compression device should be used in patients with a contraindication for heparin. Stress ulcer prophylaxis should be provided with histamine 2 (H_2) receptor antagonists.[19]

▶ STARTING A SEPSIS AND QUALITY INITIATIVE PROGRAM

The evidence for the 6- and 24-hour bundle has shown repeatedly to improve outcome in numerous follow-up studies in both adults and children.[72,73] EGDT in particular has been shown to be cost-effective by decreasing sepsis-related hospital costs by 20% even after taking into account all the training and equipment needed for this initiative.[74] If an institution averages >16 septic patients per year, then the institution will average a 32.6% reduction of cost. These cost analysis studies have been repeated and validated.[75,76]

There are multiple models an institution can adopt. A coordinated patient care model requires convergence of multiple expertise and resources to be initiated by the ED until a patient arrives to the ICU. A second model requires a rapid response team that is mobile and can move within the hospital.[77] This model covers the entire hospital and transfers to the ICU would be initiated for the management part of the bundle. A third model requires early ICU admission, and allows the ICU intensivist to start EGDT.

▶ SUMMARY

Early sepsis management is associated with morbidity, mortality, and health care resource consumption. Similar to acute myocardial infarction, stroke, and trauma, the management of sepsis is time-sensitive and requires emergent expertise in the ED.

REFERENCES

1. Rivers EP. Early goal-directed therapy in severe sepsis and septic shock: converting science to reality. *Chest.* 2006;129:217–218.
2. McCaig LF, Burt CW. National Hospital Ambulatory Medical Care Survey: 2002 emergency department summary. *Adv Data.* 2004;340:1–34.
3. Angus D, Linde-Zwirble WT, Lidicker MA, et al. Epidemiology of severe sepsis in the United States: analysis of incidence, outcome, and associated costs of care. *Crit Care Med.* 2001;29:1303–1310.
4. Wang H, Shapiro N, Angus D, et al. National estimates of severe sepsis in United States emergency departments. *Crit Care Med.* 2007;35:1928–1936.
5. Zambon M, Ceola M, Almeida-de-Castro R, et al. Implementation of the surviving sepsis campaign guidelines for severe sepsis and septic shock: we could go faster. *J Crit Care.* 2008;23:455–460.
6. Bone RC, Balk RA, Cerra FB, et al. The American College of Chest Physicians/Society of Critical Care Medicine Consensus Conference Committee: definitions for sepsis and organ failure and guidelines for the use of innovative therapies in sepsis. *Chest.* 1992;101:1644–1655.

7. Levy MM, Fink MP, Marshall JC, et al. 2001 SCCM/ESICM/ACCP/ATS/SIS international sepsis definitions conference. *Crit Care Med*. 2003;31:1250–1256.

8. Marshall JC, Vincent JL, Fink MP, et al. Measures, markers, and mediators: toward a staging system for clinical sepsis. A report of the Fifth Toronto Sepsis Roundtable. *Crit Care Med*. 2003;31:1560–1567.

9. Luzzani A, Polati E, Dorizzi R, et al. Comparison of procalcitonin and c-reactive protein as markers of sepsis. *Crit Care Med*. 2003;31:1737–1741.

10. Shapiro NI, Trzeciak S, Hollander JE, et al. A prospective, multicenter derivation of a biomarker panel to assess risk of organ dysfunction, shock, and death in emergency department patients with suspected sepsis. *Crit Care Med*. 2009;37:96–104.

11. Levy MM, Dellinger RP, Townsend SR, et al. The Surviving Sepsis Campaign: results of an international guideline-based performance improvement program targeting severe sepsis. *Crit Care Med*. 2010;(38):367–374.

12. The Surviving Sepsis Campaign. Available at: http://www.survivingsepsis.org/background/barcelona_declaration.

13. Mikkelsen ME, Miltiades AN, Gaieski DF, et al. Serum lactate is associated with mortality in severe sepsis independent of organ failure and shock. *Crit Care Med*. 2009;37:1670–1677.

14. Berkman M, Ufberg J, Nathanson LA, Shapiro NI. Anion gap as a screening tool for elevated lactate in patients with an increased risk of developing sepsis in the emergency department. *J Emerg Med*. 2009;36:391–394.

15. Nguyen HB, Rivers EP, Knoblich BP, et al. Early lactate clearance is associated with improved outcome in severe sepsis and septic shock. *Crit Care Med*. 2004;32:1637–1642.

16. Kumar A, Roberts D, Wood KE, et al. Duration of hypotension before initiation of effective antimicrobial therapy is the critical determinant of survival in human septic shock. *Crit Care Med*. 2006;34:1589–1596.

17. Larche J, Azoulay E, Fieux F, et al. Improved survival of critically ill cancer patients with septic shock. *Intensive Care Med*. 2003;29:1688–1695.

18. Vincent JL, Bihari DJ, Suter PM, et al. The prevalence of nosocomial infection in intensive care units in Europe. Results of the European Prevalence of Infection in Intensive Care (EPIC). EPIC International Advisory Committee. *JAMA*. 1995;274:639–644.

19. Dellinger RP, Levy MM, Carlet JM, et al. Surviving Sepsis Campaign: international guidelines for management of severe sepsis and septic shock: 2008. *Crit Care Med*. 2008;36:296–327.

20. Leone M, Perrin AS, Granier I, et al. A randomized trial of catheter change and short course of antibiotics for asymptomatic bacteriuria in catheterized ICU patients. *Intensive Care Med*. 2007;33:726–729.

21. Costerton JW, Stewart PS, Greenberg EP. Bacterial biofilms: a common cause of persistent infections. *Science*. 1999;284:1318–1321.

22. Carunta FA, Benea L. Spontaneous bacterial peritonitis: pathogenesis, diagnosis, treatment. *J Gastrointest Liver Dis*. 2006;15:51–56.

23. Elliott DC, Kufera JA, Myers RA, et al. The microbiology of necrotizing soft tissue infections. *Am J Surg*. 2000;179:361–366.

24. Arabi Y, Memish ZA, Balkhy Y, HH, et al. Ventriculostomy associated infections: incidence and risk factors. *Am J Infect Control*. 2005;33:137–143.

25. Marshall JC, al Naqbi A. Principles of source control in the management of sepsis. *Crit Care Clin*. 2009;25:753–768, viii–ix.

26. Dellinger RP. Cardiovascular management of septic shock. *Crit Care Med*. 2003;31:946–955.

27. Vincent JL, Gerlach H. Fluid resuscitation in severe sepsis and septic shock: an evidence-based review. *Crit Care Med*. 2004;32:S451–S454.

28. Finfer S, Bellomo R, Boyce N, French J, Myburgh J, Norton R. A comparison of albumin and saline for fluid resuscitation in the intensive care unit. *N Engl J Med*. 2004;350:2247–2256.

29. Brunkhorst FM, Engel C, Bloos F, et al. Intensive insulin therapy and pentastarch resuscitation in severe sepsis. *N Engl J Med*. 2008;358:125–139.

30. Wiedermann CJ. Systematic review of randomized clinical trials on the use of hydroxyethyl starch for fluid management in sepsis. *BMC Emerg Med*. 2008;8:1.

31. Sriskandan S, Altmann DM. The immunology of sepsis. *J Pathol*. 2008;214:211–223.

32. Vincent JL, Weil MH. Fluid challenge revisited. *Crit Care Med*. 2006;34:1333–1337.

33. Rivers EP. Fluid-management strategies in acute lung injury—liberal, conservative, or both? *N Engl J Med*. 2006;354(24):2598–2600.

34. Wiedemann HP, Wheeler AP, Bernard GR, et al. National Heart, Lung, and Blood Institute Acute Respiratory Distress Syndrome (ARDS) Clinical Trials Network. Comparison of two fluid management strategies in acute lung injuries. *N Engl J Med*. 2006;354(24):2564–2575. Epub May 21, 2006.

35. Levy MM, Macias WL, Vincent JL, et al. Early changes in organ function predict eventual survival in severe sepsis. *Crit Care Med*. 2005;33(10):2194–2201.

36. Landry DW, Levin HR, Gallant EM, et al. Vasodilation deficiency contributes to the vasodilatation of septic shock. *Circulation*. 1997;95:1122–1125.

37. Morgenthaler NG, Struck J, Alonso C, et al. Assay for the measurement of copeptin, a stable peptide derived from the precursor of vasopressin. *Clin Chem*. 2006;52:112–119.

38. Marini JJ, Wheeler AP, eds. *Critical Care Medicine: The Essentials*. 3rd ed. Philadelphia: Lippincott Williams & Wilkins; 2006.

39. Martin C, Viviand X, Leone M, Thirion X. Effect of norepinephrine on the outcome of septic shock. *Crit Care Med*. 2000;28:2758–2765.

40. Marik PE, Mohedin M. The contrasting effects of dopamine and norepinephrine on systemic and splanchnic oxygen utilization in hyperdynamic sepsis. *JAMA*. 1994;272:1354–1357.

41. Landry DW, Oliver JA. The pathogenesis of vasodilatory shock. *N Engl J Med*. 2001;345:588–595.

42. Beale RJ, Hollenberg SM, Vincent JL, Parrillo JE. Vasopressor and inotropic support in septic shock: an evidence-based review. *Crit Care Med*. 2004;32:S455–S465.

43. Jakob S. Clinical review: splanchnic ischaemia. *Crit Care.* 2002;6:306–312.

44. Sakr Y, Reinhart K, Vincent JL, et al. Does dopamine administration in shock influence outcome? Results of the Sepsis Occurrence in Acutely Ill Patients (SOAP) Study. *Crit Care Med.* 2006;34:589–597.

45. Parrillo JE, Dellinger RP, eds. *Critical Care Medicine: Principles of Diagnosis and Management in the Adult.* 3rd ed. Philadelphia: Mosby Elsevier; 2008.

46. De Backer D, Creteur J, Silva E, Vincent JL. Effects of dopamine, norepinephrine, and epinephrine on the splanchnic circulation in septic shock: which is best? *Crit Care Med.* 2003;31:1659–1667.

47. Levy B. Use of pressors in the management of septic shock. *Lancet.* 2007;370:1827. Author reply 8.

48. Dellinger RP, Levy MM, Carlet JM, et al. Surviving Sepsis Campaign: international guidelines for management of severe sepsis and septic shock: 2008. *Crit Care Med.* 2008;36:296–327.

49. Landry DW, Levin HR, Gallant EM, et al. Vasopressin deficiency contributes to the vasodilation of septic shock. *Circulation.* 1997;95:1122–1125.

50. Ertmer C, Morelli A, Bone HG, et al. Dobutamine reverses the vasopressin-associated impairment in cardiac index and systemic oxygen supply in ovine endotoxemia. *Crit Care.* 2006;10:R144.

51. Russell JA, Walley KR, Singer J, et al. Vasopressin versus norepinephrine infusion in patients with septic shock. *N Engl J Med.* 2008;358:877–887.

52. Rivers E, Nguyen B, Havstad S, et al. Early goal-directed therapy in the treatment of severe sepsis and septic shock. *N Engl J Med.* 2001;345:1368–1377.

53. Gattinoni L, Brazzi L, Pelosi P, et al. A trial of goal-oriented hemodynamic therapy in critically ill patients. SvO$_2$ Collaborative Group. *N Engl J Med.* 1995;333(16):1025–1032.

54. Chawla LS, Zia H, Gutierrez G, et al. Lack of equivalence between central and mixed venous oxygen saturation. *Chest.* 2004;126(6):1891–1896.

55. Tamion F, Le Cam-Duchez V, Menard JF, et al. Serum erythropoietin levels in septic shock. *Anaesth Intensive Care.* 2005;33(5):578–584.

56. Oelkers W. Adrenal insufficiency. *N Engl J Med.* 1996;335:1206–1212.

57. Lefering R, Neugebauer E. Steroid controversy in sepsis and septic shock: a met analysis. *Crit Care Med.* 1995;23:1294–1303.

58. Sprung CL, Caralis PV, Marcial EH, et al. The effect of high-dose corticosteroids in patients with septic shock. *N Engl J Med.* 1984;311:1137–1143.

59. Annane D, Sebille V, Charpentier C, et al. Effect of treatment with low doses of hydrocortisone and fludrocortisone on mortality in patients with septic shock. *JAMA.* 2002;288:862–871.

60. Sprung CL, Annane D, Keh D, et al. Hydrocortisone therapy for patients with septic shock. *N Engl J Med.* 2008;358:111–124.

61. Sakles JC, Laurin EG, Rantapaa AA, et al. Airway management in the emergency department: a one-year study of 610 tracheal intubations. *Ann Emerg Med.* 1998;31:325–332.

62. Watt I, Ledingham IM. Mortality amongst multiple trauma patients admitted to an intensive therapy unit. *Anesthesia.* 1984;39:973–981.

63. Wagner RL, White PF, Kan PB, et al. Inhibition of adrenal steroidogenesis by the anesthetic etomidate. *N Engl J Med.* 1984;310:1415–1421.

64. Benard GR, Vincent JL, Laterre PF, et al. Efficacy and safety of recombinant human activated protein C for severe sepsis. *N Engl J Med.* 2001;344:699–709.

65. Fourrier F. Recombinant human activated protein C in the treatment of severe sepsis: an evidence based review. *Crit Care Med.* 2004;32(S):S434–S441.

66. Yan SB, Helterbrand JD, Hartman DL, et al. Low levels of protein C are associated with poor outcome in severe sepsis. *Chest.* 2001;120:915–922.

67. Vincent JL, Bernard GR, Beale R, et al. Drotrecogin alfa (activated) treatment in severe sepsis from the global open-label trial ENHANCE: further evidence for survival and safety and implications for early treatment. *Crit Care Med.* 2005;33:2266–2277.

68. Bernard GR, Artigas A, Brigham KL, et al. The American–European consensus conference on ARDS. Definitions, mechanisms, relevant outcomes, and clinical trial coordination. *Am J Respir Crit Care Med.* 1994;149:818–824.

69. The Acute Respiratory Distress Syndrome Network. Ventilation with lower tidal volumes as compared with traditional tidal volumes for acute lung injury and the acute respiratory distress syndrome. *N Engl J Med.* 2000;342:1301–1308.

70. Van den Berghe G, Wouters P, Weekers F, et al. Intensive insulin therapy in critically ill patients. *N Engl J Med.* 2001;345:1359–1367.

71. Van den Berghe G, Wilmer A, Hermans G, et al. Intensive insulin therapy in the medical ICU. *N Engl J Med.* 2006;354:449–461.

72. Rivers EP, Coba V, Whitmill M. Early goal-directed therapy in severe sepsis and septic shock: a contemporary review of the literature. *Curr Opin Anaesthesiol.* 2008;21:128–140.

73. Gao F, Melody T, Daniels DF, Giles S, Fox S. The impact of compliance with 6-hour and 24-hour sepsis bundles on hospital mortality in patients with severe sepsis: a prospective observational study. *Crit Care.* 2005;9:R764–R770.

74. Huang DT, Angus DC, et al. Cost-effectiveness of early goal-directed therapy in the treatment of severe sepsis and septic shock. *Crit Care.* 2003;7:S116.

75. Shapiro NI, Howell MD, Talmor D, et al. Implementation and outcomes of the Multiple Urgent Sepsis Therapies (MUST) protocol. *Crit Care Med.* 2006;34(4):1025–1032.

76. Trzeciak S, Dellinger RP, Abate NL, et al. Translating research to clinical practice: a 1-year experience with implementing early goal-directed therapy for septic shock in the emergency department. *Chest.* 2006;129(2):225–232.

77. Frank ED. A shock team in a general hospital. *Anesth Analg.* 1967;46(6):740–745.

CHAPTER 37

Nosocomial and Health Care-Associated Pneumonia

Michael T. McCurdy

► INTRODUCTION

Whether in the emergency department or in the intensive care unit (ICU), pneumonia is a disease with which all treating clinicians must be familiar. In order to accurately recognize and appropriately manage pneumonia, one must first understand its varying classifications, affiliated pathogens, available diagnostic methods, treatment options, and methods of prevention.

► DEFINITION

Pneumonia classically has been dichotomized as either community-acquired pneumonia (CAP) or nosocomial pneumonia (NP), depending on where the patient becomes infected. NP must occur at least 48 hours after hospital admission and not be incubating at the time of admission.[1] NP developing in an individual after requiring at least 48 hours of mechanical ventilation is termed ventilator-associated pneumonia (VAP). NP can also be categorized according to the timing of its onset following hospital admission. Early onset NP occurs within the first 4 days of hospitalization and can be due to antibiotic-susceptible bacteria found in the community (e.g., *Pneumococcus, H. influenzae, Moraxella*).[2] Late-onset NP occurs after at least 5 hospital days, is generally caused by multidrug-resistant (MDR) organisms (e.g., *P. aeruginosa, Acinetobacter* spp.), and has a higher associated mortality.[3] These definitions are clinically relevant because each is associated with a distinct set of typical infecting organisms, management strategies, and outcomes.

However, as the lines between typical outpatient and inpatient settings blur (e.g., due to increased utilization of outpatient dialysis, surgical, and rehabilitation centers), these standard definitions inadequately account for the evolving landscape of causative bacteria resulting in pneumonia. The type of pneumonia infecting individuals with exposure to health care settings is now termed health care–associated pneumonia (HCAP). Although this type of pneumonia typically presents in individuals technically living in the community, the bacterial flora and clinical outcomes affiliated with HCAP are generally similar to those of NP. Therefore, assessing a patient's risk factors for HCAP is essential for its prompt identification and subsequent antibiotic selection (Table 37-1).

► TABLE 37-1. NOSOCOMIAL PNEUMONIA (NP) AND HEALTH CARE–ASSOCIATED PNEUMONIA (HCAP) RISK FACTORS FOR MULTIDRUG RESISTANCE

- Presence of risk factors for both NP and HCAP:
  - Antimicrobial therapy in preceding 90 days
  - Current hospitalization of ≥5 days
  - High frequency of antibiotic resistance in community or specific ICU
  - Immunosuppressive disease and/or therapy
- Presence of risk factors for HCAP:
  - Hospitalization for ≥2 days in preceding 90 days
  - Residence in a nursing home or extended care facility
  - Home infusion therapy (including antibiotics)
  - Chronic dialysis within 30 days
  - Home wound care
  - Family member with multidrug-resistant pathogen

► EPIDEMIOLOGY

Pneumonia exacts a great toll on the physical and financial health of both individuals and society. Compared with the estimated 10% mortality with CAP, one review of over 4,500 hospitalized patients demonstrated mortalities of 19.8% with HCAP and 18.8% with NP.[4] NP, and in particular VAP, has an expectedly high mortality due to the invasive organisms infecting a very ill patient population. Some hypothesize that the similarly elevated mortality rate with HCAP may be due to the late recognition, and therefore inadequate antibiotic regimen for HCAP by clinicians not familiar with its risk factors.[4]

Occurring in 9–27% of all intubated patients,[5] VAP accounts for approximately 90% of cases of NP[6] and is the most lethal form of all hospital-acquired infections.[7] VAP mortality typically ranges from 20% to 70%[8,9] but commonly is >70% when caused by invasive MDR organisms.[8] Although an accurate assessment of its lethality is difficult due to the numerous variables among studies on the topics of VAP (e.g., heterogeneity of patient populations, duration of mechanical ventilation prior to VAP onset, diagnostic methods used, infecting pathogens, time until appropriate antibiotic administration), its estimated in-hospital attributable mortality is 30%.[8] Of note, these multiple confounders plague many of the attempted comparisons made among studies on the topic.

On average, each episode of NP increases the patient's hospital length of stay (LOS) by at least a week,[10] and each VAP significantly increases the time on mechanical ventilation, ICU LOS, and hospital LOS. Additionally, VAP increases the cost of hospitalization by at least $40,000.[11]

► PATHOPHYSIOLOGY

To best develop strategies to diagnose, treat, and prevent NP, it is essential to first understand its underlying pathophysiology. HCAP and non-VAP NP generally originate from initial nasopharyngeal or oropharyngeal colonization of bacterial pathogens via either airborne passage or direct inoculation from an affected source.[12] Potential sources include contact with medical staff or aspiration of gastrointestinal (GI) flora. Antibiotics that are often administered during a typical hospitalization eliminate indigenous GI bacteria, thus promoting the colonization of resistant strains. Additionally, acid-suppressive medications used for gastric ulcer prophylaxis increase gastric bacterial growth when gastric pH >4.6.[13,14] The growing reservoir of increasingly resistant bacteria within the GI tract is particularly dangerous for individuals susceptible to aspiration, such as those with altered mental status, poor cough reflex,

swallowing difficulties, or other circumstances diminishing proper airway protection. In fact, more than half of all critically ill patients routinely aspirate.[15]

In the presence of factors that adversely alter the body's antimicrobial milieu and normal host defenses, colonizing bacteria can subsequently gain access to the lower respiratory system, where they multiply and invade the affected area of lung. The pathogenesis of VAP shares some characteristics with those aforementioned pneumonias, but only VAP involves the presence of an endotracheal tube (ETT) in the upper airway, which directly bypasses normal airway protective mechanisms.

Intubation is the most important risk factor for the development of VAP.[16] Although bacteria can access the lungs via inhalation into the respiratory tract from a colonized ventilator apparatus (e.g., humidifiers, filters, suction catheters), hematogenous spread, or direct extension from a parapneumonic process, tracheal colonization most commonly results from the leakage of bacteria-laden secretions pooling in the subglottic space around the cuff of the ETT.[17] The insertion of nasal tubes (e.g., nasotracheal, nasogastric) can also displace bacteria colonizing the maxillary sinuses into the subglottic space, serving as a further risk factor for bacterial entry into the airway.[18] Certain bacteria form a gelatinous substance called biofilm along the inner and outer sides of the ETT.[19] Biofilm, which is found more frequently in individuals with VAP,[20] may maintain a steady bacterial load that can serve as a source for recurrent pneumonia.[21]

► MICROBIOLOGY

Because of the relative ease of obtaining culture specimens from mechanically ventilated patients, more microbiologic data are available for VAP compared with other types of pneumonias. However, due to shared risk factors for multidrug resistance, the causative bacteria for both NP (including VAP) and HCAP are considered to be quite similar.[1] In addition to the potential for infection from highly resistant organisms, individuals developing early onset NP (i.e., within 4 days of hospital admission) are also at risk for bacterial infection from community-acquired etiologies. Despite the possibility of infections from these more easily treated bacteria, patients with NP or HCAP should initially receive broad-spectrum antibiotics, making the treatment for community-acquired infections a moot point until culture data return.

Aerobic gram-negative bacilli (e.g., *P. aeruginosa, E. coli, K. pneumoniae, Enterobacter* spp., *Acinetobacter* spp.) are the most frequently implicated sources of NP, estimated to cause up to 60% of cases of VAP.[5] Gram-positive cocci (e.g., *S. aureus, Streptococcus* spp.)

account for most of the remaining cases of VAP.[4] Moreover, up to half of *S. aureus*–induced cases of NP and HCAP are due to methicillin-resistant *S. aureus* (MRSA) strains.[4,22] Various combinations of bacteria have been noted to coexist in up to 40% of cases of VAP.[23] Viruses and fungi are exceedingly rare causes of VAP in immunocompetent patients.[1] Although a considerable array and combination of bacteria may cause NP and HCAP, the typical microbial flora of the two types of pneumonia is quite similar and often resistant to multiple antibiotics. Therefore, acquisition of appropriate cultures prior to initiation of antibiotics is important to be able to later tailor the antibiotic regimen to cover only the infecting pathogens. Additionally, every community, hospital, and ICU has its own bacterial resistance patterns that continue to evolve along with antibiotic prescribing practices, so the initial antibiotic regimen must be suited to current local susceptibilities.[24] Inadequately covering MDR bacteria in the treatment of NP or HCAP translates into increased mortality, particularly when those pathogens are *Pseudomonas*, *Acinetobacter*, or MRSA.[25,26]

▶ DIAGNOSIS

Three objectives exist when evaluating for the possibility of NP: confirm its presence, grade its severity, and identify its microbiologic cause.[9] The diagnosis of HCAP, NP, and VAP remains an ongoing contentious topic due to the lack of a diagnostic gold standard and a host of confounding variables among studies assessing different diagnostic techniques. The diagnosis of NP can be made clinically, microbiologically, or using some combination of the two methods.

A clinical diagnosis of NP may be made by the presence of a new or progressive infiltrate on chest radiography plus $\geq$ 2 clinical criteria that the infiltrate has an infectious origin (Table 37-2).[1,27] A more complex 12-point scoring system called the clinical pulmonary infection score (CPIS) was developed in the early 1990s,[28] but its inaccuracy (sensitivity 60–77%,

specificity 42–75%) makes its use impractical.[29,30] The currently recommended, broadly defined clinical diagnostic approach to NP gains sensitivity at the expense of specificity to avoid missing this potentially fatal disease. Unfortunately, this approach still inadequately identifies all cases of NP, as evidenced by one study demonstrating a sensitivity of 69% for the diagnosis of VAP when using two out of the three aforementioned clinical criteria compared with immediate postmortem lung tissue culture and histology.[30] Complicating the matter further, however, is that diagnostic inconsistencies evident even with autopsy, histology, and lung aspirate cultures prevent the adoption of a diagnostic gold standard for VAP, and, therefore, NP and HCAP.[31,32]

Microbiologic diagnostic methods attempt to regain a suitable degree of specificity via the acquisition and culture of causative pathogens. Despite numerous studies attempting to answer this diagnostic question, the most accurate method of obtaining a bacterial specimen still is unclear. Many argue for culturing upper airway secretions from the trachea due the method's greater sensitivity, less invasive nature, and lower associated costs. One trial of 740 patients suspected of having late-onset VAP were randomized to either endotracheal aspiration without quantitative culture or bronchoalveolar lavage (BAL) with quantitative culture.[33] Although the authors concluded that there was no significant benefit in clinical outcomes or antibiotic use with either diagnostic method, $\geq$40% of the screened patients were excluded for having a chronic disease, being immunocompromised, or having carbapenem-resistant bacteria. Due to the exclusion of a patient population that is so commonly encountered in the ICU setting, the applicability of the study's results is lessened. Others advocate culturing specimens from the lower airway due to enhanced specificity, which allows for more precise antibiotic de-escalation or cessation, and subsequently less antibiotic resistance in the future. In a multicenter study of over 400 patients suspected of having VAP, those who were randomized to fiberoptic-directed lower respiratory tract sampling with quantitative culture, as opposed to endotracheal aspiration without quantitative culture, experienced fewer deaths at 14 days (16.2% vs. 25.8%; $P = .022$) and decreased antibiotic use at 28 days (11.5 vs. 7.5 antibiotic-free days; $P < .001$).[34] This reduction in 2-week mortality in patients receiving the more invasive diagnostic strategy is puzzling because adverse antibiotic reactions are rare and antibiotic stewardship would be expected to translate into longer-term, not short-term, benefits. One can postulate that the benefit of the more invasive, although more specific, test may force the clinician to more aggressively search for, identify, and then appropriately treat an alternative infectious source instead of continuing to treat an infection that would have been misdiagnosed as VAP based on the nonspecific criteria

▶ **TABLE 37-2. CLINICAL DIAGNOSIS OF NOSOCOMIAL PNEUMONIA (NP) AND HEALTH CARE–ASSOCIATED PNEUMONIA (HCAP)**

- Presence of a new or progressive radiographic infiltrate
- Plus at least two (out of the following three) clinical features:
  - Fever >38°C
  - Leukocytosis >12,000 WBC/μL or leukopenia <4,000 WBC/μL
  - Purulent tracheobronchial secretions

of a radiographic opacity, two clinical criteria, and a positive culture from an endotracheal aspirate.

Even those who believe that lower airway cultures more accurately reflect true infection disagree about what methods to use in obtaining airway secretions and how to most appropriately interpret culture data to distinguish colonization from infection. Techniques to acquire lower airway secretions can be categorized as either bronchoscopic or "blind." Bronchoscopic modalities (which can also include the use of biopsy) utilize visually directed sampling, whereas blind ones entail the nondirected insertion of a catheter to some predetermined distance, usually until the catheter meets resistance. Lower airway secretions can be sampled with either a BAL, which involves flushing and subsequently aspirating a total of $\geq$120 mL of sterile saline through the tip of a bronchoscope or catheter that is wedged into a peripheral airway, or a protected specimen brush (PSB), which requires rubbing the airway wall with a brush that is otherwise contained within a protective sheath when it passes through the bronchoscope or catheter.

Quantitative cultures use a predefined logarithmic threshold of bacterial growth to attempt to differentiate colonization from infection. This diagnostic threshold for VAP varies according to the sampling method used: endotracheal aspirate 10^6 CFU/mL; BAL 10^4 CFU/mL; and PSB 10^3 CFU/mL.[1,35] Because of inconsistencies among obtained sputum samples inherent to differing patient characteristics, type of bacteria, receipt of antibiotics prior to culture, techniques used to acquire sputum, volume of lavage fluid actually instilled and later aspirated, anatomic location of the sampled fluid, methods of bacterial analysis, and lack of a diagnostic gold standard for NP, the very development of arbitrary quantitative diagnostic thresholds is considered flawed math by some experts.[36] Additionally, the accurate comparison of these thresholds among studies, which are plagued by so many confounding variables and technical differences, is exceedingly difficult.

Despite these diagnostic controversies, the diagnosis of NP should include the use of clinical criteria (radiographic evidence of a new or worsening infiltrate plus $\geq$2 abnormalities of: temperature, WBC count, or sputum) to initiate a diagnostic workup and antimicrobial treatment, followed by bacterial cultures from either the upper or lower airway, with or without quantitative cultures, to complete it.[1]

▶ TREATMENT

The cornerstones of treatment for NP are to obtain appropriate cultures, select initial antibiotics to treat the most likely pathogens based on the patient's risk factors and local susceptibility patterns, give empirical broad-spectrum antibiotics promptly, and de-escalate or stop empirical antibiotics based on the results of adequate culture data and clinical response. Although the same concept holds true for the treatment of HCAP, initially assessing a patient's risk factors for resistant organisms is of paramount importance to properly identify those individuals from the community with HCAP who require broad-spectrum antimicrobial therapy instead of treatment for CAP. Any delay in the administration of appropriate antibiotics results in increased mortality.[37–39]

Initial broad-spectrum antibiotics should be determined by an individual's risk for MDR pathogens (Table 37-1). In the absence of MDR risk factors and severe pneumonia, monotherapy can be instituted with a second- or third-generation cephalosporin (e.g., ceftriaxone), a β-lactam/β-lactamase inhibitor (e.g., ampicillin/sulbactam, piperacillin/tazobactam), ertapenem, or a fluoroquinolone (e.g., moxifloxacin, levofloxacin).[1] Either a fluoroquinolone or the combination of clindamycin and aztreonam can be used in those who are allergic to penicillin. In the presence of MDR risk factors, combination therapy is important, not for synergy, but because it allows for a wider coverage of bacteria that are often resistant to one of the drug classes instituted. Therefore, therapy should include an antipseudomonal cephalosporin (e.g., cefepime, ceftazidime), carbapenem (e.g., imipenem, meropenem, doripenem), or β-lactam/β-lactamase inhibitor (e.g., piperacillin/tazobactam), *plus* either an antipseudomonal fluoroquinolone (e.g., ciprofloxacin, levofloxacin) or an aminoglycoside (e.g., gentamicin, tobramycin, amikacin), *plus* coverage for MRSA (e.g., linezolid, vancomycin). Confirmed infection with *P. aeruginosa*, however, warrants a 5-day combination of a β-lactam and an aminoglycoside, which can then be narrowed per culture data.[1] For particularly drug-resistant gram-negative bacteria, polymyxin B and colistimethate (colistin) are treatment options. Additionally, the adjunctive use of inhaled antibiotics (e.g., aminoglycosides, colistin) shows promise, although limited data exist to routinely recommend it.[40,41]

Patients with VAP responding appropriately to the initial antibiotic regimen should exhibit clinical improvement within the first 6 days of the start of therapy, but some degree of recovery is usually seen well before then.[1] If such resolution of disease severity is not seen within the first few days of antibiotics, then alternative pathogens and diagnoses should be aggressively sought. Successful attempts have been made at reducing the duration of therapy from what had historically required 10–14 days of antibiotics. For example, one trial of over 400 patients diagnosed with VAP by BAL and randomized to either an 8- or 15-day course of antibiotics had no significant difference in 28-day mortality

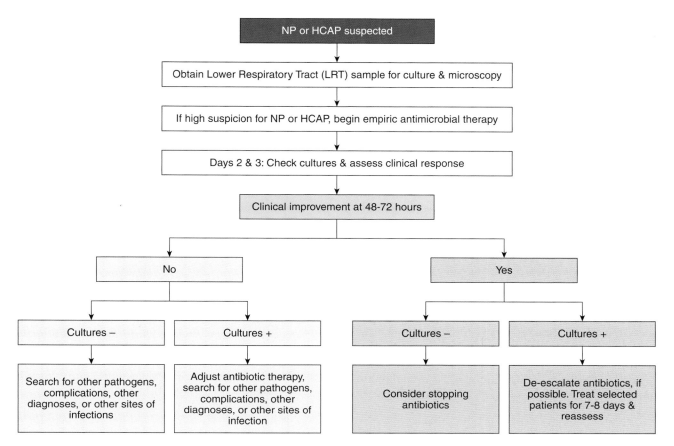

Figure 37-1. Nosocomial pneumonia (NP) and health care–associated pneumonia (HCAP) management algorithm. Adapted from the American Thoracic Society's Executive Summary on "Guidelines for the Management of Adults with Hospital-acquired, Ventilator-associated, and Healthcare-associated Pneumonia (*Am J Resp Crit Care Med* 2005; 171:388–416.)

but much less antibiotic use and MDR emergence, prompting recommendations for a shorter course of therapy.[1,42] Another study supports the use of even a 7-day course of antibiotics, which also showed no difference in hospital mortality or LOS (Figure 37-1).[43]

▶ PREVENTION

Preventing NP hinges on properly addressing its underlying pathophysiology. Strategies used to prevent VAP include: utilize the least invasive method suitable for respiratory support, minimize the duration of mechanical ventilation, avoid unnecessary medications (e.g., stress ulcer prophylaxis, antibiotics), prevent the accumulation of secretions, inhibit bacterial colonization of airway equipment and pooled secretions, prevent the passage of secretions to the lower airway, enhance immune defenses, and enhance health care providers' compliance with these preventive measures.[44]

Because intubation is the biggest risk factor for the development of NP, a key component of prevention is the avoidance of intubation altogether. Early use of

noninvasive positive pressure ventilation (NPPV), for example, bilevel positive airway pressure (BiPAP) or continuous positive airway pressure (CPAP), may obviate the need for intubation in certain circumstances.[45] For those who require mechanical ventilation, aggressive ventilator weaning strategies should be instituted with the goal of prompt extubation,[46] and for those unable to be extubated within a timely manner, early tracheostomy should be considered.[47] Care should be exerted to minimize the chance of accidental extubation, as that significantly increases the development of VAP.[48,49] Due to the risk of nasal and sinus carriage of potential pathogens, mechanically ventilated patients should be intubated via the orotracheal route when possible.[50] A simple measure such as maintaining patients in the semirecumbent position (i.e., >30° above horizontal) is effective in reducing the chance of aspirating colonized gastric secretions.[51,52] Moreover, acid-suppressive medications, particularly proton pump inhibitors, are associated with an approximately 30% increased odds of developing NP, so these should be used only when indicated.[53]

A trial of almost 6,000 ICU patients randomized to oral bacterial decontamination with topical antibiotics, digestive tract decontamination with topical antibiotics and 4 days of cefotaxime, or standard care demonstrated that both oral and gastric bacterial decolonization significantly reduced 28-day mortality (26.6% vs. 26.9% vs. 27.5%, respectively; $P < .05$).[54] Some experts recommend oral decontamination with antiseptics in lieu of antibiotics in facilities with high antibiotic resistance, which is supported by studies that demonstrate a decreased incidence of VAP with the institution of oral chlorhexidine cleansing.[55] To prevent leakage of colonized subglottic secretions around the ETT, endotracheal cuff pressures should remain between 20 and 30 cm H_2O[56,57] and continuous aspiration of those secretions with special ETTs has proven to be advantageous.[58] By inhibiting bacterial colonization, silver-coated ETTs significantly decrease the incidence of VAP when compared with uncoated ETTs (4.8% vs. 7.5%; $P = .03$).[59] When attempting to prevent NP, each of these interventions has modest effects when used alone; however, when implemented as a "ventilator bundle," more dramatic effects have been demonstrated.[60] The proactive application of preventive measures for NP can dramatically reduce mortality and health care expenditures savings for the individuals and society alike.

REFERENCES

1. American Thoracic Society, Infectious Diseases Society of America. Guidelines for the management of adults with hospital-acquired, ventilator-associated, and health-care-associated pneumonia. *Am J Respir Crit Care Med.* 2005;171:388–416.

2. Friedman ND, Kaye KS, Stout JE, et al. Health care-associated bloodstream infections in adults: a reason to change the accepted definition of community-acquired infections. *Ann Intern Med.* 2002;137:791–797.

3. Moine P, Timsit JF, Lassence A, et al. Mortality associated with late-onset pneumonia in the intensive care unit: results of a multi-center cohort study. *Intensive Care Med.* 2002;28:154–163.

4. Kollef MH, Shorr A, Tabak YP, et al. Epidemiology and outcomes of health-care-associated pneumonia. *Chest.* 2005;128:3854–3862.

5. Chastre J, Fagon JY. Ventilator-associated pneumonia. *Am J Respir Crit Care Med.* 2002;165:897–903.

6. Mehta RM, Niederman MS. Nosocomial pneumonia in the intensive care unit: controversies and dilemmas. *J Intensive Care Med.* 2003;18:175–188.

7. Ibrahim EH, Tracy L, Hill C, et al. The occurrence of ventilator-associated pneumonia in a community hospital: risk factors and clinical outcomes. *Chest.* 2001;120:555–561.

8. Heyland DK, Cook DJ, Griffith L, et al. The attributable morbidity and mortality of ventilator associated pneumonia in the critically ill patient. The Canadian Critical Trials Group. *Am J Respir Crit Care Med.* 1999;159:1249–1256.

9. Liapikou A, Valencia M, Torres A. Diagnosis and treatment of nosocomial pneumonia. In: Lucangelo U, Pelosi P, Zin WA, Aliverti A, eds. *Respiratory System and Artificial Ventilation.* Milan, Italy: Springer-Verlag; 2008:167–188.

10. Fagon JY, Chastre J, Hance AJ, et al. Nosocomial pneumonia in ventilated patients: a cohort study evaluating attributable mortality and hospital stay. *Am J Med.* 1993;94:281–288.

11. Rello J, Ollendorf DA, Oster G, et al., VAP Outcomes Scientific Advisory Group. Epidemiology and outcomes of ventilator-associated pneumonia in a large US database. *Chest.* 2002;122:2115–2121.

12. Alcon A, Fabregas N, Torres A. Pathophysiology of pneumonia. *Clin Chest Med.* 2005;26(1):35–46.

13. Torres A, El-Ebiary M, Soler N, et al. Stomach as a source of colonization of the respiratory tract during mechanical ventilation in association with VAP. *Eur Respir J.* 1996;8:1729–1735.

14. Bonten MJM, Gaillard CA, van der Geest S, et al. The role of intragastric acidity and stress ulcer prophylaxis on colonization and infection in mechanically ventilated patients: a stratified, randomised, double blind study of sucralfate versus antacids. *Am J Respir Crit Care Med.* 1995;152:1825–1834.

15. Scheld WM. Developments in the pathogenesis, diagnosis and treatment of nosocomial pneumonia. *Surg Gynecol Obstet.* 1991;172(suppl):42–53.

16. Diaz E, Rodriguez A, Rello J. Ventilator associated pneumonia: issues related to the artificial airway. *Respir Care.* 2005;50:900–906.

17. Cook D, De Jonghe B, Brochard L, Brun-Buisson C. Influence of airway management on ventilator-associated pneumonia: evidence from randomized trials. *JAMA.* 1998;279:781–787.

18. Holzapfel L, Chastang C, Demingeon G, et al. A randomized study assessing the systemic search for maxillary sinusitis in nasotracheally mechanically ventilated patients: influence of nosocomial maxillary sinusitis on the occurrence of ventilator-associated pneumonia. *Am J Respir Crit Care Med.* 1999;159:695–701.

19. Consterton JW. Introduction to biofilm. *Int Antimicrob Agents.* 1999;11:217–221.

20. Koerner RJ. Contribution of endotracheal tubes to the pathogenesis of ventilator-associated pneumonia. *J Hosp Infect.* 1997;35:83–89.

21. Feldman C, Kassel M, Cantrell J, et al. The presence and sequence of endotracheal tube colonization in patients undergoing mechanical ventilation. *Eur Respir J.* 1999;13:546–551.

22. Weber DJ, Rutala WA, Sickbert-Bennett EE, et al. Microbiology of ventilator-associated pneumonia compared with that of hospital-acquired pneumonia. *Infect Control Hosp Epidemiol.* 2007;28:825–831.

23. Fagon JY, Chastre J, Comart Y, et al. Nosocomial pneumonia in patients receiving continuous mechanical ventilation: prospective analysis of 52 episodes with use of a protected specimen brush and quantitative culture techniques. *Am Rev Respir Dis.* 1989;139:877–884.

24. Rello J, Sa-Borges M, Correa H, et al. Variations in etiology of ventilator-associated pneumonia across four

treatment sites. Implications for antimicrobial prescribing practices. *Am J Respir Crit Care Med.* 1999;160:608–613.

25. Kollef MH. Inadequate antimicrobial treatment: an important determinant of outcome for hospitalized patients. *Clin Infect Dis.* 2000;31(suppl 44):S131–S138.

26. Valles J, Pobo A, Garcia-Esquirol O, et al. Excess ICU mortality attributable to VAP: the role of early vs. late onset. *Intensive Care Med.* 2007;33:1363–1368.

27. Tablan OC, Anderson LJ, Besser R, Bridges C, Hajjeh R, CDC, Healthcare Infection Control Practices Advisory Committee. Guidelines for preventing health-care-associated pneumonia, 2003: recommendations of CDC and the Healthcare Infection Control Practices Advisory Committee. *MMWR Recomm Rep.* 2004;53(RR-3):1–36.

28. Pugin J, Auckenthaler R, Mili N, et al. Diagnosis of ventilator-associated pneumonia by bacteriologic analysis of bronchoscopic and non-bronchoscopic "blind" bronchoalveolar lavage fluid. *Am Rev Respir Dis.* 1991;143:1121–1129.

29. Fartoukh M, Maitre B, Honoré S, et al. Diagnosing pneumonia during mechanical ventilation: the clinical pulmonary infection score revisited. *Am J Respir Crit Care Med.* 2003;168:173–179.

30. Fabregas N, Ewig S, Torres A, et al. Clinical diagnosis of ventilator associated pneumonia revisited: comparative validation using immediate post-mortem lung biopsies. *Thorax.* 1999;54:867–873.

31. Chinsky KD. Ventilator-associated pneumonia: is there any gold in these standards? *Chest.* 2002;122:1883–1885.

32. Marquette CH, Copin MC, Wallet F, et al. Diagnostic testes for pneumonia in ventilated patients: prospective evaluation of diagnostic accuracy using histology as a diagnostic gold standard. *Am J Respir Crit Care Med.* 1995;151:1878–1888.

33. The Canadian Critical Care Trials Group. A randomized trial of diagnostic techniques for ventilator-associated pneumonia. *N Engl J Med.* 2006;355:2619–2630.

34. Fagon JY, Chastre J, Wolff M, et al. Invasive and non-invasive strategies for management of suspected ventilator-associated pneumonia: a randomized trial. *Ann Intern Med.* 2000;132:621–630.

35. Chastre J, Combes A, Luyt CE. The invasive (quantitative) diagnosis of ventilator-associated pneumonia. *Respir Care.* 2005;50:797–807.

36. Fujitani S, Yu VL. Quantitative cultures for diagnosing ventilator-associated pneumonia: a critique. *Clin Infect Dis.* 2006;43:S106–S113.

37. Alvarez-Lerma F. Modification of empiric antibiotic treatment in patients with pneumonia acquired in the intensive care unit. ICU-Acquired Pneumonia Study Group. *Intensive Care Med.* 1996;22:387–394.

38. Kollef MH, Sherman G, Ward S, Fraser VJ. Inadequate antimicrobial treatment of infections: a risk factor for hospital mortality among critically ill patients. *Chest.* 1999;115:462–474.

39. Luna CM, Aruj P, Niederman MS, et al, for the GANAR group. Appropriateness and delay to initiate therapy in ventilator-associated pneumonia. *Eur Respir J.* 2006;27:158–164.

40. Czosnowski QA, Wood GC, Magnotti LJ, et al. Adjunctive aerosolized antibiotics for treatment of ventilator-associated pneumonia. *Pharmacotherapy.* 2009;29:1054–1060.

41. Luyt CE, Combes A, Nieszkowska A, et al. Aerosolized antibiotics to treat ventilator-associated pneumonia. *Curr Opin Infect Dis.* 2009;22:154–158.

42. Chastre J, Wolff M, Fagon J et al. Comparison of 8 vs. 15 days of antibiotic therapy for ventilator-associated pneumonia in adults. *JAMA.* 2003;290:2588–2598.

43. Ibrahim EH, Ward S, Sherman G, et al. Experience with a clinical guideline for the treatment of ventilator-associated pneumonia. *Crit Care Med.* 2001;29:1109–1115.

44. Kollef MH. Prevention of hospital-associated pneumonia and ventilator-associated pneumonia. *Crit Care Med.* 2004;32:1396–1405.

45. Evans TW, Albert RK, Angus DC, et al. International consensus conferences in intensive care medicine: non-invasive positive pressure ventilation in acute respiratory failure. *Am J Respir Crit Care Med.* 2001;163:283–291.

46. Girard TD, Kress JP, Fuchs BD, et al. Efficacy and safety of a paired sedation and ventilator weaning protocol for mechanically ventilated patients in intensive care (Awakening and Breathing Controlled trial): a randomized controlled trial. *Lancet.* 2008;371:126–134.

47. Freeman BD, Borecki I B, Coopersmith CM, Buchman TG. Relationship between tracheostomy timing and duration of mechanical ventilation in critically ill patients. *Crit Care Med.* 2005;33:2513–2520.

48. Torres A, Gatell JM, Aznar E, et al. Re-intubation increases the risk of nosocomial pneumonia in patients needing mechanical ventilation. *Am J Respir Crit Care Med.* 1996;153:137–141.

49. de Lassence A, Alberti C, Azoulay E, et al. Impact of unplanned extubation and reintubation after weaning on nosocomial pneumonia risk in the intensive care unit: a prospective multicenter study. *Anesthesiology.* 2002;97:148–156.

50. Holzapfel L, Chevret S, Madinier G, et al. Influence of long-term oro- or nasotracheal intubation on nosocomial maxillary sinusitis and pneumonia: results of a prospective, randomized clinical trial. *Crit Care Med.* 1993;21:1132–1138.

51. Kollef MH. Ventilator-associated pneumonia: a multivariate analysis. *JAMA.* 1993;270:1965–1970.

52. Drakulovic MB, Torres A, Bauer TT, et al. Supine body position as a risk factor for nosocomial pneumonia in mechanically ventilated patients: a randomized trial. *Lancet.* 1999;354:1851–1858.

53. Herzig SJ, Howell MD, Ngo LH, et al. Acid-suppressive medication use and the risk for hospital-acquired pneumonia. *JAMA.* 2009;301:2120–2128.

54. De Smet AMGA, Kluytmans JAJW, Cooper BS, et al. Decontamination of the digestive tract and oropharynx in ICU patients. *N Engl J Med.* 2009;360:20–31.

55. Koeman M, van der Ven AJ, Hak E, et al. Oral decontamination with chlorhexidine reduces the incidence of ventilator-associated pneumonia. *Am J Respir Crit Care Med.* 2006;173:1348–1355.

56. Rello J, Soñora R, Jubert P, et al. Pneumonia in intubated patients: role of respiratory airway care. *Am J Respir Crit Care Med.* 1996;154:111–115.

57. Seegolin RD, Van Hesselt GL. Endotracheal cuff pressure and tracheal mucosal blood flow: endoscopic study of effects of four large volume cuffs. *BMJ.* 1984;288:965–968.

58. Berra L, De Marchi L, Panigada M, et al. Evaluation of continuous aspiration of subglottic secretion in an in vivo study. *Crit Care Med.* 2004;32:2071–2078.

59. Kollef MH, Afessa B, Anzueto A, et al. Silver-coated endotracheal tubes and incidence of ventilator-associated pneumonia: the NASCENT randomized trial. *JAMA.* 2008;300:805–813.

60. Marra AR, Rodrigues Cal RG, Silva CV, et al. Successful prevention of ventilator-associated pneumonia in an intensive care setting. *Am J Infect Control.* 2009:37: 619–625.

CHAPTER 38

Infectious Endocarditis

Joseph R. Shiber

► INTRODUCTION

Endocarditis, inflammation of the endocardial surface of the heart, can have numerous etiologies including mechanical irritation, neoplastic, autoimmune, or infectious diseases.[1–4] This chapter will focus on the infectious causes that are typically bacteria, mycobacteria, and fungi. Although the cardiac valves are most commonly involved, the mural endocardium, septal defects, chordae tendineae, and even intracardiac medical equipment (pacemaker/defibrillator leads or septal occluder devices) can also be sites of infection.[1–6] Infectious endocarditis (IE) has an incidence of 3.6/100,000 per year and accounts for 1/1,000 hospital admissions in the United States. There is a 2:1 male to female ratio with current overall in-patient mortality between 11% and 26%, although this figure may be drastically different for the various subsets of IE patients.[1,3,7]

► CLASSIFICATIONS

The first published description of the valvular cardiac lesions due to IE was over 300 years ago by Lazarus Riverius, while about 200 years ago Jean Baptiste Boulaud defined the anatomy of the endocardium; 150 years ago, the association of preexisting rheumatic valvular damage and bicuspid aortic valves with IE was noted by Sir James Paget.[8,9] In 1905 when blood cultures came into clinical practice, the antemortem diagnostic rate for IE was approximately 50%.[9] IE has had numerous classification schemes over the last century starting with Sir William Osler who divided IE into "simple" and "malignant" categories based on the length of time from symptom onset to death along with the associated complications. These categories evolved into the following IE classification in the preantibiotic era: (1) acute (onset of symptoms to death <6 weeks, caused by a highly virulent organism capable of infecting a normal heart); (2) subacute (onset of symptoms to death 6 weeks to 3 months, caused by a less virulent organism that infects hearts with preexisting endocardial damage); (3) chronic (>3 months from symptom onset to death, caused by an indolent microbe capable of infecting only abnormal hearts or immunosuppressed patients).[9,10] Current classifications include diagnostic status (definite or probable), anatomic site (right- or left-sided cardiac valves), valve type (native or prosthetic), microbe (bacterial or fungal species), and patient population (intravenous [IV] drug abusers [IVDA], elderly, nosocomial infection). Prosthetic valve IE is further divided into early (<2 months after surgery), intermediate (2 months to 1 year), and late (>1 year after surgery) cases; the early cases are typically nosocomial while the intermediate and late cases are community acquired.[10–12] Another classification that reflects the early description by Osler is simple (infection limited to valve cusps and leaflets) or advanced (deep tissue infection including perivalvular structures, cardiac abscess or pseudoaneurysm formation, and systemic infectious emboli). These various categories of IE differ in incidence, presentation, microbial etiology, and outcome.[1,3,10,13]

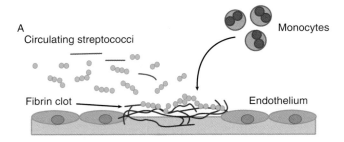

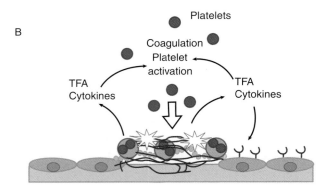

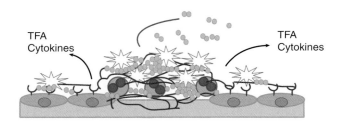

Figure 38-1. Pathogenesis of bacterial valve colonization. Viridans group streptococci adhere to fibrin–platelet clots that form at the site of damaged cardiac endothelium (A). The fibrin-adherent streptococci activate monocytes to produce tissue factor activity (TFA) and cytokines (B). These mediators activate the coagulation pathway, resulting in further recruitment of platelets and growth of the vegetation (C). (Reproduced with permission from McPhee SJ, Ganong WF. *Pathophysiology of Disease: An Introduction to Clinical Medicine.* 5th ed. New York, NY: McGraw-Hill Inc; 2006.)

▶ ETIOLOGY

The disease process of IE and vegetation formation requires multiple steps (see Figure 38-1) starting with endothelial damage from high-velocity jets of blood due to congenital or acquired cardiac abnormalities, or mechanical damage from intracardiac devices or blood-borne debris.[1,10] Platelets and fibrin then form a sterile thrombus at the site of endothelial damage; certain disease states, such as malignancy, uremia, and autoimmune diseases, can form sterile cardiac vegetations without overt endothelial damage. The initially sterile site is seeded by transient bacteremia and then matures with additional fibrin deposition and bacterial proliferation. The vegetation has no vasculature, so it is relatively protected from activated phagocytes or antibiotic penetration.[10,11]

In developing countries, rheumatic heart disease is still the main risk for IE; as treatment of streptococcal pharyngitis improved in the United States and Europe, there has been less cardiac sequelae, so in these areas congenital (bicuspid aortic valve, hypertrophic obstructive cardiomyopthy, mitral valve prolapse with regurgitation) and degenerative cardiac diseases (aortic valve calcification) are the leading risk factors for IE. Other recognized risks include diabetes mellitus, hemodialysis, immunosuppression, and previous IE. Approximately 50% of cases have no known prior valve abnormality but likely had microscopic valvular lesions that were vulnerable to highly virulent organisms such as *Staphylococcus aureus* or *Streptococcus pneumoniae*.[2,3,7]

▶ MICROBIOLOGY

While streptococcal species are still the leading infectious agents for IE worldwide, their incidence has been declining with better oral hygiene and dental care plus appropriate antibiotic prophylaxis. On the other hand, *S. aureus* IE has been increasing in incidence and is the leading cause in intensive care unit (ICU) cases and in IVDA. In non-IVDA native valve endocarditis (NVE), streptococcal species (*viridans, mutans, mitis, sanguis*) typically from the mouth and nasopharynx account for 17–36% of cases; *Streptococcus bovis* accounts for 6% and is associated with gastrointestinal (GI) lesions in the elderly. *S. aureus* accounts for up to 30% of the cases in this category, with the skin as the major source, but in half of the cases there is no obvious portal of entry so that nasal carriage is also a source. *Enterococcus* species cause 8–11% of the NVE in non-IVDA patients, who are mostly older with GI/genitourinary (GU) lesions or recent procedures. The *Haemophilus, Actinobacillus, Cardiobacterium, Eikenella,* and *Kingella* (HACEK) group only accounts for 3% of cases in this population; although gram-negative bacilli (GNB) are leading causes of sepsis, their lack of avid adherence to endothelium diminishes the risk of IE during bacteremia. *S. pneumoniae* causes a small number of cases of NVE in a subset of non-IVDA patients with diabetes mellitus, malignancy, chronic obstructive pulmonary disease (COPD), or alcoholism; the lungs are

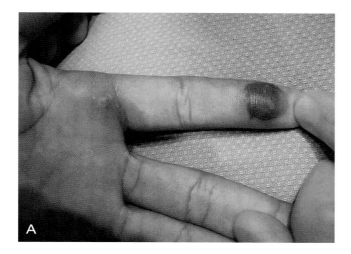
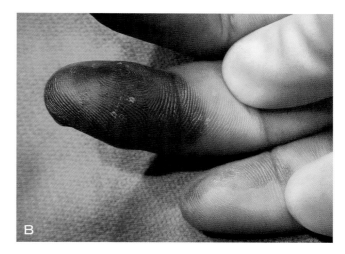

Figure 38-2. Photographs of a young man with *Streptococcus pyogenes* endocarditis demonstrating: (A) two septic emboli of the left index finger (metacarpal head and finger tip); the large pustular lesion was aspirated by the author immediately prior to the photograph and demonstrated the organism by Gram stain. (B) Septic emboli with necrosis of the tips of the right middle and ring finger.

the source, and meningitis is associated in 40–60% of patients. Fungal or polymicrobial IE is uncommon in NVE who are not IVDA.[1,2,7,14]

In the IVDA population, there is a 2–5% per year risk of IE; it is higher with cocaine than heroin due to the shorter duration of cocaine that requires more frequent injections but not heating of the drug, which may decrease the bacterial counts with heroin "cooking." *S. aureus* is the number one microbe in this group, with the majority being methicillin-sensitive. Fungus, predominantly *Candida* and *Aspergillus* species, accounts for about 10% of IE cases in drug abusers. *Pseudomonas aeruginosa* can also be responsible for IE when unboiled tap or toilet water is used to rinse drug paraphernalia or to dissolve drugs for injection. Polymicrobial IE is unique to this population where it accounts for 2–5% of cases. Human immunodeficiency virus (HIV) infection is an independent risk factor for IE in the IVDA and is associated with increased mortality as the CD4 cell count is decreased below 200 cells/mm³. It should be noted that IE is usually not considered a complication of acquired immune deficiency syndrome (AIDS) and is quite rare in non-IVDA patients with HIV infection. When this patient type develops IE, atypical organisms such as *Salmonella* are often responsible.[15–17]

▶ PRESENTATION

The typical presentation of fever and cardiac murmur with skin and conjunctival lesions may not necessarily be present, and in cases of very acute IE due to aggressive organisms, the classic cutaneous and retinal immunologic findings will be absent. Although 85% of

patients with IE have a murmur, they may not have a murmur at initial presentation but only develop it during the course of their illness. Obvious signs of bacterial emboli (see Figure 38-2A and B) are indicative of IE on physical examination when present in approximately 50% of cases.[1,5]

▶ COMPLICATIONS

At least one complication occurs in 57% of cases, with 26% having two and 14% having three or more complications. Complications of IE are divided into the two categories of cardiac and extracardiac, with the overwhelming majority of complications occurring early in the course of illness. Cardiac complications are secondary to local destruction and emboli and include valve cusps and leaflets, chordae tendineae, atrioventricular (AV) nodal and His–Purkinje conductive tissue, myocardium (abscess, septal or free wall perforation, aneurysm), pericardium (purulent pericarditis or hemopericardium leading to tamponade), and coronary arteries (due to emboli). Congestive heart failure (CHF) is the most common complication of IE, occurring due to valvular regurgitation; myocardial failure is not a typical feature. Extracardiac complications include systemic embolization and organ failure. The emboli may be sterile and cause ischemia or infarction at the target organ or they may be septic and form an abscess; alternatively, a bland infarct may be seeded by ongoing bacteremia and lead to an abscess. The most frequent sites of embolization are the brain, spleen, kidneys, skin, liver, and mesenteric and iliac arteries. A mycotic aneurysm may result at any arterial site of emboli.[1,10,18]

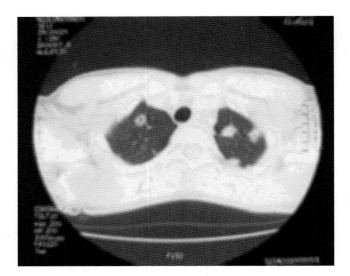

Figure 38-3. Chest CT of IVDA patient with tricuspid valve endocarditis due to *Staphylococcus aureus* showing multiple pulmonary emboli, some with early cavitation. A left-sided empyema was also present requiring thoracostomy tube drainage.

With right-sided IE, pulmonary emboli may occur leading to septic emboli (see Figure 38-3), empyema, and right heart dysfunction. Organ failure during the course of IE is most commonly due to hemodynamic deterioration and hypoperfusion, again from valvular CHF. The exception is acute renal failure, which may be multifactorial due to acute tubular necrosis from ischemia or drugs (aminoglycosides, vancomycin, IV contrast), glomerulonephritis, or renal infarcts from emboli (see Figure 38-4). Embolization risk is highest for large vegetations (>1 cm diameter) particularly if involving the anterior leaflet of the mitral valve.[2,7]

With left-sided IE, CHF due to severe valvular incompetence is the most common serious complication. It occurs more frequently with aortic than mitral valve infection since the left ventricle is less tolerant of the sudden volume overload of acute regurgitation than is the left atrium. Central nervous system (CNS) complications occur in 20–40% of left-sided IE cases; they occur early and are the first sign of IE in 47% of patients, but the risk of further complications drops drastically after initiation of appropriate antibiotics. CNS complications are due to emboli to the cerebral arteries (the middle cerebral artery in >90% of episodes) leading to ischemia or infarction secondary to vessel occlusion. The resulting transient ischemic attack (TIA)/cerebrovascular accident (CVA) is the most common CNS complication of IE representing 40–50% all CNS events. Brain abscess due to septic emboli (see Figure 38-5) only accounts for 5% of CNS events while meningitis accounts for 5–40%. Intracranial hemorrhage represents 10% of CNS complications of IE and can be caused by rupture of a mycotic aneurysm, septic erosion of a vessel without aneurysm (known as acute necrotizing arteritis), or hemorrhagic transformation of a recent ischemic stroke.[1,18]

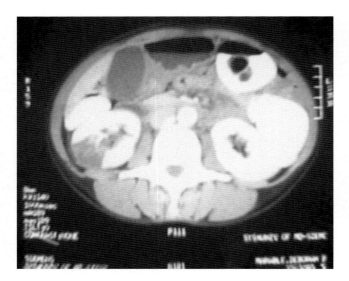

Figure 38-4. Abdominal CT scan with IV contrast: wedge-shaped right renal infarct in a patient with *Staphylococcus aureus* endocarditis of her mitral valve; splenic infarcts were also present.

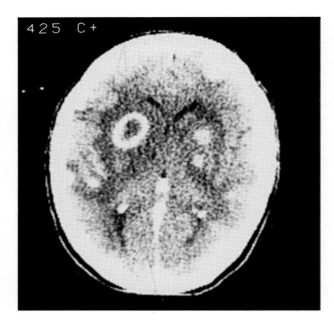

Figure 38-5. Multiple brain abscesses associated with bacterial endocarditis (*S. aureus*) in a 55-year-old man. The large abscess in the right hemisphere shows a characteristic ring enhancement. (Reproduced with permission from Ropper AH, Samuels MA. *Adams & Victor's Principles of Neurology.* 9th ed. New York, NY: McGraw Hill Inc; 2009. Figure 32-1A.)

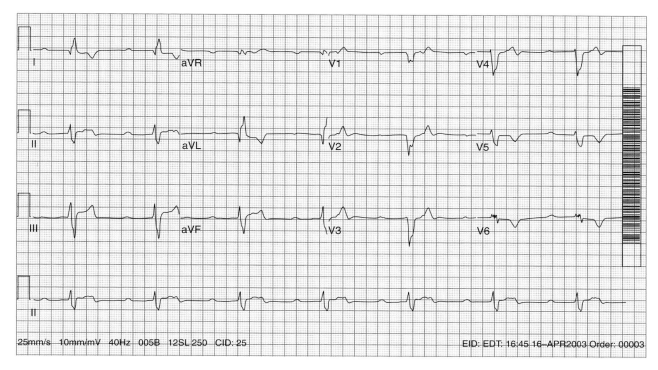

Figure 38-6. EKG: second-degree heart block (2:1 conduction) with a ventricular conduction delay due to *Staphylococcus aureus* endocarditis of the aortic valve with a ring abscess in a hemodialysis patient. The patient progressed to third-degree block requiring temporary transvenous pacing.

► ICU ADMISSIONS

IE patients may require admission to an ICU due to septic shock, cardiogenic shock, respiratory failure, pulmonary edema from acute valve dysfunction, acute renal failure requiring renal replacement therapy, acute CNS events (stroke, intracranial hemorrhage, encephalitis), or symptomatic bradycardia/heart block requiring cardiac pacing (see Figure 38-6). While simple IE cases can be treated by an in-patient physician, these complicated cases necessitate a multidisciplinary approach by the coordinated care of intensivists, infectious disease specialists, neurologists, cardiologists, and cardiac surgeons.[19,20]

DRUG USERS

The incidence of IE in IVDA is 1.5–20/1,000 addicts, with 80% involving the right heart as compared with only 9% right heart infection in non-IVDA native valve IE patients. This high proportion of right-sided disease in drug users is thought to result from microscopic endocardial damage due to impurities in illicit drug preparations and repeated bacteremia from unsterile injections. The most frequent underlying cardiac abnormality that predisposes IVDA patients to IE is a previous episode of IE. Right-sided IE is also associated with cardiac pacing

and implanted defibrillators, where the vegetations are usually confined to the leads but there is tricuspid valve involvement in 10% of cases.[7,15,17]

PROSTHETIC VALVE

Prosthetic valve endocarditis (PVE) accounts for up to one quarter of all IE cases, and the percentage has been increasing as more valve replacements are performed. The risk of IE for patients with prosthetic valves is 1% at 1 year and 2–3% at 5 years. The early risk is higher with mechanical valves than for biologic valves, but the risk appears to become equivalent later in the postoperative dates. PVE of mechanical valves typically has involvement of the cusps, sewing ring, and valve annulus, while with biologic valves the infection is mostly limited to the cusps.[2,5,7]

NOSOCOMIAL ENDOCARDITIS

A relatively new category of endocarditis is nosocomial IE (NIE) defined as occurring greater than 48 hours after hospital admission or within 4–8 weeks of an invasive procedure performed in the hospital, which includes early prosthetic valve infections. The incidence of NIE is estimated to be 0.8 per 10,000 hospital admissions, and it accounts for 14–25% of all IE cases. Considered a subset of NIE is ICU-acquired IE that has an estimated incidence of 5 per 1,000 ICU admissions. Elderly (age >65) patients more often develop NIE than do younger (age <65) patients and have twice the in-patient mortality; their risk factors are diabetes mellitus, and GI or GU cancers. The source of infection is a central venous catheter in 9–48% of cases, a peripheral venous catheter in 6–22% of cases, a pulmonary artery catheter in 2–9% of cases, and GU tract surgery or instrumentation in 20–30% of cases. *S. aureus* is the most prevalent microbe causing 52–57% of cases (an intravascular device is the source in 91% of these patients); 13–25% of hospitalized patients experiencing staphylococcal bacteremia will develop IE. Coagulase-negative *Staphylococcus* causes 40% of cases (associated with prosthetic valves in 89%), *Enterococcus* species causes 5–30% of cases, and GNB cases are rare except for *P. aeruginosa* in hemodialysis patients. This organism has the capability to adhere to endocardium unlike most GNB that are often responsible for bacteremia and sepsis but not IE due to low adherence factors. Although fungal NIE is still relatively rare (less than 10% of all IE cases), its incidence is increasing; the hallmarks of fungal IE are bulky vegetations with emboli to major arteries.[10,13,14]

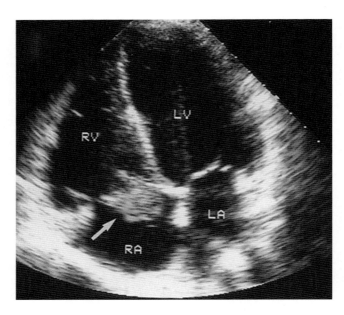

Figure 38-7. Apical four-chamber view demonstrating a large tricuspid valve vegetation (*arrow*). LA, left atrium; LV, left ventricle; RA, right atrium; RV, right ventricle. (Reproduced with permission from Fuster V, O'Rourke RA, Walsh RA, Poole-Wilson P. *Hurst's the Heart.* 12th ed. New York, NY: McGraw-Hill Inc; 2008. Figure 16-94A.)

▶ DIAGNOSIS

Previous diagnostic criteria for IE, such as the Von Reyn criteria, have been replaced by the more sensitive and specific Duke criteria that include echocardiographic data that previously were not included. Recent updates to the Duke criteria have made evidence of *S. aureus* bacteremia a major criterion. For suspected cases of IE, at least three sets of blood cultures should be done at individual venipuncture sites during the first 24 hours after presentation; there should be at least 1 hour between first and last sets being drawn. This protocol is intended to reduce the chance of identifying contaminated samples while enhancing the ability to detect persistent bacteremia, the hallmark of IE. Only 5–7% of patients not recently on antibiotics have negative blood culture results. In these patients, antibiotic binding resins can be used to enhance the culture yield as well as polymerase chain reaction (PCR) testing can be done on vegetation or embolic samples, since PCR will yield positive results even after several weeks of antibiotic treatment.[1,2,21]

▶ ECHOCARDIOGRAPHY

Transthoracic echocardiography (TTE) has a sensitivity of 46–65% for detecting left heart vegetations as compared with 90–93% for transesophageal echocardiography (TEE); the sensitivity for detecting left heart

regurgitation is also 58–63% for TTE and 88–98% for TEE, but the two modalities are equal for detecting right heart IE. The risk of a false-negative study TTE is increased by obesity, COPD, prosthetic valves, and vegetation size <5 mm. TTE is often of limited utility in the ICU due to restrictions on patient positioning, surgical wounds interfering with optimal ultrasound probe contact, and mechanical ventilation resulting in poor image resolution. Based on these data, it is considered reasonable for low-risk suitable patients to have a TTE as an initial study but to use TEE for high-risk or complicated patients including any suspected PVE. Although there are pathognomonic echocardiographic findings, such as leaflet perforation, periannular or myocardial abscess, or new prosthetic valve dehiscence, neither mode can reliably differentiate the classic sonographic finding of IE, an oscillating intracardiac mass representing a vegetation (see Figure 38-7), from other noninfective lesions such as tumors, thrombus marantic endocarditis, or myxomatous valvular degeneration. Other diagnostic tests that are considered helpful in IE are a chest radiograph, an electrocardiogram, and a urinalysis.[22–24]

▶ MEDICAL TREATMENT

The treatment for IE is based on the principal of sustained antimicrobial activity with high serum concentrations in order to eradicate dormant microbes in vegetations and distant emboli. Prolonged IV bactericidal antibiotic regimens are the standard treatment. Blood cultures should be drawn every 24–48 hours after initiation of therapy until cultures are negative; this result marks the beginning of the time course of the regimen. Initial antibiotic regimens are described for the distinct patient population and should be adjusted based on microbe sensitivity and minimum inhibitory concentration. An initial choice of a cell wall active drug (β-lactam or vancomycin) plus an aminoglycoside will give synergistic coverage against *Staphylococcus*, *Streptococcus*, and *Enterococcus* species that account for over 80% of all IE; this strategy has been shown to reduce the duration of bacteremia but not to change clinical outcomes.[2,4]

Streptococcus viridans IE cases typically respond clinically to antibiotic treatment more quickly than does IE due to *S. aureus* or *Enterococcus*. For IE due to les virulent organisms, fever often resolves after 2–5 days of appropriate antibiotics. Persistent fever beyond the first week of treatment often indicates complicated disease, while recurrence of fever in weeks 3–4 is more often due to drug hypersensitivity, particularly with high β-lactams, but emboli may still occur. All patients should receive their first 2 weeks of therapy as in-patients to monitor for complications during this highest-risk period. Stable patients without complication may be considered for outpatient IV therapy to complete their regimen after this time. There is no benefit of additional oral antibiotics after completing a full IV course. Follow-up cultures should be done to ensure treatment success without relapse that most commonly occurs within 2 months of the conclusion of the antibiotic regimen. The relapse, or treatment failure rate, is <2% for *S. viridans*, 8–20% for *Enterococcus*, and 11% for *S. aureus*. There is no proven benefit at preventing emboli by giving aspirin or heparin, but since these agents increase the risk of intracranial hemorrhage, they should be avoided. Anticoagulation can be used judiciously for a prosthetic valve patient, but it should be held for 2 weeks if an embolic CNS event occurs.[2,4,11]

▶ SURGICAL TREATMENT

Although there have not been any controlled studies, it does appear that combined medical and surgical treatment yields a better outcome than medical treatment alone for complicated left-sided IE, particularly if *S. aureus* is the cause. More than 25% of all IE patients receive cardiac surgery during their acute illness and 20–40% receive it later. Despite the goal of sterilizing the tissue of the surgical field prior to procedure, there is little correlation between length of preoperative antibiotics and outcome. It may be a more productive goal of performing valve surgery early so as to prevent the

possible complications that may occur and thereby increase the operative risks. The strongest indications for surgical treatment are CHF due to acute valvular dysfunction or prosthesis dehiscence, prosthetic valve obstruction, periannular or myocardial abscess, mycotic aneurysm, fungal IE, or *S. aureus* PVE. Combined medical and surgical therapy lowers the mortality rate of NVE patients with moderate–severe CHF to 11–35% as compared with 56–86% with medical therapy alone. Persistent bacteremia after 1 week on appropriate antibiotics or ongoing systemic emboli is also considered indications for surgical treatment. Unstable septic shock or severe uncorrected coagulopathy is a contraindication for valve surgery. Operative mortality is significantly higher if pulmonary edema or cardiogenic shock due to valvular dysfunction has developed. If the patient has had an ischemic CNS embolic event, surgery can be done early (within 72 hours) in efforts to prevent further emboli or surgery should be delayed 2–3 weeks to decrease the risk of hemorrhagic transformation due to heparin exposure; it is recommended to delay surgery for a minimum of 4 weeks after an intracranial hemorrhage. These recommendations to postpone surgery are only valid if CHF or cardiogenic shock has not developed. Tricuspid valvulectomy without replacement is highly effective treatment for IE but invariably leads to severe and permanent right ventricular dysfunction. The postoperative antibiotic regimen should complete a full course or be at least 7–15 days if the valve cultures are negative; if the valve cultures are positive, then a full antibiotic course should be given starting at the date of surgery.[25–30]

▶ MORTALITY

While the overall in-patient mortality is 16% for all IE cases, there is quite a range in mortality depending on the disease category. The mortality is 26% for complicated left-sided NVE, 44% for PVE, 45–54% for IE patients requiring ICU admission, and highest at 68% for NIE; the lowest risk mortality at <10% is in IVDA with isolated right-sided disease. Factors indicating a poor prognosis are CHF, septic shock, CNS events, acute renal failure, immunocompromise, higher Acute Physiology and Chronic Health Evaluation (APACHE) II score, and *S. aureus* as the infectious agent.[2,4,5,20]

▶ PROPHYLAXIS

New recommendations for IE prophylaxis have limited treatment to the highest-risk groups (see Table 38-1): prosthetic valves, previous IE, valvulopathy after cardiac transplant, complex cyanotic congenital heart disease, and surgical systemic–pulmonary shunts. It also

▶ **TABLE 38-1. DISEASE PREVENTION: ENDOCARDITIS**

Organization (Date)	Population	Recommendations	Comments	Source
AHA (2007)	Persons at highest risk for adverse sequelae from endocarditis[a]	Give antibiotic prophylaxis[b] before certain dental[c] as well as certain other procedures[d]	1. New emphasis is on providing prophylaxis to patients at greatest risk of complications of endocarditis, rather than at greatest lifetime risk of endocarditis 2. General consensus suggests few cases of infective endocarditis can be prevented by preprocedure prophylaxis with antibiotics	*Circulation.* 2007;116:1736

Reproduced with permission from Gonzales R, Kutner JS. *Current Practice Guidelines in Primary Care, 2009.* New York, NY: McGraw-Hill Inc; 2009. Available at: http://www.accessmedicine.com/guidelines.aspx.
[a]Patients with prosthetic valve, previous endocarditis, selected patients with congenital heart disease (unrepaired cyanotic CHD, completely repaired congenital heart defect with prosthetic material or device during first 6 months after procedure, repaired cyanotic CHD with residual defects at or near repair site), and cardiac transplant recipients who develop valvulopathy.
[b]Standard prophylaxis regimen: amoxicillin (adults 2.0 g; children 50 mg/kg orally 1 hour before procedure). If unable to take oral medications, give ampicillin (adults 2.0 g IM or IV; children 50 mg/kg IM or IV within 30 minutes of procedure). If penicillin-allergic, give clindamycin (adults 600 mg; children 20 mg/kg orally 1 hour before procedure) or azithromycin or clarithromycin (adults 500 mg; children 15 mg/kg orally 1 hour before procedure). If penicillin-allergic and unable to take oral medications, give clindamycin (adults 600 mg; children 20 mg/kg IV within 30 minutes before procedure). If allergy to penicillin is not anaphylaxis, angioedema, or urticaria, options for nonoral treatment also include cefazolin (1 g IM or IV for adults, 50 mg/kg IM or IV for children), and for penicillin-allergic oral therapy includes cephalexin 2 g PO for adults or 50 mg/kg PO for children.
[c]All dental procedures that involve manipulation of gingival tissue or the periapical region of teeth or perforation of oral mucosa.
[d]Antibiotic prophylaxis may be reasonable for procedures in the respiratory tract or infected skin, skin structures, or musculoskeletal tissue. Antibiotic prophylaxis solely to prevent endocarditis is *not* recommended for GU or GI procedures.

limited the procedures requiring prophylaxis to gingival or periapical dental work or incision through infected skin or soft tissue.[31]

REFERENCES

1. McDonald JR. Acute infective endocarditis. *Infect Dis Clin North Am.* 2009;23:643–664.
2. Baddour LM, Wilson WR, Bayer AS, et al. Infective endocarditis: diagnosis, antimicrobial therapy, and management of complications: a statement for healthcare professionals from the Committee on Rheumatic Fever, Endocarditis, and Kawasaki Diseases, Council on Cardiovascular Diseases in the Young, and Councils on Clinical Cardiology, Stroke, and Cardiovascular Surgery and Anesthesia, American Heart Association: endorsed by the Infectious Diseases Society of America. *Circulation.* 2005;111:e394–e434.
3. Wolff M, Timsit JF. Infectious endocarditis. In: Fink MP, Abraham E, Vincent JL, Kochanek PM, et al, eds. *Textbook of Critical Care.* Philadelphia: Elsevier; 2005:871–878.
4. Mylonakis E, Calderwood SB. Infective endocarditis in adults. *N Engl J Med.* 2001;345:1218–1230.
5. Nishimura RA, Carabello BA, Faxon DP, et al. ACC/AHA 2008 guideline update on valvular heart disease: focused update on infective endocarditis: a report of the American College of Cardiology/American Heart Association Task Force on Practice Guidelines: endorsed by the Society of Cardiovascular Anesthesiologists, Society for Cardiovascular Angiography and Interventions, and Society of Thoracic Surgeons. *Circulation.* 2008;118:887–896.
6. Slesnick TC, Nugent AW, Fraser CD Jr, et al. Incomplete endothelialization and late development of acute bacterial endocarditis after implantation of an Amplatzer septal occluder device. *Circulation.* 2008;117:e326–e327.
7. Prendergast BD. The changing face of infective endocarditis. *Heart.* 2006;92:879–885.
8. Osler W. Gulstonian lectures on malignant endocarditis. *Br Med J.* 1885;1:467–579.
9. Levy DM. Centenary of William Osler's 1885 Gulstonian lectures and their place in the history of bacterial endocarditis. *J R Soc Med.* 1985;78:1039–1047.
10. Hill EE, Herijgers P, Herregods MC, et al. Evolving trends in infective endocarditis. *Clin Microbiol Infect.* 2006;12:5–12.
11. Moreillon P, Que YA. Infective endocarditis. *Lancet.* 2004;363:139–149.
12. Devlin RK, Andrews MM, von Reyn CF. Recent trends in infective endocarditis: influence of case definitions. *Curr Opin Cardiol.* 2004;19:134–139.
13. Giamarellou H, Antoniadou A. Infectious endocarditis. In: Fink MP, Abraham E, Vincent JL, et al, eds. *Textbook of Critical Care.* Philadelphia: Elsevier; 2005:1341–1344.
14. Durante-Mangoni E, Bradley S, Selton-Suty C, et al. Current features of infective endocarditis in elderly

patients: results of the International Collaboration on Endocarditis Prospective Cohort Study. *Arch Intern Med.* 2008;168:2095–2103.

15. Miro JM, del Rio A, Mestres CA. Infective endocarditis in intravenous drug abusers and HIV-1 infected patients. *Infect Dis Clin North Am.* 2002;16:273–295.

16. Reyes MP, Ali A, Mendes RE, et al. Resurgence of *Pseudomonas endocarditis* in Detroit, 2006–2008. *Medicine.* 2009;88:294–301.

17. Losa JE, Miro JM, Del Rio A, et al. Infective endocarditis not related to intravenous drug abuse in HIV-1 infected patients. *Clin Microbiol Infect.* 2003;9:45–54.

18. Mocchegiani R, Nataloni M. Complications of infective endocarditis. *Cardiovasc Hematol Disord Drug Targets.* Epub 2009;9(4):240–248.

19. Mourvillier B, Trouillet JL, Timsit JF, et al. Infective endocarditis in the intensive care unit: clinical spectrum and prognostic factors in 228 consecutive patients. *Intensive Care Med.* 2004;30:2046–2052.

20. Karth GD, Koreny M, Binder T, et al. Complicated infective endocarditis necessitating ICU admission: clinical course and prognosis. *Crit Care.* 2002;6:149–154.

21. Li JS, Sexton DJ, Mick N, et al. Proposed modifications to the Duke criteria for the diagnosis of infective endocarditis. *Clin Infect Dis.* 2000;30:633–638.

22. Alam M. Transesophageal echocardiography in critical care units: Henry Ford hospital experience and review of the literature. *Prog Cardiovasc Dis.* 196;38: 315–328.

23. Morguet AJ, Werner GS, Andreas S, et al. Diagnostic value of transesophageal compared with transthoracic echocardiography in suspected prosthetic valve endocarditis. *Herz.* 1995;20: 390–398.

24. Humpl T, McCrindle BW, Smallhorn JF. The relative roles of transthoracic compared with transesophageal echocardiography in children with suspected infective endocarditis. *J Am Coll Cardiol.* 2003;41:2068–2071.

25. Makota H, Hashimoto K, Mashiko K, et al. Active infective endocarditis: management and risk analysis of hospital death from 24 years experience. *Circ J.* 2008;72: 2062–2068.

26. Grunenfelder J, Akins CW, Hilgenberg AD, et al. Long term results and determinants of mortality after surgery for native and prosthetic valve endocarditis. *J Heart Valve Dis.* 2001;10:694–702.

27. Dreyfus G, Serraf A, Jebara VA, et al. Valve repair in acute endocarditis. *Ann Thorac Surg.* 1990;49:706–713.

28. Rubinovitch B, Pittet D. Infective endocarditis: too ill to be operated? *Crit Care.* 2002;6:106–107.

29. Arbulu A, Holmes RJ, Asfaw I. Tricuspid valvulectomy without replacement: twenty years experience. *J Thorac Cardiovasc Surg.* 1991;102:917–922.

30. Gammie JS. An outstanding series of tricuspid valve operations for infective endocarditis. *Ann Thorac Surg.* 2007;84:1949.

31. Wilson W, Taubert KA, Gewitz M, et al. Prevention of infective endocarditis: guidelines from the American Heart Association: a guideline from the American Heart Association Rheumatic Fever, Endocarditis, and Kawasaki Disease Committee, Council on Cardiovascular Disease in the Young, and Council on Clinical Cardiology, Council on Cardiovascular Surgery and Anesthesia, and the Quality Care and Outcomes Research Interdisciplinary Working Group. *Circulation.* 2007;116: 1736–1754.

CHAPTER 39

Clostridium Difficile Infection (CDI)

Claudio D. Tuda

Clostridium difficile infection (CDI) is the most commonly recognized cause of infectious diarrhea in hospitals and long-term care facilities.[1] The incidence of CDI is difficult to establish because it is not a reportable disease in the United States. It is estimated that there are at least 500,000 cases in US hospitals and nursing homes per year resulting in 30,000 deaths.[2] Approximately 4.6 cases per 10,000 patient admissions was the incidence noted in data from the Canadian surveillance studies conducted in hospitals in 1997 and 2005.[3] A recent European hospital-based survey showed a similar incidence of 4.1 cases per 10,000 patient days.[4]

The number of patients discharged from the hospital and transferred to long-term care facilities with the diagnosis of CDI doubled between 2000 and 2003. Close to 2% of them carried the diagnosis of CDI.

► EPIDEMIOLOGY

The epidemiology of CDI is changing, especially in the last few years. In 2001, the number of patients discharged from the hospital with the diagnosis of CDI increased at a very rapid rate.[5] The number of patients older than 65 years was substantially larger than the group aged 45–64 years, representing a 5-fold increase in the number of cases in this age group. The outbreaks in Canada and the United States were considered very severe between 2002 and 2006.[6,7] These outbreaks were associated with the use of fluoroquinolones. The strains of the outbreaks in Canada and United States were identical.[8] This strain is known by its restriction analysis pattern, B1, by its pulsed-field gel electrophoresis (PFGE) pattern, North American PFGE type 1 (NAPI), or its ribotype name 027. It is now designated and known as NAPI/B1/027.[9] This strain accounted for almost all of the infections. The strain has some genetic characteristics that included gene coding for toxins A and B and an 18-base pair deletion in *tcdC*, a putative negative regulator of expression of toxins A and B. The presence of one or two of these genetic markers is one of the reasons for the increased virulence. The patients infected with the NAPI/B1/027 developed a more severe disease than the patients infected with other strains. This strain, NAPI/B1/027, has spread to 40 states in the United States and 7 Canadian provinces and has caused outbreaks in Europe and Asia, as well.[10–12]

The main means of transmission is person to person through the fecal–oral route, usually in in-patients in hospitals and nursing homes.[13] The prevalence of asymptomatic colonization in nursing homes is estimated to be between 5% and 7%[14] and in hospitals between 7% and 26%.[13] There is a significant increased risk of colonization with longer hospitalizations.

The incubation period from the time of exposure to the development of symptoms is not very well known, but in studies it has been estimated to be 2–3 days.[13] Those persons who are colonized with *C. difficile* and remain asymptomatic over longer periods of time appear to have a lower rather than increased risk of development of CDI. This is believed to be due to the boosting of serum antibody levels against *C. difficile* toxins A and B.[15].

The contamination of the environment has a rather important role in the transmission of *C. difficile* in hospitals. When bedpans, commodes, and shared thermometers are inadequately cleaned, they become a transmitting source in health care settings.[16] The hands of health care workers have been recognized as one of the most important modes in the transmission of *C. difficile*.[13]

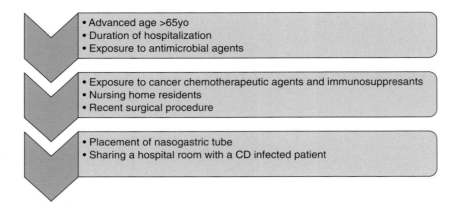

- Advanced age >65yo
- Duration of hospitalization
- Exposure to antimicrobial agents

- Exposure to cancer chemotherapeutic agents and immunosuppressants
- Nursing home residents
- Recent surgical procedure

- Placement of nasogastric tube
- Sharing a hospital room with a CD infected patient

Figure 39-1. Risk factors for CDI.

The main risk factors for the development of CDI (Figure 39-1) have been clearly established, and **advanced age** (>65) is one of the most important of all.[9] **Duration of hospitalization also** has been identified, and clearly, the risk of acquisition of CDI increases with the length of stay.[13]

Exposure to antimicrobial agents is probably the most important modifiable risk factor. Almost every single antimicrobial agent has been linked to the development of CDI. Cephalosporins, broad-spectrum penicillins, clindamycin, and fluoroquinolones play a very important role. The risk of developing CDI with the use of antibiotics is increased due to the influence of the antibiotics, which suppress the normal bowel flora and allow *C. difficile* to develop. Longer exposure to antimicrobials and the use of multiple antimicrobials clearly increases the risk of CDI, but even in situations of limited exposure, such as single-dose surgical antibiotic prophylaxis, the risk is also increased.[17] Another risk factor to consider is the **cancer chemotherapeutic agents**. This is believed to be due in part to the antimicrobial activity of certain chemotherapeutic agents.[18] Tube feedings or previous gastric surgery have also been linked to the development of CDI.[19] The use of proton pump inhibitors was initially associated with the development of CDI, but recent controlled studies have shown this association is perhaps inaccurate and is most likely due to the severity of illness and duration of institutional stay rather than a direct result of the use of acid-suppressant agents.[20,21]

▶ PATHOPHYSIOLOGY

The disruption of the normal colonic flora is the main precipitating factor for the development of CDI. Antibiotics commonly cause disruption of the colonic microflora.[22] After the disruption of the colonic microflora, colonization of *C. difficile* is achieved through the ingestion of heat-resistant spores.[23] Clinical manifestations of CDI or an asymptomatic carrier state may develop, depending on the host factors.[23] The patients with the highest risk to develop more severe disease are those who recently have had surgery and those who have received immunosuppressive therapy. These patients seem to have an inability to mount an appropriate IgG immune antibody response against *C. difficile* toxin A. When a patient has the ability to mount an adequate immune response, there are decreased morbidity and mortality, and a lower chance of recurrence.

C. difficile causes toxin-mediated colitis. It produces two exotoxins: toxin A and toxin B. Toxin A activates macrophages and mast cells. The inflammatory cascade leads to increased mucosal permeability and fluid secretion.

On the contrary, the toxin B has a potent cytotoxic activity in vitro but low enterotoxic activity. The leukocyte chemotaxis and upregulation of cytokines caused by these toxins are responsible for the severe colonic inflammatory response that is clinically evident with a very high WBC count. Pseudomembrane is the result of progressive worsening of the colitis with focal ulceration and accumulation of purulent material and necrotic debris.[22]

▶ CLINCAL PRESENTATION AND DIAGNOSIS

The clinical presentation is quite variable, and the spectrum ranges from no symptoms to fulminant colitis.[1]

A very detailed history emphasizing prior exposure to antibiotic in the preceding 3–6 months is a very important piece of information.

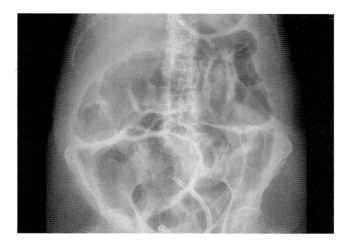

Figure 39-2. Significant dilatation of the colon. Presence of ileus.

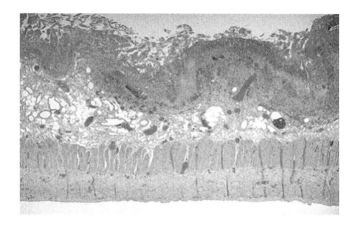

Figure 39-4. Scanning magnification reveals total denudation of the colonic mucosa with extensive replacement by firbrinopurulent exudate (H&E × 400).

Diarrhea is present in almost every case, but in some patients may be initially absent, especially in severely ill patients. With the presence of an ileus, leukocytosis is perhaps the most common laboratory finding. A sudden rise of the WBC to >30,000 mm³ is an important indicator of impending fulminant colitis.[24] Abdominal x-ray may show an ileus, a distended colon, and, sometimes, evidence of colitis or toxin megacolon (Figure 39-2). The use of flexible sigmoidoscopy is a tool that can provide an immediate diagnosis (Figure 39-3).[25] The finding of pseudomembranes is pathognomonic for this disease (Figures 39-4 to 39-6).

CT scan of the abdomen can also be very helpful with distinctive findings such as the presence of pancolitis (Figure 39-7).[25]

The Infectious Disease Society (IDSA) and the Society for Healthcare Epidemiology of America (SHEA) recently published the *Clinical Practice Guidelines* and addressed the best testing strategy for diagnosis of CDI.[26] Testing of stool from asymptomatic patients is not clinically useful, including use as a test of cure. Stool culture is the most sensitive test and is essential for epidemiologic purposes but is not clinically practical due to the slow turnaround time. Enzyme immunoassay (EIA) testing for *C. difficile* toxins A and B is rapid but is less sensitive than the cell cytotoxic assay, and it is a suboptimal approach for diagnosis. EIA sensitivity is 63–94% and the specificity 75–100%. Toxin testing is most important clinically but is hampered by its lack of sensitivity. These tests (EIA) have been adopted by >90% of the laboratories in

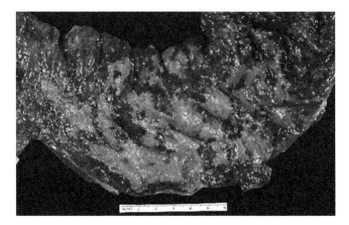

Figure 39-3. Macroscopic examination reveals the variegated appearance of the colonic mucosa due to the alternating areas of ulceration (single arrow) and membranouslike deposition of necrotic debris (double arrow).

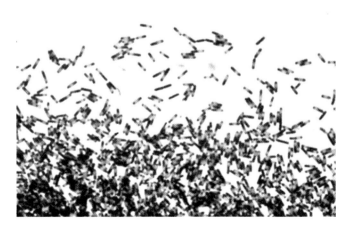

Figure 39-5. Oil immersion (×10,000) power of Gram stain from culture material shows *C. difficile* organisms with the characteristic uneven staining.

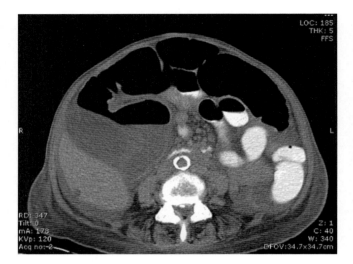

Figure 39-6. Pancolitis that is more evident in the descendent colon, with significant surrounding stranding and free fluid. Transverse and cecum distended with air.

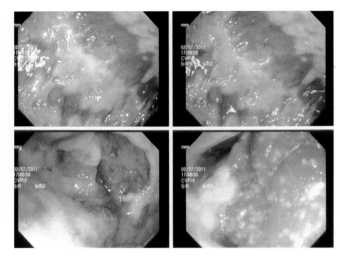

Figure 39-7. Severe *C. difficile colitis.* Edematous, gray, dusky, erythematous, thick pseudomembranes.

the United States because of their easy use and lower labor costs compared with the cell cytotoxin assay. One potential strategy to overcome this problem is a two-step approach that uses EIA detection of glutamate dehydrogenase (GDH) as initial screening and then uses the cell cytotoxin assay or toxigenic culture as the confirmatory test for the GDH-positive stools. The sensitivity of the GDH detection assay is 85–95% and the specificity 89–99%. PCR testing appears to be a rapid, sensitive, and specific modality, but more data are needed at this time.[26]

▶ TREATMENT

The treatment modality has been stratified according to the severity of the disease (Figure 39-8).[26,27]

Severe CDI is suggested by the presence of fever, rigors, abdominal pain, WBC >15,000 mm^3 or rise in serum creatinine ≥50% above the baseline, CT evidence of colitis, or endoscopic visualization of pseudomembranous colitis. Mild to moderate CDI (no features of severe CDI) may be treated with oral metronidazole 500 mg three times daily for 10–14 days. Severe CDI should be treated with oral vancomycin 125 mg four times daily for 10–14 days. Severe, complicated CDI is suggested by the presence of rising lactic acid levels, hypotension, megacolon, ileus, and shock. In cases of complicated CDI, vancomycin 500 mg, oral or nasogastric administration, four times daily plus intravenous metronidazole 500 mg three times daily should be administered. Intracolonic administration of vancomycin 500 mg four to six times daily should be given if ileus is present or suspected. Early surgical opinion is suggested in this situation.[26,27]

The symptoms improve rapidly, with resolution of the fever in the first 48 hours and diarrhea within the first 4 or 5 days when the treatment is effective.

Up to one quarter of the patients may experience recurrence that is usually due to reinfection or the germination of spores in the colon after the treatment.[1]

Most of the recurrences will respond to another course of treatment with the same medications. Some patients may experience multiple episodes of recurrences. The management in these cases remains controversial, and multiple approaches have been used, including longer courses of antibiotics, with tapering doses over a period of weeks,[27] even stool transplant from healthy donors to replenish the normal colonic flora. A recent published study has shown that fidaxomicin was associated with a significantly lower rate of recurrence when compared with vancomycin.[28]

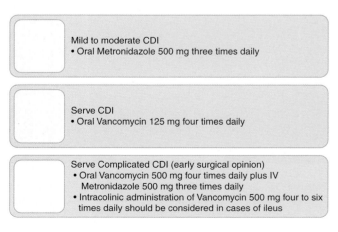

Figure 39-8. Treatment guidelines.

Mild to moderate CDI
• Oral Metronidazole 500 mg three times daily

Serve CDI
• Oral Vancomycin 125 mg four times daily

Serve Complicated CDI (early surgical opinion)
• Oral Vancomycin 500 mg four times daily plus IV Metronidazole 500 mg three times daily
• Intracolinic administration of Vancomycin 500 mg four to six times daily should be considered in cases of ileus

Evidence supporting the use of probiotics in CDI is limited[29] and is not routinely recommended. Intravenous immunoglobulin (IVIG) has been used to treat severe CDI. A recent study reported a high mortality rate (57%) in 21 patients treated with IVIG for severe CDI. The authors suggested that the role of IVIG is limited in cases of CDI in which extracolonic dysfunction is manifested (SIRS), and its use may be less beneficial.[30] Human monoclonal antibodies is another treatment modality that has been assessed in phase II trials. They were administered as an adjuvant to standard therapy, and the treatment was associated with a 72% reduction in recurrence when compared with placebo.[31]

Active vaccination with a *C. difficile* toxoid vaccine is underway in the United States. The estimated completion date is December 2011.[32]

Newer options for the treatment of CDI (as mentioned earlier) include fidaxomicin, a poorly absorbed antibiotic with potent activity against *C. difficile* and limited activity against normal fecal flora. Recent published trial reported fidaxomicin 200 mg twice daily is at least as effective as vancomycin 125 mg four times daily. Recurrence rates were significantly lower with fidaxomicin (13% vs. 25%).[28]

Tigecycline has been used off-label in patients with severe CDI; five successful cases have been reported in the literature.[33] Rifaximin 400 mg twice daily has been used off-label to treat patients with multiple recurrences with a success rate of 86%. The main concern is the rapid development of resistance.[34] Nitazoxanide is a compound used for parasitic infections. A small trial suggested that it is comparable to vancomycin. It is expensive but may have a role for refractory or recurrent CDI.[35] Newer treatment alternatives under investigation for treatment of CDI include ramoplanin, oritavancin, Rifalazil, REP3123, and NVB302.[36]

REFERENCES

1. Bartlett JG. Clinical practice. Antibiotic-associated diarrhea. *N Engl J Med.* 2002;346:334–349.
2. Rupnik M, Wilcox MH, Gerding DN. *Clostridium difficile* infection: new developments in epidemiology and pathogenesis. *Nat Rev Microbiol.* 2009;7:526–536.
3. Gravel D, Miller M, Simor A, et al. Healthcare-associated *Clostridium difficile* infection in adults admitted to acute care hospitals in Canada: a Canadian nosocomial infection surveillance program study. *Clin Infect Dis.* 2009;48:568–576.
4. Bauer MP, Notermans DW, van Benthem BHB, et al. First results of the European *Clostridium difficile* infection survey (ECDIS). In: 19th European Congress of Clinical Microbiology and Infectious Diseases (ECCMID); May 16–19, 2009; Helsinki.

5. McDonald LC, Owings M, Jernigan DB. *Clostridium difficile* infection in patients discharged from US short-stay hospitals, 1996–2003. *Emerg Infect Dis.* 2006;12:409–415.
6. Muto CA, Pokrywka M, Shutt K, et al. A large outbreak of *Clostridium difficile*-associated disease with an unexpected proportion of deaths and colectomies at a teaching hospital following increased fluoroquinolone use. *Inf Control Hosp Epidemiol.* 2005;26:273–280.
7. Pepin J, Alary ME, Valiquette L, et al. Increasing risk of relapse after treatment of *Clostridium Difficile* colitis in Quebec, Canada. *Clin Infect Dis.* 2005;40:1591–1597.
8. Loo VG, Poirier L, Miller MA, et al. A predominant clonal multi-institutional outbreak of *Clostridium difficile*-associated diarrhea with high morbidity and mortality. *N Engl J Med.* 2005;353:2442–2449.
9. McDonald LC, Killgore GE, Thompson A, et al. An epidemic, toxin gene-variant strain of *Clostridium difficile.* *N Engl J Med.* 2005;353:2433–2441.
10. Centers for Disease Control and Prevention. Data and statistics about *Clostridium difficile* infections. Available at: http://www.cdc.gov.
11. Eggertson L. Quebec strain of *C. difficile* in 7 provinces. *Can Med Assoc J.* 2006;174:607–608.
12. Kuijper EJ, Barbut F, Brazier JS, et al. Update of *Clostridium difficile* infection due to PCR ribotype 027 in Europe, 2008. *Euro Surveill.* 2008;13(31):pii:18942.
13. McFarland LV, Mulligan ME, Kwok RY, et al. Nosocomial acquisition of *Clostridium difficile* infection. *N Engl J Med.* 1989;320:204–210.
14. Rivera EV, Woods S. Prevalence of asymptomatic *Clostridium difficile* colonization in a nursing home population: a cross sectional study. *J Gend Specif Med.* 2003;6:27–30.
15. Kyne L, Warny M, Qamar A, et al. Association between antibody response to toxin A and protection against recurrent *Clostridium difficile* diarrhoea. *Lancet.* 2001;357:189–193.
16. Mayfield JL, Leet T, Miller J, et al. Environmental control to reduce transmission of *Clostridium difficile.* *Clin Infect Dis.* 2000;31:995–1000.
17. Privitera G, Scarpellini P, Ortisi G, et al. Prospective study of *Clostridium difficile* intestinal colonization and disease following single-dose antibiotic prophylaxis in surgery. *Antimicrob Agents Chemother.* 1991;35:208–210.
18. Anand A, Glatt AE. *Clostridium difficile* infection associated with antineoplastic chemotherapy: a review. *Clin Infect Dis.* 1993;17:109–113.
19. Bliss DZ, Johnson S, Savik K, et al. Acquisition of *Clostridium difficile* and *Clostridium difficile*-associated diarrhea in hospitalized patients receiving tube feeding. *Ann Intern Med.* 1998;129:1012–1019.
20. Dial S, Delaney JA, Barkun AN, et al. Use of gastric acid-suppressive agents and the risk of community-acquired *Clostridium difficile*-associated disease. *JAMA.* 2005;294:2989–2995.
21. Shah S, Lewis A, Leopold D, et al. Gastric acid suppression does not promote clostridial diarrhea in the elderly. *QJM.* 2000;93:175–181.
22. Hurley BW, Nguyen CC. The spectrum of pseudomembranous enterocolitis and antibiotic-associated diarrhea. *Arch Intern Med.* 2002;162:2177–2184.

23. Kelly CP, Lamont JT. *Clostridium difficile* infection. *Annu Rev Med.* 1998;49:375–390.

24. Dallal RM, Harbretch BG, Boujoukas AJ, et al. Fulminant *Clostridium difficile*: an underappreciated and increasing cause of death and complications. *Ann Surg.* 2002;235:363–372.

25. Kyne L, Farrell RJ, Kelly CP. *Clostridium difficile. Gastroenterol Clin North Am.* 2001;30:753–777.

26. Cohen SH, Gerding DN, Johnson S, et al. Clinical practice guidelines for *Clostridium difficile* infection in adults: 2010 update by the Society for Healthcare Epidemiology of America (SHEA) and the Infectious Disease Society of America (IDSA). *Infect Control Hosp Epidemiol.* 2010;31(5):431–455.

27. Bauer MP, Kuijper EJ, van Diesel JT. European Society of Clinical Microbiology and Infectious Diseases (ESCMID): treatment guidance document for *Clostridium difficile infection* (CDI). *Clin Microbiol Infect.* 2009;15:1067–1079.

28. Louie TJ, Miller MA, Mullane K. Fidaxomicin versus vancomycin for *Clostridium difficile infection. N Engl J Med.* 2010;364(5):422–431.

29. McFarland LV. Evidence based review of probiotics for antibiotic-associated diarrhea and *Clostridium difficile* infections. *Anaerobic.* 2009;15:274–280.

30. Abougergi MS, Broor A, Cui W. Intravenous immunoglobulin for the treatment of severe *Clostridium difficile* colitis: an observational study and review of the literature. *J Hosp Med.* 2010;5:e1–e9.

31. Lowy I, Molrine DC, Ledv BA, et al. Treatment with monoclonal antibodies against *Clostridium difficile* toxins. *N Engl J Med.* 2010;362:197–205.

32. Sougioultzis S, Kyne L, Drudy D, et al. *Clostridium difficile* toxoid vaccine in recurrent *C. difficile*-associated diarrhea. *Gastroenterology.* 2005;128:764–770.

33. Herpers BL, Vlaminckx B, Burkharat O, et al. Intravenous tigecycline as adjunctive or alternative therapy for severe refractory *Clostridium difficile* infection. *Clin Infect Dis.* 2009;48:1732–1735.

34. Garey KW, Jiang ZD, Bellard A, et al. Rifaximin in treatment of recurrent *Clostridium difficile*-associated diarrhea: an uncontrolled pilot study. *J Clin Gastroenterol.* 2009;43:91–93.

35. Musher DM, Logan N, Mehendiratta V, et al. *Clostridium difficile* colitis that fails conventional metronidazole therapy: response to nitazoxanide. *J Antimicrob Chemother.* 2007;59:705–710.

36. Johnson AP. New antibiotics for severe selective treatment of gastrointestinal infection caused by *Clostridium difficile. Expert Opin Ther Patents.* 2010;20:1389–1399.

SECTION IX

Toxicologic Conditions

CHAPTER 40

Approach to Poisoning

Mohan Punja and Robert J. Hoffman

► INTRODUCTION

Patients with poison exposure and toxicity may present with a spectrum of various clinical signs, symptoms, and problems. Most of these are very straightforward and easily anticipated, but others may be unpredictable or associated with exposure to unidentified substances that hinder the clinician from knowing what to expect. There are, however, general principles that may be employed as a framework on which approach to most poisonings may be based. These are employed when managing adverse effects from poisoning by known or unidentified substances. Less than 5% of poisonings require use of specific antidotes; thorough general supportive care is the most important approach in caring for most poisoned patients.[1]

The initial principles of management of poisoned patients generally follow the protocol used for the management of urgent and emergent problems. There are some slight differences if the "airway, breathing, circulation" approach is used, with some specific amendments relevant to poison exposures and toxicity. "Airway, breathing, circulation, disability, dextrose, exposure, ECG" comprise the general "A, B, C, D, D, E, E" mantra of poison management. This may differ from other emergency department (ED) management in that "disability" and "exposure," necessary for patients with trauma, are not essential in most poisoned patients, but can reveal some valuable diagnostic information.

► HISTORY

Critical to proper management of poisoning is recognition that poison exposure occurred. When evaluating a poisoned patient, a good approach is to identify the reason of exposure (i.e., intentional, unintentional, misadventure), the type of substance involved (i.e., prescription, over-the-counter, herbal, illicit drug), the formulation (i.e., immediate vs. sustained release), the dose of the substance, the amount of substance involved, the route of exposure (i.e., ingestion, inhalation, intravenous, dermal), the time of exposure (hours since exposure, acute vs. chronic), any potential coingestion, and the severity of exposure.

Obtaining a medical history from the poisoned patient may be difficult, and, therefore, other people such as family members, friends, prehospital personnel, the patient's physician or therapist, or previous medical records may provide crucial information to aid in management. Thorough medical knowledge of all ailments, medical history, medication history, and other medications or substances the patient had access to often provides useful information.

After initial assessment, stabilization, and physical exam, further management may include (1) decontamination, (2) prevention of absorption, (3) administration of antidote, and (4) enhanced elimination of the toxic substance.

► PHYSICAL EXAMINATION

Examination of patients with poison exposure and toxicity is often more focused than a general physical examination, with particular attention to areas that are expected to yield useful information (Table 40-1).

Assessment of vital signs, neurologic status, pupils, skin, bowel, and bladder permits the recognition of a *toxidrome*. A toxidrome, or toxicologic syndrome, is a constellation of signs and symptoms that herald toxicity

▶ **TABLE 40-1. COMMON FINDINGS IN POISONING**

Clinical and/or laboratory findings in poisoning

Agitation	Anticholinergics,[a] ethanol and sedative–hypnotic withdrawal, hypoglycemia, phencyclidine, sympathomimetics[b]
Alopecia	Alkylating agents, radiation, selenium, strontium, thallium
Ataxia	Benzodiazepines, carbamazepine, carbon monoxide, ethanol, hypoglycemia, lithium, mercury, phenytoin, nitrous oxide
Blindness or decreased visual acuity	Caustics (direct), cocaine, cisplatin, mercury, methanol, quinine, thallium
Blue skin	Amiodarone, FD&C #1 dye, methemoglobin, silver, sulfhemoglobin
Constipation	Anticholinergics,[a] botulism, lead, opioids, thallium (severe)
Tinnitus, deafness	Aminoglycosides, cisplatin, heavy metals, loop diuretics, quinine, salicylates
Diaphoresis	Amphetamines, cholinergics,[c] ethanol and sedative–hypnotic withdrawal, hypoglycemia, opioid withdrawal, salicylates, serotonin syndrome, sympathomimetics[b]
Diarrhea	Arsenic and other metals/metalloids, boric acid (blue-green), botanical irritants, cathartics, cholinergics,[c] colchicine, iron, lithium, opioid withdrawal, radiation
Dysesthesias, paresthesias	Acrylamide, arsenic, ciguatera, cocaine, colchicine, n-hexane, thallium
Gum discoloration	Arsenic, bismuth, hypervitaminosis A, lead, mercury
Hallucinations	Anticholinergics,[a] dopamine agonists, ergot alkaloids, ethanol, ethanol and sedative–hypnotic withdrawal, LSD, phencyclidine, sympathomimetics,[b] tryptamines (e.g., AMT)
Headache	Carbon monoxide, hypoglycemia, monoamine oxidase inhibitor/food interaction (hypertensive crisis), nitrites, serotonin syndrome
Metabolic acidosis (elevated anion gap)	Cyanide, ethylene glycol, ketoacidosis (diabetic, starvation, alcoholic), iron, isoniazid, lactic acidosis, metformin, methanol, paraldehyde, phenformin, protease inhibitors, salicylates, toluene, uremia
Miosis	Cholinergics,[c] clonidine, opioids, phencyclidine, phenothiazines
Mydriasis	Anticholinergics,[a] botulism, methanol, opioid withdrawal, sympathomimetics[b]
Nystagums	Barbiturates, carbamazepine, carbon monoxide, ethanol, lithium, monoamine oxidase inhibitors, phencyclidine, phenytoin, quinine
Purpura	Anticoagulant rodenticides, clopidogrel, corticosteroids, heparin, pit viper venom, quinine, salicylates, warfarin
Radiopaque ingestions	Arsenic, "body packer," chloral hydrate, enteric-coated tablets, halogenated hydrocarbons, metals (e.g., iron, lead)
Red skin	Anticholinergics,[a] boric acid, disulfiram interaction, hydroxocobalamin, scombroid, vancomycin
Rhabdomyolysis	Carbon monoxide, doxylamine, HMG CoA reductase inhibitors, sympathomimetics,[b] Tricholoma mushrooms
Salivation	Arsenic, caustics, cholinergics,[c] ketamine, mercury, phencylidine, strychnine
Seizures	Bupropion, carbon monoxide, cyclic antidepressants, ethanol and sedative–hypnotic withdrawal, Gyromitra mushrooms, hypoglycemia, isoniaziad, theophylline
Tremor	Antipsychotics, arsenic, carbon monoxide, cholinergics,[c] ethanol, lithium, mercury, methyl bromide, sympathomimetics,[b] thyroid replacement
Weakness	Botulism, diuretics, magnesium, neuromuscular blockers, paralytic shellfish, steroids, toluene
Yellow skin	Acetaminophen (late), Amanita mushrooms, β-carotene, dinitrophenol, pyrrolizidine alkaloids

Reproduced with permission from Nelson LS, Lewin NA, Howland ME, Hoffman RS, Goldfrank LS, Flomenbaum NE. *Goldfrank's Toxicological Emergencies.* 9th ed. New York: McGraw-Hill Companies Inc; 2010:40. Table 4-2.
[a]Anticholinergics: for example, antihistamines, atropine, cyclic antidepressants, and scopolamine.
[b]Sympathomimetics: for example, amphetamines, β-adrenergic agonists, cocaine, ephedrine, and methylxanthines.
[c]Cholinergics: for example, muscarinic mushrooms, organic phosphorus compounds, and carbamates, including Alzheimer's drugs and physostigmine, plocarpine, and other direct-acting cholinergics.

from a category of poisons. Recognition of the presence of a toxidrome is useful in managing patients with exposure to unidentified substances and is also useful after known exposure to a category of substances known to cause a specific toxidrome.

Traditionally there are four described toxidromes: adrenergic/sympathomimetic, anticholinergic, cholinergic, and opioid. There is also a well-recognized pattern of clinical findings associated with sedative–hypnotic substances. The classes of substances causing toxidromes include:

- **Adrenergic (sympathomimetic):** sympathomimetic agents capable of α- and/or β-adrenergic agonism, for example, cocaine, amphetamines, theophylline, caffeine, pseudoephedrine, ephedrine, epinephrine, norepinephrine, and methylenedioxymethamphetamine (MDMA) (ecstasy).

► TABLE 40-2. **COMMON FINDINGS IN TOXIDROMES AND POISONINGS**

| Group | Vital Signs | | | | | | | | |
	BP	P	R	T	Mental Status	Pupil Size	Peristalsis	Diaphoresis	Other
Anticholinergics	−/↑	↑	±	↑	Delirium	↑	↓	↓	Dry mucous membranes, flush, urinary retention
Cholinergics	±	±	−/↑	−	Normal to depressed	±	↑	↑	Salivation, lacrimation, urination, diarrhea, bronchorrhea, fasciculations, paralysis
Ethanol or sedative–hypnotics	↓	↓	↓	−/↓	Depressed	±	↓	−	Hyporeflexia, ataxia
Opioids	↓	↓	↓	↓	Depressed		↓	−	Hyporeflexia
Sympathomimetics	↑	↑	↑	↑	Agitated	↑	−/↑	↑	Tremor, seizures
Withdrawal from ethanol or sedative–hypnotics	↑	↑	↑	↑	Agitated, disoriented, hallucinations	↑	↑	↑	Tremor, seizures
Withdrawal from opioids	↑	↑	−	−	Normal, anxious	↑	↑	↑	Vomiting, rhinorrhea, piloerection, diarrhea, yawning

↑, increase; ↓, decrease; ±, variable; −, change unlikely; BP, blood pressure; P, pulse; R, respirations; T, temperature. Reproduced with permission from Nelson LS, Lewin NA, Howland ME, Hoffman RS, Goldfrank LS, Flomenbaum NE. *Goldfrank's Toxicological Emergencies.* 9th ed. New York: McGraw-Hill Companies Inc; 2010:40. Table 3-2.

- **Anticholinergic:** substances that block cholinergic receptors, for example, atropine, scopolamine, antihistamines, phenothiazines, cyclic antidepressants, and cyclobenzaprine.
- **Cholinergic:** substances that afflict cholinergic receptors, for example, organophosphate pesticides and nerve agents, physostigmine, rivastigmine, and nicotine.
- **Opioid:** substances that afflict opioid receptors, for example, heroin, morphine, hydromorphone, methadone, diphenoxylate, clonidine, and tramadol.
- **Sedative–hypnotic:** substances that increase GABA activity, for example, benzodiazepines, barbiturates, alcohols, GHB, and zolpidem.

It is important to note that patients presenting with potential toxicity may have mixed clinical picture and may not entirely fall under a specific toxidrome. This is particularly true for patients presenting with polydrug overdoses, or in cases in which an ingested drug has been adulterated with another toxidrome-causing substance (Table 40-2).

► **LABORATORY AND DIAGNOSTIC ASSAYS**

The investigations and assays most useful in management of poisoned patients are commonplace in emergency medicine and critical care. Although it is possible to assay for hundreds of substances capable of causing toxicity, the most frequently indicated investigations are familiar to the ED and critical care physicians and are readily available in any setting where emergency and critical care are delivered.

ELECTROCARDIOGRAM

Electrocardiograms are indicated in patients with exposure to substances capable of inducing dysrhythmia, exposure to unidentified substances, and exposures with intent of self-harm. Most often, ECGs obtained in the ED setting for nonpoisoned patients are for the purpose of detecting ischemic changes. For patients with poison exposures and toxicity, evaluation for changes in cardiac conduction, conduction intervals, and dysrhythmia is of greatest interest. Ischemia is certainly of interest if present, but this is not the primary focus of ECG evaluation in patients with poison exposure and toxicity.

The triad of pseudo right bundle branch block consisting of R wave in AVR, S wave in lead I, and S wave in AVL, are highly sensitive indicators of sodium channel blockade resulting from tricyclic antidepressant exposure.[2] If these findings are present, prolongation of QRS duration to 100 and 150 milliseconds is predictive of seizure and ventricular dysrhythmia, respectively.[3,4]

Dysrhythmias may result from toxins too numerous to list. Characteristic changes with ventricular bradydysrhythmia are seen with digoxin and other cardiac glycoside toxicity. Nonspecific ST changes throughout all leads and, occasionally bradycardia accompany lithium toxicity.

Poison-induced dysrhythmias may require very different management from the same dysrhythmia that occurs due to other means. In such cases, use of the "standard" management will be ineffective, and occasionally use of the standard management algorithm will increase morbidity and mortality. Some of these managements are described by the American Heart Association.[5] Patients with poison-induced cardiac dysrhythmias should be managed by clinicians familiar with and preferably experienced with these clinical scenarios. (See also the chapter "The Critically Ill Poisoned Patient.")

LABORATORY—ROUTINELY INDICATED ASSAYS

Serum glucose measurement and serum electrolyte analysis are the two most indicated lab assays in the management of poisoned patients. These tests allow detection of hypoglycemia, which may result from a variety of poisons, including both agents known to cause hypoglycemia and substances that may cause hyperglycemia and a subsequent hypoglycemic response. Any patient with altered mental status, including depressed or altered sensorium, coma, or agitation, should have immediate bedside assessment of the blood glucose level. This assay provides a result that is immediately interpretable, meaningful to the treating clinicians, and allows an anticipated, appropriate response with administration of dextrose or glucagon. Serum chemistry assessment allows detection of anion gap metabolic acidosis, alterations of sodium, potassium, and serum bicarbonate, and alterations of the other measured substances.

The anion gap is calculated by the following formula: $[Na^+] - [Cl^- + HCO_3^-]$, and the normal value is generally accepted to be between 6 and 14 mEq/L.[6] Discovery of an anion gap in the poisoned patient should prompt investigation of the cause if unknown. Such causes may be exogenous or endogenous etiologies as represented by the MUDPILES mnemonic: methanol, uremia, diabetic ketoacidosis, paraldehyde/phenformin, iron/inhalants (carbon monoxide, cyanide, and hydrogen sulfide), isoniazid/ibuprofen, lactic acidosis, ethylene glycol/ethanol ketoacidosis, and salicylates/solvents (benzene, toluene)/sympathomimetics/starvation ketoacidosis. Measurement of the serum osmolar gap is occasionally useful in the patient with suspected toxic alcohol ingestion, but has many limitations. The measured serum osmolarity is compared with the calculated serum osmolarity to derive the gap that represents other osmotically active substances. The formula is: $Osm_{calc} = 2[Na^+] + (BUN/2.8) + (glucose/18) + (ethanol/4.6)$. Methanol, ethylene glycol, and numerous other drugs, chemicals, and disease states may contribute to this gap. There is a wide, poorly defined range of "normal" osmolar gap, usually ranging from -5 to $+15$ mOsm/kg.[7,8] Given that the patients' baseline osmolar gap is rarely known, it is difficult to reliably determine if an unmeasured osmotically active substance is present. Thus, the change in this gap as the toxic alcohol is metabolized, in conjunction with the anion gap and any laboratory levels of alcohols, is more important; a "normal" osmolar gap does not rule out exposure to a toxic alcohol.

Additional laboratory assays that are commonly useful include serum acetaminophen level, salicylate level, ethanol level, and blood gas analysis. Serum acetaminophen assays are indicated for any patient with potentially toxic exposure to acetaminophen and any patient with exposure with intent of self-harm, regardless of whether acetaminophen exposure is reported,[9] and may be useful in patients with elevation of hepatic transaminases after exposure to unidentified substances.

Serum salicylate levels may aid in detection of undisclosed salicylate exposure. Salicylate toxicity may be identified by clinical findings,[10] but these may be obscured by polydrug exposure, other medical ailments, or lack of clinician exposure to salicylate-poisoned patients.[11] We advocate routine use of serum salicylate screening in patients with unidentified exposures or exposures with intent of self-harm.

Serum ethanol levels may provide insight into causality of depressed mental status. Although wide variability in patient tolerance to ethanol makes interpretation of serum ethanol level and correlation with degree of depression of consciousness less than fully accurate,[12] this assay is a staple of ED assessment of patients with depressed consciousness.

Readers are advised to interpret serum ethanol level with caution. Overlooking other emergent causes of depressed or altered mental status, such as intracranial hemorrhage, encephalitis, or sepsis, by inappropriately attributing the mental state to ethanol exposure is a very common error in emergency medicine. This error routinely results in morbidity and mortality, and is a common cause for legal cases brought against treating physicians. The presence of a serum ethanol level capable of causing intoxication should not cause the clinician to discontinue investigating potential emergent causes of altered or depressed mental status.

Blood gas analysis is useful for a variety of reasons, including to elucidate the type and degree of acidosis or alkalosis, detect dyshemoglobinemias through carboxyhemoglobin or methemoglobin level, and determine oxygen extraction and utilization in poisonings that may result in blockade of oxidative phosphorylation, such as by cyanide. In nearly all cases, with the most common exception of cardiac arrest, venous blood gas sampling has been shown to be nearly equivalent to arterial sampling. The simplest correction or correlation of pH between venous and arterial blood gas samples is performed by adding 0.03 to the venous pH to obtain the arterial pH.[13,14] In most cases venous blood gas sampling is adequate,[13,14] and arterial blood sampling should only be performed when necessary. An exception to this general rule is evaluation for cyanide or other disruptors of oxidative phosphorylation, in which comparison of simultaneously obtained arterial and venous blood gas samples is used to assess oxygen extraction across the capillary and tissue bed.

Serum creatine phosphokinase may be obtained when a patient exhibits signs of altered temperature regulation and muscle tone such as in the serotonin and neuroleptic malignant syndromes or the sympathomimetic toxidrome. Additionally, many common drugs have the potential to cause rhabdomyolysis, the most well known of which are statins, steroids, theophylline, and doxylamine. Any condition that has the potential to cause trauma or prolonged immobilization, such as the abuse of rapid-onset sedatives, may damage muscle, thereby releasing potentially dangerous amounts of potassium and creatine phosphokinase.

LABORATORY—QUANTITATIVE ASSAYS

Generally, on exposure to a substance for which a serum concentration, or "level," may be obtained, such information may potentially be highly useful for management and/or prognosis. Occasionally these are critical to select a specific management, especially hemodialysis, other method of enhanced elimination, or antidote administration.

LABORATORY—DRUG OF ABUSE SCREENING

Laboratory screening for drugs of abuse, commonly amphetamines, cannabinoids (marijuana), cocaine, PCP, and opioids, is the toxicology lab screening that is least useful, most overutilized, and most misunderstood and misinterpreted toxicologic lab assay.[15–17] Other than for forensic purposes, lab assay for drugs of abuse is not routinely indicated for patients with exposure to drugs or abuse or for patients with unidentified exposures. As these screenings are only qualitative, they confirm only that exposure to the substance in question that occurred within the previous days or week, depending on the substance. Many such assays are not complete for the respective drug category. A screening assay specific for amphetamine might not detect methamphetamine or MDMA (ecstasy), which are much more widely abused than amphetamine. A typical opioid screening will detect natural opioids but not synthetic opioids, such as methadone, fentanyl, propoxyphene, tramadol, etc. Many commonly abused drugs, such as ketamine and GHB, are not detected by any routine laboratory screening. Many medications known to cause false-positive drug of abuse screening exist. Screening for cocaine is the most accurate of the commonly used drug of abuse screening tests, but the tested metabolite benzoylecgonine typically is detectible in urine for 2–3 days after a single exposure.[18]

Failure to understand the limitations of drug of abuse screening leads uninformed clinicians to obtain this test, and often to misinterpret the results.

Malicious exposures, exposures in children incapable of volitionally using drugs, and other circumstances for which forensic evidence of drug abuse exposure would be useful should be obtained in consultation with physicians with forensic experience and law enforcement officials.

IMAGING

Occasionally, imaging may be useful in evaluation. Some radiodense materials, such as lead, heavy metals, enteric-coated tablets, and ingested packages containing drugs such as cocaine or heroin, may be identified by plain radiography. In some circumstances, abdominal x-ray may reveal radiopaque materials, such as hydrocarbons, that may cause a characteristic "double bubble" sign in the stomach. Two heavy metals particularly amenable to detection by plain films are nonchewable iron tablets and ingested lead containing foreign bodies. The sensitivity of plain x-ray to identify ingested drug packages is very high, and classic findings may include visualization of staples used to hold packs closed, "rosettelike finding" of air trapped in knots where packets are tied, and the "double condom" sign in which air is seen trapped between layers of latex (Figures 40-1 and 40-2).[19]

Computerized tomography (CT) may also be indicated to identify ingested substances such as ingested drug packages or radiodense materials. In the case of rupture of ingested packages, CT scanning should be performed after surgery to document complete gastrointestinal tract clearance.[19]

Imaging is useful to evaluate for the consequences of poisoning; examples are chest radiograph that may identify pneumonitis associated with hydrocarbon or other aspiration, abdominal radiograph showing bowel obstruction or perforation, or CT that may provide information about the extent and severity of injury from caustic ingestion.

Endoscopy may provide direct imaging of the airway or GI tract and may be particularly useful in patients with caustic exposures to aid in diagnosis, discharge,

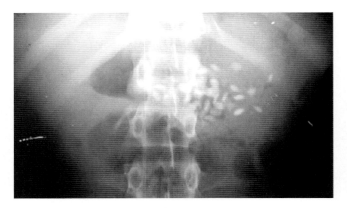

Figure 40-1. Iron tablet overdose. The identification of the large amount of radiopaque tablets corroborates the diagnosis in a patient with a suspected iron overdose. (Image contributed by the Toxicology Fellowship of the New York City Poison Center.)

and prognosis. We recommend endoscopy with all intentional caustic ingestions and most nonalkali exposures. In children, stridor, or the combination of drooling and vomiting, should prompt endoscopy.[20] When indicated, endoscopy should be performed within 8–12 hours and no later than 24 hours.

▶ DECONTAMINATION, PREVENTING DRUG ABSORPTION, AND ENHANCED ELIMINATION

Decontamination to prevent adverse effects of poison exposure has long been advocated as a poison management strategy. The concept that removing a poison from the body may avert illness is easily understood by laypersons and clinicians alike, and this strategy seems to make common sense. Despite this, repeated and rigorous testing of gastrointestinal decontamination methods has routinely failed to demonstrate any convincing benefit. Gastrointestinal decontamination plays an increasingly small and marginal role in the management of poisoned patients. External decontamination of the skin and eyes continues to play a vital role in some poison management.

EXTERNAL AND OCULAR DECONTAMINATION

When a toxin is on a patient's body, external decontamination should be performed to protect staff from becoming ill and to limit ongoing toxicity to the patient. This is best performed at a designated shower or mass casualty decontamination area near the entrance of the ED. The patient should be completely disrobed; jewelry, watch, etc., should be removed and the entire

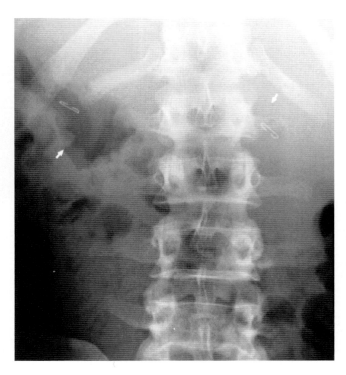

Figure 40-2. A patient in police custody was brought to the emergency department for allegedly ingesting drug packets. The patient admitted swallowing several plastic bags that were stapled closed. (Image contributed by the Toxicology Fellowship of the New York City Poison Center.)

body or exposed area thoroughly washed. For ocular exposures, the eyes are irrigated with copious isotonic solution (such as normal saline or lactated Ringer's) for at least 30 minutes or until a normal ocular pH is obtained. For full efficacy, a Morgan lens should be used in the affected eye, and ocular anesthetic such as tetracaine or proparacaine should be instilled prior to the procedure.[21]

GI DECONTAMINATION

Multiple methods of gastrointestinal decontamination are available to reduce the bioavailability of an ingested toxin. Most of these methods are outdated and provide little clinical benefit; however, there may be scenarios appropriate for their use.

Emesis induced by syrup of ipecac is not recommended for routine use,[22] and we recommend against its use except in the specific scenario of the alert, conscious patient within an hour of a large ingestion of a potentially fatal toxin (not a corrosive substance or hydrocarbon) that is not adsorbed to activated charcoal (AC). Gastrointestinal lavage is the passage of large-bore orogastric tube to administer liquid and aspirate a toxic substance in the stomach. Due to serious risks and limited benefit, there is no place for the routine use of lavage, but use in the critically ill patient with toxic ingestion, depressed mental status, and instability presenting within 1 hour of ingestion may be appropriate.[23,24] Use of nasogastric lavage to aspirate liquid poisons does not carry the risk of orogastric lavage and has been demonstrated to reduce poison absorbed.[23] Nasogastric aspiration of liquid poison may be performed in patients presenting after ingestion of liquid poison who are still anticipated to have poison remaining in the stomach.

Whole bowel irrigation (WBI) is a method of emptying the gastrointestinal tract in order to limit further absorption of a toxin. This is typically done using a warmed polyethylene glycol–electrolyte solution (PEG–ES) at rates of 0.5–1L/h in the adults, which often requires the placement of a nasogastric or orogastric tube.[25] WBI may be performed in select situations, for example, large and potentially fatal ingestions of substances not bound by charcoal such as iron or lead, sustained-release preparations, or in the body packing of illicit substances. It is contraindicated in bowel obstruction, perforation, gastrointestinal hemorrhage, hemodynamic instability, unstable airway, or potential for deterioration of the airway.[25]

Of all methods of gastrointestinal decontamination, AC has the most potential benefit but is still not recommended for routine use in the poisoned patient.[26]

AC may be used at 1 g/kg up to 100 g, and is best performed within 1 hour of ingestion with limitations similar to WBI. It decreases the bioavailability of a wide variety of toxins but is not useful for the ingestions of alcohols, corrosives (acids/alkalis), magnesium, potassium, or metals such as iron and lithium. A majority of the adverse effects related to AC are from aspiration or direct administration of charcoal into the lungs.[27] Clinicians may sedate and intubate a patient in order to administer WBI or AC, but in doing so must recognize that the risk for aspiration, though small, still exists.

ENHANCED ELIMINATION

Enhancing elimination of a toxin is indicated in patients who have decreased elimination of a drug (i.e., renal failure with ingestion of drug that is mainly eliminated in the urine) or in toxins that have a prolonged elimination half-life. Multidose AC may be used in the appropriately alert patient with potential severe toxic or fatal ingestions of carbamazepine, dapsone, phenobarbital, quinine, phenytoin and theophylline, or in cases of ingestion of long-acting or enteric formulations, and in bezoar formation.[28] After the initial dose of AC, administer 0.25–0.5 g/kg Q 2–6 hours for up to 12 hours.

Urine alkalinization is method of enhancing elimination of weakly acidic toxins by trapping them in an

► **TABLE 40-3. SELECTED NORMAL AND TOXIC LAB VALUES FOR COMMON SUBSTANCES, AND POTENTIAL ACTIONS TO BE TAKEN**

Substance	Therapeutic or Normal Level	Toxic or Actionable Level	Action
Acetaminophen	10–30 μg/mL	>150 μg/mL or if toxic on Rumack–Matthew nomogram	N-Acetylcysteine
Caffeine	1–10 μg/mL	>25 μg/mL chronic >90 μg/mL acute	Multiple dose activated charcoal Dialysis
Carboxyhemoglobin	0–2% Up to 10% in smokers	>15% (dependent on pt symptoms/pregnancy)	Oxygen + hyperbaric oxygen chamber
Cyanide	<1 μg/mL		Cyanide antidote kit
Digoxin	0.8–2.0 ng/mL	>2.0 ng/L	DigiFab
Ethylene glycol	0 mg/dL	>25 mg/dL	Fomepizole and/or dialysis
Iron	80–180 μg/dL	>500 μg/dL	Deferoxamine
Lead	<10 μg/dL	>25 μg/dL	Deferoxamine, calcium EDTA, dimercaprol, or succimer
Lithium	0.6–1.2 mEq/L	>2.5 mEq/L chronic >4.0 mEq/L acute	Hemodialysis
Methanol	0 mg/dL	>25 mg/dL	Fomepizole and/or hemodialysis
Methemoglobin	<1%	>15–20%	Methylene blue
Phenobarbital	15–40 mg/L	>100 μg/mL	Hemoperfusion Exchange transfusion in infants
Phenytoin	10–20 mg/L	>30 mg/L	Multidose activated charcoal
Salicylates	15–30 mg/dL	>30 mg/dL chronic >60 mg/dL acute	Urine alkalinization Hemodialysis
Theophylline	5–15 μg/mL	>25 μg/mL chronic >90 μg/mL acute	Multidose activated charcoal Hemoperfusion/dialysis

alkaline urine compartment. This is only recommended as first line for the treatment of moderately severe salicylate poisoning and as second line in the ingestion of fluoride, methotrexate, phenobarbital, 2,4-dichlorophenoxyacetic acid, and mecoprop.[29] A urine pH of 8.0 can be achieved by an initial bolus one to two ampules of sodium bicarbonate followed by an infusion of two to three ampules in 1 L of D5W at 1.5 times maintenance with concurrent aggressive repletion of potassium.

Hemodialysis and charcoal hemoperfusion are the most invasive and expensive methods of enhancing elimination of toxins and have the added advantage of improving acid–base and electrolyte imbalances. Salicylate, methanol, ethylene glycol, theophylline, caffeine, carbamazepine, lithium, and procainamide (refer to Table 40-3) are amenable to dialysis.

ANTIDOTES

Although most management of the poisoned patient is supportive care, the judicious use of an antidote is sometimes the only therapy capable to prevent morbidity or mortality. Examples of this are the administration or hydroxocobalamin or sodium thiosulfate for cyanide poisoning, oxygen for carbon monoxide toxicity, digoxin Fab, fomepizole and/or ethanol for toxic alcohol poisoning, or N-acetylcysteine for acetaminophen toxicity, and calcium for calcium channel blocker overdose.

Critically ill patients who present with symptoms justifying reasonable suspicion for poison exposure can also be treated empirically. Examples of such include empirical use of naloxone in patients with respiratory depression and pinpoint pupils or use of pyridoxine for the child in status epilepticus whose household member is being treated for tuberculosis with isoniazid.

Antivenom exists for the hematologic, neurologic, and cytotoxic effects of the two main categories of snakes in the United States (Elapidae and Crotalinae). There are other antivenoms for scorpions and spiders that are available in specific geographic areas of the United States where they are relevant. There are also antivenins for rare, nonindigenous exotic snakes that are imported and used in zoos and research facilities and occasionally used to treat envenomation from exotic animals illicitly imported and kept as pets. These exotic antivenins tend to be available at facilities that must be prepared for such envenomations, such as zoos or the hospitals that serve them.

REFERENCES

1. Bronstein AC, Spyker DA, Cantilena LR, et al. 2008 annual report of the American Association of Poison Centers' National Poison Data System (NPDS): 26th annual report. *J Clin Toxicol.* 2009;47:911.

2. Liebelt EL, Francis PD, Woolf AD. ECG lead aVR versus QRS interval in predicting seizures and arrhythmias in acute tricyclic antidepressant toxicity. *Ann Emerg Med.* 1995;26(2):19.

3. Liebelt EL, Ulrich A, Francis PD, et al. Serial electrocardiogram changes in acute tricyclic antidepressant overdoses. *Crit Care Med.* 1997;25(10):1721.

4. Boehnert M, Lovejoy FH. Value of the QRS duration versus the serum drug level in predicted seizures and ventricular arrhythmias after acute OD of TCAs. *N Engl J Med.* 1985;313:474.

5. American Heart Association. 2005 American Heart Association guidelines for cardiopulmonary resuscitation and emergency cardiovascular care. Part 10.2: toxicology in ECC. *Circulation.* 2005;112:IV-126.

6. Ishihara K, Szerlip HM. Anion gap acidosis. *Semin Nephrol.* 1998;18(1):83.

7. Glasser L, Sternglanz PD, Combie J, et al. Serum osmolality and its applicability to drug overdose. *Am J Clin Pathol.* 1973;60(5):695.

8. Hoffman RS, Smilkstein MJ, Howland MA, et al. Osmol gaps revisited: normal values and limitations. *J Toxicol Clin Toxicol.* 193;31(1):81.

9. Sporer KA, Khayam-Bashi H. Acetaminophen and salicylate serum levels in patients with suicidal ingestion or altered mental status. *Am J Emerg Med.* 1996;14(5):443.

10. Mongan E, Kelly P, Nies K, et al. Tinnitus as an indication of therapeutic serum salicylate levels. *JAMA.* 1973;226(2):142.

11. McGuigan MA. A two-year review of salicylate deaths in Ontario. *Arch Intern Med.* 1987;147(3):510.

12. Sullivan JB, Hauptman M, Bronstein AC. Lack of observable intoxication in humans with high plasma alcohol concentrations. *J Forensic Sci.* 1987;32(6):1660.

13. Barker SJ, Curry J, Redford D. Measurement of carboxyhemoglobin and methemoglobin by pulse oximetry: a human volunteer study. *Anesthesiology.* 2006;105:892.

14. Kelly AM, McAlpine R, Kyle E. Venous pH can safely replace arterial pH in the initial evaluation of patients in the emergency department. *Emerg Med J.* 2001;18:340.

15. Kellermann AL, Fihn SD, LoGerfo JP, et al. Impact of drug screening in suspected overdose. *Ann Emerg Med.* 1987;16:1206.

16. Mahoney JD, Gross PL, Stern TA, et al. Quantitative serum toxic screening in the management of suspected drug overdose. *Am J Emerg Med.* 1990;8:16.

17. Brett A. Toxicologic analysis in patients with drug overdose. *Arch Intern Med.* 1988;148:2077.

18. Perrone J, De Roos F, Jayaraman S, et al. Drug screening versus history in detection of substance use in ED psychiatric patients. *Am J Emerg Med.* 2001;19:49.

19. Traub SJ, Hoffman RS, Nelson LS. Body packing—the internal concealment of illicit drugs. *N Engl J Med.* 2003;349:2519.

20. Crain EF, Gershel JC, Mezey AP. Caustic ingestions: symptoms as predictors of esophageal injury. *Am J Dis Child.* 1984;138(9):863.

21. Kuckelkorn R, Schrage N, Keller G, et al. Emergency treatment of chemical and thermal eye burns. *Acta Ophthalmol Scand.* 2002;80(1):4.

22. American Academy of Clinical Toxicology, European Association of Poisons Centres and Clinical Toxicologists. Position paper: ipecac syrup. *J Toxicol Clin Toxicol.* 2004;42(2):133.

23. American Academy of Clinical Toxicology, European Association of Poisons Centres and Clinical Toxicologists. Position paper: gastric lavage. *J Toxicol Clin Toxicol.* 2004;42(7):993.

24. Kulig K, Bar-Or D, Cantril SV, et al. Management of acutely poisoned patients without gastric emptying. *Ann Emerg Med.* 1985;14(6):562.

25. American Academy of Clinical Toxicology, European Association of Poisons Centres and Clinical Toxicologists. Position paper: whole bowel irrigation. *J Toxicol Clin Toxicol.* 2004;42(6):843.

26. American Academy of Clinical Toxicology, European Association of Poisons Centres and Clinical Toxicologists. Position paper: single dose activated charcoal. *Clin Toxicol.* 2005;43:61.

27. Sabga E, Dick A, Lertzman M, Tenenbein M. Direct administration of charcoal into the lung and pleural cavity. *Ann Emerg Med.* 1997;30:695.

28. American Academy of Clinical Toxicology, European Association of Poisons Centres and Clinical Toxicologists. Position paper and practice guidelines on the use of multi-dose activated charcoal in the treatment of acute poisoning. *J Toxicol Clin Toxicol.* 1999;37(6):731.

29. Proudfoot AT, Krenzelok EP, Vale JA. Position paper on urine alkalinization. *J Clin Toxicol.* 2004;42(1):1.

CHAPTER 41

The Critically Ill Poisoned Patient

Robert J. Hoffman

▶ INTRODUCTION

The 2001 publication by the American Heart Association, *TOX-ACLS Toxicologic-Oriented Advanced Life Support*,[1] marked wide recognition that critical illness resulting from poisoning may require very different management from similar illness occurring in the nonpoisoned patient. That publication made specific suggestions for management of dysrhythmias and other toxicity caused by cocaine, calcium channel blockers and β-blockers, opioids, tricyclic antidepressants, and drug-induced cardiovascular shock. In 2010, the updated American Heart Association ACLS guidelines contained specific evaluation and recommendations regarding poisoning with these same aforementioned toxins, as well as cyanide, digoxin, and antidotal therapy with flumazenil and lipid emulsion.[2] The relevance of those publications is recognition that proper management of many clinical problems caused by toxins differs or deviates from management of the same clinical problem occurring in the nonpoisoned patient.

The main focus of this chapter is on the most commonly encountered problems in the clinical management of poisoned patients. We present a general approach to management and discuss the unique management issues involving poisoning. This chapter cannot cover all poisoning circumstances that require unique management, but it does cover the most common problems relevant to intensivists.

Although the severe consequences of poisoning and toxicity may cause a wide array of clinical problems, the majority of critical illnesses resulting from poisoning involve the following problems: (1) airway or respiratory compromise, (2) cardiovascular depression manifested as hypotension and/or bradycardia, (3) cardiovascular stimulation manifested as hypertension, tachycardia, and/or tachydysrhythmia, (4) hyperthermia, and (5) seizure and status epilepticus (Table 41-1).

▶ COMPROMISED AIRWAY AND RESPIRATION

As with other clinical circumstances, airway management is nearly universally the primary concern in management of the poisoned patient. Airway compromise, respiratory depression, and/or respiratory compromise must be immediately addressed, and, when possible, their underlying etiology corrected or addressed.

ENDOTRACHEAL INTUBATION AND UNIQUE CONSIDERATIONS

The decision to perform endotracheal intubation in the poisoned patient is based on expectation of lack of continuing airway patency and prognostic factors. Although Glasgow Coma Score (GCS) was not developed to be used as a guide to airway and respiratory status, in many poisonings it can predict the need for endotracheal intubation and/or mechanical ventilation. Patients with a GCS of 6 or less as a result of poisoning often require endotracheal intubation.[3]

There are numerous exceptions to the principle of GCS <6 being predictive of need for intubation, including toxicity from dissociative agents that cause depressed mental status or coma but do not typically compromise airway and respiration.[4] Such agents include ketamine, phencyclidine (PCP), and dextromethorphan; agents that cause waxing and waning respiratory comprise primarily clonidine; γ-hydroxybutyrate (GHB) and its

▶ **TABLE 41-1. UNIQUE MANAGEMENT OF SELECTED TOXINS AND ASSOCIATED ILLNESSES**

Toxin	Effect	Pathophysiology	Unique Therapy
Multiple toxins	Toxin-induced seizure	Multiple pathways	Use benzodiazepines, barbiturates, empirical pyridoxine, or propofol. Do not administer phenytoin
Carbon monoxide	Metabolic acidemia, cardiovascular depression, dysrhythmia, seizure, cardiac arrest	Binds hemoglobin and myoglobin preventing oxygen delivery, binds cytochrome oxidase	Oxygen therapy, hyperbaric oxygen therapy
Caustic exposure	Airway compromise due to burn	Direct tissue injury and inflammation	Emergently secure a definitive airway by endotracheal intubation
Clonidine	Apnea, respiratory depression, cardiovascular depression	Opioidlike effect	Physical stimulation of patient when apneic. High-dose naloxone infusion
Cyanide	Metabolic acidemia, cardiovascular depression, dysrhythmia, seizure, cardiac arrest	Blocks oxidative phosphorylation	Antidotal use of hydroxocobalamin or cyanide antidote kit (nitrites and sodium thiosulfate)
Methemoglobinemia	Metabolic acidemia, cardiovascular depression, dysrhythmia, seizure, cardiac arrest	Alters hemoglobin, preventing oxygen delivery	Methylene blue
Organophosphate	Apnea, bronchorrhea, bronchospasm, cardiovascular depression	Muscarinic cholinergic agonism	Prolonged paralysis may result from neuromuscular blockade due to diminished pseudocholinesterase
Organophosphates	Cholinergic syndrome, bradycardia, bronchorrhea, bronchospasm, cardiovascular depression, dysrhythmia, seizure, cardiac arrest	Inhibits acetylcholinesterase, cholinergic excess	Decontamination outside of clinical care area supersedes A, B, C and resuscitation. Allowing contaminated patient into clinical treatment area risks ongoing patient toxicity and potential poisoning of staff caring for patient
Salicylate	Hyperventilation	Centrally mediated and compensatory to metabolic acidemia	Even brief interruption of hyperventilation may result in rapid or immediate death. Initial respiratory rate and volume initially 150% of normal
Stimulants, hallucinogens	Cardiovascular stimulation; hyperthermia secondary to psychomotor agitation		Use benzodiazepines for agitation, cardiovascular stimulation
Theophylline, caffeine	Cardiovascular depression, dysrhythmia	β-Adrenergic agonism, adenosine antagonism	Short-acting β-blocker administration to treat refractory hypotension
Tricyclic antidepressants	Cardiovascular depression, dysrhythmia	Multiple effects	Use of direct-acting pressors. Use of sodium bicarbonate to reduce sodium channel blockade

congeners may also fit into this category. This latter group may result in apnea and/or respiratory depression that is reversible with stimulation of the patient.

An exceptional circumstance warranting rapid securing of the airway is airway compromise secondary to caustic exposure. Due to the potential for rapid deterioration and loss of ability to secure an airway later, it is advisable to endotracheally intubate patients with caustic exposure and stridor, aphonia, or dysphonia in a manner similar to that conducted for an airway burn.[5]

Certain toxins require specific considerations when performing endotracheal intubation. Poisoning with organophosphate pesticides deactivates pseudocholinesterase, resulting in an extremely prolonged half-life of paralytic agents used for neuromuscular blockade.[6] This should be taken into consideration when administering these medications and when selecting agents based on their half-life and duration of action.

Salicylate toxicity results in metabolic acidemia with respiratory alkalemia due to salicylate stimulation of central respiratory drive and compensatory increase in respiratory drive.[7] In salicylate-poisoned patients, increased minute ventilation is achieved through tachypnea and/or hyperpnea. Interrupting this for even the brief time required to perform endotracheal intubation may result in rapid or immediate seizure or cardiovascular collapse.[8] Endotracheal intubation in a patient with salicylate toxicity should be undertaken only when necessary, and performed by a clinician with the highest capability to complete the procedure rapidly. Immediately after endotracheal intubation, the patient should be ventilated at both a rate and volume 150% of the rate and volume typically used. Serial blood gas analysis will allow rate and volume settings to be adjusted. Failure to maintain hyperventilation may result in rapid or immediate death.

A unique exception to the "airway, breathing, circulation" paradigm familiar to emergency medicine and critical care clinicians is physical decontamination of patients. Allowing a contaminated patient to enter clinical areas without proper decontamination is a well-documented risk to caregivers and other patients, and is capable of rendering an emergency department's critical care unit incapable of providing effective care. Even the presence of patients with detectable odors due to minimally toxic substances has well-recognized potential to be disruptive and generate unease, panic, and hysteria, causing vague, nonspecific but incapacitating symptoms in a manner best described as hysteria or mass hysteria.[9] Accordingly, any patient contaminated with highly toxic substances capable of cross-contaminating staff or clinical areas, such as organophosphate pesticides and certain hydrocarbons, absolutely must be decontaminated in a "hot" or "warm" zone outside the "cool" zone in which only decontaminated patients are managed and in which clinical care is provided. It is an appropriate practice for a contaminated patient to be kept outside of the emergency department, even if unstable, apneic, or in a state of cardiovascular collapse, before being brought inside a clinical care area without decontamination.

When securing the airway in a setting with clinicians wearing personal protective equipment, consider use of a laryngeal mask airway rather than endotracheal intubation, as LMA placement is less impacted by wearing cumbersome PPE suits.[10]

POISONS AFFECTING RESPIRATORY DRIVE AND VENTILATION

Numerous drugs and medications may cause hypoventilation by blunting central respiratory drive, most notably sedative–hypnotic medications such as benzodiazepines, barbiturates, and alcohol, and opioids such as morphine, heroin, and fentanyl.

▶ **TABLE 41-2. DRUGS AND MEDICATIONS CAUSING HYPOVENTILATION**

Baclofen	γ-Hydroxybutyrate
Barbiturates	and analogs
Botulinum toxin	Isopropanol
Carbamates	Methanol
Clonidine	Neuromuscular blockers
Conium maculatum	Nicotine
(Poison Hemlock)	Opioids
Colchicine	Organic phosphorous
Cyclic antidepressants	compounds
Elapid envenomation	Sedative–hypnotics
Electrolyte abnormalities	Strychnine
Ethanol	Tetanus toxin
Ethylene glycol	Tetrodotoxin

Reproduced with permission from Nelson LS, Lewin NA, Howland ME, Hoffman RS, Goldfrank LS, Flomenbaum NE. *Goldfrank's Toxicological Emergencies*. 9th ed. New York: McGraw-Hill Companies Inc; 2010. Table 21-1.

In addition to central blunting of respiratory drive, hypoventilation may occur as a result of impaired chest wall movement. This may be due to weakness or paralysis, as occurs from exposure to botulinum toxin, pesticides and other organophosphates, and neuromuscular blockers, or from hypokalemia and hypermagnesemia. Chest wall rigidity can cause hypoventilation, and may result from tetanus, strychnine, or fentanyl exposure. For fentanyl chest wall rigidity, also termed "wooden chest," use of naloxone in standard or high doses may be attempted. Chest wall rigidity from tetanus or strychnine may be relieved with neuromuscular blockers (Table 41-2).

By far the most common effect, if any, toxin exposure will have on respiratory status is to induce respiratory depression. Certain unique toxins, however, result in increase in central respiratory drive. Caffeine and theophylline, which are used therapeutically to increase respiratory drive in neonatal apnea syndrome,[11] salicylates, and cocaine result in increased respiratory rate by stimulation of central respiratory drive. Salicylates additionally have metabolic effects that cause peripheral effects that increase respiratory drive.

POISONS AFFECTING CELLULAR RESPIRATION

Certain poisons affect respiration on the cellular or molecular level. This may commonly result from alteration of hemoglobin to form methemoglobin or carboxyhemoglobin, both of which are incapable of normal oxygen delivery. Cellular or molecular impairment of respiration may also occur by interference with oxidative phosphorylation, such as by poisoning with cyanide, carbon monoxide, or hydrogen sulfide.

Methemoglobin

Methemoglobinemia results from oxidative stress on hemoglobin that results in iron oxidation to the ferric (Fe^{3+}) rather than standard ferrous (Fe^{2+}) state.[12] This derivative of hemoglobin binds H_2O rather than oxygen, and does not deliver oxygen to tissues. Methemoglobinemia presents clinically with expected results of hypoxia: tachypnea, dyspnea, and severe cyanosis. Pulse oximetry readings in this condition are inaccurate due to inability of standard pulse oximeters to interpret methemoglobin light absorption, as standard pulse oximeters are only intended to quantify oxyhemoglobin and deoxyhemoglobin. Methemoglobinemia typically results in pulse oximetry readings that range from 75% to 85% on standard pulse oximeters. Co-oximeters are capable of precisely measuring oxyhemoglobin, deoxyhemoglobin, methemoglobin, and carboxyhemoglobin, and can accurately quantify the precise methemoglobin level.[13] They are laboratory devices that interpret blood gas samples, not to be confused with pulse oximeters, which are bedside devices that estimate hemoglobin saturation using light absorption. Normal methemoglobin levels are 0.5–3%. Methemoglobin levels >10% may be associated with symptomatic illness, and levels >50% may result in rapid death. Treatment of methemoglobinemia involves administration of high-flow oxygen and chemical reduction of the methemoglobin back to hemoglobin using methylene blue.

In the normal state, small quantities of methemoglobin may be converted back to hemoglobin through an NADH-dependent reaction catalyzed by cytochrome b_5 reductase. This is the mechanism by which nontoxic quantities of methemoglobin that form during day-to-day exposure to oxidants correct methemoglobinemia. During severe methemoglobinemia, this reaction is insufficient, and an alternative metabolic pathway that does not function without the aid of an exogenously administered reducing agent is needed. The reducing agent used therapeutically is methylene blue, and it works by action through the hexose monophosphate shunt to reduce methemoglobin, yielding normal, functional hemoglobin.

Optimal methylene blue dosing is unknown, and numerous varied recommended doses exist. Methylene blue may result in hemolysis in G6PD-deficient persons, and should be avoided or used with extreme caution in them. Dosing of methylene blue is 1–2 mg/kg given IV over 5 minutes.[14] Response is usually very rapid, but if methemoglobin levels remain elevated, 1 hour later methylene blue may be readministered at the same dose. Methylene blue interferes with pulse oximetry reading, and continued use of co-oximetry by measurement of venous blood gas samples is required to monitor methemoglobin levels. Dapsone toxicity may cause prolonged methemoglobinemia due to the long half-life of dapsone. Repeated treatments with methylene blue, not to exceed 5 mg/kg/24 hours, may be required in symptomatic patients.

Carbon Monoxide

Carbon monoxide is a by-product of combustion. Carbon monoxide poisoning typically results from closed-space fires or by exposure to exhaust from combustion engines. Carbon monoxide binds hemoglobin with an affinity approximately 250 times greater than that of oxygen.[15] Carbon monoxide binding of hemoglobin results in carboxyhemoglobin, which is a nonfunctional form of hemoglobin that does not transport oxygen.

Clinical problems resulting from acute carbon monoxide poisoning include headache, nausea, vomiting, disorientation, altered mental status or coma, syncope, seizure, and cardiac arrest. Chronic carbon monoxide poisoning presents differently, often with headache and malaise that may be misdiagnosed as a viral syndrome.

Carboxyhemoglobin is not detected by standard bedside pulse oximetry. Pulse oximeters misinterpret carboxyhemoglobin as oxyhemoglobin, and therefore give a falsely normal pulse oximetry reading in patients with carbon monoxide poisoning. Co-oximetry measurement of carboxyhemoglobin level in venous or arterial blood gas is required to quantify degree of carbon monoxide binding of hemoglobin. There is no "normal" carboxyhemoglobin level, but average persons have levels <3% that may result from exposure to automobile exhaust and other sources. Smokers have notably higher carbon monoxide levels[16] based on how heavily they smoke, and they may have baseline carboxyhemoglobin levels as high as 10%.

Symptomatic illness from carbon monoxide poisoning may occur acutely with any level of carboxyhemoglobin, but is typical at levels >10%. Depending on health of the patient, severe illness and injury may occur with carboxyhemoglobin levels as low as 10%, although healthy individuals usually tolerate higher levels. Significant acute carbon monoxide poisoning results from levels >25%, and levels >45% are immediately life threatening.[17]

Treatment of carbon monoxide toxicity involves administering supplemental oxygen. This may be normobaric, or if possible hyperbaric oxygen. Hyperbaric oxygen does not have notable immediate benefit to the patient, but is administered to prevent the potentially devastating neurologic sequelae of poisoning.[18] These sequelae include a Parkinson-like syndrome and extreme neuropsychiatric disability that may render the patient incapable to work, study, or pursue the usual activities of daily living.

Cyanide

Cyanide toxicity results from cyanide binding to cytochrome a_3, which interferes with oxidative phosphorylation. This prevents cellular respiration, in effect suffocating the tissues on a cellular level. Cyanide exposure may result from inhalation of smoke in closed-space fires.[19,20] Fires have been recognized to often produce copious quantities of cyanide that result from burning of plastic, polyurethane, rubber, silk, wool, and many other materials typically contained in homes and offices. Cyanide poisoning may result iatrogenically from prolonged use of nitroprusside, which contains cyanide and the antiquated antineoplastic agent laetrile. Certain plants, such as pits or seed from peaches, apricots, plums, pears, apples, and bitter almond, are cyanogenic. Cyanide is used commonly in the jewelry industry and in some fields such as photography. Homicidal and suicidal use of cyanide is well reported.

Cyanide toxicity presents clinically with acute onset of severe illness after exposure. This is typically syncope, coma, seizure, cardiac dysrhythmia, or cardiac arrest. Due to inability to use oxygen in oxidative phosphorylation, fair-skinned patients typically have a flushed, pink appearance. Lab corroboration of cyanide toxicity may be obtained by comparing arterial and venous blood gas samples drawn simultaneously and by noting a lack of oxygen extraction across the capillary bed.[21] Metabolic acidemia is always present and usually severe. In the setting of closed-space fires, lactate concentration >10 mmol/L is pathognomonic or cyanide toxicity.[19] This appears to be true regardless of the presence of carbon monoxide poisoning or the extent of body surface burn.[19]

Serum cyanide levels are rarely clinically available, but are of use if they can be obtained rapidly. Cyanide levels <1.0 mg/L correlate with tachycardia and flushing, 1.0–2.5 mg/L with altered mental status, seizure, and hypotension, and levels >3.0 mg/L are typically rapidly fatal.

Treatment for cyanide toxicity involves use of hydroxocobalamin, which is the optimal antidote, or use of all or part of the cyanide antidote kit, which is a combination of amyl nitrite pearls, sodium nitrite, and sodium thiosulfate.[22,23]

Cyanide antidote therapy should be given to any patient with known or suspected exposure to cyanide or from a closed-space fire if he or she has metabolic acidemia, elevation of lactate concentration, loss of consciousness or altered mental status, shock, cardiac dysrhythmia, or cardiac arrest.

Hydroxocobalamin, a vitamin B_{12} precursor, directly binds cyanide to form vitamin B_{12}, which is harmless and excreted in the urine. Dosing of hydroxocobalamin is 70 mg/kg, to a maximum dose of 5 g, given IV over 30 minutes. In cases of cardiac arrest, it can be given as an IV push. The dose can be repeated to a maximum total of 15 g. Use of hydroxocobalamin may subsequently interfere with pulse oximetry readings and co-oximetry readings, rendering it difficult or impossible to know oxygen saturation, leaving only measurements of P_{O_2} as a guide.[24] These interferences may last as long as several days.

Use of the cyanide antidote kit involves three parts: amyl nitrite inhalation pearls, sodium nitrite for IV administration, and sodium thiosulfate for IV administration. Nitrates are used to induce methemoglobinemia. These are only used in cyanide toxicity not resulting from closed-space fires and smoke inhalation. After closed-space fire, carbon monoxide poisoning may concomitantly be present, and decrease oxygen-carrying capacity by causing formation of methemoglobin is contraindicated. For patients who possibly have carbon monoxide poisoning, only the sodium thiosulfate portion of the kit is administered.[22] This works by enhancing formation of cyanomethemoglobin through the enzyme rhodanese.

Use of the various portions of the kit are as follows: amyl nitrite pearl is crushed and inhaled for 1 minute until IV access is obtained. The sodium nitrite dose is 10 mL of the 3% solution included in the kit; pediatric dosing is 0.33 mL/kg. Hypotension may result from nitrite use. Nitrites are intended to cause methemoglobinemia; if methemoglobin level >10–15% is not induced by the initial dosing of sodium nitrite, half of the original dose may be administered 30–60 minutes after the first dose.

Sodium thiosulfate is administered as 12.5 g IV, which is the full 50-mL bottle of 25% sodium thiosulfate solution included in the kit. The pediatric dose is 1.65 mL/kg of the same 25% solution. Repeat dosing of sodium thiosulfate may be given as one half of the original dose 30–60 minutes after the initial dose.

▶ CARDIOVASCULAR DEPRESSION

Cardiovascular depression in the form of hypotension and/or bradycardia may result from exposure to cardioselective medications, such as digoxin, β-adrenergic antagonists, calcium channel antagonists, and clonidine, and also occurs from numerous other toxins. As a preterminal event, cardiovascular depression may result secondary to toxicity from any poison, including cardiovascular stimulants. Treatment of cardiovascular depression from certain toxins, particularly cardioselective medications, may require very specific, unique therapy.

Asymptomatic hypotension and/or bradycardia, particularly in the absence of end-organ manifestations, do not necessarily indicate treatment. The lower limit at which clinicians are comfortable allowing heart rate

▶ **TABLE 41-3. DRUGS AND MEDICATIONS CAUSING BRADYCARDIA**

α_1-Adrenergic agonists (reflex bradycardia)
  Phenylephrine
  Phenylpropanolamine
α_2-Adrenergic agonists (centrally acting)
  Clonidine
  Methyldopa
β-Adrenergic antagonists
Antidysrhythmics
  Amiodarone
  Sotalol
Calcium channel blockers
Cardioactive steroids
Cholinergics
  Carbamates or organic phosphorous compounds
  Edrophonium
  Neostigmine
  Physostigmine
Opioids
Sedative–hypnotics
Sodium channel openers
  Aconitine
  Andromedotoxin
  Ciguatoxin
  Veratridine

Reproduced with permission from Nelson LS, Lewin NA, Howland ME, Hoffman RS, Goldfrank LS, Flomenbaum NE. *Goldfrank's Toxicological Emergencies.* 9th ed. New York: McGraw-Hill Companies Inc; 2010:333. Table 23-2. Chapter Hemodynamic Principles.

or blood pressure to remain varies. Generally, maintaining the heart rate at 45 beats/min or greater, systolic blood pressure >90 mm Hg, and diastolic blood pressure >40 mm Hg are limits above which vital signs should be maintained.

Intravenous fluid bolus, atropine, and pressors may be used to treat cardiovascular depression with exceptions noted here. Bradycardia resulting from most cardioactive medications infrequently responds to atropine because homeostatic mechanisms will have already decreased or removed vagal tone in an attempt to compensate. Use of atropine is not contraindicated for medications such as digoxin, β-adrenergic antagonists, calcium channel antagonists, and clonidine, but more effective and definitive therapy should not be delayed due to atropine administration.

Pressors similarly may lack their typical effectiveness when used in poisoned patients. As with all patients, care should be exercised in balancing attempts to maintain central arterial or venous pressure with end-organ or extremity capillary perfusion pressure to prevent paradoxical hypoperfusion of organs, digits, and extremities with high-dose pressor infusions (Tables 41-3 and 41-4).

TRICYCLIC ANTIDEPRESSANT HYPOTENSION

If an indirect or mixed-acting pressor is used without success, particularly in cases of hypotension from tricyclic antidepressants, norepinephrine should be initiated. The pathophysiology of cyclic antidepressant poisoning may result in catecholamine depletion to a degree that no quantity of an indirect-acting agent such as dopamine will be effective, and norepinephrine or epinephrine may be necessary.

DIGOXIN CARDIOVASCULAR DEPRESSION

Specific unique therapies for cardioactive medication toxicity may be indicated. Cardiotoxicity from digoxin, digitoxin, or other cardioactive steroids such as bufotoxin may be treated with digoxin-specific Fab.[25] Although this antidote is produced for digoxin, cross-specificity with digitoxin, bufotoxin from toad species, oleandrin from oleander, and other botanical cardiac glycosides typically respond to digoxin-specific Fab. Empirical dosing for acute digitoxin toxicity is 10–15 vials in adults or children. In cases of oleander, toad, or other related poisoning, the typical dose for acute digoxin toxicity may be used, and additional doses may be needed.

β-BLOCKER CARDIOVASCULAR DEPRESSION

β-Blocker toxicity typically does not respond significantly to IV fluid, atropine, or pressors. Glucagon is often effective as a result of its activity, since it is independent and unaffected by blockade of the β-adrenergic receptors.[26] An empirical dose of glucagon is 5 mg SC or IV in adults, 1 mg in children <20 kg, or 2 mg in children >20 kg. If effective, glucagon may be administered again as necessary. If glucagon therapy proves to be ineffective, more than two consecutive attempts to restore cardiovascular function should not be attempted using this therapy.

CALCIUM CHANNEL BLOCKER CARDIOVASCULAR DEPRESSION

Calcium channel antagonists are unique cardiotoxins. Due to calcium channel blockade, patients with calcium channel antagonist overdose often maintain normal mentation even in the state of extremely low systolic and mean arterial blood pressure. This phenomenon is so characteristic and notable that normal mental status in the presence of extreme hypotension/bradycardia should be considered highly suggestive of calcium channel antagonist toxicity.

▶ TABLE 41-4. **HEART RATE AND ECG ABNORMALITIES OF DRUGS CAUSING HYPOTENSION**

Heart Rate	Characterstics EGC Abnormalities		
	Sinus Rhythm	Heart Block or Prolonged Intervals	Dysrhythmia

Bradycardia	α_2-Adrenergic agonists
	Opioids
	Sedative–hypnotics
		β-Adrenergic antagonists
		Calcium channel blockers
		Cholinergics
		Cardioactive steroids
		Magnesium (severe)
		Methadone
		Propafenone
		Sotalol
			Digoxin
			Plant toxins
			   Aconitine
			   Andromedotoxin
			   Veratrine
			Propafenone
			Propoxyphene
			Sotalol

Tachycardia	Angiotensin-converting enzyme inhibitors Anticholinergics Arterial dilators Bupropion Cocaine Disulfiram Diuretics Iron Yohimbine	Anticholinergics Antidysrhythmics Antihistamines Arsenics Bupropion Cocaine Cyclic antidepressants Phenothiazines Quinine/chloroquine	Anticholinergics Antidysrhythmics Antihistamines Arsenics Chloral hydrate Cocaine Cyclic antidepressants Methylxanthines Noncyclic antidepressants Phenothiazines Sympathomimetics

Reproduced with permission from Nelson LS, Lewin NA, Howland ME, Hoffman RS, Goldfrank LS, Flomenbaum NE. *Goldfrank's Toxicological Emergencies.* 9th ed. New York: McGraw-Hill Companies Inc; 2010:336. Table 23-6. Chapter Hemodynamic Principles.

Therapy for calcium channel antagonists includes administration of high-dose calcium. Calcium gluconate or calcium glubionate is effective and its concentration is safe to be used in peripheral veins. Calcium chloride contains three times the elemental calcium of calcium gluconate and therefore has some advantage in use. Extreme caution must be exercised to avoid extravasation of calcium chloride. An antidotal therapy used regularly for the past decade that is highly effective in treating calcium channel antagonist-induced cardiovascular depression is insulin–euglycemia.[27]

Pathophysiologically, the healthy myocardium uses free fatty acids for energy. Myocardium that is unhealthy, stressed, or in a shock state will utilize glucose for energy, and it is believed that this is the mechanism by which insulin–glucose infusion aids calcium channel blocker–induced cardiovascular depression.

HYPERINSULINEMIA/ EUGLYCEMIA THERAPY

Insulin–euglycemia therapy involves initiating a 1-U/kg bolus of regular insulin with 0.5 g/kg of dextrose. If the blood glucose is >400 mg/dL prior to the insulin bolus, no glucose bolus is necessary. After the initial bolus, an insulin infusion of 0.5–1.0 U/kg/h with a continuous dextrose infusion beginning at 0.5 g/kg/h should be started. This dextrose is best infused at D25 or

D50 given by central venous access to limit free water administration. The dextrose infusion may be titrated to give more or less dextrose as needed to maintain acceptable serum glucose.

Cardiac function should be reassessed every 20–30 minutes. In cases of persistent cardiovascular depression, the insulin infusion may be increased in increments of 0.5 U/kg/h every 30 minutes if needed to a maximum dose of 2.5 U/kg/h. Increasing the insulin infusion dose will require increase in the amount of dextrose infused.

The initial response to insulin–euglycemia therapy is typically not seen immediately, and it may take 20–40 minutes after initiation of therapy to detect clinical response in cases in which the therapy is successful.

It is critical to monitor the blood glucose frequently during this therapy, every 30 minutes at minimum until stable, and then every 1 hour after the insulin infusion, glucose infusion, and blood glucose are stable. It is also necessary to monitor the serum potassium, since some degree of hypokalemia is expected. Stable hypokalemia at levels down to 2.5 mEq/L does not require supplemental potassium administration.

LIPID EMULSION THERAPY

Lipid emulsion therapy may be used in treatment of lipophilic cardiotoxins of all types: calcium channel blocker, β-blocker, local anesthetic, tricyclic antidepressants, and others.[28] Lipid emulsion is administered as an initial bolus of intralipid or other lipid emulsion in a 20% concentration in a 1.5 mL/kg followed by 0.25 mL/kg/min or 15 mL/kg/h to run for 30 or 60 minutes. Occasionally a prolonged infusion in a dose of 1–2 g/kg per day or 5–10 mL/kg per day is necessary. Although propofol contains lipid, it should never be used as the agent to provide the lipid for this antidotal therapy. The quantity of propofol to lipid is such that an extremely toxic overdose of propofol would be necessary to deliver an adequate dose of lipid for lipid emulsion therapy.

CLONIDINE CARDIOVASCULAR DEPRESSION

Clonidine is an α-agonist with opioidlike effects, and toxicity often mimics the opioid toxidrome of miosis, coma, and apnea.[29] In known or suspected clonidine toxicity, high-dose naloxone may be used if the patient is not opioid tolerant. Opioid-tolerant patients are expected to have severe opioid withdrawal as a result of naloxone administration. This may result in severe vomiting and aspiration if depressed mental status is present. If high-dose naloxone is effective at improving respiratory effort or cardiovascular depression resulting from clonidine, an infusion of two-thirds of the dose that achieved clinical response given hourly is recommended. This may be titrated as needed.

CAFFEINE AND THEOPHYLLINE HYPOTENSION

Therapy of hypotension resulting from severe theophylline or caffeine toxicity is best carried out by typical use of IV fluid and pressors. If this is unsuccessful, administration of a short-acting β-adrenergic antagonist, such as esmolol, may be highly effective in reducing or eliminating hypotension.[30]

It is useful to discuss the underlying pathophysiology by which a β-blocker is used to treat hypotension: Hypotension from theophylline or caffeine results from excess β-stimulation, including $β_2$, which causes hypotension. This hypotension may involve a characteristically widened pulse pressure, in which the difference between systolic and diastolic pressures may be 150% or greater than the diastolic pressure. Blockade of $β_2$ agonism in such cases may result in rapid and complete resolution of hypotension as well as typical metabolic effects of theophylline toxicity such as hyperglycemia and hypokalemia.[29] Esmolol is preferred due to a titratable effect; long-acting β-blockers are not recommended.

▶ CARDIOVASCULAR STIMULATION

Cardiovascular stimulation in the form of hypertension, tachycardia, and/or tachydysrhythmia commonly results from a variety of poisonings. Cocaine toxicity is the commonly encountered situation requiring unique therapy to control cardiovascular stimulation.

Cocaine causes release of large quantities of catecholamines in a dose-dependent manner. Therefore, the primary pharmacologic treatment of cocaine toxicity, including cardiovascular stimulation and cocaine chest pain, is benzodiazepines, often required in very large doses. Benzodiazepines counteract this effect and typically result in abatement of hypertension, tachycardia, as well as psychomotor agitation.

After liberal administration of benzodiazepines, use of antihypertensives may be required. During the initial years of the introduction of crack cocaine into the United States, numerous case reports followed by large case series documented a paradoxical rise in blood pressure in cocaine-intoxicated patients treated with β-blockers. Some of these resulted in catastrophic or fatal intracranial hemorrhage and other sequelae of severe hypertension. The mechanism by which β-blockers may cause increased rather than decreased blood pressure in cocaine-intoxicated patients is by removal of β-adrenergic tone, leaving unopposed α-adrenergic tone and extreme vasoconstriction. For this reason, β-blockers should generally be avoided in management of cocaine-induced cardiovascular stimulation. If benzodiazepine therapy is inadequate to control cardiovascular stimulation, use of phentolamine is preferred to treat hypertension. Other therapies may include use of nitrites such as nitroglycerine or nitroprusside, calcium channel blockers, and both conduction-modulating agents such as verapamil or diltiazem and newer agents such as nifedipine, nicardipine, and others.

Some centers do not adhere to the admonishment to avoid β-blocker use. In such settings, labetalol is often used because it has some degree of α- as well as β-blockade. Use of other β-blockers should only follow or accompany concomitant use of an α-blocking agent such as phentolamine.

Sympathetic nervous system stimulation by cholinergic poisons such as pesticides is a less commonly encountered situation requiring unique care. Acetylcholine excess may cause muscarinic excess, secondary bradycardia/hypotension, or nicotinic excess with secondary stimulation of the sympathetic chain ganglia and tachycardia/hypertension. It may also cause alternation between cardiovascular stimulation and depression. For this reason, management of cardiovascular stimulation secondary to cholinergic poisons such as organophosphates should be managed by use of short-acting, titratable medications such as esmolol or nitroprusside. Such use allows rapid cessation of the medication if the

▶ **TABLE 41-5.** **DRUGS AND MEDICATIONS CAUSING HYPERTENSION**

Hypertensive Effects Mediated by α-Adrenergic Receptor Interaction	Hypertensive Effects Not Mediated by α-Adrenergic Receptor Interaction
Direct α-receptor agonists	β-Andrenergic receptor
Clonidine[b]	agonists[a]
Epinephrine	Nonselective
Ergotamines	Isoproterenol
Methoxamine	Cholinergics[b]
Norepinephrine	Corticosteroids
Phenylephrine	Nicotine[b]
Tetrahydrozoline	Thromboxane A_2
Indirect-acting agonists	Vasopressin
Amphetamines	
Cocaine	
Dexfenfluramine	
Monoamine oxidase	
inhibitors	
Phencyclidine	
Yohimbine	
Direct- and indirect-acting	
agonists	
Dopamine	
Ephedrine	
Metaraminol	
Naphazoline	
Oxymetazoline	
Phenylpropanolamine	
Pseudoephedrine	

Reproduced with permission from Nelson LS, Lewin NA, Howland ME, Hoffman RS, Goldfrank LS, Flomenbaum NE. *Goldfrank's Toxicological Emergencies.* 9th ed. New York: McGraw-Hill Companies Inc; 2010:335. Table 23-5. Chapter Hemodynamic Principles.
[a]These can also cause hypotension.
[b]These may cause transient hypertension followed by hypotension.

patient transitions from a state of cardiovascular stimulation to cardiovascular depression (Table 41-5).

▶ HYPERTHERMIA

Pathophysiologically, there are several ways in which poison exposure and toxicity may result in hyperthermia. By alteration of normal mental state, cognition, and psychomotor agitation, patients may be unaware of own temperatures or that of their surroundings. They may fail to avoid exercise or activity in hot ambient environments, become unable to leave the environment, or continue to exert themselves while restrained. Examples include becoming comatose in a closed automobile during daytime, and comatose on a hot surface such as asphalt, where heat gain by conduction may occur quickly. Commonly, this may occur with drugs of abuse such as ethanol, cocaine, opioids, and PCP.

Psychomotor agitation associated with drugs of abuse may also result in significant heat production.

Such cases are understandably more common in warmer months, summer in the Northern hemisphere and winter in the Southern hemisphere. A clear relationship between deaths from cocaine hyperthermia and ambient temperature exists: Deaths from cocaine hyperthermia in New York City, for example, dramatically peak during the warmest summer months and are rare during other times.[31] This is likely true for other drugs that cause psychomotor agitation and hyperthermia, as well.

Other pathophysiologic mechanisms for hyperthermia include uncoupling of oxidative phosphorylation, such as with salicylate or dinitrophenol toxicity; increased metabolism, such as from thyroid hormone or thyroid extract toxicity; impaired sweating, such as from antihistamines and anticholinergics; vasoconstriction due to α-adrenergic agonism, such as from amphetamines, cocaine, pseudoephedrine, and other sympathomimetics. Malignant hyperthermia (MH), resulting from ryanodine receptor dysfunction, as well as serotonin syndrome (SS) and neuroleptic malignant syndrome (NMS), is discussed later in this chapter.

Although different pathophysiology underlies the manner in which hyperthermia is reached, the initial acute treatments are similar. The temperature at which permanent neurologic injury will occur in any patient cannot be known, but a core temperature of 107°F or 42°C warrants active cooling, preferably by immersion in ice or an ice bath. Tepid sponging, mist spray and fans, or other less effective measures should only be used in the extraordinary instance when true ice immersion cannot be achieved.

A simple method of ice immersion is placing the patient in a partially closed body bag enclosed with ice. Covering the patient in ice and wrapping in a sheet or blanket is also suitable, understanding that this will quickly result in water pooling on the floor surrounding the patient as the ice melts. If a cholera bed is available, this aids in collection of melting ice water and is preferable from a nursing and housekeeping perspective. Using immersion makes cardiopulmonary monitoring more difficult.

Typically patients with hyperthermia resulting from psychomotor agitation, hypermetabolism, or uncoupled oxidative phosphorylation do not typically feel uncomfortable in an ice pack or ice bath. After some period of time when the temperature decreases, they may communicate that they feel cold or uncomfortable, and this often correlates with reaching a goal temperature of 100–102°F. Care should be taken to carefully monitor patients to avoid overcooling below normal body temperature.

Treatment of psychomotor agitation should include chemical restraint by benzodiazepine administration. Use of haloperidol is contraindicated for this purpose as it lowers seizure threshold, results in increased incidence of cardiac dysrhythmia, and impairs heat dissipation. In cases of true MH, dantrolene is indicated. Dantrolene is often errantly used for hyperthermia from causes other than MH, in which there is no potential benefit and thus the small risk of use is not justified. Use of COX inhibitors such as aspirin, acetaminophen, ibuprofen, ketorolac, naproxen, or others plays no role whatsoever in toxin-induced hyperthermia.

HYPERTHERMIC SYNDROMES: SEROTONIN SYNDROME, NEUROLEPTIC MALIGNANT SYNDROME, AND MALIGNANT HYPERTHERMIA

SS, NMS, and MH are toxin-induced illnesses that result in hyperthermia by different mechanisms (Table 41-6). These syndromes have significant overlap in clinical presentation, but careful evaluation can clearly differentiate between them. Hotline numbers for the Neuroleptic Malignant Syndrome Information Service are 1-888-667-8367 and 1-315-464-4001. Another hotline to aid in management of MH is the Malignant Hyperthermia Association of the United States, which can be reached at 1-800-644-9737 or 1-315-434-7079. These services are intended to provide advice about diagnosis and management of NMS and MH, respectively. They are supported by medical toxicologists and are able to

assist in differentiating NMS, MH, and SS, and to make treatment recommendations.

Onset of illness and progression of illness are distinct for SS, NMS, and MH. SS develops over hours and universally <24 hours after exposure to the serotonin agonist. SS is rapidly progressive, and can quickly transition from mild illness to critical instability or death in hours. This helps differentiate from NMS, which develops over days, and for which both the progression and resolution occur over a more prolonged time period. MH develops more acutely than both SS and NMS, within minutes to hours, and nearly universally within 12 hours of exposure to the causal medication(s). It may rapidly progress and rapidly dissipate. As a result, initial diagnosis and treatment of MH infrequently involves emergency medicine or critical care physicians, usually occurs in operating rooms or postoperative recovery rooms, and is overseen by anesthesiologists managing the patient at that time.

Serotonin Syndrome

SS results from excess serotonergic agonism, typically as a result of exposure to two or more serotonin agonists or massive exposure to a single serotonin agonist. It characteristically causes mental status changes, autonomic hyperactivity, and neuromuscular abnormalities. Alteration of mental status usually does not involve coma or impaired consciousness. Typically it is anxiety,

▶ **TABLE 41-6. COMPARISON OF FINDINGS IN SEROTONIN SYNDROME, NEUROLEPTIC MALIGNANT SYNDROME, AND MALIGNANT HYPERTHERMIA**

Illness	Onset	Mental Status	Muscular Changes	Vital Signs	Offending Agent(s)	Treatment
Serotonin syndrome	Hours	Confused, agitated	Twitching, fasciculation, shivering, hyperreflexia	Severe hyperthermia, hypertension, tachycardia, hypotension, and bradycardia when deteriorating	Serotonergic medications and drugs of abuse	Cyproheptadine, active cooling
Neuroleptic malignant syndrome	Days	Catatonic, mute	Catatonic, lead-pipe rigidity	Mild hyperthermia <102.5°F	Neuroleptic antipsychotic agents, withdrawal of anti-Parkinson dopamine agonists	Bromocriptine
Malignant hyperthermia	Minutes to hours	Poorly defined, patient usually sedated or anesthetized	Rigidity, may not be present if already paralyzed	Elevated EtCO$_2$ Severe hyperthermia	Inhalational anesthetics, succinylcholine	Dantrolene, active cooling

disorientation, psychomotor agitation, and hyperalertness, with patients startling easily. The neuromuscular findings may be hyperreflexia, clonus, tremor, muscle rigidity, myoclonus, hyperreflexia, and a unique form of shivering that is sometimes rhythmic and progressive along the torso, similar to that of a dog shaking water from its coat. Autonomic manifestations are tachycardia and hypertension, with hyperthermia.

To fulfill Hunter criteria to diagnose SS, the patient must have been exposed to a serotonergic medication or drug, and have any of the following: (1) spontaneous clonus; (2) inducible clonus plus agitation or diaphoresis; (3) ocular clonus plus agitation or diaphoresis; (4) tremor and hyperreflexia; (5) hypertonia; (6) temperature >38°C plus ocular clonus or inducible clonus.

Laboratory abnormalities include myoglobinuria, elevated creatine phosphokinase (CPK), and hyperkalemia. In suspected cases, obtain blood gas analysis with lactate concentration, serum electrolytes, liver function tests, and CBC.

Treatment of SS includes maintaining vital signs within acceptable limits, including cooling to <39°C (102.2°F), and use of benzodiazepines, as well as possibly cyproheptadine. Benzodiazepines treat agitation, serve as muscle relaxants, and are useful because the CNS side effects of benzodiazepines do not overlap with CNS changes that result from SS. Lorazepam 0.05–0.1 mg/kg IV is given every 20–30 minutes until clinical effect is reached, followed by repeat administration at the appropriate dose in 2- to 6-hour periods. Diazepam 0.1–0.5 mg/kg may also be used, with initial doses repeated every 10–15 minutes and repeat dosing every 1–2 hours as needed. If benzodiazepines fail to sedate thoroughly, cyproheptadine is given empirically in adults as a 12-mg initial dose followed by 2 mg every 2 hours until symptoms resolve. Dosing would be modified on a weight basis in children.

Cyproheptadine is only available in a PO formulation, but can be crushed and injected down a nasogastric tube to patients with altered mental status. Medications such as chlorpromazine and olanzapine should not be used, since they lower seizure threshold and increase risk of developing NMS.

Neuroleptic Malignant Syndrome

NMS is an extrapyramidal syndrome associated with hyperthermia, muscle rigidity, autonomic instability, and altered mental status. This occurs predominantly with use of antipsychotics and less commonly when anti-Parkinson dopamine agonists are withdrawn.

NMS occurs in particular with potent antipsychotics such as haloperidol and fluphenazine, and with depot formulations such as long-acting depot haloperidol injection, but it has been reported to occur from all classes of neuroleptic drugs, as well as new atypical antipsychotic agents.

Epidemiologically, NMS occurs more commonly in males and in younger patients, but can occur in any gender or age patient. NMS is an idiosyncratic reaction, meaning it is not dose dependent. It may occur with the first dose of medication or may occur in a patient who has been receiving the medication for years without any adverse side effects. NMS occurs more frequently within the first 2 weeks of initiating a neuroleptic or antipsychotic treatment, with depot injection use, and with rapid dose escalation. The pathophysiology and etiology of NMS are unknown, but are widely believed to be mediated by central dopamine antagonism.

As mentioned, NMS may be differentiated from SS by timing of onset. NMS symptoms typically develop over several days, whereas SS develops over hours. Because NMS occurs in patients with psychiatric illness and is slower in onset, there is more likely to be delayed or missed diagnosis. Hyperthermia, altered mental status, autonomic instability, and muscle rigidity are universally present in patients with NMS.

Hyperthermia is usually not as extreme as with SS or NMS, with temperatures typically in the range of 38–39°C (100.4–102.2°F) and uncommonly greater than 40°C (104°F). Muscular rigidity with NMS is more catatonic, lead-pipe rigidity, whereas SS is associated with fasciculation, twitching, shivering, and hyperreflexia. Mental status changes are also more similar to those of catatonic states, and patients may be mute, stuporous, or comatose.

Lab testing is critical in management of NMS. Elevations of CPK may be severe. Rhabdomyolysis and myoglobinuric renal failure may result. Expectedly, associated electrolyte abnormalities may include hyperkalemia and mild elevations of lactate. Low serum iron concentration has >95% sensitivity in detecting NMS.[32]

Management of NMS includes immediate discontinuation of the offending drug and supportive care with correction of dehydration and electrolyte imbalance. Cooling to decrease temperature to acceptable range may be carried out by the physical methods mentioned earlier in this section. Pharmacologic treatment for NMS should be administered. Hyperthermia from NMS is usually less severe than SS, and typically will not require the aggressive measures to lower temperature that are commonly needed for SS.

Pharmacologic therapy for NMS includes bromocriptine, which agonizes dopamine receptors. This is only available as a PO formulation, and may be crushed and given by nasogastric tube. Dosing is 2.5 mg PO Q 6–8 hourly. It is recommended to continue this for 10–14 days after the symptoms of NMS have resolved. Amantadine may be used instead of bromocriptine. Benzodiazepines may also be used for muscle relaxation and to relieve psychomotor agitation. Lorazepam

2 mg IV/PO Q 6 h is typically effective, but this dose may be increased as necessary.

NMS resolution typically takes days to weeks, on average 5–15 days, to resolve. This is in contrast to SS, for which onset and resolution are often within hours.

Malignant Hyperthermia

MH is a hypermetabolic crisis typically encountered in the setting of anesthesia administration, and may be seen in genetically susceptible patients who receive inhalational anesthetics and/or succinylcholine. As previously mentioned, MH is rarely encountered in the emergency department or ICU setting, and is typically managed in the operative and postoperative setting. Because MH is the toxin-induced hyperthermic crisis that develops most rapidly, within minutes to hours, and is most likely to result in severe morbidity or mortality, clinicians who administer succinylcholine or manage postoperative patients should be aware of this entity and its management.

MH involves excessive release of calcium from the sarcoplasmic reticulum of myocytes, and an ensuing hypermetabolism that results in hypercarbia, mixed respiratory and metabolic acidosis, rhabdomyolysis, and hyperthermia that is sometimes severe, with temperatures rapidly rising up to 113°F. It is widely misunderstood and misstated that hyperthermia rapidly develops in patients with MH: in fact, hyperthermia and rhabdomyolysis may be the last of the clinical symptoms to become apparent, occurring after muscle rigidity, hypercarbia, and mixed respiratory and metabolic acidemia.

The earliest clinical indication of MH is often hypercarbia. There is no absolute P_{CO_2} that is diagnostic, but a Pa_{CO_2} >60–65 or end-tidal CO_2 >55–60 in the absence of other obvious cause should be considered suggestive in postoperative patients. This hypercapnia may be managed by increasing minute ventilation, although the increases required by mechanical ventilation are often greater than would normally be expected. If the patient is not already being mechanically ventilated, he or she should be endotracheally intubated and mechanically ventilated with 100% FiO_2, with a minute ventilation that corrects the P_{CO_2} as reasonably as possible.

It is appropriate to correct hypercarbia, but investigation for other evidence of MH should be initiated. This includes physical exam to detect increased muscle tone; evaluation of arterial blood gas; urinary myoglobin, serum CPK, and serum potassium that may be associated with rhabdomyolysis; PT/PTT, INR, and fibrin split products to detect disseminated intravascular coagulation; and rectal or core temperature monitoring. Although hyperthermia is often not present when MH is initially suspected, when elevation of temperature does begin, it may be rapid, with temperatures rising as much as 2°F every 5 minutes.

At any time when MH is strongly suspected, any possible inciting medications should be discontinued and dantrolene administration should begin. Despite any other supportive care given, without dantrolene patients are extremely unlikely to survive MH.[33] Prior to the development of dantrolene, 70% of cases of MH were fatal. With current supportive care and dantrolene administration in the United States, approximately 10% of cases are fatal.

Supportive care includes correcting hypercarbia, providing 100% oxygen to support the hypermetabolic state, correcting hyperkalemia and treating rhabdomyolysis, managing disseminated intravascular coagulation if it occurs, and, last, management of hyperthermia.

Use of active cooling as described in the beginning of this section is recommended in conjunction with dantrolene administration.

▶ TOXIN-INDUCED SEIZURE

Seizure may be the consequence of numerous pathophysiologic events, most commonly metabolic and neurochemical. Management of seizure or status epilepticus resulting from poisoning varies significantly from management of epilepsy or trauma-associated seizure.[34] The initial management of toxin-induced seizures should include rapid bedside assessment of blood glucose and assessment for hypoxia.

Management of toxin-induced seizures differs from epileptic or traumatic seizures in that phenytoin use is contraindicated.[33] Specifically, phenytoin results in increases in severe seizure activity and increased incidence of cardiac dysrhythmia and death. Although the sodium channel blocking activity of phenytoin is effective in decreasing activity of epileptogenic foci or focal activity of traumatized brain, toxin-induced seizure activity is the culmination of diffuse and global cerebral dysfunction, for which sodium channel blockade both is unhelpful and may worsen seizure activity. It is ill-advised to treat toxin-induced seizure with phenytoin, as doing so is expected to be ineffective and, more important, to increase morbidity and mortality.

A management protocol for toxin-induced seizures can be summarized as follows: administration of a benzodiazepine, such as lorazepam 0.05–0.1 mg/kg every 10–15 minutes or diazepam 0.1–0.2 mg/kg every 5–10 minutes to a maximum of three doses. Further dosing is not detrimental, but use of benzodiazepines should be considered inadequate if three doses have not successfully terminated seizures, and escalation to more intensive therapy is warranted.

Benzodiazepine use should be followed by empirical dosing of pyridoxine (vitamin B_6) to treat potential effect of isoniazid or other hydralazine-induced seizure. Dosing is 1 g pyridoxine for every 1 g of isoniazid or other hydrazine ingested. Empirical dosing is 2–4 g in adults or 70 mg/kg in children. Because pyridoxine is not often immediately accessible at the dose required, this may be ordered from the pharmacy and progression down the treatment algorithm continues, with pyridoxine administered as soon as it is available.

The traditional algorithm for management of seizures or status epilepticus has been three doses of a benzodiazepine, after which use of a barbiturate begins (Figure 41-1). Due to the advent of highly effective medications such as propofol and valproic acid, these newer medications may be used instead of barbiturates after initial use of benzodiazepines fails. Decision to use barbiturates or newer medications such as propofol or valproic acid is based on clinician preference and comfort.

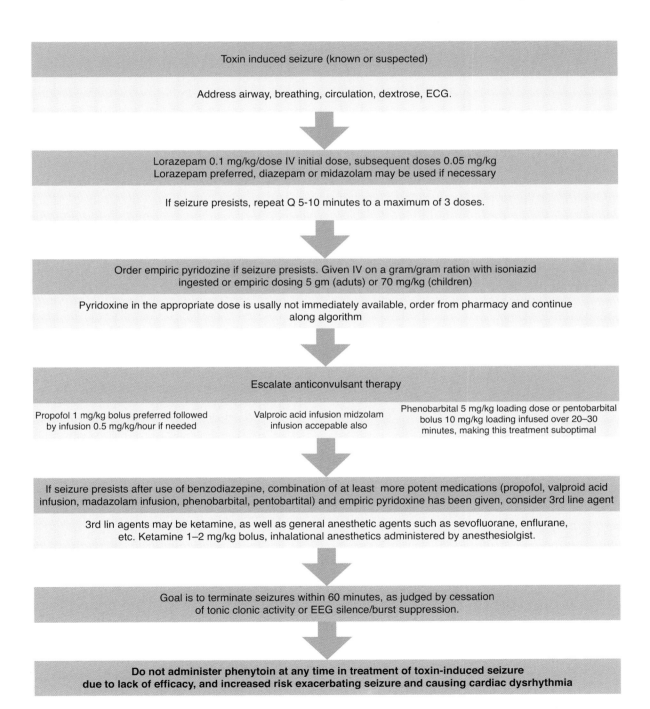

Figure 41-1. Management of toxin-induced seizure.

PROPOFOL

Propofol is extraordinarily rapid in its ability to terminate seizure activity, and its activity as both a GABA agonist and NMDA antagonist makes it the most useful and preferred agent for toxin-induced status epilepticus. We recommend propofol for use after failure of benzodiazepine therapy by administration of 1 mg/kg IV followed by repeated boluses of titration of propofol infusion at 0.1–0.3 mg/kg/min titrated to clinical effect.

BARBITURATE

Barbiturate loading would be with pentobarbital 5 mg/kg IV or phenobarbital 10–20 mg IV, typically loaded over 20 minutes.

VALPROIC ACID OR MIDAZOLAM

Valproic acid works by GABA agonism; dosing is 25 mg/kg infused over 5–10 minutes. Midazolam is also a GABA agonist; loading and infusion dosing are: loading dose 0.15 mg/kg IV followed by infusion of 1 mcg/kg/min. Every 5 minutes of seizure activity, double infusion rate to maximum rate of 16 mcg/kg/min. If continuous seizure, this would take 20 minutes to reach the maximum infusion dose rate.

Respiratory depression and need for endotracheal intubation should be anticipated when administering a barbiturate subsequent to a benzodiazepine or with any therapeutic propofol use. For this reason, administration of propofol with planned endotracheal intubation is reasonable. Unless continuous EEG monitoring is available, use of any long-acting paralytic agent is not recommended, since it may mask seizure activity and prevent appropriate escalation of pharmacologic therapy if seizures continue. Due to brief duration of activity, succinylcholine may be used as a paralytic if there are no contraindications such as significant hyperkalemia.

THIRD-LINE ANTICONVULSANTS

Other medications that may be employed are third-line agents levetiracetam[35] and ketamine.[36]

Levetiracetam mechanism of action is unknown, and therefore less desirable for use in toxin-induced seizures, as there is potential, such as with phenytoin, to exacerbate seizures or to increase morbidity and mortality. Levetiracetam dosing is 20–40 mg/kg IV diluted in 100 mL of saline and infused over 15 minutes.

Ketamine is an NMDA antagonist with potential to dissipate seizures by a different mechanism of action, NMDA antagonism, than other medications reviewed here, most of which work by GABA agonism. Little data on ketamine therapy for status epilepticus exist. Dosing is initial 1 mg/kg IV bolus, followed by 0.05–0.1 mg/kg/min infusion. Further treatment may involve general anesthetic agents administered by an anesthesiologist.

Management of seizures from other toxin-induced phenomena such as hyponatremia or hypocalcemia may be carried out in the typical fashion.

REFERENCES

1. Albertson TE, Dawson A, Delatorre F, et al. TOX-ACLS: toxicologic-oriented advanced cardiac life support. *Ann Emerg Med.* 2001;37(4 suppl):S78–S90.
2. Vanden Hoek TL, Morrison LJ, Shuster M, et al. Cardiac arrest in special situations: 2010 American Heart Association guidelines for cardiopulmonary resuscitation and emergency cardiovascular care. *Circulation.* 2010;122:S829–S861.
3. Kelly CA, Upex A, Bateman DN. Comparison of consciousness level assessment in the poisoned patient using the alert/verbal/painful/unresponsive scale and the Glasgow Coma Scale. *Ann Emerg Med.* 2004;44: 108–113.
4. Fulton J, Greller HA, Hoffman RS, et al. GCS and AVPU: the alphabet soup doesn't spell "c-o-m-a" in toxicology. *Ann Emerg Med.* 2005;45:224–225.
5. Fulton JA. Caustics. In: Nelson LS, Lewin NA, Howland MA, et al, eds. *Goldfrank's Toxicologic Emergencies.* 9th ed. New York, NY: McGraw-Hill; 2010.
6. Sener EB, Ustun E, Kocamanoglu S, Tur A. Prolonged apnea following succinylcholine administration in undiagnosed acute organophosphate poisoning. *Acta Anaesthesiolo Scand.* 2002;46(8):1046–1049.
7. Flomenbaum NE. Salicylates. In: Nelson LS, Lewin NA, Howland MA, et al, eds. *Goldfrank's Toxicologic Emergencies.* 9th ed. New York, NY: McGraw-Hill; 2010.
8. Stolbach A, Hoffman RS, Nelson LS. Mechanical ventilation was associated with acidemia in a case series of salicylate-poisoned patients. *Acad Emerg Med.* 2008;15:866–869.
9. Amin Y, Hamdi E, Eapen V. Mass hysteria in an Arab culture. *Int J Soc Psychiatry.* 1997;43(4):303–306.
10. Castle N, Owen R, Hann M, et al. Impact of chemical, biological, radiation, and nuclear personal protective equipment on the performance of low- and high-dexterity airway and vascular skills. *Resuscitation.* 2009;80(11):1290–1295.
11. Eventov-Friedman S, Rozin I, Shinwell ES. Case of chest-wall rigidity in a preterm infant caused by prenatal fentanyl administration. *J Perinatol.* 2010;30(2):149–150.
12. Price DP. Methemoglobinemia. In: Nelson LS, Lewin LA, Howland MA, et al, eds. *Goldfrank's Toxicologic Emergencies.* 9th ed. New York, NY: McGraw Hill; 2010.
13. Ziljlstra WG, Buursma A, Zwart A. Performance of an automated six-wavelength photometer (Radiometer OSM3) for routine measurement of hemoglobin derivatives. *Clin Chem.* 1988;34:149–152.

14. Howland MA. Methylene blue. In: Nelson LS, Lewin LA, Howland MA, et al, eds. *Goldfrank's Toxicologic Emergencies*. 9th ed. New York, NY: McGraw Hill; 2010.

15. Hardy KR, Thom SR. Pathophysiology and treatment of carbon monoxide poisoning. *J Toxicol Clin Toxicol*. 1994;32:613–629.

16. Low ECT, Ong MCC, Tan M. Breath carbon monoxide as an indication of smoking habit in the military setting. *Singapore Med J*. 2004;45:578–582.

17. Tomaszewski C. Carbon monoxide. In: Nelson LS, Lewin LA, Howland MA, et al, eds. *Goldfrank's Toxicologic Emergencies*. 9th ed. New York, NY: McGraw Hill; 2010.

18. Weaver LK, Hopkins RO, Chan KJ, et al. Hyperbaric oxygen for acute carbon monoxide poisoning. *N Engl J Med*. 2002;347:1057–1067.

19. Baud FJ, Barriot T, Toffis V, et al. Elevated blood cyanide concentrations in victims of closed-space fires. *N Engl J Med*. 1991;325:1761–1766.

20. Walsh DW, Eckstein M. Hydrogen cyanide in fire smoke: an underappreciated threat. *Emerg Med Serv*. 2004;33:160–163.

21. Johnson RP, Mellors JW. Arteriolization of venous blood gases: a clue to the diagnosis of cyanide poisoning. *J Emerg Med*. 1988;6:401–404.

22. Howland MA. Sodium thiosulfate. In: Nelson LS, Lewin LA, Howland MA, et al, eds. *Goldfrank's Toxicologic Emergencies*. 9th ed. New York, NY: McGraw Hill; 2010.

23. Howland MA. Hydroxocobalamin. In: Nelson LS, Lewin LA, Howland MA, et al, eds. *Goldfrank's Toxicologic Emergencies*. 9th ed. New York, NY: McGraw Hill; 2010.

24. Lee J, Mukai D, Kreuter K, et al. Potential interference by hydroxocobalamin on cooximetry hemoglobin measurements during cyanide and smoke inhalation treatments. *Ann Emerg Med*. 2007;49:802–805.

25. Howland MA. Digoxin-specific antibody fragments. In: Nelson LS, Lewin LA, Howland MA, et al, eds. *Goldfrank's Toxicologic Emergencies*. 9th ed. New York, NY: McGraw Hill; 2010.

26. Howland MA. Glucagon. In: Nelson LS, Lewin LA, Howland MA, et al, eds. *Goldfrank's Toxicologic Emergencies*. 9th ed. New York, NY: McGraw Hill; 2010.

27. Howland MA. Insulin–euglycemia therapy. In: Nelson LS, Lewin LA, Howland MA, et al, eds. *Goldfrank's Toxicologic Emergencies*. 9th ed. New York, NY: McGraw Hill; 2010.

28. Bania TC. Intravenous fat emulsions. In: Nelson LS, Lewin LA, Howland MA, et al, eds. *Goldfrank's Toxicologic Emergencies*. 9th ed. New York, NY: McGraw Hill; 2010.

29. Seger DL. Clonidine toxicity revisited. *J Toxicol Clin Toxicol*. 2002;40:145–155.

30. Gaar GC, Banner W Jr, Laddu AR. The effects of esmolol on the hemodynamics of acute theophylline toxicity. *Ann Emerg Med*. 1987;16:1334–1339.

31. Bohnert ASB, Prescott MR, Vlahov D, Tardiff KJ, Galea S. Ambient temperature and risk of death from accidental drug overdose in New York City, 1990–2006. *Addiction*. 2010;105:1049–1054.

32. Rosebush P, Stewart T. A prospective analysis of 24 episodes of neuroleptic malignant syndrome. *Am J Psychiatry*. 1989;146:717–725.

33. Larach MD, Brandon BW, Allen GC, et al. Cardiac arrests and deaths associated with malignant hyperthermia in North America from 1987 to 2005: a report from the North American Malignant Hyperthermia Registry of the Malignant Hyperthermia Association of the United States. *Anesthesiology*. 2008;108:603–611.

34. Sharma AN, Hoffman RJ. Toxin-related seizures. *Emerg Med Clin North Am*. 2011;29:125–139.

35. Knake S, Gruener J, Hattemer K, et al. Intravenous levetiracetam in the treatment of benzodiazepine refractory status epilepticus. *J Neurol Neurosurg Psychiatry*. 2008;795:588–589.

36. Lowenstein DH. The management of refractory status epilepticus: an update. *Epilepsia*. 2006;47:35–40.

CHAPTER 42

Acetaminophen Overdose

Seth R. Podolsky

▶ INTRODUCTION & BACKGROUND

Acetaminophen is the most widely used analgesic and a commonly used antipyretic. It has been available as an over-the-counter formulation for more than 40 years and is exceptionally safe when used according to manufacturer directions. Unfortunately, toxic levels can make it a silent and lethal killer, as overdose may initially present with few, if any, symptoms.[1-3] If not promptly discovered and treated, acetaminophen toxicity can lead to liver failure and death (unless a successful liver transplant is performed).[4-10]

Acetaminophen is packaged under multiple names and is a component of many different medicinal products around the globe. In the United States it is commonly sold as the brand name Tylenol®, while in the United Kingdom it is generally sold under the alternate generic names of paracetamol and N-acetyl-p-aminophenol (APAP).[11]

In the United States, acetaminophen is available in varied doses and forms. Pill forms are made in 325- and 500-mg immediate release, as well as 650-mg extended release. For both products, the adult dose should not exceed 4 g per day.[12] Pediatric formulas vary in both dosing and form, including concentrated drops, liquid suspensions, suppositories, and dissolving or chewable tablets.[11,12] Pediatric doses (child and infant) should not exceed 90 mg/kg per day or 15 mg/kg per dose every 4 hours.[11]

Acetaminophen is found in many over-the-counter and prescription medicines (i.e., Sudafed PE® Severe Cold: acetaminophen, diphenhydramine, and phenylephrine; Percocet®: acetaminophen and oxycodone; Fioricet®: acetaminophen, butalbital, and caffeine). Unintentional overdose may occur with these multidrug products, as the general public is unaware of the multiple names.

Acetaminophen overdose may be acute or chronic (Figure 42-1). An acute overdose is generally defined as a toxic dose (>150 mg/kg) ingested in less than 8 hours. A chronic overdose is generally defined as a toxic dose taken over more than 8 hours. Overdose may be accidental, as is frequently the case with pediatric overdoses, or it may also be intentional, as is the case with suicide attempt.

Overdose is defined as anything over the recommended 4 g per day. However, for the average adult (70 kg), the acetaminophen ingestion necessary for hepatotoxicity is much higher—150 mg/kg, or approximately 10.5 g. Thus, approximately 20 extra strength (500 mg each) pills are potentially lethal for the average patient.[1,13] Since acetaminophen is readily available over-the-counter, it is an easy overdose agent for suicide attempts.

Additionally, pediatric dosing (child and infant formulas) is easy to confuse and can often lead to therapeutic error. Pediatric dosing is particularly problematic since the infant's formula (100 mg/mL) is more than three times as concentrated when compared with the

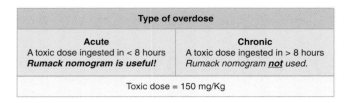

Type of overdose	
Acute	**Chronic**
A toxic dose ingested in < 8 hours	A toxic dose ingested in > 8 hours
Rumack nomogram is useful!	*Rumack nomogram **not** used.*
Toxic dose = 150 mg/Kg	

Figure 42–1. Acute versus chronic overdose.

children's formula (32 mg/mL).[11] Thus, equal volumes contain significantly different milligrams of acetaminophen, creating a high potential for overdose.

The risk of hepatotoxicity after an acute acetaminophen overdose is determined using the Rumack–Matthew nomogram (Figure 42-2).[1,3,13–17] This easy-to-use graph allows providers to assess risk based on plasma acetaminophen concentration and time postingestion. The antidote, *N*-acetylcysteine (NAC), is administered if there is a possible risk of hepatotoxicity.[1,3,13–24] This is discussed in detail further in this chapter.

▶ EPIDEMIOLOGY

Acetaminophen is a frequently used analgesic throughout the world, particularly in the United States, Canada, and Europe.[20,25,26] In the United States, it is the most commonly used prescription and over-the-counter drug, taken either alone or as a multidrug product, with over 50 million people using it every week.[26] In the United States it is the most common type of medicine associated with poisoning, and the second most common medicine related to overdose-related deaths (of which half are due to ingestions of a multidrug product that contains acetaminophen).[25]

In 2009, Poison Control Centers responded to 258,016 calls involving acetaminophen (234,084 in combination with another drug, and 23,932 calls regarding acetaminophen alone.[25] Additionally that year, acetaminophen (alone or in combination) was responsible for 410 deaths—nearly 15% of all poison related deaths in the United States.[25]

Acetaminophen overdose places a large burden on the health care system, as it is responsible for over 70,000 visits to health care facilities.[25–27] If untreated within 24 hours, acetaminophen poisoning has significant morbidity and mortality risks. Patients who initially present with hepatic failure have a mortality rate of 20–40%.[27]

Acetaminophen overdose is now the number one cause of acute liver failure in the United States.[28–32] This morbidity and mortality can be avoided when promptly treated.[27,33,34] As discussed below, the antidote, NAC, is nearly 100% effective if given within 8 hours, is often useful up to 12–24 hours, and occasionally may even prove useful after 24 hours.[17–24]

▶ PATHOPHYSIOLOGY

Acetaminophen is rapidly absorbed in the gastrointestinal tract. Peak serum levels occur within 4 hours, and possibly as soon as 2 hours, after ingestion. The drug is primarily metabolized by the liver.[1,3,5–10,29]

The drug itself does not directly damage the liver. Rather, damage is caused by acetaminophen metabolism when *N*-acetyl-*p*-benzoquinone imine (NAPQI), a hepatotoxic metabolite, is produced (Figure 42-3).[1,3,5–10,29]

Therapeutic acetaminophen doses create approximately 5% of the metabolite NAPQI. These small amounts of NAPQI are rapidly detoxified by glutathione into cysteine and mercapturic acid conjugates.[1,3,5–10,29] However, in the setting of acetaminophen overdose, glutathione stores are depleted and there is an accumulation of NAPQI that causes hepatic injury and cell death.

The American College of Emergency Physicians (ACEP) defines hepatotoxicity after acetaminophen overdose as any increase in the aspartate aminotransferase (AST) level.[34] Severe hepatotoxicity is generally defined as an AST level >1,000 IU/L.[34] Acute liver failure is defined as severe hepatotoxicity with hepatic encephalopathy (Figures 42-4 and 42-5).[34]

If glutathione can be replenished, then NAPQI can be metabolized into a nontoxic form that is then excreted via the kidneys. Cysteine is the rate-limiting substrate necessary for the creation of glutathione (which is formed via the synthesis of cysteine, glutamate, and glycine). NAC is a substance that provides an absorbable form of cysteine that can then be hydrolyzed to synthesize glutathione. This additional glutathione is then used to detoxify the enormous levels of NAPQI created during acetaminophen overdose.

There are several factors that appear to lessen hepatotoxicity. Acute ethanol ingestion is reported to reduce the hepatotoxic effects of acetaminophen by nearly 50%, although this protective effect is without clear mechanism.[35] Others suggest that coingestion of opioid analgesics is a protective factor in the development of hepatic encephalopathy (OR 0.26; CI 0.07, 0.96).[36] Phenytoin, initially thought to cause hepatotoxicity, is now suggested to be hepatoprotective by increasing glucuronidation that facilitates the metabolism of acetaminophen into nontoxic metabolites.[37] These studies are clinically limited; thus, further research is necessary to fully understand the above relationships and the underlying mechanisms of action.

Multiple factors appear to worsen hepatotoxicity during acetaminophen overdose. These include cirrhosis, chronic alcohol abuse, coingestions, certain preventable conditions, other medications, and dehydration and/or malnutrition.[31,38]

Nearly one third of all patients who overdose on acetaminophen ingest other substances (often alcohol and/or opiates). Certain coingestions appear to be independent

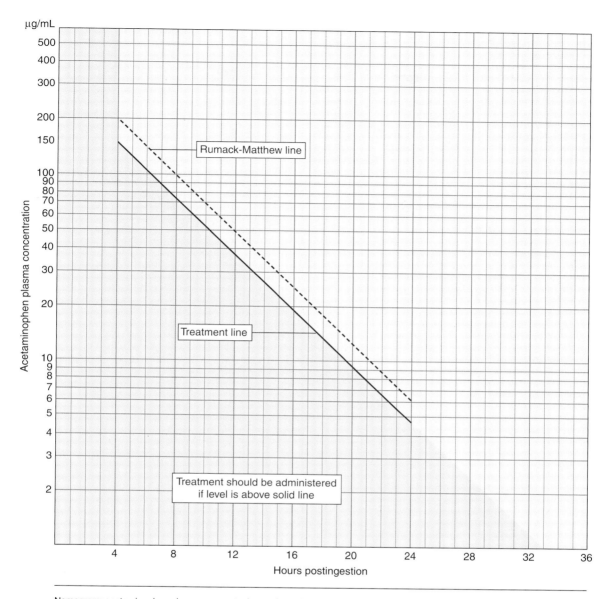

Figure 42–2. Rumack–Matthew nomogram. *Guidelines for the management of acetaminophen overdose* (www.tylenolprofessional.com). (Adapted with permission from Rumack BH, Matthew H. Acetaminophen poisoning and toxicity. Pediatrics. 1975;55:871.)

risk factors for the development of hepatic encephalopathy, renal dysfunction, and death or liver transplantation.[36] Preventable conditions also appear to increase mortality among patients found to be hepatotoxic secondary to acetaminophen overdose. These include attempted suicide, substance abuse, and trauma.[30,31]

The relation between chronic, heavy alcohol abuse and acetaminophen use has been debated for decades.

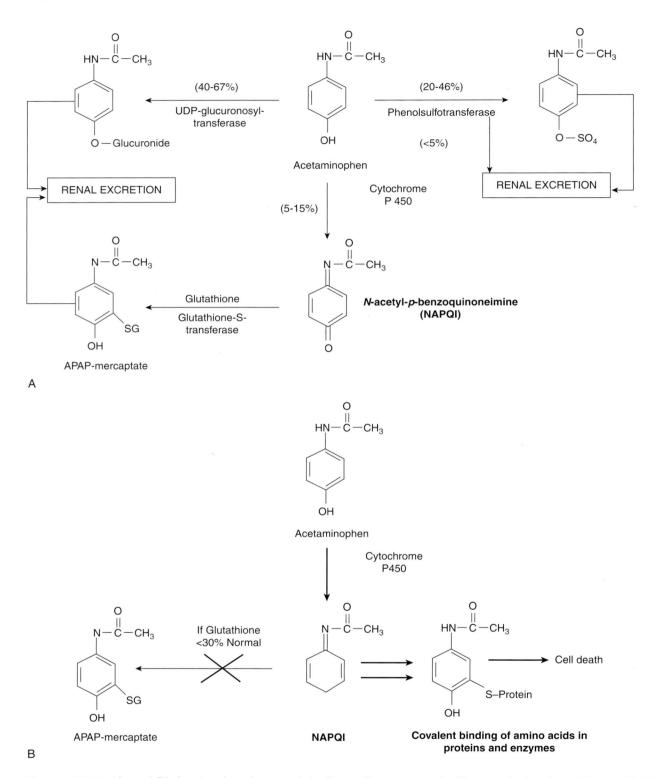

Figure 42–3. (A and B) Acetaminophen metabolism. (Reproduced with permission from Tintanelli JE, Kelen GD, Stapczynski JS. *Tintinalli's Emergency Medicine: A Comprehensive Guide.* 6th ed. New York, NY: McGraw-Hill Inc; 2004:1089. Figure 171-1.)

Stages of acetaminophen toxicity			
Stage	Time	Liver effects	Signs & Symptoms
1	0-24 hrs	Preclinical	• General malaise • Nausea and vomiting • Diffuse abdominal pain • Possibly asymptomatic • Minimal signs and symptoms • Normal liver function tests, possibly
2	24-72 hrs	Hepatotoxicity	• RUQ pain, possibly • Clinically asymptomatic, possibly • AST and ALT begin to rise, and possibly bilirubin • Coagulopathy studies (PT, PTT, INR) may increase, if severe injury

3	72-96 hrs	Hepatic failure with encephalopathy	• Liver function tests peak
			• Clinical signs and symptoms of liver failure are evident, including:
			  • Jaundice
			  • Vomiting
			  • GI upset
			  • Coagulopathy
			  • Encephalopathy
			  • Metabolic acidosis
			  • Pancreatitis, possibly
			  • Acute renal failure, possibly

4	> 96 hrs	Survival or death	• Full resolution of hepatotoxicity, <u>or</u> • Multi-organ failure and death

Figure 42–4. Stages of acetaminophen toxicity.

While alcoholics are likely to be at a greater risk for hepatotoxicity following acetaminophen overdose, there is little to no evidence to suggest such toxicity when taking therapeutic doses of acetaminophen.[37] Dehydration and/or malnutrition may compound the relationship between alcoholism and acetaminophen toxicity during acute ingestions; however, further research is needed to better understand these potential risk factors.[31,37]

► HISTORY

Any patient presenting to the Emergency Department receives a primary survey: airway, breathing, circulation, disability/dextrose, and exposure. In a poisoned patient, the resuscitation and diagnosis occur simultaneously by utilizing all members of the health care team. It is imperative to receive a thorough history from emergency medical services (EMS) personnel, as well as family, friends, and/or bystanders.

The history should be obtained from both the patient and a corroborator. Questions should address the time of ingestion, the specific substances, the route of ingestion (PO, IV, PR, inhaled), and the exact amounts. Regardless of historical source, it is imperative to count pills if the bottles (prescription or OTC) are available. Specific to acetaminophen overdose:

- *Were there coingestions?*
- *Were extended-release tablets involved?*
- *Did the patient intend to hurt himself or herself or was the ingestion accidental?*
- *Was the ingestion acute (i.e., all at once) or was it chronic (generally >8 hours)?*

The history and physical exam must focus on coingestions, self-harm, homicidal intent, and psychiatric illness. Keep in mind that any attempted suicide must consider acetaminophen overdose among possible coingestions.

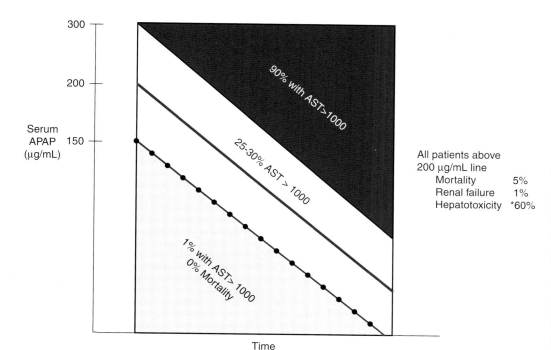

All patients above
200 μg/mL line
  Mortality   5%
  Renal failure   1%
  Hepatotoxicity *60%

Figure 42–5. Outcome of acetaminophen-poisoned patients (based on AST). *Defined as AST > 1000. (Adapted with permission from Smilkstein MJ, Knapp GL, Kulig KW, et al. Efficacy of oral *N*-acetylcysteine in the treatment of acetaminophen overdose. *New Engl J Med.* 1988;319:1557.)

► STAGES OF ACETAMINOPHEN TOXICITY

The clinical presentation and progression of acetaminophen overdose are generally categorized into four stages (Figure 42-4):

Stage 1 (0–24 hours): *Preclinical toxic effects* with minimal signs and symptoms, possibly asymptomatic, and often normal liver function tests. The vague, nonspecific symptoms of this stage might include nausea and vomiting, diffuse abdominal pain, and general malaise.

Stage 2 (24–72 hours): *Hepatic injury (hepatotoxicity)*. Patients may begin to develop RUQ pain, although sometimes they are clinically asymptomatic. AST and ALT begin to rise, and possibly bilirubin. If injury is severe, then coagulopathy studies (PT, PTT, INR) may increase.

Stage 3 (72–96 hours): *Hepatic failure with encephalopathy*. Liver function tests peak, and clinical signs and symptoms of liver failure are evident, including jaundice, vomiting and gastrointestinal pain, coagulopathy, encephalopathy, metabolic acidosis, and possibly acute renal failure and/or pancreatitis.

Stage 4 (>96 hours): *Survival or death*. Either there is full resolution of hepatotoxicity or fulminant liver failure progresses to multiorgan failure and death.

► PHYSICAL EXAM

Patients presenting with acetaminophen overdose must be completely undressed and examined from head to toe. It is useful to use security and/or police at the bedside for staff safety and the collection of patient belongings. This includes a thorough inspection of substances or objects that might be in pockets or hidden in/on the patient's body. Providers should be extremely cautious for dirty needles, sharp objects, and/or other contaminants.

As part of the primary survey, a blood glucose check is essential, as is an inspection of the oropharynx. It may be useful to inspect the rectal cavity for any retained substances (i.e., tablets, drug balloons, or other paraphernalia) and/or gastrointestinal bleeding.

An acute acetaminophen overdose will generally have few, if any, symptoms. Those symptoms that do exist may be vague and nonspecific, and may include mild abdominal pain or cramping, nausea and vomiting, and general malaise. Massive, acute overdose may, on occasion, present initially with metabolic acidosis and coma, even before the development of hepatotoxicity. Usually such presentation is caused by coingestions, frequently alcohol and/or opiates.

Coingestions often create additional signs and symptoms elicited during the physical exam of an acetaminophen overdose. Classic toxidromes may be encountered when additional substances are ingested: opioid, sympathomimetic, cholinergic, anticholinergic, or others.

Delayed presentation of acute acetaminophen overdose may present with more severe symptoms of hepatotoxicity, such as jaundice, RUQ pain and tenderness, and possibly altered mental status.

► LABORATORY DATA & RELATED STUDIES

Applicable laboratory data and related studies should be ordered as listed in Figure 42-6. The Rumack–Matthew nomogram is the most important tool used to guide clinical decisions about the treatment of acute acetaminophen overdose up to 24 hours after ingestion. It has potential use for the ingestion of extended-release preparation, as discussed later in the chapter. The nomogram may not be used under the following circumstances[34]:

- Unknown time or duration of ingestion;
- Chronic ingestion (repeated supratherapeutic);
- Delayed presentation (>24 hours after ingestion).

The following serum acetaminophen levels are toxic according to the nomogram (Figure 42-2):

- 4-hour level >150 mcg/mL.
- 6-hour level >110 mcg/mL;
- 8-hour level >75 mcg/mL;
- 24-hour level >4.5 mcg/mL.

► TREATMENT GUIDELINES

There are four general treatment modalities for acetaminophen overdose: (1) decrease absorption, (2) increase elimination, (3) antidote, and (4) liver transplantation.[20,39]

In the Emergency Department, one must first complete a primary survey and ensure that airway, breathing, and circulation are appropriately established. Oxygen, IV access, cardiac monitor, and pulse oximetry are ordered as needed.

Nasogastric tubes (NGT) are of limited clinical benefit, if any, in the setting of acetaminophen overdose.[20,39,40] Some facilities continue to use this practice, although it is not supported by evidence-based guidelines. Given the risk for inducing vomiting, and potentially compromising the airway, most physicians have abandoned the use of an NGT. There is a limited argument for the continued use of an NGT if the ingestion occurs less than 1 hour prior to arrival or if dangerous coingestants were consumed. Under these circumstances, it is argued that gastric lavage may remove some of the pill fragments remaining in the stomach, thereby preventing further absorption.

Laboratory data & related studies	
Lab Test	**Expected Findings**
Acetaminophen level	Check at 4-hours post-ingestions. Toxic *if > 150 micrograms per deciliter* Repeat at 8-hours if extended release tablets with a normal 4-hour level. Toxic *if > 75 micrograms per deciliter*
Electrolytes, BUN/Cr, and glucose	Metabolic acidosis (with large ingestions).
Liver function tests	AST usually rises first, then ALT and bilirubin.
Coagulation studies	Rise with hepatotoxicity and liver failure.
Urinalysis and UhCG	Proteinuria and hematuria, if acute tubular necrosis, in conjunction with liver failure.
If suicide attempt and/or altered mental status then consider: • Aspirin level • Alcohol level • Complete blood count (CBC) • Arterial/venous blood gas (pH and lactate may predict mortality) • Electrocardiogram (prolonged QT, or other changes, seen with co-ingestions) • Radiology studies, as indicated	

Figure 42–6. Laboratory data and related studies.

The medications used to treat acetaminophen overdose consist of activated charcoal (decreases adsorption and enhances elimination) and NAC (antidote to increase elimination), with antiemetics used as clinically indicated.

Gastrointestinal decontamination is primarily achieved with activated charcoal. There is moderate evidence that significant benefit occurs if this is given within 1 hour of the ingestion.[20,40] Super activated charcoal may offer some detoxification benefit when given within 3 hours postingestion; however, this is not typically stocked in many Emergency Departments.[41] There is no clinical benefit to the use of syrup of ipecac and it should no longer be used in acetaminophen overdose.[39] Antiemetics are used symptomatically to prevent aspiration and airway compromise.

The most important treatment in acetaminophen overdose is the antidote NAC—manufactured under the brand names Mucomyst® and Acetadote®.[17,20,22,24,33] It works via the pathways discussed above (Figure 42-3).

When given within 8–10 hours postingestion, there is no difference in the efficacy between the oral and IV preparations.[18,22] Historically, the oral preparation was used; however, the IV preparation was approved by the Food and Drug Administration (FDA) in 2004, and has subsequently become the primary preparation.[42] Many institutions now use the IV form because of decreased treatment time, a decreased likelihood of complications secondary to vomiting, and a decreased hospital stay and associated costs.[20] IV NAC should also be used if treatment is more than 10 hours postingestion or if underlying conditions prevent oral use.[18,19] There

is some evidence that patients with asthma or atopic dermatitis should receive oral therapy because of the decreased risk of anaphylactoid reaction; however, this is not necessarily the current standard of care.[18,42,43]

Over the past decade, a significant change in treatment has occurred as the IV form of NAC has become the standard over PO. This decreases total time of treatment and also reduces risk of aspiration from vomiting (Figures 42-7 to 42-9).

The IV dosing for adults (patients >40 kg) consists of the following protocol: Acute ingestions (8–10 hours after ingestion) receive an IV loading dose of 150 mg/kg (body weight) diluted in 250 mL of D5W infused over 1 hour. Two maintenance doses are then initiated as follows: The first maintenance dose (started immediately after the loading dose) is 50 mg/kg diluted in 500 mL of D5W infused IV over 4 hours. The second maintenance dose (started immediately after the first maintenance dose) is 100 mg/kg diluted in 1,000 mL of D5W infused over 16 hours. The total of the three doses administered is 300 mg/kg over 21 hours.

The oral (PO) loading dose for adults is 140 mg/kg (body weight) once, and then maintenance doses (start 4 hours after loading dose) of 70 mg/kg repeated every 4 hours for a total of 17 additional doses. Total of 18 doses administered equaling 1,330 mg/kg over 72 hours.[33,44–45]

The IV dosing for adult chronic ingestion, or late presentation (>8 hours after ingestion), is an IV loading dose of 140 mg/kg (body weight) diluted in 500 mL D5W infused over 1 hour. Maintenance doses are then initiated as follows: 70 mg/kg diluted in 250 mL of D5W infused IV over at least 1 hour. This maintenance dose is repeated

Intravenous (IV) NAC dosing for adult and pediatrics Total of 3-doses over 21-hours				
Dose	Time	Amount	Diluent	Infusion Rate
1st	Immediate IV loading dose	150 mg/Kg	Adult 250 mL of D5W Pediatric 3 mL/Kg of D5W	Over 1-hour
2nd	Immediately after 1st dose	50 mg/Kg	Adult 500 mL of D5W Pediatric 1 mL/Kg of D5W	Over 4-hours
3rd	Immediately after 2nd dose	100 mg/Kg	Adult 1 L of D5W Pediatric 2 mL/Kg of D5W	Over 16-hrs

Oral (PO) NAC dosing for adult and pediatrics Total of 18-doses over 72-hours				
Dose	Time	Amount	Route	Considerations
1st	Immediate PO loading dose	140 mg/Kg	Oral	Anti-emetic may be helpful
2nd – 18th	Every 4-hours after loading dose	70 mg/Kg	Oral	Anti-emetic may be helpful

Figure 42–7. NAC dosing (PO and IV) for adult and pediatrics.

every 4 hours for at least 12 doses. Total treatment time is at least 48 hours.[46] If fluid restriction is required, then the total volume of D5W may be decreased.

The IV dosing for pediatrics (patients <40 kg) is the same as the adult protocol, except the volume of D5W is decreased (Figure 42-7). The oral (PO) dosing protocol for pediatrics is the same as the adult protocol above.

All patients treated with NAC must be admitted to the hospital for further treatment and evaluation. Any patient presenting with an overdose secondary to a suicide attempt must be evaluated by Psychiatry.

► RENAL INSUFFICIENCY AND HEPATIC FAILURE

Dose-dependent hypokalemia has been observed, although it tends to be more profound at higher levels of acetaminophen toxicity.[47,48] It is unclear if this is related to acetaminophen or other confounding factors. One study suggests a renal effect (of unclear etiol-

ogy) that causes kaliuresis within the first 24 hours after ingestion.[48] This occurs regardless of NAC treatment and is independent of vomiting. The treatment is to replace potassium accordingly.

Renal insufficiency occurs in 1–2% of patients, generally among the more severe ingestions.[49] One study suggests nephrotoxicity is higher in adolescents, possibly as high as 9%, although further research is indicated.[50]

Fulminant liver failure may lead to significant acidosis, coagulopathy, cerebral edema, and/or multiorgan system failure.[51] Each of these findings must be addressed accordingly, and is frequently resolved in the Intensive Care Unit (ICU) setting. Referral to a liver transplant center is required.

► SPECIAL CONSIDERATIONS

Pediatric patients are treated similarly to adults, except the D5W is decreased during the administration of IV NAC.

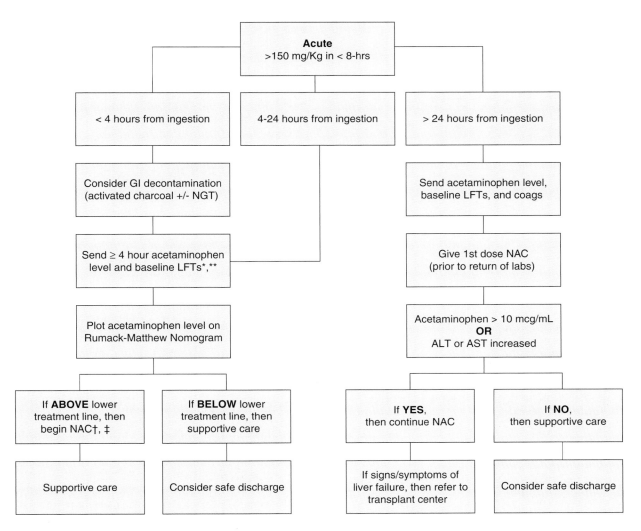

Guidelines For The Management Of Acetaminophen Overdose at www.tylenolprofessional.com states:
* Plasma acetaminophen levels drawn less than 4 hours post-ingestion may not represent peak levels.
** With the extended-release preparation, plasma acetaminophen levels drawn less than 8 hours post-ingestion may not represent peak levels. Draw a second level 4 to 6 hours after the initial level was drawn. Acetylcysteine treatment should be initiated and continued until acetaminophen assay results are available.
† Acetylcysteine can be withheld until acetaminophen assay results are available as long as initiation of treatment is not delayed beyond 8 hours post-ingestion. If more than 8 hours post-ingestion, start acetylcysteine treatment immediately.
‡ With the extended-release preparation, provide acetylcysteine treatment if either level plots above the lower treatment line.

Figure 42–8. Treatment guidelines for acute acetaminophen ingestion.

Pregnant patients are treated similarly to nonpregnant patients.[19,20,52] There is no increased risk of adverse pregnancy unless there is severe maternal toxicity.[19]

Extended-release tablets (650-mg pill) are composed of half immediate-release acetaminophen (325 mg/pill) and half extended-release acetaminophen (325 mg/pill). Therefore, there may be a delayed rise in serum acetaminophen levels.[20,53,54] If the initial 4-hour serum acetaminophen level is *above* the nontoxic range on the Rumack–Matthew nomogram, then treatment with NAC should be immediately initiated. However, if the initial 4-hour serum acetaminophen level is *below* the nontoxic range on the Rumack–Matthew nomogram, then

research suggests that a second serum acetaminophen level and AST/ALT should be repeated 4–6 hours after the first (8–10 hours postingestion) and treated accordingly based on results.[20,53,54] Treatment with NAC should be initiated if the serum acetaminophen level is >10 mcg/mL or if serum AST or ALT is elevated.

Delayed presentation (ingestion >24 hours prior to presentation) requires the immediate initiation of NAC. Laboratory tests should be ordered as listed above, including acetaminophen level and liver function tests Figure 42-6. Treatment with NAC should be continued if the serum acetaminophen level is >10 mcg/mL or if serum AST or ALT is elevated (Figure 42-8).

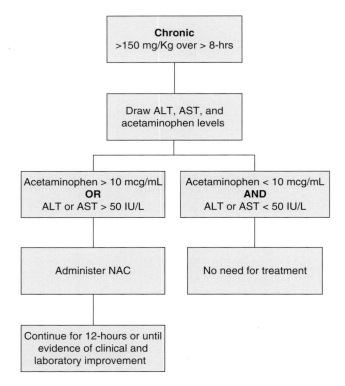

Figure 42–9. Treatment guidelines for chronic acetaminophen ingestion.

Chronic ingestion (toxic overdose taken over >8 hours) requires laboratory tests as above, including liver function tests Figure 42-6. The Rumack–Matthew nomogram may *not* be used in this scenario. NAC should be initiated if the serum acetaminophen level is >10 mcg/mL *or* if serum AST or ALT is >50 IU/L. It should be continued for 12 hours or until evidence of clinical and laboratory improvement substantiates cessation. Treatment with NAC should be considered if the patient has a history of chronic overdose or exhibits signs and symptoms consistent with toxicity (Figure 42-9).[46]

Safe discharge from the Emergency Department may occur (on rare occasion) if the following criteria are met:

- No coingestions;
- No significant medical problems;
- Observation for 4–6 hours with a normal reevaluation;
- Safe acetaminophen levels based on the Rumack–Matthew nomogram;
- Psychiatry evaluation and clearance, if suggestion of intentional overdose.

► PREVENTION

Patients are often unaware that acetaminophen is commonly present in other medicine they are taking—either prescribed or over-the-counter.[55] There is evidence to suggest that the removal of acetaminophen from multi-drug products (e.g, percocet, vicodin, etc.) may reduce unintentional overdose. Also, multiple studies suggest that limiting the quantity of acetaminophen available in a single purchase generally reduces associated morbidity and mortality from acute and chronic toxicity.[56,57] Presently, the FDA and Congress are considering both of these strategies.

► CONCLUSION

Acetaminophen is the most widely used analgesic, and a commonly used antipyretic, that is a potentially silent and lethal killer. If not promptly discovered and treated, acetaminophen overdose may lead to liver failure and death. However, if treated early with the antidote NAC, then survival is nearly 100%. IV NAC is now the preferred route of treatment for both adults and pediatrics. Given the high morbidity and mortality associated with acetaminophen overdose, it is essential that the Emergency Medicine physician have a high index of suspicion for any potentially lethal overdose.

REFERENCES

1. Rumack BH, Matthew H. Acetaminophen poisoning and toxicity. *Pediatrics*. 1975;55(6):871–876.
2. Peterson RG, Rumack BH. Toxicity of acetaminophen overdose. *JACEP*. 1978;7(5):202–205.
3. Rumack BH, Peterson RG. Acetaminophen overdose: incidence, diagnosis, and management in 416 patients. *Pediatrics*. 1978;62(5 pt 2 suppl):898–903.
4. Boyer TD, Rouff SL. Acetaminophen-induced hepatic necrosis and renal failure. *JAMA*. 1971;218(3):440–441.
5. Jollow DJ, Mitchell JR, Potter WZ, et al. Acetaminophen-induced hepatic necrosis. II. Role of covalent binding in vivo. *J Pharmacol Exp Ther*. 1973;187(1):195–202.
6. Mitchell JR, Jollow DJ, Potter WZ, et al. Acetaminophen-induced hepatic necrosis. I. Role of drug metabolism. *J Pharmacol Exp Ther*. 1973;187(1):185–194.
7. Mitchell JR, Jollow DJ, Potter WZ, et al. Acetaminophen-induced hepatic necrosis. IV. Protective role of glutathione. *J Pharmacol Exp Ther*. 1973;187(1):211–217.
8. Potter WZ, Davis DC, Mitchell JR, et al. Acetaminophen-induced hepatic necrosis. III. Cytochrome P-450-mediated covalent binding in vitro. *J Pharmacol Exp Ther*. 1973;187(1):203–210.
9. Jollow DJ, Thorgeirsson SS, Potter WZ, et al. Acetaminophen-induced hepatic necrosis. VI. Metabolic disposition of toxic and nontoxic doses of acetaminophen. *Pharmacology*. 1974;12(4–5):251–271.
10. Potter WZ, Thorgeirsson SS, Jollow DJ, et al. Acetaminophen-induced hepatic necrosis. V. Correlation of hepatic necrosis, covalent binding and glutathione depletion in hamsters. *Pharmacology*. 1974;12(3):129–143.
11. Acetaminophen. In: *Physicians' Desk Reference*. 63rd ed. Montvale, NJ: Thomson PDR; 2009:1915–1916.

12. Krenzelok EP. The FDA Acetaminophen Advisory Committee meeting—what is the future of acetaminophen in the United States? The perspective of a committee member. *Clin Toxicol.* 2009;47(8):784–789.

13. Rumack BH, Peterson RC, Koch GG, et al. Acetaminophen overdose. 662 cases with evaluation of oral acetylcysteine treatment. *Arch Intern Med.* 1981;141(3 spec no):380–385.

14. Rumack BH. Acetaminophen overdose. *Am J Med.* 1983;75(5A):104–112.

15. Rumack BH. Acetaminophen overdose in young children. Treatment and effects of alcohol and other additional ingestants in 417 cases. *Am J Dis Child.* 1984;138(5):428–433.

16. Rumack BH. Acetaminophen: acute overdose toxicity in children. *Drug Intell Clin Pharm.* 1985;19(12):911–912.

17. Rumack BH. Acetaminophen overdose in children and adolescents. *Pediatr Clin North Am.* 1986;33(3):691–701.

18. Kanter MZ. Comparison of oral and i.v. acetylcysteine in the treatment of acetaminophen poisoning. *Am J Health Syst Pharm.* 2006;63(19):1821–1827.

19. Kozer E, Koren G. Management of paracetamol overdose: current controversies. *Drug Saf.* 2001;24(7):503–512.

20. Zed PJ, Krenzelok EP. Treatment of acetaminophen overdose. *Am J Health Syst Pharm.* 1999;56(11):1081–1091. Quiz 1091–1093.

21. Dean BS, Bricker JD, Krenzelok EP. Outpatient *N*-acetylcysteine treatment for acetaminophen poisoning: an ethical dilemma or a new financial mandate? *Vet Hum Toxicol.* 1996;38(3):222–224.

22. Linden CH, Rumack BH. Acetaminophen overdose. *Emerg Med Clin North Am.* 1984;2(1):103–119.

23. Lindgren K, Lattrez J, Nguyen C, et al. Intravenous *N*-acetylcysteine (NAC) protocols recommended by North American Poison Centers. *J Toxicol Clin Toxicol.* 2004;42(5):733.

24. Prescott LF, Park J, Ballantyne A, et al. Treatment of paracetamol (acetaminophen) poisoning with *N*-acetylcysteine. *Lancet.* 1977;2(8035):432–434.

25. Bronstein AC, Spyker DA, Cantilena Jr. LR, et al. 2009 Annual Report of the American Association of Poison Control Centers' National Poison Data System (NPDS): 27th Annual Report. *Clin Toxicol.* 2010;48(10):0979–1178.

26. Kaufman DW, Kelly JP, Rosenberg L, et al. Recent patterns of medication use in the ambulatory adult population of the United States: the Slone survey. *JAMA.* 2002;287(3):337–344.

27. Heard KJ. Acetylcysteine for acetaminophen poisoning. *N Engl J Med.* 2008;359(3):285–292.

28. Larson AM. Acetaminophen hepatotoxicity. *Clin Liver Dis.* 2007;11(3):525–548.

29. Larson AM, Polson J, Fontana RJ, et al. Acetaminophen-induced acute liver failure: results of a United States multicenter, prospective study [see comment]. *Hepatology.* 2005;42(6):1364–1372.

30. Myers RP, Li B, Fong A, et al. Hospitalizations for acetaminophen overdose: a Canadian population-based study from 1995 to 2004. *BMC Public Health.* 2007;7:143.

31. Myers RP, Shaheen AA, Li B, et al. Impact of liver disease, alcohol abuse, and unintentional ingestions on the outcomes of acetaminophen overdose. *Clin Gastroenterol Hepatol.* 2008;6(8):918–925. Quiz 837.

32. Simpson KJ, Bates CM, Henderson NC, et al. The utilization of liver transplantation in the management of acute liver failure: comparison between acetaminophen and non-acetaminophen etiologies. *Liver Transpl.* 2009;15(6):600–609.

33. Smilkstein MJ, Knapp GL, Kulig KW, et al. Efficacy of oral *N*-acetylcysteine in the treatment of acetaminophen overdose. Analysis of the national multicenter study (1976 to 1985) [see comment]. *N Engl J Med.* 1988;319(24):1557–1562.

34. Wolf SJ, Heard K, Sloan EP, et al. Clinical policy: critical issues in the management of patients presenting to the emergency department with acetaminophen overdose. *Ann Emerg Med.* 2007;50(3):292–313.

35. Sivilotti ML, Yarema MC, Juurlink DN, et al. Predicting hepatotoxicity following acetaminophen overdose: a nomogram for the post-N-AC era. *J Toxicol Clin Toxicol.* 2003;41(5):724.

36. Schmidt LE, Dalhoff K. Concomitant overdosing of other drugs in patients with paracetamol poisoning. *Br J Clin Pharmacol.* 2002;53(5):535–541.

37. Rumack BH. Acetaminophen hepatotoxicity: the first 35 years. *J Toxicol Clin Toxicol.* 2002;40(1):3–20.

38. Sivilotti ML, Good AM, Yarema MC, et al. A new predictor of toxicity following acetaminophen overdose based on pretreatment exposure. *Clin Toxicol.* 2005;43(4):229–234.

39. Brok J, Buckley N, Gluud C. Interventions for paracetamol (acetaminophen) overdose. *Cochrane Database Syst Rev.* 2006; Apr 19;(2):CD003328.

40. Buckley NA, Whyte IM, O'Connell DL, et al. Activated charcoal reduces the need for *N*-acetylcysteine treatment after acetaminophen (paracetamol) overdose. *J Toxicol Clin Toxicol.* 1999;37(6):753–757.

41. Sato RL, Wong JJ, Sumida SM, et al. Efficacy of superactivated charcoal administered late (3 hours) after acetaminophen overdose. *Am J Emerg Med.* 2003;21(3):189–191.

42. Smilkstein MJ, Bronstein AC, Linden C, et al. Acetaminophen overdose: a 48-hour intravenous *N*-acetylcysteine treatment protocol. *Ann Emerg Med.* 1991;20(10):1058–1063.

43. Sandilands EA, Bateman DN. Adverse reactions associated with acetylcysteine. *Clin Toxicol.* 2009;47(2):81–88.

44. Woo OF, Mueller PD, Olson KR, et al. Shorter duration of oral *N*-acetylcysteine therapy for acute acetaminophen overdose. *Ann Emerg Med.* 2000;35(4):363–368.

45. Betten DP, Cantrell FL, Thomas SC, et al. A prospective evaluation of shortened course oral *N*-acetylcysteine for the treatment of acute acetaminophen poisoning. *Ann Emerg Med.* 2007;50(3):272–279.

46. Dart RC, Erdman AR, Olson KR, et al. Acetaminophen poisoning: an evidence-based consensus guideline for out-of-hospital management. *Clin Toxicol.* 2006;44:01–18.

47. Waring WS, Stephen AF, Malkowska AM, et al. Acute acetaminophen overdose is associated with dose-dependent hypokalaemia: a prospective study of 331 patients. *Basic Clin Pharmacol Toxicol.* 2008;102(3):325–328.

48. Pakravan N, Bateman DN, Goddard J. Effect of acute paracetamol overdose on changes in serum and urine electrolytes. *Br J Clin Pharmacol.* 2007;64(6):824–832.

49. Mazer M, Perrone J. Acetaminophen-induced nephrotoxicity: pathophysiology, clinical manifestations, and management. *J Med Toxicol.* 2008;4(1):2–6.

50. Boutis K, Shannon M. Nephrotoxicity after acute severe acetaminophen poisoning in adolescents. *J Toxicol Clin Toxicol.* 2001;39(5):441–445.

51. Roth B, Woo O, Blanc P. Early metabolic acidosis and coma after acetaminophen ingestion. *Ann Emerg Med.* 1999;33(4):452–456.

52. Wilkes JM, Clark LE, Herrera JL. Acetaminophen overdose in pregnancy. *South Med J.* 2005;98(11):1118–1122.

53. Graudins A, Pham HN, Salonikas C, et al. Early presentation following overdose of modified-release paracetamol (Panadol Osteo) with biphasic and prolonged paracetamol absorption. *N Z Med J.* 2009;122(1300):64–71.

54. Tan C, Graudins A. Comparative pharmacokinetics of Panadol Extend and immediate-release paracetamol in a simulated overdose model. *Emerg Med Australas.* 2006;18(4):398–403.

55. Fosnocht D, Taylor JR, Caravati EM. Emergency department patient knowledge concerning acetaminophen (paracetamol) in over-the-counter and prescription analgesics. *Emerg Med J.* 2008;25(4):213–216.

56. Gunnell D, Murray V, Hawton K. Use of paracetamol (acetaminophen) for suicide and nonfatal poisoning: worldwide patterns of use and misuse. *Suicide Life Threat Behav.* 2000;30(4):313–326.

57. Andrew E, Bøe GH, Haga C, et al. Poisonings from analgesics in Norway with emphasis on paracetamol. An epidemiological study. *J Toxicol Clin Toxicol.* 2004;42(4):520.

CHAPTER 43

Salicylate Overdose

(Shawn) Xun Zhong and Andrew Stolbach

Salicylates have been used since the 19th century.[1] Today, salicylates are used therapeutically throughout the world. The most commonly encountered salicylate is acetylsalicylic acid (aspirin). Other medications include the liniment methyl salicylate (oil of wintergreen) and bismuth subsalicylate, the active ingredient in Pepto-Bismol. Because salicylates are ubiquitous, there is great potential for toxicity, intentional or accidental. In 2008, there were over 19,000 aspirin-alone exposures reported and about 2,000 aspirin coingestions reported to the National Poison Data System.[2]

▶ PHARMACOKINETICS

At therapeutic concentrations, salicylate ingested is rapidly absorbed into the bloodstream with a peak serum concentration in 1 hour. When gastric contents are present, absorption may be delayed. Eighty to 90% of plasma salicylate is bound to protein, especially albumin. Most salicylate is biotransformed by the hepatic endoplasmic reticulum but about 10% is eliminated unchanged in the urine. Salicylates and its metabolized products are renally eliminated in a pH-dependent manner. The difference between alkaline and acidic urine can cause free excretion to vary from higher than 30% to 2%.[3]

In overdoses, plasma peak concentrations are often delayed up to 35 hours, especially when ingesting extended-release and/or enteric-coated tablets.[4,5] Bezoar may also form, extending the time of absorption and making the time of peak concentration impossible to predict in any given overdose. As salicylate concentration rises above normal, protein binding and hepatic metabolization are saturated. As a result of the saturation, salicylate metabolism changes from first- to zero-order kinetics,[6] and a larger portion of the unmetabolized salicylate is excreted in the urine (see Figure 43-1).[3]

▶ PATHOPHYSIOLOGY OF SALICYLATE POISONING

In plasma, salicylates are in equilibrium between the protonated (uncharged) and unprotonated (charged) forms. Salicylic acid is a weak acid (pK_a 3.5), which means that a majority of the drug exists in the protonated (uncharged) form. In its uncharged form, it can move easily across membranes and deposit into various tissues, most importantly the CNS. At acidic pH, the equilibrium is shifted farther toward the protonated (uncharged form), increasing the amount of salicylate able to diffuse across the membranes. Conversely, at high serum pH, equilibrium is shifted toward the unprotonated (charged) form. In this charged form, it cannot cross membranes and becomes "trapped" (see Figure 43-2).[7]

Salicylates affect many organ systems. Gastrointestinal effects are prominent, especially in the acute toxicity. Patients may present with nausea and vomiting from gastric mucosal irritation (from decreased prostaglandin production) and from direct salicylate effects on the medullary chemoreceptor zone. Perforation can occur but is uncommon in acute toxicity.

Salicylates affect the CNS. In the brain, salicylates stimulate the medullary respiratory center causing hyperpnea, tachypnea, and respiratory alkalosis.[8] In severe toxicities, cerebral edema, seizures, and coma can occur.

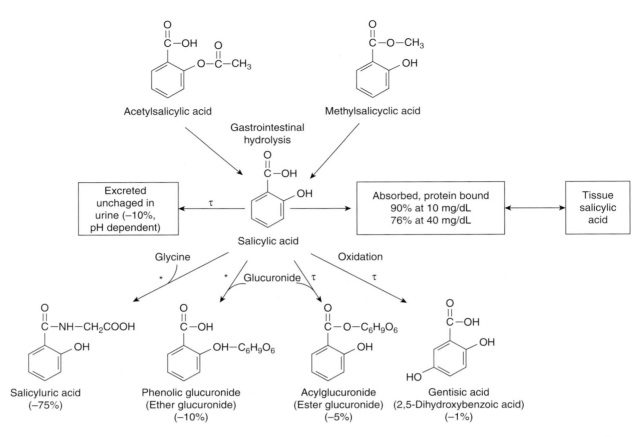

Figure 43-1. Salicylate metabolism. (Reproduced with permission from Goldfrank LR, Nelson LS, Howland MA, et al. *Salicylates in Goldfrank's Toxicological Emergencies.* 8th ed. McGraw-Hill Companies Inc; 2006. Figure 35-1.)

Prior to alkalinization

Tissues pH 6.8	Plasma pH 7.1	Urine pH 6.5
HA	HA	HA
H⁺ + A⁻	H⁺ + A⁻	H⁺ + A⁻

After alkalinization

Tissues pH 6.8	Plasma pH 7.4	Urine pH 8.0
HA	HA	HA
H⁺ + A⁻	H⁺ + A⁻	H⁺ + A⁻

Figure 43-2. Alkalinization shifts equilibrium toward the plasma and urine and away from the tissues. (Reproduced with permission from Goldfrank LR, Nelson LS, Howland MA, et al. *Salicylates in Goldfrank's Toxicological Emergencies.* 8th ed. McGraw-Hill Companies Inc; 2006. Figure 35-2.)

Salicylates disrupt respiration and metabolism. In severe toxicity, acute lung injury may occur. However, the most important effect is on the mitochondria. Salicylates uncouple oxidative phosphorylation, which means the energy generated from the electronic transport chain is dissipated as heat and not available for ATP formation. Heat generation manifests as hyperthermia and lack of ATP for cellular energy leads to increased anaerobic metabolism and production of pyruvate and lactic acid.[9] Lipid metabolism is also stimulated, leading to generation of ketones and anion gap acidosis.[10] Salicylates also inhibit ATP-dependent reactions resulting in increased oxygen consumption and carbon dioxide production. The increased lipid and glycogen metabolism is especially important in those with poor glycogen storage, for example, infants and chronic alcoholics.

► HISTORY

A careful history should be taken to the amount of salicylate the patient ingested and the presence of coingestants. The clinician should identify comorbid

▶ TABLE 43-1. **SALICYLATE OVERDOSE SYMPTOMS**

Organ System	Minor/Moderate Symptoms	Severe Symptoms
Neurologic	Anxiety, difficulty concentrating, hallucinations, vertigo, lethargy, tremors, delirium	Seizures, coma, cerebral edema
Cardiovascular	Tachycardia	Hypotension, dysrhythmias, asystole
Pulmonary	Tachypnea (from stimulation of respiratory center), hyperpnea	Noncardiogenic pulmonary edema, respiratory arrest, apnea
Gastrointestinal	Nausea, vomiting (from stimulation of chemoreceptor in brain), abdominal pain (many focused on epigastric region), delayed gastric emptying	GI bleed, bowel perforation
ENT	Tinnitus	Deafness
Psychiatric	Exacerbation of underlying psychiatric illness	
Hematologic	Inhibition of platelet function and disturbances in clotting factors	
Metabolic	Hyperthermia, hypoglycemia, hyperglycemia	

conditions that might complicate treatment, such as a history of liver disease, renal failure, or congestive heart failure. The chronicity of ingestion is vital when determining therapy. Acute overdoses are more likely in young patients and intentional overdoses. Ingestions of more than 300 mg/kg is considered serious while greater than 500 mg/kg can be potentially fatal. Chronic toxicity is more likely in the elderly and from unintentional overuse. In contrast with acute ingestion, which is usually easily identified by history, chronic ingestion may not be apparent in the history. In some cases, patients have been hospitalized for days before chronic salicylate poisoning is identified.[11–13] The mortality rate for acute overdoses is about 1% compared with 25% for chronic toxicities.

▶ CLINICAL MANIFESTATIONS

As expected, salicylate toxicity can present with various clinical findings (see Table 43-1). Patients can report anxiety, difficulty with concentration, hallucinations, lethargy, or even at the end of the spectrum with coma and seizures. On physical examination, patients may be tachycardiac, tachypneic, hyperpneic, and hyperthermic. In acute ingestions, nausea and vomiting may be prominent.

▶ DIAGNOSTIC TESTING

Traditionally, a serum salicylate concentration of up to 30 mg/dL is considered therapeutic. Tinnitus, an early sign of toxicity, occurs at about 35 mg/dL. However, salicylate concentrations should be interpreted in context of the chronicity of ingestion. In acute toxicity, there is a large amount of salicylate in the GI tract and blood and proportionally less in the tissues. In contrast, in chronic salicylate poisoning, in which there is

a high tissue burden, patients may exhibit toxicity at lower serum salicylate concentrations. Serum salicylate concentration may not correlate with the CSF salicylate concentration, which is why clinical symptoms are more important than serum concentrations. A toxicity nomogram was once proposed for salicylate poisoning but is not recommended as it does not accurately predict poisoning.[14]

Salicylate poisoning causes both primary metabolic acidosis and primary respiratory alkalosis. Respiratory alkalosis predominates early in poisoning. As toxicity worsens, a metabolic acidosis develops. Pure metabolic acidosis is unusual in adults unless combined with coingestions of respiratory depressants. Serum pH of 7.4 or less in salicylate poisoning is a marker of severe toxicity.

Electrolyte and fluid abnormalities may occur in salicylate toxicity, as a result of both poisoning and therapy. Emesis and diaphoresis can causes severe hypovolemia. Hypokalemia can result from vomiting and alkalinization, and serum calcium levels may drop from alkalinization. In severe salicylate poisonings, serum glucose concentration can be high from glycogenolysis and gluconeogenesis in the earlier stages and low from impaired gluconeogenesis and increased usage in later stages. However, be mindful that salicylate toxicity can decrease CNS glucose concentration despite a normal peripheral glucose concentration.[15]

▶ MANAGEMENT

As with most emergency critical care, the clinician should ensure that the airway is stable. However, intubation in a severe salicylate overdose can be dangerous. The presence of hyperpnea and tachypnea should not necessarily be interpreted as "respiratory distress" requiring intubation. Rather, intubation and mechanical ventilation should be reserved for patients who are no longer protecting their airway, are failing to oxygenate, or have serum pH indicating that they are failing to maintain respiratory alkalosis. In severe poisonings, patients are dependent on tachypnea and hyperpnea to breathe off carbon dioxide and maintain near-normal pH. If ventilation is abruptly decreased, a sudden rise in carbon dioxide and drop in serum pH may occur, resulting in passage of more salicylate into the tissues and worsening poisoning. In a case series, mechanical ventilation was associated with worsening of pH in salicylate-poisoned patients.[16]

If intubation is necessary, an experienced operator should perform the procedure. To minimize hypoventilation, a rapid-onset sedative and paralytic should be used, and patients should be hyperventilated throughout until initiation of laryngoscopy. Once intubated, patients should be hyperventilated to maintain the respiratory alkalosis compensating for the metabolic acidosis. Patients should be sedated to prevent breath-stacking and ventilatory asynchrony. CPAP mode of ventilation should be considered because it will allow the patient to breathe at his or her own rate. As the sedative and paralytic effects dissipate, patient's tachypnea and hyperpnea may return and may cause "breath stacking" and ventilatory asynchrony. Frequent blood gases should be obtained and serum pH should be maintained between 7.5 and 7.6.

GASTRIC DECONTAMINATION AND ACTIVED CHARCOAL

Gastric lavage should be only considered if a dangerous amount of tablets is still in the stomach. This is usually only within 60 minutes of ingestion, so gastric lavage is rarely used. The risk of aspiration usually outweighs the benefits of possible extraction of tablets still in the stomach. If performed, lavage should be followed by activated charcoal.[17]

Ipecac should not be used, and was shown to be inferior to activated charcoal in lowering the absorption of salicylates.[18]

Activated charcoal should be administered in all patients who are not at risk of pulmonary aspiration. It reduces the absorption of therapeutic aspirin doses by 50–80%.[19] Adding sorbital to activated charcoal may prevent salicylate absorption.[20] It is not clear whether there is increased benefit to multiple-dose activated charcoal.[21–24] In theory, multiple-dose activated charcoal will decrease absorption of salicylate still present in the GI tract from bezoar formation or enteric-coated formulations. We recommend charcoal with sorbital on initial presentation followed by charcoal without sorbital at 4-hour intervals until salicylate poisoning has resolved.

Whole bowel irrigation (oral administration of polyethylene glycol electrolyte lavage solution) does not increase the clearance of absorbed salicylate.[24,25]

ALKALINIZATION

Since an increase in pH shifts the equilibrium of salicylate to the ionized state, alkalinization of blood will limit salicylates from entering other organs (most importantly the brain). This phenomenon has been described as "ion trapping" because ionized salicylate is trapped in the plasma, and thus cannot pass into tissues. Serum alkalinization results in urine alkalinization, which may increase elimination by trapping ionized salicylate in the renal tubules. In support of this concept, it has been shown that elimination of salicylates is dependent on urinary pH.[26,27] Excretion increases from 2% in acidic urine to 31% in alkaline urine. As expected, the half-life of salicylate also decreases and total body clearance of salicylate increases under alkaline conditions.[27]

Alkalinization should be considered in patients with serum salicylate concentration greater than 35 mg/dL and suspected salicylate toxicity until blood pH is available to properly guide treatment. Alkalemia should be achieved with intravenous sodium bicarbonate. The goal should be plasma pH between 7.45 and 7.55 and urinary pH of 7.5–8.0. (We recommend adding 150 mEq of sodium bicarbonate to 1 L of D5W and administering at 150–200 mL/h or twice maintenance rate.) In a critically ill patient receiving bicarbonate therapy, frequent serum and urinary pH should be obtained to determine bicarbonate dosage. Carbonic anhydrase inhibitors, which alkalinize urine, should not be used as they create a metabolic acidosis.

Potassium and calcium are important electrolytes to monitor in salicylate toxicities. Hypokalemia can result from induced alkalemia, urinary potassium loss, diarrhea if cathartic is used, and metabolic alkalosis from vomiting. In the presence of hypokalemia, alkalosis therapy may be hindered. Hypocalcemia can result from bicarbonate therapy and must be repleted quickly.

EXTRACORPOREAL TREATMENT

Extracorporeal treatment is usually reserved for correcting fluid, electrolyte, acid–base, and urea abnormalities along with clearing unwanted solute. In salicylate overdose, extracorporeal treatment is usually reserved for patients with severe toxicity or those who cannot tolerate conventional therapy. It is recommended for patients with CNS toxicity, acute lung injury or pulmonary edema, renal insufficiency, refractory acidosis,

▶ **TABLE 43-2. SALICYLATE METABOLISM**

- CNS disturbances: altered mental status, seizures, coma, cerebral edema
- Renal insufficiency
- Refractory serum acidosis despite aggressive medical therapy
- Clinical deterioration despite aggressive medical therapy
- Plasma salicylate concentration >100 mg/dL (7.2 mmol/L) in acute ingestions or >60 mg/dL (4.3 mmol/L) in chronic ingestions (some clinicians set concentrations lower, especially for chronic ingestions)
- Consideration for mechanically ventilated patients and hepatic dysfunction

or clinical deterioration despite medical therapy. In the absence of these conditions, extracorporeal treatment should be performed for serum salicylate concentration >100 or >60 mg/dL in chronic poisonings (see Table 43-2).[28] The serum salicylate concentration indication for extracorporeal treatment in chronic ingestions is set lower, since many cases of fatal cases report lower serum concentrations, some in the 50- to 70-mg/dL range.[29] A patient on mechanical ventilation should also be considered, since mechanical ventilation alone may be inadequate to maintain respiratory alkalosis. Finally, hepatic dysfunction may require extracorporeal treatment as salicylates are metabolized by the liver.

Hemodialysis is the extracorporeal technique of choice. Hemoperfusion provides better clearance but hemodialysis has the added benefit of correcting electrolyte imbalances and acid–base disorders. Hemodialysis and hemoperfusion can be done in series but are rarely used in reality.[30] In hemodynamically unstable patients who cannot tolerate large fluid shifts caused by hemodialysis, continuous venovenous hemodiafiltration can be used.[31] Extracorporeal treatments should be used in conjunction with other therapies and other therapies should not be held while waiting for extracorporeal treatment.

REFERENCES

1. Patrono C, Rocca B. Aspirin, 110 years later. *J Thromb Haemost.* 2009;7:258–261.
2. 2008 annual report of the American Association of Poison Control Centers' National Poison Data System (NPDS): 26th annual report. *Clin Toxicol.* 2009;47:911–1084.
3. Bruton LL, Lazo JS, Parker KL. *Goodman & Gillman's The Pharmacological Basis of Therapeutics.* 11th ed. McGraw-Hill Companies Inc; 2006.
4. Wortzman DJ, Grunfled A. Delayed absorption following enteric-coated aspirin overdose. *Ann Emerg Med.* 1987;16(4):434–436.
5. Rivera W, Kleinschmidt KC, Velez LI, et al. Delayed salicylate toxicity at 35 hours without early manifestations following a single salicylate ingestion. *Ann Pharmacother.* 2004;38(7–8):1186–1188.
6. Levy G. Clinical pharmacokinetics of salicylates: a reassessment. *Br J Clin Pharmacol.* 1980;10(suppl 2): 285S–290S.
7. Temple AR. Acute and chronic effects of aspirin toxicity and their treatment. *Arch Intern Med.* 1981;141:364–369.
8. Tenney SM, Miller RM. The respiratory and circulatory action of salicylate. *Am J Med.* 1955;19:498–508.
9. Krebs HG, Woods HG, Alberti KG. Hyperlactatemia and lactic acidosis. *Essays Med Biochem.* 1975;1:81–103.
10. Rothschild BM. Hematologic perturbations associated with salicylate. *Clin Pharmacol Ther.* 1979;26:145–150.
11. Anderson RJ, Potts DE, Gabow PA, et al. Unrecognized adult salicylate intoxication. *Ann Intern Med.* 1976;85(6):745–748.
12. Bailey RB, Jones SR. Chronic salicylate intoxication: a common cause of morbidity in the elderly. *J Am Geriatr Soc.* 1989;37(6):556–561.
13. Chui PT. Anesthesia in a patient with undiagnosed salicylate poisoning presenting as intraabdominal sepsis. *J Clin Anesth.* 1999;11(3):251–253.
14. Dugandzic RM, Tierney MG, Dickinson Ge, et al. Evaluation of the validity of the Done nomogram in the management of acute salicylate intoxication. *Ann Emerg Med.* 1989;18:1186–1190.
15. Thurston JH, Pollock PG, Warren SK, et al. Reduced brain glucose with normal plasma glucose in salicylate poisoning. *J Clin Invest.* 1970;49(11):2139–2145.
16. Stolbach AI, Hoffman RS, Nelson LS. Mechanical ventilation was associated with acidemia in a case series of salicylate-poisoned patients. *Acad Emerg Med.* 2008; 15(9):866–869.
17. Burton BT, Bayer MJ, Barron L, et al. Comparison of activated charcoal and gastric lavage in the prevention of aspirin absorption. *J Emerg Med.* 1984;1(5):411–416.
18. Curtis RA, Barone J, Giacona N. Efficacy of ipecac and activated charcoal/cathartic. Prevention of salicylate absorption in a simulated overdose. *Arch Intern Med.* 1984;144(1):48–52.
19. Levy G, Tsuchiya T. Effect of activated charcoal on aspirin absorption in man. *Clin Pharmacol Ther.* 1972;13: 317–322.
20. Keller RE, Schwab RA, Krenzelok EP. Contribution of sorbitol combined with activated charcoal in prevention of salicylate absorption. *Ann Emerg Med.* 1990;19:654–656.
21. Barone JA, Raia JJ, Huang YC. Evaluation of the effects of multiple-dose activated charcoal on the absorption of orally administered salicylate in a simulated toxic ingestion model. *Ann Emerg Med.* 1988;17:34–37.
22. Hillman RJ, Prescott LF. Treatment of salicylate poisoning with repeated oral charcoal. *BMJ.* 1986;291:1472.
23. Kirshenbaum LA, Mathews SC, Sitar DS, et al. Does multiple-dose charcoal therapy enhance salicylate excretion? *Arch Intern Med.* 1990;150:1281–1283.
24. Mayer AL, Sitar DS, Tenebein M. Multiple-dose charcoal and whole-bowel irrigation do not increase clearance of absorbed salicylate. New York, New York. *Arch Intern Med.* 1992;152:393–396.

25. Tenenbein M. Whole-bowel irrigation as a gastrointestinal decontamination procedure after acute poisoning. *Med Toxicol.* 1988;3:77–84.

26. Prescott LF, Balali-Mood M, Critchley JA, et al. Diuresis or urinary alkalinization for salicylate poisoning? *BMJ.* 1982;285:1383–1386.

27. Vree TB, Van Ewijk-Beneken Kolmer EW, Verwey-Van Wissen CP, et al. Effect of urinary pH on the pharmacokinetics of salicylic acid, with its glycine and glucuronide conjugates in humans. *Int J Clin Pharmacol Ther.* 1994; 32:550–558.

28. Fertel BS, Nelson LS, Goldfarb DS. The underutilization of hemodialysis in patients with salicylate poisoning. *Kidney Int.* 2009;75(12):1349–1353.

29. Watson WA, Litovitz TL, Rodgers GC, et al. 2004 annual report of the American Association of Poison Control Centers Toxic Exposure Surveillance System. *Am J Emerg Med.* 2005;23:589–666.

30. DeBroe ME, Verpooten GA, Christiaens ME, et al. Clinical experience with prolonged combined hemoperfusion–hemodialysis treatment of severe poisoning. *Artif Organs.* 1981;5:59–66.

31. Wrathall G, Sinclair R, Moore A, et al. Three case reports of the use of haemodiafiltration in the treatment of salicylate overdose. *Hum Exp Toxicol.* 2001;20:491–495.

SECTION X

Ultrasonography in Critical Care

CHAPTER 44

Point-of-Care Echocardiography in the Emergency Department

Stephen J. Leech, Falk Eike Flach, and L. Connor Nickels

▶ OVERVIEW

Point-of-care echocardiography is ideally suited to the care of the critical patient in the emergency department or intensive care unit. It is highly accurate, noninvasive, portable, rapidly performed, easily repeatable, and simple to learn. It can provide critical information in real time that otherwise may not be available, particularly in the setting of life-threatening emergencies. Point-of-care echocardiography increases patient safety, improves diagnostic accuracy, reduces diagnostic uncertainty, improves efficiency, and saves lives.

The purpose of this chapter is to provide a general understanding of point-of-care echocardiography, as it is applied and accepted in the emergency department and ICU setting. We present an overview of how echocardiography can be utilized in the management of the critically ill patient. This chapter is not intended as a complete reference and assumes a basic understanding of ultrasound physics, image generation, ultrasound modes, terminology, and system operation.

▶ SCOPE OF PRACTICE

Point-of-care ultrasound developed originally in Japan and Europe, and came into emergency medicine practice in United States in the 1990s. Point-of-care echocar-

diography is considered core content of the specialty of emergency medicine by the American Board of Emergency Medicine.[1] The American Medical Association supports the use of ultrasound by appropriately trained clinicians in varied specialties, and supports specialty-specific guidelines for training, education, and oversight.[2]

Point-of-care echocardiography is not the same as a comprehensive echocardiogram or an ultrasound study done in a traditional imaging suite. It is performed, interpreted, and integrated into patient care in real time at the bedside. Our goal is to immediately impact patient care by quickly and accurately performing a brief or focused exam designed to answer simple yes/no questions. Our exam will focus on immediate life-threatening conditions and to assess response to resuscitative measures. Point-of-care echocardiography has evolved over the past two decades into a bedside diagnostic tool, a method to safety guide invasive procedures, and a way to noninvasively assess and monitor ongoing resuscitation. The most current *American College of Emergency Physicians (ACEP) Emergency Ultrasound Guidelines* provide a comprehensive overview of the scope of practice, and training and credentialing guidelines, and serve as an excellent reference for any department starting and developing a point-of-care ultrasound program.[3]

► ECHOCARDIOGRAPHY— CLINICAL INDICATIONS

Echocardiography is an essential skill for emergency physicians and is especially well suited to the critically ill patient. Using simple qualitative echocardiography, emergency physicians can rapidly and definitively assess for cardiac activity in cardiac arrest, evaluate for pericardial effusion and tamponade, estimate left ventricular systolic function, noninvasively estimate preload and right ventricular filling pressure, identify acute right heart strain, direct resuscitation and medical decision making, and immediately differentiate treatable causes of PEA and shock. This chapter will focus on image acquisition, image interpretation, and integration of this information obtained into the care of the critically ill patient.

► ECHOCARDIOGRAPHY— TECHNICAL CONSIDERATIONS

Echocardiography is a technically challenging study to perform for many reasons. The heart is surrounded by the bony ribs and sternum, as well as the air-filled lungs that expand and compress with a varying respiratory rate. Both of these impede image acquisition by reflecting and scattering the sound waves, respectively. In addition, differences in body habitus, particularly obesity and deformities of the chest wall, and chronic disease conditions, such as emphysema, may make performing the study more difficult. The left lateral decubitus position is preferred for obtaining high-quality images, but many critical patients cannot be optimally positioned. Despite these inherent challenges, echocardiography rapidly provides critical, high-yield information, making it an invaluable tool.

The heart sits inside the left chest cavity at an oblique angle with the long axis of the heart running along a plane from the right shoulder to the left hip. The great vessels and base are cephalad and the apex is caudad. The right side of the heart is anterior inferior and the left side of the heart is posterior superior. Knowing this basic anatomy will improve image acquisition and help to explain orientation of structures.

The phased array transducer is the transducer of choice for echocardiography (Figure 44-1). Its small footprint and wide field of view allow easy manipulation and imaging between intercostal spaces. Image resolution is worse than transducers with similar frequencies, but temporal resolution (frame rate) is more important in the dynamic imaging of echocardiography.

Standard cardiac orientation orients the image toward the patient's head or left side, with the image indicator appearing in the upper right of the ultrasound screen. Views will be obtained with the transducer indicator oriented to the patient's head or left side. This leftward orientation is the opposite of abdominal

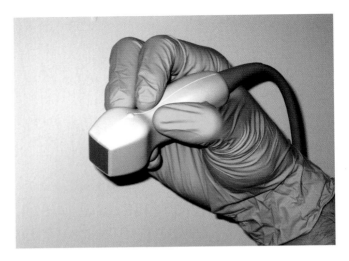

Figure 44-1. Phased array transducer. Its small footprint and superior frame rate make it the transducer of choice for echocardiography.

sonography, in which the image is oriented toward the patient's head or right side. Most ultrasound systems have a cardiac or echo preset that will automatically orient the image. The techniques and images in this chapter are presented in the traditional leftward or cardiac orientation.

Echocardiography is a dynamic medium, and still images do not convey the same amount of detail and information as live imaging. Most modern ultrasound systems have the capability to store digital video clips, which is the preferred image storage modality.

► ECHOCARDIOGRAPHY— IMAGING WINDOWS AND VIEWS

Many imaging windows and views have been described in echocardiography. We present a series of five views that allow for a rapid and comprehensive evaluation. These include the subxiphoid four-chamber view, subxiphoid longitudinal inferior vena cava (IVC) view, parasternal long-axis view, parasternal short-axis view, and apical four-chamber view. Additional views, such as the apical five-chamber view, will be discussed when evaluating left ventricular systolic function. The authors recommend obtaining as many views as is possible on each patient. Each view has strengths and weaknesses, and additional views may add additional critical information. One view may be sufficient in certain settings, such as cardiac arrest, but generally two to five views allow for a more accurate and comprehensive assessment.

SUBXIPHOID FOUR-CHAMBER VIEW

To obtain the subxiphoid four-chamber view, place the transducer in subxiphoid region, point the transducer

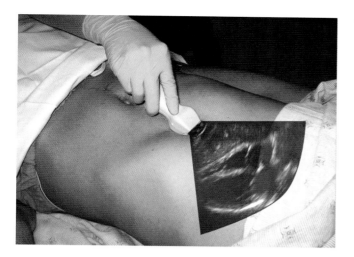

Figure 44-2. Subxiphoid four-chamber probe placement. Proper probe positioning for the subxiphoid four-chamber view is with the transducer below the xiphoid process in the epigastrium, pointing toward the left shoulder at a shallow angle, while the transducer indicator faces the patient's left side.

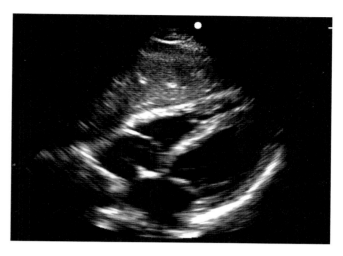

Figure 44-3. Subxiphoid four-chamber view of a normal heart. Note the right ventricle and right atrium in the near field and the larger left ventricle and atrium in the far field. The bright echogenic pericardium can be seen wrapping from the right atrium around the apex to the left atrium.

indicator toward patient's left side, and aim the ultrasound beam toward patient's left shoulder at a shallow angle (Figure 44-2). Identify the liver, cardiac silhouette, right ventricle, left ventricle, right atrium, left atrium, and pericardial space (Figure 44-3). Adjust the image by tilting, rocking, rotating, or sliding the transducer in order to align the beam angle so that all structures are in view.

This view is the easiest four-chamber view to obtain, and provides a great global overview. It allows for evaluation of pericardial effusion and evaluation of chamber size comparison, and is the best view during cardiopulmonary resuscitation because it does not interfere with resuscitative efforts including chest compressions, central lines, and pacer pads. This is generally the easiest view to obtain in patients with emphysema or other chest deformities.

Common mistakes when performing this view include too steep an angle of the ultrasound beam, as well as not enough depth to visualize the entire heart. A tip to allow a shallow angle of approach is to grasp the transducer from above, which allows a shallower angle without the operator's hand in the way. Stomach gas may obscure this view, which may be improved with either steady transducer pressure or having the patient take and hold a deep breath. Becoming familiar with the various troubleshooting techniques will allow for more efficient imaging.

SUBXIPHOID LONGITUDINAL IVC VIEW

To obtain the subxiphoid longitudinal IVC view, place the transducer in subxiphoid region, point the trans-

ducer indicator toward patient's head, and sweep into the patient's right upper quadrant to find IVC running through liver in a longitudinal plane (Figure 44-4). Identify the liver, IVC running through the liver, junction

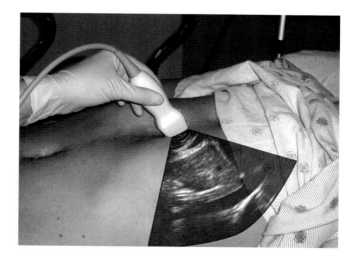

Figure 44-4. Subxiphoid IVC probe placement. Proper probe positioning for the subxiphoid IVC view is with the transducer below the xiphoid process, angled slightly upward, while the transducer indicator faces the patient's head. Once in this position, sweep laterally into the right upper quadrant until the IVC can be seen running through the liver into the right atrium. Alternatively, this view can be achieved by obtaining a subxiphoid four-chamber view with the right atrium in the center of the screen and then rotating the transducer 90° counterclockwise.

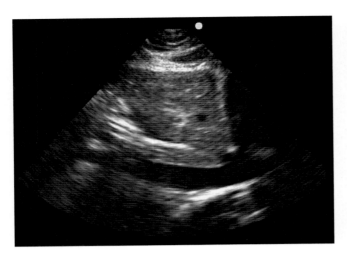

Figure 44-5. Subxiphoid IVC view of a healthy subject. Note the IVC is seen running through the liver, with thin walls, and joining the right atrium. Within the liver, the hepatic vein can be seen emptying into the IVC. The proper location for measuring IVC diameter is just distal to this junction.

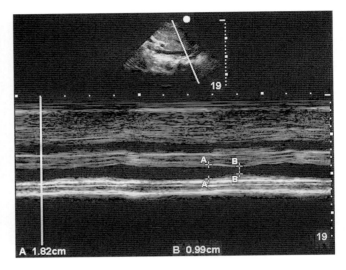

Figure 44-6. Subxiphoid IVC M-mode view showing normal IVC diameter (1.5–2.5 cm) with normal respiratory collapse (~50%).

of the IVC and hepatic veins, junction of the IVC and right atrium, right atrium, right ventricle, and pericardial space (Figure 44-5). Adjust the image by tilting, rocking, rotating, or sliding the transducer, in order to align the beam angle so that all structures are in view. The IVC may also be imaged in cross-section, but the longitudinal view is the authors' preference.

This view allows noninvasive assessment of central venous pressure during normal respiration, using both IVC diameter and respiratory change. M-mode is useful to obtain both maximal and minimal diameters of the IVC during the respiratory cycle (Figure 44-6).

A common mistake when performing the subxiphoid longitudinal IVC view is failing to tilt the transducer to shallow the angle of the ultrasound beam. When measuring the IVC diameter, it is important to have the long axis of the IVC perpendicular to the ultrasound beam. In addition, the IVC and abdominal aorta may be confused. The IVC is more to the patient's right, runs through the liver, has thin walls, generally exhibits respiratory variation, and enters the right atrium. The aorta is more to the patient's left, runs posterior to the liver, has thick echogenic walls, and has the celiac and SMA vessels exiting anteriorly.

PARASTERNAL LONG-AXIS VIEW

To obtain the parasternal long-axis view, place the transducer perpendicular to chest wall in the left fourth to sixth parasternal space, and point the transducer indicator toward patient's right shoulder (Figure 44-7).

Identify the right ventricle, left ventricle, left atrium, mitral valve, aortic valve, aortic root, and descending thoracic aorta posterior to the left atrium (Figure 44-8). Adjust the image by tilting, rocking, rotating, or sliding the transducer, in order to align the beam angle so that all the structures are in view. Rolling the patient into the left lateral decubitus position may allow for better image quality.

This is the best view for measurement of aortic root diameter, which should be less than 3.8 cm in diameter.

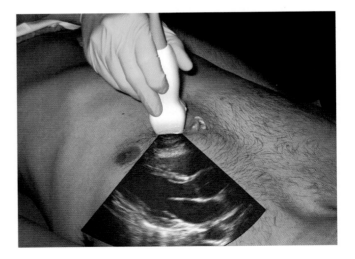

Figure 44-7. Parasternal long-axis probe placement. Proper probe positioning for the parasternal long-axis view is with the transducer in the fourth to sixth intercostal space immediately to the left of the sternum, while the transducer indicator is pointing toward the patient's right shoulder.

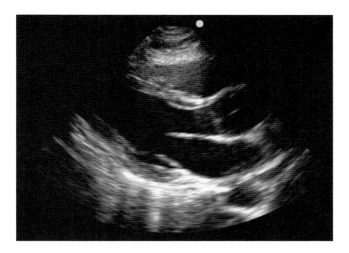 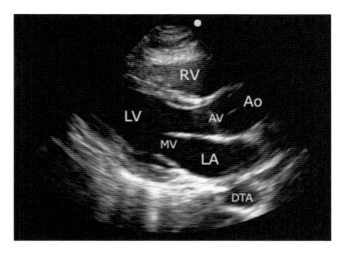

Figure 44-8. Parasternal long-axis view of a normal heart. The RV is the most anterior chamber and the RA is not in view. A true long-axis view of the left ventricle displays both the aortic and mitral valves simultaneously. The mitral valve is open; the heart is in mid-diastole. Note the descending aorta posterior to the left ventricle. Just anterior to the aorta, the bright echogenic pericardium wraps around the heart in a clockwise fashion.

In order to perform Doppler estimation of cardiac output, the left ventricular outflow tract (LVOT) diameter (LVOT D) should be measured in this view. This is also an excellent view for estimation of left ventricular systolic function using qualitative methods.

PARASTERNAL SHORT-AXIS VIEW

To obtain the parasternal short-axis view, place the transducer perpendicular to the chest wall in the left fourth to sixth parasternal space, and point the transducer indicator toward the patient's left shoulder (Figure 44-9). This view can also be obtained by rotating the transducer 90° clockwise from the parasternal long-axis view. Identify the right ventricle, left ventricle, and papillary muscles indenting the left ventricle (Figure 44-10). The papillary muscles serve as a landmark to make sure the section in view is through the left ventricle, and not the left atrium or aortic root. To obtain this view, the operator may have to tilt the transducer slightly downward, toward the patient's left hip, along the long axis of the heart. Rolling the patient into the left lateral decubitus position may allow for better image quality.

This is an excellent view for estimation of left ventricular systolic function, and the best view for identification of regional left ventricular systolic dysfunction.

APICAL FOUR-CHAMBER VIEW

To obtain the apical four-chamber view, place the transducer at the point of maximum impulse (PMI), point the transducer indicator toward the patient's left axilla, and aim the ultrasound beam toward patient's right shoulder at a shallow angle (Figure 44-11). Alternatively, the apical window can be found by finding the apex of the heart in the parasternal long-axis view toward the left of the screen. The transducer is moved over the apex in real time, and then rotated toward the patient's left axilla and the beam angle flattened. This is the most

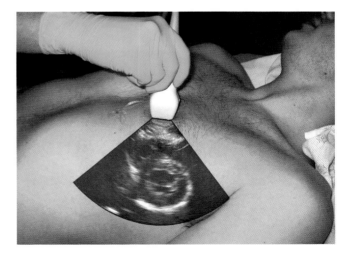

Figure 44-9. Parasternal short-axis probe placement. Proper probe positioning for the parasternal short-axis view is with the transducer in the fourth to sixth intercostal space immediately to the left of the sternum, while the transducer indicator is pointing toward the left shoulder. Alternatively, this view can be achieved by obtaining a parasternal long-axis view and then rotating the transducer 90° clockwise.

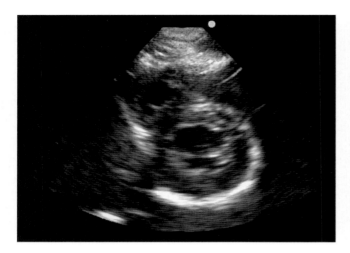
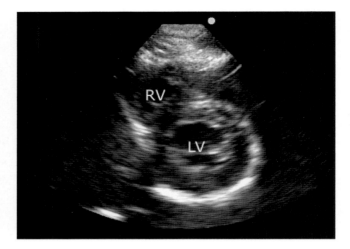

Figure 44-10. Parasternal short-axis view at the level of the papillary muscles of a normal heart. This marks the portion of the left ventricle immediately distal to the mitral valve, which is where left ventricular function is assessed. This view is also excellent for identifying regional wall motion abnormalities.

challenging basic view to obtain, and rolling the patient into the left lateral decubitus position usually allows for better image quality. Identify the left ventricle, mitral valve, left atrium, right ventricle, tricuspid valve, and right atrium (Figure 44-12).

This is the best view for assessment of valvular pathology, as well as comparing relative right and left ventricular sizes. The normal right ventricle to left ventricle ratio is <0.6 to 1 measured across valve leaflets. A good rule of thumb for qualitative inspection is that the image should be "1/3 right ventricle, 2/3 left ventricle." This view is also excellent for Doppler interrogation of

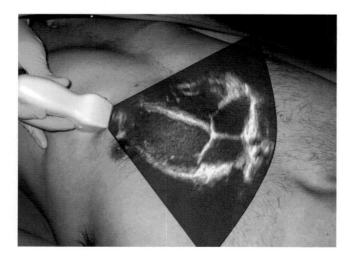

Figure 44-11. Apical four-chamber probe placement. Proper probe positioning for the apical four-chamber view is with the probe overlying the PMI, pointing at a shallow angle toward the right shoulder, while aiming the transducer indicator toward the left axilla.

inflow and outflow velocities for advanced echocardiographic applications.

▶ TRAINING

One prospective study showed that a focused 6-hour training course significantly improved emergency medicine residents' theoretical and practical knowledge of bedside echocardiography.[4] This study enrolled 21 emergency medicine residents who underwent 5 hours of didactics and 1 hour of hands-on instruction on echocardiography. Subjects underwent preexposure and postexposure testing of their theoretical and practical knowledge. Practical scores significantly increased from 56% to 94%, and theoretical scores significantly improved from 54% to 76%. This study suggests that skills necessary for competent bedside echocardiography can quickly be learned and applied.

Current ACEP guidelines recommend performing at least 25 proctored exams prior to using bedside echocardiography independently in patient care decisions.[3] The exception to this would be in a case where delaying treatment or further interventions in order to obtain some other reference standard would cause undue harm to the patient.

▶ CLINICAL SCENARIOS

ECHOCARDIOGRAPHY IN CARDIAC ARREST

Echocardiography is an excellent adjunct in the setting of cardiac arrest. It enables one to differentiate organized and agonal cardiac contraction from cardiac standstill, providing prognostic information. In addition, it allows

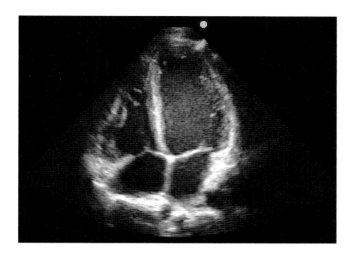
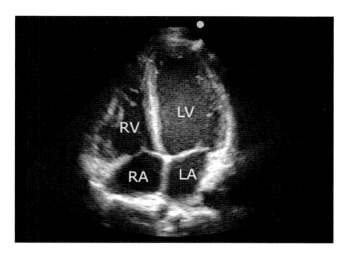

Figure 44-12. Apical four-chamber view of a normal heart. Note the normal right to left ventricular size ratio of less than of 0.6 to 1.

rapid diagnosis and treatment of reversible causes of cardiac arrest, such as hypovolemia, tamponade, left ventricular dysfunction secondary to myocardial infarction, and acute right heart strain due to pulmonary embolus.

There is a strong association between cardiac standstill on echocardiogram and mortality. One prospective observational trial enrolled 169 patients in cardiac arrest.[5] All 136 patients with cardiac standstill on initial bedside echocardiogram died in the emergency department. Another prospective observational study of 70 patients in cardiac arrest showed 100% mortality for patients with cardiac standstill.[6] An additional prospective observational study of patients in cardiac arrest enrolled 20 patients, and found 100% mortality for patients in cardiac standstill.[7] If replicated in larger studies, these results imply that substantial hospital resources and manpower could be saved by using echocardiography to identify cardiac standstill during resuscitation. At the time of this writing, a multicenter prospective study is underway to confirm these findings with sufficient power.

Cardiac standstill carries a grave prognosis and can be considered a marker for termination of resuscitative efforts in certain settings. Individual reflections from slow-moving red blood cells may be seen, or blood may be seen clotting in the heart, which is a late finding (Figure 44-13).

The presence of cardiac activity during any point of the resuscitative effort is strongly associated with survival to hospital admission. In a prospective observational trial on 102 patients in cardiac arrest, patients with cardiac activity at any point of the resuscitation survived at a much higher rate, 27% versus 3%.[8] A similar study showed that 12 out of 18 patients (67%) with PEA and cardiac contractions survived to hospital admission.[5]

A third study showed that 8 out of 11 patients (73%) with PEA and cardiac contractions survived to hospital admission.[6]

Any cardiac motion corresponding with electrical impulses should be considered to be cardiac activity, and aggressive attempts at resuscitation should be continued. The presence of cardiac activity predicts return of spontaneous circulation.

Another benefit of bedside ultrasound during cardiac arrest is the ability to identify reversible causes, such as pericardial tamponade. In a prospective observational study of patients in cardiac arrest of 20 patients, the authors demonstrated pericardial effusions in 8 of 12 patients with cardiac motion, including 3 cases of tamponade.[7] Finding a treatable cause of cardiac arrest,

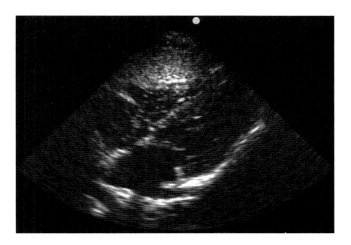

Figure 44-13. Subxiphoid four-chamber view showing cardiac arrest with lack of cardiac contraction and characteristic reflection of swirling; slow-moving red blood cell reflectors seen within the right atrium and ventricle.

such as a large pericardial effusion, should prompt immediate definitive treatment. In this case, pericardiocentesis is indicated, preferably under ultrasound guidance. The findings of tamponade physiology are discussed later in the chapter.

As previously mentioned, the subxiphoid four-chamber view is an excellent view during cardiac arrest. It does not interfere with chest compressions or other resuscitative efforts, and provides an excellent global view of the heart. From this window, the heart can be quickly assessed for the presence of cardiac contraction, pericardial effusion and tamponade, left ventricular function, as well as right ventricular size, to detect right ventricular dilation in suspected pulmonary embolus or a flat right ventricle in suspected hypovolemia. Alternatively, the parasternal long axis can be used. Imaging should occur during pulse checks to minimize interruptions in CPR.

ECHOCARDIOGRAPHY TO IDENTIFY PERICARDIAL EFFUSION AND TAMPONADE PHYSIOLOGY

Emergency physicians can rapidly and accurately identify pericardial effusion and tamponade physiology using point-of-care echocardiography.

Several studies have shown emergency physicians can accurately identify pericardial effusion and tamponade physiology. One prospective observational enrolled 515 patients at high risk for pericardial effusion and found 103 positive studies.[9] All studies were performed and interpreted by emergency physicians and subsequently reviewed by a cardiologist. Sensitivity and specificity of bedside echocardiography performed by emergency physicians for pericardial effusion were 96% and 98%, respectively. Another study showed that patients with unexplained new-onset dyspnea may benefit from emergency physician–performed echocardiography to rule out pericardial effusion.[10] This prospective, observational trial enrolled 103 patients with new-onset dyspnea unexplained by pulmonary, infectious, hematologic, traumatic, psychiatric, cardiovascular, or neuromuscular disease after ED evaluation. Fourteen of 103 patients had effusions, with 4 classified as large.

In penetrating chest trauma, echocardiography has been shown to reduce time to diagnosis and decrease mortality. In one retrospective study, the authors reviewed the records of 49 patients with penetrating cardiac injury.[11] Survival was 100% in the echo group, compared with 57% in the nonecho group. The average time to diagnosis and disposition for surgical intervention was significantly shorter at 15 minutes for the echo group versus 42 minutes for the nonecho group A prospective multicenter study enrolled 261 patients, with 29 true positives confirmed in the operating room.[12]

Bedside echocardiography had a sensitivity of 100% and a specificity of 97% for the diagnosis of hemopericardium, and mean time from ED arrival to operative intervention in positive cases was 12 minutes. Due to its excellent test characteristics and time savings, the authors recommended bedside echocardiography as the initial diagnostic modality of choice in penetrating chest trauma.

A pericardial effusion appears as an anechoic fluid collection in the pericardial space. Typically, effusions are circumferential, but may be loculated in postoperative patients and patients with inflammatory conditions. In these cases, there may be some echoes present within the effusion. The absence of pericardial effusion essentially rules out tamponade as a cause of hypotension.

Pericardial effusions are seen in many sizes. A small effusion may only be seen in the dependent portion of the pericardium, and generally measures less than 5 mm. Moderate pericardial effusions are generally circumferential, and measure between 5 and 10 mm. Large pericardial effusions are circumferential and measure greater than 10 mm. Swinging of the heart in the pericardial sac may be seen, and often manifests as electrical alternans on electrocardiography (Figures 44-14 to 44-18).

Pitfalls in diagnosing pericardial effusions do exist. The most common are mistaking a normal fat pad or pleural effusion for a pericardial effusion. These pitfalls can be avoided with careful scanning, observing the heart in multiple views, and identifying key landmarks.

A pericardial fat pad can often have a similar appearance to an effusion (Figure 44-19). Typically, a fat pad is only present anteriorly, has internal echoes,

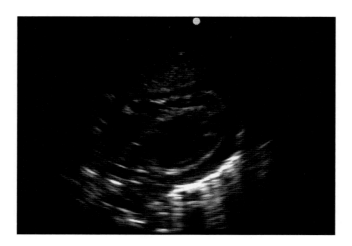

Figure 44-14. Subxiphoid four-chamber view showing a moderate pericardial effusion with an anechoic fluid stripe circumferentially surrounding the heart.

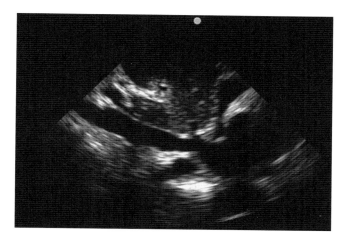

Figure 44-15. Subxiphoid IVC view demonstrating a large pericardial effusion between liver and RV. In this case, there was normal IVC diameter and respiratory change, without evidence of tamponade physiology.

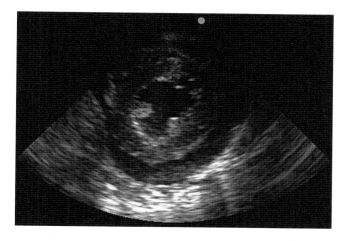

Figure 44-17. Parasternal short-axis view of the left ventricle at the level of the papillary muscles showing a large pericardial effusion with an anechoic fluid stripe circumferentially surrounding the heart.

and moves with the heart. Using multiple views will allow the user to distinguish an anatomic fat pad from an abnormal pericardial effusion.

A left-sided pleural effusion is commonly mistaken for a pericardial effusion. Pericardial effusions are typically circumferential, where a pleural effusion is only seen posterior to the heart. Key landmarks for identifying pericardial from pleural fluid are the left atrium and descending thoracic aorta on the parasternal long-axis view. Pericardial fluid will appear between the left atrium and descending aorta, whereas pleural effusion will be seen posterior to the descending aorta (Figure 44-20).

When a pericardial effusion is identified, tamponade must be considered. Tamponade is a time-critical clinical diagnosis of hypoperfusion in the setting of a pericardial effusion. Increasing pressure in the non-distensible pericardium limits right ventricular filling and venous return, leading to circulatory collapse. Tamponade is difficult to diagnose solely on clinical findings. A recent case series showed that pericardial tamponade can often present without the classic findings of Beck's triad, and mimic more common disease processes.[13]

Qualitative echocardiography can show evidence of "tamponade physiology." Findings consistent with

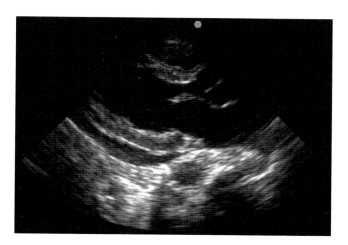

Figure 44-16. Parasternal long-axis view showing a moderate-sized pericardial effusion with an anechoic fluid stripe layering out posterior to the myocardium and anterior to the descending aorta.

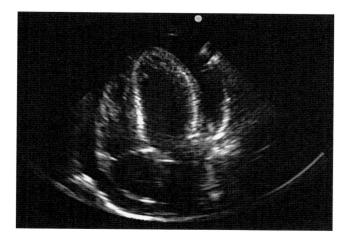

Figure 44-18. Apical four-chamber view showing a large pericardial effusion with an anechoic fluid stripe circumferentially surrounding the heart. Note no evidence of either RA or RV collapse, ruling out tamponade physiology.

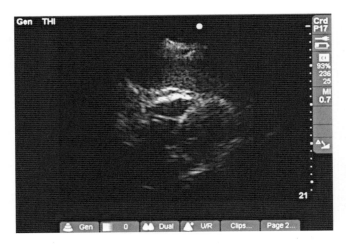

Figure 44-19. Subxiphoid four-chamber view showing a small pericardial fat pad anteriorly between the liver and RV. Note the internal echoes, and absence of any collection posterior to the LV. In real time, a fat pad can be seen stretching and moving with the heart.

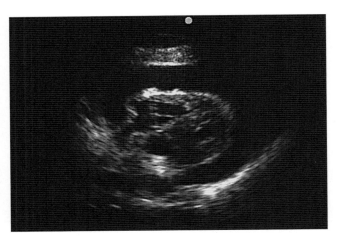

Figure 44-21. Subxiphoid four-chamber view showing RA atrial collapse. Note the large pericardial effusion surrounding the entire heart. The elevated pericardial pressure is causing RA collapse in late diastole, consistent with tamponade physiology.

tamponade physiology include early diastolic collapse of the right ventricle, late diastolic collapse of the right atrium, as well as dilation of the IVC with loss of normal respiratory variation (Figures 44-21 to 44-24).

Doppler echocardiography can also be used to diagnose tamponade in the setting of pericardial effusion. Normal cardiac filling is influenced by respiratory phase, with filling reduced in inspiration due to negative intrathoracic pressure. This phenomenon leads to the presence of pulsus paradoxus. In tamponade, cardiac filling is further impaired, and this can be demonstrated using pulsed wave spectral Doppler interrogation of mitral inflow velocities. This is best seen in the apical four-chamber view. To obtain this information, place the pulsed wave spectral Doppler gate in the LV to measure mitral inflow velocity. Normal E-wave (early diastolic) velocity decreases with inspiration, but usually less than 10–15%. With tamponade, LV inflow is further restricted, leading to an exaggerated inspiratory decrease of greater than 25% in maximal E-wave velocity (Figure 44-25).[14]

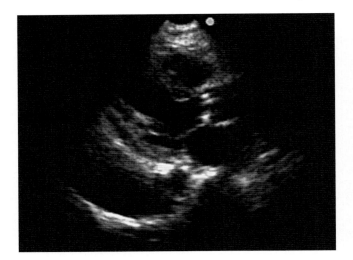

Figure 44-20. Parasternal long-axis view showing a large pleural effusion with an anechoic fluid stripe layering out posterior to the LV and descending aorta. Compare this image with Figure 44-16 to see the difference between locations of a pericardial and pleural effusion.

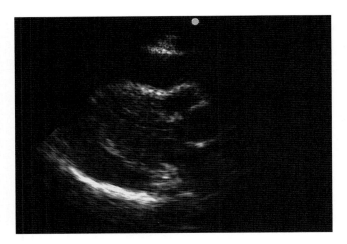

Figure 44-22. Parasternal long-axis view showing right ventricular collapse. Note the large pericardial effusion surrounding the heart. The elevated pericardial pressure is causing RV collapse in early diastole, consistent with tamponade physiology.

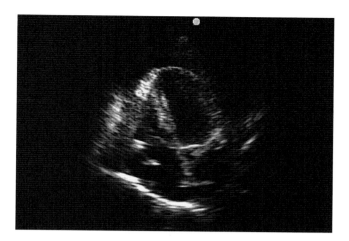

Figure 44-23. Apical four-chamber view showing right atrial collapse. Note the large pericardial effusion surrounding the entire heart. The elevated pericardial pressure is causing RA collapse in late diastole, consistent with tamponade physiology.

One prospective observational study in 56 consecutive patients with pericardial effusion study compared qualitative findings of tamponade and Doppler findings of tamponade.[15] Sixteen patients were found to have tamponade and underwent drainage. A 22% decrease in peak mitral inflow velocity during inspiration had sensitivities and specificities of 77% and 80%, respectively. Right ventricular collapse performed quite similarly with sensitivities and specificities of 75% and 85%, respectively.

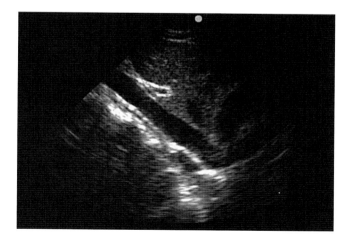

Figure 44-24. Subxiphoid IVC view with effusion, dilated IVC, and lack of respiratory variation. Note the dilated IVC running through the liver joining with the right atrium. In tamponade, right atrial filling pressures are elevated, increasing IVC diameter, as well as reducing respiratory variation.

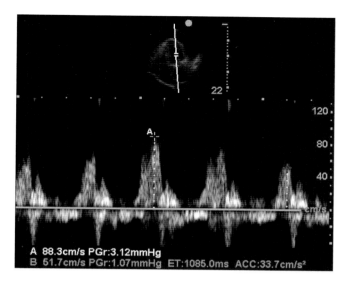

A 88.3cm/s PGr:3.12mmHg
B 51.7cm/s PGr:1.07mmHg ET:1085.0ms ACC:33.7cm/s²

Figure 44-25. Apical four-chamber with effusion, mitral inflow Doppler decrease >25%. Doppler waveform of mitral inflow velocity obtained from an apical four-chamber view with the Doppler gate in the left ventricle just beyond the mitral leaf leaflets. The maximum inflow velocity of the E wave (passive ventricular filling) is measured during expiration (A) and inspiration (B), and decreases by more than 25% with inspiration, indicating the presence of tamponade physiology.

ECHOCARDIOGRAPHY TO ESTIMATE LEFT VENTRICULAR SYSTOLIC FUNCTION

Emergency physicians can accurately estimate left ventricular systolic function using point-of-care echocardiography. Both qualitative and quantitative estimation methods will be reviewed. Simple qualitative methods are fast, easy to learn, and accurately correlate with quantitative methods.

Several studies have shown that emergency physicians can accurately estimate left ventricular systolic function. A prospective observational study enrolled a convenience sample of 51 patients with symptomatic hypotension.[16] Patients underwent bedside echocardiography by emergency physicians and were classified to have normal, depressed, or severely depressed ejection fraction. A blinded cardiologist interpreted these images and served as the gold standard, while a second cardiologist reviewed the studies to determine interobserver reliability between cardiologists. Pearson's correlation coefficient between emergency physicians and the cardiologist was 0.86, compared with 0.84 between the cardiologists. Classification of ejection fraction between EP and cardiology showed a weighted κ of 0.61, representing substantial agreement. Another prospective observational study enrolled 115 patients in whom emergency physicians performed bedside echocardiography and classified ejection fraction as poor, moderate, and normal.[17] The cardiology department performed and interpreted a comprehensive echocardiogram, which served as the gold standard. Results showed a Pearson's correlation coefficient of 0.71, with an overall agreement of 86%. The highest agreement was found in the normal category (92.4%), followed by the poor category (70.4%). While emergency physicians perform well overall when classifying ejection, they perform best when ejection fraction is clearly normal or poor, which represents the most clinically relevant determination. Another study showed that intensivists could classify left ventricular function appropriately in the critically ill patient.[18] This prospective observational study enrolled 44 patients, who underwent echocardiography by intensivists, followed by the cardiology department, which was used as the gold standard. Intensivists classified left ventricular function as grossly normal or abnormal with excellent agreement and κ of 0.72. Intensivists also correctly placed ejection fraction into one of the three categories (normal, mild to moderately depressed, severely depressed) in 36 of 44 patients for a κ of 0.68.

One study showed that emergency physicians preferred the parasternal long-axis view over all other cardiac views studied, except the parasternal short-axis view.[19] This prospective observational study enrolled 70 patients in a surgical intensive care unit on whom the following views were obtained: parasternal long axis, parasternal short axis, subxiphoid four chamber, subxiphoid short axis, and apical four chamber. Sonographers rated their preference for each window obtained on a 5-point Likert scale. Parasternal long-axis view was preferred over all other views ($P < .05$), except the parasternal short-axis view ($P = .23$). Since time needed for a study to be completed is an important factor in the evaluation of the critically ill, this should be considered when choosing the initial view for determining left ventricular function in this patient population.

Qualitative Estimation of Left Ventricular Systolic Function

Qualitative estimation of left ventricular systolic function can be performed by analysis of left ventricular end-diastolic diameter, change in left ventricular diameter during systole, change in thickness of left ventricular walls during systole, and rate and force of valve motion. Each of these criteria will be covered in further detail.

Normal left ventricular end-diastolic diameter is generally less than 5 cm. An LV end-diastolic diameter greater than 6 cm is consistent with dilated cardiomyo-

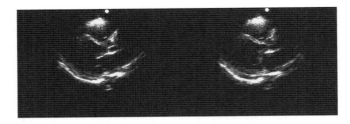

Figure 44-26. Parasternal long-axis view, dilated LV, poor EF. Parasternal long-axis view during (a) diastole and (b) systole, showing severely reduced left ventricular systolic function. Note the dilated left ventricle, incomplete excursion of the anterior mitral valve leaflet during diastole, minimal change in the left ventricular diameter between diastole and systole, and poor ventricular wall thickening during systole.

pathy. Furthermore, it indicates high left ventricular diastolic pressure and diminished left ventricular squeeze (Figure 44-26).

Left ventricular diameter should change by about 40% from end diastole to end systole (Figure 44-27). This may be more accurately seen using M-mode (Figure 44-28). The left ventricular walls thicken during systole by about 40%. This can also be more accurately seen and measured using M-mode (Figures 44-28 to 44-31).

The rate and force of valvular motion can also be used to estimate LV systolic function. The parasternal long-axis view, having both the mitral and aortic valves in view, is ideal for assessing rate and force of valvular opening. In early diastole, LV pressure is low, and the mitral valve should open wide and fast, with the anterior leaflet almost touching the intraventricular septum (Figure 44-32). The distance between the anterior MV leaflet and septum at their closest point is known as the E-point septal separation (EPSS). When LV pressures remain high with poor LV function, the

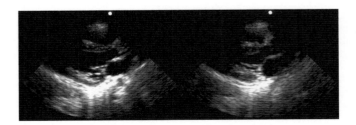

Figure 44-27. Parasternal long-axis view, normal LV, normal EF. Parasternal long-axis view during (a) end diastole and (b) end systole, demonstrating good left ventricular systolic function. Note normal ventricular cavity size, change in LV diameter, and left ventricular wall muscle thickening.

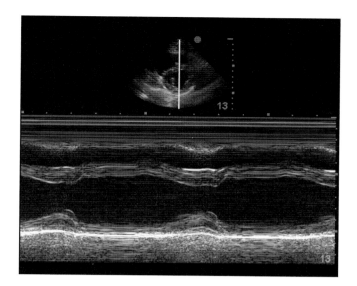

Figure 44-28. Parasternal short-axis view, normal EF, M-mode. Parasternal short-axis M-mode view at the level of the papillary muscles with M-mode with marker bisecting the left ventricle. Note the reduction in LV diameter of ~40% from end diastole to end systole, as well as normal ventricular wall thickening during systole.

mitral valve opens more slowly and not as wide (Figure 44-33). The mitral valve can be assessed with M-mode, and this more accurately depicts mitral valve opening (Figures 44-34 and 44-35).

Quantitative Estimation of Left Ventricular Systolic Function

Several methods exist to quantitatively measure left ventricular systolic function. These methods can be time consuming. Furthermore, qualitative estimation by an experienced sonographer has been shown to be as accurate as a measured quantitative estimation.

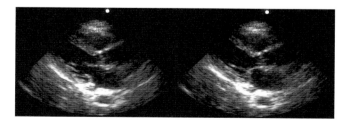

Figure 44-29. Parasternal long-axis view, depressed EF. Parasternal long-axis view during (a) diastole and (b) systole, demonstrating moderately reduced ventricular function. Note the incomplete excursion of the anterior mitral valve leaflet during diastole, less than 40% reduction in LV diameter during systole, and poor ventricular wall thickening during systole.

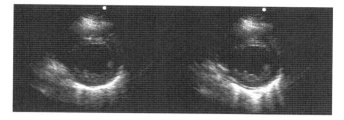

Figure 44-30. Parasternal short-axis view, dilated LV, poor EF. Parasternal short-axis view at the level of the papillary muscles showing poor left ventricular systolic function. Note almost no change in left ventricular cavity size or muscle wall thickness from (a) end diastole to (b) end systole.

An estimated ejection fraction can be calculated using LV measurements obtained when measuring fractional shortening. Fractional shortening is determined by the following formula: (LV end-diastolic diameter − LV end-systolic diameter)/LV end-diastolic diameter. The normal range for fractional shortening is 30–45%. M-mode using either the parasternal long- or short-axis views can be used to accurately measure fractional shortening. Most ultrasound systems can calculate fractional shortening using built-in calculator packages from left ventricular measurements. Fractional shortening can be used to calculate a measured ejection fraction (Figure 44-36). Ejection fraction is calculated from fractional shortening from the following formula: EF = ([LV end-diastolic diameter]^3 − [LV systolic diameter]^3)/

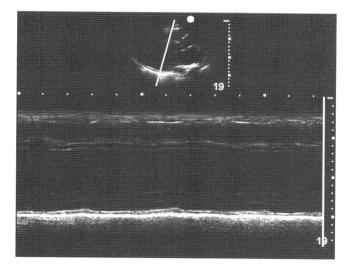

Figure 44-31. Parasternal long-axis M-mode view, poor EF. Parasternal long-axis M-mode view at the level of the papillary muscles with M-mode with marker bisecting the left ventricle. Note the severely reduced left ventricular systolic function as evidenced by the dilated left ventricle, minimal change in LV diameter, and poor ventricular wall thickening during systole.

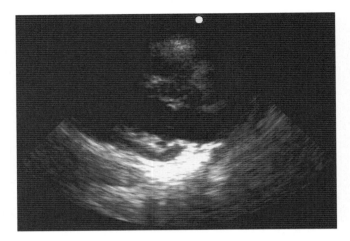

Figure 44-32. Parasternal long-axis view, normal EF, normal MV valve motion. Parasternal long-axis view during mid-diastole showing maximal mitral valve opening in a heart with normal systolic function. Note the anterior mitral valve leaflet almost touching the septum.

(LV end-diastolic diameter)^3. This is best performed in the parasternal long- or short-axis views. This technique is easy to learn and perform, but has several drawbacks. Measurements must be completely perpendicular to the ventricle, accurate, and avoid overestimating or underestimating the measurements, as any measurement error is compounded as measurements are cubed in the calculation. In addition, this measurement assumes a symmetrically contracting ventricle that is uniform in shape. Any area of hypokinesis will lead to overestimation of ejection fraction.

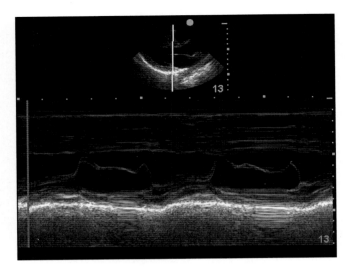

Figure 44-34. Parasternal long-axis M-mode view, normal EF, normal EPSS. Parasternal long-axis M-mode view with M-mode with marker across the anterior mitral valve leaflet, with the movement of the anterior mitral valve leaflet plotted versus time. The first peak in its excursion represents the E point; it corresponds to mitral valve inflow secondary to ventricular relaxation. The second peak, the A point, is secondary to mitral valve inflow from atrial contraction. Note the normal EPSS within the normal range of less than 0.85 cm.

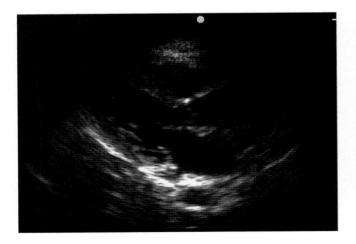

Figure 44-33. Parasternal long-axis view, low EF, abnormal MV valve motion. Parasternal long-axis view during mid-diastole showing maximal mitral valve opening in a heart with abnormal systolic function. Note the anterior mitral valve leaflet is greater than 1 cm from the septum, indicating elevated LV pressure and diminished LV function.

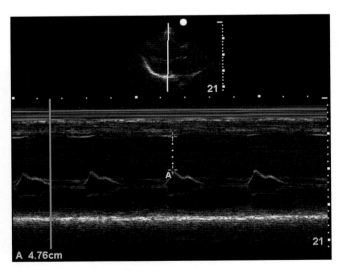

Figure 44-35. Parasternal long-axis M-mode view, poor EF, abnormal EPSS. Parasternal long-axis M-mode view with M-mode with marker across the anterior mitral valve leaflet, with the movement of the anterior mitral valve leaflet plotted versus time. Note the markedly increased EPSS. This is most commonly secondary to reduced left ventricular function, but can also be seen in mitral stenosis and aortic regurgitation.

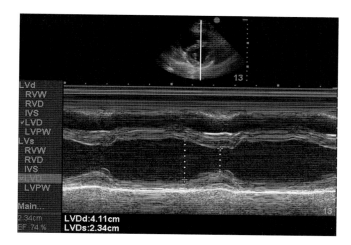

Figure 44-36. Parasternal short-axis M-mode view, normal EF. Parasternal short-axis M-mode view at the level of the papillary muscles with M-mode with marker bisecting the left ventricle. Using the LV end-diastolic (LVDd) and end-systolic diameters (LVDs), both fractional shortening and ejection fraction can be calculated.

Left ventricular systolic function can also be estimated using Simpson's method of discs. To perform this method, obtain an apical four-chamber view. End diastole should be identified and the image frozen. The LV volume can be traced using a caliper along the endocardial border. LV volume in diastole will be calculated by forming several small discs in the LV cavity (Figure 44-37). Once the LV end-diastolic volume is calculated, obtain a view of the LV at end systole. Again, trace the endocardial border to obtain LV end-systolic volume. Once the end-diastolic and end-systolic volumes are calculated, ejection fraction will be calculated by the following formula: EF = (end-diastolic LV volume − end-systolic LV volume)/end-diastolic LV volume. For increased accuracy, the procedure would be repeated in the apical two-chamber view, obtained by rotating the transducer 90° counterclockwise from the

apical four-chamber view. This method, although accurate, has a few drawbacks. It can be time consuming, the endocardial border can be difficult to clearly visualize, and errors can be made in identifying which frames represent end diastole and end systole.

Doppler echocardiography can also be used to quantitatively estimate stroke volume and cardiac output using the velocity–time integral (VTI) of left ventricular outflow, along with the LVOT D and heart rate. This method compares favorably with traditional pulmonary artery catheter thermodilution methods. First, obtain a parasternal long-axis view and identify the aortic root and aortic valve leaflets. Measure the LVOT D when the aortic valve is open where the valve leaflets attach. The US system will use this measurement to calculate the LVOT cross-sectional area (Figure 44-38). Next, obtain an apical five-chamber view. This view is very similar to the apical four-chamber view, with the probe in the same position and orientation. The transducer is angled slightly anteriorly toward the chest wall to bring the LVOT into view. Using spectral pulsed wave Doppler, obtain a Doppler tracing of LVOT outflow (Figure 44-39). The LVOT outflow waveform will be the tracing under the baseline. It is very important to have the Doppler gate as perpendicular to the LVOT as possible to avoid measurement error. Using the calculator package, trace the LVOT outflow curve. The area under this curve will be the VTI, and most systems will calculate this value automatically (Figure 44-40). Stroke volume is calculated as LVOT VTI times LVOT cross-sectional area, and cardiac output can be calculated by multiplying stroke volume and heart rate. Some US systems allow continuous tracing and instantaneous calculation of VTI, stroke volume, and cardiac output

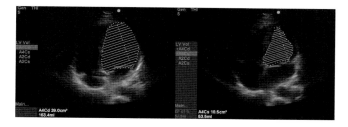

Figure 44-37. Apical four-chamber view showing use of Simpson's method of discs to calculate left ventricular ejection fraction. End-diastolic volume (a) is estimated at 163 mL, and end-systolic volume (b) is estimated at 53 mL, yielding ejection fraction of 67%.

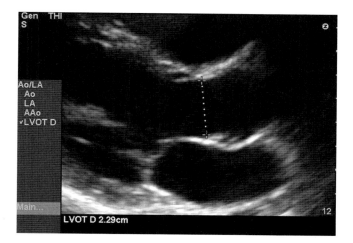

Figure 44-38. Parasternal long-axis view demonstrating correct measurement of LV outflow tract diameter at the aortic valve leaflet point of attachment. The US system will use this measurement to calculate LV outflow tract area.

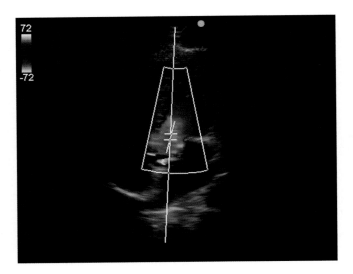

Figure 44-39. Apical five-chamber view showing the spectral Doppler gate within the left ventricular outflow tract. Note the blue color indicating flow away from the transducer and the vector adjustment of the Doppler gate to be with the LV outflow tract.

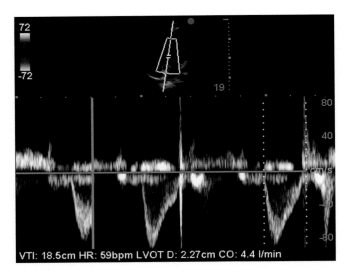

VTI: 18.5cm HR: 59bpm LVOT D: 2.27cm CO: 4.4 l/min

Figure 44-40. LVOT spectral Doppler waveform. Doppler waveform of the LV outflow tract obtained from an apical five-chamber view. Note the normal finding of minimal variation between peak aortic outflow velocities with respiration. Aortic outflow is plotted under the baseline, as the velocities are moving away from the transducer. The area under the curve is the velocity–time integral (VTI). Using the VTI and LVOT area, the US system can calculate stroke volume. When heart rate is added, cardiac output (CO) can be calculated and is displayed at the bottom of the screen.

in real time. Drawbacks to this technique include needing to obtain an apical view, as well as not having the proper perpendicular angle when obtaining the Doppler tracing. In addition, the aortic root and LVOT may be difficult to identify in some patients.

ECHOCARDIOGRAPHY TO ESTIMATE CENTRAL VENOUS AND RV FILLING PRESSURES

Emergency physicians can accurately estimate central venous and right ventricular filling pressure using point-of-care echocardiography. Key methods for estimation of volume status include assessment of IVC diameter and IVC collapsibility index. These measures can be helpful in differentiating hypovolemia, patients in septic shock who will respond to fluid resuscitation, fluid overload states such as CHF, tamponade physiology, and elevated RV pressures in suspected pulmonary embolus.

The IVC is a capacitance vessel, and its volume and pressure dynamics are related to CVP. The standard location to measure the IVC diameter is just distal to the IVC and hepatic vein junction, as the IVC is fixed at the diaphragm, which limits evaluation for respiratory variation. The normal diameter of the IVC in adults is between 1.5 and 2.5 cm. Patients with low volume will tend to have IVC diameters less than 1.5 cm, while patients with volume overload will tend to have IVC diameters greater than 2.5 cm. With inspiration, thoracic pressure becomes negative, leading to increased venous return and a smaller IVC diameter. This can be accentuated and more accurately measured using M-mode (Figures 44-41 and 44-42). The ratio of maximal IVC diameter to minimal IVC diameter during inspiration is the IVC collapsibility index, also known as caval index. Normal variation with inspiration is about a 50% reduction in IVC diameter. CVP is estimated using both the IVC diameter and percent change during respiration. This estimation correlates with CVP best at the extremes, which is the most clinically relevant scenario. Using this

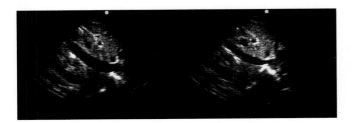

Figure 44-41. Subxiphoid IVC view, normal IVC diameter and respiratory change. Subxiphoid IVC view showing the IVC in (a) expiration and (b) inspiration, with normal IVC diameter and inspiratory collapse of approximately 50%.

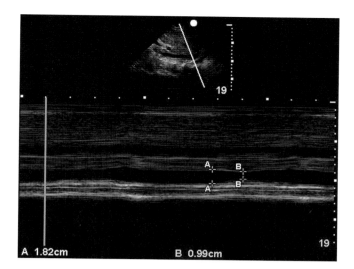

Figure 44-42. Subxiphoid IVC M-mode view showing the IVC in (a) expiration and (b) inspiration, with normal IVC diameter and normal inspiratory collapse of approximately 50%.

technique, emergency physicians can rapidly and accurately diagnose the low and high CVP noninvasively.

A recent prospective observational study enrolled 102 patients undergoing right heart catheterization and echocardiography.[20] Initially receiver operating characteristics were analyzed to determine optimal cutoffs, which were then prospectively studied. An IVC diameter of 2 cm correctly predicted RAP above or below 10 with a sensitivity and specificity of 73% and 85%, respectively, and a collapsibility of 40% performed similar with sensitivities and specificities of 73% and 84%, respectively. A recent study showed that greater than 50% collapse of the IVC with inspiration was sensitive and specific for a central venous pressure measurement less than 8 mm Hg.[21] This prospective observational study enrolled 73 patients who were undergoing central venous catheterization. Ultrasound measurements of the IVC during inspiration and expiration were performed and caval index was calculated. They found greater than 50% collapse was associated with central venous pressure less than 8 mm Hg with a sensitivity of 91%, a specificity of 94%, positive predictive value of 87%, and negative predictive value of 96%.

Several studies have shown that a flat IVC and elevated collapsibility index is an accurate and sensitive marker of hypovolemia. One study showed that IVC diameter correlated with hypovolemia in trauma patients.[22] This prospective observational study enrolled 35 victims of trauma, 10 patients found to be in shock, defined as an SBP <90 mm Hg on arrival or within 12 hours of arrival, and a control group of 25 hemodynamically stable patients. The mean diameter of the IVC was much smaller at 7.7 mm in the shock group, com-

pared with 13.4 mm in the control group. Subjects were also divided into two groups based on IVC diameter. Those with an IVC diameter of 9 mm or less had significantly larger blood transfusion volume, 11.3 U versus 0.3 U. Another study by the same authors showed that in patients being resuscitated with hemorrhagic shock, IVC diameter could predict recurrence of shock.[23] This prospective observational study enrolled 30 patients with hemorrhagic shock, who after enrollment were fluid resuscitated until SBP was above 90 mm Hg. All patients then had IVC diameter recorded using bedside sonography. Patients were subsequently divided into two groups: those who remained stable after initial resuscitation (13 patients) and those who experienced recurrence of hypotension (17 patients). These two groups had no significant differences in vital signs after fluid resuscitation. However, those who experienced recurrence of shock had significantly smaller IVC diameters, 6.5 ± 0.5 mm versus 10.7 ± 0.7 mm ($P < .05$). Although larger studies are needed to confirm these results, this implies that IVC diameter may be a useful adjunct in predicting the clinical course of trauma patients. Another study showed that IVC diameter was consistently decreased even by a small amount of blood loss.[24] This prospective observational study enrolled 31 healthy volunteers at a blood donation center. IVC diameter was measured before and after donation of 450 mL of blood. Mean IVC diameter before donation was 17.4 mm (95% CI 15.2–19.7 mm) and decreased to 11.9 mm after donation (95% CI 10.3–13.6 mm). A flat, collapsable IVC should prompt aggressive fluid resuscitation (Figures 44-43 and 44-44).

Additional studies have shown that a dilated IVC and low collapsibility index is an accurate marker of volume overload. One prospective observational study enrolled 75 patients hospitalized for acute decompen-

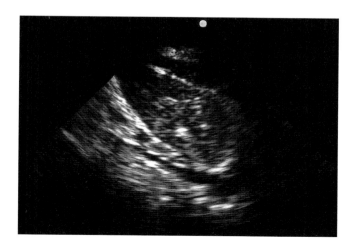

Figure 44-43. Subxiphoid IVC view showing a flat IVC with a diameter <1.5 cm, indicating low CVP.

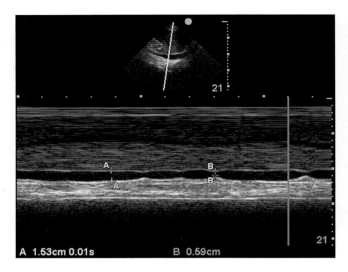

A 1.53cm 0.01s   B 0.59cm

Figure 44-44. Subxiphoid IVC M-mode view showing flat IVC with a diameter <1.5 cm, with respiratory collapse of >50%, indicating decreased CVP.

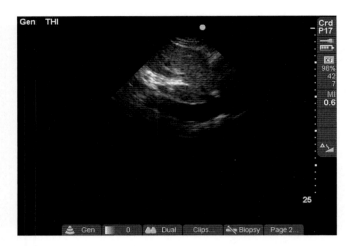

Figure 44-45. Subxiphoid IVC view showing a dilated IVC with a diameter >2.5 cm, indicating elevated CVP.

sated CHF.[25] The authors found that predischarge IVC diameter, collapsibility index, and BNP were predictive of the need for readmission. Another study showed that the IVC caval index can identify patients with right heart failure.[26] This cohort study enrolled 95 patients without right heart failure and 32 patients with documented right heart failure. The caval index was measured in both groups and results of receiver operator characteristics were analyzed. A cutoff caval index value of 0.22 yielded a sensitivity of 78% and specificity of 98% for the presence of right heart failure. Another study showed the IVC caval index to be useful in the emergency department to diagnose congestive heart failure.[27] This prospective observational study enrolled 46 patients presenting to the emergency department with dyspnea. IVC caval index was determined prior to initiation of therapy, and patients with a final diagnosis of CHF were compared with those who had an alternative final diagnosis. Respiratory variation in patients with CHF was smaller than in those without CHF—9.6% versus 46%. Receiver operating characteristic curve analysis with a cutoff of 15% yielded a sensitivity of 92% with 84% specificity (Figures 44-45 and 44-46).

Two studies evaluated the ability of IVC diameter and caval index to predict fluid responsiveness in patients in septic shock. One prospective observational study enrolled 23 patients with sepsis and respiratory failure on mechanical ventilation.[28] IVC diameter at end expiration and end inspiration was measured and the distensibility index was calculated ($[D_{max} - D_{min}]/D_{min}$). Cardiac index was calculated using Doppler flow before and after patients received a fluid challenge. IVC distensibility above 18% identified fluid responders, those

with an increase in cardiac index of at least 15%, with a sensitivity and specificity of 90%. Similar results were found in another study.[29] This prospective observational trial enrolled 39 mechanically ventilated patients in septic shock. IVC distensibility was calculated as the difference between expiratory and inspiratory diameters divided by their mean. Cardiac index was measured before and after a fluid challenge. IVC distensibility above 12% distinguished between responders (those with an increase in cardiac index of at least 15% following fluid challenge) and nonresponders with positive and negative predictive values of 93% and 92%, respectively.

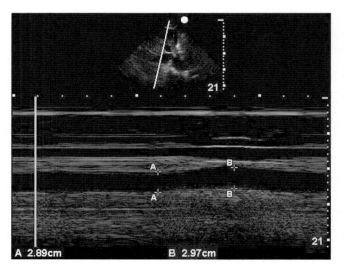

A 2.89cm   B 2.97cm

Figure 44-46. Subxiphoid IVC M-mode view showing dilated IVC with a diameter >2.5 cm, with no respiratory variation, indicating elevated CVP.

EVALUATION OF ACUTE RIGHT HEART STRAIN

Emergency physicians can identify acute right heart strain using point-of-care echocardiography. This can be very clinically helpful in the setting of massive or submassive pulmonary embolism to direct the proper course of treatment.

A recent study showed that emergency echocardiogram could support the diagnosis of pulmonary embolism.[30] The authors conducted a prospective observational trial enrolling 124 patients with a suspected diagnosis of pulmonary embolism who then underwent emergent echocardiography. A study was considered positive if it displayed any two of the following signs: right ventricular dilatation, abnormal septal motion, right ventricular hypokinesis, elevated pulmonary artery or right ventricular pressures, moderate to severe tricuspid regurgitation, or visualization of a clot within the right ventricle or pulmonary artery. CT, MRI, and VQ scan identified 27 cases of pulmonary embolism. Echocardiography performed with a sensitivity and specificity of 41% and 91%, respectively. This study shows that a positive study in a high-risk patient should prompt treatment, but a negative study should not be used to rule out pulmonary embolism.

There are several helpful simple findings to identify acute right ventricular strain on bedside echocardiography. These include a dilated RV, septal shift of the intraventricular septum during diastole, RV hypokinesis, and intracardiac thrombus. Each of these findings will be discussed in further detail.

The normal RV to LV ratio is less than 0.6 to 1. This is best seen and measured in the apical four-chamber view, and the standard location for measurements is at the tricuspid and mitral valve leaflets (Figure 44-47).

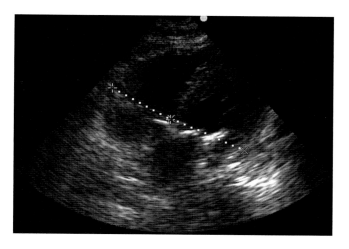

Figure 44-47. Apical four-chamber view showing right ventricular dilation. Note the right ventricle and left ventricle are almost equal in size and end diastole.

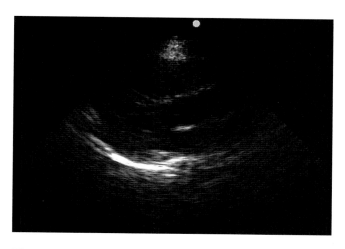

Figure 44-48. Parasternal long-axis view showing right ventricular dilation. Note the right ventricle that measures more than 3 cm in this view. Septal flattening and bowing of the septum to the left is also seen.

Additional views may also show RV enlargement. The subxiphoid four-chamber view may also be used, although the transducer angle may overestimate or underestimate RV diameter. In the parasternal long-axis view, the RV diameter should be less than 2.5–3 cm (Figure 44-48). A good rule of thumb for simple qualitative visual inspection is that the image should be "1/3 RV, 2/3 LV." As pressure builds, the RV may become larger than the LV.

When RV filling pressure exceeds LV filling pressure, the septum will paradoxically bow into the LV cavity during diastole. This finding is known as septal shift, and can be best visualized in the subxiphoid four-chamber or apical four-chamber views. Assess the septum for shift during diastole by watching for paradoxical motion while the tricuspid and mitral valves are open (Figure 44-49). In the parasternal short-axis view, septal shift causes a flattening and bowing of the intraventricular septum. This causes a finding known as the "D sign," as the LV cavity takes on a "D"-shaped appearance, instead of the "O"-shaped appearance normally seen (Figure 44-50).

Another finding of acute RV strain is RV hypokinesis, especially of the midventricular walls. The RV typically pumps against lower pressure, and acute pressure overload causes pump failure. This finding is best seen in the subxiphoid four-chamber or apical four-chamber views. This finding is also known as McConnell's sign. In addition, the RV may lose its typical triangular or wedge-shaped appearance, and take on more of an ovoid shape.

Occasionally, mobile intracardiac thrombus is directly visualized on echocardiography. This represents

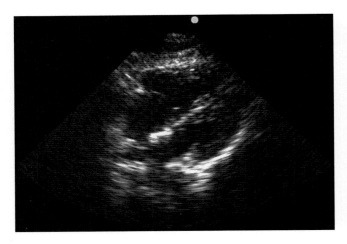

Figure 44-49. Subxiphoid four-chamber view showing right ventricular dilation and septal shift. Note the RV:LV ratio is elevated above 0.6:1. The TV and MV are open, indicating the heart is in diastole. There is flattening of the septum toward the LV in diastole, indicating elevated right ventricular pressure.

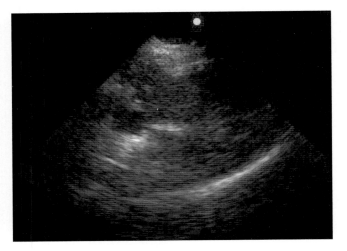

Figure 44-51. Subxiphoid four-chamber view showing right ventricular dilation and echogenic clot inside the RV. The clot was seen to be freely mobile in real time, and represents a pulmonary embolus in transit. This patient presented in PEA, was treated with TPA, and had return of spontaneous circulation.

a pulmonary embolus in transit, and should prompt aggressive treatment (Figures 44-51 and 44-52).

Chronic cor pulmonale can be differentiated from acute cor pulmonale by assessment of RV wall thickness and RV contractility. Over time, the RV can adapt to elevated pressures by hypertrophy of the ventricular walls. Normal RV wall thickness is less than 0.5 cm, and measurements greater than this suggest RV hypertrophy. In addition, the chronically overloaded RV regains

the ability to contract forcefully, and RV hypokinesis is not seen in chronic cor pulmonale.

DIFFERENTIATION OF PEA AND SHOCK STATES

Using the techniques illustrated in this chapter, emergency physicians can use echocardiography to differentiate shock states. This was best illustrated in a

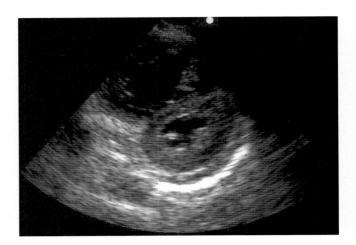

Figure 44-50. Parasternal short-axis view showing right ventricular dilation and septal shift. Note the characteristic D sign, with flattening of the septal wall during diastole secondary to increased right ventricular pressure. This gives the left ventricle a "D" shape, as opposed to its usual rounded "O" shape.

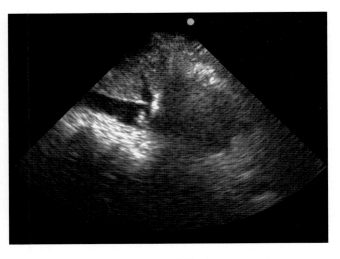

Figure 44-52. Subxiphoid IVC view showing an echogenic clot in the IVC at the level of the hepatic vein junction. The clot was seen to be freely mobile in real time, moving between the IVC and RA.

prospective study that showed using bedside ultrasound improved diagnostic accuracy in medical patients with undifferentiated hypotension.[31] The authors conducted a randomized controlled trial, enrolling 184 nontrauma patients with hypotension and at least one clinical sign of shock. Patients were randomized to receive an immediate ultrasound exam versus an ultrasound exam delayed by 15–30 minutes. The ultrasound exam consisted of a five-view echocardiogram (parasternal long- and short-axis, apical four-chamber, subxiphoid four-chamber, and IVC views), as well as a view of the hepatorenal recess to evaluate for free intraperitoneal fluid and a transverse view of the abdominal aorta to evaluate for the presence of an AAA. This exam took less than 5 minutes to complete. At 15 minutes, in the immediate ultrasound group physicians entertained a smaller number of viable diagnoses (median 4 vs. 9, $P < .0001$), and ranked the correct final diagnosis as the most like one more frequently (80% vs. 50%, difference 30%). This study is a great example of how to use echocardiography in the critically ill patient and shows how using echocardiography can rapidly cone the differential diagnosis and allow greater certainty when faced with an undifferentiated hypotensive patient.

► CONCLUSION

With relatively brief training, emergency physicians can learn to perform and interpret echocardiography. Using this technology, emergency physicians can rapidly and definitively assess for cardiac activity in cardiac arrest, immediately differentiate treatable causes of PEA and shock, evaluate for pericardial effusion and tamponade, estimate left ventricular systolic function, identify acute right heart strain, noninvasively estimate preload and right ventricular filling pressure, and direct resuscitation and medical decision making with improved diagnostic accuracy.

REFERENCES

1. ABEM. 2009 model of the clinical practice of emergency medicine. Available at: http://www.abem.org/public/portal/alias__Rainbow/lang__en-US/tabID__3590/DesktopDefault.aspx. Accessed April 16, 2010.
2. AMA Policy H-230.960. Privileging for ultrasound imaging. Available at: www.ama-assn.org&uri=/ama1/pub/upload/mm/PolicyFinder/policyfiles/HnE/H-230.960. HTM. Accessed April 16, 2010.
3. *ACEP Emergency Ultrasound Guidelines*. October 2008. Available at: http://www.acep.org/acepmembership.aspx?id=30276. Accessed April 16, 2010.
4. Jones AE, Tayal VS, Kline JA. Focused training of emergency medicine residents in goal-directed echocardiography: a prospective study. *Acad Emerg Med*. 2003;10(10):1054–1058.
5. Blaivas M, Fox JC. Outcome in cardiac arrest patients found to have cardiac standstill on the bedside emergency department echocardiogram. *Acad Emerg Med*. 2001;8(6):616–621.
6. Salen P, Melniker L, Chooljian C, et al. Does the presence or absence of sonographically identified cardiac activity predict resuscitation outcomes of cardiac arrest patients? *Am J Emerg Med*. 2005;23(4):459–462.
7. Tayal VS, Kline JA. Emergency echocardiography to detect pericardial effusion in patients in PEA and near-PEA states. *Resuscitation*. 2003;59(3):315–318.
8. Salen P, O'Connor R, Sierzenski P, et al. Can cardiac sonography and capnography be used independently and in combination to predict resuscitation outcomes? *Acad Emerg Med*. 2001;8(6):610–615.
9. Mandavia DP, Hoffner RJ, Mahaney K, Henderson SO. Bedside echocardiography by emergency physicians. *Ann Emerg Med*. 2001;38(4):377–382.
10. Blaivas M. Incidence of pericardial effusion in patients presenting to the emergency department with unexplained dyspnea. *Acad Emerg Med*. 2001;8(12):1143–1146.
11. Plummer D, Brunette D, Asinger R, Ruiz E. Emergency department echocardiography improves outcome in penetrating cardiac injury. *Ann Emerg Med*. 1992;21(6):709–712.
12. Rozycki GS, Feliciano DV, Ochsner MG, et al. The role of ultrasound in patients with possible penetrating cardiac wounds: a prospective multicenter study. *J Trauma*. 1999;46(4):543–551. Discussion 551–552.
13. Jacob S, Sebastian JC, Cherian PK, Abraham A, John SK. Pericardial effusion impending tamponade: a look beyond Beck's triad. *Am J Emerg Med*. 2009;27(2):216–219.
14. Burstow DJ, Oh JK, Bailey KR, Seward JB, Tajik AJ. Cardiac tamponade: characteristic Doppler observations. *Mayo Clin Proc*. 1989;64(3):312–324.
15. Materazzo C, Piotti P, Meazza R, Pellegrini MP, Viggiano V, Biasi S. Respiratory changes in transvalvular flow velocities versus two-dimensional echocardiographic findings in the diagnosis of cardiac tamponade. *Ital Heart J*. 2003;4(3):186–192.
16. Moore CL, Rose GA, Tayal VS, Sullivan DM, Arrowood JA, Kline JA. Determination of left ventricular function by emergency physician echocardiography of hypotensive patients. *Acad Emerg Med*. 2002;9(3):186–193.
17. Randazzo MR, Snoey ER, Levitt MA, Binder K. Accuracy of emergency physician assessment of left ventricular ejection fraction and central venous pressure using echocardiography. *Acad Emerg Med*. 2003;10(9):973–977.
18. Melamed R, Sprenkle MD, Ulstad VK, Herzog CA, Leatherman JW. Assessment of left ventricular function by intensivists using hand-held echocardiography. *Chest*. 2009;135(6):1416–1420. Epub February 18, 2009.
19. Mark DG, Ku BS, Carr BG, et al. Directed bedside transthoracic echocardiography: preferred cardiac window for left ventricular ejection fraction estimation in critically ill patients. *Am J Emerg Med*. 2007;25(8):894–900.
20. Brennan JM, Blair JE, Goonewardena S, et al. Reappraisal of the use of inferior vena cava for estimating right atrial pressure. *Am Soc Echocardiogr*. 2007;20(7):857–861.
21. Nagdev AD, Merchant RC, Tirado-Gonzalez A, Sisson CA, Murphy MC. Emergency department bedside

ultrasonographic measurement of the caval index for noninvasive determination of low central venous pressure. *Ann Emerg Med.* 2010;55(3):290–295.

22. Yanagawa Y, Nishi K, Sakamoto T, Okada Y. Early diagnosis of hypovolemic shock by sonographic measurement of inferior vena cava in trauma patients. *J Trauma.* 2005;58(4):825–829.

23. Yanagawa Y, Sakamoto T, Okada Y. Hypovolemic shock evaluated by sonographic measurement of the inferior vena cava during resuscitation in trauma patients. *J Trauma Inj Infect Crit Care.* 2007;63(6):1245–1248. Discussion 1248.

24. Lyon M, Blaivas M, Brannam L. Sonographic measurement of the inferior vena cava as a marker of blood loss. *Am J Emerg Med.* 2005;23(1):45–50.

25. Goonewardena SN, Gemignani A, Ronan A, et al. Comparison of hand-carried ultrasound assessment of the inferior vena cava and N-terminal pro-brain natriuretic peptide for predicting readmission after hospitalization for acute decompensated heart failure. *JACC Cardiovasc Imaging.* 2008;1(5):595–601.

26. Goei R, Ronnen HR, Kessels AH, Kragten JA. Right heart failure: diagnosis via ultrasonography of the inferior vena cava and hepatic veins. *Rofo.* 1997;166(1):36–39.

27. Blehar DJ, Dickman E, Gaspari R. Identification of congestive heart failure via respiratory variation of inferior vena cava diameter. *Am J Emerg Med.* 2009;27(1):71–75.

28. Barbier C, Loubières Y, Schmit C, et al. Respiratory changes in inferior vena cava diameter are helpful in predicting fluid responsiveness in ventilated septic patients. *Intensive Care Med.* 2004;30(9):1740–1746.

29. Feissel M, Michard F, Faller JP, Teboul JL. The respiratory variation in inferior vena cava diameter as a guide to fluid therapy. *Intensive Care Med.* 2004;30(9):1834–1837.

30. Jackson RE, Rudoni RR, Hauser AM, Pascual RG, Hussey ME. Prospective evaluation of two-dimensional transthoracic echocardiography in emergency department patients with suspected pulmonary embolism. *Acad Emerg Med.* 2000;7(9):994–998.

31. Jones AE, Tayal VS, Sullivan DM, Kline JA. Randomized, controlled trial of immediate versus delayed goal-directed ultrasound to identify the cause of nontraumatic hypotension in emergency department patients. *Crit Care Med.* 2004;32(8):1703–1708.

CHAPTER 45

Ultrasound-Guided Critical Care Procedures

Ashika Jain, Lawrence E. Haines, and Eitan Dickman

▶ INTRODUCTION

The use of bedside ultrasonography has become an integral tool for evaluating and managing the critically ill patient. Improved image quality and increased portability of ultrasound machines have augmented the utility of physician-performed bedside ultrasonography in the emergency department and the intensive care unit. Not only is ultrasound useful diagnostically, but it can also shine a light into the darkness of invasive procedures traditionally performed with a landmark or "blind" technique. While initially the ultrasound-guided procedure may take more time as the practitioner's skills are developing, the ultimate benefits of fewer complications, less time to completion, and fewer attempts to complete the procedure make this technique worthwhile to master.[1],[2]

Increased utilization of bedside sonography in the critical care arena has generated a large amount of research in the field. This has led to a paradigm shift in the way that procedures are performed at the bedside. Emblematic of this shift is the document released in 2001 by the Agency for Research and Health Care Quality, *Making Health Care Safer: A Critical Analysis of Patient Safety Practices*, which states that the body of evidence supports the use of ultrasound guidance for placement of central venous catheters.[3]

The performance of multiple critical care procedures may be improved with the addition of sonographic guidance. This chapter provides information about how ultrasound can be used to guide the following invasive procedures: central venous access, arterial line placement, pericardiocentesis, thoracentesis, paracentesis, lumbar puncture, endotracheal tube placement confirmation, and thoracostomy tube placement confirmation.

▶ PROBE SELECTION

There are multiple transducers to choose from when performing a sonographic study. Selecting the correct probe can make the difference between a good image that is helpful and an image that is of poor quality and misleading. As a general rule, the higher the frequency, the better the resolution. The tradeoff is that high-frequency sound waves cannot penetrate deep into the tissues of the body. A high-frequency linear transducer

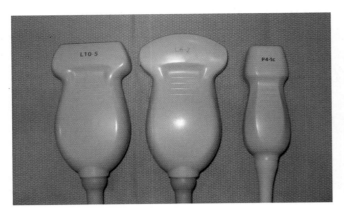

Figure 45-1. The three most commonly used probes. On the left is the high-frequency linear probe. In the center is a low-frequency curvilinear probe and to the right is a phased array probe.

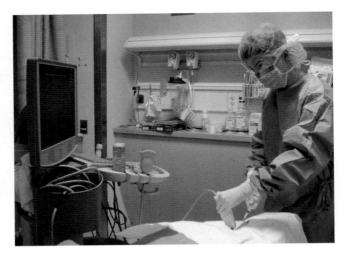

Figure 45-2. Optimal relationship between practitioner, patient, and ultrasound machine. Note the machine is in the same line of sight as the patient.

is used to image superficial structures and is ideal for sonographic guidance when obtaining vascular access, performing lumbar puncture, and confirming placement of a thoracostomy or endotracheal tube. The curvilinear probe (2.5–5 MHz) is most often used for evaluating deep structures in the abdomen and pelvis. Because of its lower frequency, it results in good sound-wave penetration, but with a relative loss of resolution. The phased array probe (1–4 MHz) is ideal for intercostal imaging since it has a small footprint, a narrow superficial field of view, and a wider deep field of view (Figure 45-1).

► SETUP

When performing an ultrasound-guided procedure, the ultrasound machine should be positioned in such a way as to allow for easy visibility of the ultrasound screen by the practitioner. The ultrasound machine should be placed alongside the patient's bed directly in line with the operator's line of vision. This allows for minimal eye movement while looking at the ultrasound screen and performing the procedure. The machine should also be placed in a position so that there is enough cord slack to allow for adequate maneuvering of the transducer during the procedure (Figures 45-2 and 45-3).

► STERILITY

When performing any invasive procedure, standard aseptic technique should be observed. Sterile gown, mask, cap, and gloves should be donned for all ultrasound-guided procedures. The addition of the ultrasound probe into the sterile field has the potential to compromise the sterility of the procedure. Therefore, transducer covers are essential to keeping the field

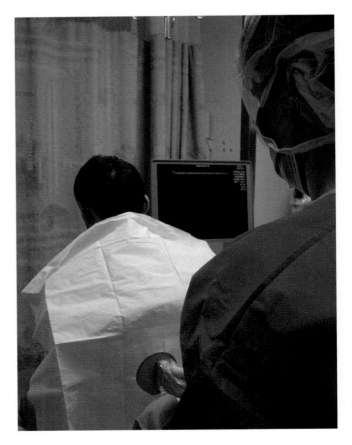

Figure 45-3. Note the relationship between patient and ultrasound machine.

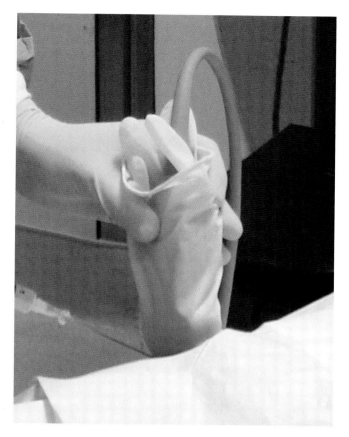

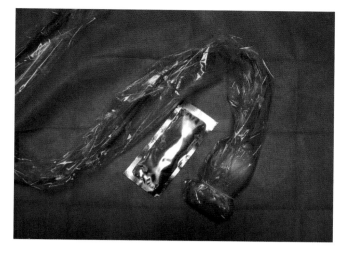

Figure 45-5. A commercially available sterile probe sheath, which covers the cord as well.

Figure 45-4. Sterile probe cover using a sterile glove. The glove must be pulled tight to prevent air pockets from disrupting the ultrasound image. Caution must be taken with the nonsterile cord when working in a sterile field.

sterile. There are many commercially available sterile covers that are particularly useful as the sterile cover usually extends to cover the cord as well. Alternatively, a sterile glove or occlusive dressing can also be used to cover the probe. However, care must be taken so the nonsterile cord will not contaminate the field. A nonsterile conducting medium (gel) can be placed between the probe and the sterile cover, but a sterile conducting medium such as sterile ultrasound gel, povidone iodine solution, or surgical lubricating jelly is placed between the probe cover and the skin (Figures 45-4 and 45-5).

▶ DYNAMIC VERSUS STATIC

Ultrasound guidance may be dynamic or static. With dynamic ultrasound guidance, the procedure is performed using continuous imaging. This is recommended for vascular access in order to ensure proper trajectory of the needle during the procedure. With static imaging, the anatomy is sonographically visualized and the needle entry point is marked on the skin. The transducer is

then removed, the area is appropriately cleansed, and the procedure is performed in the traditional manner. The ultrasound probe does not need to be in a sterile sheath when using static imaging.

▶ SINGLE- VERSUS TWO-OPERATOR TECHNIQUE

When first learning how to perform ultrasound-guided procedures, a two-person technique may be easier if dynamic ultrasound guidance is utilized. Using this approach, one person holds the transducer and guides the other person who performs the procedure. Once proficiency is obtained, a single-person technique can be employed, in which the transducer is held in the nondominant hand and the needle is held in the dominant hand.

▶ CENTRAL VENOUS ACCESS

Central venous access is frequently necessary to adequately manage the critically ill patient. Over 5 million central venous catheters are placed annually by physicians.[4,5] Central venous catheters allow measurement of hemodynamic variables that cannot be measured accurately by noninvasive means and allow delivery of medications and nutritional support that cannot be given safely through peripheral intravenous catheters. Other indications for central venous access include lack of peripheral access and the need for aggressive fluid resuscitation. Many factors can make obtaining central venous access more difficult including body habitus, hypovolemia, congenital anomalies, poor vascular access due to history of intravenous drug use, and the presence of indwelling catheters. Typical sites for central venous access are the internal jugular vein, the supraclavicular and infraclavicular approaches to the subclavian vein, and the femoral vein.

Mechanical complications (e.g., arterial puncture, hematoma, pneumothorax, hemothorax) are reported to occur in 5–19% of patients, infectious complications (catheter colonization and associated blood stream infections) in 5–26%, and thrombotic complications (deep venous thrombosis) in 2–26%.[6–9] Furthermore, coagulopathy, anatomic anomalies, anatomic deformity due to trauma, and operator inexperience can all contribute to a failure to cannulate a central vein. When compared with a traditional landmark approach, the use of ultrasound guidance has been shown to significantly reduce the mechanical complications.[10–12] In a review of the literature, central venous catheter placement under ultrasound guidance was shown to decrease placement failure by 64%, complications by 78%, and multiple placement attempts by 40%.[13] Achieving these lower rates of complication takes time and practice as placing an ultrasound-guided catheter requires developing additional hand–eye coordination.

As discussed above, appropriate positioning of the patient and the ultrasound machine is crucial for success. When cannulating the internal jugular or the subclavian vein, placing the patient in Trendelenburg will help to engorge the vein of interest and will allow for easier sonographic visualization and better blood return once the vein is punctured. For the femoral vein, reverse Trendelenburg will assist in this regard. One study described humming to be as effective as the Valsalva maneuver and Trendelenburg position for ultrasonographic visualization of the internal jugular vein and common femoral vein.[14]

Using the high-frequency linear array transducer, the area of interest should be prescanned to identify all pertinent structures as well as any structures in the field that should be avoided. In addition, confirmation that the desired vein is easily compressible demonstrates lack of an occult deep venous thrombosis. Recognizing the difference between the artery and the vein is extremely important in order to avoid arterial puncture. Veins are more easily compressible and have thinner walls than arteries. Doppler can be employed if there is doubt. Arteries will demonstrate characteristic arterial pulsations, whereas veins will demonstrate continuous flow.

For the short-axis approach, the depth of the center of the vessel from the skin surface should be measured. Once the depth is ascertained, the same distance is measured distally from the middle of the probe on the skin surface. This is where the needle should enter at a 45° angle. By triangulation, the needle tip should pierce the vessel. The needle is introduced into the ultrasound field under the center of the long face of the probe and is seen as a hyperechoic dot in

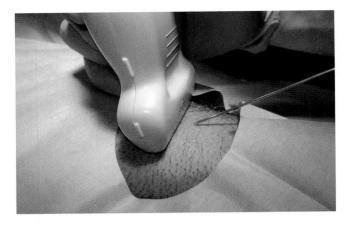

Figure 45-6. Needle–probe relationship in short axis.

cross-section. The true depth of the needle may be difficult to appreciate when using a transverse orientation. The transducer may need to be moved in a caudal or cephalad direction in order to find the needle tip. There are multiple visualization techniques that can be utilized to monitor needle placement and movement. Whether by direct visualization of the needle tip, seeing "ring-down" artifact, or noting tissue movement as the needle moves, one must be cognizant of needle location at all times, particularly when operating near other critical structures (Figures 45-6 to 45-9).[2,10]

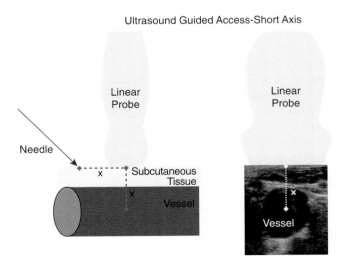

Figure 45-7. Short-axis schematic. The distance from the center of the target vessel to the skin surface is measured. This same distance is measured back from the middle of the transducer, and this is where the needle should penetrate the skin at a 45° angle.

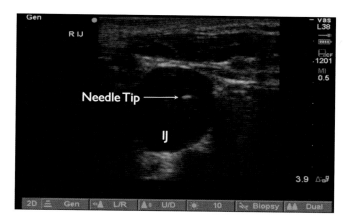

Figure 45-8. Needle tip in the right internal jugular vein (IJ) in short-axis view.

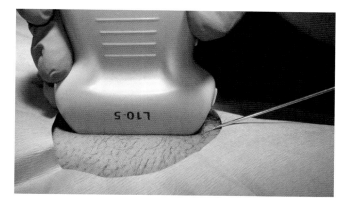

Figure 45-10. Needle–probe relationship in long axis.

For the long-axis approach, the needle is introduced in the same plane as the long axis of the ultrasound transducer. The entire length and the depth of the needle are appreciated using this technique. However, the needle must be kept directly under the center of the transducer as there will be complete loss of visualization of the needle if either the needle or the transducer is moved out of plane.[15] This is because the width of the beam generated by the transducer is very narrow. Recent evidence supports the use of the longitudinal approach over the transverse approach as it is associated with lower rates of posterior wall puncture rates when attempting to cannulate the internal jugular vein (Figures 45-10 and 45-11).[16]

INTERNAL JUGULAR VEIN

The internal jugular vein lies deep to the sternocleidomastoid muscle and is usually lateral and superficial to the carotid artery. Placing a catheter in this vein allows for central venous pressure monitoring and has the advantage of lower rates of pneumothorax when compared with attempting to cannulate the subclavian vein.[5] In addition, catheters in the internal jugular vein have a lower infection rate than catheters in the femoral vein.[17]

To place a catheter in the internal jugular vein using sonographic guidance, place the patient in the Trendelenburg position. The ultrasound machine is positioned next to the patient's bed with the screen facing the head of the bed. With the probe, it is best to find an area where the carotid artery and the internal jugular vein are not in the same vertical plane. This will minimize the chance of arterial puncture via the posterior venous wall.[11,13,18,19] Once the vessel is visualized and the surrounding anatomy appreciated, vessel cannulation proceeds as described above (Figure 45-12).

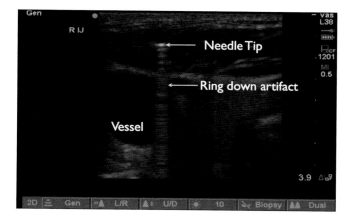

Figure 45-9. Ring-down artifact seen in a short-axis view of a needle near the right internal jugular vein.

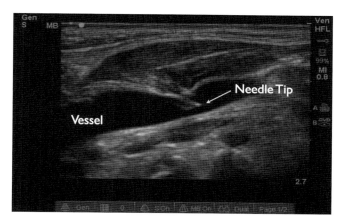

Figure 45-11. Longitudinal view of needle entering vessel.

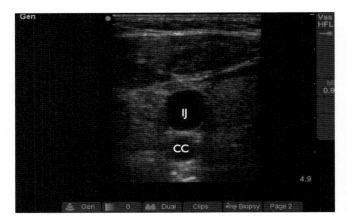

Figure 45-12. Example of a poor location for ultrasound-guided central venous access. The internal jugular vein (IJ) is positioned directly over the common carotid artery (CC), which increases the potential for arterial puncture during the procedure.

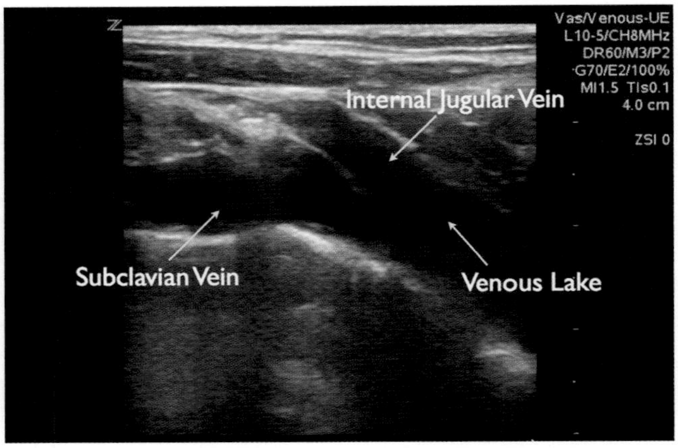

Figure 45-13. Longitudinal view of supraclavicular approach for subclavian vein access. Venous lake formed by confluence of internal jugular vein and subclavian vein.

SUBCLAVIAN VEIN

When compared with other possible sites for central venous catheterization, the subclavian vein has the lowest rates of infection but also the highest rates of pneumothorax.[5,20] For this procedure, the ultrasound machine should be positioned on the side of the bed opposite to the subclavian vein that will be cannulated. This will allow for easy visualization of the screen while placing the catheter. The subclavian vein crosses under the clavicle just medial to the midclavicular point. It is often difficult to visualize the subclavian vein at this location due to the strong echogenicity and posterior shadowing of the clavicle. To avoid this, one must visualize the vein more proximally or more distally with respect to the clavicle. It is possible to visualize the "venous lake" where the subclavian vein joins the internal jugular vein using the supraclavicular approach. It is also possible to visualize the subclavian vein inferior and lateral to the first rib where it is the proximal axillary vein (Figures 45-13 and 45-14). The vein may be cannulated in either of these locations. Due to the proximity of the subclavian vein to the lung pleura, a longitudinal approach is advised so that the entire needle can be visualized throughout the procedure.

FEMORAL VEIN

Routine use of the femoral vein for central venous catheter placement should be avoided in adults due to higher rates of line sepsis and deep venous thrombosis formation when compared with other sites.[5,7,21] How-

ever, the femoral vein is readily accessible in an emergent situation and can be useful as a compressible site in the setting of coagulopathy.[5] To optimize positioning, the patient should be placed in reverse Trendelenburg with the leg externally rotated at the hip so as to increase the diameter of the femoral vein.[22] The ultrasound machine should be placed at the side of the bed at shoulder level with the screen facing toward the patient's feet. Beginning the procedure in a transverse orientation just inferior to the inguinal ligament allows both the artery and vein to be visualized (Figure 45-15). The area where the greater saphenous vein drains into the common femoral vein usually provides the largest target. Usually, the vein will lie medial to the artery. In the femoral region, the vein and artery

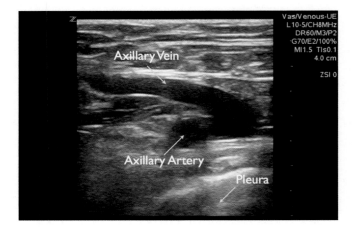

Figure 45-14. Longitudinal view of lateral subclavian/axillary vein approach.

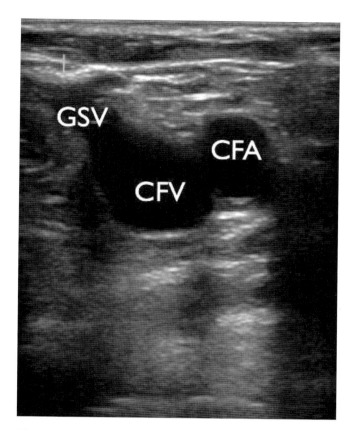

Figure 45-15. Transverse image of femoral vessels. CFV is the common femoral vein, CVA is the common femoral artery and GSV is the greater saphenous vein.

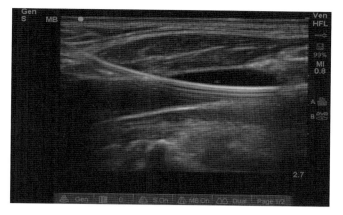

Figure 45-16. Longitudinal view of a guidewire being introduced into the vessel. Note ring-down artifact from the guidewire.

are adjacent to each other in the very proximal thigh, whereas more distally, the vein will be deep to the artery. Find the location where the artery and vein lie next to each other in order to avoid arterial puncture (Figure 45-16).[23]

▶ PERIPHERAL INTRAVENOUS ACCESS

Peripheral intravenous access is routinely performed in order to obtain blood for diagnostic tests as well as administration of fluids and medications. There are many factors that can make obtaining intravenous access challenging including obesity, intravenous drug use, and multiple previous peripheral access attempts.[24,25] Ultrasound-guided peripheral vascular access is a safe and rapid method of obtaining vascular access and provides an alternative to either central venous access or multiple "blind" attempts.[26] Furthermore, it has been shown that there is no increased risk of infection when performing ultrasound-guided peripheral access as compared with traditionally placed catheters.[27]

The high-frequency linear array transducer is utilized for obtaining vascular access of the superficial veins. Veins are round or oval anechoic structures that are easily collapsible with slight pressure of the probe on the skin. Color Doppler can be utilized to aid in differentiating an artery from a vein. The skin should be appropriately cleansed. The use of sterile ultrasound gel has not been shown to change infection rates.[27] Once a suitable vein is identified, the static or dynamic technique employing either a transverse or longitudinal approach can be used to cannulate the vein. Frequently, by the time ultrasound is brought to the bedside, the patient has already undergone multiple attempts at vascular access. As a result, the external jugular vein and the veins in the proximal arm are often utilized to gain vascular access. If the brachial or the cephalic veins are cannulated, it may be necessary to use a longer (2.5 in) catheter as these veins may be beyond the reach of a standard intravenous catheter (Figures 45-17 and 45-18).[28]

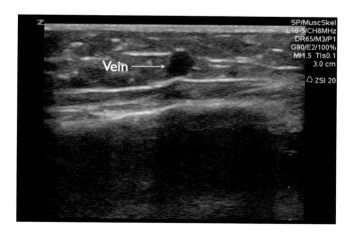

Figure 45-17. Short-axis view of a peripheral vein.

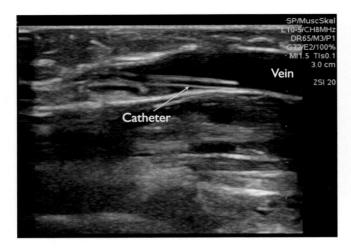

Figure 45-18. Longitudinal view of a catheter within a peripheral vein.

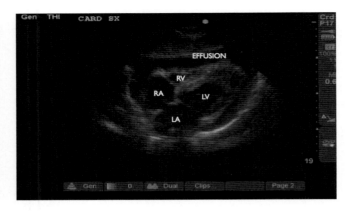

Figure 45-19. Tamponade. Subxiphoid view of pericardial effusion with collapse of the right ventricle. RA, right atrium; RV, right ventricle; LA, left atrium; LV, left ventricle.

▶ ARTERIAL CATHETER PLACEMENT

Arterial catheter placement in a peripheral artery can be challenging, especially in a hypotensive patient with a weak or absent peripheral pulse. In the intensive care unit, the need for continuous blood pressure monitoring and frequent evaluation of arterial blood gas can make arterial catheters crucial to patient care. Traditionally, the arterial catheter is inserted via a technique using palpation of the pulse to guide the needle insertion. Difficulty with locating the artery or inserting the catheter subjects patients to multiple painful attempts. The use of ultrasound for arterial catheter insertion has been shown to increase first-pass success, thereby reducing time to insertion and the number of attempts.[29]

The linear high-frequency ultrasound transducer is used to identify the thick-walled pulsatile artery that is less compressible than the adjacent thin-walled and easily compressible veins. The addition of pulsed wave or color Doppler can be used to visualize the characteristic pulsatile arterial blood flow. Once the artery is identified, the catheter can be placed dynamically to monitor first the needle and then the guidewire entering the artery in real time. In cases where the radial artery cannot be cannulated, ultrasound guidance can also be used to cannulate the brachial, femoral, dorsalis pedis, or axillary artery.[30,31]

▶ PERICARDIOCENTESIS

Cardiac tamponade is a life-threatening condition that can be remedied with pericardiocentesis. Traditionally, pericardial effusion and tamponade were diagnosed clinically using Beck's triad (hypotension, muffled

heart sounds, and jugular venous distention), along with pulsus paradoxus, and a pericardial friction rub. However, many of these findings either occur late in the disease process or may be difficult to appreciate. Echocardiography has become the standard of care to diagnose a pericardial effusion and tamponade, and can also be used to localize the area with the largest fluid collection in anticipation of pericardiocentesis.[32] Emergent pericardiocentesis should be performed when the patient sustains cardiac arrest or hemodynamic instability in the setting of a large pericardial effusion. Major complications of pericardiocentesis include cardiac chamber laceration, intercostal vessel injury, pneumothorax, sustained ventricular tachycardia, and death.[33,34] Ultrasound guidance can make this dangerous, yet life-saving procedure, significantly safer.[33]

The patient should first be imaged using standard cardiac windows with the phased array transducer. This also allows for evaluation of global cardiac function. Cardiac tamponade can be diagnosed on ultrasound by observing right ventricular collapse during early diastole or invagination of the free wall of the right atrium during end diastole. A plethoric inferior vena cava with little change in diameter during respiration as well as alterations in transvalvular flow velocities may also be visualized (Figure 45-19).[35]

The subxiphoid and the parasternal approaches are most commonly used for pericardiocentesis The decision to use one rather than the other lies mainly with operator experience and where the largest amount of fluid is. The subxiphoid approach is most often used with the static technique, while the parasternal approach is more commonly performed as a dynamic ultrasound-guided procedure (Figure 45-20).

For a parasternal approach, the patient can be supine, with the upper body elevated 30–45°, or the

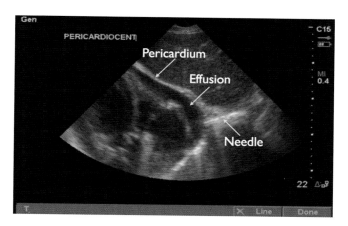

Figure 45-20. Pericardiocentesis with needle entering largest pocket of fluid.

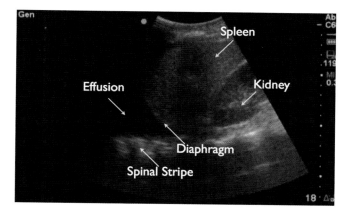

Figure 45-21. Pleural effusion with the hyperechoic line representing the spinal stripe extending beyond the diaphragm, indicative of an effusion.

patient can be placed in the left lateral decubitus position. The patient should be prepped and draped using standard sterile technique. The ultrasound transducer can then be placed in the parasternal long-axis orientation at the third or fourth intercostal space just to the left of the sternum to visualize the largest pocket of fluid that is usually between the probe and the anterior wall of the heart. The distance from the skin to the pericardial space should be measured to judge how far the needle will be advanced in order to enter the pericardial space.[36] Care must be taken to avoid the left internal mammary artery that lies 3–5 cm lateral to the sternal border. Once the ideal entry path has been determined, local anesthesia should be infiltrated at the entry site and along the proposed path for the needle. The longitudinal approach is recommended for this procedure so that the needle can be visualized throughout the procedure. The needle should be large bore, 18 gauge or greater, and preferably sheathed with a Teflon catheter to allow for continuous drainage of the effusion. A thoracentesis tray usually contains this type of catheter. As the needle is inserted, the tip should be followed carefully with continuous sonographic visualization. Once a "flash" of fluid is obtained, the needle can be advanced a few millimeters and the fluid can then be aspirated with the needle or the Teflon sheath can be advanced while the needle is removed for continuous drainage.[37]

When employing a subxiphoid approach, either static or dynamic sonographic guidance can be used. For the static technique, the probe is positioned in the subxiphoid region. The effusion should be visualized with the largest pocket centered on the screen. The entry point, direction of the needle, and depth necessary to reach the fluid should be noted. After the probe is removed, the needle can be introduced as described above.[36,38]

► THORACENTESIS

Pleural effusion is a relatively common entity among critically ill patients and thoracentesis is the most common interventional thoracic procedure.[39] The etiology of the collection can be elusive and pathologic examination of a fluid sample is often diagnostic. Potential complications of thoracentesis include pain, pneumothorax, vasovagal reactions, reexpansion pulmonary edema, inadvertent liver or splenic laceration, as well as infection and hemothorax.[39,40] Ultrasound can be used not only to detect an effusion but also to guide drainage, which may be necessary to perform emergently if the pleural fluid is causing respiratory distress. Ultrasound is more sensitive than chest radiography for detecting pleural effusions. It has also been shown to increase the success rate of thoracentesis and to decrease the rate of complications,[39,40] including pneumothorax and lacerations of the liver and spleen.[41]

To detect a pleural effusion by ultrasound, place the patient in a supine position with the head of the bed at 45°. The low-frequency curved abdominal probe should be placed longitudinally in the posterior axillary line just inferior to the nipple so that the curved hyperechoic line of the diaphragm above the liver or spleen can be visualized. A pleural effusion will be represented by an anechoic collection of fluid superior to the diaphragm. When no effusion is present, the spinal stripe will terminate at the diaphragm as the ultrasound waves are refracted by the air-filled lungs. However, when an effusion is present, the fluid collection allows for visualization of structures normally obscured by the lungs, namely, the thoracic spine superior to the diaphragm. Visualizing the hyperechoic spinal stripe superior to the diaphragm indicates that fluid is present in the chest, as does an anechoic collection with sharp angles superior to the diaphragm (Figure 45-21). Once an effusion has been detected, a more thorough evaluation of the chest should be performed. The movement of the lung with the respiratory cycle and the location of the diaphragm and abdominal organs should be noted so as to avoid these structures when a thoracentesis is performed.

With a cooperative awake patient, the patient can be placed in the sitting position at the edge of the bed with his or her arms folded on a tray table. The posterior hemithorax should be scanned with a small footprint phased array or a microconvex probe from the inferior scapular border to the upper lumbar region, and then from the paraspinal region to the posterior axillary line in order to delineate the extent of the fluid collection and the area of the largest pocket.[41] A hyperechoic line, representing the pleura, should be visible between the ribs. Noting the depth of the pleura will be useful to determine the length the needle will need to traverse to successfully aspirate fluid.[35] After the effusion is mapped out, the critical structures of the diaphragm and the lung are located, and the entry point is determined and marked. A static approach is employed and the procedure proceeds in the normal fashion. Care must be taken to ensure that the needle is placed superior to the diaphragm. The hyperechoic diaphragm should be visualized and the needle should be introduced at least two rib spaces above this structure to ensure that the peritoneal cavity is not violated. The procedure can also be performed dynamically, visualizing the needle as it enters the pleural space. If a thoracostomy tube is to remain in the thoracic cavity, a location in the midaxillary line will be more comfortable for the patient when lying in the supine position.

A sedated or intubated patient requiring a thoracentesis should be placed in the supine position with the arm abducted and the stretcher in the reverse Trendelenburg position. The puncture site will be in the lateral chest in the midaxillary line similar to the location commonly used for chest tube placement. Ultrasound can help to target the largest fluid pocket and to avoid critical structures. If the patient is mechanically ventilated, temporarily decreasing the tidal volume during the procedure may reduce the incidence of pneumothorax. While pneumothorax is a significant complication in the mechanically ventilated patient, the incidence is decreased with use of ultrasound.[43,44]

▶ PARACENTESIS

Paracentesis is performed in the critically ill patient with ascites for diagnostic or therapeutic reasons, or both. US guidance has been shown to confer a much higher success rate when compared with a landmark-based technique (95% vs. 65%).[35] An additional benefit of ultrasound guidance is visualizing little or no free fluid in the abdomen in a patient with a markedly distended

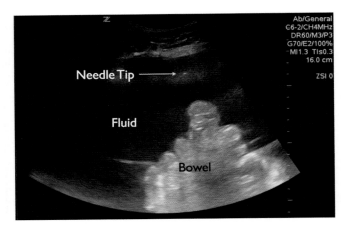

Figure 45-22. Paracentesis. Needle tip in abdominal fluid.

abdomen that was thought to be due to ascites. This discovery can spare the patient an invasive procedure.

With the patient supine or in a slightly left lateral oblique position and the head of the bed slightly raised, the lower abdomen should be scanned in two orthogonal planes with the low-frequency curved transducer. The left lower quadrant has been traditionally preferred as a gas-filled cecum or an appendectomy scar inhibiting the free flow of fluid may be present in the right lower quadrant, although ultrasound guidance allows for identification and avoidance of these structures so either lower quadrant may be utilized. The largest fluid collection site should be noted and the entry point marked. A fluid collection at least 3 cm in diameter is considered adequate for drainage. Static guidance is most commonly used for this procedure, although one may use dynamic guidance to observe the needle entering the peritoneum (Figure 45-22).

Structures to note and avoid when scanning the abdomen are the inferior epigastric artery in the abdominal wall, the bladder, and the intestines. The thickness of the abdominal wall and the depth of the fluid collection should be noted as well. Also note that a large loop of fluid-filled bowel should not be mistaken for a fluid collection. Fluid-filled bowel has a hyperechoic wall surrounding it and exhibits peristalsis, whereas peritoneal fluid will be located outside the intestinal walls.

▶ ENDOTRACHEAL INTUBATION

Unrecognized esophageal intubation is relatively infrequent, although in those rare occurrences, morbidity and mortality are significantly increased.[44] There are multiple methods employed at the bedside to confirm endotracheal intubation including direct visualization of the tube passing between the vocal cords, chest rise after intubation, auscultation over both lungs, and end-tidal carbon dioxide monitoring. However, any single method is not entirely reliable. Confirmatory methods may be inaccurate, especially in patients suffering from cardiac arrest or traumatic injury or those who have recently vomited or bled.[44,45]

Ultrasound has recently been shown to be useful as a bedside adjunct for confirming endotracheal intubation. Using the high-frequency linear array transducer, ultrasonography should be performed dynamically during the intubation procedure. Just prior to intubation, the vocal cords can be visualized as a triangular structure. The probe is held transversely over the cricothyroid membrane. As the endotracheal tube is passed, a brief "snow storm" should be seen, after which the transcricothyroid membrane should appear round with posterior hypoechoic shadowing.[44,46] If the tube has instead passed through the esophagus, the unintubated trachea produces a reverberating type of artifact knows as "ring down". Usually, the esophagus is not visualized sonographically, as it is collapsed. However, in the setting of an esophageal intubation, the esophagus may be noted to be distended by the endotracheal tube. In addition, confirmation of bilateral lung sliding should be performed by placing the linear transducer longitudinally over both hemithoraces in order to check for pleural sliding. The presence of bilateral sliding provides confirmation of an endotracheal intubation and helps to differentiate a right mainstem intubation from a main tracheal intubation. The bilateral absence of lung sliding may indicate an esophageal intubation (Figure 45-23 and 45-24).[44,46–49]

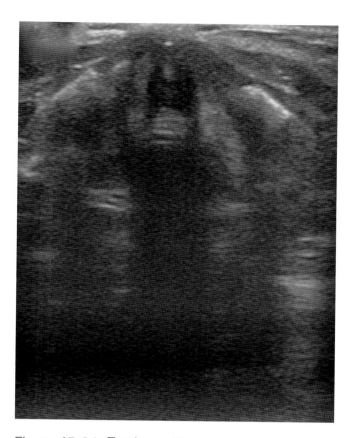

Figure 45-24. Trachea with endotracheal tube in place demonstrating posterior shadowing from the tube and loss of ring-down artifact.

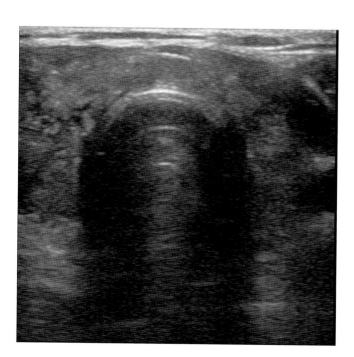

Figure 45-23. Trachea before intubation with ring-down artifact.

► CHEST TUBE PLACEMENT

Subcutaneous placement of the chest tube is a known complication of tube thoracostomy. While chest radiography is routinely used, differentiating tubes that are extrathoracic but appear intrathoracic in the anteroposterior radiographic view can be challenging. Computed tomography of the chest is more sensitive and specific in identifying correct tube placement. However, this imaging modality requires a patient to be moved to the radiology suite, which may be inadvisable in an unstable patient. Ultrasonography has recently emerged as a sensitive and specific modality for verifying intrathoracic versus extrathoracic tube thoracostomy placement.

Using a linear array high-frequency transducer placed in a transverse orientation relative to the chest tube, the tube will appear as a hyperechoic arc. Starting at the site where the tube pierced the skin, the tube is followed and the disappearance of the arc indicates that the tube entered the pleural space. Visualization of the arc superior to the thoracostomy site for the length of the tube indicates that the tube is in the subcutaneous tissue.[50]

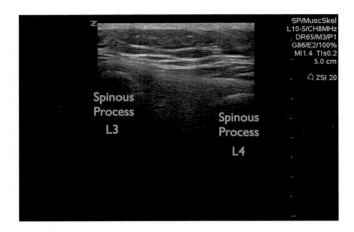

Figure 45-25. Static longitudinal view of L3–L4 interspinous space.

► LUMBAR PUNCTURE

Lumbar puncture is a commonly performed procedure used to aid in the diagnosis of meningitis, subarachnoid hemorrhage, and other neurologic emergencies. Traditionally, the procedure relies on identification of bony landmarks. However, these landmarks may be difficult to palpate or identify due to body habitus, contractions, or inability to properly position the patient. Furthermore, using Tuffier's line between the iliac crests to identify safe lumbar interspaces may be inaccurate.[51] Ultrasound guidance has been shown to increase the success of lumbar puncture in patients with elevated body mass index[52] and may be helpful after multiple failed attempts in the nonobese patient.

To perform the procedure, the patient is placed in the lateral decubitus or the sitting position. The linear high-frequency probe is preferred. In an obese patient, a low-frequency probe may be used if deeper sonographic penetration is necessary to visualize the bones. The probe is placed at the top of the gluteal fold in a longitudinal orientation and the hyperechoic bony sacrum should be visualized. Moving superiorly, the first break in the hyperechoic line is the L5–S1 disc space. The L5 spinous process appears as a hyperechoic convex line. Moving the transducer superiorly, the three lower spinous processes and the intervening disc spaces can be mapped out. The probe can be moved laterally to find the lateral margins of the spinous processes as they disappear from view. Also, the probe can be turned 90° to better appreciate the lateral margins of the spinous processes (Figure 45-25).[53,54]

With indelible ink, the central line of the spine and each spinous process can be drawn on the skin. These marks can be used to proceed with the lumbar puncture in the traditional manner using the pen marks instead of the bony landmarks as a guide.

► CONCLUSION

There is a growing body of literature demonstrating the value of ultrasonography in the care of the critically ill patient. Ultrasound is widely available, portable, repeatable, relatively inexpensive, pain-free, and safe. It should be considered in conjunction with traditional methods when performing invasive procedures.

REFERENCES

1. Mandavia DP, Aragona J, Chan L, et al. Ultrasound training for emergency physicians—a prospective study. *Acad Emerg Med.* 2000;7:1008–1014.
2. Palepu GB, Deven J, Subrahmanyam M. Impact of ultrasonography on central venous catheter insertion in intensive care. *Indian J Radiol Imaging.* 2009;19:191–198.
3. Shojania KG, Duncan BW, McDonald KM, et al. Making health care safer: a critical analysis of patient safety practices. *Evid Rep Technol Assess (Summ).* 2001;43:i–x, 1–668.
4. DeFrances CJ, Hall MJ. 2002 National Hospital Disaster Survey. *Adv Data.* 2004;342:1–30.
5. McGee DC, Gould MK. Preventing complications of central venous catheterization. *N Engl J Med.* 2003;348: 1123–1133.
6. Merrer J, De Jonghe B, Golliot F, et al. Complications of femoral and subclavian venous catheterization in critically ill patients: a randomized controlled trial. *JAMA.* 2001;286:700–707.
7. Sznajder JI, Zveibil FR, Bitterman H, et al. Central vein catheterization: failure and complication rates by three percutaneous approaches. *Arch Intern Med.* 1986;146:259–261.
8. Mansfield PF, Hohn DC, Fornage BD, et al. Complications and failures of subclavian-vein catheterization. *N Engl J Med.* 1994;331:1735–1738.
9. Leung J, Duffy M, Finckh A. Real-time ultrasonographically-guided internal jugular vein catheterization in the emergency department increases success rates and reduces complications: a randomized, prospective study. *Ann Emerg Med.* 2006;48:540–547.
10. Theodoro D, Bausano B, Lewis L, Evanoff B, Kollef M. A descriptive comparison of ultrasound-guided central venous cannulation of the internal jugular vein to landmark-based subclavian vein cannulation. *Acad Emerg Med.* 2010 Apr;17(4):416–422.
11. Miller AH, Roth BA, Mills TJ, Woody JR, Longmoor CE, Foster B. Ultrasound guidance versus the landmark technique for the placement of central venous catheters in the emergency department. *Acad Emerg Med.* 2002;9:800–805.
12. Randolph AG, Cook DJ, Gonzales CA, Pribble CG. Ultrasound guidance for placement of central venous catheters: a meta-analysis of the literature. *Crit Care Med.* 1996 Dec;24(12):2053–2058.
13. Slama M, Novara A, Safavian S. Improvement of internal jugular vein cannulation using an ultrasound-guided technique. *Int Care Med.* 1997;23:916–919.

14. Lewin MR, Stein J, Wang R. Humming is as effective as Valsalva's maneuver and Trendelenburg's position for ultrasonographic visualization of the jugular venous system and common femoral veins. *Ann Emerg Med.* 2007;50:73–77.

15. Stone MB, Moon C, Sutijono D, et al. Needle tip visualization during ultrasound-guided vascular access: short-axis vs long-axis approach. *Am J Emerg Med.* 2010;28:343–347.

16. Blaivas M. Video analysis of accidental cannulation with dynamic ultrasound guidance for central venous access. *J Ultrasound Med.* 2009;28:1239–1244.

17. Timsit JF. What is the best site for central venous catheter insertion in critically ill patients? *Crit Care.* 203;7:397–399.

18. Denys BG, Uretsky BF, Reddy PS. Ultrasound-assisted cannulation of the internal jugular vein. A prospective comparison to the external landmark-guided technique. *Circulation.* 1993;87:1557–1562.

19. Hrics P, Wilber S, Blanda MP, Gallo U. Ultrasound-assisted internal jugular vein catheterization in the ED. *Am J Emerg Med.* 1998;16:401–403.

20. Lorente L, Henry C, Martín MM, et al. Central venous catheter-related infection in a prospective and observational study of 2,595 catheters. *Crit Care.* 2005;9:631–635.

21. McKinley S, Mackenzie A, Finfer S, et al. Incidence and predictors of central venous catheter related infection in intensive care patients. *Anaesth Intensive Care.* 1999;27:164–169.

22. Werner SL, Jones RA, Emerman CL. Effect of hip abduction and external rotation on femoral vein exposure for possible cannulation. *J Emerg Med.* 2008;35:73–75.

23. Hilty WM, Hudson PA, Levitt MA, et al. Real-time ultrasound-guided femoral vein catheterization during cardiopulmonary resuscitation. *Ann Emerg Med.* 1997;29:331–336.

24. Constantino TG, Parikh AK, Satz WA, et al. Ultrasonography-guided peripheral intravenous access versus traditional approaches in patients with difficult intravenous access. *Ann Emerg Med.* 2005;46:456–461.

25. Juvin P, Blarel A, Fabienne B, et al. Is peripheral line placement more difficult in obese than in lean patients? *Anesth Analg.* 2003;96:1218.

26. Dargin JM, Rebholz CM, Lowenstein RA, et al. Ultrasonography-guided peripheral intravenous catheter survival in ED patients with difficult access. *Am J Emerg Med.* 2010;28:1–7.

27. Adhikari S, Blaivas M, Morrison D. Comparison of infection rates among ultrasound-guided versus traditionally placed peripheral intravenous lines. *J Ultrasound Med.* 2010;29:741–747.

28. Gregg SC, Murthi SB, Sisley AC, Stein DM, Scalea TM. Ultrasound-guided peripheral intravenous access in the intensive care unit. *J Crit Care.* 2010 Sep;25(3):514–519. Epub 2009 Oct 15.

29. Levin PD, Sheinin O, Gozal Y. Use of the ultrasound in the insertion of radial artery catheters. *Crit Care Med.* 2003;31(2):481–484.

30. Maher JJ, Dougherty JM. Radial artery cannulation guided by Doppler ultrasound. *Am J Emerg Med.* 1989;7:260–262.

31. Sandhu NS. The use of ultrasound for axillary artery catheterization through the pectoral muscles: a new anterior approach. *Anesth Analg.* 2004;99:562–565.

32. American College of Emergency Physicians. ACEP emergency ultrasound guidelines—2001. *Ann Emerg Med.* 2001;38:470–481.

33. Tsang T, Enriquez-Sarano M, Freeman W, et al. Consecutive 1127 therapeutic echocardiographically guided pericardioscenteses: clinical profile, practice patterns, and outcomes spanning 21 years. *Mayo Clin Proc.* 2002;77:429–436.

34. Wong B, Murphy J, Chang CJ, et al. The risk of pericardiocentesis. *Am J Cardiol.* 1979;44:1110–1114.

35. Dewitz A, Jones R, Goldstein J. In Ma OJ, Mateer JR, Blaivas M, eds. *Emergency Ultrasound: Additional Ultrasound Guided Procedure.* New York: McGraw Hill; 2008:507–551.

36. Salem K, Mulji A, Lonn E. Echocardiographically guided pericardiocentesis—the gold standard for the management of pericardial effusion and cardiac tamponade. *Can J Cardiol.* 1999;15:1251–1255.

37. Fagan SM, Chan KL. Pericardiocentesis: blind no more! *Chest.* 1999;116:275–276.

38. Lindenberger M, Kjellberg M, Karlsson E, et al. Pericardiocentesis guided by 2D echocardiography: the method of choice for treatment of pericardial effusion. *J Int Med.* 2003;253:411–417.

39. Mynarek G, Brabrand K, Jakonsen JA, et al. Complications following ultrasound guided thoracocentesis. *Acta Radiol.* 2004;5:519–522.

40. Jones PW, Moyers JP, Rogers JT, et al. Ultrasound-guided thoracentesis—is it a safer method? *Chest.* 2003;123:418–423.

41. Diacon AH, Brutsche MH, Soler M. Accuracy of pleural puncture sites: a prospective comparison of clinical examination with ultrasound. *Chest.* 2003;123:436–441.

42. Mayo PH, Goltz HR, Tafreshi M, et al. Safety of ultrasound-guided thoracentesis in patients receiving mechanical ventilation. *Chest.* 2004;125:1059–1062.

43. Pihlajamaa K, Bode MK, Puumalainen T. Pneumothorax and the value of chest radiography after ultrasound-guided thoracocentesis. *Acta Radiol.* 2004;8:828–832.

44. Park SC, Ryu JH, Yeom SR, et al. Confirmation of endotracheal intubation by combined ultrasonographic methods in the emergency department. *Emerg Med Australas.* 2009;21:293–297.

45. Grmec S. Comparison of three different methods to confirm tracheal tube placement in emergency intubation. *Intensive Care Med.* 2002;28:701–704.

46. Drescher MJ, Conard FU, Schamban NE. Identification and description of esophageal intubation using ultrasound. *Acad Emerg Med.* 2000;7:722–725.

47. Sustić A. Role of ultrasound in the airway management of critically ill patients. *Crit Care Med.* 2007;35:S173–S177.

48. Ma G, Davis DP, Schmitt J, et al. The sensitivity and specificity of transcricothyroid ultrasonography to confirm endotracheal tube placement in a cadaver model. *J Emerg Med.* 2007;32:405–407.

49. Weaver B, Lyon M, Blaivas M. Confirmation of endotracheal tube placement after intubation using the ultrasound sliding lung sign. *Acad Emerg Med.* 2006;13:239–244.

50. Salz TO, Wilson SR, Leibmann O, et al. An initial description of a sonographic sign that verifies intrathoracic chest tube placement. *Am J Emerg Med.* 2010;28:626–630.

51. Broadbent CR, Maxwell WB, Ferrie R, et al. Ability of anesthetists to identify a marked lumbar interspace. *Anaesthesia.* 2000;55:1122–1126.

52. Nomura JY, Leech SJ, Shenbagamurthi S, et al. A randomized controlled trial of ultrasound-assisted lumbar puncture. *J Ultrasound Med.* 2007;26:1341–1348.

53. Watson MJ, Evans S, Thorp JM. Could ultrasonography be used by an anaesthetist to identify a specified lumbar interspace before spinal anaesthesia? *Br J Anaesth.* 2003;90:509–511.

54. Sandoval M, Shestak W, Sturmann K, et al. Optimal patient position for lumbar puncture, measured by ultrasonography. *Emerg Radiol.* 2004;10:179–181.

SECTION XI

Special Considerations

CHAPTER 46

Classification of Shock

Tiffany M. Osborn and David A. Farcy

▶ INTRODUCTION

Critical illness is defined as "any patient who is physiologically unstable, requiring constant and minute-to-minute titration of therapy according to the evolution of the disease process."[1] It is a continuum often culminating in rapid decline, shock, organ failure, and, frequently, patient demise. Traditionally, shock is defined as a clinical diagnosis identified through physical manifestations observed by medical staff.[2] Complementing clinical acumen is the recognition of accumulating oxygen debt due to perturbations of microvascular circulation. Early phases of evolving shock may manifest through biochemical markers with minimal physical alterations.[3-5] Although typically considered an intensive care unit (ICU) ailment, shock develops well before ICU admission with patients often initially presenting to the emergency department (ED). Effective, timely shock treatment requires a continuum of care beginning with prehospital providers, continuing within the ED, and concluding within the ICU.[6,7] Thus, shock treatments should be defined by level of care rather than location of care.[8]

With the ever-increasing incidence of the critically ill and injured initially presenting through the ED, active emergency medicine participation in the continuum of care is essential. The number one reason for ED overcrowding is reported as a severe lack of accessible ICU beds.[9] Lambe et al noted a 59% increase of ED critical care volume with an 8% decrease in nonurgent patients[10] (Figure 46-1). This is mirrored nationally with 23% of ED patients triaged as requiring immediate or emergent (within 15 minutes) care. One of every 10 patients hospitalized from the ED is directly admitted to the ICU.[11] Underscored is the clinical reality that emergency medicine physicians are seeing a higher volume of patients, with more patients severely ill than in the past.

ED epidemiology of shock remains speculative as it is typically veiled within other diagnoses. However, shock is a significant contributor to ED critical care volume; an estimated 1.1 million patients present to the ED with potential shock each year.[12] From 1999 to 2002, the prevalence of patients requiring emergent resuscitation increased from 17% to 22%.[11,13] Mortality is high, ranging from 23% to 80%, depending on the type of shock, patient age, and comorbidities.[14-17] As Americans age, the incidence of shock is expected to increase with estimates of one half of patients initially presenting to the ED.[15]

▶ STRUCTURE AND FUNCTION

Traditionally, the diagnosis of shock is made based on clinical signs and symptoms such as hypotension, tachycardia, weak pulse, and cold, clammy skin. Unfortunately, due to diverse circumstances, many of these signs and symptoms—or their absence—prove to be unreliable gauges of the presence and/or degree of shock. Furthermore, different etiologies of shock often result in differing degrees of signs and symptoms. For instance, due to pathologic vasodilatation and excessive organ dysfunction, sepsis will account for a much more complicated array of signs and symptoms than those attributed to hemorrhage. Moreover, otherwise healthy individuals possess the ability to sustain a considerable loss of volume before exhibiting such obvious signs and symptoms, while a less healthy patient, or one with significant preexisting comorbidities, may not be able to endure even a small volume loss without demonstrating serious signs and symptoms. In short, depending on the patient's age, comorbidities, and clinical circumstances, shock may exist prior to the onset of evident signs and symptoms.

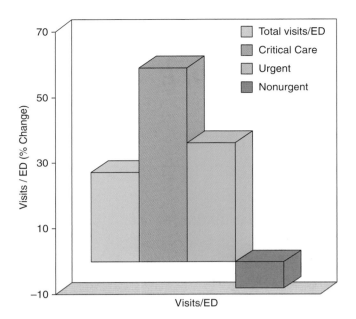

Figure 46-1. ED volume trends in California from 1990 to 1999. Critically ill ED visits increased by 59% as nonurgent visits decreased by 8% ($P < .001$) throughout the state of California.

Therefore, shock is not defined by clinical condition, but rather by biochemical outcome resulting from ineffective tissue perfusion, that is, inadequate delivery of oxygen and substrates for normal cellular function.[18,19]

Understanding shock requires understanding the concepts of oxygen delivery. Oxygen delivery (DO_2) is the total amount of oxygen bound to hemoglobin (Hg) and delivered to the peripheral tissues per minute. It is calculated as follows (see Figure 46-2):

$$DO_2 = CO \times CaO_2 \times 10$$

Cardiac output (CO) is the most important determinant of oxygen delivery. As illustrated in Figures 46-3 to 46-6, CO has the ability to compensate for increases in metabolic needs or decreases in O_2-carrying capacity. However, CO is a product of both heart rate and stroke volume (SV), and SV is affected by a multiplicity of factors. Thus, CO can be difficult to predict and manipulate.

- DO_2 = Oxygen delivery (DO_2) = Arterial oxygen content (CaO_2) × cardiac output (CO) × 10.
- $DO_2 = CO \times CaO_2 \times 10$
- $CO = HR \times SV$
- CaO_2 = Arterial oxygen content (CaO_2) = The amount of Hb available to bind O_2, the amount of oxygen saturated Hb (SaO_2), and the amount of dissolved oxygen (PaO_2) in arterial blood. PaO_2 is usually ignored because the number is so small.
- $CaO_2 = (Hb \times SaO_2 \times 1.38) + (0.0031 \times PaO_2)$
- $DO_2 = CO \times (Hb \times SaO_2 \times 1.38) + (0.0031 \times PaO_2)$

Figure 46-2. Calculation 1.

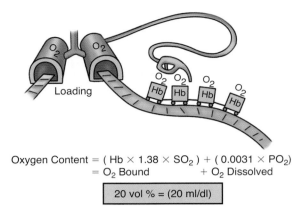

Oxygen Content = (Hb × 1.38 × SO_2) + (0.0031 × PO_2)
                      = O_2 Bound   + O_2 Dissolved

20 vol % = (20 ml/dl)

Figure 46-3. Oxygen delivery. Oxygen content is a function of bound oxygen (Hb) and unbound or dissolved oxygen. (Reproduced with permission from Edwards Lifesciences, Irvine, California.)

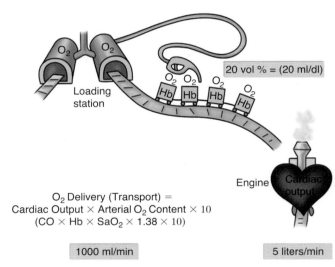

O_2 Delivery (Transport) =
Cardiac Output × Arterial O_2 Content × 10
(CO × Hb × SaO_2 × 1.38 × 10)

1000 ml/min   5 liters/min

Figure 46-4. Oxygen delivery. Oxygen delivery is a function of cardiac output (CO), oxygen saturation (SaO_2), and hemoglobin (Hb). A disruption in any one of those components may adversely impact oxygen delivery. (Reproduced with permission from Edwards Lifesciences, Irvine, California.)

Hg is another significant contributor to oxygen delivery. As Hg is easily manipulated through transfusion, it becomes an important factor in regulating oxygen delivery. A schematic of a train may represent the impact of these components on the DO_2 system. How much oxygen is delivered to the tissues through the microvasculature depends on how many oxygen-carrying units (Hg) are present, how many of those Hb units are effectively carrying oxygen, and how effectively the heart is working to transport the oxygenated units. In cases with accumulating oxygen debt, demonstrated through elevated lactate and/or decreased

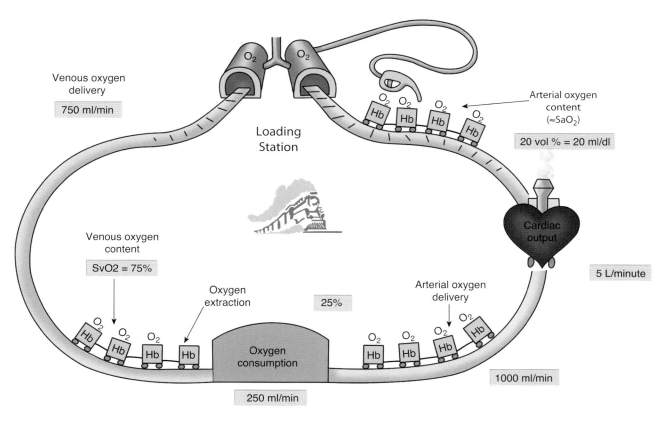

Figure 46-5. Oxygen delivery. At the level of the microvasculature, oxygen is extracted from the Hb and consumed by the tissues. Normally about 25% is extracted so that the oxygen saturation at the level of the heart (pulmonary artery, SvO_2; superior vena cava, $ScvO_2$) is about 75%. When SvO_2 or $ScvO_2$ is <70%, oxygen debt is occurring. (Reproduced with permission from Edwards Lifesciences, Irvine, California.)

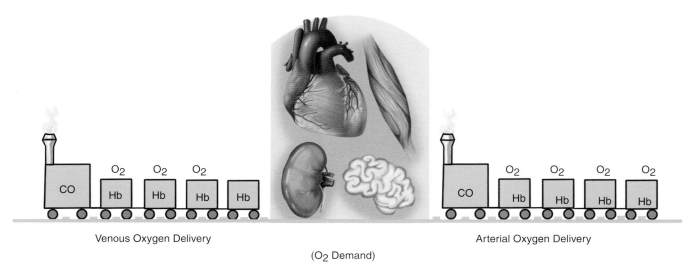

Figure 46-6. Oxygen delivery. Oxygen consumption by the tissues is the difference between the amount of oxygen carried to the tissues (arterial oxygen delivery) and the amount of oxygen returning to the heart (venous oxygen delivery). (Reproduced with permission from Edwards Lifesciences, Irvine, California.)

central venous oxygen saturation ($ScvO_2$), individual patient requirements must be assessed by considering the previously discussed components of oxygen delivery ($DO_2 = CO \times CaO_2 \times 10$):

1. Is there sufficient oxygenation?
2. Is there sufficient preload—does the patient require further fluid resuscitation?
3. Is there sufficient afterload for end-organ perfusion?
4. Is the concentration of oxygen-carrying units optimal? This is best assessed via a postresuscitation Hb, as the initial value may be significantly hemoconcentrated.

Arterial oxygen saturation (SvO_2), measured as blood is ejected from the left side of the heart, is approximately 100%. As oxygenated blood circulates through the microvasculature, an estimated 25% of delivered oxygen is extracted by the peripheral tissues. This is best measured by evaluating the SvO_2 through a pulmonary artery catheter. However, because of efficacy and safety questions surrounding pulmonary artery catheters,[20] the measurement of $ScvO_2$ has been proven a functional surrogate,[19] and because of logistics, $ScvO_2$ is a more practical and less morbid alternative in the ED and even ICU setting.

$ScvO_2$ is measured through a central line placed into the superior vena cava (SVC). This translates into the oxygen saturation report from a venous blood gas taken from the distal port of a typical internal jugular (IJ) or subclavian (SC) central line, or from an electronic readout from a central line with an appropriate sensor. $ScvO_2$ provides a measurement of global tissue hypoxia. For patients in shock, $ScvO_2$ is typically 5–7% higher than SvO_2. Thus, $ScvO_2$ measurements below 70% may represent significant unresolved oxygen debts.[19] $ScvO_2$ can be measured by individual blood draws from a typical SVC central line or one may use a central line that allows continuous monitoring of $ScvO_2$.

CLINICAL IMPLICATIONS OF SHOCK PATHOPHYSIOLOGY

Traditionally systolic blood pressure (SBP) or mean arterial pressure (MAP) is used to denote shock (<90 or 65 mm Hg, respectively). This is based on the misconception that peripheral blood pressure universally equates to end-organ perfusion. Traditionally, shock has been defined or diagnosed at the point at which it could easily be identified via vital sign aberrations. However, shock does not commence when blood pressure deteriorates; blood pressure deteriorates when the body can no longer compensate physiologically for oxygen debt not yet identified and/or addressed. Cryptic shock, also described as normotensive shock, refers to

a physiologic state at the microvascular level resulting in accumulating oxygen deficit. Cryptic shock confers a high risk of morbidity and/or mortality.[21–24] Biomarkers, in conjunction with vital signs and physical exam, assist in early identification. If developing shock is arrested prior to decompensation, significant mortality benefit is achieved. This concept is already established in hemorrhagic/traumatic,[25–28] cardiovascular,[29–32] septic,[21,33–35] and general critical shock presenting to the ED.[36–37]

► PHYSICAL EXAM, PRESENTING SIGNS AND SYMPTOMS

The presenting signs and symptoms of specific types of shock are presented elsewhere in this text. As with any emergent patient, whether in the ED, ICU, or deteriorating in a less monitored setting, airway, breathing, and circulation should be quickly assessed on presentation and intervened upon as necessary.

Vital signs should be checked frequently. This is a reality that cannot be overstated; in a scenario in which the patient is unstable, vital signs are, by definition, changing unpredictably. In the presence of such a dynamic situation, the repeated monitoring of vital signs may often translate into the difference between recovery and significant morbidity and/or mortality.

An initial set of vital signs should include blood pressure, temperature, heart rate, respiratory rate, oxygen saturation, fingerstick glucose, and ECG. The patient should be placed onto a cardiac monitor with frequent reassessments. A rectal temperature should be considered in all patients. Any vital sign abnormality is a clear indicator that further workup is warranted.

Any patient with clear or suspected shock requires a thorough physical exam, including the often omitted skin, back, urogenital system, and all orifices. Potential etiologies of shock should be considered during each component of the physical exam. Other chapters will discuss specific elements; the following list is only a general reminder of elements to include or consider:

1. General appearance—"How does the patient look when I walk into the room?" The patient's general appearance will direct the immediate plan of action.
2. Mental status and full neurologic exam—Altered mental status refers to a wide spectrum from confusion to coma. Mild, new confusion may be an early indicator of an ominous process, especially in the elderly. A complete neurologic exam should be performed. When the neurologic exam is limited, radiographic assessment may be required.
3. Head, ears, eyes, nose, and throat—An oral process is a potential septic source frequently overlooked.

4. Neck—Hypotension with full neck veins requires consideration of a cardiac etiology, and hypotension with flat neck veins may indicate a systemic origin. Furthermore, consideration should be given to an infectious or traumatic process contributing to the presentation. Swelling that causes tracheal deviation may be due to a pharyngeal abscess. In the setting of trauma, tracheal deviation may be due to hemorrhage, and crepitus may be due to a laryngeal fracture. Furthermore, a cervical spine fracture may lead to neurogenic shock.

5. Chest/heart/lungs—Potential etiologies that may manifest acutely as shock include but are not limited to acute myocardial infarct, pericardial tamponade, myocarditis, tension pneumothorax, and/or pneumonia.

6. Abdominal exam—An extensive evaluation in conjunction with the history for physical manifestations of multiple diseases is important. Considerations include but are not limited to vascular insufficiency, bowel perforation, cholangitis, hemorrhage, and perforated stomach ulcer. Radiographic exam is often necessary. Notably an unimpressive abdominal exam does not rule out a significant insult; notoriously, the elderly may present with a seemingly unimposing exam while harboring significant pathophysiology.

7. Urogenital exam—A complete urogenital exam will prevent missing important causes of toxic shock syndrome such as intrauterine devices and tampons, or sepsis due to Fournier's gangrene in a diabetic patient.

8. Back—If the back has not been evaluated, only half of the patient has been examined. In patients using intravenous drugs, consider an epidural abscess.

9. Rectal exam—Evaluation may include but should not be limited to perirectal abscess, blood, and foreign body.

10. Skin—Septic shock may be from an unrecognized infected joint, decubitus ulcer, or endocarditis. Especially in obese patients in whom heart sounds can be difficult to auscultate, it is even more important to check hands, feet, and nail beds.

▶ DIFFERENTIAL DIAGNOSIS

CLASSIFICATION OF SHOCK

The clinical utility of the differential diagnosis of shock is based on understanding differences in effective tissue perfusion. Shock can be divided into four categories: hypovolemic, distributive, cardiogenic, and obstructive shock. Poor venous return is the base etiology of hypovolemic (absolute reduced intravascular volume) and distributive (ineffective vasomotor tone, relative reduced intravascular volume) shock. Cardiogenic shock is due to pump failure, so while there may be adequate intravascular volume, there is inadequate circulating volume. Finally, obstructive shock is due to a structural impediment of blood flow through the cardiac circuit. Additionally, there are mixed forms of shock with various overlaps of the above categories.[2,18]

Hypovolemic Shock

Hypovolemic shock is due to decreased intravascular volume, leading to decreased preload and therefore CO, resulting in reduced oxygen delivery. Potential etiologies include dehydration, hemorrhage, vomiting, severe burns, and iatrogenic sources such as diuretics and vasodilators. Hypovolemic shock can be recognized clinically by tachycardia, tachypnea, hypotension, narrow pulse pressure, altered mental status, decreased venous pressure, decreased urine output, and capillary refill. These signs and symptoms are derived from the lack of baroreceptor activation, which tends to increase heart rate and contractility coupled with a lack of stretch receptor activation in the atria leading to reduced release of atrial natriuretic peptide. Other acute changes that occur include activation of the renin–angiotensin–aldosterone system, mediated by the kidney. Angiotensin causes two main responses: vasoconstriction of the arteriolar smooth muscle and secretion of aldosterone, which promotes sodium reabsorption and water retention that results in extreme thirst. Often, these clinical symptoms are not recognized until 10–20% of whole blood volume has been lost. Importantly, it is possible for children to compensate for loss of volume for a longer period of time than adults (blood pressure maintenance despite hypovolemia). However, when decompensation commences, clinical decline is extremely rapid, often with poor outcomes. Fluid replacement and blood transfusions are the ultimate treatments for hypovolemic shock.

Cardiogenic Shock

Cardiogenic shock results from significant "pump failure" that may occur due to valvular pathology, myocardial insult, or pericardial pathology.[18] Depending on patient reserve, for myocardial etiologies, cardiogenic shock may occur when 40% of the myocardium is compromised, due usually to toxins, ischemia, immune, or inflammatory processes.[38] The reduction in effective CO results in decreased DO_2. The clinical manifestation may appear similar to hypovolemia (see above), except the patient may have jugular venous distension (due to increased jugular venous pressure) and a pulmonary exam consistent with edema (due to fluid backup resulting from inefficient pumping of the heart).

Additionally, there may be cardiac sounds such as a new murmur or ECG changes that may guide resuscitation. Diagnosis of cardiogenic shock can be made by clinical findings (as above); radiologic findings, which may show poor ventricular function or ventricular septal rupture on echocardiography; or ECG findings, which may demonstrate arrhythmias or signs of ischemia.

Initial treatment for cardiogenic shock often consists of carefully chosen combinations of vasopressors and inotropic agents. Vasopressors cause vasoconstriction while inotropic agents increase the force of cardiac contraction, depending on which receptors are stimulated by these medications. The goal is to increase perfusion of the ischemic myocardium. In the particular case of cardiogenic shock, however, extreme heart rates must be avoided due to increased myocardial oxygen consumption, which may further impair cardiac function and worsen the cardiogenic shock. In addition, there is the potential for increasing permanent damage to the heart (by increasing infarction size or causing valvular dysfunction). Short-acting inotropes, such as dobutamine, dopamine, or norepinephrine, should be considered, while longer-acting agents such as milrinone should be used with caution. (Please refer to Chapter 16 for further details.) Cautious fluid administration might be considered as required to maintain preload and thereby CO, but must be monitored carefully. In cases of myocardial infarction, rapid definitive treatment of coronary artery reperfusion should be sought. When rapid transport to a cardiac catheterization laboratory is not possible, chemical thrombolysis and/or mechanical device support such as an intra-aortic balloon pump (IABP) should be considered. Additionally, in appropriate cases a left ventricular assist device (LVAD) may be a necessary bridge to cardiac transplant.

Obstructive Shock

Obstructive shock is an extracardiac obstruction resulting in decreased diastolic filling or decreased ejection fraction. Usually both diastolic filling and decreased ejection are involved, with one predominating. Decreased CO occurs from decreased diastolic filling such as occurs in restrictive pericarditis and cardiac tamponade. Decreased CO is also seen—immediately—with large pulmonary emboli. A large pulmonary embolus (or multiple smaller ones) decreases the cross-sectional area of blood flow from the right ventricle to the left atrium causing right ventricular overload and leading to right ventricular failure. The clinical presentation is similar to that of cardiogenic shock with hypotension and IJ distension but without pulmonary edema.

Distributive Shock

Distributive shock is due to significant vasodilatation that causes decreased preload. In the arterial bed, it manifests through decreased arterial resistance, causing hypotension. Distributive shock may arise from circumstances such as sepsis, anaphylaxis, adrenal insufficiency, and neurogenic shock.

Despite the various etiologic agents, sepsis is the most prominent example.

Initially, septic shock typically presents as hypovolemia due to both vasodilatation (distributive shock) and leaking capillary membranes (hypovolemic shock). However, a distinguishing clinical feature is significantly more intravenous fluid requirement. It is not uncommon for distributive shock patients to have a 6- to 10-L fluid deficit and still require vasopressors to maintain a reasonable mean arterial blood pressure (MAP ≥65mm Hg).[39] Once the fluid deficit is abated, the typical manifestations of distributive shock, such as high CO, low systemic vascular resistance (SVR), and hypotension, emerge.

Interestingly, although the patient in distributive shock exhibits a high CO, it is paradoxically in conjunction with depressed myocardium. Inflammatory mediators cause myocardial depression so that the heart pumps less efficiently. The myocardial depression results in a depressed biventricular ejection fraction. In response to volume loading, the stroke work index is further reduced. However, it appears that simultaneously the ventricles dilate. The dilatation, in conjunction with an increased heart rate, provides the increased cardiac index (CI). This may actually be protective, as nonsurvivors who were unable to attain left ventricular dilatation have been observed to die from a cardiogenic form of septic shock.[40]

Although distributive shock manifests with a normal or increased CO, it is functionally ineffective due to maldistribution of blood flow caused by shunting either from or within an organ, such that the organ, either in part or whole, may be compromised. A common clinical example is a septic patient who has normal or increased CO but is in acute renal failure. Clinically, distributive shock may manifest as a hyperdynamic, high-flow state with hyperdynamic heart sounds, prominent and rapid pulses, quick capillary refill, and a wide pulse pressure.

Mixed Shock

Although it would be helpful if all patients presented in a specific isolated type of shock, frequently there is significant overlap requiring solid clinical acumen. The most challenging clinical example is septic shock, which may manifest with multiple components of the various forms of shock listed above.

- Hypovolemic shock—Septic shock patients presenting with a lactate ≥4 commonly have a 6- to 10-L fluid deficit. Aggressive fluid administration is a mainstay of initial treatment, underscoring the importance of measuring central venous pressure

(CVP) on presentation and using this measurement to guide the amount of fluid resuscitation.

- Distributive shock—Bacterial-derived mediators such as endotoxin, along with components of the inflammatory cascade, cause distributive shock with low SVR early in the disease presentation and normal to high CO in later stages.
- Cardiogenic shock—Although the typical description of septic shock is high CO in the face of a low SVR, early septic shock frequently manifests as a low CO/CI state consistent with hypodynamic, cardiogenic shock. In the early goal-directed therapy (EGDT) study of Rivers et al, the average time to enrollment was 1 hour with the CI ranging between 1.7 and 2.9.[21] Depressed myocardium persisted even after fluid resuscitation, implying myocardial dysfunction rather than a factor of decreased preload as the etiology of a low CI. The high CO state arises after the compensatory dilatation of the ventricles as described earlier in the section "Distributive Shock."[40,41]

The inflammatory response of any of these forms of shock, especially distributive, may result in multiple organ dysfunction syndrome (MODS). Often at this time, the only therapeutic options left are supportive with many patients refractory to the support.

▶ INTERVENTIONS, PROCEDURES, AND DIAGNOSTIC TESTING

Interventions and procedures are based on the type of shock suspected. All require confirmation that oxygen delivery is meeting demand. However, not all facilities are equipped to deal with patients in shock. Thus, transfer to an ICU or to an ED that has more resources may be necessary.

Noninvasive tests depend on the type of shock suspected. Most cases will require ECG, x-ray, pulse oximetry, and continuous vital sign monitoring. The role of ultrasound is rapidly expanding beyond the standard extended focused assessment for trauma (EFAST), which is sensitive and reliable in the assessment of trauma patients. Ultrasound applications such as the ability to look at the ventricle size, estimate the ejection fraction, and determine the collapsibility of the inferior vena cava are sensitive in cases of differentiated and undifferentiated shock.[42–49] If the patient is sufficiently stable to leave the department, further noninvasive diagnostic testing is based on suspected shock etiology such as CT for blunt trauma or PE.

Laboratory testing should also be based on the type of shock but generally includes chemistry, complete blood count (CBC), coagulation profile, troponin, lactate, arterial blood gas, central venous blood gas (if continuous $ScvO_2$ monitoring is not available), urinalysis, and cultures of blood and urine. Additional labs may include liver function tests, thyroid function tests, base deficit, toxicology screening for medications or drugs of abuse, and an ethanol level.

Depending on the cause of the shock, potential invasive procedures include:

- General practice for all forms of shock:
  1. Central line placement for administration of vasopressors, measurement of CVP, measurement of $ScvO_2$ (preferably SC line or IJ line), need for multiple ports, or an inability to establish sufficient peripheral intravenous accesses.
  2. Arterial line placement for continuous arterial blood pressure monitoring should be considered in all hypotensive patients requiring vasopressors.
- Cardiogenic shock should be considered for rapid transfer to the cardiac catheterization lab; however, these patients may additionally require a balloon pump as a bridge to percutaneous cardiac intervention or bypass surgery if not readily available.
- Obstructive shock interventions are based on potential etiology:
  1. Pericarditis or cardiac tamponade: Pericardiocentesis, traditional or guided by real-time cardiac ultrasound or echocardiography.
  2. Massive pulmonary embolus: Thrombectomy, emergent thoracotomy, and cardiopulmonary bypass.

▶ TREATMENT AND DISPOSITION

CRYPTIC SHOCK: SUPPORT FOR EARLY RECOGNITION AND TREATMENT

Shock must be recognized before it can be treated. Fulminant or late forms of shock manifesting with hypotension are not difficult to identify. Diagnosing shock before physiologic deterioration is a far greater challenge. However, significant improvements in morbidity and mortality can be achieved with early recognition of biochemical or cryptic shock that manifests as physiologic deterioration on a microvascular level, prior to deterioration of global parameters such as blood pressure (Figure 46-7).

- Cryptic shock in severe sepsis and septic shock: The EGDT trial demonstrated an absolute mortality benefit of 16% when septic patients who were hypotensive after a fluid bolus OR and had a lactate ≥4 mmol/dL were treated under a protocol that normalized CVP, blood pressure, $ScvO_2$, and

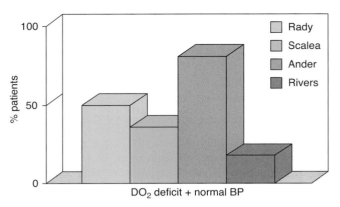

Rivers: *NEJM. 2001*	Severe sepsis or septic shock,	18%: MAP > 100; lactate > 4: mortality difference 40%
Ander: *Am J Cardiology. 1998*	Acute on chronic CHF: stratified by lactate	Normal MAP: 81% _lactate (5.6) _ScvO₂ (36%)
Rady: *AJEM. 1996*	ED: Resuscitation shock to MAP > 70	50% normal vitals • ScvO₂ < 65%; Lactate > 2
Scalea: *J Trauma. 1990*	Resuscitation ED trauma to "normal vital signs"	36%: ScvO₂ < 65% • _blood loss/Tx; Injury

Figure 46-7. Summary table of data supporting cryptic shock: abnormal biomarkers in the face of normal vital signs.

lactate. The authors then sought to evaluate what happened to patients who "looked good" with a normal blood pressure at presentation but had abnormal biomarkers. A subgroup analysis of EGDT trial showed that for patients who were normotensive (MAP >100 mm Hg) with abnormal biomarkers (lactates ≥4 mm Hg and ScvO₂ <70%) but for whom practitioners were able to achieve biomarker normalization within 6 hours, the mortality benefit was 40%.[48]

Authors who stratified infected ED patients by lactate found that an initially elevated lactate was associated with ICU admission from the ED, transfer to the ICU after admission to the floor, and increased in-hospital mortality.[49]

Another study evaluated infected patients presenting to the ED with lactate ≥4 mmol/dL. Twenty-nine percent of this population was normotensive, yet mortality, if lactate was not normalized within 6 hours, was 55%. For every 10% decrease in lactate, there was a corresponding 11% decrease in mortality.[33]

- Cryptic shock in congestive heart failure (CHF): In another study, patients with end-stage CHF with

an ejection fraction ≤30% presenting in decompensated CHF were stratified by lactate. They were then treated by protocol using ScvO₂ as a real-time guide to management instead of traditional use of vital signs alone. The treatment group was compared with a control group of clinic patients with known, stable, end-stage CHF (EF <30%) for 3 months. There was *no statistical difference in vital signs*, or Killip and New York Heart Association criteria, among the three groups.

The authors found that 50% of their patient population with normal vital signs (as designated by the control group) had evidence of ongoing biochemical shock with significantly lower presenting ScvO₂ and higher lactate. Both values significantly improved with protocol-directed treatment based on ScvO₂ and lactate rather than vital signs alone.[32,50]

- Cryptic shock in general shock patients: Rady and Rivers evaluated patients presenting to the ED in shock. After triage, the patients were resuscitated to an MAP >70 mm Hg and CVP ≥15 mm Hg. After achieving MAP and CVP goals, ScvO₂ and lactate were measured. They found 50% of patients with an MAP >70 mm Hg and SBP >100 mm Hg had an ScvO₂ <65% and a lactate >2. This level of anaerobic metabolism supported a continued process of biochemical shock in the face of traditionally "normal" blood pressure. Additional resuscitation led to a significant increase of ScvO₂ (52–65%; $P <$ .05) and decreased lactate (4.6–2.6; $P <$ .005) while MAP and SBP remained unchanged.[36]
- Cryptic shock in trauma patients—*The Golden Hour and Silver Day*[25]: Occult shock in trauma patients has been extensively studied. Scalea et al demonstrated that biochemical markers of hypoxia were present in trauma patients with "normal" vital signs. Thirty-nine percent of patients with normal vital signs had evidence of tissue hypoxia (ScvO₂ <65%, lactate >2.5 mmol/dL). The occult hypoxia group had more extensive injuries and greater blood loss, and required significantly more transfusions.[23]

Another study evaluated lactate clearance in critically injured trauma patients who had an elevated lactate, SBP greater than 100, pulse rate less than 120, and urine output greater than 1 mL/kg/h. Sixty-eight percent of patients had occult hypoperfusion (elevated lactate with normal blood pressure) during the first 24 hours. Of those with occult hypoperfusion, if the lactate was cleared within 24 hours, multisystem organ failure, respiratory compromise, and mortality were significantly reduced ($P <$ .05). The authors concluded that early identification and aggressive resuscitation based on biomarker normalization improved survival and reduced morbidity in the critically injured patient.[25] Other studies have since confirmed the concept of resuscitation to normalization of biomarkers in trauma patients.[51–60]

Primary Survey

As with all ED patients, especially those who present as critically ill or injured, the first step is assessing airway, breathing, and circulation. Simultaneously, large-bore IV access should be established, oxygen should be administered, and continuous vital sign monitoring and pulse oximetry are applied. With establishment of IV access, blood can be drawn and held for laboratory and point-of-care testing. Laboratory evaluation should be targeted to the type of shock suspected but should include lactic acid. (*Note:* Lactate is metabolized by the liver. A patient with liver insufficiency or failure may have an elevated lactate due to reduced clearance rather than oxygen debt. Furthermore, due to shunting, liver failure patients frequently demonstrate an elevated $ScvO_2$. Therefore, a high lactate and high $ScvO_2$ may not provide information about oxygen debt. However, a high lactate and low $ScvO_2$ may signify the presence of oxygen debt.)

- Airway: *If in doubt, secure the airway.* A patient in shock usually has multiple reasons for intubation and mechanical ventilation. Ventilatory failure should be recognized early through the clinical presentation. In shock, the decision to intubate is made by the clinician, not the lab. Thus, a blood gas is not required. The decision to intubate may fall into one of the following four categories:

  1. Respiratory failure: Respiratory muscle fatigue may manifest as inability to speak in complete sentences, labored breathing, either rapid or slow respiratory rate, diaphoresis, pale or cyanotic skin, paradoxical abdominal breathing, or the use of accessory muscles.
  2. Mental status change: If the patient is obtunded with a GCS <8, or is combative or uncooperative, intubation should be considered.
  3. Potential for decline or unsupervised location: If the patient is hypermetabolic or has potential to decline, early intubation is the best course of action. This includes the necessity to send the patient out of the department for diagnostic testing or for transfer to another unit or hospital. Additionally, if the physician is in a low-coverage, high-acuity situation in which other patients require significant time, this should be considered similar to an unsupervised or low supervision state, and the patient should be intubated.

  4. Significant oxygen debt, multisystem organ failure or insufficiency: The increased metabolic demand of failing respiratory muscles consumes a disproportionate component of "whole-body oxygen delivery." Thus, supporting ventilation assists in oxygen delivery to other high-need areas.[2]

- Breathing: During the primary survey, an assessment of breathing only involves auscultation. Adventitious breath sounds may suggest cardiogenic or obstructive shock, absent breath sounds in the face of shock may suggest a tension pneumothorax and therefore obstructive shock, and an area of decreased breath sounds may suggest a consolidation and therefore pneumonia in septic shock. For patients intubated during the primary survey, it is important to confirm endotracheal placement by ensuring that the endotracheal tube (ETT) was seen passing through the vocal cords, auscultation, appearance of condensation in the ETT, end-tidal CO_2 detection, maintenance of oxygen saturation with manual or ventilator-delivered breaths, and CXR. Other methods such as bronchoscopy, ultrasound, or esophageal detector devices may be used as well. Direct visualization, however, remains the "gold standard" for confirming tube placement.
- Circulation: Specific causes of shock may be suggested by findings such as muffled heart sounds and electrical alternans (pericardial tamponade), or murmurs (valve pathology, papillary muscle rupture). Furthermore, injuries such as flail chest or penetrating wounds may also suggest certain injuries or, more likely, the need for definitive treatment in an OR. Pulses in all extremities should be checked for quality and symmetry. Vital signs should be rechecked frequently.
- Neurologic exam, including neurologic assessments of the extremities as deficits, may indicate a neurogenic cause of the shock.
- Full-body exposure with special attention given to clues to the etiology of the shock.

With hypotensive patients, although early consideration should be given to administering a vasopressor, it is important to remember that for a vasopressor to be effective, there must be sufficient intravascular volume "to press." Fluid is the fundamental component for the initial therapy for shock. With appropriate volume resuscitation, the CI may improve by 25–40%,[61] and up to half of patients presenting with hypotension due to distributive shock may resolve with fluid replacement alone.[62] How much fluid and how fast it may be given are based on shock etiology and individual patient response. Cardiogenic shock due to an ischemic left ventricle will require smaller, frequent boluses such as 250 cm^3 every 30 minutes while monitoring for inotropic failure and treating with vasopressors or inotropic agents as needed. However, cardiogenic shock due to right ventricular failure will need significantly more fluid at a faster rate, though again dependent on patient response. Starting fluid resuscitation at 500 cm^3 every 30 minutes for hypovolemic or distributive shock is a reasonable starting point, but it should be increased or decreased based on patient conditions or response.

Optimally, adequate fluid resuscitation occurs prior to administering vasopressors or inotropes. In extreme cases, the physician may choose to administer vasopressors in conjunction with giving fluid and then titrating down the pressor dose as volume is replenished. Note that oxygen debt and end-organ perfusion can be worsened in underresuscitated patients receiving vasopressors.

Secondary Survey

Obtain history from any available source. If the patient is unable to give an adequate history, speak with the EMTs and any friends or family.

Do a complete physical exam.

Assess results from interventions done in the primary survey; decide on further interventions and formulate a differential diagnosis.

Airway: If the patient has been intubated and placed on mechanical ventilation, or even if the patient has been placed on noninvasive ventilation with a rate, consider the following:

- Tidal volume: Traditionally, tidal volumes of 15 cm^3/kg were used. Recent data support the use of 6 cm^3/kg in acute respiratory distress syndrome (ARDS).[63] Because many emergently intubated patients are at high risk for ARDS, this recommendation is a good starting point for all respiratory failure patients.
- Weaning: Since mechanical ventilation is not a therapy in and of itself but is, instead, a support therapy, consideration should be given to weaning, as soon as mechanical ventilation is initiated. An initial blood gas should be checked for pH and PCO_2, checking for carbon dioxide retention. Minute ventilation can then be titrated by adjusting the tidal volume, rate, and pressure support (for patients with spontaneous breaths). FiO_2 can be weaned by pulse oximetry. If the patient is unstable and in current oxygen debt, wean the oxygen as permitted keeping the SaO_2 100%. When oxygen debt has been resolved, wean as permitted keeping $SaO_2 \geq 93\%$. Goal FiO_2 is 30–40%.

- If intubated, consider an oral gastric tube for gastric decompression and a Foley catheter for bladder decompression pending urologic exam.

Circulation: If the patient remains hypotensive after appropriate fluid boluses:

- Fluid optimization: For patients who remain hypotensive despite sufficient IV fluid, there are additional considerations. First, it is important to consider how much fluid has been given. Certainly, for patients who have received <20 mL/kg, absent signs of fluid overload, it is prudent to continue administering IV fluid. However, at some point the question must be asked as to whether sufficient fluid has been administered or should vasopressors be initiated. If vasopressors have been started and the patient remains hypotensive, should they be increased, or a second agent added, or does the patient have an unmet fluid requirement? Volume status is very difficult to assess clinically in the critically ill patient and often is inaccurate. Currently the most clinically practical and dynamic bedside method of monitoring fluid requirement in the ED is through CVP. While central access is being obtained, crystalloid or colloid equivalent should continue to be administered peripherally as a 500-cm^3 bolus every 30 minutes, depending on patient dynamics, until a goal CVP of >8 mm Hg is achieved.[64] CVP measurements can be determined from femoral, IJ, or SC central lines. In the supine patient, a femoral line is almost as accurate as an IJ or SC central line, although this is not true if the head of the bed is placed at 30°. Furthermore, $ScvO_2$ measurements are also more accurate when taken from an IJ or SC central line since they include venous drainage from the head. However, $ScvO_2$ values can be obtained from a femoral central line. While not as accurate, the trend can be monitored and monitoring the trend can be as accurate as monitoring the trend of an IJ or SC central line. However obtained, the CVP and $ScvO_2$ values will be critically important in optimizing therapy if initial fluid boluses are not sufficient, and therefore an SC or IJ line is preferable when possible.
- MAP optimization: If a patient remains hypotensive (MAP <65 mm Hg) after receiving adequate volume resuscitation (CVP >8 mm Hg), a vasopressor should be added to titrate the MAP $\geq$65 mm Hg. The MAP may be measured via a standard arterial line in either a femoral or radial location. An arterial line is recommended in hypotensive patients, especially if vasopressors are required, as noninvasive BP monitoring in hypotensive or tachycardic patients may be less accurate.[39,64-68]

- After CVP and MAP have been optimized, $ScvO_2$ and serum lactate must be reassessed. If the values have normalized, treatment goals are complete. If they remain abnormal, oxygen debt and shock persist. To optimize DO_2, the components of oxygen delivery must be reevaluated:

$$DO_2 = CO \times (Hb \times SaO_2 \times 1.38)$$
$$CO = SV \times HR$$

If SaO_2, preload (CVP >8 mm Hg), and afterload (MAP >65) have been addressed, attention can be turned to Hg and CO. A repeat hematocrit (HCT) should be evaluated, as the pre-resuscitation analysis may be hemoconcentrated, and the administration of IV fluids may not yield a low HCT. If the HCT <30%, the patient should be transfused red blood cells until an HCT goal of ≥30% is achieved. If the goal CVP, MAP, and HCT have been achieved and the $ScvO_2$ remains <70%, an inotropic agent should be considered to enhance forward flow and tissue oxygenation. The physician may choose to evaluate myocardial function by direct observation such as with a pulmonary artery catheter or echocardiography if immediately available. However, if there is any significant delay, inotropes should be initiated empirically.

Due to the short half-life, dobutamine is the most readily available and most commonly used inotropic agent. It should be considered if the CVP, MAP, and HCT goals have been met and the $ScvO_2$ remains <70% despite resuscitation and vasopressor support. It is not advocated in tachycardic patients (HR >120).

At the end of the secondary survey, the patient should be reevaluated, checking all endpoint parameters and labs. This should be repeated as often as necessary.

DISPOSITION

As soon as a shock patient is identified, the ICU should be notified and admission or transfer should be initiated. However, due to stressed ICU resources, the critically ill or injured patient may reside in the ED longer than optimal or appropriate. The emergency physician should have a clear understanding of the care required, balanced with the resources available for optimal patient care and disposition.

REFERENCES

1. Brilli R. Critical care delivery in the intensive care unit: defining clinical roles and the best practice model. *Crit Care Med.* 2001;29:2007–2019.
2. Holmes CL, Walley KR. The evaluation and management of shock. *Clin Chest Med.* 2003;24(4):775–789.
3. Rivers E. The outcome of patients presenting to the emergency department with severe sepsis or septic shock. *Crit Care.* 2006;10(4):154.
4. Rivers EP, Nguyen HB. Goal-directed therapy for severe sepsis. Reply. *N Engl J Med.* 2002;346(13):1025–1026.
5. Shapiro NI, Trzeciak S, Hollander JE, et al. A prospective, multicenter derivation of a biomarker panel to assess risk of organ dysfunction, shock, and death in emergency department patients with suspected sepsis. *Crit Care Med.* 2009;37(1):96–104. 110.1097/CCM.1090b1013e318192fd318199d.
6. Safar P. Critical care medicine—quo vadis? *Crit Care Med.* 1974;2(1):1–5.
7. Huang DT, Osborn TM, Gunnerson KJ, et al. Critical care medicine training and certification for emergency physicians. *Ann Emerg Med.* 2005;46(3):217–223.
8. Johnson S. Personal communication regarding care of septic patients. In: *Conversation after a Cryptic Shock Presentation by Dr. Rivers edn.* 2003.
9. USGA Office. *Hospital Emergency Departments—Crowded Conditions Vary among Hospitals and Communities.* Report to the Ranking Minority Member, Committee on Finance, US Senate; 2003.
10. Lambe S, Washington DL, Fink A, et al. Trends in the use and capacity of California's emergency departments, 1990–1999. *Ann Emerg Med.* 2002;39(4):389–396.
11. McCaig LF, Burt CW. National Hospital Ambulatory Medical Care Survey: 2002 emergency department summary. *Adv Data.* 2004;(340):1–34.
12. McCaig LF, Ly N. National Hospital Ambulatory Medical Care Survey: 2000 emergency department summary. *Adv Data.* 2002;(326):1–31.
13. McCaig LF. National Hospital Ambulatory Medical Care Survey: 1998 emergency department summary. *Adv Data.* 2000;(313):1–23.
14. Dellinger RP. Cardiovascular management of septic shock. *Crit Care Med.* 2003;31(3):946–955.
15. Angus DC, Linde-Zwirble WT, Lidicker J, Clermont G, Carcillo J, Pinsky MR. Epidemiology of severe sepsis in the United States: analysis of incidence, outcome, and associated costs of care. *Crit Care Med.* 2001;29(7):1303–1310.
16. Osborn TM, Tracy JK, Dunne JR, Pasquale M, Napolitano LM. Epidemiology of sepsis in patients with traumatic injury. *Crit Care Med.* 2004;32(11):2234–2240.
17. Prasad A, Lennon RJ, Rihal CS, Berger PB, Holmes DR Jr. Outcomes of elderly patients with cardiogenic shock treated with early percutaneous revascularization. *Am Heart J.* 2004;147(6):1066–1070.
18. Parrillo JE. Approach to the patient with shock. In: Goldman L, Ausiello D, eds. *Cecil Medicine.* 23rd ed. Philadelphia, PA: Saunders Elsevier; 2007;107:742–749.
19. Rivers EP, Ander DS, Powell D. Central venous oxygen saturation monitoring in the critically ill patient. *Curr Opin Crit Care.* 2001;7(3):204–211.
20. Harvey S, Harrison DA, Singer M, et al. Assessment of the clinical effectiveness of pulmonary artery catheters in management of patients in intensive care (PAC-Man): a randomised controlled trial. *Lancet.* 2005;366(9484):472–477.

21. Rivers E, Nguyen B, Havstad S, et al. Early goal-directed therapy in the treatment of severe sepsis and septic shock. *N Engl J Med*. 2001;345(19):1368–1377.

22. Nguyen HB, Corbett SW, Steele R, et al. Implementation of a bundle of quality indicators for the early management of severe sepsis and septic shock is associated with decreased mortality [see comment]. *Crit Care Med*. 2007;35(4):1105–1112.

23. Scalea TM, Hartnett RW, Duncan AO, et al. Central venous oxygen saturation: a useful clinical tool in trauma patients. *J Trauma Inj Infect Crit Care*. 1990;30(12):1539–1543.

24. Scalea TM, Simon HM, Duncan AO, et al. Geriatric blunt multiple trauma: improved survival with early invasive monitoring. *J Trauma Inj Infect Crit Care*. 1990;30(2):129–134. Discussion 134–136.

25. Blow O, Magliore L, Claridge JA, Butler K, Young JS. The golden hour and the silver day: detection and correction of occult hypoperfusion within 24 hours improves outcome from major trauma. *J Trauma*. 1999;47(5):964–969.

26. Scalea TM, Maltz S, Yelon J, Trooskin SZ, Duncan AO, Sclafani SJ. Resuscitation of multiple trauma and head injury: role of crystalloid fluids and inotropes. *Crit Care Med*. 1994;22(10):1610–1615.

27. Abou-Khalil B, Scalea TM, Trooskin SZ, Henry SM, Hitchcock R. Hemodynamic responses to shock in young trauma patients: need for invasive monitoring. *Crit Care Med*. 1994;22(4):633–639.

28. Abramson D, Scalea TM, Hitchcock R, Trooskin SZ, Henry SM, Greenspan J. Lactate clearance and survival following injury. *J Trauma*. 1993;35(4):584–588. Discussion 588–589.

29. Rady MY, Edwards JD, Rivers EP, Alexander M. Measurement of oxygen consumption after uncomplicated acute myocardial infarction. *Chest*. 1993;104(3):930–934.

30. Rady M, Jafry S, Rivers E, Alexander M. Characterization of systemic oxygen transport in end-stage chronic congestive heart failure. *Am Heart J*. 1994;128(4):774–781.

31. Jaggi M, McGeorge FT, Charash DS, et al. Occult cardiogenic shock in end-stage heart failure patients presenting to the emergency department. *Clin Intensive Care*. 1995;6(2):104.

32. Ander DS, Jaggi M, Rivers E, et al. Undetected cardiogenic shock in patients with congestive heart failure presenting to the emergency department. *Am J Cardiol*. 1998;82(7):888–891. In process citation.

33. Nguyen HB, Rivers EP, Knoblich BP, et al. Early lactate clearance is associated with improved outcome in severe sepsis and septic shock. *Crit Care Med*. 2004;32(8):1637–1642.

34. Donnino MW, Nguyen HB, Jacobsen G, Tomlanovich M, Rivers EP. Cryptic septic shock: a sub-analysis of early goal-directed therapy. *Chest*. 2003;124:90S.

35. Donnino M, Nguyen B, Rivers EP. Severe sepsis and septic shock: a hemodynamic comparison of early and late phase sepsis. *Chest*. 2002;122:5S.

36. Rady MY, Rivers EP, Nowak RM. Resuscitation of the critically ill in the ED: responses of blood pressure, heart rate, shock index, central venous oxygen saturation, and lactate. *Am J Emerg Med*. 1996;14(2):218–225.

37. Knoblich BRE, Nguyen B, Rittinger W, et al. Lactic acid clearance (lactime) in the emergency department: implications for the development of multisystem organ failure and death. *Acad Emerg Med*. 1999;6(5):479.

38. Kline JA. Shock. In: Marx J, ed. *Rosen's Emergency Medicine: Concepts and Clinical Practice*. 5th ed. Philadelphia, PA Mosby; 2002.

39. Hollenberg SM, Ahrens TS, Annane D, et al. Practice parameters for hemodynamic support of sepsis in adult patients: 2004 update. *Crit Care Med*. 2004;32(9): 1928–1948.

40. Court O, Kumar A, Parrillo JE, Kumar A. Clinical review: myocardial depression in sepsis and septic shock. *Crit Care*. 2002;6(6):500–508.

41. Krishnagopalan S, Kumar A, Parrillo JE. Myocardial dysfunction in the patient with sepsis. *Curr Opin Crit Care*. 2002;8(5):376–388.

42. Jones AE, Tayal VS, Sullivan DM, Kline JA. Randomized, controlled trial of immediate versus delayed goal-directed ultrasound to identify the cause of nontraumatic hypotension in emergency department patients. *Crit Care Med*. 2004;32(8):1703–1708.

43. Brooks A, Davies B, Smethhurst M, Connolly J. Emergency ultrasound in the acute assessment of haemothorax. *Emerg Med J*. 2004;21(1):44–46.

44. Ong AW, McKenney MG, McKenney KA, et al. Predicting the need for laparotomy in pediatric trauma patients on the basis of the ultrasound score. *J Trauma*. 2003;54(3):503–508.

45. Blaivas M. Triage in the trauma bay with the focused abdominal sonography for trauma (FAST) examination. *J Emerg Med*. 2001;21(1):41–44.

46. Dulchavsky SA, Schwarz KL, Kirkpatrick AW, et al. Prospective evaluation of thoracic ultrasound in the detection of pneumothorax. *J Trauma*. 2001;50(2):201–205.

47. Tumbarello C. Ultrasound evaluation of abdominal trauma in the emergency department. *J Trauma Nurs*. 1998;5(3):67–72. Quiz 79–80.

48. Oxygen-dependent killing of bacteria by phagocytes [letter]. *N Engl J Med*. 1978;298(26):1478.

49. Ebarb J, Sculley K, Nguyen H, Sawyer RG, Barlotta K, Osborn TM. Lactate as a prognostic indicator in sepsis syndrome. *Intensive Care Med*. 2005;31(suppl 1):S48.

50. Rady M, Rivers EP, McGeorge F. Continuous central venous oximetry for the evaluation and treatment of acute cardiac failure in the emergency department. *Int J Int Care*. 1994;1:64–65.

51. Kincaid EH, Miller PR, Meredith JW, Rahman N, Chang MC. Elevated arterial base deficit in trauma patients: a marker of impaired oxygen utilization [see comments]. *J Am Coll Surg*. 1998;187(4):384–392.

52. Kremzar B, Spec-Marn A, Kompan L, Cerovic O. Normal values of SvO_2 as therapeutic goal in patients with multiple injuries. *Intensive Care Med*. 1997;23(1): 65–70.

53. Porter JM, Ivatury RR. In search of the optimal end points of resuscitation in trauma patients: a review. *J Trauma*. 1998;44(5):908–914.

54. Botha AJ, Moore FA, Moore EE, Peterson VM, Goode AW. Base deficit after major trauma directly relates to neutrophil CD11b expression: a proposed mechanism of shock-induced organ injury [see comments]. *Intensive Care Med*. 1997;23(5):504–509.

55. Davis JW. The relationship of base deficit to lactate in porcine hemorrhagic shock and resuscitation [see comments]. *J Trauma*. 1994;36(2):168–172.

56. DeAngeles DA, Scott AM, McGrath AM, et al. Resuscitation from hemorrhagic shock with diaspirin cross-linked hemoglobin, blood, or hetastarch. *J Trauma*. 1997;42(3):406–412. Discussion 412–414.

57. Landow L. The relationship between base deficit and lactate concentration in resuscitation [letter; comment]. *J Trauma*. 1994;37(5):869–870.

58. Leppaniemi A, Soltero R, Burris D, et al. Early resuscitation with low-volume PolyDCLHb is effective in the treatment of shock induced by penetrating vascular injury. *J Trauma*. 1996;40(2):242–248.

59. Marshall HP Jr, Capone A, Courcoulas AP, et al. Effects of hemodilution on long-term survival in an uncontrolled hemorrhagic shock model in rats. *J Trauma*. 1997;43(4):673–679.

60. Schultz SC, Hamilton IN Jr, Malcolm DS. Use of base deficit to compare resuscitation with lactated Ringer's solution, Haemaccel, whole blood, and diaspirin cross-linked hemoglobin following hemorrhage in rats. *J Trauma*. 1993;35(4):619–625. Discussion 625–626.

61. Packman MI, Rackow EC. Optimum left heart filling pressure during fluid resuscitation of patients with hypovolemic and septic shock. *Crit Care Med*. 1983;11(3):165–169.

62. Sugerman HJ, Diaco JF, Pollock TW, Miller LD. Physiologic management of septicemic shock in man. *Surg Forum*. 1971;22:3–5.

63. de Durante G, del Turco M, Rustichini L, et al. ARDS-Net lower tidal volume ventilatory strategy may generate intrinsic positive end-expiratory pressure in patients with acute respiratory distress syndrome. *Am J Respir Crit Care Med*. 2002;165(9):1271–1274.

64. Dellinger RP, Carlet JM, Masur H, et al. Surviving Sepsis Campaign guidelines for management of severe sepsis and septic shock. *Crit Care Med*. 2004;32(3):858–872.

65. Beale RJ, Hollenberg SM, Vincent JL, Parrillo JE. Vasopressor and inotropic support in septic shock: an evidence-based review. *Crit Care Med*. 2004;32(11 suppl):S455–S465.

66. Hynson JM, Katz JA, Mangano DT. On the accuracy of intra-arterial pressure measurement: the pressure gradient effect. *Crit Care Med*. 1998;26(10):1623–1624.

67. Hynson JM, Sessler DI, Moayeri A, Katz JA. Thermoregulatory and anesthetic-induced alterations in the differences among femoral, radial, and oscillometric blood pressures. *Anesthesiology*. 1994;81(6):1411–1421.

68. Hynson JM, Sessler DI, Moayeri A, McGuire J, Schroeder M. The effects of preinduction warming on temperature and blood pressure during propofol/nitrous oxide anesthesia. *Anesthesiology*. 1993;79(2):219–228. Discussion 221A–222A.

CHAPTER 47

Fluid Management

Alan C. Heffner and Matthew T. Robinson

▶ INTRODUCTION

Relative and absolute hypovolemia complicate many clinical conditions, and fluid therapy is a cornerstone of acute critical illness management. The clinician is constantly tasked with assessment of volume status, the need for fluid therapy, and selection of the appropriate fluid and dose guided to a suitable endpoint. Timely fluid therapy maintains macrocirculatory and microcirculatory support and reduces morbidity and mortality.[1-3] In contrast, both under-resuscitation and over-resuscitation adversely affect outcome; inadequate resuscitation risks leaving a patient in compensated shock, and overly aggressive fluid administration results in volume overload without improving oxygen delivery and is associated with worse clinical outcomes.[4,5] A thorough understanding of the appropriate selection, timing, and goals of fluid therapy is vital to optimize patient care.

▶ GENERAL PRINCIPLES

FLUID DISTRIBUTION AND MOVEMENT

Water is the most abundant constituent of the body, comprising between 50% and 70% of total body weight. Variations in total body water (TBW) depend primarily on lean body mass, since fat and other tissue contain very little water (Table 47-1). Water is distributed within both intracellular fluid (ICF) and extracellular fluid (ECF) compartments. The distribution of water in an average adult male is shown in Table 47-2. The intracellular space contains two thirds of the TBW, with the remainder distributed to the extracellular space, which is further divided into interstitial and intravascular spaces in a 3:1 ratio. These fluid compartments are not contiguous, but may be treated as such due to similar composition and behavior.

Water freely crosses cell membranes. Osmotic forces within fluid compartments determine water distribution within the body. Intracellular and ECF environments are iso-osmolar, but physiochemically distinct due to tight regulation of dissolved solutes and proteins. Membrane-bound sodium–potassium-ATPase pumps compartmentalize sodium and potassium to the extracellular and intracellular spaces, respectively. Active restriction of sodium to the extracellular space is the foundation for isotonic sodium-based resuscitation solutions.

▶ TABLE 47–1. **TOTAL BODY WATER ESTIMATES**

	TBW (%)
Adult	
Male	60
Female[a]	50
Elderly[a]	50
Obese[a]	50
Infant	70

Total body water (TBW) represents 50–60% of lean body weight in adults.
[a]Lower TBW proportional to skeletal muscle mass.

▶ **TABLE 47–2. SIZE AND COMPOSITION OF BODY FLUID COMPARTMENTS (VALUES BASED ON 70-KG MALE)**

Compartment	Body Weight (%)	Volume (L)	H_2O (L)	Na (mmol/L)	K (mmol/L)	Cl (mmol/L)	HCO_3 (mmol/L)
Total body	60	45	42				
ICF	40	30	28 (60%)	16	150		10
ECF	20	15	14 (40%)	140	4	103	26
Interstitial	16	12					
Plasma	4	3					
Blood	7	5					

The intravascular fluid, or plasma, differs from all other fluid compartments in that it exists as a single continuous fluid collection and contains trapped protein moieties in a higher concentration than the surrounding interstitial fluid. These trapped proteins produce the colloid oncotic pressure (COP) that favors fluid flow into the vascular space. Fluid flux across vascular endothelial membranes is governed by Starling forces (Table 47-3). In health, transcapillary hydrostatic force is nearly opposed by COP. Small net losses from the vascular space are returned to the systemic circulation via the lymphatic system. Albumin typically accounts for 80% of COP, while large cellular moieties such as red cells and platelets contribute less oncotic pressure effect. Positive hydrostatic pressure, hypoalbuminemia, and pathologic endothelial permeability are common clinical conditions that enhance fluid extravasation from the vascular compartment. The clinical consequences may be large and persistent resuscitation requirements with the cost of cumulative tissue (e.g., lung, brain, gut) edema that can adversely impact function. Alteration of COP and enhanced retention of intravascular volume is one theoretical advantage of colloid-based fluids.

EFFECTIVE CIRCULATING VOLUME

Effective circulating volume (ECV) refers to the portion of intravascular volume contributing to organ perfusion. It falls with hypovolemia but does not necessarily correlate with volume status, since organ perfusion is also dependent on cardiac output (CO), arterial tone, and circulatory distribution. As an example, ECV may be compromised by limited CO despite optimized volume status.

▶ **TABLE 47–3. STARLING'S LAW GOVERNING FLUID FLUX ACROSS VASCULAR ENDOTHELIUM**

$$V = K_f \left[(P_{capillary} - P_{interstitium}) - \sigma(COP_{capillary} - COP_{interstitium}) \right]$$

P, hydrostatic pressure; σ, reflection coefficient that reflects membrane permeability (value range 0–1). Inflammatory-mediated endothelial permeability reduces σ. COP, colloid oncotic pressure.

▶ PATHOPHYSIOLOGY

The immediate consequence of hypovolemia is impaired oxygen delivery, which triggers a swift compensatory response. CO is the most important determinant of oxygen delivery, with the flexibility to compensate for reduced oxygen-carrying capacity and/or increased metabolic demands. In the setting of hypovolemia, the body acts to defend itself through adjustments to maintain perfusion pressure and oxygen delivery (Table 47-4).

At the macrocirculatory level, volume loss leads to decreased venous return and decreased CO. Reduced stretch sensed by aortic and carotid baroreceptors leads to swift sympathetic catecholamine release, resulting in peripheral vasoconstriction, tachycardia, and enhanced cardiac contractility. These compensatory measures attempt to maintain CO in the face of a falling stroke volume. Venoconstriction shunts blood from capacitance vessels and maintains intrathoracic blood volume and cardiac preload. Organ blood flow is directly proportional to perfusion pressure in most vascular beds, and vasoconstriction maintains critical arterial pressure. Preferential perfusion simultaneously shunts limited CO to vital organs, at the expense of reduced blood flow to noncritical (hepatosplanchnic, renal, cutaneous) organs. As such, mean arterial pressure (MAP) is maintained despite hypovolemia and organ hypoperfusion.

▶ **TABLE 47–4. DETERMINANTS OF SYSTEMIC OXYGEN DELIVERY**

Oxygen Delivery **(DO_2)** = Cardiac Output **(CO)** × Oxygen carrying capacity **(CaO_2)**

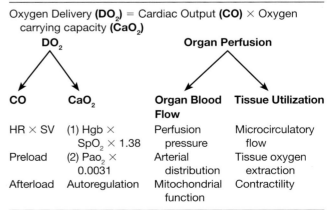

DO₂		**Organ Perfusion**	
CO	**CaO₂**	**Organ Blood Flow**	**Tissue Utilization**
HR × SV	(1) Hgb × SpO₂ × 1.38	Perfusion pressure	Microcirculatory flow
Preload	(2) Pao₂ × 0.0031	Arterial distribution	Tissue oxygen extraction
Afterload	Autoregulation	Mitochondrial function	Contractility

▶ CLINICAL PRESENTATION

SIGNS AND SYMPTOMS

Hypovolemia primarily manifests as circulatory insufficiency. Signs and symptoms reflect organ dysfunction and the counterregulatory response set in motion to offset the hypovolemic state. Classically, hypovolemia is portrayed to follow a stepwise progression of signs and symptoms based on the volume deficit. The clinical reality is that signs of hypovolemia are highly variable depending on the culprit disease, acuity of evolution, and individual physiologic reserve. Compared with hemorrhage, sepsis presents a complicated hypovolemic state in which absolute fluid deficits are compounded by pathologic vasodilation and accelerated end-organ dysfunction. Children and healthy adults with vigorous compensatory mechanisms may tolerate large volume loss in the absence of severe clinical symptoms. In contrast, patients with limited cardiac reserve may poorly tolerate even minimal fluid loss.

Delayed capillary refill, dry axilla and mucus membranes, abnormal skin turgor, and sunken eyes are classic, but imperfect, hallmarks of hypovolemia. Symptoms of reduced CO such as fatigue, dyspnea, postural dizziness, or near syncope are common but are neither specific nor sensitive. Nonfocal confusion, agitation, and lassitude are common manifestations of hypovolemia in elderly patients.[6] Organ dysfunction can be the heralding signal of hypovolemia and may occur in the absence of global hypoperfusion or hemodynamic instability. Oliguria, concentrated urine, and increased serum creatinine are examples. Electrolyte and acid–base derangements associated with hypovolemia may also produce a constellation of associated symptoms.

BLOOD PRESSURE

Shock defines a state of inadequate tissue perfusion in which tissue oxygen delivery is inadequate to meet metabolic needs. Contrary to popular belief, the term does not reflect perfusion pressure; shock may occur with low, normal, or elevated blood pressure. Inadequate perfusion in the setting of normal blood pressure is labeled *compensated shock*. Arterial pressure is intensely preserved via compensatory vasoconstriction, and normotension often masks clinical recognition of hypoperfusion and individual severity of illness. The difficulty in identifying these patients has spawned the terms *occult hypoperfusion* and *cryptic shock* to describe hemodynamically stable patients with microvascular insufficiency. Hyperlactatemia (>4 mmol/L) is an important clue to identify these patients.[7]

The majority of critically ill patients present in compensated shock with normal or near-normal blood pressures. Left unresuscitated, these patients may progress to frank hypotension. Brief episodes of hypotension are important markers of hypoperfusion and herald progressive hemodynamic deterioration.[8,9] These self-limited hypotensive episodes represent progressive exhaustion of cardiovascular compensation and are the first sign of uncompensated shock.

Uncompensated shock, characterized by hypotension, is a late finding, and develops when physiologic attempts to maintain normal perfusion pressure are overwhelmed or exhausted. As such, hypotension should always be considered pathologic. MAP of less than 65 mm Hg, systolic blood pressure less than 90 mm Hg, and/or MAP more than 20 mm Hg below baseline should raise concern. Normal blood pressure values do not reliably indicate adequate oxygen delivery, and hypotension is typically found in the late stage of shock.[10,11]

It is important to understand the limitations of blood pressure measurements in critically ill patients. Automated blood pressure cuffs rely on the oscillometric method of blood pressure determination and may overestimate true arterial blood pressure in low-flow states.[12,13] Direct auscultation with reliance on Korotkoff sounds may underestimate actual systolic blood pressure by as much as 30 mm Hg in low-flow states.[14] The potential for large measurement errors in hemodynamically unstable patients warrants consideration for invasive arterial pressure monitoring.

HEART RATE

Sinus tachycardia is nonspecific, but should prompt careful clinical consideration of volume depletion, hemorrhage, and sepsis. Heart rate typically increases in the early stages of hypovolemia to maintain CO in the face of falling stroke volume. However, heart rate response to acute volume loss is highly variable. In otherwise healthy patients, volume loss of up to 20% fails to induce a tachycardic response.[6] This compensatory response may be further blunted by comorbid disease and medications, especially β-blockers. Paradoxical and relative bradycardia occur in up to 30% of patients with traumatic and nontraumatic hemoperitoneum.[15,16]

ORTHOSTATIC BLOOD PRESSURE

The discriminative power of postural vital signs depends on appropriate testing and integration with specific clinical findings. Reassessment of supine resting blood pressure and pulse rate should be performed at least 2 minutes after standing, because all patients have a brief orthostatic response after standing. Postural pulse change greater than 30 beats/min is unusual in normovolemic patients.[6] Severe postural dizziness with intolerance of the upright position confirms hypovolemia, in contrast to subjective symptoms that do not limit standing. Postural hypotension, defined as a systolic blood pressure decline of greater than 20 mm Hg, is seen in 10–30% of normovolemic patients. The postural hemodynamic response may also be altered due to aging and medications. Up to 30% of elderly patients demonstrate an orthostatic response in the absence of volume depletion.[16]

SHOCK INDEX

The shock index (SI) is the ratio of the heart rate to systolic blood pressure. The normal range for SI is 0.5–0.7. SI >0.9 may aid identification of patients with critical illness despite seemingly normal vital signs.[17] SI identifies acute blood loss better than either HR or SBP alone.[18] Unfortunately, elevated SI is not specific for hypovolemia and may be less accurate in clinical conditions with fever-associated tachycardia.

► FLUID RESUSCITATION

Indications

Circulatory failure is the final common pathway of many diseases and carries a wide differential diagnosis (Table 47-5). Inadequate circulating volume is the most common primary etiology of shock. Immunologically mediated pathologic vasodilation compounds the fluid deficit in many clinical conditions. Acute cardiac decompensation and pulmonary embolus are two exceptional situations in which limited volume resuscitation and priority of mechanical and catecholamine resuscitation are recommended.

Volume depletion describes the state of contracted ECF with clinical implications of compromised ECV,

► **TABLE 47-5. DIFFERENTIAL DIAGNOSIS OF UNDIFFERENTIATED SHOCK AND/OR HYPOTENSION**

Hypovolemia
  Blood loss
  Fluid loss
    Gastrointestinal
    Renal
    Insensible
  Third space
Vasodilatory
  Sepsis
  Anaphylaxis
  Adrenal crisis
  Neurogenic shock
  Toxin/medication induced
Obstructive/central
  Cardiac dysfunction
  Cardiac tamponade
  Pulmonary embolus
  Tension pneumothorax

► **TABLE 47-6. ANATOMIC SITES OF NONHEMORRHAGIC VOLUME LOSS**

Gastrointestinal	Vomiting
	Diarrhea
	Drainage (e.g., ostomy, fistula, nasogastric, wound VAC)
Renal	Diuresis (e.g., medication, osmotic)
	Salt wasting
	Diabetes insipidus
Skin	Burn
	Wound
	Exfoliative rash
	Sweat
Third space sequestration	Intestinal obstruction
	Peritonitis
	Crush injury
	Pancreatitis
	Ascites
	Pleural effusion
	Capillary leak
Insensible loss	Respiration
	Fever

tissue perfusion, and function. It is distinguished from *dehydration*, which implies an intracellular water deficit characterized by plasma hypernatremia and hyperosmolarity. Hypovolemia may occur as a consequence of blood, electrolyte, and/or primary water loss (Table 47-6).

In any state of presumed or suspected volume depletion, rapid restoration of underlying fluid deficit is a first step to reverse hypoperfusion. Similarly, empirical volume therapy is a cornerstone of early resuscitative efforts in undifferentiated shock. Restoration of adequate oxygen delivery through fluid resuscitation initially relies on maximizing stroke volume. After the initial resuscitation and stabilization phase, ongoing fluid replacement can be more adequately tailored to specific clinical scenarios.

Intravenous Access

Appropriate intravenous access is vital to resuscitation. The determinants of flow through a rigid tube are shown in Table 47-7. The rate of volume infusion is determined by the dimension of the vascular catheter, and not by the size of the cannulated vein. Flow is directly proportional to the fourth power of the catheter

► **TABLE 47-7. DETERMINANTS OF FLOW THROUGH A RIGID TUBE**

Hagen–Poiseuille equation: $Q = (P_{in} - P_{out}) \times (\pi r4/8\mu L)$

Q, flow; $P_{in} - P_{out}$, pressure gradient; μ, viscosity; L, tube length; r, radius.

► TABLE 47-8. **INTRAVENOUS FLUID FLOW RATE THROUGH INTRAVENOUS AND CENTRAL VENOUS CATHETERS**

Size of Cannula	Length (mm)	Internal Diameter (mm)	Flow Rate (mL/min)
20 gauge IV	32	0.7	54
18 gauge IV	32	0.9	104
18 gauge IV	45	0.9	90
16 gauge IV	32	1.2	220
16 gauge IV	45	1.2	186
14 gauge IV	32	1.6	302
14 gauge IV	45	1.6	288
9 Fr Perc. sheath	100	2.5	838
3 mm IV tubing		3	1,030

► TABLE 47-9. **PRIORITIZED ENDPOINTS OF FLUID THERAPY**

1. Adequate intravenous access
2. Mean arterial pressure >65 mm Hg
3. Optimized oxygen delivery and organ perfusion
   a. Systemic markers
      • $ScvO_2$ >70%
      • Serum lactate clearance (>5%/h) and normalization
   b. Regional markers
      • Cutaneous temperature and perfusion
      • Urine output .0.5 mL/kg/h
      • Mental status

radius and inversely proportional to the catheter length. Therefore, doubling the catheter size results in a 16-fold increase in flow, whereas doubling the cannula length decreases flow by half.

Central venous catheters (CVCs) enable hemodynamic monitoring and provide a reliable portal for volume therapy, vasoactive drug infusion, and serial blood sampling. Due to the differential catheter lengths, infusion rates through adult CVCs are up to 75% less than with peripheral catheters of equal diameter. In some circumstances, massive volume infusion may require the use of large-bore introducer (8.5–9.5 French) catheters that support flow rates approaching that of intravenous tubing at almost 1 L/min[19] (Table 47-8). Additionally, manual compression of the fluid bag is an inefficient method of improving flow when compared with use of an external pressure bag.[20]

Endpoints of Resuscitation

Endpoints or markers of resuscitation are imperative to guide therapy during acute critical illness support (Table 47-9). Rapid restoration of perfusion pressure is a priority. Restoration of MAP to 60–65 mm Hg supports vital organ autoregulation.[21] However, normalization of traditional markers of blood pressure, heart rate, and urine output does not guarantee adequate oxygen delivery or organ perfusion.[1,10,11] Resuscitation aimed to these markers risks leaving the patient in persistent compensated shock.

Resuscitation aims to stabilize oxygen delivery to meet global and regional metabolic requirements. Central venous oxygen saturation ($ScvO_2$) and serum lactate have emerged as rapid, reliable global perfusion markers. $ScvO_2$ reflects the systemic balance of oxygen delivery and utilization. Decreasing oxygen delivery is compensated by increased tissue oxygen extraction, resulting in a fall in $ScvO_2$ below the normal 70%. $ScvO_2$ is a practical bedside measurement that is sampled from a catheter (CVC or PICC) positioned in the superior vena cava. $ScvO_2$ response is rapid and dynamic, such that monitoring provides immediate feedback on resuscitation efforts (or clinical deterioration).

Admission lactate and base deficit (BD) predict morbidity and mortality independent of hemodynamics.[7,22–24] These markers of illness severity are conversely useful as endpoints of resuscitation. Rapid lactate clearance is associated with improved outcome from critical illness and should be incorporated in the goals of resuscitation.[25–28] It is important to recognize that initial BD often correlates with serum lactate, but initial and serial measures may be confounded by underlying disease (e.g., renal insufficiency, malnutrition), resuscitation fluid (e.g., normal saline [NS]–induced acidosis), and other therapies (e.g., bicarbonate, blood products).

The optimal endpoint of resuscitation remains controversial. Novel markers such as tissue capnometry, oximetry, and near-infrared spectroscopy hold promise but their roles remain to be clarified. However, we cannot expect a single resuscitation endpoint to perform in all clinical circumstances. As such, a multimodal approach seeking to normalize a combination of both global and regional perfusion markers is most prudent (Table 47-9).

► THE EMPIRICAL VOLUME CHALLENGE

The empirical volume challenge remains the standard means of early fluid resuscitation. Volume expansion is achieved by infusing serial aliquots of isotonic fluid under direct observation and is appropriate in acute undifferentiated shock or when there is obvious or suspected hypovolemia. The use of crystalloid (10–20 mL/kg) or colloid (5–10 mL/kg) is infused quickly over 15–20 minutes, and serial boluses are titrated to the clinical endpoint objective while monitoring for adverse effects. A positive clinical response to volume loading confirms volume responsiveness but does not predict further response to therapy. This can contribute to overly aggressive volume expansion.

Total volume requirements are difficult to predict at the onset of resuscitation and are often underestimated. Classic hypovolemia that occurs with acute hemorrhage or fluid loss may stabilize rapidly with appropriate volume expansion. The 3:1 rule of hemorrhage resuscitation suggests that 3 volumetric unit of crystalloid are required to replete the ECF deficit of 1 unit of blood loss. However, experimental models confirm the experience in severely traumatized patients whose fluid requirements exceed the 3:1 suggestion.[29] Pathologic vasodilation and transcapillary leak contribute to the need for ongoing volume replacement. Crystalloid requirements average 40–60 mL/kg in the first hour of septic shock but may be as high as 200 mL/kg to normalize perfusion parameters.[30–32]

► VOLUME RESPONSIVENESS

The ability of fluid administration to improve stroke volume depends on a number of variables that include venous tone and ventricular function. Following initial resuscitation, the ability of fluid to further improve macrocirculatory flow is as low as 50%.[33,34] Volume or preload responsiveness refers to the ability to augment stroke volume with fluid administration. *In contrast to the empirical volume challenge, volume responsiveness is gauged prior to fluid administration with the information used to guide whether fluid administration is part of the solution to reverse clinical hypoperfusion.* Fluid loading in nonresponsive patients should be avoided because it delays appropriate therapy and contributes to volume overload and organ dysfunction, including hypoxemic respiratory failure and abdominal compartment syndrome.[4,5] Recent trials highlight the importance of fluid balance in organ function and morbidity.[2]

Predicting Volume Responsiveness

Invasive hemodynamic measurements are frequently used as surrogates of preload and predictors of volume responsiveness. Central venous pressure (CVP) monitoring is widely advocated. In the absence of conflicting data, a target CVP of 8–12 mm Hg is recommended to optimize preload prior to the institution of pressor and inotropic support.[1,31]

Unfortunately, cardiac pressure surrogates of preload (CVP and PAOP) reflect the net influences of intravascular volume, venous tone, cardiac function, and intrathoracic pressure. These myriad influences confound their ability to reflect intravascular volume status

or preload responsiveness of an individual patient.[33,34] There is no consistent threshold CVP to reliably estimate response to fluid administration.[35,36] Values that are considered low, normal, or high can be found in patients who respond positively to fluid. Obstructive lung disease, positive pressure ventilation, myocardial dysfunction, reflex venoconstriction, and erroneous measurements are several examples that can result in elevated CVP in a volume-responsive patient. CVP rise coupled to clinical improvement with volume loading corroborates fluid responsiveness, but does not anticipate further effect.

Volumetric measures of preload including stoke volume, right and global end-diastolic volume, and left ventricular end-diastolic area can be obtained with several monitoring techniques. These volumetric surrogates of preload are intuitively more desirable, but they too have limited predictive value because discriminatory thresholds are imprecise and infrequent in clinical practice.[33] Serial volumetric data in response to therapy may assist in individual patient management, but the dynamic nature of cardiovascular function during critical illness may confound data interpretation.

Dynamic Indices of Fluid Responsiveness

Fluid responsiveness is best predicted by dynamic indices of preload reserve. Respirophasic variation in stroke volume during positive pressure mechanical ventilation is among the most reliable signs of preload responsiveness.[33,34] Positive pressure ventilation induces cyclic alteration in preload. A resulting variation of systolic pressure, pulse pressure, and stroke volume greater than 13% identifies patients capable of augmenting stroke volume in response to fluid administration. A regular (preferably sinus) rhythm, positive pressure ventilation on >8 mL/kg tidal volume, and absence of significant patient interaction with the ventilator are important requirements for interpretation of these data.

Passive leg raising (PLR) is a provocative maneuver that tests whether a reversible volume challenge results in improved stroke volume.[37,38] This is an attractive option, since it provides immediate information to guide therapy without the administration of potentially unnecessary fluid. PLR results in the translocation of venous blood from the lower extremities to the thorax. The transient increase in preload improves stroke volume within minutes. Rapid feedback stroke volume measurement tools are required to identify the brief response to PLR. Sensitivity and specificity of PLR in predicting volume responsiveness is greater than 95% in a wide variety of patients, including ventilated and spontaneously breathing patients, and in those with irregular cardiac rhythms.[39]

▶ TABLE 47–10. **INTRAVENOUS FLUID COMPOSITION AND DISTRIBUTION**

| Solution | Electrolytes (mEq/L) | | | | | | | mOsm/L | pH | Distribution | |
	Na	K	Ca	Mg	Cl	HCO$_3$	Lactate			ECF	ICF
Crystalloid											
0.9% NaCl	154				154			308	5	100%	
Ringer's lactate	130	4	2.7		109		28	273	6.5		
150 mEq NaHCO$_3$ (three ampoules) in 1 L water	130					130		260			
3% NaCl	513				513			1,027	5		
7.5% NaCl								2,400			
0.45% NaCl	77				77			154	5	67%	33%
0.20% NaCl	34				34			77	5		
D$_5$W								278	4	33%	67%

▶ FLUID SELECTION

The goal of fluid resuscitation is intravascular expansion to optimize stroke volume. Early resuscitation and ongoing replacement of fluid deficits may be performed using a variety of fluid choices. Each possesses specific benefits and potential disadvantages in given clinical scenarios, and an understanding of fluid composition is important (Tables 47-10 and 47-11).

CRYSTALLOID

Isotonic sodium-based crystalloids preferentially distribute to the extracellular compartment, which includes the

▶ TABLE 47–11. **COMPOSITION OF COLLOID SOLUTIONS**

Solution	Na (mEq/L)	Cl (mEq/L)	K (mEq/L)	Ca (mEq/L)	Lactate (mEq/L)	Colloid	Average Molecular Weight (Da)	pH	mOsm/L	Oncotic Pressure (mm Hg)
5% albumin (plasbumin, buminate, albuminar)	130–160	130–160				Human albumin (50 g/L)	70,000	6.6	290	20
25% albumin (plasbumin, buminate, albuminar)	130–160	130–160				Human albumin (250 g/L)	70,000	6.6	310	100
Hetastarch										
Hespan®	154	154	4			HES (60 g/L)	600,000	5.9	310	30
Hextend®	143	124			28	HES (60 g/L)	670,000	5.9	307	30
Voluven®	154	154				HES (60 g/L)	130,000	4.0–5.5	308	36–37
Pentastarch										
Pentaspan	154	154				Pentastarch (100 g/L)	200,000– 300,000	5.0	326	32–36
HAES-steril® 6%	154	154				HES (60 g/L)	200,000	3.0–6.0	309	32–36
HAES-steril® 10%	154	154				HES (100 g/L)	200,000	3.0–6.0	309	25
Hexastarch										
EloHAES 6%	154	154				HES (60 g/L)	450,000	5.5	310	29–32
Dextrans										
Dextran 40®	154	154				Dextran (100 g/L)	40,000	6.7	320	68
Dextran 70®	154	154				Dextran (60 g/L)	70,000	6.3	320	70
Gelatins										
Gelofusine®	154	120	5.1	6.25		Succinylated gelatin (40 g/L)	30,000	7.4	274	30
Haemaccel®	145	145	5.1	6.25		Urea-linked gelatin (35 g/L)	35,000	7.3	325	30

vascular space. One-liter infusion of isotonic crystalloid distributes approximately one quarter into the vascular compartment. This is the basis for the 3:1 rule often cited for resuscitation in acute hemorrhagic shock. The ratio more closely approximates 7:1 or 10:1 in severe hemorrhage due to decreased COP secondary to hemorrhage, capillary leak, and crystalloid replacement. Interstitial tissue edema is the cost of such high-volume crystalloid requirement.

Fluid selection appears less important than volume dosage titrated to an appropriate therapeutic endpoint. NS (0.9%) and lactated Ringer's (LR) are the two most commonly used isotonic resuscitation solutions. Evidence of clinical superiority for either is lacking. However, the source of hypovolemia, associated electrolyte derangements, and volume requirements should impact fluid selection.

NS supplies a supraphysiologic sodium and chloride load that should be expected to induce hyperchloremic metabolic acidosis when administered in large volumes. This may be advantageous to correct volume and electrolyte disturbances in cases of metabolic alkalosis such as loss of gastric secretions (e.g., vomiting, gastric outlet obstruction, NG suctioning).

LR, or Hartmann's solution, was originally introduced in the 1930s by adding sodium lactate as a buffer to Ringer's solution for the treatment of metabolic acidosis. It is a more physiologic fluid, containing potassium and calcium in concentrations near plasma levels. Due to its more physiologic pH, it is preferred in large volume resuscitation. One caution is that calcium within the solution can bind to medications and the citrated blood anticoagulant, such that it is not a compatible transfusion fluid.

COLLOIDS

Colloid solutions are composed of electrolyte preparations fortified with large-molecular-weight molecules (MW >30,000). The presence of these large molecules contributes to total oncotic pressure, which favors retention of fluid within the vascular space. The ideal colloid solution has an oncotic pressure similar to plasma, which permits replacement of the plasma volume without distribution to other fluid compartments. The net effect and theoretical benefit of colloid infusion is intravascular expansion without accompanying expansion of the interstitial compartment. The potency of colloid solutions on plasma expansion differs with individual fluids. Higher COP provides greater expansion of the plasma volume. Albumin, dextran, and blood are naturally occurring colloids, while synthetic colloids include modified gelatins, hydroxyethyl starch (HES), and hemoglobin solutions. Albumin is the only colloid that contains molecules of uniform weight. Other colloid solutions are comprised of polymers with a wide variety of molecular sizes. However, the average molecular weight of a colloid solution is an unreliable indicator of intravascular persistence and molecular weight distribution curves provide the best indicator of intravascular effect.

ALBUMIN

Human albumin is a single polypeptide solution derived from pooled human serum albumin, and is available in 5% and 25% concentrations. Five percent albumin is iso-oncotic to plasma with greater than 70% of infused volume retained within the vascular space. It is recommended for resuscitation of patients with severe hypoalbuminemia and cirrhosis.[31,40,41] Hyperoncotic albumin (25% albumin) was initially developed in the 1940s for combat resuscitation. Infusions of hyperoncotic albumin result in vascular expansion greater than two times the administered volume.[42] Besides the obvious benefits of small volume resuscitation, improved portability, and more rapid hemodynamic stabilization, hyperoncotic albumin has additional advantages. Synergistic interaction with administered drugs and primary antioxidant effects are hypothesized explanations for the improved morbidity and mortality linked to hyperoncotic albumin for complicated hypoalbuminemic states including decompensated end-stage liver disease.[43,44] Increased COP mobilizes interstitial edema, and the effects of hyperoncotic albumin are relatively long-lasting, persisting for up to 12 hours after infusion. As such, hyperoncotic albumin is often matched with loop diuretic therapy to mobilize fluid in volume-overloaded patients.[45]

HYDROXYETHYL STARCH

HES solutions are semisynthetic polymers of nonuniform size derived from amylopectin. HES is typically available as a 6% isotonic solution. Intravascular persistence is maximized by substitution of hydroxyethyl groups, which limit degradation by amylase. Smaller polymers of less than 60 kDa are rapidly eliminated through glomerular filtration, while medium- and large-molecular-weight polymers are cleared by the reticuloendothelial system. High-molecular-weight HES reduce factor VIII and von Willebrand factor that may lead to coagulopathy. Medium- and small-molecular-weight polymers have less effect on coagulation. The overall effect of a 6% HES solution is volume expansion comparable to 5% albumin. Renal dysfunction and coagulopathy that complicated early generation synthetic colloids do not appear clinically significant with new-generation HES solutions.

GELATIN SOLUTIONS

Gelatin polypeptides are derived from bovine collagen. Urea-bridged gelatin is derived by cross-linking polypeptides derived from cattle bone, while succinylated gelatin is produced by thermal degradation of calf skin collagen. Approximately 80% of urea-bridged gelatin is smaller than 20 kDa and is therefore rapidly excreted by the kidneys, with a short intravascular persistence (2–3 hours). Gelatin solutions are generally considered to have no effect on clotting. Since gelatins are formed from degraded animal collagens, there is an inherent risk of anaphylaxis.

DEXTRANS

Dextran solutions are composed of polysaccharides of varying molecular weights. Currently available solutions are 6% dextran 70 and 10% dextran 40. Dextran 40 is hyperoncotic and therefore expands intravascular volume by more than the treatment infused. Solutions reduce blood viscosity and enhance fibrinolysis. The majority of dextran is excreted by the kidney, although dextran 40 has been associated with kidney injury, especially in the presence of preexisting renal dysfunction or hypovolemia.

COLLOID RESUSCITATION

There is no clear mortality impact of colloid resuscitation over crystalloid use across a broad range of critical illness.[46,47] However, strategic use may provide advantage in specific situations, as part of a mixed resuscitation or in attempt to avoid the risk associated with large volume crystalloid resuscitation. Vascular retention of colloids makes them efficient volume expanders. Although equally effective when titrated to the same clinical endpoints, crystalloid solutions require two to four times more volume for equivalent resuscitation.[48] Colloids therefore restore intravascular volume and tissue perfusion more rapidly if access and administration rate are limited. Furthermore, dilutional hypoalbuminemia, transcapillary fluid shift, and interstitial and pulmonary edema are limited. Albumin improves organ function and morbidity and is superior to crystalloids for intravascular volume expansion during hemodialysis, following large-volume paracentesis and in combination with antibiotic therapy for spontaneous bacterial peritonitis.[41,44,49,50] Traumatic brain injury remains one important exception in which isotonic albumin is associated with increased risk of adverse outcome compared with crystalloid resuscitation.[46,51]

HYPERTONIC SALINE

Hypertonic sodium (HS) solutions, with sodium concentrations ranging from 3% to 7.5%, rapidly expand intravascular volume by mobilizing water from interstitial and intracellular spaces. Small infusions expand plasma by several times the infused volume without resultant expansion of the interstitial fluid space and edema seen with crystalloid infusions.[52] Additional benefits include

improved cardiovascular performance secondary to positive inotropic effects and microvascular vasodilation, improved microcirculatory flow, and attenuation of the inflammatory response. This combination of effects is attractive for use in volume expansion in trauma and septic patients alike. Used alone, however, the hemodynamic effects of hypertonic crystalloid are transient. HS is generally used in combination with hyperoncotic colloid (6% dextran or 10% hetastarch). HS is safe, but there are insufficient data to conclude that hypertonic saline is better than isotonic crystalloid for the resuscitation of patients with burns, trauma, or sepsis. Multitrauma patients with traumatic brain injury remain the most common indication for HS, but outcome benefit also remains equivocal in this group.[53,54]

▶ SPECIAL CIRCUMSTANCES

MINIMAL VOLUME RESUSCITATION OF HEMORRHAGIC SHOCK

Hemorrhagic shock poses a unique challenge between balancing the timing and type of resuscitation in relation to the achievement of hemostasis. On one hand, hypotensive patients should be stabilized with rapid fluid infusion to maintain perfusion to essential organs. However, overly aggressive fluid resuscitation before control of bleeding may result in increased blood loss and mortality.[55] Factors that prevent hemostatic plug formation and allow renewed bleeding such as increased volume and blood pressure, decreased blood viscosity, and dilution of clotting factors are all associated with fluid resuscitation.

Strategic, limited volume resuscitation reemerged in the 1980s as the value of early prehospital resuscitation in penetrating trauma was questioned. A prospective trial comparing immediate and delayed fluid resuscitation in hypotensive patients with penetrating torso injuries showed improved mortality, fewer complications, and a shorter hospital length of stay with delayed resuscitation.[56,57] Limited prehospital resuscitation with judicious use of fluids may offer the optimal approach with conventional resuscitation ensuing after surgical hemostasis is achieved.[58] The degree and duration of permissive hypotension remains unclear, although current recommendations target SBP of 70 mm Hg. Patients with concomitant brain injury are not candidates for this strategy (Table 47-12).

BURN RESUSCITATION

Patients with second- and third-degree burns exhibit marked fluid shifts related to denuded skin, injured tissue, and systemic inflammatory response. Aggressive fluid resuscitation is necessary to restore intravascular volume and maintain end-organ perfusion. Early anticipation of

▶ **TABLE 47-12. SOURCES OF LIFE-THREATENING HEMORRHAGE TO CONSIDER A STRATEGY OF LIMITED VOLUME RESUSCITATION PENDING SURGICAL BLEEDING CONTROL**

Penetrating torso trauma
Ruptured abdominal aortic aneurysm
Major hemothorax
Major hemoperitoneum
Traumatic aortic injury
Severe pelvic fracture
Gastrointestinal bleeding
Ectopic pregnancy
Postpartum hemorrhage

▶ **TABLE 47-13. PARKLAND BURN RESUSCITATION FORMULA TO GUIDE ACUTE FLUID THERAPY**

Parkland formula:
24-Hour fluid requirement = 4 mL × weight (kg) × body surface area burn (%)
1/2 fluid calculation administered over the first 8 h from injury
Second 1/2 fluid calculation administered over the subsequent 16 h
Maintenance fluid calculations should be added to burn resuscitation estimates
Burn formulas estimate fluid requirements over the initial 24 h of burn therapy
Volume requirements may substantially exceed formula approximation

these large fluid requirements prevents underresuscitation. Initial fluid requirements are most commonly calculated according to the Parkland formula (Table 47-13).

Formula calculations are based on the time of injury as opposed to the time to medical attention, and should incorporate prehospital fluid administration. LR is the preferred crystalloid solution. Several formulas exist but no single method is clearly superior.[59] All formulas are intended to provide an initial *guide* for resuscitation requirements. Actual fluid needs may vary significantly, necessitating modifications based on individual status.[60] Strict adherence to a calculated goal may result in overresuscitation or underresuscitation. Overresuscitation is common and contributes to increased pulmonary complications and morbidity. Maintenance fluid requirements should be allocated in addition to burn formula replacement. Urine output greater than 1 mL/kg/h is a traditional endpoint of acute burn resuscitation and may be augmented by perfusion endpoints discussed above.

▶ MAINTENANCE FLUID THERAPY

In contrast to resuscitation therapy, the goal of maintenance fluid therapy is normal body fluid composition and volume. Fluid orders anticipate daily fluid requirement, ongoing losses, and coexisting electrolyte abnormalities. Although often ordered concurrently, daily physiologic fluid estimate (true maintenance) should be consciously distinguished from therapy aimed to slowly replace an existing fluid deficit.

Routine water and electrolyte maintenance are based on normal energy expenditure, sensible loss from urine and stool, and insensible loss from the respiratory tract and skin. Calculations assume euvolemia and are adjusted for body mass (Table 47-14). Greater per kilogram fluid requirements in children are proportionate to TBW and metabolism. All maintenance prescriptions should be individualized; energy expenditure, fluid losses, and electrolyte status vary with disease and dictate rate and electrolyte modifications. For example,

exfoliative skin disease, increased work of breathing, and fever enhance insensible loss. Measurable nasogastric, fistula, ostomy, and urinary drainage can be estimated or replaced by drainage volume. Limitation of fluid and potassium is an important disease-specific modification for patients with renal insufficiency.

Hypotonic solutions with or without dextrose and potassium are popular fixed-combination maintenance solutions. Hospitalized patients often suffer impaired free water excretion due to nonosmotic antidiuretic hormone (ADH) release, making them vulnerable to hyponatremia. Serum sodium concentration provides a simple and accurate marker of hydration status. Isotonic maintenance solutions should be considered in patients (including children), especially those with serum sodium <138 mEq/L.[61-63] Glucose infusions are best formulated by adding dextrose to an electrolyte solution (e.g., LR, NS, 0.45 NS) rather than using 5% dextrose (D_5W), which behaves as electrolyte free water on sugar metabolism.

▶ **TABLE 47-14. MAINTENANCE FLUID ESTIMATE**

Body Weight (kg)	Daily Maintenance (mL/day)	Hourly Maintenance (mL/h)
1–10	100 mL/kg	5 mL/kg/h
10–20	1,000 mL plus 50 mL/kg	40 mL/h plus 2 mL/kg/h
20–80	1,500 mL plus 20 mL/kg[a]	60 mL/h plus 1 mL/kg/h[a]

Sodium and chloride: 2–3 mEq per 100 mL water. Potassium: 1–2 mEq per 100 mL water. D5 1/4 normal saline with 20 mEq KCl is a common maintenance solution for most euvolemic pediatric patients and provides 20% of daily calories at routine maintenance rate. Comorbid conditions and/or electrolyte abnormalities may require modification.
[a]To maximum 2,400 mL/day or 100 mL/h.

► KEY TEACHING POINTS

1. The critical window to reverse organ hypoperfusion is measured in hours, emphasizing the need for rapid recognition and correction of shock.
2. The majority of ED patients who require resuscitation present in compensated shock with normal blood pressure.
3. Early recognition of circulatory insufficiency must be coupled with timely resuscitation to impact patients.
4. Normalization of vital signs does not insure adequate systemic perfusion or completion of resuscitation.
5. The clinical endpoint used to guide dosage of fluid resuscitation is more important than the individual product (i.e., crystalloid vs. colloid) selection.
6. Overly aggressive fluid resuscitation and positive fluid balance negatively impact patient morbidity.
7. Dynamic markers of volume responsiveness are important guides for fluid therapy.

REFERENCES

1. Rivers E, Nguyen B, Havstad S, et al. Early goal-directed therapy in the treatment of severe sepsis and septic shock. *N Engl J Med.* 2001;345(19):1368–1377.
2. Murphy CV, Schramm GE, Doherty JA, et al. The importance of fluid management in acute lung injury secondary to septic shock. *Chest.* 2009;136(1):102–109.
3. Jones AE, Brown MD, Trzeciak S, et al. The effect of a quantitative resuscitation strategy on mortality in patients with sepsis: a meta-analysis. *Crit Care Med.* 2008;36(10):2734–2739.
4. Wiedemann HP, Wheeler AP, Bernard GR, et al. Comparison of two fluid-management strategies in acute lung injury. *N Engl J Med.* 2006;354(24):2564–2575.
5. Balogh Z, McKinley BA, Cocanour CS, et al. Supranormal trauma resuscitation causes more cases of abdominal compartment syndrome. *Arch Surg.* 2003;138(6):637–642.
6. McGee S, Abernethy WB III, Simel DL. The rational clinical examination. Is this patient hypovolemic? *JAMA.* 1999;281(11):1022–1029.
7. Howell MD, Donnino M, Clardy P, Talmor D, Shapiro NI. Occult hypoperfusion and mortality in patients with suspected infection. *Intensive Care Med.* 2007;33(11):1892–1899.
8. Jones AE, Aborn LS, Kline JA. Severity of emergency department hypotension predicts adverse hospital outcome. *Shock.* 2004;22(5):410–414.
9. Jones AE, Yiannibas V, Johnson C, Kline JA. Emergency department hypotension predicts sudden unexpected in-hospital mortality: a prospective cohort study. *Chest.* 2006;130(4):941–946.
10. Rady MY, Rivers EP, Nowak RM. Resuscitation of the critically ill in the ED: responses of blood pressure, heart rate, shock index, central venous oxygen saturation, and lactate. *Am J Emerg Med.* 1996;14(2):218–225.
11. Wo CC, Shoemaker WC, Appel PL, Bishop MH, Kram HB, Hardin E. Unreliability of blood pressure and heart rate to evaluate cardiac output in emergency resuscitation and critical illness. *Crit Care Med.* 1993;21(2):218–223.
12. Gravlee GP, Brockschmidt JK. Accuracy of four indirect methods of blood pressure measurement, with hemodynamic correlations. *J Clin Monit.* 1990;6(4):284–298.
13. Pytte M, Dybwik K, Sexton J, Straume B, Nielsen EW. Oscillometric brachial mean artery pressures are higher than intra-radial mean artery pressures in intensive care unit patients receiving norepinephrine. *Acta Anaesthesiol Scand.* 2006;50(6):718–721.
14. Cohn JN. Blood pressure measurement in shock. Mechanism of inaccuracy in ausculatory and palpatory methods. *JAMA.* 1967;199(13):118–122.
15. Demetriades D, Chan LS, Bhasin P, et al. Relative bradycardia in patients with traumatic hypotension. *J Trauma.* 1998;45(3):534–539.
16. Carlson JE. Assessment of orthostatic blood pressure: measurement technique and clinical applications. *South Med J.* 1999;92(2):167–173.
17. Rady MY, Smithline HA, Blake H, Nowak R, Rivers E. A comparison of the shock index and conventional vital signs to identify acute, critical illness in the emergency department. *Ann Emerg Med.* 1994;24(4):685–690.
18. Birkhahn RH, Gaeta TJ, Terry D, Bove JJ, Tloczkowski J. Shock index in diagnosing early acute hypovolemia. *Am J Emerg Med.* 2005;23(3):323–326.
19. Jayanthi NV, Dabke HV. The effect of IV cannula length on the rate of infusion. *Injury.* 2006;37(1):41–45.
20. Stoneham MD. An evaluation of methods of increasing the flow rate of i.v. fluid administration. *Br J Anaesth.* 1995;75(3):361–365.
21. LeDoux D, Astiz ME, Carpati CM, Rackow EC. Effects of perfusion pressure on tissue perfusion in septic shock. *Crit Care Med.* 2000;28(8):2729–2732.
22. Weil MH, Afifi AA. Experimental and clinical studies on lactate and pyruvate as indicators of the severity of acute circulatory failure (shock). *Circulation.* 1970;41(6):989–1001.
23. Husain FA, Martin MJ, Mullenix PS, Steele SR, Elliott DC. Serum lactate and base deficit as predictors of mortality and morbidity. *Am J Surg.* 2003;185(5):485–491.
24. Davis JW, Parks SN, Kaups KL, Gladen HE, O'Donnell-Nicol S. Admission base deficit predicts transfusion requirements and risk of complications. *J Trauma.* 1996;41(5):769–774.
25. Nguyen HB, Rivers EP, Knoblich BP, et al. Early lactate clearance is associated with improved outcome in severe sepsis and septic shock. *Crit Care Med.* 2004;32(8):1637–1642.
26. Donnino MW, Miller J, Goyal N, et al. Effective lactate clearance is associated with improved outcome in post-cardiac arrest patients. *Resuscitation.* 2007;75(2):229–234.
27. Jones AE, Shapiro NI, Trzeciak S, Arnold RC, Claremont HA, Kline JA. Lactate clearance vs central venous oxygen saturation as goals of early sepsis therapy: a randomized clinical trial. *JAMA.* 2010;303(8):739–746.
28. Jansen TC, van Bommel J, Schoonderbeek FJ, et al. Early lactate-guided therapy in intensive care unit patients: a multicenter, open-label, randomized controlled trial. *Am J Respir Crit Care Med.* 2010;182(6):752–761.
29. Moore FA, McKinley BA, Moore EE. The next generation in shock resuscitation. *Lancet.* 2004;363(9425):1988–1996.

30. Carcillo JA, Davis AL, Zaritsky A. Role of early fluid resuscitation in pediatric septic shock. *JAMA*. 1991;266(9):1242–1245.

31. Dellinger RP, Levy MM, Carlet JM, et al. Surviving Sepsis Campaign: international guidelines for management of severe sepsis and septic shock: 2008. *Crit Care Med*. 2008;36(1):296–327.

32. Brierley J, Carcillo JA, Choong K, et al. Clinical practice parameters for hemodynamic support of pediatric and neonatal septic shock: 2007 update from the American College of Critical Care Medicine. *Crit Care Med*. 2009;37(2):666–688.

33. Michard F, Teboul JL. Predicting fluid responsiveness in ICU patients: a critical analysis of the evidence. *Chest*. 2002;121(6):2000–2008.

34. Marik PE, Baram M, Vahid B. Does central venous pressure predict fluid responsiveness? A systematic review of the literature and the tale of seven mares. *Chest*. 2008;134(1):172–178.

35. Osman D, Ridel C, Ray P, et al. Cardiac filling pressures are not appropriate to predict hemodynamic response to volume challenge. *Crit Care Med*. 2007;35(1):64–68.

36. Kumar A, Anel R, Bunnell E, et al. Pulmonary artery occlusion pressure and central venous pressure fail to predict ventricular filling volume, cardiac performance, or the response to volume infusion in normal subjects. *Crit Care Med*. 2004;32(3):691–699.

37. Boulain T, Achard JM, Teboul JL, Richard C, Perrotin D, Ginies G. Changes in BP induced by passive leg raising predict response to fluid loading in critically ill patients. *Chest*. 2002;121(4):1245–1252.

38. Monnet X, Rienzo M, Osman D, et al. Passive leg raising predicts fluid responsiveness in the critically ill. *Crit Care Med*. 2006;34(5):1402–1407.

39. Coudray A, Romand JA, Treggiari M, Bendjelid K. Fluid responsiveness in spontaneously breathing patients: a review of indexes used in intensive care. *Crit Care Med*. 2005;33(12):2757–2762.

40. Hollenberg SM, Ahrens TS, Annane D, et al. Practice parameters for hemodynamic support of sepsis in adult patients: 2004 update. *Crit Care Med*. 2004;32(9):1928–1948.

41. Dubois MJ, Orellana-Jimenez C, Melot C, et al. Albumin administration improves organ function in critically ill hypoalbuminemic patients: a prospective, randomized, controlled, pilot study. *Crit Care Med*. 2006;34(10):2536–2540.

42. Lamke LO, Liljedahl SO. Plasma volume expansion after infusion of 5%, 20% and 25% albumin solutions in patients. *Resuscitation*. 1976;5(2):85–92.

43. Jacob M, Chappell D, Conzen P, Wilkes MM, Becker BF, Rehm M. Small-volume resuscitation with hyperoncotic albumin: a systematic review of randomized clinical trials. *Crit Care*. 2008;12(2):R34.

44. Sort P, Navasa M, Arroyo V, et al. Effect of intravenous albumin on renal impairment and mortality in patients with cirrhosis and spontaneous bacterial peritonitis. *N Engl J Med*. 1999;341(6):403–409.

45. Martin GS, Moss M, Wheeler AP, Mealer M, Morris JA, Bernard GR. A randomized, controlled trial of furosemide with or without albumin in hypoproteinemic patients with acute lung injury. *Crit Care Med*. 2005;33(8):1681–1687.

46. Finfer S, Bellomo R, Boyce N, French J, Myburgh J, Norton R. A comparison of albumin and saline for fluid resuscitation in the intensive care unit. *N Engl J Med*. 2004;350(22):2247–2256.

47. Alderson P, Schierhout G, Roberts I, Bunn F. Colloids versus crystalloids for fluid resuscitation in critically ill patients. *Cochrane Database Syst Rev*. 2000;(2):CD000567.

48. Trof RJ, Sukul SP, Twisk JW, Girbes AR, Groeneveld AB. Greater cardiac response of colloid than saline fluid loading in septic and non-septic critically ill patients with clinical hypovolaemia. *Intensive Care Med*. 2010;36(4):697–701.

49. Vincent JL, Navickis RJ, Wilkes MM. Morbidity in hospitalized patients receiving human albumin: a meta-analysis of randomized, controlled trials. *Crit Care Med*. 2004;32(10):2029–2038.

50. Runyon BA. Management of adult patients with ascites due to cirrhosis. *Hepatology*. 2004;39(3):841–856.

51. Myburgh J, Cooper DJ, Finfer S, et al. Saline or albumin for fluid resuscitation in patients with traumatic brain injury. *N Engl J Med*. 2007;357(9):874–884.

52. Bunn F, Roberts I, Tasker R, Akpa E. Hypertonic versus near isotonic crystalloid for fluid resuscitation in critically ill patients. *Cochrane Database Syst Rev*. 2004;(3):CD002045.

53. Bulger EM, May S, Brasel KJ, et al. Out-of-hospital hypertonic resuscitation following severe traumatic brain injury: a randomized controlled trial. *JAMA*. 2010;304(13):1455–1464.

54. Simma B, Burger R, Falk M, Sacher P, Fanconi S. A prospective, randomized, and controlled study of fluid management in children with severe head injury: lactated Ringer's solution versus hypertonic saline. *Crit Care Med*. 1998;26(7):1265–1270.

55. Solomonov E, Hirsh M, Yahiya A, Krausz MM. The effect of vigorous fluid resuscitation in uncontrolled hemorrhagic shock after massive splenic injury. *Crit Care Med*. 2000;28(3):749–754.

56. Bickell WH, Wall MJ Jr, Pepe PE, et al. Immediate versus delayed fluid resuscitation for hypotensive patients with penetrating torso injuries. *N Engl J Med*. 1994;331(17):1105–1109.

57. Dutton RP, Mackenzie CF, Scalea TM. Hypotensive resuscitation during active hemorrhage: impact on in-hospital mortality. *J Trauma*. 2002;52(6):1141–1146.

58. Stern SA. Low-volume fluid resuscitation for presumed hemorrhagic shock: helpful or harmful? *Curr Opin Crit Care*. 2001;7(6):422–430.

59. Ipaktchi K, Arbabi S. Advances in burn critical care. *Crit Care Med*. 2006;34(9 suppl):S239–S244.

60. Blumetti J, Hunt JL, Arnoldo BD, Parks JK, Purdue GF. The Parkland formula under fire: is the criticism justified? *J Burn Care Res*. 2008;29(1):180–186.

61. Moritz ML, Ayus JC. Water water everywhere: standardizing postoperative fluid therapy with 0.9% normal saline. *Anesth Analg*. 2010;110(2):293–295.

62. Choong K, Kho ME, Menon K, Bohn D. Hypotonic versus isotonic saline in hospitalised children: a systematic review. *Arch Dis Child*. 2006;91(10):828–835.

63. Hoorn EJ, Geary D, Robb M, Halperin ML, Bohn D. Acute hyponatremia related to intravenous fluid administration in hospitalized children: an observational study. *Pediatrics*. 2004;113(5):1279–1284.

CHAPTER 48

Nutritional Support in Critical Care

Colleen Casey

Nutrition support is a significant component of patient care for hospitalized patients, particularly in the critical care setting. Critical illness is often characterized by a hypermetabolic and systemic inflammatory response including increased infectious morbidity, increased length of hospital stay, multiorgan dysfunction, and finally increased mortality. Historically, nutrition has been a secondary or supportive part of the care for critically ill patients with the goals of preserving lean body mass, maintaining immune function, and averting metabolic complications of critical illness (blunting the catabolic effect of critical illness). Recently these goals have evolved to focus on applying nutrition as a therapy with current goals being to attenuate metabolic response to stress, prevent oxidative cellular injury, and favorably modulate immune response.[1,2] The importance of nutrition support as a therapy is becoming more readily apparent with advances in evidence-based medicine. However, there are many factors to consider when determining an appropriate comprehensive nutrition therapy plan for each critically ill patient.

Consulting a registered dietitian or nutrition support team for expert care is paramount to maximizing nutritional support and its associated benefits for the critically ill patient. Early involvement of these practitioners in patient care allows for management of aspects of nutrition support as large in scope as meeting macronutrient needs (the necessary calorie and protein provision for recovery) to the finest nuances of micronutrient, vitamin, and mineral provision. The nutrition support practitioner adjusts the nutrition support regimen throughout the changing and, at times, complex course of the critically ill patient. He or she tailors the frequency of intervention and reassessment to meet the needs of each individual patient as the patient progresses through critical illness.

▶ ASSESSMENT OF NUTRITION STATUS

Assessment of nutrition status involves several components:

- Subjective information
- Anthropometrics
- Physical exam
- Laboratory values
- Calculation of calorie and protein requirements

Subjective information can include, but is not limited to, diet and weight history, social history as it relates to nutrient intake, chronic diseases that may alter nutrient intake, absorption, and utilization, use of medications, etc. Physical assessment will include subjective global assessment of the patient.

Anthropometrics not only gives us a sense of one's weight in relation to height by determining ideal body weight (IBW) and body mass index (BMI), but also helps us begin to determine our patient's nutritional state by revealing if one is overweight, obese, or with baseline malnutrition (see Table 48-1). Determination of IBW and %IBW is important in the formulation of nutrition therapy goals as they are applied to many predictive equations commonly utilized in critical care to estimate patients' calorie and protein requirements.

The Hamwi method is a common and practical method of determining IBW[3]:

- Male: 106 lb for first 5 ft in height, plus 6 lb for each additional inch of height.
- Female: 100 lb for first 5 ft in height, plus 5 lb for each additional inch of height.

▶ TABLE 48-1. **MALNUTRITION CLASSIFICATION**

Malnutrition Classification	IBW Assessment (%)	BMI Assessment
Severe malnutrition	<69	<16
Moderate malnutrition	70–79	16–17
Mild malnutrition	80–90	17–18.5
Normal weight	91–110	18.5–24.9
Overweight	111–129	25–29.9
Obese	≥130	≥30
Class I obesity/mild obesity		30–34.9
Class II obesity/ moderate obesity		35–39.9
Class III obesity/severe obesity		≥40

Some additional factors to consider when determining IBW of critically ill patients include amputations (Figure 48-1) and history of spinal cord injury[4-7]:

- Paraplegia: IBW = metropolitan life insurance height and weight table value with 5–10% subtracted.
- Quadriplegia: IBW = metropolitan life insurance height and weight table value with 10–15% subtracted.

BMI is determined by the following formula: weight (kg)/(height)^2 (m^2).

LABORATORY VALUES

Laboratory assessment can help determine whether there is organ system dysfunction, overall fluid imbalance, and/or micronutrient or macronutrient deficiencies when utilized in conjunction with overall assessment of the critically ill patient. Some serum protein values commonly obtained in the critical care setting include the negative acute-phase reactants albumin and prealbumin, and positive acute-phase reactant C-reactive protein. In healthy individuals, visceral proteins albumin and prealbumin serve as markers of nutritional status. However, albumin and prealbumin are primarily synthesized in the liver during times of anabolism, thus becoming better markers of inflammation and severity of illness than of nutritional status in the critically ill.

Albumin is not an ideal marker of nutrition status in an acute care setting due to its relatively lengthy half-life of approximately 20 days.

Factors impacting albumin include:

Increased level:

- Dehydration

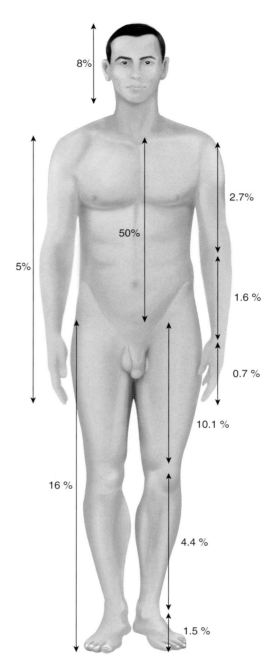

FIGURE 48-1. IBW adjustment for amputations. (Reprinted with permission from © American Dietetic Association. All rights reserved. License #ADAT4816.) (*ADA Times*, May/June 2008.)

Decreased level:

- Liver disease
- Protein-losing enteropathy/nephropathy
- Third spacing (ascites, anasarca, effusions, burns)
- Hemodilution
- Acute catabolic states (stress, trauma, infection, burns, surgery)
- Malignancy

Prealbumin is the preferred marker of nutrition status in an acute care setting due to its 2- to 3-day half-life. It can increase by as much as 4 mg/dL within 8 days with adequate nutrition support.[8]

Factors impacting prealbumin include:

Increased level:

- Renal failure
- Corticosteroid use
- Pregnancy
- Alcoholism (associated with acute alcohol abuse)

Decreased level:

- Liver disease (cirrhosis)
- Protein-losing enteropathy/nephropathy
- Nephrotic syndrome
- Hemorrhage
- Acute catabolic states (stress, trauma, infection, burns, surgery)
- Malignancy

C-reactive protein is elevated by inflammation. Thus, it is a useful tool to assess the overall status of a critically ill patient when prealbumin and/or albumin are not normalizing with the provision of presumably adequate nutrition support in the absence of any known stressors listed above. An elevated C-reactive protein value indicates that prealbumin and albumin continue to be markers of the inflammatory state of illness rather than nutritional status.

Nitrogen balance study can offer an alternative means of assessing protein needs when traditional serum protein markers (such as albumin and prealbumin) are not clinically relevant. It determines the amount of nitrogen necessary to maintain nitrogen equilibrium by assessing urinary losses in a 24-hour urine collection. Urinary urea nitrogen reflects muscle catabolism, hence lean body mass. However, in the critical care population, nitrogen balance is typically negative for up to 3 weeks postinsult or postinjury due to overall stress response.

Requirements for an accurate study include:

- Creatinine clearance >50 mL/min.
- 24-Hour urine collection for urine urea nitrogen (UUN).
- Measured creatinine clearance (from urine sample) may be obtained and compared with a calculated creatinine clearance to evaluate the validity of the urine sample and urea nitrogen result.

Factors impacting outcome include:

- Tendency to overestimate intake (i.e. if nutrition intake inaccurately recorded)
- Underestimating losses (i.e., unquantified gastrointestinal losses, or losses from chest tubes or wounds drains)

- Not considering specific amino acid source (l-arginine 5.1 g/protein to 1 g nitrogen)
- Renal insufficiency
- Inadequate urine collection
- Possible hematuria

Goals for nitrogen balance may include:

- Equilibrium −1 to +1
- Anabolism +2 to +4
- Decreased negative nitrogen balance (when anabolism not possible for critically ill patient):

Nitrogen balance = nitrogen intake − nitrogen losses

$$\text{Nitrogen balance} = \left[\frac{\text{protein (g per day)}}{6.25}\right] - [\text{UUN (g per day)} + 4^*]$$

The following assumptions should be applied to the above formula:

- $\text{UNN (g per day)} = \left[\frac{\text{UUN (mg/dL)}}{100}\right] \times \text{urine (L per day)}$
- Non-UUN = ~1–2 g
- Fecal nitrogen = ~1–2 g
- Miscellaneous losses from desquamation of skin, epithelial surfaces, sweat, etc. = ~1 g
- UUN >30 (g/24 hours) uses a factor of +6 insensible losses (patients with extraordinary losses)
- *Typical factor = +4 (*routine insensible losses*)

Using nitrogen balance study, one would increase protein delivery by 6.25 g for each gram of nitrogen under desired balance. However, clinical status may prevent protein increase to meet desired balance in patients with organ dysfunction or fluid restrictions.[9,10]

CALCULATION OF CALORIE AND PROTEIN REQUIREMENTS

Calculation of energy requirements most often involves the use of indirect calorimetry, predictive equations, or kilocalories per kilogram calculations. For purposes of this section, the terms calorie and kilocalorie are equivalent.

Indirect calorimetry is the "gold standard" for determining calorie requirements in the critically ill and is the standard against which predictive equations are compared. It is particularly useful in determining caloric needs in complex patient populations such as trauma, burns, obesity, sepsis, cancer, prolonged mechanical ventilation, amputations, patients with unreliable anthropometrics, COPD, major surgical procedure, acute pancreatitis, hypermetabolism/hypometabolism, paralysis/quadriplegia, and failure to respond to nutrition therapy.

Indirect calorimetry measures oxygen consumption (VO_2) and carbon dioxide production (VCO_2):

- Respiratory quotient (RQ) can be calculated by dividing VCO_2 by VO_2.
- Resting energy expenditure (REE) is calculated by the abbreviated Weir equation:

$$REE = 3.9(VO_2) \text{ [L per day]} + 1.1(VCO_2) \text{ [L per day]}$$

Factors impacting the accuracy of indirect calorimetry include:

- Inspired oxygen (FiO_2 >60%)
- Air leaks (endotracheal tube cuff, chest tube, bronchopulmonary fistula)
- Hemodialysis (HD) (loss of CO_2 via dialysis coil)
- Metabolic acidosis (increases VCO_2 and alters RQ)
- Disconnection from ventilator results in hypoxemia, bradycardia, or any other adverse effect
- Canopy inappropriate for patient (i.e., claustrophobia)
- Obtaining readings in a non–steady state (Table 48-2)

An RQ of 0.8–0.95 is indicative of a patient utilizing a mixed fuel or receiving an appropriate calorie provision for maintenance of current state. However, it is important to note that for malnourished critically ill or unstable patients, overall status may prevent increasing calorie provision for repletion. Maintenance may be the only feasible and desirable acute goal.[11–14]

For patients or institutions where indirect calorimetry is not feasible, practical, or available, predictive equations provide a widely utilized alternative. There are more than 200 predictive equations.[1,2] A recent systemic review summarized by Frankenfield et al evaluated seven commonly utilized equations with validation studies and the Fick method.[15] The review included some more commonly utilized equations: Harris–Benedict equation, Harris–Benedict equation (with injury and activity factors), Ireton–Jones equation (1992 version), Ireton-Jones equation (1997 version), Penn State equation (1998 version), Penn State equation (2003 version), and Swinamer equation. The accuracy of all predictive equations is affected by the individuals comprising the patient population to which they are applied, and no single equation can be applied to all critical care patients.

Perhaps the simplest of calculations to determine calorie goals is kilocalories per kilogram calculations. In guidelines jointly established by the Society for Critical Care Medicine (SCCM) and American Society for Parenteral and Enteral Nutrition (ASPEN) in 2009, this method was reviewed and the recommendation of providing 25–30 kcal/kg per day in enterally fed nonobese critically ill patients received a grade E recommendation.[1,2,16] In the critically ill obese patient, permissive underfeeding or hypocaloric enteral feeding was recommended with a goal of meeting 60–70% of calorie requirements. Recommendations were for 11–14 kcal/kg actual body weight or 22–25 kcal/kg IBW and ≥2.0 g/kg IBW of protein for Class I and Class II obesity (BMI 30–40). For Class III obesity (BMI >40), ≥2.5 g/kg IBW of protein was recommended. This recommendation received a grade D recommendation with the rationale or goal being to yield weight loss while maintaining nitrogen balance (Table 48-3).[1,2]

Protein is the most important macronutrient in the critical care setting for wound healing, maintaining lean body mass, and immune function. In nonobese patients (BMI <30), the recommendation to meet these goals is 1.2–2 g/kg protein per day with needs further escalating in significantly catabolic states such as burns and trauma. This recommendation received a grade E rating.[1,2]

▶ TABLE 48-3. GRADING SYSTEM USED FOR SCCM/ASPEN GUIDELINE

Grade of recommendation

A: supported by at least two Level I investigations
B: supported by one Level I investigation
C: supported by Level II investigations only
D: supported by at least two Level III investigations
E: supported by Level IV or V evidence

Level of evidence

I: large, randomized trials with clear-cut results; low risk of false-positive (α) error or false-negative (β) error
II: small, randomized trials with uncertain results; moderate to high risk of false-positive (α) and/or false-negative (β) error
III: nonrandomized, contemporaneous controls
IV: nonrandomized, historical controls
V: case series, uncontrolled studies, and expert opinion

Large studies warranting Level I evidence are defined as those with greater than or equal to 100 patients or those which fulfilled endpoint criteria determined by power analysis. Meta-analyses were used to organize information and draw conclusions about overall treatment effect from multiple studies on a particular subject. The grade of recommendation, however, was based on the level of evidence of the individual studies. Data from Ref.[16]

▶ TABLE 48-2. TRADITIONAL INTERPRETATION OF RESPIRATORY QUOTIENTS (RQ)

Substrate Utilization	RQ
Lipogenesis	1.0–1.2
Carbohydrate	0.9
Protein	0.82
Mixed substrate	0.85
Lipolysis	0.7
Ketosis	<0.7
Non–steady state hyperventilation	>1.0
Non–steady state hypoventilation	0.7
Alcohol	0.67
Starvation	0.65–0.67

► ROUTE OF NUTRITION SUPPORT

ENTERAL NUTRITION

Enteral nutrition (EN) is the preferred route of nutrition support over parenteral nutrition (PN). Few studies show an effect on mortality; however, the most commonly seen benefit is reduction in infectious morbidity (when comparing EN and PN). Additional benefits include reduced length of hospital stay, decreased cost of nutrition support,[1,2,17] and return of cognitive function in brain injury.[1,2,18]

EN should be initiated within 24–48 hours of admission and advanced toward goal in the following 48–72 hours (receiving grade C and E recommendations, respectively, in the SCCM/ASPEN guideline).[1,2] The rationale is that early initiation of enteral feedings is associated with decreased gut permeability and beneficial modulation of the body's immune and inflammatory responses to insult. It should also be noted that enteral feeding protocols increase percentage of goal calories delivered to the patient with a grade C recommendation for implementing these types of protocols. While trickle feeding may prevent intestinal atrophy, an overall goal of receiving >50–65% of calorie goal during the first week of hospitalization is warranted to achieve other ICU goals for nutrition support (maintaining lean body mass, etc.). The SCCM/ASPEN guideline gives the latter goal a grade C recommendation.[1,2]

EN should be deferred in the hemodynamically unstable patient until stabilization or resuscitation is achieved due to potential for subclinical intestinal ischemia/reperfusion injury, although less than 1% actually results in ischemic bowel. Consideration for gastric or small intestinal feeding with caution is appropriate in patients with stabilizing or tapering pressors in conjunction with ongoing GI and abdominal assessment.[1,2,19]

Both gastric and small bowel enteral feeding are appropriate in the ICU setting, with the exception of small bowel feeding being recommended for patients with known intolerance of gastric feedings or at high aspiration risk. Three meta-analyses found no difference in mortality when comparing gastric and postpyloric feeding in the ICU with only one of the meta-analyses showing a significantly lower rate of ventilator-associated pneumonia with postpyloric feeding. This difference was attributed to the inclusion of one study that was excluded from the remaining two meta-analyses.[1,2]

Real or perceived high gastric residuals may be an additional reason to pursue postpyloric feeding if the finding results in tube feeding being held. Holding EN for gastric residuals <500 mL is not warranted in the absence of additional GI symptoms of intolerance and may contribute to ileus resulting from cumulative NPO time. There is no correlation between gastric residual volume and incidence of aspiration, regurgitation, or overall gastric emptying.[1,2,20–24]

Elevating the head of the bed 30–45° in all intubated enterally fed patients and utilizing prokinetic agents or narcotic antagonists are additional measures that can be taken to reduce aspiration risk.[1,2,25,26] Erythromycin and metoclopramide have been shown to improve gastric outcome, but have little effect on overall patient outcomes. Naloxone was shown to decrease gastric residual volume, increase total EN received, and decrease incidence of ventilator-associated pneumonia in one study.[27]

Blue food coloring and glucose oxidase strips should not be used in the critical care setting to assess for aspiration. Blue dye is an insensitive marker and associated with mitochondrial toxicity and patient death in the critical care setting. The US Food and Drug Administration issued a mandate against the use of blue food coloring as a marker for aspiration of EN in September 2003. Glucose oxidase strips have poor sensitivity/specificity as they rely on the inaccurate notion that glucose in tracheal secretions is exclusively from aspirated EN.[1,2,28]

The presence of bowel sounds is not necessary for the initiation of enteral feeding. Bowel sounds are only indicative of contractility and do not relate to mucosal integrity, barrier function, or digestive/absorptive capacity. Perceived presence of bowel sounds is variable among care providers and can be unnoticed due to noise from patient care equipment and other individuals at the bedside. Evidence shows that 70–85% of ICU patients can reach and tolerate EN goals within 72 hours of admission when enteral feeding protocols are utilized (regardless of the presence of bowel sounds, flatus, or stool).[1,2]

In planning enteral formula selection, use of immunomodulating formulas should be considered in burns, trauma, head and neck cancer, major elective surgery, and critically ill mechanically ventilated patients with caution in severe sepsis. This earns a grade A and B recommendation in the SCCM/ASPEN guideline for surgical ICU and medical ICU patients, respectively.[1,2] Immunomodulating formulas are supplemented with a variety of combinations of omega-3 fatty acids, arginine, glutamine, antioxidants, and ribonucleotides. The overall outcomes on meta-analyses reveal decreased length of hospital stay, decreased duration of mechanical ventilation, and decreased infectious morbidity in the appropriate patient populations.[1,2,29,30] The initial hypothesis that arginine-enhanced formulations may increase patient risk by increasing nitric oxide production in severe sepsis is not widely supported. Arginine is now considered safe in mild to moderate sepsis with caution in severe sepsis.[1,2,31] Immunomodulating formulas are not recommended for indiscriminate use due to increased financial expense of these formulas and decreased effect on outcomes outside of the targeted patient groups above. The SCCM/ASPEN guideline also

▶ TABLE 48-4. **OSMOLALITY (mOsm/kg) OF SOME LIQUID MEDICATIONS**

Commercially Available Product	Average Osmolality
Acetaminophen elixir, 65 mg/mL	5,400
Acetaminophen/codeine elixir	4,700
Amantadine HCl solution, 10 mg/mL	3,900
Aminophylline liquid, 21 mg/mL	450
Amoxicillin suspension, 25 mg/mL	1,541
Amoxicillin suspension, 50 mg/mL	2,250
Ampicillin suspension, 50 mg/mL	2,250
Cephalexin suspension, 50 mg/mL	1,950
Cimetidine solution, 60 mg/dL	5,550
Co-trimoxazole suspension	2,200
Dexamethasone Intensol solution, 1 mg/mL	3,100
Digoxin elixir, 50 µg/mL	1,350
Diphenhydramine HCl elixir, 2.5 mg/mL	850
Diphenoxylate/atropine suspension	8,800
Docusate sodium syrup, 3.3 mg/mL	3,900
Erythromycin ethyl succinate suspension, 40 mg/mL	1,750
Ferrous sulfate liquid, 60 mg/mL	4,700
Furosemide solution, 10 mg/mL	2,050
Haloperidol concentrate, 2 mg/mL	500
Hydroxyzine HCl syrup, 2 mg/mL	4,450
Kaolin–pectin suspension	900
Lactulose syrup, 0.67 g/mL	3,600
Magnesium citrate solution	1,000
Milk of magnesia suspension	1,250
Multivitamin liquid	5,700
Nystatin suspension, 100,000 U/mL	3,300
Phenytoin sodium suspension, 25 mg/mL	1,500
Promethazine HCl syrup, 1.25 mg/mL	3,500
Sodium citrate liquid	2,050
Sodium phosphate liquid, 0.5 mg/mL	7,250
Theophylline solution, 5.33 mg/mL	700

gives a grade A recommendation for formulas with anti-inflammatory lipid profiles (omega-3 fish oils and borage oil) combined with antioxidants in acute respiratory distress syndrome (ARDS) and acute lung injury (ALI) due to significantly reduced length of ICU stay, duration of mechanical ventilation, organ failure, and mortality. At least 50–65% of goal calories should be received from immunomodulating formulas to achieve the above benefits.[1,2,32–34]

Enteral formulas containing soluble fiber or small peptide formulas should be considered in the presence of ongoing diarrhea when infectious causes (*C. difficile*) and hyperosmolar agents (medications) have been eliminated (Table 48-4).[1,2,35]

PARENTERAL NUTRITION

PN should only be considered for use when EN is not an option. When evaluating the ICU population as a whole, the SCCM/ASPEN guideline recommends no PN even if EN is not feasible or available in the first 7 days of admission (grade C). In the previously well-nourished patient population, PN is recommended only after the first 7 days without the option of EN (grade E). In patients with evidence of protein calorie malnutrition, PN should be initiated as soon as possible following admission and adequate resuscitation when EN is not an option. (Protein calorie malnutrition was typically defined as loss of at least 10–15% of recent usual weight, or being less than 90% of IBW [grade C].) The above recommendations regarding the ICU population as a whole and the well-nourished portion of the ICU are based on two major meta-analyses that found overall reduced infectious morbidity and complications when patients were left without nutrition support and a significant increase in mortality when PN was initiated within the first 7 days. Adverse clinical outcomes increase when patients remain greater than 7 days without nutrition support or PN. The same meta-analyses showed reversed findings for the protein calorie malnourished group in the first 7 days (increased complications and risk of mortality).

The SCCM/ASPEN guideline goes on to state a consensus that if a patient is to undergo major upper GI surgery and EN is not an option, then PN should be initiated under very specific circumstances:

- The malnourished patient should receive PN 5–7 days preoperatively and therapy should continue postoperatively.
- In well-nourished patients, PN should be delayed 5–7 days postoperatively.
- PN should not be initiated if total duration of therapy is anticipated to be less than 7 days.

Finally, the guideline recommends initiating supplemental PN when unable to meet 100% of targeted calorie goal after 7–10 days of EN alone (grade E) with the notation that initiating supplemental PN prior to 7–10 days does not improve outcome and may be harmful (grade C). This is based on the outcomes of the two meta-analyses discussed above.[1,2]

In terms of maximizing the benefit of PN for patients receiving this therapy, a few steps are recommended:

- Permissive underfeeding to 80% of calorie need until patient stabilizes (grade E).
- Omit soy-based lipids in the first week of ICU admission (grade D).
- Utilize a protocol for moderately strict control of serum glucose (grade B) with a potential goal range of 110–150 mg/dL (grade E).
- Utilize parenteral glutamine in critical care (grade C).
- In patients transitioning to EN, do not discontinue PN until ≥60% needs are met with EN (grade E).[1,2]

The rationale for permissive underfeeding above is to essentially avoid complications of overfeeding and insulin resistance. Avoidance of soy-based lipids would allow one to avoid the inflammatory effects of omega-6 lipids; however, it would require total avoidance of IV lipids in the United States as soy-based lipids are the only form available and meeting FDA approval. One should also consider whether the benefit of omitting IV lipid could be limited in patients receiving propofol for sedation (presently a 10% soy-based lipid solution). The current recommendation for moderate glucose control (110–150 mg/dL) is a liberalization of earlier recommendations and evidence showing improved outcomes with serum glucoses ranging 80–110 mg/dL in critical care in order to minimize mortality associated with incidence of hypoglycemia.[1,2,36] Parenteral glutamine has been shown to decrease infectious complications, length of ICU stay, and mortality in the critically ill. However, the dipeptide glutamine that this research is primarily based on is not commercially available in the United States or FDA approved. l-Glutamine is the only parenteral source in the United States, with limited availability, due to stability issues. The final point above pertaining to the transition from PN to EN as a primary nutrition therapy is in keeping with meeting the previously discussed goal of meeting at least 50–65% of caloric needs in the ICU.

ADJUNCTIVE THERAPY

Probiotics have been shown to improve outcome by decreasing infection in critically ill transplant, severe trauma, and major abdominal surgery patients. The SCCM/ASPEN guideline gives this a grade C recommendation due to the heterogeneity of the patient population and variability in probiotics utilized, but notes that the recommendation could be as high as a grade B in specific diagnoses.[1,2]

Antioxidant vitamins and minerals should be given to critically ill patients requiring specialized nutrition therapy (a combination of vitamins C and E, trace elements zinc, copper, and specifically selenium) particularly in burns, trauma, and mechanical ventilation. This is the result of a meta-analysis showing significant reduction in mortality when utilized and receives a grade B recommendation in the SCCM/ASPEN guideline.[1,2,37] Parenteral selenium was found to decrease mortality in sepsis and septic shock.[1,2,38,39]

Enteral glutamine supplementation is recommended in burns, trauma, and mixed ICU patients when not already provided in the EN formula. Enteral glutamine has been shown to decrease ICU and hospital length of stay in burn and mixed ICU patients and decrease mortality in burn patients. The SCCM/ASPEN guideline recommends 0.3–0.5 g/kg per day glutamine given in two to three divided doses per day (grade B).[1,2,40–42]

▶ GUIDELINES FOR SPECIFIC DISEASE STATES

The use of high-fat, low-carbohydrate formulas for the purpose of altering RQ and reducing CO_2 production in acute respiratory failure is not recommended. Presently, there is no consensus regarding route, source, and amount of fat to provide. Existing evidence shows that the fat to carbohydrate ratio may only be of significance in the setting of overfeeding.[1,2]

Standard ICU goals for calorie and protein should be utilized in the face of acute renal failure and standard enteral formulations utilized also. If there are significant electrolyte abnormalities, an electrolyte-restricted specialty formula designed for renal failure can be utilized. Acute renal failure rarely exists in an ICU setting as isolated organ failure and the overall diagnoses and status of the patient should be considered when assessing macronutrient needs. Diets containing <1 g/kg per day of protein have been shown to increase lean tissue loss in the ICU. Patients receiving HD or continuous renal replacement therapy (CRRT) may require up to 2.5 g/kg per day of protein to achieve positive nitrogen balance.[1,2,43]

Traditional markers of assessing nutrition status in critically ill patients with cirrhosis or liver failure should be utilized with caution. Complications of ascites, intravascular dryness, and overall liver synthesis of visceral proteins affect weight-based estimations of needs and laboratory values. Indirect calorimetry is ideal for determining energy needs. EN is the preferred route of nutrition in acute or chronic liver disease due to decreased rates of infection and metabolic complications as compared with PN. Protein restriction should be avoided and protein should be provided in amounts similar to the general ICU population. Specialty enteral formulas (containing branched-chain amino acids) should be reserved for encephalopthic patients unresponsive to luminal antibiotics and lactulose.[1,2,44]

Patients with severe acute pancreatitis (as defined by Atlanta Classification, Acute Physiology and Chronic Health Evaluation, or Ranson criteria) should have a nasoenteric feeding tube placed and EN initiated as soon as volume resuscitation is complete. Three meta-analyses reveal improved outcomes with early EN and reduction in the following when compared with PN: infectious morbidity, hospital length of stay, need for surgical intervention, multiple organ failure, and mortality.[1,2,45,46] Patients may be fed via gastric or postpyloric access.[1,2,47] The SCCM/ASPEN guideline gives the following recommendations to enhance tolerance of EN:

- Provide early EN to minimize the duration of ileus (grade D).
- Position EN infusion more distally in the GI tract (grade C).

- Change from intact EN formulation to small peptide and medium-chain triglyceride or nearly fat-free elemental formula (grade E).
- Switch from bolus to continuous infusion (grade C).[1,2]

The relative ease of achieving nasal gastric feeding access, as compared with postpyloric, can aid the delivery of early EN and improve the likelihood of EN tolerance. Although evidence does show overall tolerance of gastric feeding in severe acute pancreatitis, pancreatic exocrine stimulation is more likely with proximal feeds (as compared with feeding ≥40 cm below the ligament of Treitz that causes little to no stimulation). A small randomized trial demonstrated decreased bicarbonate, volume, and enzyme output production from the pancreas when jejunal bolus feedings were transitioned to continuous infusion, but it is unknown whether the same benefits would occur with gastric EN.

Lastly, patients with severe acute pancreatitis should be considered for PN therapy (grade C) only after the first 5 days of hospital admission when EN is not feasible (grade E). This is based on a study showing significant reductions in overall length of hospital stay, overall complications, and mortality when PN is delayed until 24–48 hours after full liquid resuscitation and the latter recommendation was based on the expert opinion of the panel.[1,2,48]

REFERENCES

1. McClave SA, Martindale RG, Vanek VW, et al. Guidelines for the provision and assessment of nutrition support therapy in the adult critically ill patient: Society of Critical Care Medicine (SCCM) and American Society for Parenteral and Enteral Nutrition (A.S.P.E.N.). *J Parenter Enteral Nutr.* 2009;33:277–316.
2. McClave SA, Martindale RG, Vanek VW, et al. Guidelines for the provision and assessment of nutrition support therapy in the adult critically ill patient: Society of Critical Care Medicine (SCCM) and American Society for Parenteral and Enteral Nutrition (A.S.P.E.N.). *Crit Care Med.* 2009;37:1–30.
3. Hamwi GJ. Changing dietary concepts. In: Danowski TS, ed. *Diabetes Mellitus: Diagnosis and Treatment.* Vol. 1. New York, NY: American Diabetes Association; 1964:73–78.
4. Kearns PJ, Thompson JD, Werner PC, et al. Nutritional and metabolic response to acute spinal cord injury. *J Parenter Enteral Nutr.* 1992;16:11–15.
5. Shigal HM, Roza A, Leduc B, et al. Body composition in quadriplegic patients. *J Parenter Enteral Nutr.* 1986;10:364–368.
6. Peiffer SC, Blust P, Leyson JF. Nutritional assessment of the spinal cord injured patient. *J Am Diet Assoc.* 1981;78:501–505.
7. Varella L, Jastremski CA. Neurological impairment. In: Gottschlich MM, ed. *The Science and Practice of Nutrition Support: A Case-Based Core Curriculum.* Dubuque, IA: Kendall/Hunt Publishing Company; 2001;421–444.
8. Beck FK, Rosenthal TC. Prealbumin: a marker for nutritional evaluation. *Am Fam Physician.* 2002;65:1575–1578.
9. Mandt Shopbell J, Hopkins B, Politzer Shronts E. Nutrition screening and assessment. In: Gottschlich MM, ed. *The Science and Practice of Nutrition Support: A Case-Based Core Curriculum.* Dubuque, IA: Kendall/Hunt Publishing Company; 2001:107–140.
10. Wooley JA, Frankenfield D. Energy. In: Gottschlich MM, ed. *The A.S.P.E.N. Nutrition Support Core Curriculum: A Case-Based Approach—The Adult Patient.* Silver Spring, MD: ASPEN; 2007:22.
11. McClave SA, Spain DA, Skolnick JL, et al. Achievement of steady state optimizes results when performing indirect calorimetry. *J Parenter Enteral Nutr.* 2003;27:16–20.
12. McClave SA, Lowen CC, Kleber MJ, et al. Clinical use of the respiratory quotient obtained from indirect calorimetry. *J Parenter Enteral Nutr.* 2003;27:21–26.
13. AARC clinical practice guideline: metabolic measurement using indirect calorimetry during mechanical ventilation. *Respir Care.* 1994;39:1170–1175.
14. Wooley JA, Sax HC. Indirect calorimetry: applications to practice. *Nutr Clin Pract.* 2003;18:434–439.
15. Frankenfield D, Hise M, Malone A, et al. Prediction of resting metabolic rate in critically ill adult patients: results of a systematic review of the evidence. *J Am Diet Assoc.* 2007;107:1552–1561.
16. Dellinger RP, Carlet JM, Masur H, et al. Surviving Sepsis Campaign Management Guidelines Committee: Surviving Sepsis Campaign guidelines for management of severe sepsis and septic shock. *Crit Care Med.* 2004;32:S445–S447.
17. Heyland DK, Dhaliwal R, Drover JW, et al. Canadian Critical Care Clinical Practice Guidelines Committee: Canadian clinical practice guidelines for nutrition support in mechanically ventilated, critically ill adult patients. *J Parenter Enteral Nutr.* 2003;27:355–373.
18. Taylor SJ, Fettes SB, Jewkes C, et al. Prospective, randomized, controlled trial to determine the effect of early enhanced enteral nutrition on clinical outcome in mechanically ventilated patients suffering head injury. *Crit Care Med.* 1999;27:2525–2531.
19. Zaloga GP, Roberts PR, Marik P. Feeding the hemodynamically unstable patient: a critical evaluation of the evidence. *Nutr Clin Pract.* 2003;18:285–293.
20. Burd RS, Lentz CW. The limitations of using gastric residual volumes to monitor enteral feedings: a mathematical model. *Nutr Clin Pract.* 2001;16:349–354.
21. McClave SA, Snider HL, Lowen CC, et al. Use of residual volume as a marker for enteral feeding intolerance: prospective blinded comparison with physical examination and radiographic findings. *J Parenter Enteral Nutr.* 1992;16:99–105.
22. Pinilla JC, Samphire J, Arnold C, et al. Comparison of gastrointestinal tolerance to two enteral feeding protocols in critically ill patients: a prospective, randomized controlled trial. *J Parenter Enteral Nutr.* 201;25:81–86.
23. Lin HC, Van Citters GW. Stopping enteral feeding for arbitrary gastric residual volume may not be

physiologically sound: results of a computer simulation model. *J Parenter Enteral Nutr.* 1997;21:286–289.

24. Montejo JC, Minabres E, Bordeje L, et al. Gastric residual volume during enteral nutrition in ICU patients: the REGANE study. *Intensive Care Med.* March 16, 2010;36:1386–1393. (published online ahead of print).

25. Ibanez J, Penafiel A, Raurich JM, et al. Gastroesophageal reflux in intubated patients receiving enteral nutrition: effect of supine and semirecumbent positions. *J Parenter Enteral Nutr.* 1992;16:419–422.

26. Torres A, Serra-Batlles J, Ros E, et al. Pulmonary aspiration of gastric contents in patients receiving mechanical ventilation: the effect of body position. *Ann Intern Med.* 1992;116:540–543.

27. Meissner W, Dohrn B, Reinhart K. Enteral naloxone reduces gastric tube reflux and frequency of pneumonia in critical care patients during opioid analgesia. *Crit Care Med.* 2003;31:776–780.

28. Maloney JP, Ryan TA. Detection of aspiration in enterally fed patients: a requiem for bedside monitors of aspiration. *J Parenter Enteral Nutr.* 2002;26:S34–S41.

29. Consensus recommendations from the U.S. summit on immune-enhancing enteral therapy. *J Parenter Enteral Nutr.* 2001;25:S61–S63.

30. Heyland DK, Novak F, Drover JW, et al. Should immunonutrition become routine in critically ill patients? A systematic review of the evidence. *JAMA.* 2001;286:944–953.

31. Caparros T, Lopez J, Grau T. Early enteral nutrition in critically ill patients with a high-protein diet enriched with arginine, fiber, and antioxidants compared with a standard high-protein diet. The effect on nosocomial infections and outcome. *J Parenter Enteral Nutr.* 2001;25:299–308.

32. Gadek JE, DeMichele SJ, Karlstad MD, et al. Effect of enteral feeding with eicosapentaenoic acid, gamma-linolenic acid, and antioxidants in patients with acute respiratory distress syndrome. *Crit Care Med.* 1999;27:1409–1420.

33. Singer P, Theilla M, Fisher H, et al. Benefit of an enteral diet enriched with eicosapentaenoic acid and gamma-linolenic acid in ventilated patients with acute lung injury. *Crit Care Med.* 2006;34:1033–1038.

34. Pontes-Arruda A, Aragao AM, Albuquerque JD. Effects of enteral feeding with eicosapentaenoic acid, gamma-linolenic acid, and antioxidants in mechanically ventilated patients with severe sepsis and septic shock. *Crit Care Med.* 2006;34:2325–2333.

35. Beckwith MC, Feddema SS, Barton RG, et al. A guide to drug therapy in patients with enteral feeding tubes: dosage form selection and administration methods. *Hosp Pharm.* 2004;39:225–237.

36. Van den Berghe G, Wouters P, Weekers F, et al. Intensive insulin therapy in the critically ill patients. *N Engl J Med.* 2006;354:449–461.

37. Heyland DK, Dhaliwal R, Suchner U, et al. Antioxidant nutrients: a systematic review of trace elements and vitamins in the critically ill patient. *Intensive Care Med.* 2005;31:327–337.

38. Crimi E, Liguori A, Condorelli M, et al. The beneficial effects of antioxidant supplementation in enteral feeding in critically ill patients: a prospective, randomized, double-blind, placebo-controlled trial. *Anesth Analg.* 2004;99:857–863.

39. Angstwurm MW, Engelmann L, Zimmermann T, et al. Selenium in intensive care (SIC): results of a prospective randomized, placebo-controlled, multiple-center study in patients with severe systematic inflammatory response syndrome, sepsis, and septic, shock. *Crit Care Med.* 2007;35:118–126.

40. Jones C, Palmer TE, Griffiths RD. Randomized clinical outcome study of critically ill patients given glutamine-supplemented enteral nutrition. *Nutrition.* 1999;15:108–115.

41. Houdijk AP, Rijnsburger ER, Jansen J, et al. Randomised trial of glutamine-enriched enteral nutrition on infectious morbidity in patients with multiple trauma. *Lancet.* 1998;352:772–776.

42. Garrel DR, Patenaude J, Nedelec B, et al. Decreased mortality and infectious morbidity in adult burn patients given enteral glutamine supplements: a prospective, controlled, randomized clinical trial. *Crit Care Med.* 2003;31:2444–2449.

43. Wooley JA, Btaiche IF, Good KL. Metabolic and nutritional aspects of acute renal failure in critically ill patients requiring continuous renal replacement therapy. *Nutr Clin Pract.* 2005;20:176–191.

44. Plauth M, Cabre E, Riggio O, et al. ESPEN guidelines on enteral nutrition: liver disease. *Clin Nutr.* 2006;25:285–294.

45. McClave SA, Chang WK, Dhaliwal R, et al. Nutrition support in acute pancreatitis: a systematic review of the literature. *J Parenter Enteral Nutr.* 2006;30:143–156.

46. Gupta R, Patel K, Calder PC, et al. A randomised clinical trial to assess the effect of total enteral and total parenteral nutritional support on metabolic, inflammatory and oxidative markers in patients with predicted severe acute pancreatitis (APACHE II > or = 6). *Pancreatology.* 2003;3:406–413.

47. Eatock FC, Chong P, Menezes N, et al. A randomized study of early nasogastric versus nasojejunal feeding in severe acute pancreatitis. *Am J Gastroenterol.* 2005;100:432–439.

48. Xian-Li H, Qing-Jui M, Kian-Guo L, et al. Effect of total parenteral nutrition (TPN) with and without glutamine dipeptide supplementation on outcome in severe acute pancreatitis (SAP). *Clin Nutr Suppl.* 2004;1:43–47.

CHAPTER 49

Percutaneous Tracheostomy for the Intensivist

Jonathan L. Marinaro, Rajeev P. Misra, and Dan Hale

▶ INTRODUCTION

Percutaneous dilatational tracheostomy (PDT) is one of the most commonly performed ICU procedures. For clinicians performing PDT, knowledge of the pertinent anatomy, the ideal population for PDT, techniques of the percutaneous method, potential complications, and postprocedural tracheostomy care are crucial to assure excellent patient care. As this book is directed to the EM intensivist, this chapter will focus on PDT for the nonsurgeon.

Within the specialty of critical care and the field of medicine as a whole, there is an ever-growing body of literature to support or refute treatment modalities, procedures, and management decisions. In the evaluation of any literature, knowing the limitations, evaluating the methodology, and understanding the difficulty of performing prospective studies must be taken into account before being too dogmatic about an approach to a clinical issue of procedural or managerial significance.

▶ ANATOMY AND ANATOMIC ISSUES FOR PATIENT SELECTION

The airway is divided into the upper and lower airways. The upper airway consists of the nasopharynx, oropharynx, and laryngopharynx. The lower airway begins at the vocal cords and consists of the larynx (which includes the cricoid cartilage [the only complete cartilaginous ring in the trachea] and cricoid membrane) and the elements of the tracheobronchial tree. The adult trachea is 12 cm in length and the external diameter of the trachea in the coronal plane is 2.3 cm.[1] The trachea has a series of 20 "U"-shaped cartilaginous rings; each tracheal ring is 4 mm wide and separated by a 2-mm membranous segment.[2] The female trachea is smaller in diameter and length. The general shape of the trachea is ovoid with posterior flattening; yet as one ages, the trachea becomes narrower and deeper (laterally narrower and deeper anterior–posteriorly). The trachea is approximately 18–32 mm deep from the skin, and the posterior wall of the trachea is 40–56 mm deep from skin.[3]

On bronchoscopic evaluation of the trachea, the cartilaginous rings are seen anteriorly and the longitudinal folds of dense elastic fibers are present posteriorly. Distally, the carina can be seen branching into the right and left main bronchi.

Paramount to performing PDT is the assessment of externally pertinent anatomy (Figures 49-1 and 49-2). Identifying the patient with a short neck, assessing the landmarks in the obese patient, and evaluating potential

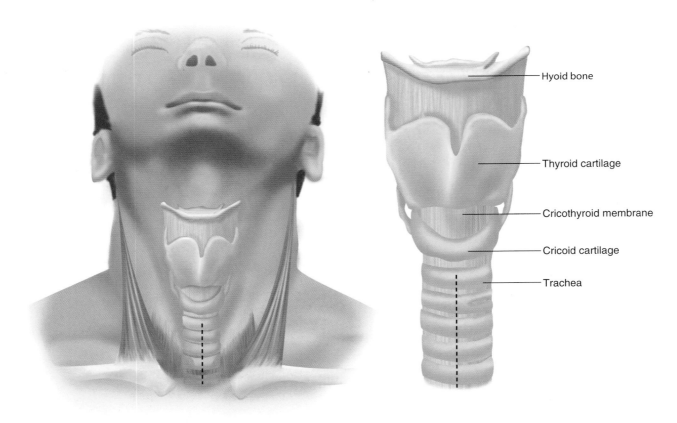

Figure 49-1. The skin incision is made in the midline, beginning below the cricoid cartilage and extending down toward the suprasternal notch. An incision made with these landmarks will lie over the second to fourth tracheal rings. (Reproduced with permission from Reichman EF, Simon RR. *Emergency Medicine Procedures.* New York, NY: McGraw-Hill Inc; 2004. Figure 15-9.)

vascular contraindications must be completed prior to deciding on PDT. In addition, issues of previous tracheal surgery and cervical spine injury are important anatomic considerations.

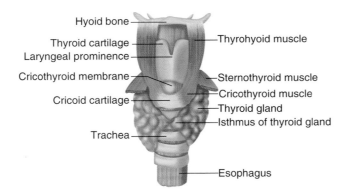

Figure 49-2. The framework of the airway in the neck. (Reproduced with permission from Reichman EF, Simon RR. *Emergency Medicine Procedures.* New York, NY: McGraw-Hill Inc; 2004. Figure 15-3.)

The short neck is defined as patients with less than 3 cm from the sternal notch to the thyroid apophysis (the vocal cords are located posterior to the thyroid apophyseal cartilage).[4] This shortened area between the vocal cords and sternal notch may make the procedure more complex with less area in which to work, and potentially increases the risk. Body mass index (BMI) and a resultant thick neck have been evaluated as a possible contraindication for PDT. Byhahn et al evaluated patients with BMI ≥27.5 kg/m² in 73 obese patients and had a 9.6% serious complication rate.[5] They found obese patients had a 2.7-fold increased risk for perioperative complications, and a 4.9-fold increased risk for serious complications. Contradicting the data of Byhahn et al, Heyrosa et al performed tracheostomy on 143 patients with BMI>35 (89 PDT and 53 Open Tracheostomy) and concluded PDT in obese patients was as safe as open tracheostomy at their institution. Both open tracheostomy and PDT had 6.5% complication rates.[6] Mansharamani et al also challenged the BMI dogma and evaluated PDT in obese patients.[7] The mean weight was 132 ± 40.8 kg (range 76.8–206 kg), and the mean BMI was 45.9 ± 12.4 kg/m² (range 28.1–61.8 kg/m²). Caution with these data is warranted. There were only

13 patients in this series; 3 required extra long 8-mm internal diameter tracheostomy tube and another required a 9-mm tube. Two patients had complications: cuff leak with need for tracheostomy replacement on day 2 and paratracheal insertion that was readily identified and corrected. Interestingly, no study has looked at neck size in particular, only the surrogate of BMI. Given the conflicting data, remembering that PDT is an elective procedure and should have equal or less morbidity than the open procedure is paramount. Therefore, if a patient has poorly identifiable anatomy, it may be wise to consider open tracheostomy.

Because bleeding is the most commonly reported complication in percutaneous tracheostomy, vascular abnormalities overlying the percutaneous route must be evaluated.[8] The assessment of this can be based on anatomic understanding of potential vasculature in the area, visual assessment of large pretracheal veins, and ultrasonographic evaluation.

Common sources of bleeding include the thyroid gland, aberrant anterior jugular veins, and unnamed venous vasculature. Visual assessment of large vessels overlying the insertion site should occur, but the addition of ultrasound to this assessment has been proposed and early literature supports ultrasound evaluation prior to incision. In a series of 72 PDT performed with preprocedural ultrasound, the puncture site was actually changed based on the ultrasound findings in 24% of the patients. None of the cases was complicated by bleeding or posterior tracheal injury.[9,10]

Additional anatomic considerations that must be considered are previous tracheostomy and cervical spine injury. Several small case series conclude that prior tracheostomy is not a contraindication to PDT.[11–13] Cervical spine injury is another potential anatomic contraindication to the procedure. In patients with cervical spine fracture, there are two separate risks. Initial risks are in the displacement of the fracture due to the force exerted and positioning for PDT. Mayberry et al performed PDT on patients with cleared and noncleared cervical spines.[14] Thirteen patients had cervical spine fractures, five had halo or operative stabilization, and seven were managed only with a collar prior to the procedure. Neck extension for the procedure was not utilized. There were no spinal cord injuries associated with PDT in this population, and, although not statistically significant, the complication rate was actually lower in noncleared group when compared with the cleared group. The group of seven with nonstabilized neck injuries had a 100% success rate. Ben Nun et al evaluated 38 patients with cervical spine fracture and, utilizing the modified Griggs procedure, had no PDT-related neurologic deterioration.[15] The second risk is in the postoperative patient who undergoes anterior cervical spine surgery. Without distinction of open tracheostomy versus PDT, Berney et al evaluated whether tracheostomy within 4 days of anterior cervical surgery increased infection rates.[16] Their data reported no increase in cross-contamination of wounds. O'Keeffe et al, in a smaller study with 6- to 10-day interval between surgical fixation and tracheostomy, found no cross-infection.[17] These small studies suggest the safety of performing tracheostomy in patients with cervical spine fractures and in patients within 7 days of anterior spinal fixation surgery. The authors would like to impress on the reader that, despite these data, the critical care clinician should consider which PDT procedure should be used and have a discussion with the spine service to identify the degree of instability.

► TRAUMATIC BRAIN INJURY (TBI)

TBI patients are a subset of critically ill patients who frequently require tracheostomy. These patients have a lower tolerance for hypoxia and hypercarbia, both of which can occur during bronchoscopy and PDT.[18–20] As hypoxia and hypercarbia may increase intracranial pressure (ICP), thereby decreasing cerebral perfusion pressure (CPP), there are concerns about PDT in TBI patients. Milanchi et al, using paralytics and the Ciaglia method, found no statistically significant change in CPP and ICP during PDT. One quarter of their patients had ICP readings greater than 20 during the 48-hour study period indicating that at least a portion of patients may have had some cerebral compliance issues that could have been exacerbated. The study of Milanchi et al ($n = 52$ had ICP monitoring) agreed with those of Borm and Gleixner ($n = 14$ had ICP monitoring), Escarment et al ($n = 35$ unclear how many had ICP monitoring), and Imperiale et al ($n = 65$ had ICP monitoring; "PercuTwist" method) but differed from that of Stocchetti et al ($n = 30$ with ICP monitoring; 10 PDT, 10 surgical tracheostomy, and 10 Fantoni method,) who had a statistically significant increase in ICP during all three techniques, yet the greatest frequency in ICP increases occurred in patients with PDT.[19,21–24]

Conclusions that can be reached from these papers are that tracheostomy and PDT in particular are acceptable in TBI patient without intracranial hypertension. If a patient has increased ICPs and there is a consensus that cerebral compliance is tenuous, waiting until a period of stability would seem a sensible plan. Outside of loss of airway, there is no emergent indication for tracheostomy, and allowing brain pressures to stabilize may incur less cerebral morbidity.

► ANTICOAGULATION CONSIDERATIONS

As mentioned previously, bleeding is the most frequent complication of PDT and therefore evaluation of coagulation studies and withholding anticoagulation would seem to be intrinsic to a successful, low-risk procedure. This too has been challenged. Beiderlinden et al in 2007 evaluated 415 patients.[25] A total of 137 patients had coagulation abnormalities. Fifty-eight patients had a platelet count less than 50,000/mm³, 75 had a PTT >50 seconds, and 19 patients had a PT >50% of normal values. Twenty-seven patients had two abnormal values. When the authors divided these patients into acute and chronic bleeding, they found no significant difference in coagulation variables between the acute bleeding group (defined as occurring during and immediately after the procedure) and the group without any acute bleeding complications. In evaluating chronic bleeding (defined as persisting for more than 24 hours after tube placement), Beiderlinden et al found that a PTT greater than 50 seconds predicted a 4-fold increase in chronic bleeding and platelet count <50,000/mm³ predicted a 5-fold increase in chronic bleeding. In patients with two or more coagulation variable abnormalities, there was a substantial increase in bleeding (OR = 9.5). In addition, 189 patients had prophylactic low-dose heparin and normal coagulation variables. There was no statistically significant increase in bleeding when compared with the group without heparinization and normal coagulation studies ($P = 0.55$). In the study of Beiderlinden et al, thrombocytopenia was the strongest single risk factor for chronic bleeding. In contrast, Kluge et al found that platelet counts less than 50,000/mm³ were safe.[26] The study of Kluge et al is confounded by the infusion of platelets just prior to the procedure; therefore, whether these patients truly had low platelets is unknown. In the study of Beiderlinden et al, the thrombocytopenic patients were not treated and as a result definitely had platelets less than 50,000/mm³.

As with many aspects of medicine, the proceduralist's training and past complications will flavor their threshold for proceeding in certain situations. Performing invasive procedures in coagulopathic or heparinized patients is one such situation. Although the study of Beiderlinden et al is well done and provides interesting data, the question that must be asked is whether missing a single dose of heparin or infusion of plasma or platelets to correct a marginal coagulopathy portends an increased risk of complications such as venous thromboembolism, transfusion reactions, or immunomodulation. Critical care lacks an actuarial chart, and, for that reason, until more prospective data are secured, these decisions will be very practitioner dependent.

▶ VENTILATORY CONSIDERATIONS

The decision to perform tracheostomy is rooted in improving pulmonary function. Since these patients, at best, have some degree of pulmonary dysfunction and may have high levels of ongoing oxygenation and

ventilation support, previous recommendations for performing tracheostomy suggested only performing the procedure in the setting of low FiO_2 and low positive end-expiratory pressure (PEEP). The PDT procedure inflicts periods of derecruitment (as does the open tracheostomy) and obstruction of the airway unique to PDT. Although in experienced hands these periods are brief, they are not without risk in the unstable patient. Patients who cannot tolerate hypercarbia, hypoxia, or brief loss of airway for cardiovascular reasons are better served by open procedure or delaying the procedure for a period of greater stability.

Excluding the periprocedural risks of performing tracheostomy on patients with respiratory failure, benefits of tracheostomy on the pulmonary function cannot be ignored. Tracheostomy tubes improve patient comfort and decrease sedative requirements. They can reduce dead space by up to 50% (150 mL) and the decreased length can ease work of breathing leading to facilitation of ventilator weaning.[27]

▶ INDICATIONS AND TIMING FOR TRACHEOSTOMY

As stated above, choosing to perform tracheostomy on an unstable patient may be fraught with risks but a tracheostomy can lessen ventilator days, reduce ventilator-acquired pneumonia incidence, shorten ICU stays, and prevent subglottic stenosis, all of which must be weighed in the risk/benefit analysis. To appropriately perform this analysis, the indications to perform tracheostomy need to be reviewed and the data surrounding the timing of tracheostomy must be evaluated.

Indications for tracheostomy in critical care are different than indications for anatomic considerations such as upper airway obstruction due to trauma, malignancy, vocal cord paralysis, or congenital abnormalities. Critical care indications do have crossover with anatomic reasons as many of our patients are from this latter population, but intensivists would not perform those tracheostomies. This section will focus on the benefits of tracheostomy in the avoidance of laryngeal injury from prolonged translaryngeal intubation and shortening the period until liberation from mechanical ventilation.

Prolonged intubation is one of the well-known indications for tracheostomy and is cited as an indication by the American Academy of Otolaryngology.[28] This recommendation is due to laryngeal injury rates as high as 94%[29] and chronic injury occurring in up to 19% of patients.[30] The long-term sequelae of intubation include stenosis, granulomas, and ulcerations causing chronic hoarseness and, rarely, upper airway obstruction due to stenosis. Tracheal stenosis occurs at the endotracheal tube cuff site in one third of the reported postintubation cases. Loss of regional blood flow from high cuff pressures on the tracheal wall creates the ischemic region that leads to scarring. This ischemic injury begins within the first few hours of intubation, and healing of the damaged region by secondary intention can result in densely fibrotic circumferential stenosis over a period of 3 weeks to 6 months. Large-volume, low-pressure cuffs have markedly reduced the occurrence of cuff injury. Tracheal capillary pressure is between 20 and 30 mm Hg, and perfusion impairment occurs at 22 mm Hg and is completely compromised at 37 mm Hg. The recommended cuff pressures are between 10 and 18 mm Hg (15–25 cm H_2O) at all times, and twice-daily evaluation of cuff pressures to limit the occurrence of this devastating sequelae of intubation must be assured.[31] Post-tracheostomy tracheal stenosis is also a well-described occurrence. Unlike stenosis secondary to intubation, this can occur due to abnormal wound healing with overgrowth of granulation tissue around the stoma site. It can also occur from granulation at the tip of the tracheotomy tube, or from collapse of the anterior tracheal wall above the tracheotomy stoma. The excess granulation tissue can result from cartilage injury during the procedure or due to unsupported weight of ventilator tubing creating mechanical strain and ischemia on the cartilaginous ring. Wound infection is an additional cause of post-tracheostomy stenosis.[32]

The most debated indication for tracheostomy is timing: early versus late, and whether early tracheostomy will shorten ventilator days and ICU stay, and decrease pneumonia rates. In 1989 vague guidelines were published, stating that patients with greater than 21 days anticipated intubation should have tracheostomy and less than 10 days should have translaryngeal intubation.[33] Between 10 and 21 days, there were no specific recommendations. Since then, multiple studies have attempted to identify whether early tracheostomy may prevent morbidity (see Table 49-1). When evaluating the data, it is important to realize that the definition of early and late tracheostomy can vary widely. Although there are a number of differences between the studies, it seems that duration of mechanical ventilation is statistically shortened with early tracheostomy[34] and in one study early tracheostomy had shorter weaning times.[35] Length of stay (LOS) in the ICU and/or hospital was also significantly shortened with early tracheostomy in multiple studies. Pneumonia occurrence was found to be reduced by 80% in study of Rumbak et al and by 36% in Moller's study. Bourderka found no difference in pneumonia rates but did find a delay in the development of pneumonia in the early tracheostomy group. Sugerman and Hsu were not able to identify a decreased pneumonia rate.[35,36]

Although each of these studies has its limitations due to number of subjects, length of time in the early and late groups, and heterogeneity of population, it is important to realize that in certain populations there are expert recommendations for early tracheostomy. Per Eastern Association for the Surgery of Trauma (EAST) guidelines, a Level II recommendation is that patients with severe head injury will benefit from early tracheostomy by shortened ventilator days and ICU LOS.[38] The guidelines further state that early tracheostomy may decrease the total days of mechanical ventilation and ICU LOS in trauma patients without head injuries and may decrease the rate of pneumonia in trauma patients. Their Level III recommendation is that early tracheostomy be considered in all trauma patients anticipated to require mechanical ventilation for >7 days.[38] As the data cited are limited, prospective large studies are needed to continue the improvement on the 1989 recommendations and move critical care practitioners closer to guidelines such as those from EAST that offer narrower parameters within which to make decisions.

▶ PROCEDURAL CONSIDERATIONS

Bronchoscopy is a useful adjunct in performing PDT for a number of reasons. Most importantly, any iatrogenic injuries sustained during the procedure can be immediately identified. Inadvertent puncture of the membranous (posterior) portion of the trachea is one such injury that can be avoided. Additionally, a true midline location and directionality for the placement of the wire can be confirmed by direct visualization. Last, appropriate placement of the tracheostomy device itself can be visually confirmed. One pitfall of bronchoscopic guidance is that it requires the endotracheal tube tip to be withdrawn to the level of the subglottic larynx. This can create a major cuff leak (since the cuff is no longer past the cords in the trachea) and occasionally loss of airway requiring reintubation. For reasons of patient safety and risk management, most would argue that bronchoscopic guidance and having intubation supplies nearby have become the standard of care.

▶ TECHNIQUES FOR PDT

The basis for almost all percutaneous procedures performed is the modified Seldinger technique, which was originally utilized for percutaneous nephrostomy tube placement. As a general principle, a needle is used to gain access to a lumen, and through this needle a guidewire is placed into the lumen. The technique for PDT is no different.

CIAGLIA SEQUENTIAL DILATORS

The first step is assessment of anatomic landmarks.[39] The sternal notch, cricoid, and thyroid cartilage are the key landmarks to be identified. Once the skin has

▶ TABLE 49-1. SUMMARY OF EARLY VERSUS LATE TRACHEOSTOMY TRIALS

Study	Type of Study	Sample Size, Early/Late	Timing (Days), Early/Late	Duration of MV (Days), Early/Late	ICU LOS (Days)	Hospital LOS (Days)	Pneumonia Morbidity (%)	Mortality ICU, Early/Late (%)	Mortality Hospital, Early/Late (%)
Flaaten	Retrospective	230/231	<6/>6	4.7/14.7 (median)	6.8/12.7 (median)	ND	ND	7/14.7	22.2/32.5
Barquist	Prospective, randomized	29/31	<8/>28	21.5/21.2 (NS)	25.0/24.7 (NS)	ND	96.5/90.3 (NS)	6.9/16.1 (NS)	ND
Moller	Retrospective	81/104	<7/>7	12.2 ± 0.9/21.9 ± 1.3	16.7 ± 1.0/26.0 ± 1.3	23.8 ± 1.2/33.4 ± 1.7	27.2/42.3	ND	ND
Rumbak	Prospective, randomized	60/60	<2/14–16	7.6 ± 2.0/17.4 ± 5.3	4.8 ± 1.4/16.2 ± 3.8	ND	5.0/25.0	ND	31.7/61.7
Hsu	Retrospective	163	<21/>21	19.0/44.3	10.8/14.2	ND	43.6/60.4 (NS)	14.5/28.3	44.5/54.7 (NS)
Arabi	Prospective database	29/107	<7/>7	9.6 ± 1.2/18.7 ± 1.3	10.9 ± 1.2/21 ± 1.3	101 ± 19/105 ± 7 (NS)	ND	3/1 NS	17/14 (NS)
Sugerman	Prospective, randomized	127/28	3–5/10–14	ND	20 ± 2/24 ± 2 (NS)	ND	49/57 (NS)	ND	24/18 (NS)
Bouderka	Randomized controlled trial	ND	ND	14.5 (SD = 7.3) vs. 17.5 (10.6)	ND	ND	ND	ND	ND
Rodriguez	Randomized controlled trial	ND	≤7 vs. ≥8	12 (SD = 1) vs. 32 (3)	16 (1) vs. 37 (4)	ND	78 vs. 96	ND	ND

ND, no data; SD, standard deviation; NS, nonsignificant. Adapted with permission from Groves DS, Durbin CG Jr. Tracheostomy in the critically ill: indications, timing and techniques. *Curr Opin Crit Care.* 2007;13(1):90–97.

been prepped with chlorhexidine solution and the neck draped with sterile towels, the appropriately sized tracheostomy appliance is inspected and the balloon's integrity tested. Beginning at the cricoid cartilage, after infiltration of local anesthetic, a 1- to 2-cm vertical or horizontal incision is carried caudally using #15 scalpel. Blunt dissection using a hemostat is performed through the strap muscles, until the pretracheal space is entered. This is the authors' technique, but many intensivists do not use blunt dissection and perform PDT as purely percutaneous. At this time, the fiberoptic bronchoscope should be inserted. Under direct visualization, after deflation of the ETT cuff, the tube should be withdrawn so that the light from the bronchoscope is visible in the incision site at the level of the second and third or first and second tracheal rings. It is important to remember that in patients who are difficult to oxygenate, this maneuver will likely result in desaturation, and ventilator adjustments will need to be made accordingly.

Utilizing a saline-filled syringe with an 18-gauge catheter over needle, the trachea is pierced below the cricoid cartilage through the incision. Under direct bronchoscopic guidance, the needle should be visualized passing between either the second and third or first and second tracheal rings. Aspiration of the syringe will confirm intratracheal placement by the presence of air bubbles. Bronchoscopy will ensure that the needle does not pierce the posterior wall of the trachea and is anterior midline in position. Removing the syringe and 18-gauge needle, the catheter is advanced caudally; the flexible guidewire provided in the kit is then visualized by the bronchoscope and passed. The catheter is removed, and the dilators are passed over the wire into the trachea, under direct visualization, from smallest to largest. The largest dilator used is just smaller than the inner diameter of the tracheostomy appliance, instead of a cannula, and is actually placed inside the tracheostomy tube's lumen. Once the tracheostomy tube is completely inserted, the dilator and guidewire are removed, the cuff is inflated, the tracheostomy is connected to the ventilator circuit, and the appliance is sutured into place and secured with tracheostomy ties. At this point, when the new airway has been confirmed, the endotracheal tube is removed completely as well as the bronchoscope.

BLUE RHINO™

The Blue Rhino™, or Ciaglia one-step technique, for PDT has rapidly become the most commonly utilized technique for PDT in the United States. All steps are identical to the sequential dilator technique up to and including placement of the flexible guidewire. The outside of the Blue Rhino™ dilator is hydrophilic and becomes very slippery when wet. Over the wire, a 14

French introducer sheath is placed, and over the sheath/wire combination, the Blue Rhino™ dilator is placed. This dilator has positioning marks, and is curvilinear. Curvilinear pressure is applied toward the mediastinum, creating an appropriately sized tracheostomy opening in a single pass. After this, a curvilinear dilator is placed within the tracheostomy tube; it is placed over the catheter/wire complex, and then the dilator is removed with the wire. As with the previous technique, we recommend bronchoscopic guidance. After this, the tracheostomy tube is secured in a standard fashion. Cook Medical provides an outstanding video of their Blue Rhino PDT at their Web site (http://www.cookmedical.com/cc/educationResource.do?id=Educational_Video).

GRIGGS

The Griggs technique was developed as an alternative to the sequential dilator technique in 1990.[40] The technique does not differ until after the insertion of the guidewire, at which point the operator utilizes a sharp-tipped tracheal spreader, which has been designed to slip over the guidewire. These tracheal spreaders are used to create both the soft tissue tract through the skin and the tracheal opening through which the tracheostomy tube will pass. Following this, a tracheostomy tube with an introducing sheath is passed over the wire, the wire and sheath are removed, and the device is secured into place.

PERCUTWIST™

Another technique, the PercuTwist™, which utilizes "controlled rotating dilatation," was described by Frova and Quintel in 2002.[41] A limited number of studies exist that evaluate the efficacy and safety of this technique, although one study, which compared Griggs, Ciaglia, and PercuTwist head-to-head, suggests that the PercuTwist™ is not only safe but also significantly faster to perform than the other techniques with a comparable rate of complications.[42] As with all of the previously mentioned techniques, the trachea is punctured with a needle between the cricoid and first tracheal ring under direct bronchoscopic guidance, and a flexible guidewire is passed through the needle toward the carina. A smaller (8–10 mm) skin incision is made, and the PercuTwist hydrophilically coated dilator screw is inserted over the guidewire after being lubricated with water. The clockwise rotation of the screw is stopped after the maximum diameter of the screw has been visualized within the tracheal lumen. After this, the tracheostomy tube, with an introducer sheath through its lumen, is passed over the guidewire, and secured into place. At this point, the wire and introducer sheath are removed.

► FANTONI TRANSLARYNGEAL TRACHEOSTOMY

An alternative exists to entering the trachea from the outside. Fantoni and Ripamonti have developed a retrograde percutaneous translaryngeal tracheostomy (TLT), colloquially known as the Fantoni procedure. This is the least commonly described technique in the literature, and the authors do not have any experience with this technique at our institution. The trachea is punctured at the usual site; however, the guidewire is passed cephalad and removed through the mouth, and then attached to the dilator/tracheostomy tube complex. This particular dilator has a sharp metal tip; by pulling on the guidewire with one hand, and providing countertraction with the other, the metal tip easily punctures the skin, opening the trachea from the inside out. The device is pulled until it is perpendicular to the skin and rotated 180° so that when it is readvanced into the trachea, it will be directed toward the carina. The cannula is removed so that only the tracheostomy tube remains, which is then secured into place. The major advantage of this technique, as described in the literature, is that it has been safely used in children and infants.[43] One possible disadvantage is that stomal metastases of head and neck cancers have been reported, as the device must pass through the oropharynx and vocal cords. It is, therefore, not a true percutaneous technique.[44] In a recent comparison of Blue Rhino and TLT, complications were not correlated with choice of technique, but the Blue Rhino™ was found to be cheaper and faster due to its simplicity.

► COMPLICATION OF THE DPT

Complications of percutaneous tracheostomy must be taken in the context of a comparison to surgical tracheostomy. In a large meta-analysis performed by Delaney et al, PDT was found to have a reduced incidence of infection, and subgroup analysis suggested that there were less periprocedural and long-term complications as compared with open tracheostomy.[45] Both procedures have complications that the practicing ICU clinician must be aware of; yet the addition of bronchoscopy to the PDT has decreased risks and has become part of the standard of care as mentioned previously.

During the procedure, there are multiple risks including loss of airway, hemorrhage, injury to trachea and paratracheal structures, and cardiac arrest. Loss of airway can be a complication that is anticipatable and easily dealt with when proper equipment and personnel who can intubate are readily available. Hemorrhage can be limited by utilizing the data listed for coagulation studies and understanding potential vascular interference via knowledge, clinical exam, and potentially ultrasound. Tracheal, laryngeal, and paratracheal injuries can best be avoided by understanding the anatomy and utilizing proper technique, with particular focus on midline entry into the trachea, adequate preparation of the skin, and proper technique in applying dilatational pressure in the correct plane. Cardiac arrest that occurs during the procedure may be a result of loss of airway during the procedure, or the patient being insufficiently stable to undergo the procedure. As mentioned previously, there are no critical care indications for tracheostomy that cannot wait.

Immediately after the procedure, subcutaneous emphysema (SE), pneumomediastinum (PM), pneumothorax (PTX), tube obstruction, infection, and hemorrhage can occur. SE may be a result of too tight a closure around the tracheostomy tube or prolonged duration of procedure after the point of tracheal perforation and before placement of the tube. This highlights why taking a "time-out" to assure all important tubes and equipment are in the room prior to incision is important. PTX or PM can occur when there is injury to the pleural domes. This rare complication may lead to tension PTX and therefore supports the need for postprocedure chest radiograph. Tube obstruction can have a number causes including mucous plugging and abrasion of the inner lining of the trachea. The authors have had an instance of PDT in which the friable tissue lining the trachea became a flap that partially obstructed the trachea. That flap caused high peak pressures, and was readily identified and relieved on postprocedural bronchoscopy. The solution to this problem continues to be technique and patient selection.

Infectious complications such as wound infections can be limited by both the PDT technique (as opposed to open surgical tracheostomy) and proper technique including chlorhexidine scrub, wearing mask, hat, and sterile gloves. Post-PDT cellulitis can be managed with antibiotics and increasing the size of the incision around the tracheostomy tube. Close postprocedural evaluation of any surgical intervention should be maintained, and evaluating all tubes, drains, and line sites daily is part of providing good critical care.

Delayed hemorrhage can occur and may be related to vasoconstrictor properties of injected anesthesia that has worn off or, rarely, from the potentially lethal erosion of major thoracic vasculature (0.4% of all tracheostomies), specifically the innominate artery (brachiocephalic artery). Briefly, tracheoinnominate (TI) fistula must be rapidly identified and evaluated if there is any chance to prevent the mortality from this complication.

TI fistula will present most frequently (70% of the time) during the first 3 weeks but can arise as early as 30 hours and as late as several years after the tracheostomy.[46–48] Approximately 50% of patients present with a massive hemorrhage, whereas the other half may report a small "herald" bleed[49] or a pulsating tube.[48]

The most frequent site of fistula formation is at the level of the endotracheal cuff, but one third result from pressure necrosis from the angle or the tip of the cannula. Other predisposing factors include the presence of an anomalous innominate artery, infection, and the use of steroids. Overinflation of the tracheostomy is the first maneuver that should be attempted in the face of a bedside massive hemorrhage. This technique can be successful in 85% of the cases.[49] Otherwise, a cuffed endotracheal tube should be inserted under direct laryngoscopy into the glottis and beyond the TI fistula. Finger pressure, directed anteriorly, as the artery is anterior to the trachea, is then applied on the innominate artery through the stomal opening after removal of the tracheostomy tube. For those patients presenting with sentinel bleed, preparation should be made for transfer to the operating room and emergency chest exploration. A diagnostic flexible bronchoscopy might be attempted first, but a rigid bronchoscopy is recommended for a better visualization and superior ability to suction blood clots. The rigid bronchoscope also allows the operator to stop the bleeding by applying the tube firmly against the innominate artery. The postoperative death rate is relatively high, as only 25% of those who survive the surgery are discharged alive.

Delayed complications that manifest can be less dramatic than loss of airway or TI fistula but must be respected as a serious cause of morbidity and mortality. As mentioned previously, tracheal stenosis, granulation tissue, and laryngeal injury can develop from prolonged intubation or tracheostomy and may or may not be primarily preventable. Although tracheoesophageal fistula is a complication, it can be prevented by avoiding trauma to the posterior wall of the trachea during the procedure and abstaining from prolonged large-bore feeding tubes in the esophagus. This rare complication can be initially managed by the intensivist by placing an ETT or new tracheostomy tube distal to the defect yet not too deep to be main-stemmed. Once the airway has been stabilized, a thoracic surgery consult for surgical or nonsurgical management decisions must be undertaken.[50]

▶ MANAGEMENT OF THE NEW TRACHEOTOMY TUBE

Accidental decannulation (dislodgment) in the first few days after surgery is an emergency. Since the tracheostomy site does not mature until approximately 5–7 days postprocedure, these patients should go to the operating room for replacement or an attempt to secure the airway from the translaryngeal route should be made. Attempting to replace a new tracheostomy tube into an unmatured site runs the risk of paratracheal placement, loss of airway, and death. If the patient has a disruption

between the upper and lower airways (i.e., post-tumor resection), making mask ventilation and translaryngeal intubation impossible, ventilating through the stoma may be the only choice. This increases the chance of altering the anatomy with subcutaneous air and making the operative replacement significantly more difficult. To prevent accidental tracheal decannulation, make sure the tube is properly secured, minimize manipulation of the tube and traction on the tube from oxygen or ventilator tubing, and instruct the patient to move cautiously until the tract is healed.

▶ TRACHEOTOMY TUBE CARE

Knowing how to properly care for a patient with a tracheostomy is vital because inappropriate or inadequate care may lead to complications and even death. Although details vary depending on the type of tracheostomy tube, tracheostomy care includes cleaning or changing the inner cannula, changing the dressing and tracheostomy tube holder, and suctioning if needed. Most tracheostomy tubes have disposable inner cannulas, which are replaced and secured using aseptic technique. Thoroughly assess the skin around the tracheostomy for evidence of skin breakdown related to the tracheostomy tube, tube securement device, or mucus and secretions. The area around the tracheostomy tube should be cleaned with a noncytotoxic cleanser. If you see skin breakdown, consult a wound team for a plan of care. Absorbing secretions helps prevent maceration and skin breakdown. Place a prepackaged, sterile tracheostomy dressing under the tube flanges. Always use a manufactured, one-layer split sponge rather than cutting a gauze pad. Never place anything with loose fibers around the stoma or tracheostomy tube because they can cause irritation, and the loose fibers could be aspirated.[51] Maintaining humidification is another key to avoiding potential issues. Normally, the nasopharynx humidifies inhaled air. Because the tracheostomy tube bypasses the upper airway, you need to provide adequate humidity to keep the airway moist. In hospitalized patients, this can be accomplished by a heat and moisture exchanger (HME) on a mechanical ventilator or a T-piece or tracheostomy mask.

Weaning the tracheostomy patient off ventilatory support is the first step for reaching the goal of decannulation. When the patient no longer requires ventilatory support, aerosol tracheostomy collar trials (TCT) should be initiated, and the cuff must be deflated for TCT. The patient should slowly be weaned down on the oxygen requirement as tolerated. If the patient has a cuffed tube, the tube should be downsized with a cuffless tracheostomy tube. When the patient is able to ventilate and oxygenate adequately, capping trials should be initiated. If the capping trials are tolerated without any issues for 24 hours, decannulation can be performed. The stoma should be bandaged until closure. The decannulated patient should be followed by the team for 24 hours postdecannulation.

► ACKNOWLEDGMENT

The authors would like to extend their appreciation to Natahnee Winder, who assisted with proofreading and collecting data for this chapter.

REFERENCES

1. Grillo HC, Dignan EF, Miura T. Extensive resection and reconstruction of mediastinal trachea without prosthesis or graft: an anatomical study in man. *J Thorac Cardiovasc Surg.* 1964;48:741–749.

2. Randestad A, Lindholm CE, Fabian P. Dimensions of the cricoid cartilage and the trachea. *Laryngoscope.* 2000;110(11):1957–1961.

3. Vicent J-L. *Intensive Care Medicine: Annual Update 2008.* Belgium, Germany: Springer Science and Business Media Inc; 2008.

4. Mateu A, Ricart A, Diaz-Prieto A, et al. Tracheostomy in intubated patients. *Clin Pulm Med.* 2008;15(5):267–273.

5. Byhahn C, Lischke V, Meininger D, et al. Peri-operative complications during percutaneous tracheostomy in obese patients. *Anaesthesia.* 2005;60(1):12–15.

6. Heyrosa MG, Melniczek DM, Rovito P, et al. Percutaneous tracheostomy: a safe procedure in the morbidly obese. *J Am Coll Surg.* 2006;202(4):618–622.

7. Mansharamani NG, Koziel H, Garland R, et al. Safety of bedside percutaneous dilatational tracheostomy in obese patients in the ICU. *Chest.* 2000;117(5):1426–1429.

8. Diaz-Reganon G, Minambres E, Ruiz A, et al. Safety and complications of percutaneous tracheostomy in a cohort of 800 mixed ICU patients. *Anaesthesia.* 2008;63(11):1198–1203.

9. Hatfield A, Bodenham A. Portable ultrasonic scanning of the anterior neck before percutaneous dilatational tracheostomy. *Anaesthesia.* 1999;54(7):660–663.

10. Muhammad JK, Patton DW, Evans RM, et al. Percutaneous dilatational tracheostomy under ultrasound guidance. *Br J Oral Maxillofac Surg.* 1999;37(4):309–311.

11. Bass SP, Field LM. Repeat percutaneous tracheostomy. *Anaesthesia.* 1994;49(7):649.

12. Mazzon D, Zanardo G, Dei Tos AP. Repeat percutaneous tracheostomy with the Ciaglia technique after translaryngeal tracheostomy. *Intensive Care Med.* 1999;25(6):639.

13. Meyer M, Critchlow J, Mansharamani N, et al. Repeat bedside percutaneous dilational tracheostomy is a safe procedure. *Crit Care Med.* 2002;30(5):986–988.

14. Mayberry JC, Wu IC, Goldman RK, et al. Cervical spine clearance and neck extension during percutaneous tracheostomy in trauma patients. *Crit Care Med.* 2000;28(10):3436–3440.

15. Ben Nun A, Orlovsky M, Best LA. Percutaneous tracheostomy in patients with cervical spine fractures—feasible and safe. *Interact Cardiovasc Thorac Surg.* 2006;5(4):427–429.

16. Berney S, Opdam H, Bellomo R, et al. An assessment of early tracheostomy after anterior cervical stabilization in patients with acute cervical spine trauma. *J Trauma.* 2008;64(3):749–753.

17. O'Keeffe T, Goldman RK, Mayberry JC, et al. Tracheostomy after anterior cervical spine fixation. *J Trauma.* 2004;57(4):855–860.

18. Friedman Y, Mayer AD. Bedside percutaneous tracheostomy in critically ill patients. *Chest.* 1993;104(2):532–535.

19. Stocchetti N, Parma A, Lamperti M, et al. Neurophysiological consequences of three tracheostomy techniques: a randomized study in neurosurgical patients. *J Neurosurg Anesthesiol.* 2000;12(4):307–313.

20. Dosemeci L, Yilmaz M, Gurpinar F, et al. The use of the laryngeal mask airway as an alternative to the endotracheal tube during percutaneous dilatational tracheostomy. *Intensive Care Med.* 2002;28(1):63–67.

21. Imperiale C, Magni G, Favaro R, et al. Intracranial pressure monitoring during percutaneous tracheostomy "percutwist" in critically ill neurosurgery patients. *Anesth Analg.* 2009;108(2):588–592.

22. Borm W, Gleixner M. Experience with two different techniques of percutaneous dilational tracheostomy in 54 neurosurgical patients. *Neurosurg Rev.* 2003;26(3):188–191.

23. Escarment J, Suppini A, Sallaberry M, et al. Percutaneous tracheostomy by forceps dilation: report of 162 cases. *Anaesthesia.* 2000;55(2):125–130.

24. Milanchi S, Magner D, Wilson MT, et al. Percutaneous tracheostomy in neurosurgical patients with intracranial pressure monitoring is safe. *J Trauma.* 2008;65(1):73–79.

25. Beiderlinden M, Eikermann M, Lehmann N, et al. Risk factors associated with bleeding during and after percutaneous dilational tracheostomy. *Anaesthesia.* 2007;62(4):342–346.

26. Kluge S, Meyer A, Kuhnelt P, et al. Percutaneous tracheostomy is safe in patients with severe thrombocytopenia. *Chest.* 2004;126(2):547–551.

27. Jaeger JM, Littlewood KA, Durbin CG Jr. The role of tracheostomy in weaning from mechanical ventilation. *Respir Care.* 2002;47(4):469–480. Discussion 481–482.

28. Archer S, Baugh R, Nelms C. Tracheostomy. In: *2000 Clinical Indicators Compendium.* Alexandria: American Academy of Otolaryngology-Head and Neck Surgery; 2000:45.

29. Colice GL, Stukel TA, Dain B. Laryngeal complications of prolonged intubation. *Chest.* 1989;96(4):877–884.

30. Heffner J. Tracheotomy: indication and timing. *Respir Care.* 1999;44(7):807–815.

31. Russell C, Matta B. *Tracheostomy: A Multiprofessional Handbook.* Cambridge, London: Greenwich Medical Media Limited, 2006.

32. Zias N, Chroneou A, Tabba MK, et al. Post tracheostomy and post intubation tracheal stenosis: report of 31 cases and review of the literature. *BMC Pulm Med.* 2008;8:18.

33. Plummer AL, Gracey DR. Consensus conference on artificial airways in patients receiving mechanical ventilation. *Chest.* 1989;96(1):178–180.

34. Groves DS, Durbin CG Jr. Tracheostomy in the critically ill: indications, timing and techniques. *Curr Opin Crit Care.* 2007;13(1):90–97.

35. Hsu CL, Chen KY, Chang CH, et al. Timing of tracheostomy as a determinant of weaning success in critically

ill patients: a retrospective study. *Crit Care*. 2005;9(1): R46–R52.

36. Sugerman, H J, Wolfe L, Pasquale MD et al. Multicenter, Randomized, Prospective Trial of Early Tracheostomy. *J Trauma*. 1997;43(5):741–747.

37. Engels PT, Bagshaw SM, Meier M, et al. Tracheostomy: from insertion to decannulation. *Can J Surg*. 2009;52(5): 427–433.

38. Holevar M, Dunham JC, Clancy TV, et al. Practice Management Guidelines for the Timing of Tracheostomy: The EAST Practice Management Guidelines Work Group. *J Trauma*. 2009;67(4):870–874.

39. Ciaglia P, Firsching R, Syniec C. Elective percutaneous dilatational tracheostomy. A new simple bedside procedure; preliminary report. *Chest*. 1985;87(6):715–719.

40. Griggs W, Worthley L, Gilligan J, et al. A simple percutaneous tracheostomy technique. *Surg Gynecol Obstet*. 1990;170(6):543–545.

41. Frova G, Quintel M. A new simple method for percutaneous tracheostomy: controlled rotating dilation. A preliminary report. *Intensive Care Med*. 2002;28(3):299–303.

42. Yurtseven N, Aydemir B, Karaca P, et al. PercuTwist: a new alternative to Griggs and Ciaglia's techniques. *Eur J Anaesthesiol*. 2007;24(6):492–497.

43. Fantoni A, Ripamonti D. A non-derivative, non-surgical tracheostomy: the translaryngeal method. *Intensive Care Med*. 1997;23(4):386–392.

44. Aust W, Sandner A, Neumann K, et al. Stomal metastases after translaryngeal tracheotomy (TLT) according to Fantoni: a rare complication. *HNO*. 2007;55(2): 114–117.

45. Delaney A, Bagshaw SM, Nalos M. Percutaneous dilational tracheostomy versus surgical tracheostomy in critically ill patients: a systematic review and meta-analysis. *Crit Care*. 2006;10(2):R55.

46. Gelman JJ, Aro M, Weiss SM. Tracheo-innominate artery fistula. *J Am Coll Surg*. 1994;179(5):626–634.

47. Cokis C, Towler S. Tracheo-innominate fistula after initial percutaneous tracheostomy. *Anaesth Intensive Care*. 2000;28(5):566–569.

48. Ridley RW, Zwischenberger JB. Tracheoinnominate fistula: surgical management of an iatrogenic disaster. *J Laryngol Otol*. 2006;120(8):676–680.

49. Jones JW, Reynolds M, Hewitt RL, et al. Tracheo-innominate artery erosion: successful surgical management of a devastating complication. *Ann Surg*. 1976;184(2): 194–204.

50. Chua AP, Dalal B, Mehta AC. Tracheostomy tube-induced tracheoesophageal fistula. *J Bronchol Intervent Pulmonol*. 2009;16(3):191–192.

51. Dennis-Rouse MD, Davidson JE. An evidence-based evaluation of tracheostomy care practices. *Crit Care Nurs Q*. 2008;31(2):150–160.

CHAPTER 50

Therapeutic Hypothermia: History, Data, Translation, and Emergency Department Application

David F. Gaieski and Munish Goyal

▶ INTRODUCTION

Therapeutic hypothermia (TH) has become standard of care for the management of comatose patients with return of spontaneous circulation (ROSC) after cardiac arrest. The 2010 American Heart Association (AHA) guidelines for management of post–cardiac arrest patients "recommend that comatose (i.e., lack of meaningful response to verbal commands) adult patients with ROSC after out-of-hospital ventricular fibrillation (VF) cardiac arrest should be cooled to 32°C to 34°C (89.6°F to 93.2°F) for 12 to 24 hours (Class I, LOE B). Induced hypothermia also may be considered for comatose adult patients with ROSC after in-hospital cardiac arrest of any initial rhythm or after out-of-hospital cardiac arrest with an initial rhythm of pulseless electric activity or asystole (Class IIb, LOE B)."[1] Very few recommendations in the AHA guidelines are assigned a Class I recommendation, and, as practitioners at the portal of entry for the majority of cardiac arrest patients, emergency physicians (EPs) need to be familiar with this therapy and the rationale for the level of recommendation assigned to TH.

Why is TH needed to improve outcomes after cardiac arrest? When a person suffers a cardiac arrest, no effective cardiac contractility occurs, resulting in ischemia, or lack of perfusion. Chest compressions provide some degree of circulation during arrest and can deliver up to 40% of the cardiac output produced by a spontaneously beating heart. The ischemia that occurs during cardiac arrest triggers a number of pathologic processes including the production of reactive oxygen species, initiation of a profound inflammatory cascade, development of metabolic acidosis with accompanying elevated lactate levels, and endothelial and mitochondrial dysfunction, to name some of the dozens of derangements that ensue. When ROSC occurs, ischemic tissues are reperfused with blood, and this reperfusion produces its own injury pattern. The combination of ischemia and reperfusion produces the post–cardiac arrest syndrome (PCAS), a unique disease state requiring specialized care. This was first described as a specific disease entity by Negovsky in 1972 when he stated that postresuscitation syndrome was a unique disease entity with unique pathophysiology that needed to be understood if it was to be treated appropriately.[2] Currently, TH is the best-studied and most effective therapy for treating patients with PCAS.[3] In this chapter, we will discuss the epidemiology of cardiac arrest, the rationale for using TH, data supporting its use, practical aspects of implementation, and future directions for the therapy.

▶ EPIDEMIOLOGY

Although the United States has no standardized, mandatory reporting system, it is estimated that 400,000 cardiac arrests occur each year in the United States, 75% as out-of-hospital cardiac arrests (OHCA) and 25% as in-hospital arrests.[4] Viewed from a different perspective, one arrest arrives in an ED in the United States every 2 minutes. Europe also has approximately 400,000 arrests per year.[5] In Japan, where a universal cardiac arrest reporting system exists, more accurate numbers are available; in 2007, approximately 78,000 OHCA occurred nationwide.[6] Survival from cardiac arrest is abysmal—approximately 7% of OHCA in the United States survive to hospital discharge.[4] However, survival varies significantly depending on prehospital, intra-arrest, and postarrest variables including initial arrest rhythm, whether the arrest was witnessed by a bystander, whether bystander cardiopulmonary resuscitation (CPR) was performed, ambulance response times, availability of automated external defibrillators (AED), and quality of postarrest care. In the United States, survival rates vary from 0.2% in Detroit to 17% in the greater Seattle area.[7,8] One of the main variables affecting outcome is delivery of quality postarrest care, centered on induced hypothermia. The need for high-quality postarrest care was emphasized in a 2003 publication from the National Registry of Cardiopulmonary Resuscitation (NRCPR), a registry of in-hospital cardiac arrests. Reporting on 14,792 arrests, ROSC was achieved in 39% of the patients, who had a subsequent mortality rate of 68%.[9]

▶ HISTORY

Physicians have been interested in using induced hypothermia for clinical purposes for millennia. Hippocrates wrote about packing injured patients in ice and questioned whether this simple technique would improve outcomes. In 1814, Baron Larrey, Napoleon's chief battlefield surgeon, made observations on the effect of cold on injured soldiers. While Napoleon's army retreated from Moscow after the Russian campaign, a policy of placing injured officers near the fire while keeping injured foot soldiers in the cold was enforced. Larrey noted that injured foot soldiers appeared to do better with similar injuries than the injured officers and commented, "Cold acts on living parts such that they may remain in a state of asphyxia without losing their lives." This statement summarizes early ideas of the mechanism of action of induced hypothermia: lowering temperature lowered metabolism, decreasing oxygen and glucose consumption and allowing injured cells time to recover.

Fay, a neurosurgeon at Temple University Hospital in Philadelphia, Pennsylvania, was the first to publish studies of the clinical application of induced hypothermia. In 1940, he reported treating cancer patients with TH.[10,11] In 1959, in the journal *Anesthesia and Analgesia*, Benson et al from Johns Hopkins University Hospital in Baltimore, Maryland, published results of a case series of 27 perioperative cardiac arrests, some of which were treated with TH.[12] The stated rationale for using TH was similar to that observed by Baron Larrey almost 150 years earlier: "Hypothermia has been shown to protect the brain against anoxia. There is a reduction in the cerebral oxygen consumption and cerebral blood flow with body cooling." Nineteen of the arrests were resuscitated with sustained ROSC. Twelve of the 19 were treated with TH. Fifty percent (6/12) of the patients treated with TH survived, all neurologically intact, while only 14% (1/7) of the patients who were not cooled survived. They concluded that, "The improvement in survival rate from 14% to 50% with use of hypothermia is clinically significant and warrants the use of cooling in all patients who have had cardiac arrest with demonstrable neurological injury."[12]

In 1964, in an article published in the *Journal of the Iowa Medical Society*, Safar advocated treating postarrest patients with a comprehensive management strategy centered on induced hypothermia that included attempts to gauge the cause of arrest, support ventilations and circulation, prevent seizures, and monitor closely.[13] He recommended early institution of hypothermia, stating, "start within 30 minutes if no signs of CNS recovery." There are no published case reports documenting clinical experience of Safar and colleagues with TH at the University of Pittsburgh in the 1960s. It is generally believed that they cooled patients to 30°C using ice packs and treated post–cardiac arrest patients as well as patients with other causes of brain injury including traumatic brain injury, ischemic stroke, hepatic encephalopathy, and comatose meningitis. After treating a number of patients, they abandoned the clinical use of TH and began to study its application more closely in animal models of cardiac arrest. Reasons cited for stopping clinical application of TH included coagulopathy, arrhythmias, and hypotension. These potential side effects of TH will be addressed later in this chapter.

▶ PILOT STUDIES

Insights from animal experiments including the potential efficacy of hypothermia performed at 33°C instead of lower temperatures, the complexity of ischemia–reperfusion injury, the multiple physiologic processes affected by hypothermia, the need for adequate mean arterial pressure (MAP) to maintain cerebral perfusion, and a focus on patients who remained comatose after ROSC from OHCA led to reinvestigation of the utility of employing TH in humans.[14–16] The first prospective study of TH in humans was published in the *Annals of Emergency Medicine* in 1997.[17] The objective of this pilot study was to investigate the effect of induced hypothermia to 33°C begun in the ED and continued for 12 hours in the intensive care unit (ICU) on outcomes in patients with anoxic brain injury after OHCA. Twenty-two comatose OHCA VF patients treated with TH to 33°C for 12 hours were compared with 22 matched historic controls obtained from chart review. Primary endpoints were survival and good neurologic outcomes. Survival was 23% in normothermic controls versus 55% in patients treated with hypothermia (*P* < .05), and good neurologic outcomes occurred in 14% versus 50%, respectively (*P* < .05).[17]

In 2000, in the *Journal of the American College of Cardiology*, Nagao et al from Tokyo, Japan, published their results treating comatose survivors of cardiac arrest with TH with or without emergency cardiopulmonary bypass (ECPB).[18] A convenience sample of 50 patients with an initial rhythm of VF presenting to the ED in ongoing cardiac arrest was treated with standard CPR. If ROSC was achieved and systolic blood pressure (SBP) could be maintained above 90 mm Hg, then hypothermia was induced. If ROSC was not achieved, patients were placed on ECPB as a rescue strategy, followed by treatment with TH if blood pressure was adequate. Of the 23 patients treated with TH, 12 (53%) had good neurologic outcomes. These pilot studies led investigators to pursue true, randomized controlled trials of TH in comatose survivors of OHCA.

► RANDOMIZED TRIALS AND LANDMARK STUDIES

In 2001, Hachimi-Idrissi et al published a randomized trial of cooling with a helmet device to achieve a target temperature of 34°C.[19] Thirty patients who remained comatose after ROSC from asystole or pulseless electrical activity (PEA) cardiac arrests were randomized to either normothermia (14 patients) or hypothermia (16 patients). The study was designed to test the feasibility of inducing TH using a helmet cooling device, not the efficacy of TH in this patient population. The hypothermia patients reached target core (bladder) temperatures in a mean of 180 minutes from start of therapy. Survival was low in both arms of the study: 3/16 (18.8%) survived in the hypothermia group; 1/14 (7.1%) survived in the normothermia group. Rates of good neurologic outcome were also low: 2/16 (12.5%) patients who were cooled and none of the patients who were not cooled.

Bernard et al followed up their pilot study of TH with a pseudo-randomized trial of TH compared with normothermia, which was published in *The New England Journal of Medicine* in 2002.[20] Seventy-seven patients who remained comatose after resuscitation from OHCA caused by VF were randomly assigned to treatment with hypothermia or normothermia depending on the day of the week. On odd-numbered days patients were treated with induced hypothermia and on even-numbered days with normothermia. Hypothermia therapy was begun by paramedics in the field, who removed the patient's clothing and applied cold packs. The target temperature was 33°C, and hypothermia was maintained for 12 hours. The primary outcome measure was survival to hospital discharge with good neurologic function. Twenty-six percent (9/34) of patients treated with normothermia had good neurologic outcomes versus 49% (21/43) of patients treated with hypothermia (*P* = .046). When adjusted for potential confounders including age and time to ROSC, the survival benefit with good neurologic outcome associated with TH remained (OR = 5.25; 95% confidence interval 1.47–18.76; *P*-value = .011) (see Figure 50-1).

In the same issue of *The New England Journal of Medicine*, the Hypothermia After Cardiac Arrest (HACA) Study Group published the results of a larger, randomized, prospective trial comparing hypothermia to normothermia in patients who remained comatose after being resuscitated from OHCA caused by VF.[21] The target temperature range was 32–34°C for 24 hours. The primary outcome measure was good neurologic outcome at 6 months. Secondary endpoints included mortality at 6 months and the rate of complications during the first 7 days. Good

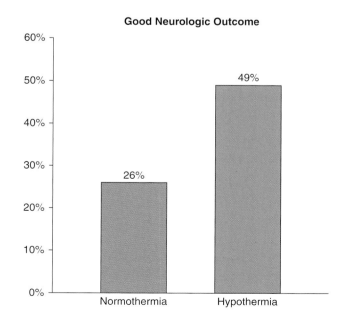

Figure 50-1. Bernard trial outcomes.

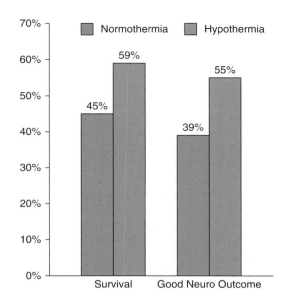

Figure 50-2. HACA trial outcomes.

outcomes occurred in 55% (75/136) of the TH patients versus 39% (54/137) of the normothermia patients (RR = 1.40; 95% confidence interval 1.08–1.81). Mortality was reduced from 55% in the normothermia group to 41% in the TH group, which was statistically significant. Despite concerns of infection, bleeding, and dysrhythmias, there were no statistically significant differences in the rate of complications between the two groups (see Figure 50-2).

► CALL FOR ADOPTION OF THERAPEUTIC HYPOTHERMIA

In 2003, the International Liaison Committee on Resuscitation evaluated the results of these randomized trials and concluded that TH should be used to treat comatose patients resuscitated from OHCA caused by VF.[22] In 2005, the AHA guidelines for postresuscitation support recommended that "unconscious adult patients with ROSC after out-of-hospital cardiac arrest should be cooled to 32°C to 34°C (89.6°F to 93.2°F) for 12 to 24 hours when the initial rhythm was VF (Class IIa). Similar therapy may be beneficial for patients with non-VF arrest out of hospital or for in-hospital arrest (Class IIb)."[23] The central question accompanying these recommendations is the following: When TH is applied in a heterogeneous group of health care settings, will the benefit observed for the therapy in the randomized trials be maintained?

► DATA FROM IMPLEMENTATION STUDIES AND DATABASES

Multiple implementation studies have been published since the randomized controlled trials of TH were published in 2002.[24–29] These implementation studies have had varying inclusion criteria including differences in age, the presence of a witness, the presenting rhythm, and duration of downtime. They have used different cooling techniques and maintained hypothermia for varying lengths of time. These diverse implementation studies were summarized in a meta-analysis published by Sagalyn et al in *Critical Care Medicine* in 2009.[30] They examined all nonrandomized studies of adults resuscitated from cardiac arrest, with or without historic controls, published after the Bernard and HACA studies appeared in early 2002. Thirteen studies were included in the analysis with a total of 924 TH patients and 336 normothermic, historic controls. The meta-analysis concluded: "The survival and neurological outcomes benefit from therapeutic hypothermia are robust when compared over a wide range of studies of actual implementation." The odds ratio for survival when treated with TH was 2.5 (95% confidence interval 1.8–3.3) and for favorable neurologic outcome was also 2.5 (95% confidence interval 1.9–3.4).[30]

Two large multi-institutional databases have also been published. The first, published by Arrich and The European Resuscitation Council Hypothermia After Cardiac Arrest Registry Study Group in 2007, was an outgrowth of the HACA trial. A total of 587 patients were included, 462 of whom were treated with TH and 123 with normothermia.[31] Survival was 57% in patients treated with TH versus 32% in normothermic patients (*P* < .001); favorable neurologic outcomes were achieved in 45% of TH patients versus 32% of normothermic patients (*P* = .02). The second, from Nielsen et al, summarized 4 years of data from cases entered into the "Hypothermia Network," a 34-center, 7-country registry of OHCA patients who remained comatose after resuscitation and were treated with TH.[32] Nine hundred and eighty-six patients were included; the median time from collapse to ROSC was 20 minutes (IQR 14–30), the median time from collapse to initiation of TH was 90 minutes (IQR 60–165), and the median time from collapse to target temperature was 260 minutes (IQR 178–400). The presenting rhythm was VF/VT in 686 patients, of whom 412 (61%) survived to 6-month follow-up and 380 (56%) had good neurologic outcomes. Of the 217 patients who presented with asystole, 54 (25%) survived to 6 months and 46 (21%) had good outcomes. For the 66 patients presenting with PEA, 18 (27%) survived to 6 months and 15 (23%) had good outcomes.

► BUNDLES OF POSTARREST CARE

These nonrandomized results provide strong, ancillary support to the findings of the randomized trials and suggest that TH should be used to treat the majority of comatose survivors of cardiac arrest regardless of initial rhythm or location of arrest. The totality of the findings from the randomized trials, implementation studies, and databases has informed the changes in the 2010 AHA recommendations about post–cardiac arrest care.[1] As the authors acknowledged in the introduction: "There is increasing recognition that systematic post–cardiac arrest care after … ROSC can improve the likelihood of patient survival with good quality of life."[1] They recommend that TH be combined with other interventions to optimize outcomes in PCAS patients. These other interventions include optimization of cardiopulmonary function and vital organ perfusion, early percutaneous coronary intervention, goal-directed critical care, and neurologic support.

▶ DETAILS OF THERAPEUTIC HYPOTHERMIA

Hypothermia therapy can be divided into three distinct phases: induction, maintenance, and rewarming.[33] Induction involves bringing the patient from the presenting temperature to target temperature. This can be accomplished by a number of methods: infusion of chilled intravenous fluids, application of ice bags, application of surface cooling equipment, insertion of intravascular cooling catheters, and other, novel equipment. In the Hypothermia Network Registry, the most common methods used to induce hypothermia were chilled fluids, used in 80% of the patients, and ice bags, used in 43%[32] (see Figure 50-3). Induction should begin as close to ROSC as possible and occur at as fast a rate as possible. Shivering is the major complication that can occur during induction of TH and can be controlled with a number of different agents including meperidine, magnesium, buspirone, or paralytics. Benzodiazepines and neuromuscular blocking agents were used in all of the patients in both of the TH randomized controlled trials to control shivering and induce sedation. In addition, as the patient's core temperature drops, metabolism slows (decreasing approximately 8%/1°C), oxygen and glucose consumption fall, and ventilator settings need to be adjusted to compensate for decreased carbon dioxide production.[33] Continuous core temperature measurement should be established during the induction phase. Place of an esophageal or urinary bladder probe should be considered, particularly if using a device that allows temperature autoregulation via a feedback loop.

During the maintenance phase, patients are kept at the target temperature for a specified period of time. The optimal length of time to maintain hypothermia is unknown. In the Bernard trial, patients were maintained for 12 hours; in the HACA trial, TH was maintained for 24 hours; in the Hypothermia Network Registry, 93% of the patients received TH for 24 hours.[20,21] The period of injury after ischemia and reperfusion may last up to 7 days, and longer periods of TH may produce better outcomes.[33] In the maintenance phase, several clinical problems need to be addressed: many patients develop postarrest myocardial stunning with accompanying decrease in ejection fraction; TH causes a cold-induced diuresis, and many patients require additional volume infusion to maintain adequate intravascular volume; electrolyte changes include hypokalemia, hypomagnesemia, and hyperglycemia.[33]

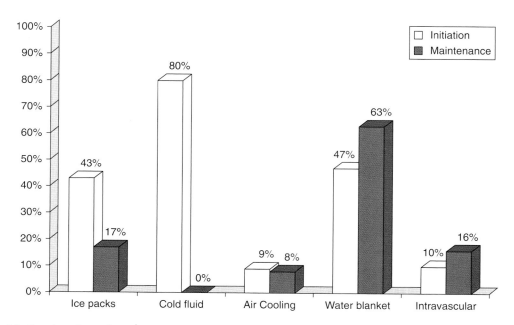

Figure 50-3. Methods of cooling from Nielsen study.

The goal of the rewarming phase is to safely return the patient to normothermia in a controlled fashion. This can be facilitated by using a cooling device with a feedback mechanism and an automatic rewarming program. During the rewarming phase, the patient begins to vasodilate, potentially causing decreased intravascular volume, requiring infusion of additional intravenous fluid. Potassium moves from intracellular compartments to the intravascular compartment and patients can become hyperkalemic; similarly, insulin resistance decreases and patients on continuous insulin infusions can become hypoglycemic. Ventilator settings need to be changed to account for the increased carbon dioxide production as metabolism increases.[33]

▶ EMERGENCY DEPARTMENT-SPECIFIC CONCERNS

The role EPs play in the management of PCAS patients varies from institution to institution, depending on hospital resources, patient flow, and ED capabilities. Many OHCA patients have ROSC prior to ED arrival; others receive CPR in the ED, and a percentage of them attain ROSC while in the ED. EPs can maximize ROSC by delivering high-quality CPR including early defibrillation,[34] quality chest compressions,[35] discovery of reversible causes, and prioritization of interventions such as vascular access, intubation, and termination of resuscitation efforts.[36] Rapid identification of patients who qualify for TH and other aspects of postarrest care is a central task of EPs.[13,20,21] In addition to assessing for persistent coma after ROSC, this may involve, as dictated by the clinical scenario, obtaining basic labs to evaluate coagulation function and head CT to ensure no intracranial hemorrhage. In addition, in the vast majority of cases, induction of TH in patients who remain comatose after resuscitation from OHCA will fall under the auspices of EPs. This may be as simple as identification of qualifying patients, application of ice bags, infusion of chilled saline through peripheral IVs, and rapid transfer to an ICU for definitive management. On the other hand, it may include the first hours of comprehensive postarrest care including induction of TH, placement of arterial and central venous catheters, hemodynamic optimization, initiation of neurologic monitoring, ventilator management, electrolyte management, and bedside echocardiography. Comprehensive PCAS management programs need to be developed with champions from EMS, the ED, cardiology, critical care, neurology, and, potentially, rehabilitation medicine.[3,29] It is imperative to delineate the responsibilities of each group of providers, given the potential rapid transition of these critically ill patients and number of interventions that need to be performed in the proximal phase.

▶ FUTURE DIRECTIONS

The number of PCAS patients qualifying for TH and other aspects of postarrest care who present to different hospitals around the country varies from a few a year to several a month. Studies have demonstrated that outcomes from cardiac arrest vary depending on hospital type with lower survival rates at more rural, nonteaching, and smaller hospitals than at urban, teaching, and larger hospitals.[37,38] Therefore, postarrest care may be optimized if regionalization occurs by diverting patients from low-volume hospitals to those treating a larger number of PCAS patients. In Arizona, the state EMS system has instituted a program of comprehensive cardiocerebral resuscitation, including TH delivered at cardiac arrest receiving hospitals. Using this approach, they have increased survival from 3.8% to 9.1%.[36]

When a cardiac arrest patient does not have ROSC, there are limited options to the physicians attempting to resuscitate the patient. After a period of unsuccessful resuscitation, the EP can halt further resuscitation efforts and pronounce the patient dead. The only alternatives available at this time are continued CPR by conventional means including chest compressions, drug administration, and defibrillation; or placing a patient on ECPB to provide circulation and ventilation for the patient until heart function recovers. During the time the patient is on ECPB, reversible causes of arrest can be addressed. Feasibility studies from Tokyo, Taipei, Seoul, and Los Angeles have demonstrated promising outcomes using ECPB; however, no randomized, prospective studies have been conducted and survivors may reflect selection bias, a Hawthorne effect, or an epiphenomenon of the timing of the intervention.

▶ CONCLUSIONS

TH is now recognized as the standard of care for patients who remain comatose after resuscitation from cardiac arrest (see Figure 50-4). An organized program of TH needs to be integrated into a comprehensive plan

2010 AHA Recommendations for Therapeutic Hypothermia	
Rhythm	**Recommendation**
Out-of-Hospital Ventricular Fibrillation	Class I, Level of Evidence B
In-Hospital Arrest	Class IIb, Level of Evidence B
Pulseless Electrical Activity, Asystole	Class IIb, Level of Evidence B

Figure 50-4. 2010 American Heart Association recommendations for therapeutic hypothermia.

for management of PCAS patients. EPs must develop these programs in concert with colleagues from EMS, neurology, cardiology, intensive care, and rehabilitation medicine. Clear delineation of who will be cooled, how they will be cooled, and the division of labor among the different care providers is vital to ensure a successful TH program.

REFERENCES

1. Peberdy MA, Callaway CW, Neumar RW, et al. Part 9: post-cardiac arrest care: 2010 American Heart Association guidelines for cardiopulmonary resuscitation and emergency cardiovascular care. *Circulation.* 2010;122:S768–S786.
2. Negovsky VA. The second step in resuscitation—the treatment of the 'post-resuscitation disease'. *Resuscitation.* 1972;1(1):1–7.
3. Neumar RW, Nolan JP, Adrie C, et al. Post cardiac arrest syndrome. Epidemiology, pathophysiology, treatment, and prognostication. A consensus statement from the International Liaison Committee on Resuscitation. *Circulation.* 2008;118: 2452–2483.
4. Lloyd-Jones D, Adams R, Carnethon M, et al. Heart disease and stroke statistics 2009 update: a report from the American Heart Association Statistics Committee and Stroke Statistics Subcommittee. *Circulation.* 2009;119:e21–e181.
5. de Vreede-Swagemakers JJ, Gorgels AP, Dubois-Arbouw WI, et al. Out-of-hospital cardiac arrest in the 1990's: a population-based study in the Maastricht area on incidence, characteristics and survival. *J Am Coll Cardiol.* 1997;30(6):1500–1505.
6. Kitamura T, Iwama T, Kawamura T, et al. Nationwide public-access defibrillation in Japan. *N Engl J Med.* 2010;362:994–1004.
7. Dunne RB, Compton S, Zalenski RJ, et al. Outcomes from out-of-hospital cardiac arrest in Detroit. *Resuscitation.* 2007;72:59–65.
8. Nichol G, Thomas T, Callaway CW, et al. Regional variation in out-of-hospital cardiac arrest incidence and outcome. *JAMA.* 2008;300(12):1423–1431.
9. Peberdy MA, Kaye W, Ornato JP, et al. Cardiopulmonary resuscitation of adults in the hospital: a report of 14720 cardiac arrests from the National Registry of Cardiopulmonary Resuscitation. *Resuscitation.* 2003;58(3):297–308.
10. Fay T. Clinical report and evaluation of low temperature in treatment of cancer. *Proc Interstate Postgrad Med Assoc North Am.* 1940:292–297.
11. Smith L, Fay T. Observations on human beings with cancer maintained at reduced temperatures of 75–90°F. *Am J Clin Pathol.* 1940;10:1–11.
12. Benson D, Williams GR, Spencer FC, et al. The use of hypothermia after cardiac arrest. *Anesth Analg.* 1959;38: 423–428.
13. Safar PJ. Community-wide cardiopulmonary resuscitation. *J Iowa Med Soc.* 1964;54:629–635.
14. Safar P. Effects of the postresuscitation syndrome on cerebral recovery from cardiac arrest. *Crit Care Med.* 1985;13(11):932–935.
15. Sterz F, Safar P, Tisherman S, et al. Mild hypothermic cardiopulmonary resuscitation improves outcome after prolonged cardiac arrest in dogs [see comment]. *Crit Care Med.* 1991;19(3):379–389.
16. Illievich UM, Zornow MH, Choi KT, et al. Effects of hypothermic metabolic suppression on hippocampal glutamate concentrations after transient global cerebral ischemia. *Anesth Analg.* 1994;78(5):905–911.
17. Bernard SA, Jones BM, Horne MK. Clinical trial of induced hypothermia in comatose survivors of out-of-hospital cardiac arrest. *Ann Emerg Med.* 1997;30:146–153.
18. Nagao K, Hayashi N, Kanmatsuse M, et al. Cardiopulmonary cerebral resuscitation using emergency cardiopulmonary bypass, coronary reperfusion therapy and mild hypothermia in patients with cardiac arrest outside the hospital. *J Am Coll Cardiol.* 2000;36(3):776–783.
19. Hachimi-Idrissi S, Corne L, Ebinger G, et al. Mild hypothermia induced by a helmet device: a clinical feasibility study. *Resuscitation.* 2001;51:275–281.
20. Bernard SA, Gray TW, Buist MD, et al. Treatment of comatose survivors of out-of-hospital cardiac arrest with induced hypothermia [see comment]. *N Engl J Med.* 2002;346(8):557–563.
21. Hypothermia after Cardiac Arrest Study Group. Mild therapeutic hypothermia to improve the neurologic outcome after cardiac arrest [see comment] [erratum appears in *N Engl J Med.* 2002;346(22):1756]. *N Engl J Med.* 2002;346(8):549–556.
22. Nolan JP, Morley PT, Vanden Hoek TL, et al. Therapeutic hypothermia after cardiac arrest: an advisory statement by the Advanced Life Support Task Force of the International Liaison Committee on Resuscitation. *Circulation.* 2003;108:118–121.
23. American Heart Association. 2005 American Heart Association guidelines for cardiopulmonary resuscitation and emergency cardiovascular care: part 7.5. Post resuscitation support. *Circulation.* 2005;112:IV-84–IV-88.
24. Al-Senani FM, Graffagnino C, Grotta JC, et al. A prospective, multicenter pilot study to evaluate the feasibility and safety of using the CoolGard System and Icy catheter following cardiac arrest. *Resuscitation.* 2004;62:143–150.
25. Busch M, Soreide E, Lossius HM, et al. Rapid implementation of therapeutic hypothermia in comatose out-of-hospital cardiac arrest survivors. *Acta Anaesthesiol Scand.* 2006;50(10):1277–1283.
26. Oddo M, Schaller MD, Feihl F, et al. From evidence to clinical practice: effective implementation of therapeutic hypothermia to improve patient outcome after cardiac arrest [see comment]. *Crit Care Med.* 2006;34(7): 1865–1873.
27. Hovdenes J, Laake JH, Aaberge L, et al. Therapeutic hypothermia after out-of-hospital cardiac arrest: experiences with patients treated with percutaneous coronary intervention and cardiogenic shock [see comment]. *Acta Anaesthesiol Scand.* 2007;51(2):137–142.
28. Gaieski DF, Band RA, Abella BS, et al. Early goal-directed hemodynamic optimization combined with therapeutic hypothermia in comatose survivors of out-of-hospital cardiac arrest. *Resuscitation.* 2009;80:418–424.
29. Sunde K, Pytte M, Jacobsen D, et al. Implementation of a standardised treatment protocol for post resuscitation

care after out-of-hospital cardiac arrest. *Resuscitation.* 2007;73(1):29–39.

30. Sagalyn E, Band RA, Gaieski DF, et al. Therapeutic hypothermia after cardiac arrest in clinical practice: review and compilation of recent experiences. *Crit Care Med.* 2009;37S:S223–S226.

31. Arrich J, The European Resuscitation Council Hypothermia After Cardiac Arrest Registry Study Group. Clinical application of mild therapeutic hypothermia after cardiac arrest. *Crit Care Med.* 2007;35:1041–1047.

32. Nielsen N, Hovdenes J, Nilsson F, et al. Outcome, timing and adverse events in therapeutic hypothermia after out-of-hospital cardiac arrest. *Acta Anaesthesiol Scand.* 2009;53:926–934.

33. Polderman K, Herold I. Therapeutic hypothermia and controlled normothermia in the intensive care unit: practical considerations, side effects, and cooling methods. *Crit Care Med.* 2009;37:1101–1120.

34. Caffrey SL, Willoughby PJ, Pepe PE, et al. Public use of automated external defibrillators. *N Engl J Med.* 2002; 347:1242–1247.

35. Abella BS, Alvarado JP, Myklebust H, et al. Quality of cardiopulmonary resuscitation during in-hospital cardiac arrest. *JAMA.* 2005;293:305–310.

36. Bobrow BJ, Clark LL, Ewy GA, et al. Minimally interrupted cardiac resuscitation by emergency medical services for out-of-hospital cardiac arrest. *JAMA.* 2008;299(10): 1158–1165.

37. Lurie KG, Idris A, Holcomb JB. Level 1 cardiac arrest centers: learning from the trauma surgeons [see comment]. *Acad Emerg Med.* 2005;12(1):79–80.

38. Carr BG, Schwab CW, Branas CC, et al. Outcomes related to the number and anatomic placement of gunshot wounds. *J Trauma Inj Infect Crit Care.* 2008;64(1): 197–202. Discussion 202–203.

CHAPTER 51

Pediatric Considerations

Fernando L. Soto

► INTRODUCTION

Pediatric visits account for 20–25% of visits to emergency departments in the United States. Most of these encounters will occur in general emergency departments, which may have limited capabilities to care for the critically ill child.[1,2] The priorities in the assessment and management of the pediatric patient are similar to those of the adult patient. The quoted ABCs of airway, breathing, and circulation still apply and are first and foremost in the evaluation of the young infant and child. There are certain anatomic, physiologic, developmental, and social considerations that are unique to this population and must be taken into account during the evaluation and treatment. This chapter will focus on the key differences in the treatment of the critically ill child. A complete discussion of the many procedures, as well as the presentation of every critical condition in pediatric patients, is well outside the scope of this text. See Table 51-1 for a list of medications used in pediatric resuscitation.

► AIRWAY

RECOGNITION OF RESPIRATORY DISTRESS

Compared with adults, infants and children have anatomic and physiologic characteristics that make them more susceptible to respiratory emergencies. During the first 6 months of life, they are obligate nose breathers, and their nasal passages can easily become occluded with a simple upper respiratory illness that will lead to obstruction. They have weak abdominal muscles and diaphragm, which tire easily during respiratory conditions. In addition, they have faster metabolic rates, which require a higher oxygen demand. This higher oxygen demand, coupled with a decreased functional residual capacity, makes them more vulnerable to decreases in their oxygen levels compared with those of adults.[3] It is based on these differences that children tend to have higher respiratory rates, even at rest. One must be familiar with the normal vital signs according to the age (see Table 51-2). Associated fatigue or sweating while feeding and weight changes will prompt the examiner to think of congestive heart failure or hereditary conditions such as cystic fibrosis.[3–5]

The child's general appearance is the best guide to the level of distress. Patients with mild tachypnea who smile or feed without difficulty and are able to track the examiner (maintain eye movement) are not in extremis. Close attention should be directed to those who look ill and appear irritable or lethargic. See Table 51-3 for a list of findings in the respiratory distressed child.

INITIAL AIRWAY MANAGEMENT

Failure to adequately manage the airway is a leading cause of preventable deaths in the pediatric population. Unlike adults, in whom cardiac failure is the primary cause of cardiopulmonary arrest, acute respiratory failure is responsible for most cardiopulmonary arrests in children.[4,5] Tachypnea is present in all but the most severe respiratory arrests—which will present with no air movement at all. Many illnesses in addition to respiratory disorders in this population can initially present with tachypnea, including sepsis, diabetic ketoacidosis (DKA), and abdominal pain. See Table 51-4 for the anatomic and physiologic differences in the pediatric airways and recommended treatment strategies.

▶ TABLE 51-1. **COMMON MEDICATIONS USED IN PEDIATRIC RESUSCITATION**

Epinephrine	0.01 mg/kg (0.1 mL/kg) IV every 3–5 min (1:10,000) in active resuscitation
Atropine	0.02 mg/kg IV every 5 min (minimum dose 0.1 mg, maximum dose 1.0 mg)
Adenosine	0.1 mg/kg IV (maximum dose 6 mg). May double to 0.2 (maximum dose 12 mg)
Amiodarone	5 mg/kg bolus for pulseless VT and over 20–60 min if perfusing arrhythmia—expert consultation advised
Narcan	0.1 mg/kg/dose IM/ET/IV/IO every 2–3 min (maximum dose 2 mg/dose)
Glucose	5–10 mL/kg of D10W in neonates and infants
	2–4 mL/kg of D25W in young children
	1–2 mL/kg of D50W in older children and adults
Calcium	100 mg/kg 10% calcium gluconate or 20 mg/kg of 10% calcium chloride
Lidocaine	1 mg/kg IV, and then infusion
Bicarbonate	1 mEq/kg, may repeat every 10 min
Prostaglandin E1	0.5 µg/kg/min IV (at lowest effective dose)

AIRWAY PLACEMENT

Nasal and oral airways are used to overcome the mechanical obstruction produced by the tongue in patients with decreased level of consciousness. To place a nasopharyngeal airway, apply some lubricant to the airway and

▶ TABLE 51-2 **APPROXIMATE NORMAL VITAL SIGNS OF PEDIATRIC PATIENTS BY AGE**

Age Group	Respiratory Rate (breaths/min)	Heart Rate (beats/min)	Systolic BP (mm Hg)
<1 month	30–60	90–160	60 ± 10
1–12 months	24–30	110–180	89 ± 25
1–2 years	20–24	90–150	96 ± 30
2–4 years	20–24	75–135	99 ± 25
4–6 years	20–24	60–130	100 ± 20
6–8 years	12–20	60–120	105 ± 13
8–10 years	12–20	60–120	110 ± 15
10–12 years	12–20	60–120	112 ± 15
12–14 years	12–20	60–120	115 ± 20
14 to adult	10–16	60–120	120 ± 20

Formulas that may help treating infants and young children:
Blood pressure estimate:

70 + (2 × age) = 50th percentile
90 + (2 × age) = 90th percentile

Estimated body weight (kg) = 2 × (age in years) + 8 or (9 + age in months)/2
A patient should double birth weight by 6 months, and then triple it by 1 year of age (estimated weight in a 1-year-old ~10 kg).

▶ TABLE 51-3. **SIGNS AND SYMPTOMS IN THE CHILD WITH RESPIRATORY DISTRESS**

Finding	Comment
Grunting	Increases auto-PEEP; maintains functional residual capacity
Tripod position	Relieves airway obstruction
Retractions	Supraclavicular or abdominal
Stridor	Consider upper airway obstruction
Apneic spells	Impending respiratory arrest in infants
Coughing	Expiratory mechanism in
Head bobbing	bronchospasm or obstruction
Nasal flaring	

Key: PEEP, positive end-expiratory pressure.

insert gently, angling back toward the pharynx.[5] A few drops of a nasal decongestant such as oxymethazoline can be added and may decrease bleeding through the nares. Oropharyngeal airways (OA) can only be used in unconscious patients with an absent cough or gag reflex. Carefully measure the airway to avoid moving the epiglottis or the tongue, worsening the obstruction. To measure the airway, place the OA by the child's cheek and hold one of the OA to the corner of the mouth and the other corner to the angle of the jaw.[6]

OXYGEN ADMINISTRATION

Administration of oxygen is vital in any respiratory illness. Pediatric patients have a very small tolerance for hypoxia. Young infants may benefit from blow-by oxygen by cupping the hand or small nasal cannulas. Cannulas have the advantage of providing oxygen while creating a small amount of positive end-expiratory pressure (PEEP), both of which stimulate the infant while preventing apneic spells. The best way to deliver close to 100% oxygen is with a face mask with a reservoir such as a non-rebreather mask. This may be uncomfortable to very young children, so using alternative methods is recommended.[6,7]

MEDICATIONS

Next to oxygen, the most important pharmacologic intervention to consider in respiratory failure is epinephrine. Epinephrine is a natural endogenous catecholamine, both α- and β-agonist. At low dose, it is primarily a β-receptor agonist causing strong bronchodilation, decreasing mucosal edema, and improving cardiovascular status with a very short onset of action.[8] It may be administered intramuscularly or intravenously in anaphylactic reaction, depending on the severity of shock. The subcutaneous route is no longer used because of poor delivery. For respiratory distress, upper airway obstruction, or edema, it can be administered in nebulized form. The standard dose is racemic epinephrine

► TABLE 51-4. **STRUCTURAL DIFFERENCES IN THE PEDIATRIC AIRWAY VERSUS ADULT AIRWAY**

Anatomy	Effect	Intervention
Larger occiput relative to body	Promotes passive flexion of cervical spine leading to airway obstruction	Maintain sniffing position; avoid hyperextension. Rolled towel under shoulder may assist
Smaller airway	More susceptible to airway obstruction from edema, mucous plugs, or foreign bodies	Oral and nasal inspection and suctioning
Larynx higher and more anterior	Difficult to visualize the vocal cords during intubation	Cricoid pressure can facilitate intubation
Narrowest portion of trachea at level of the cricoid ring	Dictates size of ETT	Use cuffed ETT in children older than 8 years of age. Use cuffed or 0.5–1.0 size smaller uncuffed ETT in younger patients
Short trachea	Intubation of right mainstem bronchus more likely	Vigilance with depth of ETT insertion (formula: $3 \times$ ETT size at lip)
Relatively large tongue and a floppy epiglottis	Tongue can fall back against the posterior pharynx with loss of tone, deep sedation, or CNS dysfunction	Chin lift. Jaw thrust in suspected cervical spine injury. Use oral airway only in unconscious patients. May use nasal airway in conscious patients but avoid in suspected basilar skull fractures, CSF leaks, or coagulopathy

Key: ETT, endotracheal tube; CNS, central nervous system; CSF, cerebrospinal fluid.

0.5 mL of the 2.25% concentration. "Crash cart" epinephrine (1:1,000) may also be used by administering 5.5 mL in nebulized form. Specific pharmacologic interventions will be discussed with specific conditions below.

VENTILATION

In some situations, positioning and administration of oxygen or other medications is not enough, and assistance in ventilation may be required. Respiratory failure is described by some authors as hypoxemia (arterial Po_2 < 60 mm Hg) and hypercarbia (arterial Pco_2 > 55 mm Hg) with associated respiratory acidosis. Intubation is considered a clinical decision and should not be withheld waiting for any laboratory testing.[5] Signs of impending respiratory failure include altered sensorium or deterioration in mentation, progressive hypoxemia, severe work of breathing, silent chest, apnea. For a complete list, please refer to Table 51-5.

► TABLE 51-5. **INDICATIONS FOR ENDOTRACHEAL INTUBATION**

- Cardiac arrest (or impending arrest)
- Severe respiratory distress as evidenced by accessory muscle use and fatigue, nasal flaring, altered mentation, grunting, silent chest, bradypnea, etc.
- Unsuccessful airway management with bag–valve mask ventilation
- Hypoxemia (Po_2 < 50 mm Hg), hypercarbia (Pco_2 > 55 mm Hg)
- Coma or absent gag reflex
- Severe trauma or shock

The ability to provide proper bag–valve ventilation is a vital skill in the airway management of adult and pediatric patients. In the prehospital setting, studies have shown that bag ventilation may be as beneficial, if not more so, as endotracheal intubation.[9,10] Ventilations may be provided for a prolonged amount of time with care not to overinflate the stomach. Increasing pressure in the stomach will increase the likelihood of vomiting and, therefore, the risk for aspiration. Overinflating the stomach may also impair ventilation by increasing intra-abdominal pressure, which would not allow the diaphragm to move adequately. Adding a nasogastric tube whenever prolonged bagged ventilation is anticipated may decrease the occurrence of these complications.

► BREATHING

Pediatric patients have smaller airways, which lead to higher resistance to flow as well as a higher propensity for obstruction. They also have an increased likelihood of adenoid tissue tonsil hypertrophy. In terms of movement of the lungs, the diaphragm has a smaller zone of apposition and horizontal ribs, which are less efficient and therefore increase the work of breathing. Finally, in younger children especially, immature musculature and higher metabolic rates may predispose to respiratory failure.[4,11]

NONINVASIVE POSITIVE PRESSURE VENTILATION (NIPPV)

NIPPV is the administration of a gas mixture at a preset pressure by way of nasal prongs or a face mask. Positive pressure is provided in either continuous or variable pressure to prevent alveolar collapse and maintain an adequate functional residual capacity by decreasing the work of breathing. Based on the modality used, continuous positive airway pressure (CPAP) provides a constant pressure at end expiration or variable/bilevel positive airway pressure (VPAP or BiPAP) that provides two levels of pressure: inspiratory positive airway pressure (IPAP) and a lower expiratory positive airway pressure (EPAP). The level of pressure can be modified based on the patient's need and response. Variable modes also offer the option to activate spontaneous IPAP, which is activated at a set rate, thus time triggered (at set intervals), or spontaneous, which triggers an IPAP when spontaneous inspiratory effort is detected, or a combination of both.

NIPPV is preferred initially in carefully selected groups of patients in order to treat their hypoxemia while reversing the disease process in attempt to avoid endotracheal intubation (see Chapter 6).

Most studies for pediatric applications of NIPPV have been done in neonates, where it is used for conditions such as transient tachypnea of the newborn, apnea of prematurity, and respiratory distress syndrome. Classically, neonates were placed on a continuous NIPPV or CPAP mode. Recent work has shown that BiPAP has a faster resolution of symptoms, is better tolerated, and has fewer side effects.[12,13]

In infants and older children, it is less established. Similar indications and contraindications apply to use with children than with adults. Patients who could benefit from this modality need to be conscious, have a protected airway with an intact gag reflex, and be able to breathe spontaneously. Contraindications to this therapy are facial injuries, impending respiratory failure, altered mental status, or inability to maintain the airway.[13,14]

The pediatric patient will need some sedation for optimal management. Ketamine has been established as the sedative of choice. It enables the patient to keep the airway intact. It also has bronchodilator effects and its safety record makes it the best choice for this particular procedure.[13] Benzodiazepines are not recommended due to their effects on respiratory depression in an already compromised patient.

CPAP initial recommended setting is 10–14 cm H_2O. "Bubble CPAP," in addition to the CPAP, provides a high-frequency ventilation effect, producing small vibrations in the infant's chest at the frequency of 15–30 Hz. This modality, if used in neonates, might contribute to gas exchange, reducing the work of breathing.

For BiPAP, the initial recommended settings are an inspiratory pressure of 12–15 cm H_2O and an expiratory pressure of 6–7 cm H_2O.

INVASIVE POSITIVE PRESSURE VENTILATION

Definitive airway management entails endotracheal intubation and mechanical ventilation. In the presence of severe trauma, altered mental status leading to coma, organ failure, or respiratory depression, a definitive airway should be considered. There are some crucial differences in ventilation between children and adults. Even if you are familiar with ventilation, consulting an expert in pediatric intensive care is highly recommended whenever you reach this point.

INTUBATION

The most important considerations for a successful intubation are evaluation of the airway, anticipating complications, and having the necessary equipment. If time permits and the required equipment or staff are unavailable, assist ventilation using bag–valve ventilation until everything is ready.

There are two commonly used laryngeal blade shapes in emergency departments today: Miller, or straight blade, and the Macintosh, or curved blade. Both come in different sizes. For pediatric patients, the Miller blade is generally preferred since it can displace the large floppy epiglottis and may help reach the pediatric vocal chords, which will be superior and anterior. Either blade may be used according to the level of the practitioner's expertise and level of comfort.

Endotracheal tubes (ETTs) also come in different shapes and sizes. There are many ways to calculate the size of the ETT for your patient. A simple way to remember is by using the patient's little finger. The pinky should be as large as the airway, plus or minus a few millimeters. Applying the formula of adding 4 to the patient's age divided by 4 (**[age + 4]/4**) gives an approximation of the tube size. Multiplying the ETT size by 3 gives an approximation of the number where the tube should rest against the lip commissure. For example, a 4-0 ETT should be introduced with the 12-cm mark at the lip. Recent recommendations state that cuffed tubes should be used in children older than 8 years of age, while both types (cuffed or uncuffed) may be safely used in younger children and infants, except newborns. Under certain conditions such as increased lung resistance, cuffed tubes may actually be preferred.[5,6]

The most reliable approach in an emergency situation, which can be very stressful, is to use a length-based resuscitation system such as the commercial Broselow™ tape with color-coordinated code cart shelves. These can be used in children 12 years or younger and give information on ETT sizes, blade numbers, indwelling catheters, as well as medication dosages based on the patient's ideal weight. There is current controversy on whether the tapes accurately measure the patient's weight, since children today are heavier than their counterparts 10 or 15 years ago. Even then, it may be useful to utilize this guide. It is also important to remember that these are only guidelines and that ETTs a half a size larger or smaller should be ready and available in case there is any complication.

RAPID SEQUENCE INTUBATION (RSI)

RSI has become the cornerstone in emergency airway management. Since its advent, outcomes in emergent endotracheal intubations of children and adults have improved greatly. Careful attention should be directed to the patient with a potentially difficult airway. RSI consists of a administering a sedative agent and a paralytic agent followed by endotracheal intubation to minimize complications such as vomiting, aspiration, and hypoxia.[15,16] There are a few mnemonics out there that describe the process. It is important to remember that even if the patient is not undergoing paralysis for any particular reason, following the steps is very useful in assuring the best possible outcome. For a list of RSI medications and dosages, please see Table 51-6.

The steps in RSI include:

1. Preparation
2. Preoxygenation
3. Premedication
4. Paralyze
5. Pass the tube
6. Proof of placement
7. Postintubation care

Preparation includes anticipating equipment requirements, calculating dosages, assessing the airway, and testing the equipment. As discussed, always keep in mind the possible complications and unexpected outcomes. At this step, it is crucial to anticipate the need for other services such as anesthesia among other types of airway equipment.

Preoxygenation is performed by administering 100% oxygen for at least 3 minutes, which will "wash out the nitrogen" and provide an oxygen reserve for most patients for up to several minutes of apnea. As discussed, younger patients have a smaller reserve and will reach hypoxia faster. Oxygen can be applied by non-rebreather mask or by bag–valve ventilation. It is important to note that self-inflating bags will not provide flow unless ventilations are given. If this equipment is being used, attempts to synchronize with the patient's breathing effort will maximize oxygen delivery.

Premedication includes administration of medications to avoid increases in intracranial pressure as well as depolarizing agents and sedatives. In pediatric patients, atropine is administered to blunt the vasovagal hypotension that can occur during laryngoscopy. Intravenous lidocaine is also given, especially in head trauma patients, in order to decrease the gag reflex, thereby minimizing the rise in ICP that the procedure may cause. At this phase, a sedative may also be administered, prior to paralytics.[16]

For sedation purposes, there are many pharmacologic options. Ketamine is well studied in the pediatric population and it is safe in patients with hypotension or shock. It is also recommended in patients with respiratory conditions such as asthma, as it induces bronchodilation and increases blood flow. Although controversial, it is still not recommended in patients with increased ICP since it is thought to worsen their conditions.[17] Benzodiazepines are safe in patients who are to be intubated but should be avoided in the presence of hypotension. Etomidate is safe in patients undergoing intubation since it does not affect cerebral blood flow or blood pressure and lasts less than 20 minutes. Side effects include transient myoclonic movements. The clinical relevance of etomidate-related adrenal insufficiency has been called into question by several studies. But patient populations especially at risk are the septic shock patients in an already suppressed state, in whom it causes adrenal suppression. Largely prospective trials are needed for validation.[18] Propofol is another candidate that is neuroprotective by decreasing neuronal metabolism but may induce hypotension. The brand name Diprivan™ should be avoided in patients with egg allergy, but the generic drug is safe. Barbiturates, especially Thiopental™, have the same safety profile as propofol but with higher neuroprotective action by reducing ICP, cerebral metabolism, and cerebral oxygen demands. However, the vasodilation and myocardial depression causing hypotension and the real potential risk of bronchospasms made the barbiturates fall out of favor during RSI.

Paralyzing is the process of total muscle relaxation; yet the patient might still be conscious, thus the sedation. The two most commonly used paralytic agents are: the depolarizing agent, that is, succinylcholine, and the nondepolarizing agents, that is, rocuronium, pancuronium, and vecuronium. Succinylcholine is a fast-acting, short-lasting depolarizing agent; you can see the onset of action as the membranes get depolarized and the patient fasciculates. There is a relative contraindication in patients with an increased ICP. It is contraindicated in patients with potential hyperkalemia or causes that can cause hyperkalemia such as suspected renal failure, muscular disorders, prolonged bed rest, and subacute

► TABLE 51-6. **LIST OF RSI MEDICATIONS**

Atropine	0.02 mg/kg (min 0.1 mg, max 1.0 mg) IV, IM
Lidocaine	1 mg/kg (max dose 100 mg) IV
Thiopental	3–5 mg/kg (max dose 25–75 mg) IV
Ketamine	1–2 mg/kg IV or 3–4 mg/kg IM
Etomidate	0.3 mg/kg IV
Midazolam	0.1–0.2 mg/kg IV, IM
Propofol	2.5 mg/kg (max dose 20 mg/bolus) IV
Succinylcholine	1–2 mg/kg (max 100 mg) IV, IM
Rocuronium	0.6–1 mg/kg IV
Vecuronium	0.1–0.2 mg/kg IV

burns, since these conditions may cause a transient rise in potassium. On the other hand, rocuronium is one of many nondepolarizing agents available for RSI. It is has a very short onset of action and, since it does not depolarize the membranes, does not affect potassium or rise in increased ICP.[19]

In *passing the tube*, the best way to verify placement is by visualizing passing of the ETT through the vocal cords. In pediatric patients, the narrower part of the airway is the subglottic space, while in the adult population, it is the vocal cords. The tube should be visualized just past the cords. The previously described formula can be used to approximate position.

Placement confirmation: auscultate the epigastrium first and then verify that breath sounds are symmetric in both lung fields. The use of a colorimetric or end-tidal CO_2 detector to confirm adequate ventilation is now the recommended method and the most sensitive method for confirming tube placement.[5] A chest radiograph is always ordered to verify the depth of placement: the end of the ETT should be 2–3 cm above the carina.

Postintubation care includes placing the patient on a mechanical ventilator (see below) and introducing a nasogastric tube to decompress the stomach. Arterial blood gasses are sent 10–15 minutes after intubation to assess oxygenation and ventilation status. The head of the bed should be kept at 45° to decrease the risk of aspiration. This is also important in patients with increased ICP as this maneuver alone may greatly improve this condition. Order restrain and appropriate sedation.

MECHANICAL VENTILATION

Mechanical ventilators have many different settings that go beyond the scope of this chapter.

For infants and neonates younger than 1 year or weighing less than 10 kg, the ventilator is usually set in pressure limited cycles since most ventilators cannot deliver a restricted low tidal volume, as small as 40–60 mL. Pressure cycles have always been the preferred mode in young patients and neonates, since they deliver a set pressure, and flow stops once the pressure is reached, thus limiting barotrauma and decreasing the rate of ventilator-induced lung injury (VILI). The downside of this modality is that tidal volumes (V_t) are variable and not guaranteed, with potential for hypoxemia. In situations with decreased lung compliance a decrease in the V_t reaching the lungs is seen, whereas in situations with increased compliance the V_t will exceed the expected. To begin ventilation with this modality, pick either synchronized intermittent mandatory ventilation (SIMV) or assist control (AC) mode. The trigger will be a pressure, so set positive inspiratory pressure (PIP) between 15 and 20 cm H_2O and titrate just enough to get an adequate chest rise. Set the PEEP at 3–5 cm H_2O.[7] Maintaining oxygen saturation above 92% guarantees appropriate oxygenation.

In older children and adults, volume cycles seem to be the preferred mode; the ventilator will deliver a set V_t regardless of the pressure necessary to achieve that delivery.

The peak pressure at end inspiration, (PIP) is a function of the inflation volume, flow resistance, and the elastic recoil of the lung and chest wall, but has nothing to do with the plateau pressure that in turn is at end inspiration when there is no air flow. Plateau pressure is a surrogate for transalveolar pressure and is directly proportional to the elasticity of the lungs and chest wall. The rapid, repetitive opening of alveoli has been associated with barotraumas and VILI. For initial settings, consider: V_t of 5–8 mL/kg, the respiratory rate at 12–20 adjusted for age, with a PEEP of 3–5 cm H_2O. Different modalities and modifications should be done depending on the etiology requiring this therapy and changed according to clinical condition. See Table 51-7 for initial ventilation settings in pediatric patients. Something to remember: there are very limited evidence-based data on specific modalities. Choice of modality is user driven, and the users should use the mode they feel most comfortable with. The goal should be to ventilate and oxygenate with minimal lung damage.

▶ **TABLE 51-7. INITIAL SETTINGS ON FOR PEDIATRIC PATIENTS ON MECHANICAL VENTILATION**

Parameter	Infants (<10 kg) or those with decreased compliance	Older children and adults
Modality	Pressure-controlled	Volume-controlled: assist control (AC) or SIMV
Settings	Positive inspiratory pressure (PIP) 15–20 cm H_2O (minimal required for adequate chest rise)	Tidal volume: 5–8 mL/kg
Respiratory rate	30–40 breaths/min	Adequate for age (12–20 breaths/min)
FiO_2	Begin at 100% and decrease to lowest possible required for adequate O_2 saturation near 99%	
I:E ratio/IT	Inspiratory:expiratory ratio of 1:2 or inspiratory time of 0.5 s (may be modified as per special requirements [e.g., air trapping])	
PEEP	3–5 cm H_2O higher if poor lung compliance (i.e., ARDS) or none at all if air trapping present (i.e., asthma)	

Avoid unnecessarily high levels of oxygen by keeping the fraction of inspired oxygen (FiO_2) at the lowest level to maintain adequate oxygenation to avoid oxygen toxicity. There is a higher correlation of oxygen toxicity and FiO_2 above 70, so it is reasonable to titrate the FiO_2 using O_2 saturation or the ABG's.[18]

Acute respiratory distress syndrome is defined as a Pao_2/FiO_2 ratio of less than 200, with the presence of bilateral infiltrates on chest radiography (radiographically similar to pulmonary edema) without left atrial pressure elevation (wedge should be less than 18 mm Hg). In the advent of ARDS or to prevent it, lung-protective ventilation is recommended using V_t 4–6 mL/kg in conjunction with a higher respiratory rate to achieve an adequate minute ventilation, limiting plateau pressure to <30 cm H_2O. Hypercapnia is expected, and the term *permissive hypercapnia* is tolerated as long the arterial pH is kept above 7.20. This trial in adults and pediatric populations showed a significant decrease in mortality. Pediatric patients who have worsening hypoxemia should be referred early for extracorporeal membrane oxygenation (ECMO) (see Chapter 7).

► CIRCULATION

Shock is a state of inadequate tissue perfusion of oxygen and normal cellular function. The causes of shock include: pump failure (i.e., cardiogenic shock), hypovolemia (i.e., dehydration, bleeding), or vasodilation (i.e., anaphylaxis or sepsis). The body will adjust to maintain perfusion and O_2 delivery via the microcirculatory and macrocirculatory systems. In the event of hypovolemia, several mechanisms are employed in order to compensate for the resulting decrease in venous return that, itself, results in decreased CO. Such mechanisms include adrenal release of catecholamines, which induce tachycardia (increased heart rate), increased cardiac contractility leading to increased stroke volume (SV), and peripheral vasoconstriction. This is in response to insufficient stretch sensed by carotid and aortic baroreceptors. In reference to vasoconstriction, venoconstriction will support intrathoracic volume and produce an increase in preload, whereas arterial constriction will increase perfusion pressure that in turn directly increases organ blood flow. The renin–angiotensin system is activated to increase sodium and water reabsorption and augment systemic vascular resistance. Glucagon is excreted leading to hyperglycemia by increasing gluconeogenesis and glycogenolysis that, coupled with decreased renal blood flow and lactic acid production from anaerobic metabolism, may lead to acidosis.[19]

Prolonged failure to maintain adequate perfusion pressure to critical organs is incompatible with life. In light of this, blood perfusion may be redirected and limited to organs essential to life with nonvital organs suffering the detrimental effect of lack of blood perfusion. This is a method of maintaining mean arterial pressure (MAP) under the conditions of hypovolemia and, ultimately, organ hypoperfusion.[19–21]

Pediatric patients respond differently to shock than do adults. The first and most sensitive response to shock in a pediatric patient is tachycardia. The myocardium is underdeveloped that prevents them from modifying their SV as needed. Therefore, the only way that cardiac output is increased is by raising the heart rate. It is important to note that in children, blood pressure in itself should not be used to monitor severity of illness or response to treatment. Young patients have a very strong response to a decrease in effective circulatory volume. They have lower baseline blood pressures and are able to increase their systemic vascular resistance and heart rate to compensate. This benefit, at the same time, gives the examiner a false sense of security since hypotension may not be observed until approaching cardiac arrest. Prompt recognition and reversal of shock is warranted to avoid morbidity and mortality.[20]

CATEGORIZING AND TREATING SHOCK

The many etiologies responsible for shock can be divided into different categories based on the type of dysfunction present. Shock may be categorized as cardiogenic, hemorrhagic, neurogenic, obstructive, dissociative, or distributive in nature. See Table 51-8 for shock etiologies and their treatment.

Hemorrhagic or hypovolemic shock occurs whenever intravascular volume is depleted. It can ensue from bleeding or dehydration with associated electrolytic disturbances. In pediatric patients, the most common cause worldwide is secondary to vomiting and/or diarrhea. Other common causes include burns, trauma, and metabolic disorders such as DKA. Treatment includes isotonic volume expansion followed by blood transfusion in the trauma setting. In the presence of shock, the initial bolus is 20 mL/kg over 5–10 minutes followed by reassessment of vital signs and mental status. Studies have shown similar outcomes whenever crystalloids or colloids are used, as long as resuscitation is adequate.[22–25] In the trauma setting, blood is administered at 10-mL/kg aliquots after initial expansion of 40 mL/kg of normal saline or Ringer's lactate. Younger infants and children with cardiac or renal conditions should receive smaller boluses of 10 mL/kg with close monitoring to avoid fluid overload.

In obstructive shock, intravascular volume is normal but the flowing process is affected. Causes of obstructive shock include pericardial tamponade, pulmonary embolism, pneumothorax, or congenital heart disease (CHD) (i.e., ductal dependent lesions). Other

▶ **TABLE 51-8. DIFFERENT TYPES OF SHOCK IN CHILDREN AND THEIR TREATMENT**

Type/Clinical Scenario	Pathophysiology	Signs and Symptoms	Treatment
Hypovolemic Most common cause is vomiting and diarrhea. May be seen in any type of bleeding or TS (nephrotic syndrome, pancreatitis, burns, etc.)	↓ CO ↑ SVR IV and Int losses	↑ HR ↓ BP ↑ RR Prolonged CR Dry skin Oliguria AMS	Initial 20 mL/kg bolus × 1–2 If hemorrhagic, provide pRBCs at 10 mL/kg after second bolus Look for site of blood loss (abdomen, open wounds, large bone fractures, etc.) Administer 10 mL/kg of NSS in cases of DKA, cerebral edema, or fluid overload (e.g., renal failure, CHF, etc.)
Septic Acutely ill with suspicion or evident source of infection Three main mechanisms	↑ CO, ↓ SVR (20%)	↑ HR, ↓ BP, ↑ RR, AMS, bounding pulses, flushing, TS, edema	Repeat 20 mL/kg bolus; may need >60 mL/kg in first hour (up to 200 mL/kg in some cases).[18] Consider colloids Add inotropics as per protocol. Dopamine is first choice
	↓ CO, ↑ SVR (60%)	↑ HR, normal or ↓ BP, ↑ RR, AMS, ↓ pulses, delayed CR, TS, edema	Consider epinephrine (cold shock) or norepinephrine (warm shock) Treat hypoglycemia/hyperglycemia and hypocalcemia, and protect from hypothermia Consider steroids for catecholamine-resistant shock.
	↓ CO ↓ SVR (20%)	↑ HR, ↓ BP, ↑ RR, AMS, ↓ pulses, delayed CR, TS, edema	
Distributive **Anaphylaxis:** Hx allergy and/or exposure to allergen, vomiting, rash, flushing, etc.	↑ CO, ↓ SVR	Angioedema, rapid TS, ↓ BP, respiratory distress	Start with epinephrine, steroids, and antihistamines. May require continuous epinephrine infusion
Spinal cord injury: Patients present after contusion/transection of cervical spine (T6 or above) sympathetic loss with unopposed vagal tone	Normal CO, ↓ SVR	↓ BP, with normal to ↓ HR, paralysis with loss of vascular tone	Aggressive fluid therapy Pharmacologic support of SVR with vasopressors: norepinephrine or phenylephrine Evaluate and treat associated injuries
Cardiogenic History evident for congenital heart disease, myocarditis, dysrhythmias, etc.	↓ CO, normal to ↑ SVR	Normal to ↑ HR, ↓ pulses, delayed CR, oliguria, JVD, hepatomegaly BP normal until late in course	Pharmacologic support of CO with dobutamine, milrinone, and dopamine Judicious fluid replacement as indicated clinically. Prostaglandin E1 in cases of ductal dependent lesions

Key: CO, cardiac output; SVR, systemic vascular resistance; HR, heart rate; RR, respiratory rate; CR, capillary refill; BP, blood pressure; AMS, altered mental status; TS, third spacing; Hx, history; NSS, normal saline solution; IV and Int losses, intravascular and interstitial losses; JVD, jugular vein distension; CHF, congestive heart failure. *Note:* Signs and symptoms are not in order of progression and some may not be observed at all (i.e., low BP). **Pediatric patients will have normal BP until late in the course.**

causes of obstructive shock will be discussed elsewhere in this book.

Cardiogenic shock occurs when the pump fails to propel the blood due to intrinsic myocyte dysfunction. In pediatric patients, the common causes include infectious etiologies such as myocarditis or pericarditis, cardiac dysrhythmias, and those secondary to CHD. Depending on the etiology, different therapies are warranted. Arrhythmias should be corrected with the use of amiodarone, β-blockers, calcium channel blockers, or adenosine. Pericarditis and myocarditis may benefit from inotropic medications such as dopamine. For a list of vasopressors, see Table 51-8. CHD requires a particular set of treatments depending on the pathophysiology involved. Shock within the first 4–6 weeks should prompt examiners to consider CHD. In these situations, the administration of prostaglandin E1 may be life saving with the goal of maintaing the ductus arteriosus open.[25]

► TABLE 51-9. **MANIFESTATIONS OF ANAPHYLAXIS**

Cutaneous (80–90%)	Pruritis, flushing, warmth, urticaria, angioedema
Respiratory (90%)	Itching of mouth or throat, throat or chest tightness, nasal congestion, hoarseness, wheezing, stridor, dyspnea
Cardiovascular (30%)	Faintness, palpitations, hypotension, shock
Gastrointestinal (30%)	Nausea, cramps, diarrhea, vomiting
Other	Itchy, watery eyes, dizziness, impending sense of doom

Distributive shock involves patients with normal plasma volume that has been displaced by loss of vascular tone or increased capillary leakage. Patients with this type of shock usually have anaphylactic reactions, infectious processes such as sepsis or dengue shock syndrome, or an acute inflammatory state, all of which will increase capillary leakage as a third-spacing phenomenon.

Anaphylaxis is a common cause of distributive shock. Pediatric patients most commonly develop anaphylactic reactions from exposure to exogenous antigens such as food and medications.[26] Signs and symptoms can be cutaneous, respiratory, cardiovascular, gastrointestinal, and generalized. A list of signs and symptoms can be found in Table 51-9. It is important to note that in many instances, the urticaria and flushing may lag presentation of more severe symptoms by minutes to hours. Treatment involves epinephrine (1:1,000) 0.15 (< 30kg) or 0.3–0.5 mL (> 30 kg) delivered into the medial thigh region. Recent studies have shown that the IM route achieves a faster peak in delivery and better symptom response than subcutaneous administration. In addition, corticosteroids, H_2 blocking agents, and antihistamines should be administered. If symptoms persist, repeated doses of epinephrine should be continued every 5–15 minutes. In the presence of hypotension, epinephrine should be administered IV and an epinephrine drip considered for persistent shock. Delayed reactions may occur up to 72 hours after the initial reaction. Close observation and follow-up are advised.[27]

Neurogenic shock is observed in the setting of spine trauma at the T6 level and above. Findings include hypotension, bradycardia, and flushed extremities associated to a decreased CO. Treatment includes spine immobilization, normal saline boluses, and vasopressors such as norepinephrine or epinephrine.

In dissociative shock, there is an uncoupling between oxygen demand and energy production caused by poisoning and intoxication such as cyanide, aspirin,

or methemoglobin. The definite treatment includes IV fluid boluses and administration of a specific antidote.

IV access is vital in the treatment of any kind of shock. Placement of two peripheral lines is usually more than enough but in cases of severe shock and dehydration, it may prove difficult. Classic teaching states that in the critically ill child, inability to gain vascular access within three attempts or 90 seconds should prompt placement of an intraosseous (IO) line. Newer systems make this process easier and anticipating a difficult line may be more than enough. Through an IO, fluids and resuscitation drugs may be administered easily. For a more definite access, performing a central line using the Seldinger technique will also provide the ability to get blood for sampling. In children and infants, the preferred approach is the femoral and external jugular veins.[28]

SEPTIC SHOCK

Sepsis is defined as a suspected or confirmed source of infection in a patient with two or more of the following systems involved:

1. Temperature >38.3°C (>101°F) or <36°C (<96.8°F)
2. Heart rate >90 beats/min
3. Respiratory rate >20 breaths/min
4. Acute mental status change
5. Hyperglycemia in the absence of diabetes
6. WBC count >12,000 and <4,000/mm³, or >10% immature (bands)

Severe sepsis is defined as an acute sepsis causing organ dysfunction, hypoperfusion, or hypotension before fluid challenge, whereas septic shock is the evidence of persistent hypoperfusion after fluid challenge in a patient with severe sepsis. This has been closely studied in both the adult and the pediatric populations. In a study by Han et al, approximately 3% of pediatric transports to a pediatric emergency department had a final diagnosis of septic shock. In this article, mortality approached 25% in this population.[29] According to new pediatric guidelines, the use of resuscitation protocols as recommended by the Society of Critical Care Medicine decreased mortality to approximately 2% in previously healthy children and 10% in chronically ill children, with a number needed to treat of 3.3. Pediatric patients will require proportionally more fluid in resuscitation due to their usual hypovolemic state and earlier intubation strategies due to their low functional residual capacity.[21]

Other differences include variations in their capacity to respond to SV requirements and their cardiovascular response to septic shock. For instance, based on the formula CO = SVR × HR, if an adult faces a need for increased SV, doubling the resting heart rate from

▶ TABLE 51-10. **VASOPRESSOR THERAPY**

Inotropic Agent	Effect	Dosing (µg/kg/min)	Recommendation
Dopamine	Dopaminergic	1–5	Initial treatment of septic shock unresponsive to initial fluids, during initial resuscitation. Particularly useful when ↓ CO + ↓ SVR
	β-Adrenergic	5–15	
	α-Adrenergic	>15	
Norepinephrine	α, β	0.01–0.3	If unresponsive to dopamine infusion in the presence of warm shock (norepinephrine) or cold shock (epinephrine)
Epinephrine	β, α (higher doses)	0.01–0.3	
Dobutamine	β	5–15	Use with dopamine for initial treatment of hyperdynamic or "cold" shock (↑ SVR and ↓ CO)

Key: SVR, systemic vascular resistance; CO, cardiac output.

70 to 140 will more than double the CO. On the other hand, infants and children have, at baseline, higher resting heart rates and doubling the resting heart rate from 150 to 300 will not be as effective, shortening diastolic time leading to decreased coronary artery perfusion and cardiac preload time.[22] Further, the clinical presentation of septic shock in young children or infants will present different variations leading to cold or warm shock, whereas adults usually present with a state of elevated CO with decreased SVR. These differences may be observed in the initial physical exam but may become more evident once the initial resuscitation has taken place in the emergency department. Finally, most pediatric septic shock is linked to volume depletion, which is the reason they require comparatively more fluid than do adults, usually 40–60 mL/kg, and to some extremes up to 200 mL/kg in the first hours or resuscitation.[20]

RECOGNITION

Diagnosis in pediatric septic shock is mainly clinical. Children commonly present with tachycardia, vasodilation, and fever. In septic shock, additional findings include hypothermia or hyperthermia, changes in mental status, oliguria, prolonged capillary refill (more than 2 seconds) in cold shock, and peripheral vasodilation in warm shock. Hypotension with bounding pulses is considered warm shock; diminished peripheral perfusion with prolonged CR is considered compensated cold shock, while hypotension with associated prolonged CR is considered decompensated shock. The expected heart rate should be between 90 and 160 bpm in young infants and between 70 and 150 bpm in children. These have the same goal: to monitor with improvement in condition.[20]

The workup should be directed at finding a source. Bacterial etiologies are usually sought, but viral syndromes are seen as common agents as well. Along with the usual workup, there should be other considerations. Although the adult literature recommends that lactate be sampled and monitored as evidence of hypoper-

fusion, there is no consensus for this in the pediatric literature. This test should probably be added to the initial evaluation, but its benefit has not been clearly established. On the other hand, according to the recent literature, elevated troponin levels in pediatric patients may be useful in predicting myocardial dysfunction and a subsequent decrease in CO.[30]

The main goal of treatment in pediatric septic shock is early recognition, followed by aggressive fluid resuscitation with early administration of antibiotics. Manage the airway and get vascular access as previously discussed. Approximately 40% of CO is dedicated to the work of breathing. Intubating and sedating the patient will allow the CO to be dedicated to vital organs. Administer an initial fluid bolus of 20 mL/kg of normal saline or 5% albumin over 5–10 minutes and repeat if there is no improvement. These patients may require close to 60 mL/kg or more, in certain situations. Reassess after each bolus. Palpable hepatomegaly or rales on lung examination will be found in fluid overload. If signs of fluid overload are present, boluses should be of only 10-mL/kg aliquots and careful monitoring should take place. Diuretics, peritoneal dialysis, and continuous renal replacement therapy may be considered in patients who have undergone stabilization but are unable to manage the fluid overload.

Inotropic agents should be added to patients who present with fluid-resistant shock (Table 51-10). Fluid-refractory shock is the presence of clinical signs of shock after 60 mL/kg of fluid administration. In most patients, dopamine remains the first-line agent for fluid-refractory shock, although some studies suggest that infants younger than 6 months may not have enough norepinephrine stores due to an immature sympathetic innervention.[22,31] Adding dobutamine to this initial intervention will be beneficial. In the presence of dopamine-resistant shock, titrating epinephrine (cold shock) or norepinephrine (warm shock) is beneficial in most cases. If no central line access is available, inotropes may be administered peripherally as long as there is close monitoring of the area for any signs of necrosis (Figure 51-1).[19]

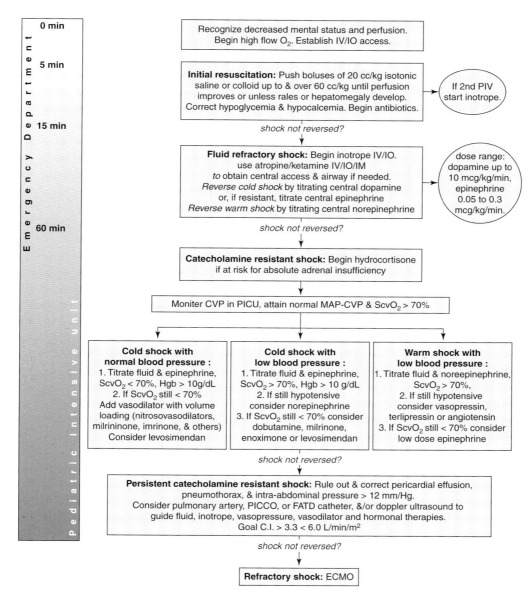

Figure 51-1. Approach to management of pediatric septic shock. (Reproduced with permission from Brierley J, Carcillo J, Choong K, et al. 2007 American College of Critical Care Medicine clinical practice parameters for hemodynamic support of pediatric and neonatal septic shock. *Crit Care Med.* 2009;37(2): 666–688. Figure 1.)

▶ FURTHER INTERVENTIONS

In the presence of catecholamine, dexamethasone at a dose of 1–2 mg/kg may be administered in patients at risk for adrenal insufficiency. Very young infants have low glycogen stores and underdeveloped thermoregulatory systems. Close attention should be paid to hypothermia and electrolyte disturbances such as hyperglycemia or hypoglycemia and hypocalcemia. Vasodilator therapies with agents such as nitroprusside, nitroglycerine, and

milrinone should be considered in patients with persistent shock despite the above interventions.

GOALS OF INTERVENTION

Therapeutic goals of intervention in septic pediatric patients in the emergency department include restoration of capillary refill to less than 2 seconds and normal mental status, pulses, and blood pressure, with an adequate urine output of >1 mL/kg/h. Even if the patient improves significantly during the first hour, admission to a pediatric intensive care unit is warranted.

▶ CONCLUSION

The differences in pediatric and adult critical care management stem from complex social, developmental, and physiologic interactions. Knowledge of these differences and adequate preparation are key in improving care for this important population.

REFERENCES

1. Gausche-Hill M, Schmitz C, Lewis RJ. Pediatric preparedness of United States emergency departments: a 2003 survey. *Pediatrics*. 2007;120(6):1229–1237.
2. Watson RS, Carcillo JA, Linde-Zwirble WT, et al. The epidemiology of severe sepsis in children in the United States. *Am J Respir Crit Care Med*. 2003;167(5):695–701.
3. Stenklyft PG, Cataletto ME, Lee BS. The pediatric airway in health and disease. In: Gausche-Hill M, Fuchs S, Yamamoto L, eds. *APLS: The Pediatric Emergency Medicine Resource*. 4th ed. Sudbury, MA: Jones and Bartlett Publishers; 2006:52–106.
4. Lee JK, Cheng T. In brief: newborn resuscitation. *Pediatr Rev*. 2006;27:e52–e53.
5. The International Liaison Committee on Resuscitation (ILCOR) consensus on science with treatment recommendations for pediatric and neonatal patients: pediatric basic and advanced life support. *Pediatrics*. 2006;117:e955–e977.
6. 2005 American Heart Association guidelines for cardiopulmonary resuscitation and emergency cardiovascular care. Part 12: pediatric advanced life support. *Circulation*. 2005;112:IV-167–IV-187.
7. Chieftez IM. Invasive and noninvasive pediatric mechanical ventilation. *Respir Care*. 2003;48(4):442–458.
8. Lei Huang L, Sun S, Fang X, et al. Simultaneous blockade of α1- and β-actions of epinephrine during cardiopulmonary resuscitation. *Crit Care Med*. 2006;34(12 suppl):S483–S485.
9. Gausche M, Lewis RJ, Stratton SJ, et al. Effect of out-of-hospital pediatric endotracheal intubation on survival and neurological outcome: a controlled clinical trial. *JAMA*. 2000;283:783–790.
10. Gerritse BM, Draaisma JM, Schalkwijk A, et al. Should EMS-paramedics perform paediatric tracheal intubation in the field? *Resuscitation*. 2008;79(2):225–229.
11. Nørregaard O. Noninvasive ventilation in children. *Eur Respir J*. 2002;20:1332–1342.
12. Lemyre B, Davis PG, De Paoli AG. Nasal intermittent positive pressure ventilation (NIPPV) versus nasal continuous positive airway pressure (NCPAP) for apnea of prematurity [*Cochrane* review]. In: *The Cochrane Library*. Issue 4. Chichester, UK: John Wiley & Sons; 2003.
13. Deis JN, Abramo TJ, Crawley L. Noninvasive respiratory support. *Pediatr Emerg Care*. 2008;24(5):331–338.
14. Carroll C, Schramm C. Noninvasive positive pressure ventilation for the treatment of status asthmaticus in children. *Ann Allergy Asthma Immunol*. 2006;96:454–459.
15. Gerardi MJ, Sacchetti A, Cantor RM, et al. Rapid-sequence intubation of the pediatric patient. Pediatric Emergency Medicine Committee of the American College of Emergency Physicians. *Ann Emerg Med*. 1996 Jul;28(1):55–74.
16. Sagarin MJ, Chiang V, Sakles JC, et al, National Emergency Airway Registry (NEAR) Investigators. Rapid sequence intubation for pediatric emergency airway management. *Pediatr Emerg Care*. 2002;18(6):417–423.
17. Green S, Coté C. Ketamine and neurotoxicity: clinical perspectives and implications for emergency medicine. *Ann Emerg Med*. 2009;54(2):181–190.
18. Rotta AT, Steinhorn DM. Is permissive hypercapnia a beneficial strategy for pediatric acute lung injury? *Respir Care Clin N Am*. 2006;12(3):371–387.
19. Brierly J, Carcillo JA, Choong K, et al. Clinical parameters for hemodynamic support of pediatric and neonatal septic shock: 2007 update from the American College of Critical Care Medicine. *Crit Care Med*. 2009;37(2):666–688.
20. Ching KY, Baum CR. Newer agents for rapid sequence intubation: etomidate and rocuronium. *Pediatr Emerg Care*. 2009;25(3):200–207.
21. Parker MM, Hazelzet JA, Carcillo JA. Pediatric considerations. *Crit Care Med*. 2004;32(11 suppl):S591–S594.
22. Carcillo JA. What's new in pediatric intensive care. *Crit Care Med*. 2006;34(9 suppl):S183–S190.
23. Ngo NT, Cao XT, Kneen R, et al. Acute management of dengue shock syndrome: a randomized double-blind comparison of 4 intravenous fluid regimens in the first hour. *Clin Infect Dis*. 2001;32(2):204–213. Epub January 15, 2001.
24. Wills B, Van Ngoc T, Van NTH, et al. Hemostatic changes in Vietnamese children with mild dengue correlate with the severity of vascular leakage rather than bleeding. *Am J Trop Med Hyg*. 2009;81:638–644.
25. Sharieff GQ, Wylie TW. Pediatric cardiac disorders. *J Emerg Med*. 2004;26(1):65–79.
26. Lieberman P. Epidemiology of anaphylaxis. *Curr Opin Allergy Clin Immunol*. 2008;8(4):316–320.
27. Lieberman P, Kemp S, Oppenheimer J, et al. The diagnosis and management of anaphylaxis: an updated practice parameter. *J Allergy Clin Immunol*. 2005;115:s483–s523.
28. Haas NA. Clinical review: vascular access for fluid infusion in children. *Crit Care*. 2004;8(6):478–484.
29. Han YY, Carcillo JA, Dragotta MA, et al. Early reversal of pediatric–neonatal septic shock by community physicians is associated with improved outcome. *Pediatrics*. 2003;112:793–799.
30. Fenton KE, Sable CA, Bell MJ, et al. Increases in serum levels of troponin I are associated with cardiac dysfunction and disease severity in pediatric patients with septic shock. *Pediatr Crit Care Med*. 2004;5(6):533–538.
31. Bhatt-Mehta V, Nahata MC, McClead RE, et al. Dopamine pharmacokinetics in critically ill newborn infants. *Eur J Clin Pharmacol*. 1991;40:593–597.

CHAPTER 52

Transportation of the Critical Care Patient[1]

Ira Nemeth and Julio R. Lairet

► INTRODUCTION

Moving a critical patient is a dangerous medical intervention. As with any medical intervention, there are risks and benefits. Over time, the risks have been mitigated by creation of specialized transport teams and equipment. The benefits still revolve around providing specialized treatments and diagnostics not available at every facility.[1] Recent literature has shown that time until definitive treatment is an important consideration. All these factors need to be taken into account by the physician when deciding when and how to transport critical patients.

Transporting critical care patients intrafacility or interfacility has some overlap. When moving a patient inside or outside of your facility, the patient needs to be packaged so that he or she is self-contained. All tubes (Foley, nasogastric, intravenous, and drainage), electronic equipment (monitors and pumps), and oxygen equipment must be secured to the patient or vehicle on which the patient is transported.[2] Equipment and medication to deal with anticipated changes in condition of failure of life supporting machines must be carried with the transporting team. While transporting inside a facility might only require a small amount of supplies, the longer a transport is in time or distance, the larger the amount of supplies to carry.

When transporting a patient between facilities, there is a broad array of specialized teams and equipment to move patients. The resources are designed to provide scene response, hospital-to-hospital transfers, or medical repatriation. The transport vehicle, skill of providers, and equipment carried in the vehicle are varied depending on the mission. Identifying the most appropriate resource requires understanding of the different types.[3] In addition, legal issues based around the Emergency Medical Treatment and Active Labor Act (EMTALA) need to be addressed prior to interfacility transfers.

Trauma was the first disease process to identify the benefits of moving critical patients to facilities that could provide definitive care. More recently, cardiac, stroke, and sepsis care have seen the benefits of getting critical patients to definitive treatment. All of these disease processes have realized the time-dependent need for highly specialized care. In many areas, emergency medical services (EMS) have developed systems to get the patients to the most appropriate facility, but sometimes this is not possible and the patients will have to be transferred from one facility to another.

► HISTORY

The use of transportation resources to support the overall care of patients has a long-standing tradition. Organized movement of people with illnesses or injuries to higher levels of care began in the Napoleonic

---

[1] The opinions or assertions contained herein are the private views of the author and are not to be construed as reflecting the views of the Department of the Air Force, the Department of Defense, or the US government.

Era.[4] As with many medical advances, military conflict has provided the impetus for improvement. During the Civil War, under the leadership of Joseph Barnes and Jonathan Letterman, the beginnings of field treatment and then transport to higher level of care in the United States were established. The Civil War experience was translated into civilian use in New York City as the first urban system in the United States to adopt this care. World War I and World War II provided many steps forward and some steps backward in the advancement of transportation care.

The next big step forward, the use of helicopters for the movement of the injured, started during the Korean War. Helicopters were used more formally in the Vietnam War. The first civilian helicopter services began in the early 1970s and were hospital-based systems.[5] These services were staffed with a doctor and a nurse. They started to bring advanced care to the prehospital arena.

In 1966, the National Academy of Science–National Research Council released their report entitled *Accidental Death and Disability: The Neglected Disease of Modern Society.* This report helped Congress pass the Highway Safety Act of 1966, which created the cabinet-level Department of Transportation (DOT). The DOT was given the responsibility for improving EMS. Many advancements have occurred in the care provided by both ground and helicopter EMS.

The recent Institute of Medicine (IOM) report titled *Emergency Medical Services at the Crossroads* made many recommendations to improve the whole EMS system including transport agencies and helicopter services, including the recommendation to extend critical care board certification to all acute care and primary care physicians who have completed an accredited fellowship. It was recommended that a subspecialty certification in EMS be created by the American Board of Emergency Medicine.[6]

▶ RISK VERSUS BENEFIT

When deciding to transfer a patient, the risks and potential benefits related to the patient's condition must be weighed. Certain medical conditions benefit from specialized facilities that frequently[7] take care of the condition. The most common conditions for which higher level of care transfers are initiated include trauma, cardiac injury, burns, acute stroke, spinal trauma, obstetric, and pediatric/neonatal-related issues. The risks are 2-fold, patient deterioration from their disease process and potential transportation-related injury.

Patient deterioration can be mitigated by appropriate stabilization prior to transfer and providing specialized care transport teams. Complete stabilization prior to transfer might not be possible and could be the reason the patient is being transferred. Specialized teams are limited and might not be readily available. Weather may hamper the ability of specialized teams to get to the facility and limit the transportation mode to slower possibilities.

The hazards of transportation are not commonly considered but need to be taken into account. Medical transport both air and ground are some of the highest risk ways to travel. The inadequacy of appropriate restraining devices, including those for pediatric patients, has been reported. Recent helicopter crashes have brought the issue of medical helicopter safety under National Traffic Safety Board (NTSB) and Congressional scrutiny.[8] Helicopter EMS crews had the highest fatality rate of all professions (Figure 52-1). Many variables including weather conditions and time of day have impact on the risk.

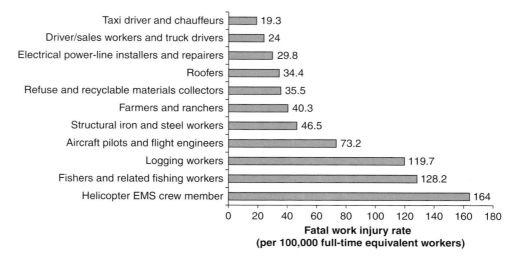

Figure 52-1. Selected occupations with high fatal injury rates, 2008.

► REGIONAL SYSTEMS

In the United States, certain systems have been established to streamline transfers. These include trauma centers, burn centers, and pediatric centers. Pediatric centers, realizing the need for highly specialized transport resources, have maintained control of the transport services, while trauma and burn centers usually leave the transport resource decision up to the transferring facility. New systems are being discussed for critical care, cardiac care, and stroke care.

Trauma systems have been established since the late 1970s to provide a regionalized approach to the care of the traumatically injured patient. The systems are based around limited but highly specialized facilities where increased volume leads to improved outcome. There are more facilities that can provide stabilization and arraign transfer to higher care if needed. Over the 30 years of trauma systems, there has been much debate about the need and benefit of helicopter transportation.[5,9–13] Many studies have shown a survival benefit from helicopter transportation but it has been difficult to separate the increased skill of the providers involved from the transport service and the mode of transport.

Trauma center transfers are designed to minimize the time to the appropriate facility. The most common cause of traumatic death is still hemorrhage. Damage control surgery and correction of coagulopathy to optimize hemorrhage control have become the practice paradigm for civilian and military trauma care. Therefore, time to surgery is an important factor and drives the need for rapid transfer to the facility that can perform the appropriate procedure. This applies in the newly forming stroke centers and cardiac centers. Cardiac centers have shown a survival benefit from percutaneous coronary intervention (PCI) initiated as close to the cardiac event as possible. However, studies have shown more complications[14] with helicopters or minimal time benefit[15] with helicopters in cardiac patients. Stroke centers also have a benefit from medication or intra-arterial procedures within certain time frames.[16]

Pediatric transfer systems have been established to provide more generalized critical care than trauma, cardiac, or stroke systems. A recent study suggested that having a more specialized transport team was more important than the time delay in response.[17] The study found a higher rate of unplanned events during transport and mortality with less specialized teams. There has been significant debate over the level of knowledge needed by the transport team. Studies have found no benefit to adding a physician to the pediatric transport team.[18,19]

In the current age of cost containment, some systems have looked at using transfers to help contain outside system costs. Kaiser Permanente implemented a plan to transfer patients with chest pain complaints from community emergency departments to one of their facilities.[20] They showed no specific deterioration in the care provided but also did not analyze the actual cost of this process.

The concept of regionalization of adult critical care that is being discussed[21] would require the identification and classification of facilities. Regionalization has the possibility for benefits in standardization and cost control. A definite volume–outcome benefit has not been proven. As transport systems are developed for this new concept, it will be important to consider the type of system to be created. Will it look like the pediatric transfer model with the receiving center providing the transport oversight or the trauma model with the sending facility responsible for choosing the transport agency? The EMTALA passed as part of the Consolidated Omnibus Budget Reconciliation Act in 1985 makes the referring provider responsible for ensuring safe and optimal transport.

► AIR TRANSPORT CONSIDERATIONS

Boyle's law describes the inverse relationship between pressure and volume in gases. Basically, gas expands as pressure decreases. This can present significant problems when transporting patients by air. As the aircraft increases its altitude, the pressure decreases. This causes problems for gas-filled structures in closed spaces and diffusion across the alveolar–capillary membrane. Pressurizing the cabin can return the pressure to sea level. There is a limit to how much pressurization can be achieved and, for certain conditions, a lower flying altitude must be maintained, resulting in longer flight times.

Gas-filled structures in closed spaces can cause significant in-flight complications but with some simple preparation these complications can be avoided. A small pneumothorax that usually would be managed conservatively will need to have a chest tube placed prior to air transport. Chest tubes need to be vented with a one-way valve or a continuous suction device that can operate in hypobaric pressures. Even the gas in the GI system can cause problems and a nasogastric or orogastric tube needs to be considered prior to transport. Any tube being held in place by balloon filled with air (endotracheal, Foley, etc.) needs to be monitored closely or filled with saline instead.

For the majority of patients, a simple volume control ventilator is sufficient for transport. However, finding a ventilator that can perform this function accurately at different barometric pressures is limited. The most commonly used ventilator is the Uni-Vent Eagle Model 754 (Impact Instrumentation, Inc, West Caldwell, New Jersey, USA).[22] The ventilator can perform volume control ventilation with up to 20 cm of PEEP and a maximum inspiratory flow rate of 60 L/min. If the patient requires more significant respiratory management, the transport options are limited to highly specialized teams. The majority of these teams are part of the military.

▶ MILITARY SYSTEM

Over the years, there have been many advances in military medicine. A significant change involves how critically injured or ill service members are transported to the United States. The movement of critical care patients within the military has evolved to a mature system, capable of transporting very ill or seriously injured patients over long distances in a timely manner. These teams are a fundamental part of the current military medical system that cares for our wounded warriors. Within the US military, there are three primary adult platforms that are used to carry out this mission. The goal of these teams is to conduct seamless ICU-level care while transporting the patient to a higher level of care.

CRITICAL CARE AIR TRANSPORT TEAMS (CCATT)

The CCATT concept was born in 1994.[23] The CCATTs are not a stand-alone platform; they augment the US Air Force Aeromedical Evacuation system, adding a critical care capability to the system. Their goal is to manage casualties who have undergone initial resuscitation but who remain critically ill while transporting them to a higher level of care.[23] A physician leads this team to ensure that the patient has continuous access to medical decision making. This enables the team to have the inherent capability to titrate therapies and ventilator settings to the patient's condition, start new therapies if required, and perform procedures when needed. The end result is an environment in which patients can continue to progress toward stability without interruption or setback during transport.[23]

CCATTs are composed of a critical care physician, who may be a general surgeon, pulmonary/critical care physician, anesthesiologist, emergency medicine physician, or a cardiologist. Completing the team are a critical care nurse and a respiratory therapist. CCATTs have the capability of caring for up to three ventilator patients or six less acute patients.[24] This capability can be expanded to five ventilator patients by augmenting the primary CCATT with the addition of a CCATT extender team, which is made up of two critical care nurses.[24]

CCATTs are experienced and current in the management of critically ill or injured patients with multisystem trauma, open/closed head injuries, shock, burns, respiratory failure, multiple organ failure, and other life-threatening complications.[23] The success of this platform is evident from the operations carried out during Operation Iraqi Freedom and Operation Enduring Freedom.

The acuity of the patients transported by CCATTs is demonstrated by the results of the recent study performed by Beninati et al, titled *Short Term Outcomes of US Air Force Critical Care Air Transport Team (CCATT) Patients Evacuated from a Combat Setting between 2007 and 2008.*[25] In this study, 656 patient moves were examined retrospectively. The distribution of the transports included 425 (64.8%) patients with traumatic injuries and 231 (35.2%) with medical complaints. When looking at the trauma subset, the mean ISS was 22 (range 1–75). The breakdown of the type of injury was also impressive, resulting in: 269 suffering polytrauma (multisystem) injuries, 80 having amputations, 90 suffering head injuries, 73 suffering burns, 121 having intra-abdominal injuries, and 98 having intrathoracic injuries. The intensity of care during transport reflects the severity of the casualties moved; 318 (48.5%) patient moves required mechanical ventilation, 68 (10.4%) received vasoactive medications, and 43 (6.6%) required blood products administration during the flight.[25]

The movement of burn casualties has its own inherent challenges due to the severity of the injury, which can include an inhalational component. As with other casualties, the movement includes two phases. The first from Iraq or Afghanistan to Germany, which is carried out by the Air Force AE system, augmented with CCATT. After arrival in Germany, the next step of transport can be carried out by either CCATT or the US Army Institute of Surgical Research Burn Flight Team (BFT), according to patient requirements.

US ARMY INSTITUTE OF SURGICAL RESEARCH BURN FLIGHT TEAM

The history of the USAISR BFT is a long one with thousands of burn patients moved to date. The team was formed in 1951 and is based out of Brooke Army Medical Center (BAMC) at Fort Sam Houston, Texas.[26,27] The team composition includes a general surgeon (team leader) experienced in burn, trauma, and surgical critical care, and two nurses, one of whom serves as the lead flight nurse. This individual is a registered nurse with significant burn and critical care experience. The second nurse of the team is a licensed vocational nurse who has completed the Army's Critical Care Nursing Program. The fourth member of the team is a Certified Respiratory Therapist who has extensive experience in using a variety of ventilators and in treating patients with severe lung disease and inhalational injury. Completing the team is an operations noncommissioned officer who is also a medical technician and both serves as the operations officer for each mission and provides assistance to the flight team as needed.[26] As with the CCATT, the BFT can be augmented with additional personnel as required by the mission.[26] A key unique aspect of the BFT over other critical care transport platforms involves continuity of care. The BFT surgeon who assesses the patient in Germany routinely becomes the attending physician for that patient during the hospitalization in the burn center.[26]

When deciding which platform will transport a burn casualty from Germany to the United States, key factors taken into account are the patient's condition, pulmonary status, and response to conventional ventilatory support.[26] The BFT personnel are versed in the management of inhalation or pulmonary injury requiring ventilatory support beyond the capabilities of traditional transport ventilators.[26] If needed, the BFT physician can perform fiberoptic bronchoscopy during the transport of the casualty. In caring for burn casualties during transport, the BFT uses both the volumetric diffusive respirator (VDR-4) and the TXP pressure control ventilator (Percussionaire Corp, Sand Point, Idaho).[26,28]

After the decision has been made to activate the BFT, the team flies from San Antonio (BAMC) to Germany while the casualty is being transported by CCATT from Iraq or Afghanistan. On arrival, the casualty is evaluated and cared for by the BFT surgeon.

ACUTE LUNG RESCUE TEAM (ALRT)

CCATT has been very effective in moving patients quickly from theater, at times in just hours after injury and surgical intervention. On occasion, some patients develop severe ARDS requiring advanced modes of ventilation. In November 2005, the ALRT was formed to fill this capability of moving these patients from Iraq and Afghanistan to Landstuhl Regional Medical Center (LRMC) in Germany. The ALRT is based at LRMC and is versed in the use of high-frequency percussive ventilation using the VDR-4 (Percussionaire Corp), and other advanced ventilator strategies such as inverse I/E ratio. The team composition includes a trauma or critical care surgeon, a pulmonary or critical care physician, a critical care nurse, and a respiratory therapist who is experienced in the use of the VDR-4 (Percussionaire Corp).[29]

Between November 2005 and March 2007, the ALRT successfully transported five patients with a mean Pao_2/FiO_2 ratio of 71, consistent with severe ARDS.[29] In the same study period, the ALRT was activated for 1% of mechanically ventilated patients brought to LRMC. While CCATT continues to be the primary platform for moving critically injured/ill patients from the theater, having the capability of the ALRT available when needed is fundamental for mission success.

The aircraft used to carry out aeromedical evacuation to include the critical care transport mission are aircraft of opportunity; their primary mission is not one of medical care. These aircraft have a variety of missions ranging from troop movements to cargo transport. Because of this, all the equipment needed to care for the patient must be brought aboard by the CCATT, USAISR BFT, and ALRT. In effect, the end result is converting the back of an aircraft into a flying ICU. The intertheater missions can be long, extending from 4.5 to 13 hours depending on the destination. Patient care priorities during transport are the same as those carried out in a trauma ICU regardless of which team carries out the mission. The ultimate goal is to maintain the same standard of care through the continuum of care.

Moving critical care patients has its own inherent challenges created by the environment such as decreased lighting, vibration, noise, lack of humidity, and temperature regulation, not to mention that the resources available in the back of the aircraft are limited to what the team brings with them. During transport, a primary focus of the team is airway protection and maintenance. Continuous ventilator monitoring is carried out through pulse oximetry and waveform end-tidal CO_2 monitoring. Arterial blood gases are performed to adjust ventilator settings as necessary during the flight. Hemodynamic status is monitored through invasive means (arterial blood pressure and CVP). When caring for casualties with a head injury, intracranial pressure is monitored with a ventriculostomy or ICP monitor. This information is vital for the team to make appropriate interventions. Blood for transfusions has to be brought on to the aircraft by the team. If needed, the teams have the ability to insert chest tubes and central lines or intubate a patient during transport. The level of care given to these casualties is extraordinary and a testament to advances within military medicine.

▶ TRANSFER CENTERS

The transfer from one facility to another requires many moving parts. We have talked about the transport agencies and options available to move specialized patients. Current market pressures provide that many facilities do not have available capacity. Finding an accepting facility can be difficult and requires significant time on the phone contacting one facility after another. Most hospitals have tried to streamline the process and consolidate the resources needed to accomplish interfacility transfers through a centralized transfer center. In a large academic institution, there can be many different services receiving transfers at the same time. One system even found it more economical to outsource this function due to its complexity.[30]

In addition to the complexity of finding an appropriate facility, there are significant EMTALA requirements that need to be met. EMTALA has obligations

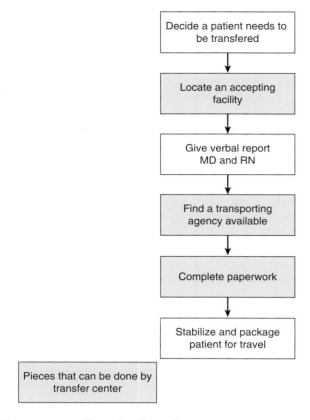

Figure 52-2. Transfer flow diagram.

for both the sending and receiving facilities. Sending facilities are required to stabilize the patient to the maximum of his or her capability prior to transferring. In addition, the sending facility is responsible for sending a copy of the patient's complete medical record, including images, and choosing the most appropriate means of transportation including qualified personnel. The receiving facility has an obligation to accept patients from other facilities if they have space available and qualified personnel who can provide the needed service. It is also required that the patient provides a written request to be transferred or a statement from the transferring physician that the medical benefits of transfer outweigh the risks involved.[31] A memorandum of transfer helps record all the different pieces required for a transfer. Having all these pieces organized and streamlined through a central transfer center will speed up the transfer. Figure 52-2 shows a simplified transfer flow pattern and identifies the pieces that a transfer center could be assigned to accomplish.

▶ SUMMARY

Critical care transport decisions are difficult and require significant thought prior to initiating. Therefore, creations of systems that are designed and take into account

these complex issues are important prior to transferring patients. There are many different options of equipment and provider skill levels available in specific teams. As a health care provider on the receiving or sending side of patient transfers, it is important to understand the teams and resources available in your region. As the volume of transfers increases, primary and backup options must be considered when creating transfer pathways.

As financial and specialization considerations make regionalization more likely in the future, it will be important to have a knowledge of critical care transport pitfalls and successes. A strong quality improvement program will help guide the formation of these systems. There is limited research on the true benefits and risks in creating systems of consolidated specialized care. However, there is no doubt that critical care transportation will be an increasing area of focus in the coming decades.

REFERENCES

1. Crippen D. Critical care transportation medicine: new concepts in pretransport stabilization of the critically ill patient. *Am J Emerg Med.* 1990;8:551–554.
2. Warren J, Fromm RE Jr, Orr RA, Rotello LC, Horst HM. Guidelines for the inter- and intrahospital transport of critically ill patients. *Crit Care Med.* 2004;32:256–262.
3. Fromm RE Jr, Varon J. Critical care transport. *Crit Care Clin.* 2000;16:695–705.
4. Blackwell TH. Emergency medical service: overview and ground transport. In: Marx JA, Hockberger RS, Walls RM, Adams J, Rosen P, eds. *Rosen's Emergency Medicine: Concepts and Clinical Practice.* 6th ed. Philadelphia: Mosby/Elsevier; 2006:2984–2993.
5. Baxt WG, Moody P. The impact of a rotorcraft aeromedical emergency care service on trauma mortality. *JAMA.* 1983;249:3047–3051.
6. Institute of Medicine (U.S.). Committee on the Future of Emergency Care in the United States Health System. *Emergency Medical Services at the Crossroads.* Washington, DC: National Academies Press; 2007.
7. van Lieshout EJ, de Vos R, Binnekade JM, de Haan R, Schultz MJ, Vroom MB. Decision making in interhospital transport of critically ill patients: national questionnaire survey among critical care physicians. *Intensive Care Med.* 2008;34:1269–1273.
8. *Helicopter Emergency Medical Services.* Washington, DC: National Transportation Safety Board; 2009.
9. Baxt WG, Moody P. The impact of a physician as part of the aeromedical prehospital team in patients with blunt trauma. *JAMA.* 1987;257:3246–3250.
10. Baxt WG, Moody P, Cleveland HC, et al. Hospital-based rotorcraft aeromedical emergency care services and trauma mortality: a multicenter study. *Ann Emerg Med.* 1985;14:859–864.
11. Thomas SH, Harrison TH, Buras WR, Ahmed W, Cheema F, Wedel SK. Helicopter transport and blunt trauma mortality: a multicenter trial. *J Trauma.* 2002;52:136–145.

12. Cunningham P, Rutledge R, Baker CC, Clancy TV. A comparison of the association of helicopter and ground ambulance transport with the outcome of injury in trauma patients transported from the scene. *J Trauma.* 1997;43:940–946.

13. Brathwaite CE, Rosko M, McDowell R, Gallagher J, Proenca J, Spott MA. A critical analysis of on-scene helicopter transport on survival in a statewide trauma system. *J Trauma.* 1998;45:140–144. Discussion 4–6.

14. Schneider S, Borok Z, Heller M, Paris P, Stewart R. Critical cardiac transport: air versus ground? *Am J Emerg Med.* 1988;6:449–452.

15. Svenson JE, O'Connor JE, Lindsay MB. Is air transport faster? A comparison of air versus ground transport times for interfacility transfers in a regional referral system. *Air Med J.* 2006;25:170–172.

16. Thomas SH, Kociszewski C, Schwamm LH, Wedel SK. The evolving role of helicopter emergency medical services in the transfer of stroke patients to specialized centers. *Prehosp Emerg Care.* 2002;6:210–214.

17. Orr RA, Felmet KA, Han Y, et al. Pediatric specialized transport teams are associated with improved outcomes. *Pediatrics.* 2009;124:40–48.

18. McCloskey KA, King WD, Byron L. Pediatric critical care transport: is a physician always needed on the team? *Ann Emerg Med.* 1989;18:247–249.

19. King BR, King TM, Foster RL, McCans KM. Pediatric and neonatal transport teams with and without a physician: a comparison of outcomes and interventions. *Pediatr Emerg Care.* 2007;23:77–82.

20. Selevan JS, Fields WW, Chen W, Petitti DB, Wolde-Tsadik G. Critical care transport: outcome evaluation after interfacility transfer and hospitalization. *Ann Emerg Med.* 1999;33:33–43.

21. Singh JM, MacDonald RD. Pro/con debate: do the benefits of regionalized critical care delivery outweigh the risks of interfacility patient transport? [Review] [73 refs]. *Crit Care.* 2009;13:7.

22. Kashani KB, Farmer JC. The support of severe respiratory failure beyond the hospital and during transportation. *Curr Opin Crit Care.* 2006;12:43–49.

23. Beninati W, Meyer MT, Carter TE. The critical care air transport program. *Crit Care Med.* 2008;36:S370–S376.

24. Force TSotA. Air Force tactics, techniques, and procedures 3-42.51. In: *Critical Care Air Transport Teams (CCATT).* Air Force Medical Service Knowledge Exchange; 2006.

25. Beninati W, Lairet J, King J, et al. Short term outcomes of US Air Force Critical Care Air Transport Team (CCATT) patients evacuated from a combat setting between 2007 and 2008. *Chest.* 2009;136:28S-g.

26. Renz EM, Cancio LC, Barillo DJ, et al. Long range transport of war-related burn casualties. *J Trauma.* 2008;64:S136–S144. Discussion S44–S45.

27. Hurd WW, Jernigan JG. *Aeromedical Evacuation: Management of Acute and Stabilized Patients.* New York: Springer; 2003.

28. Barillo DJ, Dickerson EE, Cioffi WG, Mozingo DW, Pruitt BA Jr. Pressure-controlled ventilation for the long-range aeromedical transport of patients with burns. *J Burn Care Rehabil.* 1997;18:200–205.

29. Dorlac GR, Fang R, Pruitt VM, et al. Air transport of patients with severe lung injury: development and utilization of the Acute Lung Rescue Team. *J Trauma.* 2009;66:S164–S171.

30. Strickler J, Amor J, McLellan M. Untangling the lines: using a transfer center to assist with interfacility transfers. *Nurs Econ.* 2003;21:94–96.

31. *Guide for Interfacility Patient Transfer.* Department of Transportation, National Highway Traffic Safety Administration; 2006.

CHAPTER 53

End-of-life Issues in Emergency Critical Care

Sangeeta Lamba

▶ INTRODUCTION

The majority of patients who are admitted to medical critical care units and many of those in surgical intensive care units begin their hospital course in the emergency department (ED). Thus, ED clinicians set the stage for the future management trajectory, usually initiating aggressive life-saving measures, with a curative and resuscitative approach to care.[1,2] Due to advances in technology, deaths in critical patients often result from limitation of life-supporting measures as opposed to a natural decline from disease or age.[3] This has resulted in an expansion of the mission of critical care to include provision of the best care available for dying patients and their families.[4] In 2003, an International Consensus Conference was convened to discuss some of the end-of-life challenges and to address the issues related to optimal care for dying critical care patients.[5] In order to achieve the best "quality" of life rather than just an emphasis on the "quantity" along with cure, it is essential to focus on patient comfort from the onset of care.[2,4,5]

Essential to the goal of providing good end-of-life care is understanding a few key concepts: (1) death is not a professional failure, (2) a pain-free death must be assured, (3) effective communication with family and surrogates is needed for "shared decision" making, (4) goals of care discussions aid in the "shift" from a curative to a comfort approach, and, most important, (5) a multidisciplinary team approach is absolutely essential and should include nurses, house staff, social workers, family support

teams, chaplains, and, when appropriate and available, subspecialist palliative care consult teams.[6] We further discuss the following domains frequently encountered in end-of-life care provision: (1) advance directives, (2) goals of care discussions and communication, (3) death-related issues that include delivery of bad news, death notification, and family witnessed resuscitation (FWR), (4) withdrawal of life support, and (5) palliative care with optimal symptom management at end of life.

▶ ADVANCE DIRECTIVES

Currently, decision making in critical care patients varies widely and may not always defer to patient autonomy.[5,7,8] A major study reported that physicians did not consistently document a do not resuscitate (DNR) order for patients who did not wish to have cardiopulmonary resuscitation (CPR),[7] whereas another showed that DNR orders were followed only 58% of the time.[8] Patient-value-based management and respect for patient autonomy involve a shared decision-making model that may be essential to increasing patient and family satisfaction with critical health care.

DETERMINING DECISION-MAKING CAPACITY

Determining decision-making capacity is an essential step toward assessing patient needs and values and is *decision specific*.[9] This means that the patient may have the capacity to make one particular decision but not have the same capacity for another. Physicians are responsible for judging *capacity*, whereas *competency* is assessed by a judge. A list of questions to help assess capacity include: (1) Can the patient understand and process the information? This requires him or her to relay back the content in lay terms. (2) Can the patient analyze and understand consequences? This essentially means he or she is able to weigh the risks/benefits and to communicate the reasoning behind his or her decision. (3) Can the patient communicate his or her choice? This is particularly difficult in the nonverbal, ventilator-dependent patient who may not be able to convey the elements essential to an informed consent. His or her attempts may be prone to a biased interpretation based on values of the person obtaining consent.[9] A patient for whom the answer to any of the above is "no" essentially lacks decision-making capacity.

SURROGATE DECISION MAKING FOR INCAPACITATED PATIENTS

Advance directives or surrogate decision makers come into play when a person lacks decision-making capacity. Living wills or written advance directives are rarely found to be at hand in emergent situations and, even if available, are often not specific enough to be applied to all routine, day-to-day medical decisions.[10] The main value of such documents is perhaps in the event of imminent death when a specific choice of no mechanical ventilation or no CPR is requested. In critical situations, the availability and access to a patient's designated legally authorized representative, surrogate, proxy, or durable power of attorney for health care decisions is more helpful and important for daily decision making. Using a surrogate, though, has its own limitations; some studies have found that surrogates may often fail to accurately represent the patient's wishes,[11] whereas others have shown that family members have high rates of anxiety and depression that may compromise effective decision making.[12] It is important for clinicians to guide the surrogates early, in order to make sure they understand their role in making decisions for the patient. Many have summarized that the role of a surrogate is to provide a "substituted judgment" for the incapacitated patient based on his or her knowledge of the patient and previous statements made by the patient, and should not be based primarily on the surrogate's own values.[11,12] In the event of no available pre-identified, legally authorized surrogate, family members are often involved in decision making. In many states, a hierarchy of responsibility may be as follows: spouse, adult child, parent, adult sibling, adult relative, and then a close friend. In cases of interfamily conflict, involvement of ethics committees or court action may also

become necessary. Despite a surrogate, major decisions will often also involve the approval of most close family members and effective communication therefore becomes an essential tool for the clinician.[13]

▶ GOALS OF CARE DISCUSSIONS AND COMMUNICATION

In surveys of critical care patients' families, it is reported that families consistently rate communication as among their most important concerns and often report dissatisfaction with the manner in which they were informed about the diagnosis, prognosis, and treatment and in general the quality of communication with the critical care staff.[7,10,14,15] Models of communication are being increasingly addressed in critical care literature and emphasize a "shared decision" making, proactive approach to resolving conflicts and reaching consensus (Figure 53-1).[5,13,16–19] Guidelines suggest that when organizing such goals of care family conferences, clinicians take into account the specific needs of families that have been identified in studies to include reassurance that the patient's symptoms will be managed; clear information conveyed to caregivers about the patient's

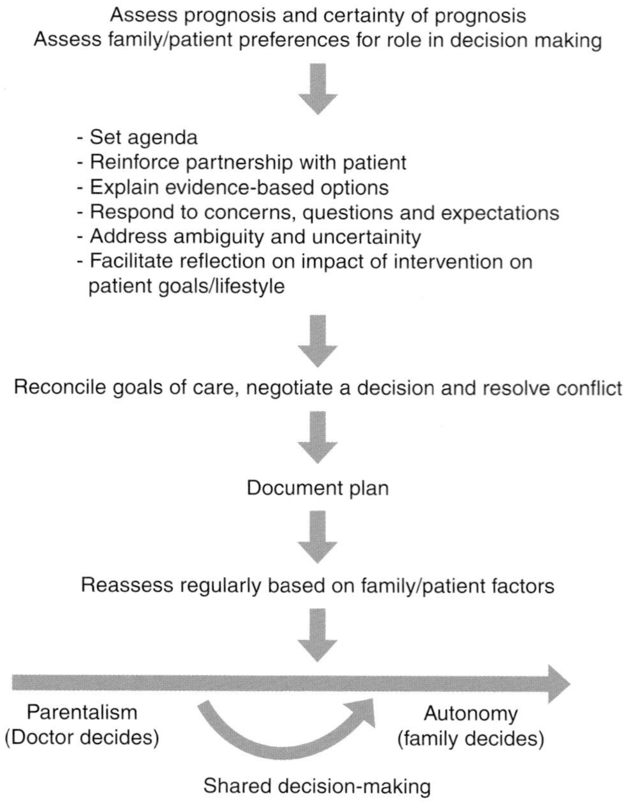

Assess prognosis and certainty of prognosis
Assess family/patient preferences for role in decision making

- Set agenda
- Reinforce partnership with patient
- Explain evidence-based options
- Respond to concerns, questions and expectations
- Address ambiguity and uncertainty
- Facilitate reflection on impact of intervention on patient goals/lifestyle

Reconcile goals of care, negotiate a decision and resolve conflict

Document plan

Reassess regularly based on family/patient factors

Parentalism (Doctor decides)   Autonomy (family decides)

Shared decision-making

Figure 53-1. Multistep approach to patient- and family centered decision making that is modified by prognosis and by family preferences. Data from[13]

► TABLE 53-1. **FAMILY CONFERENCE GUIDELINES**

1. **Why?** Clarify conference goals, review medical information. What do you hope to accomplish as a goal?
2. **Where?** A room with comfort, privacy, and circular seating
3. **Who?** Patient (if able to participate); health care proxy; family members; social support; key health care professionals
4. **Introduce**
   - Introduce self and others; review meeting goals; clarify if specific decisions need to be made
   - Establish ground rules: each person will have a chance to ask questions and express views; no interruptions; identify legal decision maker; and describe importance of supportive decision making
   - If you are new to the patient/family, spend time seeking to know the "person"—what is important in his or her life, etc.
5. **First determine what the patient/family already knows.** "Tell me your understanding of the current medical condition." Ask everyone in the room to speak
6. **Then provide review of medical status**
   - Review current status, prognosis, and treatment options
   - Ask each family member in turn if he or she has any questions about same
   - Respond to emotional reactions with empathy
   - Defer discussion of decision making until the next step
7. **Family discussion with a nondecisional patient**
   - Ask each family member in turn—What do you believe the patient would choose if the patient could speak for himself or herself?
   - Ask each family member—What do you think should be done?
   - Ask if the family would like you to leave room to let family discuss alone
   - If there is consensus, go to 9; if no consensus, go to 8
8. **When there is no consensus:**
   - Restate: What would the patient say if he or she could speak? Ask: Have you ever discussed with the patient what he or she would want in a situation like this?
   - If you, as a clinician, have a firm opinion about the best plan of care, recommend it simply and explicitly, and explain why
   - Schedule a follow-up conference later or the next day
   - Try further discussion: What values is your decision based on?
   - Identify other resources: Minister/priest; other physicians; ethics committee
9. **Conclude and wrap-up:**
   - Summarize consensus, disagreements, decisions, and plan
   - Caution against unexpected outcomes
   - Identify family spokesperson for ongoing communication
   - Document in the chart—who was present, decisions made, and follow-up plan
   - Continuity—schedule follow-up meeting for concerns

Adapted with permission from Ambuel B, Weissman DE. *Moderating an End-of-Life Family Conference, 2nd ed. Fast Facts and Concepts #16.* August 2005. Available at: http://www.eperc.mcw.edu/fastfact/ff_016.htm.

condition and treatment; a willingness of staff to listen and respond to family members and to address their emotions; value patient preferences; clear explanations about surrogate decision making; and reassurance of continuous, compassionate, and technically proficient care until death occurs.[17] Decisions should generally be made collaboratively by clinicians partnering with patients' families. Treatment choices should be crafted to meet specific, achievable goals.[20] The process is one of negotiation, and the outcome will finally be determined by the personalities and beliefs of the participants. Ultimately, it is the physician's responsibility, to decide on how reasonable a planned action may be. If a conflict cannot be easily resolved, an ethics consultation may be helpful.[4,5] Communication with family members is not different from other aspects of critical care and requires training, interdisciplinary teamwork, and implementation of effective/flexible protocols to achieve the best possible outcome (Table 53-1).[13,18,21]

► DEATH ISSUES

DELIVERY OF BAD NEWS AND DEATH NOTIFICATION

Delivery of bad news, especially death notification, is perhaps the most difficult, emotionally laden communication task that physicians perform.[22,23] Physicians often report factual medical information but avoid the most stressful issues and have trouble with empathic disclosures.[23] Stressors include the physician's fear of being blamed, the difficulty in dealing with surviving family members' emotions, and the physician's own personal fear of death.[24] ED death notifications may be especially difficult because: (1) ED deaths are often sudden/unexpected, due to an acute traumatic event, or may involve young patients, (2) there is usually no preexisting relationship between the physician and the patient or family, (3) the chaotic, public environment of the ED itself may not be suitable for the family to grieve

▶ **TABLE 53-2. GUIDELINES FOR THE APPROACH TO FAMILIES IN DEATH NOTIFICATION**

The GRIEV_ING mnemonic for death notification

G—gather; ensure that all family members are present

R—resources; private location, call for support resources available to assist the family with their grief, that is, chaplain, bereavement counselors, and friends

I—identify; identify yourself, identify the deceased or injured patient by name, and identify the level/state of knowledge of the family relative to the events and patient condition

E—educate; educate briefly as to the events that have occurred and the current status in the emergency department

V—verify; verify that their family member has died. Be clear! Use the D-words "dead" or "died"

_—space; give the family personal space and time for emotions; allow time to absorb the news

I—inquire; ask if there are any questions, and answer to the best of ability

N—nuts and bolts; inquire about organ donation, funeral services, and personal belongings. Offer the family the opportunity to view the body

G—give; give them access information. Offer to answer questions that may arise later and return their calls

Modified with permission from Hobgood et al.[26]

privately, and (4) clergy or social service support staff may not be readily available.[22,25] Various methods to inform families of the death of a loved one exist, and it is important to remember that the clinician has a responsibility toward the survivors since the words spoken to them will linger in their memories and influence the grieving process.[22,23,26] The GRIEV_ING intervention has been shown to improve physician confidence and competence in death notification. This method is outlined in Table 53-2. It may be important for each clinician to refine the particular language he or she uses in such situations, rehearse a stepwise approach to decrease his or her own stress, and review the terminology in advance when using a translator. With the rapid growth of telecommunications, it is best that phones and beepers be switched to a vibrate mode so there are no interruptions. It is also recommended that clinicians sit down to emphasize the importance of being available for questions and not rush through the delivery. Delivering the news appropriately with compassion will ease the grief period and allows loved ones to reclaim their lives.[26]

FAMILY WITNESSED RESUSCITATION

Recent literature advocates family member presence during CPR.[27–30] The perceived benefits of FWR are the following: (1) most family members prefer to be

given the option to be with the patient at time of death, (2) although such experiences are emotionally draining, they may assist in bereavement and decrease complicated grief, (3) may reduce overall fear or anxiety, (4) provide higher sense of connection with the patient, (5) remove doubt that everything possible was done for the loved one, and finally (6) provide a feeling of closure.[27–30] Provider attitudes, though, continue to represent a barrier to FWR: concerns that family involvement might cause distress for survivors, interfere in the resuscitation, distract or intimidate the team, bring greater pressure to prolong the code, cause anxiety in pronouncing death, and may lead to increased malpractice litigation, when in fact family members are probably less likely to seek medical litigation, if they feel everything possible was done.[29,30] There also appears to be more hesitation in the urban setting as compared with suburban, possibly due to lack of adequate ancillary support or underlying nature of the types of resuscitations.[30] The concerns cited with FWR include the issues of: (1) human dignity, (2) personal privacy, and (3) the provision of adequately trained staff to help relatives cope with the emotional trauma the experience of being a witness may invoke. However, most agree that a multidisciplinary, well-planned, and practiced approach is necessary and should be used to develop and enhance an institutional protocol, address staff concerns, and train family facilitators.[30]

▶ WITHDRAWAL OF LIFE SUPPORT

If analyzed closely, almost all patients who die while receiving medical attention in a critical care setting do so as a result of withholding or withdrawing of life-sustaining therapy.[3] Sometimes, the decision is made to not resuscitate the patient prior to the terminal decompensation and at other times because even multiple, vigorous resuscitation attempts have failed to halt the terminal decline and cannot be provided indefinitely.[3] The practice varies among countries and institutions.[31,32] Withdrawal of life support measures is sometimes necessary early in the care of a critical patient in the ED: for example, if a patient was initially placed on mechanical ventilation and the family wishes withdrawal after accepting the extremely poor prognosis in the case of a catastrophic intracranial bleed.

Ethically, there exists no distinction between the decisions to withdraw a specific treatment and a decision not to initiate a treatment.[31] Sometimes, initiating a time-limited course of aggressive therapy may actually be beneficial to family and caregivers, and necessary in order for them to come to terms with a critical patient's condition and to allow clinicians to adequately evaluate all treatment options.[31] As with any other treatment, if this trial does not improve status and fails to show any benefit, then there is justification for its withdrawal. CPR is the therapy most often withheld and DNR orders may precede up to 60% of all deaths.[3,7,33] Mechanical ventilation, vasoactive drugs, renal dialysis, and antibiotics are the other therapies commonly withheld. The most commonly withdrawn therapy prior to death is mechanical ventilation, followed by vasoactive drugs.[3,33–35]

Many algorithms for medical management of withdrawal of ventilator support in the ED exist.[36–39] The decision to withdraw or withhold therapy is best achieved by a consensus between the critical care team and family. Discussions with surrogates should be frank and consistent. Withholding or withdrawal of life support should be recommended, not merely listed as an option. The rationale used to come to this recommendation, including prognostication and disease-specific data, should be communicated to family in lay terms.[13,19,21] Often, multiple meetings may be necessary after the initial recommendation to reach consensus.[33] It is also advisable not to make CPR the focus of discussions, but rather to focus on the goals of care, which should define whether a therapy will be withheld or withdrawn.

Once the decision is made to withdraw mechanical ventilation and life support, all interventions should be stopped including vasopressors and antibiotics.[36,38,39] Family and caregivers should be made aware that death may not happen instantaneously and in fact some patients may survive for many hours postwithdrawal.[33] In all cases, a humane, pain-free process should be assured and the family presence at bedside encouraged. The administration of sedatives and analgesics may not hasten death; in one study, median time to death following the withholding/withdrawal of life support was 3.5 hours in patients who received such drugs compared with 1.3 hours in those who did not.[37] Both extubation and gradual weaning have been used, and patients should be premedicated and have staff present at bedside to answer concerns during and after the process.[38,39] One such protocol suggests the following steps: (1) first, discontinue all paralytics allowing full return of neuromuscular function, (2) disable all alarms, (3) titrate sedation to comfort—continuous infusions are least obtrusive, (4) reduce FiO_2 to room air and PEEP to zero over 5 minutes or less, (5) gradually reduce volume and pressure support over 20–30 minutes, and finally (6) once the patient is comfortably sedated on above settings, extubate or change to a T-piece.

Disagreements can occur among family members and also between caregivers and clinicians, especially when some may strongly believe in preserving life at all costs because of cultural or religious beliefs. Such disagreements can cause tension and moral distress among families and clinicians. Again, a multidisciplinary approach with a dedicated staff who has received prior training might facilitate and ease such decision making.

▶ PALLIATIVE CARE AND OPTIMAL SYMPTOM MANAGEMENT

The Ethics Committee of the Society of Critical Care Medicine in 2001 and the consensus conference in 2003 published guidelines based on identified end-of-life needs of patients, families, and providers.[4,5,31] Previously identified *patients'* needs at end of life are to receive adequate pain management, avoid inappropriate prolongation of dying, achieve a sense of control, relieve themselves of burdens, and strengthen their relationships with loved ones.[7,40,41] The *families'* needs are to be with their loved one during the dying process, be helpful to their loved one, be kept informed of the changing clinical status, understand the process of what and why therapy is being done, be assured of the patients' comfort, be comforted themselves, express their own emotions, be assured that their decisions regarding the patients were correct, and find meaning in the dying of their loved ones.[5,17] The needs of the *health care providers* are to establish consensus regarding the goals, have strategies for providing palliative care, gain knowledge and skills in palliation, be supported in their tasks by their institutions, and have opportunities for grieving and bereavement after patients die.[5,31]

Close attention to the principles of good pain management, communication with patient and family, and discussion of goals of care are not just for patients who are at the end of life, but are appropriate care for all critically ill patients, regardless of prognosis. In this framework, "intensive care" encompasses palliative and curative care.[2,42] With the recent growth in the palliative care field, many hospitals may have subspecialist-level, formal consultation teams to assist the critical care and ED physicians in many of the end-of-life issues discussed above.[1,2] However, most institutions still lack such support and a multidisciplinary approach to care with involvement of nursing, social workers, bereavement, and family support teams may maximize utilization of institutional resources.

Optimal symptom management at end of life should remain the focus of the clinician, whether a curative or a comfort approach to patient care is being followed.[4,5,42,43] Management of uncontrolled pain and avoidance of oligoanalgesia based on misconceptions is necessary. Cautious individual titration of opioids to analgesic effect is safe, effective, and rarely associated with addiction, clinically significant respiratory depression, rapid tolerance, or euphoria.[42,44] The use of pain assessment tools especially in the nonverbal patients, frequent reassessments, and therapy geared toward objective and subjective endpoints may facilitate this goal.

The patient must be provided with sufficient analgesia to alleviate pain and distress; if such analgesia hastens death, this "double effect" should not detract from the primary aim to ensure comfort.[5,31] The rule of double effect has been invoked to guide decision making in many end-of-life situations, for example, in *terminal or palliative sedation*, the practice of using sedatives in the terminally ill at doses that render a patient unconscious as a last resort measure to provide relief from suffering due to distressing symptoms of dyspnea or pain.[45–47] This practice is to be clearly differentiated from euthanasia or physician-assisted suicide, in which the intent is to cause death. Recently, the Supreme Court has unanimously ruled that there is no constitutional right to physician-assisted suicide. However, it went with a majority, effectively requiring all states to ensure that their laws do not obstruct the provision of adequate palliative care, especially for the alleviation of pain and other physical symptoms of people facing death.[47] One Supreme Court Justice even stated, "a patient who is suffering from a terminal illness and who is experiencing great pain has no legal barrier to obtaining medication, from qualified physicians, to alleviate that suffering, even to the point of causing unconsciousness." Unlike euthanasia, most terminal sedation protocols require titration at fixed intervals to reassess underlying symptoms and ongoing need, with the intent to provide optimal symptom relief at the *lowest* therapy dose. As always, frank and detailed conversations with family and caregivers are necessary prior to any major therapeutic interventions.[45–47]

► CONCLUSION

For provision of optimal end-of-life care to critical patients, it is recommended that clinicians: (1) refer to the basic ethical principles of patient autonomy, beneficence, and nonmaleficence, (2) recognize the necessity to shift from a curative to comfort care approach and consider limitation of life-prolonging treatments when the clinical situation is hopeless, (3) base the decision-making process to ascertain hopelessness of a clinical situation on a thorough patient evaluation and an ample time course, (4) communicate effectively with family/ surrogates for shared decision making, (5) document discussions and decisions, (6) use a multidisciplinary approach to end-of-life care, and finally (7) implement thorough palliative care and symptom management strategy once the decision to withhold or withdraw life-sustaining treatments has been made.[5]

REFERENCES

1. Meier DE, Beresford L. Fast response is key to partnering with the emergency department. *J Palliat Med.* 2007;10:641–645.
2. Lamba S, Mosenthal AC. Introduction to hospice and palliative medicine: a novel sub-specialty of emergency medicine. *J Emerg Med.* 2010 May 22. [Epub ahead of print].
3. Prendergast TJ, Claessens MT, Luce JM. A national survey of end-of-life care for critically ill patients. *Am J Respir Crit Care Med.* 1998;158:1165–1167.
4. Thompson BT, Cox PN, Antonelli M, et al. Challenges in end-of-life care in the ICU: statement of the 5th international consensus conference in critical care: Brussels, Belgium, April 2003: executive summary. *Crit Care Med.* 2004;32(8):1781–1784.
5. Carlet J, Thijs LG, Antonelli M, et al. Challenges in end-of-life care in the ICU. Statement of the 5th international consensus conference in critical care: Brussels, Belgium, April 2003. *Intensive Care Med.* 2004;30:770–784.
6. Clarke EB, Curtis JR, Luce JM, et al. Quality indicators for end-of-life care in the intensive care unit. *Crit Care Med.* 2003;31:2255–2262.
7. SUPPORT Principal Investigators. A controlled trial to improve care for seriously ill hospitalized patients. The study to understand prognoses and preferences for outcomes and risks of treatments (SUPPORT). *JAMA.* 1995;274:1591–1598.
8. Vincent JL. Forgoing life support in western European intensive care units: the results of an ethical questionnaire. *Crit Care Med.* 1999;27(8):1686–1687.
9. Applebaum PS, Grisso T. Assessing patients' capacities to consent to treatment. *N Engl J Med.* 1988;319:1635–1638.
10. Hofmann JC, Wenger NS, Davis RB, et al. Patient preferences for communication with physicians about end-of-life decisions. *Ann Intern Med.* 1997;127:1–12.
11. Seckler AB, Meier DE, Mulvihill M, Cammer Paris BE. Substituted judgment: how accurate are proxy predictions? *Ann Intern Med.* 1991;115:92–98.
12. Pochard F, Azoulay E, Chevret S, et al. Symptoms of anxiety and depression in family members of intensive care unit patients: ethical hypothesis regarding decision-making capacity. *Crit Care Med.* 2001;29:1893–1897.
13. Curtis JR, White DB. Practical guidance for evidence-based ICU family conferences. *Chest.* 2008;134(4):835–843.
14. Johnson D, Wilson M, Cavanaugh B, et al. Measuring the ability to meet family needs in an intensive care unit. *Crit Care Med.* 1998;26:266–271.
15. Levy M, McBride D. End-of-life care in the intensive care unit: state of the art in 2006. *Crit Care Med.* 2006;34:306–308.
16. Fumis RR, Nishimoto IN, Deheinzelin D. Families' interactions with physicians in the intensive care unit: the impact on family's satisfaction. *J Crit Care.* 2008;23(3):281–286.
17. Lautrette A, Ciroldi M, Ksibi H, Azoulay E. End-of-life family conferences: rooted in the evidence. *Crit Care Med.* 2006;34(11 suppl):S364–S372.
18. Ambuel B, Weissman DE. *Moderating an End-of-Life Family Conference, 2nd ed. Fast Facts and Concepts #16.* August 2005. Available at: http://www.eperc.mcw.edu/fastfact/ff_016.htm. Last accessed January 8, 2010.
19. Quill TE. Initiating end-of-life discussions with seriously ill patients. Addressing the elephant in the room. *JAMA.* 2000;284:2502–2507.
20. Siegel MD. End-of-life decision making in the ICU. *Clin Chest Med.* 2009;30(1):181–194.
21. Weissman DE. Decision making at a time of crisis near the end of life. *JAMA.* 2004;292:1738–1743.

22. Olsen JC, Buenefe ML, Falco WD. Death in the emergency department. *Ann Emerg Med.* 1998;31(6):758–765.

23. Iserson K. *Grave Words: Notifying Survivors about Sudden Unexpected Deaths.* Tucson, AZ: Galen Press; 1999.

24. Buckman R. Breaking bad news: why is it so difficult? *BMJ.* 1984;288:1597–1599.

25. Walters DT, Tupin JP. Family grief in the emergency department. *Emerg Med Clin North Am.* 1991;9:189–207.

26. Hobgood C, Harward D, Newton K, Davis W. The educational intervention "GRIEV_ING" improves the death notification skills of residents. *Acad Emerg Med.* 2005;12(4):296–301.

27. Tsai E. Should family members be present during cardiopulmonary resuscitation? *N Engl J Med.* 2002;346(13):1019–1021.

28. Doyle CJ, Post H, Burney RE, et al. Family participation during resuscitation: an option. *Ann Emerg Med.* 1987;16(6):673–675.

29. Redley B, Hood K. Staff attitudes towards family presence during resuscitation. *Accid Emerg Nurs.* 1996;4(3):145–151.

30. Macy C, Lampe E, O'Neil B, Swor R, Zalenski R, Compton S. The relationship between the hospital setting and perceptions of family-witnessed resuscitation in the emergency department. *Resuscitation.* 2006;70(1):74–79.

31. Truog RD, Cist AF, Brackett SE, et al. Recommendations for end-of-life care in the intensive care unit: the Ethics Committee of the Society of Critical Care Medicine. *Crit Care Med.* 2001;29(12):2332–2348.

32. Cook JE, Guyatt GH, Jaeschke R, et al. Determinants in Canadian health care workers of the decision to withdraw life support from the critically ill. *JAMA.* 1995;273:703–708.

33. Miller W, Levy P, Lamba S, et al. Descriptive analysis of the in-hospital course of patients who initially survive out-of-hospital cardiac arrest but die in-hospital. *J Palliat Med.* 2010;13(1):19–22.

34. Prendergast JE, Luce JM. Increasing incidence of withholding and withdrawal of life support from the critically ill. *Am J Respir Crit Care Med.* 1997;155:15–20.

35. Smedira JE, Evans BH, Grais LS, et al. Withholding and withdrawal of life support from the critically ill. *N Engl J Med.* 1999;322:309–315.

36. Truog RD, Burns JP, Mitchell C, et al. Pharmacologic paralysis and withdrawal of mechanical ventilation at the end of life. *N Engl J Med.* 2000;342:508–511.

37. Wilson JE, Smedira NG, Fink C, et al. Ordering and administration of sedatives and analgesics during the withholding and withdrawal of life support from critically ill patients. *JAMA.* 1992;267:949–953.

38. Bookman K, Abbott J. Ethics seminars: withdrawal of treatment in the emergency department, when and how? *Acad Emerg Med.* 2006;13:1328–1332.

39. Sedillot N, Holzapfel L, Jacquet-Francillon T, et al. A five-step protocol for withholding and withdrawing of life support in an emergency department: an observational study. *Eur J Emerg Med.* 2008;15:145–149.

40. Emanuel LL, Alpert HR, Baldwin DC, Emanuel EJ. What terminally ill patients care about; toward a validated construct of patients' perspectives. *J Palliat Med.* 2000;3:419–431.

41. Steinhauser KE, Clipp EC, McNeilly M, Christakis NA, McIntyre LM, Tulsky JA. In search of a good death: observations of patients, families, and providers. *Ann Intern Med.* 2000;132:825–832.

42. Mosenthal AC. Palliative care in the surgical ICU. *Surg Clin North Am.* 2005;85(2):303–313.

43. Nelson JE. Identifying and overcoming the barriers to high-quality palliative care in the intensive care unit. *Crit Care Med.* 2006;34(11 suppl):S324–S331.

44. Pain management. Accessed at http://www.cancer.gov/cancertopics/pdq/supportivecare/pain/HealthProfessional/557.cdr#Section_557. Last accessed January 8, 2010.

45. Brender E, Burke A, Glass RM. Palliative sedation. *JAMA.* 2005;294:1850.

46. Lo B, Rubenfeld G. Palliative sedation in dying patients. "We turn to it when everything else hasn't worked". *JAMA.* 2005;294:1810–1816.

47. Burt RA. The Supreme Court speaks—not assisted suicide but a constitutional right to palliative care. *N Engl J Med.* 1997;337:1234.

INDEX

Note: Page numbers followed by *f* or *t* indicate figures or tables, respectively.

Also from McGraw-Hill:

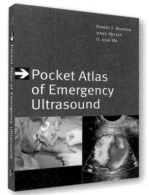

978-0-07-148480-0

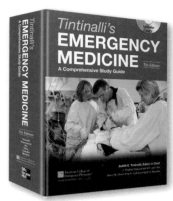

978-0-07-166807-1

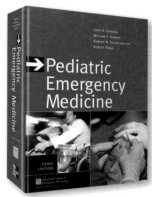

978-0-07-159737-1

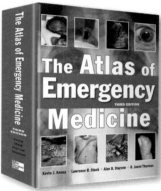

978-0-07-149618-6

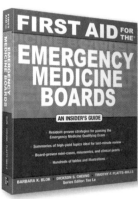

978-0-07-162592-0

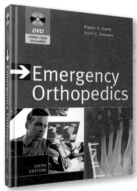

978-0-07-149617-9

Available everywhere medical books are sold

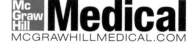

MCGRAWHILLMEDICAL.COM

For more Emergency Medicine information from McGraw-Hill:

AccessEmergency Medicine is a complete online resource that allows users to quickly find diagnosis and treatment answers with leading EM texts and videos that cover a broad spectrum of complaints encountered in the ED. Visit **www.accessemergencymedicine.com** for subscription information.

ACCESS Emergency Medicine *from McGraw-Hill*™

Meeting the Immediate Needs of the ED